Diagnostic Pathology of Pleuropulmonary Neoplasia

Annikka Weissferdt • Cesar A. Moran

Diagnostic Pathology of Pleuropulmonary Neoplasia

Springer

Annikka Weissferdt, M.D., FRCPath
Department of Pathology
The University of Texas
MD Anderson Cancer Center
Houston, TX
USA

Cesar A. Moran, M.D.
Department of Pathology
The University of Texas
MD Anderson Cancer Center
Houston, TX
USA

ISBN 978-1-4939-3992-3 ISBN 978-1-4419-0787-5 (eBook)
DOI 10.1007/978-1-4419-0787-5
Springer New York Heidelberg Dordrecht London

Printed on acid-free paper

Springer is part of Springer Science+Business Media (www.springer.com)

To my wife, Susan, and my daughters, Kate, Leticia, and Elisa Jean, for their unwavering support and understanding (CAM).
To my family (AW).

Preface

Pleuropulmonary neoplasia is a practical approach to the diagnosis of a diverse group of tumors and pseudotumoral conditions that may appear primarily in the lungs and the pleura. The text of this book has been arranged by family of tumors, which have been divided into types and, in many respects, depending on the cell of origin. In addition, we tried to provide current concepts that are being considered in the evaluation of new nomenclatures and in some cases in the classification of some tumors. Needless to say, in some areas we have taken the liberty of offering our personal opinion based on our experience and that of others from the literature. At the same time, we acknowledge that some of the current concepts may change with time, hopefully leading to further clarification. As we have discussed each entity, we have also provided matching illustrations that the reader of this text may find useful.

In addition, the text provides insights into other areas that are closely related to the diagnosis of pulmonary and pleural tumors, including diagnostic imaging, surgical approach, staging, and molecular diagnostics. For these topics, we are indebted to Dr. Patricia De Groot and Dr. Edith Marom for their chapter on diagnostic imaging, Dr. David Rice for his chapter on surgical approach and staging, and to Dr. Luisa Solis and Dr. Ignacio Wistuba for their chapter on molecular diagnosis. Last but not least, we also want to acknowledge and thank Dr. Francisco Vega for his contribution on the chapter of lymphoproliferative tumors. All these experts have clearly enhanced the usefulness of this text, and we are very grateful for their contributions.

Finally, we hope that the reader will find this book useful in his/her daily practice, not only from the histopathological aspects but also from the radiological, surgical, and molecular aspects of pulmonary and pleural tumors, which in turn should lead to a better understanding of the diverse entities herein discussed.

Houston, TX, USA — Annikka Weissferdt, M.D., FRCPath
Houston, TX, USA — Cesar A. Moran, M.D.

Contents

Contributors

Patricia M. de Groot, M.D. Department of Diagnostic Radiology, The University of Texas MD Anderson Cancer Center, Houston, TX, USA

Edith M. Marom, M.D. Department of Diagnostic Radiology, The University of Texas MD Anderson Cancer Center, Houston, TX, USA

Cesar A. Moran, M.D. Department of Pathology, The University of Texas MD Anderson Cancer Center, Houston, TX, USA

David C. Rice, M.D. Minimally Invasive Surgery Program, Thoracic Surgery, The University of Texas MD Anderson Cancer Center, Houston, TX, USA

Luisa M. Solis, M.D. Department of Pathology, The University of Texas MD Anderson Cancer Center, Houston, TX, USA

Francisco Vega, M.D., Ph.D. Department of Hematopathology, The University of Texas MD Anderson Cancer Center, Houston, TX, USA

Annikka Weissferdt, M.D., FRCPath Department of Pathology, The University of Texas MD Anderson Cancer Center, Houston, TX, USA

Ignacio I. Wistuba, M.D. Department of Pathology and Thoracic/Head and Neck Medical Oncology, The University of Texas MD Anderson Cancer Center, Houston, TX, USA

1 Diagnostic Imaging of Lung and Pleural Tumors

Patricia M. de Groot and Edith M. Marom

Introduction

Diagnosis, staging, and follow-up assessment of thoracic tumors rely heavily on imaging. Communication among clinicians and radiologists is important in optimizing imaging modality selection for these tasks. In this chapter, we present a general overview of imaging of lung and pleural tumors with an emphasis on the strengths and limitations of various imaging methods employed in the evaluation of these malignancies. We emphasize a few pathognomonic imaging findings for which a diagnostic biopsy can be avoided. Our intent is to help guide selection of appropriate imaging, thus decreasing the number of superfluous imaging studies ordered.

Overview of Diagnostic Imaging Methods

Over the past few decades, the use of computers has revolutionized medical imaging, allowing introduction and continual improvement of imaging technologies such as digitized radiography, computed tomography (CT), magnetic resonance imaging (MRI), specialized ultrasound, positron emission tomography (PET), and, most recently, combined PET-CT, which offers simultaneous morphological and physiological imaging. Each of these techniques has benefits and limitations. In some instances, different imaging methods may complement each other in clarifying a particular medical problem. In the diagnosis of tumors, the goal of imaging is to differentiate between benign and malignant tumors to correctly identify patients who need surgery. In addition to determining the resectability of tumors, imaging plays a vital role in selecting the most appropriate surgical approach and identifying tumor recurrence.

P.M. de Groot • E.M. Marom (✉)
Department of Diagnostic Radiology,
The University of Texas MD Anderson Cancer Center,
1515 Holcombe Blvd., Unit 1478, Houston, TX 77030, USA
e-mail: pdegroot@mdanderson.org; emarom@mdanderson.org

Chest Radiography

Chest radiographs effectively demonstrate pulmonary abnormalities because these abnormalities differ in density from the surrounding structures. The density of normal lungs, which contain air, differs significantly from the soft tissue density of tumors, leading to an air-tissue interface at the tumor margins. This interface is responsible for the exquisite display of lung tumors on radiographs. Chest radiography has the benefits of simplicity, low cost, lack of associated pain, and safety, with relatively little radiation exposure to the patient [1]. These benefits make chest radiography the initial imaging modality of choice, in the evaluation of symptoms suspected of originating in the lung or pleura. Although overlapping structures such as bones and crossing pulmonary vessels may mimic pulmonary nodules, the advent of digital radiography and dual energy acquisition has resulted in post-processing techniques that can be used to subtract overlying bones from the lungs and soft tissues and reduce the interference caused by overlapping structures to improve detection of pulmonary parenchymal abnormalities.

After the intraparenchymal location of a pulmonary nodule is established, the next goal of chest radiography is to determine whether it is benign or malignant. In the 1940s and 1950s, researchers attempted to identify radiographic features of benign and malignant disease. Before cross-sectional imaging emerged in the 1980s, definitive preoperative diagnosis of a solitary asymptomatic pulmonary nodule was uncommon; early exploratory thoracotomy was recommended when such indeterminate pulmonary nodules were detected [2, 3]. Although large nodules are more likely than small ones to be malignant, no size criteria allow exclusion of malignancy [4]. Two methods of distinguishing benign and malignant nodules are in use today: (1) documentation

A. Weissferdt, C.A. Moran, *Diagnostic Pathology of Pleuropulmonary Neoplasia*,
DOI 10.1007/978-1-4419-0787-5_1,

of the stability of the nodule over 2 years and (2) identification of benign-appearing calcifications. However, neither method is completely infallible. Specifically, nodule stability has robustly and scientifically proven to be unreliable, as data from the 1950s suggested that it has a positive predictive value of 65 % for benignity [5]. Also, identification of benign calcifications on radiographs has proven to be subjective [6]. However, review of prior radiographs is the most cost-efficient way to assess a pulmonary abnormality. If previous studies are not available for comparison to a current study, then shallow oblique radiographs, fluoroscopy, and/or chest CT scans are the possible next steps in investigation in determining whether a lung or pleural nodule is malignant.

CT

With its better contrast resolution, elimination of overlapping structures, and ability to obtain thin slices, CT is more sensitive than chest radiography in detecting pulmonary nodules (Fig. 1.1a, b) [7] and superior to it in determining the margins and internal characteristics of these nodules. Its disadvantages in comparison with chest radiography are a much higher cost and greater radiation exposure to the patient.

When investigating a pulmonary nodule, in the absence of prior chest radiographs that may have confirmed benignity, a patient is referred for a chest CT scan that will determine the nodule's contours and internal characteristics. Tumor margins may be spiculated, smooth and well circumscribed, or have lobulations (Fig. 1.2a–c). Spiculated margins are highly suggestive of, but not pathognomonic for, malignancy. Spiculations can reflect the presence of peritumoral fibrosis, infiltration of tumor cells into adjacent lung parenchyma, or localized lymphangitic spread [8, 9]. In a study evaluating 634 pulmonary nodules, 50 of 53 nodules (94 %) with diffuse spiculation and 134 of 165 nodules (81 %) with focal spiculation were primary lung carcinomas [10]. Conversely, 8 of 66 (12 %) smoothly marginated, nonlobulated nodules were primary lung tumors, 6 (9 %) were solitary metastases, and 52 (79 %) were benign. Lobulation of margins implies uneven growth that is often associated with malignancy [4], but it is not useful in distinguishing benign and malignant nodules. Also in the study described previously, of 350 smoothly lobulated nodules, 91 (26 %) were primary lung cancer, 57 (16 %) were metastases, and 202 (58 %) were benign [10].

Internal characteristics of pulmonary nodules may include the presence of calcification, macroscopic fat, or hypervascularity, causing intense enhancement on CT scans following administration of intravenous contrast material. Calcification is readily seen on CT scans as very high-density foci measuring more than 200 Hounsfield units (HU). Characteristics of benign calcification include central,

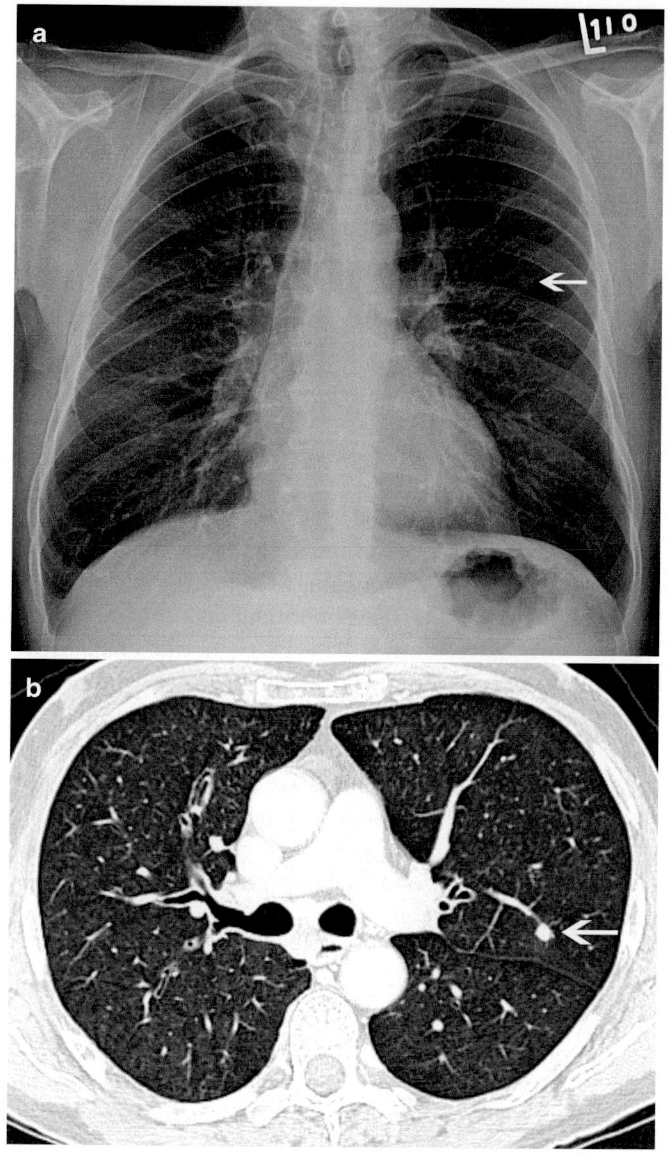

Fig. 1.1 (**a**) Routine chest radiograph showing a small nodule in the right upper lobe that is barely visible (*arrow*) in a 59-year-old man who underwent follow-up assessment after treatment of squamous cell carcinoma of the piriform sinus. (**b**) Contrast-enhanced chest CT scan with lung window settings more readily showing this small 0.6-cm nodule

diffuse, solid lamination, and a popcorn-like appearance (Fig. 1.3a–d). Solid, central, and laminated calcification typically results from a remote granulomatous infection, whereas popcorn-like calcification is seen with hamartomas. For a nodule to be considered benign, it should display one of these four patterns of calcification and must not have any other features suggestive of malignancy. If calcifications are eccentric, the nodule margins are bilobed, irregular, or spiculated; if the nodule abuts a central bronchus, the nodule should not be considered benign despite the presence of benign-appearing calcification, as calcification can be engulfed by a malignancy [10]. Also, pulmonary metastases

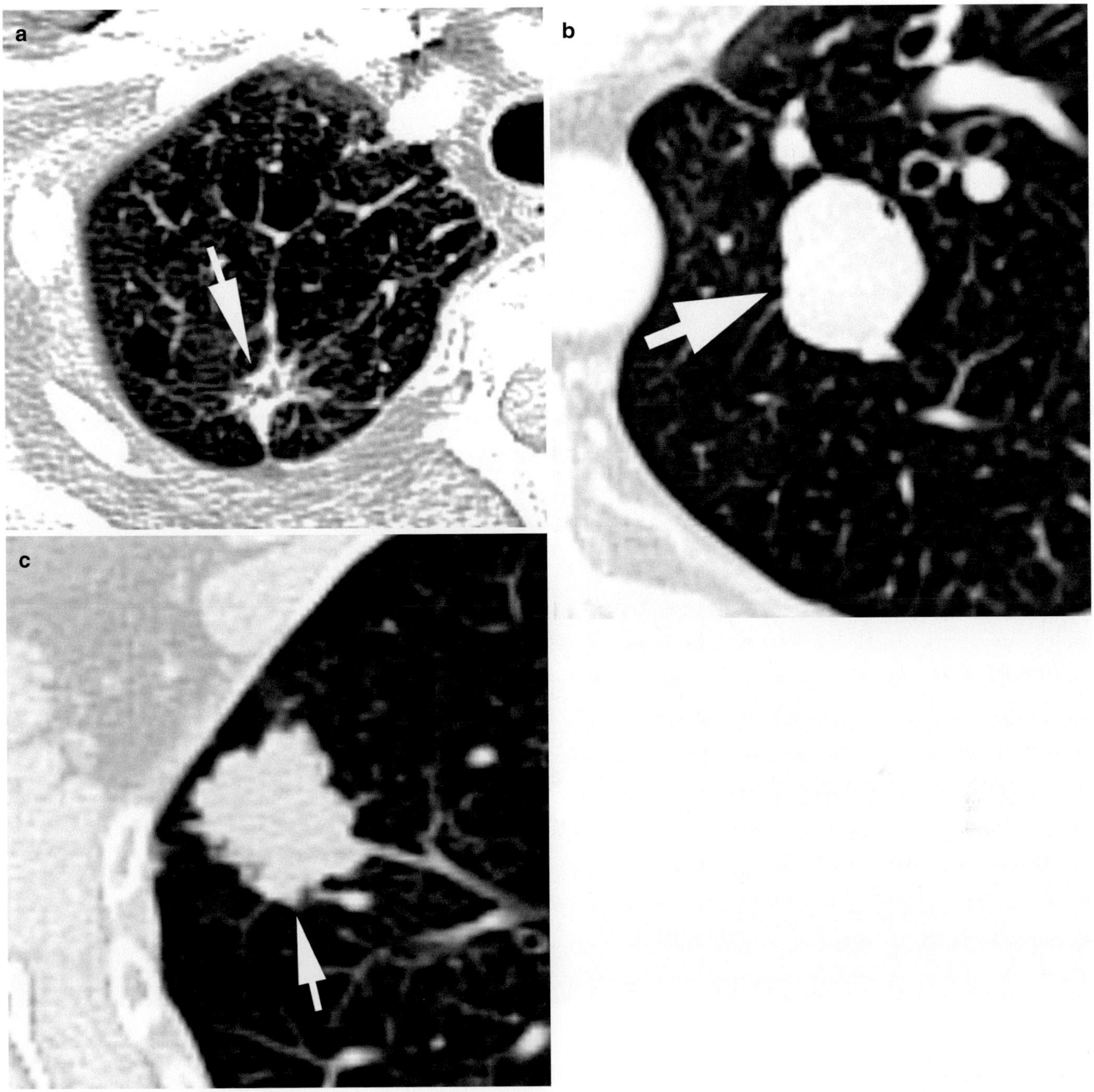

Fig. 1.2 A chest CT scan with lung window settings showing examples of pulmonary tumor margins. Tumor margins may be (**a**) spiculated as in this adenocarcinoma (*arrow*), (**b**) well circumscribed and smooth as in this carcinoid tumor with spindle cell features (*arrow*), or (**c**) lobulated as in this adenocarcinoma with mucinous features (*arrow*)

from osteosarcomas or chondrosarcomas can manifest as nodules with central or solid calcification. Therefore, nodules in patients with one of these cancers cannot be characterized as benign or malignant according to the calcification pattern (Fig. 1.4). In these patients, benignity is established by long-term nodule stability. Another type of calcification, the sand-like, amorphous form, has occurred with 6 % of lung cancers imaged using CT [11] but can also occur with benign disease. This pattern of calcification is not useful for diagnostic purposes.

Most pulmonary nodules imaged using CT are not obviously calcified. Because CT scans can objectively measure nodule density in Hounsfield units, researchers attempted to identify microscopic calcifications in such lesions not obvious to the human eye by measuring their radiodensity in Hounsfield units and establishing a threshold above which

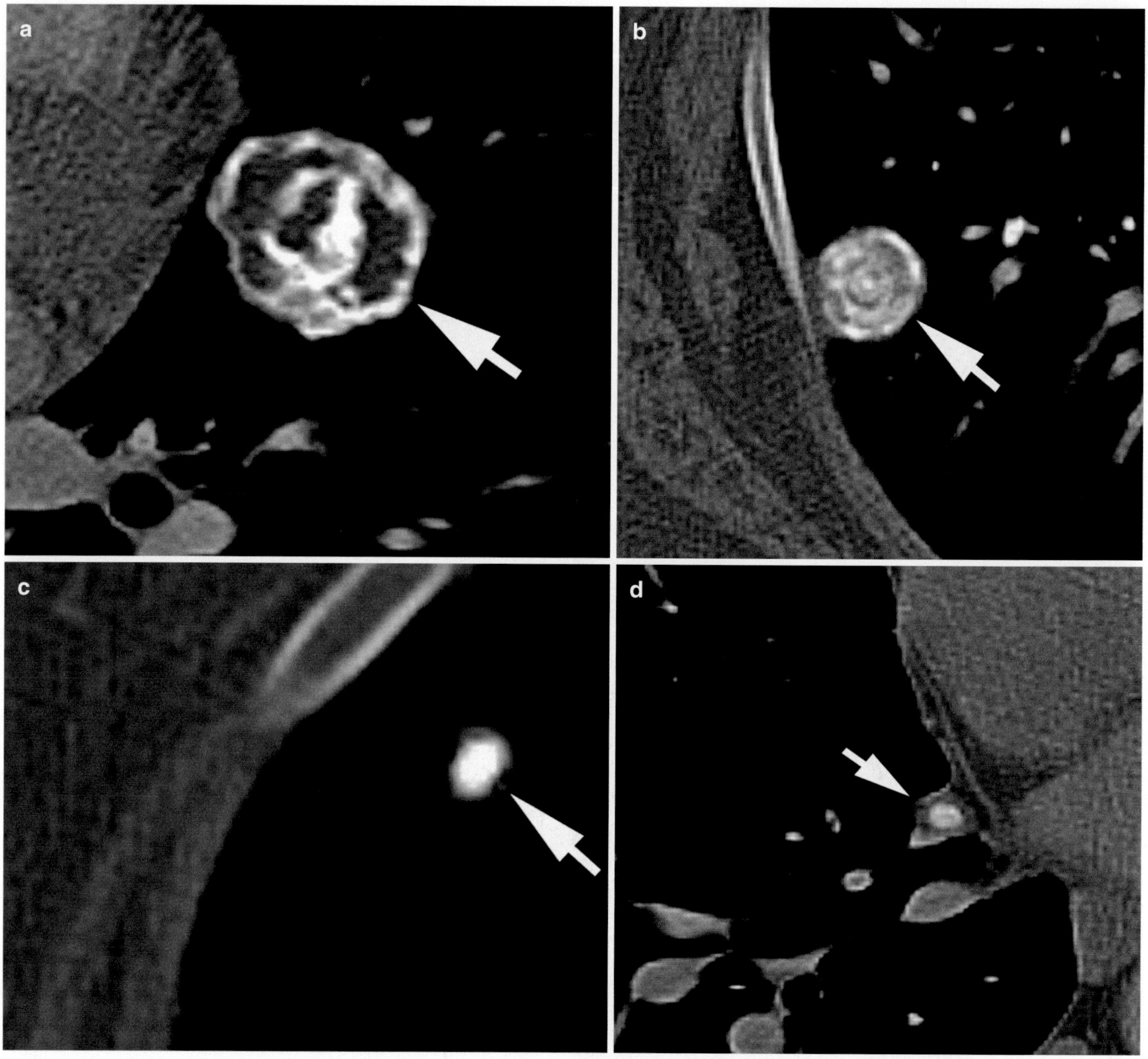

Fig. 1.3 A chest CT scan with bone window settings showing benign patterns of pulmonary nodule calcification (*arrow*). (**a**) Popcorn calcification of a hamartoma in a 27-year-old woman with Carney triad. (**b**) Pulmonary nodule with laminated calcification in a 50-year-old woman with prior histoplasmosis. (**c**) Diffuse solid calcification in a 73-year-old man with a history of histoplasmosis infection. (**d**) Central calcification in a small pulmonary nodule in a 67-year-old man with prior tuberculosis

nodules were to be considered calcified and thus benign, reducing the number of futile thoracotomies [12, 13]. However, more than 10 % of nodules with densities higher than the threshold of 185 HU (above which nodules were posited to be benign) were malignant, and the investigators abandoned the threshold method [13].

Macroscopic fat is also readily recognized on CT scans. A well-demarcated pulmonary nodule containing fat with a density of -40 to -120 HU is considered pathognomonic for a benign hamartoma (Fig. 1.5). Approximately 60 % of hamartomas on thin-section (1 mm) CT scans contain identifiable fat alone or in combination with calcification [14]. Such nodules, even if they grow slowly (doubling time >2 years), are considered benign hamartomas. However, a third of hamartomas do not exhibit calcification or fat on CT scans and thus remain indeterminate nodules.

Air bronchograms are rare in benign pulmonary nodules (6 %) but are readily identified using CT (Fig. 1.6). Their presence is almost always associated with lung cancer of any cell type but is seen most often with adenocarcinoma—both adenocarcinoma in situ (AIS) and more invasive forms [15]. CT can also differentiate among solid nodules, ground-glass

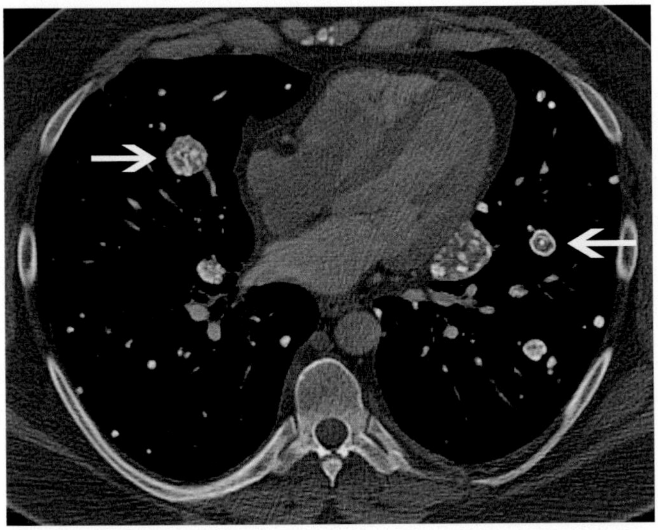

Fig. 1.4 Contrast-enhanced chest CT scan with bone window settings showing multiple bilateral calcified pulmonary metastases (*arrows*) in a 38-year-old man with a mesenchymal chondrosarcoma of the left thigh (not shown)

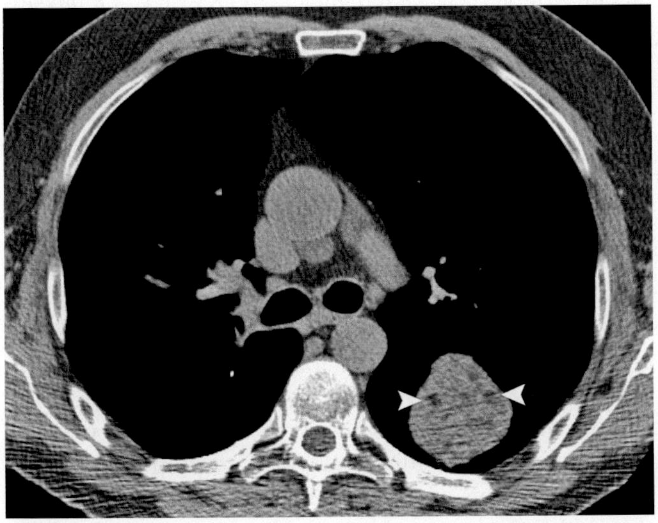

Fig. 1.5 Unenhanced chest CT scan with mediastinal windows showing a 6.5-cm mass in the superior segment of the left lower lobe in a 65-year-old man with treated right upper lobe adenocarcinoma and pulmonary hamartomas. Several foci of very low density in the mass (*arrowheads*) are consistent with macroscopic fat; they are similar to the density of subcutaneous fat and measured -122 HU, making this lesion consistent with a hamartoma. Over a 10-year observation period, this mass had a doubling time of 4 years, compatible with a benign etiology. A similar lesion was resected from the patient at the time of right upper lobectomy for carcinoma that proved to be a hamartoma

nodules (in which the pulmonary vessels can be seen through the nodule), and mixed nodules, which are combined solid and ground-glass nodules (Fig. 1.7). The malignancy rate is highest for mixed nodules (63 %) and is higher for ground-glass nodules (18 %) than for solid nodules (7 %) [16].

Despite the superior sensitivity of CT over radiography in detecting benign pulmonary nodules by identifying fat and calcium, the majority of nodules on initial CT scans remain indeterminate. For further investigation of the indeterminate nodule, studying vascular enhancement may be helpful. The vessels supplying tumors differ both quantitatively and qualitatively from those supplying benign growths and tend to be more "leaky." This inherent difference in blood supply between malignant and benign pulmonary nodules can manifest in differences in their Hounsfield unit values after intravenous contrast agent injection. This method, in which the indeterminate nodule is imaged at intervals before and after intravenous contrast administration, was perfected by Swensen et al. [17, 18]. Absence of significant lung nodule enhancement (≤15 HU) on a CT scan is suggestive of benignity. Although this method is only 77 % accurate and 58 % specific, it does

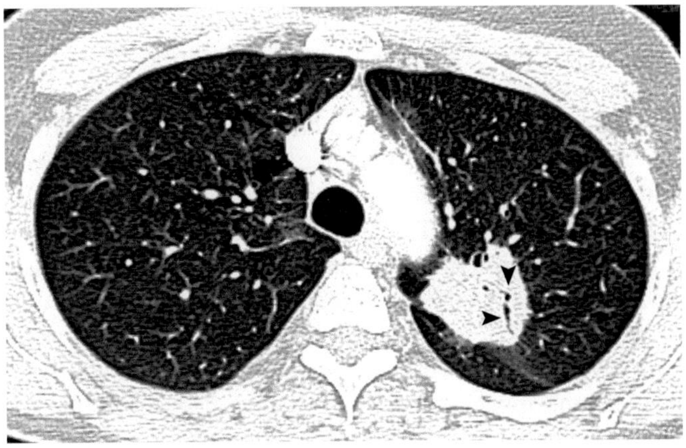

Fig. 1.6 Contrast-enhanced chest CT scan with lung window settings demonstrating a 3.4 × 3.2-cm lobulated mass in the left upper lobe of a 67-year-old woman with lung adenocarcinoma. Multiple small linear lucencies coursing through the tumor are consistent with air bronchograms (*arrowheads*)

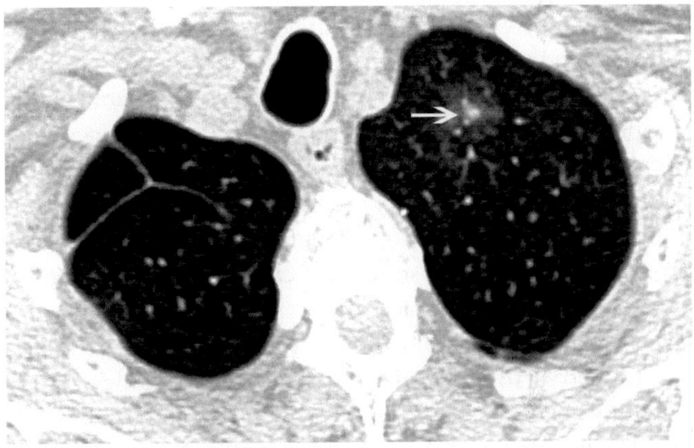

Fig. 1.7 Noncontrast thin-section chest CT scan with lung window settings demonstrating a 2.5-cm left upper lobe ground-glass nodule with a central solid component (*arrow*) in a 77-year-old woman 2 years after a right upper lobectomy for an adenocarcinoma in the right upper lobe. Similar nodules were also seen in the remainder of the lobes, which were consistent with multifocal adenocarcinoma of the lung

identify 98 % of malignant nodules and thus can be used to guide follow-up examinations and intervention.

The CT features of pulmonary nodules described herein determine the patients having nodules with benign features not requiring follow-up (benign calcifications or fat), those who would benefit from an immediate biopsy, and those who would benefit from CT-based follow-up to measure nodule growth rates. Determination of a nodule's benignity takes into account patient risk factors such as age and tobacco use, as well as the CT features that are statistically known to be strongly associated with malignancy (e.g., large tumor size, spiculation, mixed solid, and ground-glass appearance). However, radiologists and oncologists should not use the 2-year stability criterion for benignity invariably. This criterion is generally applied to nodules that are solid and larger than 1 cm in diameter. Reliably measuring the growth of nodules smaller than 1 cm can be challenging. Doubling of the volume of a nodule is equivalent to an increase in its diameter of approximately 25 %. Even using CT, visually detecting the doubling of a 4-mm nodule, which is a change in diameter from 4 to 5 mm, is difficult. Thus, small lung tumors can double in volume yet appear to be stable. Even computerized volume measurements are not always accurate with such small nodules, which can appear to change in size with changes in inspiratory effort and slice selection [19]. Ground-glass and mixed solid/ground-glass nodules are most often identified by CT scans, not chest radiographs, and a stability criterion for such nodules on CT scans, such as the 2-year stability rule used for solid nodules on chest radiographs, has yet to be established. In fact, such nodules, which often are detected incidentally or with screening chest CT studies, can have very long doubling times. For example, in a screening study in Japan [20], the mean ± standard deviation doubling times for malignant ground-glass, mixed, and solid nodules were 813 ± 375, 457 ± 260, and 149 ± 125 days, respectively. In fact, 20 % of the nodules in that study had doubling times greater than 2 years; most of those nodules were ground-glass or mixed nodules. Thus, when a ground-glass nodule smaller than 1 cm in diameter is monitored using CT to establish a benign etiology, recent management guidelines suggest a follow-up period of at least 3 years, potentially extending up to 5 years [21].

MRI

The contrast resolution of MRI is superior to that of CT. However, the spatial resolution of MRI is inferior, particularly in the thorax, primarily owing to intrinsic lung characteristics such as low proton density and numerous air-tissue interfaces, as well as examination sensitivity to artifacts from respiratory and cardiac motion. These features make identification of pulmonary nodules smaller than 1 cm difficult. However, once a malignancy is diagnosed, MRI is superior to CT in evaluation of potential soft tissue involvement by the cancer, such as invasion of the chest wall or neural and vascular structures. Small studies showed that dynamic contrast-enhanced MRIs were sensitive in the differentiating of malignant and benign solitary pulmonary nodules that were comparable with the sensitivity of dynamic contrast-enhanced CT, but the nodules investigated using MRI were usually larger than the incidental nodules discovered using CT [22–24].

Because MRI examinations usually take considerable amounts of time, they are often tailored to specific problematic locations, not to searching the entire chest for distant metastatic disease.

PET and Integrated PET-CT

PET with 2-deoxy-D-glucose labeled with ^{18}Fluorine (^{18}FDG) has emerged as a tool for evaluation of suspected and known thoracic malignancies. ^{18}FDG-PET is a physiological imaging technique with poorer spatial resolution than that of anatomic imaging methods such as chest CT and radiography. ^{18}FDG is a glucose analog labeled with a radiotracer, and PET is a technique for assessing glucose use by metabolically active tissues that preferentially take up ^{18}FDG. Many tumors have higher metabolic rates than normal tissue and therefore accumulate ^{18}FDG more intensely than do surrounding tissues. For pulmonary nodules that are indeterminate on CT scans, ^{18}FDG-PET can help identify patients who may benefit from immediate biopsy. Initial studies showed that ^{18}FDG-PET was effective in the differentiation of benign and malignant pulmonary lesions with overall sensitivity, specificity, and accuracy rates estimated to be 96, 88, and 94 %, respectively [25–31]. The combination of ^{18}FDG-PET and CT, known as integrated PET-CT, has provided significantly greater specificity than either CT or PET alone [32].

^{18}FDG-PET does have several limitations. It is neither uniformly specific nor sensitive if the target abnormality is small. In particular, nodules smaller than 1 cm in diameter are not measured accurately and sometimes fall below the resolution of the PET scan [33, 34]. Also, cell type can influence ^{18}FDG uptake. Indolent cancers such as carcinoid tumors, well-differentiated adenocarcinomas, and AIS demonstrate less ^{18}FDG avidity than do other non-small cell lung cancers (NSCLCs) and may exhibit no detectable increase in ^{18}FDG activity above background levels [28, 34–39]. In these instances, the typical morphological features of some of these tumors, such as proximity of a carcinoid tumor to a bronchus or a consolidative tumor, mixed tumor, or ground-glass AIS nodule, should be taken into account when interpreting the results of integrated PET-CT.

In integrated PET-CT studies, quantification of ^{18}FDG uptake using CT for attenuation correction can introduce an artifact related to different breathing states in the nonsimultaneously acquired CT and PET scans, the latter performed without a breath hold. Nodules in the lower lobes of the lungs, which are more affected by respiratory motion than those in the upper lobes, can erroneously exhibit lower ^{18}FDG uptake as a result [40].

Authors have reported false-positive results of studies of primary pulmonary lesions (e.g., a malignancy positive ^{18}FDG-PET result for a lesion that later proves to be benign) in patients with infectious and inflammatory processes such as tuberculosis, histoplasmosis, and rheumatoid nodules [30, 41–46]. The positive predictive value of PET in most patients is high (90 % if the patient is >60 years old) [42, 44]. Lesions with increased ^{18}FDG uptake should be considered malignant until proven otherwise and managed accordingly. A negative PET scan, that is, one in which the nodule does not show increased ^{18}FDG uptake, should serve as a tool for treatment or follow-up planning, not a definitive confirmation of benignity. If biopsy is deferred, a pulmonary abnormality with a negative PET result should be monitored using serial chest CT scans to measure any growth of the lesion. The data reported so far indicate that PET-negative lesions are indolent; thus, this approach using lack of ^{18}FDG uptake to defer immediate biopsy should not adversely affect patient outcome [34].

The use of combined PET-CT studies has enhanced the accuracy of lung cancer staging because these two studies, when integrated, complement each other by overcoming the lack of spatial resolution inherent to PET and lack of physiological information inherent to CT. Therefore, these studies, in combination with clinical and laboratory findings, can be used to determine the necessity of additional imaging studies.

Ultrasound

Ultrasound has a very limited role in the evaluation of patients with intrathoracic malignancies, as the air within the lungs interferes with sound wave transmission. However, it has better soft tissue resolution than does CT and provides real-time imaging throughout the respiratory cycle and therefore can be helpful in limited applications. For instance, regarding imaging of focal chest wall involvement by pulmonary tumors, ultrasound is superior to CT, with a sensitivity rate of 89 % (compared with 40 % for CT), and similarly specific, as both have specificity rates approaching 100 % [47]. Additionally, ultrasound can be used to locate pockets of pleural fluid for diagnostic or therapeutic thoracentesis.

Primary Malignant Lung Tumors

Lung Carcinoma

Despite the advent of new diagnostic techniques, the overall 5-year survival rate for lung cancer, which is the leading cause of cancer deaths, remains about 15 %, and most patients still present with advanced disease [48]. Because lung tumors are encased by the rib cage, early diagnosis of them using physical examination is unlikely. In addition, many lung cancers have no symptoms until they are advanced. In most cases, lung cancer appears as a pulmonary abnormality—a nodule, mass, or consolidation—on chest images. Depending on the stage of the disease, additional smaller nodules, lymphadenopathy, and/or pleural involvement may be present. Over the second half of the twentieth century, multiple studies assessed the efficacy of screening techniques—first chest radiography and later CT—in detection of lung cancer at a stage when cure or control is possible. Nonrandomized uncontrolled screening studies in the 1950s [49–52] gave way to nonrandomized controlled trials [53, 54], which showed that the screened population was more likely than the general population with lung cancer to have their cancer detected at an early stage, to have resectable disease, and to have better survival rates, but without any clear reduction in lung cancer mortality rates. This discrepancy between increased survival rates and stable mortality rates is generally attributed to a combination of lead time, length time, and overdiagnosis bias in screening studies [55].

In the 1970s, four major randomized controlled screening trials, including the Mayo Lung Project, evaluated approximately 37,000 male smokers [56–59], finding that screening chest radiography yielded no change in mortality rates and no reduction in the number of advanced cancers (i.e., no stage shift), although the screened patients had higher 5-year survival rates than the patients who were not screened. A follow-up study more than 20 years after the Mayo Lung Project confirmed the absence of a significant difference in long-term mortality rates for lung cancer [60].

In the late 1990s, advancements in CT technology began to enable detection of pulmonary nodules smaller than 1 cm in diameter in one breath hold and with reduced radiation exposure to the patient using low-dose CT (LDCT). Despite the published 10-year survival rate of 88 % in patients with stage I lung cancer [61] and the increased likelihood that cancers detected using LDCT are operable, screening LDCT in early trials yielded no decreases in the number of advanced lung cancers detected or number of deaths caused by lung cancers compared with historical models in an unscreened population with lung cancer [62].

The largest single randomized lung cancer screening study to date, the National Lung Screening Trial, was launched in 2002 to determine whether screening for lung cancer using LDCT could reduce mortality rates in patients diagnosed this way with lung cancer. It compared the effect of two screening tests, LDCT and chest radiography, on both lung-cancer-specific mortality and all-cause mortality in persons at high risk for lung cancer, including current and former heavy smokers. From August 2002 to April 2004, the researchers enrolled 53,454 participants, who underwent annual imaging for 3 consecutive years and then underwent follow-up evaluation using questionnaires. Data collection ended on December 31, 2009. This trial demonstrated a relative reduction in the mortality rate for lung cancer with LDCT screening of 20 %. Additionally, the mortality rate for any cause decreased in the LDCT group by 6.7 % [63]. The U.S. Preventive Services Task Force and American College of Radiology are expected to issue recommendations for lung cancer screening in 2012. A current initiative by the United Kingdom Lung Screen is designed to determine whether the results of the National Lung Screening Trial can be replicated in the United Kingdom, with 4,000 patients being randomized to the United Kingdom Lung Screen pilot trial and a goal of 32,000 participants in the main study [64].

Imaging of Lung Cancer Subtypes

Evidence-based guidelines for the management of lung cancer published by the American Society of Clinical Oncology (ASCO) in 2004 [65] recommend initial evaluation of lung cancer using both chest radiography and contrast-enhanced chest CT scanning. The coverage of these CT scans should include the adrenal glands and liver. A ^{18}FDG-PET scan is recommended with the absence of CT evidence of metastatic disease because ^{18}FDG-PET imaging provides improved nodal and distant metastasis staging over CT alone and frequently improves staging to a degree that changes management [66–71]. Imaging does not replace histological sampling of lung masses, but certain subtypes of lung cancer can have typical imaging features.

Primary lung malignancies are grouped into two categories: (1) NSCLC, which accounts for approximately 85 % of all lung cancers and includes several subtypes, such as squamous cell cancer, adenocarcinoma, and carcinoid tumors, and (2) small-cell lung cancer (SCLC).

NSCLC

Squamous cell carcinoma typically originates in the central lung and may cause partial or complete obstruction of a bronchus. Thus, patients with this cancer frequently present with postobstructive pneumonia or atelectasis, which is readily identified on chest radiographs (Fig. 1.8a–d) [72–74]. Less often, patients present with bronchial impaction and distal bronchiectasis associated with air trapping and hyperinflation [73–75]. Approximately one-third of all squamous cell carcinomas originate beyond the segmental bronchi [73, 74]. Because most squamous cell carcinomas grow slowly and become symptomatic because of their central location, extrathoracic metastases are encountered less often in imaging at presentation compared to adenocarcinoma [73]. Also, squamous cell carcinomas are more likely to cavitate than are the other histological subtypes of lung cancer [73]. Cavitation occurs in 10–30 % of squamous cell cancers and is more common in large peripheral masses and poorly differentiated tumors (Fig. 1.9a, b) [73].

Adenocarcinomas typically manifest as peripheral pulmonary nodules or masses. Historically, these nodules typically had soft tissue attenuation and irregular or spiculated margins (Fig. 1.10) [73, 74]. With the expanding use of CT, however, an increasing number of adenocarcinomas present as ground-glass or mixed ground-glass/solid nodules. Investigators have found an association between the spectrum of CT appearances of adenocarcinoma and the classification system proposed by Noguchi and colleagues, in which small (≤2 cm in diameter) peripheral adenocarcinomas are classified into six types based on their growth patterns:

- Type A—localized bronchioloalveolar cell carcinoma (BAC)
- Type B—localized BAC with foci of structural collapse of alveoli
- Type C—localized BAC with active fibroblastic proliferation
- Type D—poorly differentiated adenocarcinoma
- Type E—tubular adenocarcinoma
- Type F—papillary adenocarcinoma with a compressed growth pattern [76–78]

Authors have reported ground-glass attenuation of nodular opacities more often with type A–C than type D–F tumors, whereas they reported soft tissue attenuation more often with type B–F than with type A tumors [76]. The soft tissue attenuation component tends to be absent or account for less than a third of the opacity with type A tumors and account for more than two-thirds of the opacity in type D–F tumors. Mixed nodules with both ground-glass and solid components are more likely to be invasive and at a high stage than are pure ground-glass nodules [79, 80].

Reclassification of lung adenocarcinoma in 2011 by an international multidisciplinary panel consisting of the International Association for the Study of Lung Cancer, American Thoracic Society, and European Respiratory Society introduced new terminology for the different classifications of adenocarcinoma to provide uniformity in the lexicon and diagnostic criteria for this disease [81]. As a result, the terms BAC and mixed-subtype adenocarcinoma are no longer used.

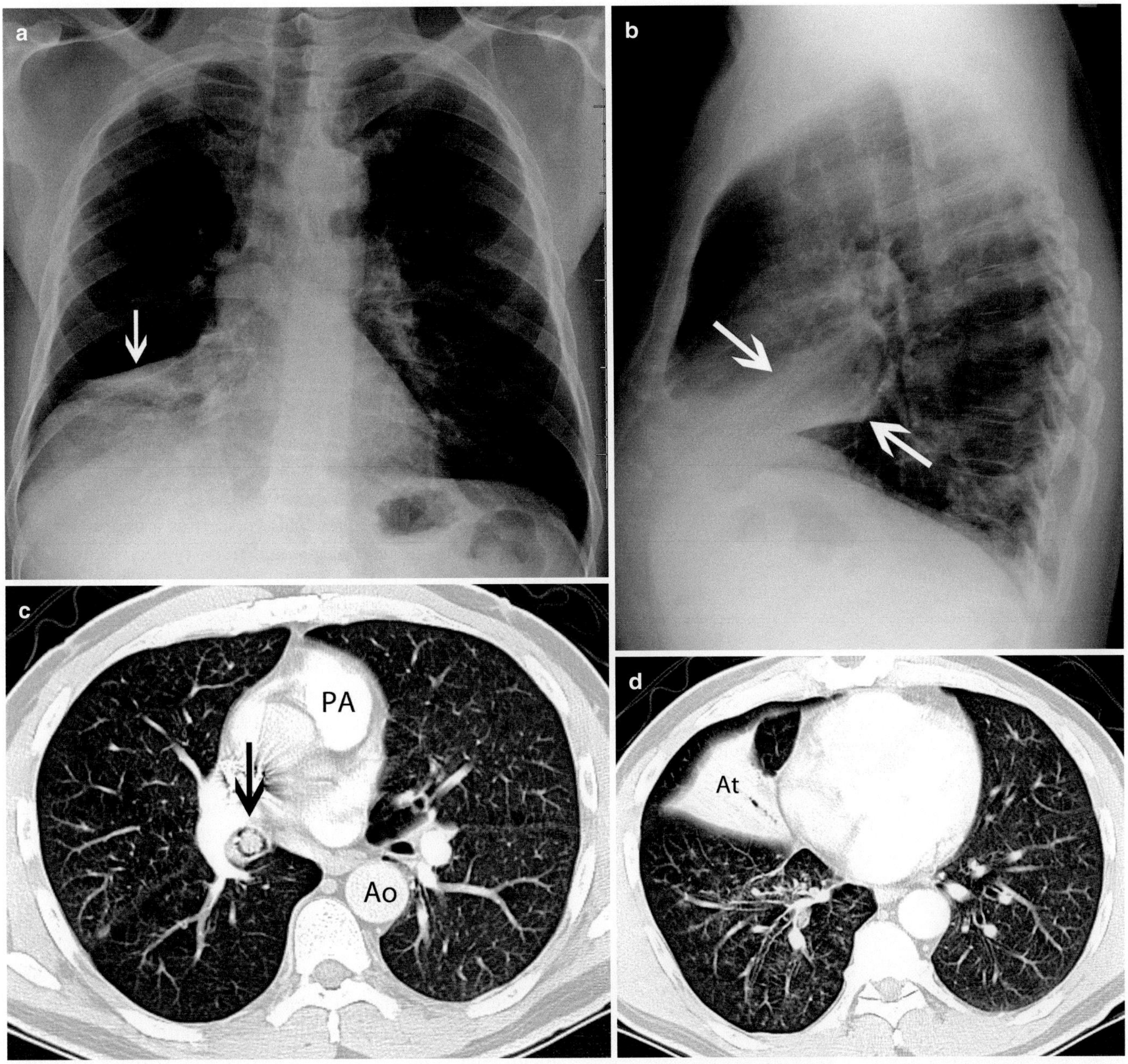

Fig. 1.8 (**a**) Posterior-anterior and (**b**) lateral chest radiographs demonstrating a consolidated collapsed right middle lobe (*arrows*) in a 54-year-old man with endobronchial squamous cell carcinoma of the lung and resultant lobar collapse. (**c, d**) Corresponding contrast-enhanced chest CT scans with lung window settings demonstrating a nodular growth almost filling the lumen of the right bronchus intermedius (*arrow*), resulting in right middle lobe atelectasis (*At*). *PA* pulmonary artery, *Ao* descending aorta

Lung adenocarcinoma is now classified into three main groups. The first group consists of preinvasive lesions and includes atypical adenomatous hyperplasia and AIS (previously BAC) of both the nonmucinous and mucinous type [81]. This group correlates with Noguchi type A and B tumors. Radiologically, the appearance of these tumors ranges from pure ground-glass nodules to ground-glass nodules with internal foci of alveolar collapse.

The second group is minimally invasive adenocarcinoma, a tumor with a predominantly lepidic pattern and invasion of up to 5 mm [81]. These tumors appear as ground-glass nodules with small internal solid foci (i.e., subsolid nodules). Patients with either preinvasive or minimally invasive adenocarcinomas have disease-specific survival rates near 100 % when the tumors are completely resected.

The third group is invasive adenocarcinoma, which includes several histological subtypes according to the predominant cell pattern, including the lepidic, acinar, papillary, micropapillary, and solid patterns [81]. Some invasive adenocarcinomas with lepidic patterns are included in the

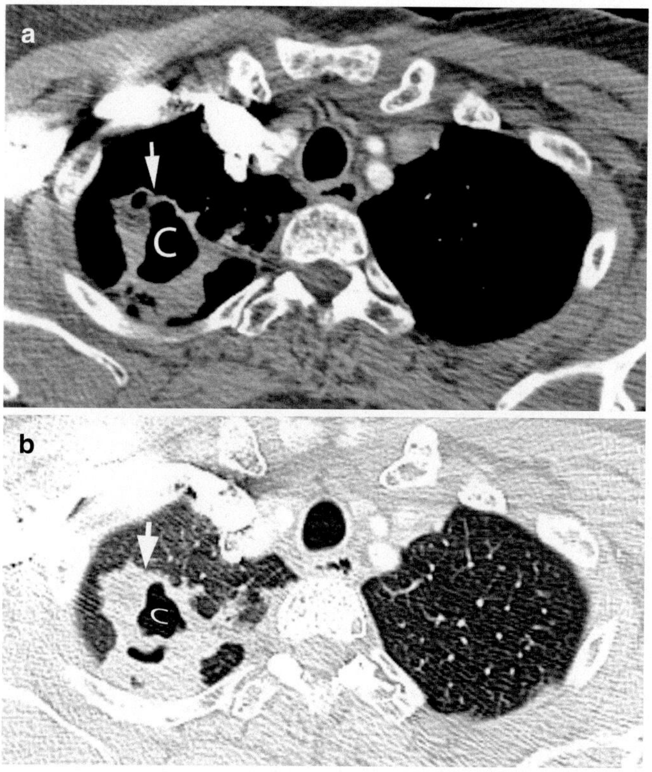

Fig. 1.9 Contrast-enhanced chest CT scan with (**a**) mediastinal window and (**b**) lung window settings showing a 4.0×4.9-cm right apical mass (*arrow*) with central cavitation (*C*) and irregularly thickened walls in a 62-year-old woman with squamous cell carcinoma

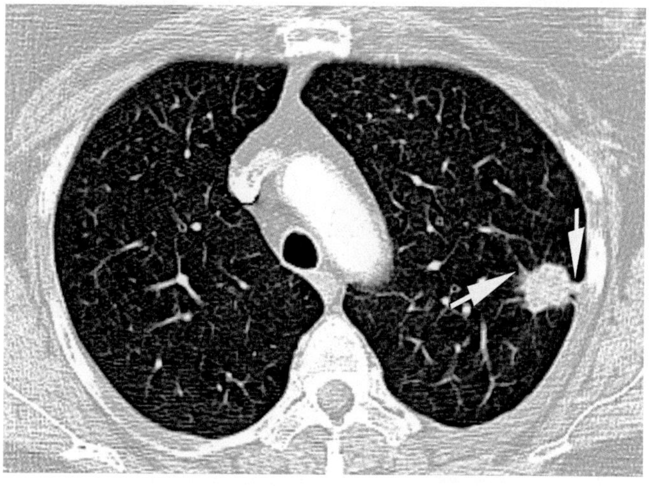

Fig. 1.10 Contrast-enhanced chest CT scan with lung window settings demonstrating a 1.9×2.1-cm peripheral nodule in the left upper lobe, with small linear extensions to the adjacent pleural surface and lung (*arrows*), giving it a spiculated appearance, in a 51-year-old woman with primary adenocarcinoma of the lung

Noguchi type C category; the others are included in the Noguchi type D–F categories. The radiological appearances of the invasive adenocarcinomas are usually of a solid nodule with spiculated margins, but distinction between the different subtypes in this invasive group by radiology is not possible.

AIS and minimally invasive adenocarcinomas manifesting as peripheral ground-glass and/or subsolid nodules have appeared as multiple tumors in up to 30 % of reported cases (Fig. 1.11) [76, 82]. These tumors are better seen on chest CT scans and are often not apparent on chest radiographs. Their size may remain stable for many years, with doubling times longer than 2 years. Cystic changes and cavitation occur rarely (≤7 % of cases) [83, 84]. When a nodule of this type exhibits multiple small, focal low-attenuation regions (pseudocavitation) or air bronchograms, the diagnosis of adenocarcinoma should be considered [9, 82, 84, 85]. The mucinous form of AIS infrequently manifests as ill-defined consolidation but should be suspected if the patient's "pneumonia" does not resolve with antibiotic-based treatment. On ^{18}FDG-PET-CT scans, AIS and minimally invasive adenocarcinomas can exhibit low FDG activity, specifically lower than that expected for a malignancy [36, 86, 87].

Large cell carcinoma usually occurs as a peripheral, rapidly growing, poorly marginated mass typically larger than 7 cm in diameter [72–74, 88–90]. Cavitation is uncommon in this tumor.

Carcinoid tumors most often occur as central endobronchial masses with or without associated atelectasis or consolidation; less often, they occur as well-demarcated pulmonary nodules (Fig. 1.12) [91, 92]. These tumors are usually less than 3 cm in diameter, although authors have reported tumors up to 10 cm in diameter [91, 93–95]. Calcification is seen in 25 % of carcinoids on CT scans [92]. Carcinoids can exhibit low ^{18}FDG uptake on PET-CT scans [34, 35, 96], which is attributed to low metabolic activity rates in these often indolent tumors.

SCLC

Primary SCLCs are typically small, centrally located, and associated with marked hilar and mediastinal adenopathy that often engulfs the primary lesion until it is no longer identifiable (Fig. 1.13a, b) [72, 74, 89, 97]. With the increased use of CT and screening CT scans in particular, the number of SCLCs diagnosed as small, early-stage peripheral solitary pulmonary nodules without intrathoracic adenopathy has increased. Historically, as reported in the literature, only 5 % of patients with SCLC have had early-stage disease at presentation [97, 98].

Staging of Lung Cancer

NSCLC

Accurate staging of lung cancer is important to management of and prognosis for this disease. The primary goal of radiological staging is to distinguish potentially resectable (stage I–IIIA) and unresectable (stage IIIB and IV) disease.

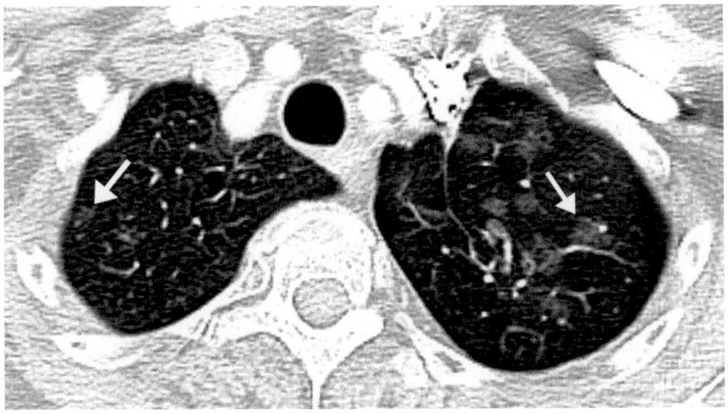

Fig. 1.11 Contrast-enhanced chest CT scan with lung window settings showing multiple ground-glass nodules (*arrows*) compatible with multifocal adenocarcinoma, which was confirmed via biopsy, in a 75-year-old woman 6 years after left upper lobectomy for adenocarcinoma

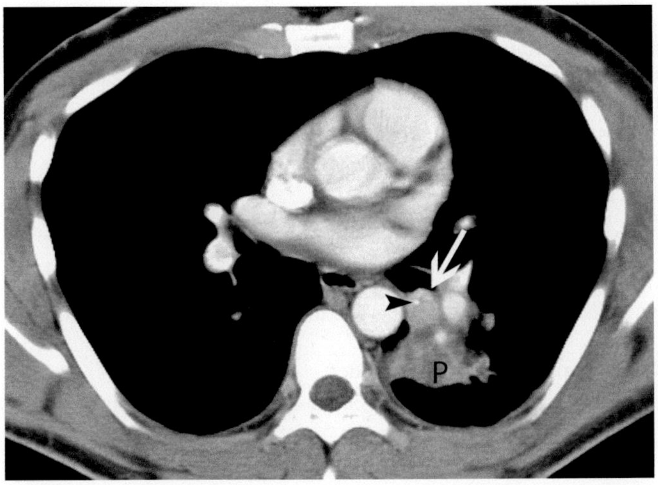

Fig. 1.12 Contrast-enhanced chest CT scan with mediastinal window settings showing a small endobronchial tumor (*arrow*) obstructing the left lower lobe superior segmental bronchus, resulting in postobstructive pneumonia (*P*) of that segment, in a 30-year-old man with a carcinoid tumor. A punctuate calcification is present in the tumor (*arrowhead*)

Tumor-nodes-metastasis (TNM) staging assesses the primary tumor (T), spread of the tumor into locoregional lymph nodes (N), and distant metastasis of the tumor (M). The original use of TNM staging was with conventional anatomic assessment based on tumor size and morphology, which did not take into account information such as metabolic activity seen on ^{18}FDG-PET scans. However, information from PET scans is now being integrated into TNM staging.

The current staging system for NSCLC is the seventh edition of the TNM system (Tables 1.1 and 1.2) and is based on analysis of long-term survival data on more than 100,000 patients in a study conducted under the auspices of the International Association for the Study of Lung Cancer [99].

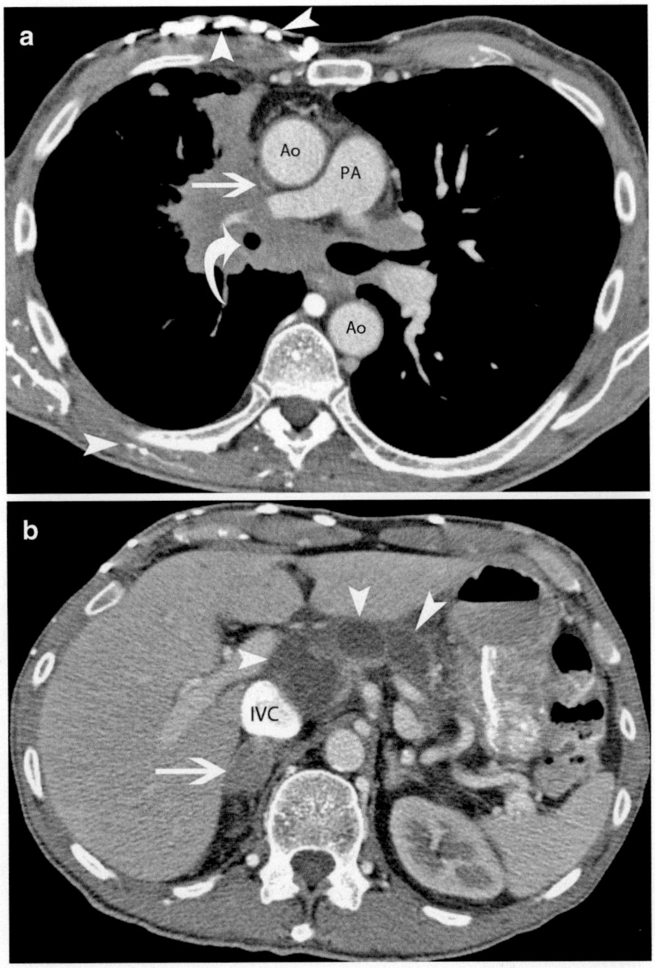

Fig. 1.13 (**a**) Contrast-enhanced chest CT scan with mediastinal window settings showing a confluent right upper lobe tumor and mediastinal and right hilar lymphadenopathy compressing the superior vena cava (*arrow*) in a 66-year-old man with lung SCLC. Numerous dilated collateral vessels in the right anterior chest wall are brightly opacified by the intravenous contrast agent injected from the right arm (*arrowheads*). Also, the bronchus intermedius is markedly narrowed (*curved arrow*) by the tumor encasement. (**b**) CT scan of the upper abdomen in the same patient demonstrating a right adrenal nodule (*arrow*) as well as numerous low-density mesenteric nodal metastases (*arrowheads*), which are compatible with extensive stage SCLC. *Ao* aorta, *PA* pulmonary artery, *IVC* inferior vena cava

Primary Tumor (T Status)

The T status is determined by the size and location of the primary tumor and its degree of invasion into surrounding structures. It is assessed primarily using CT, as the inferior spatial resolution of PET does not lend itself to T staging, which is based on morphological tumor features. However, some evidence indicates that the amount of ^{18}FDG uptake correlates with the prognosis [100–103] and that patients whose primary tumors have high ^{18}FDG avidity, even at an early stage, have shorter survival durations.

Table 1.1 TNM descriptors of NSCLC (International staging system for lung cancer, seventh edition)

T (primary tumor)	
TX	Primary tumor cannot be assessed; tumor proven by the presence of malignant cells in sputum or bronchial washings but not visualized using imaging or bronchoscopy
T0	No evidence of primary tumor
Tis	Carcinoma in situ
T1	Tumor ≤3 cm in greatest dimension surrounded by lung or visceral pleura without bronchoscopic evidence of invasion more proximal than the lobar bronchus (i.e., not in the main bronchus)[a]
T1a	Tumor ≤2 cm in greatest dimension
T1b	Tumor >2 cm but ≤3 cm in greatest dimension
T2	Tumor >3 cm but ≤7 cm in greatest dimension or tumor with any of the following features (T2 tumors with these features are classified as T2a if ≤5 cm) Involves main bronchus, ≥2 cm from the carina Invades visceral pleura Associated with atelectasis or obstructive pneumonitis that extends to the hilar region but does not involve the entire lung
T2a	Tumor >3 cm but ≤5 cm in greatest dimension
T2b	Tumor >5 cm but ≤7 cm in greatest dimension
T3	Tumor >7 cm; tumor that directly invades any of the following: chest wall (including superior sulcus tumors), diaphragm, phrenic nerve, mediastinal pleura, and parietal pericardium; tumor in the main bronchus <2 cm from the carina[a] but without involvement of the carina; tumor-associated atelectasis or obstructive pneumonitis of the entire lung or a separate tumor nodule or nodules in the same lobe
T4	Tumor of any size that invades any of the following: mediastinum, heart, great vessels, trachea, recurrent laryngeal nerve, esophagus, vertebral body, and carina; separate tumor nodule or nodules in a different ipsilateral lobe
N (regional lymph nodes)	
NX	Regional lymph nodes cannot be assessed
N0	No regional lymph node metastasis
N1	Metastasis in ipsilateral peribronchial and/or ipsilateral hilar lymph nodes and intrapulmonary nodes, including involvement via direct extension
N2	Metastasis in an ipsilateral mediastinal and/or subcarinal lymph node or nodes
N3	Metastasis in a contralateral mediastinal, contralateral hilar, ipsilateral or contralateral scalene, or supraclavicular lymph node or nodes
M (distant metastasis)	
MX	Distant metastasis cannot be assessed
M0	No distant metastasis
M1a	Separate tumor nodule or nodules in a contralateral lobe; tumor with pleural nodules or malignant pleural (or pericardial) effusion[b]
M1b	Distant metastasis

Used with permission from Goldstraw et al. [99]

[a]Uncommon superficial spreading tumors of any size with their invasive components limited to the bronchial wall, which may extend proximally to the main bronchus, are also classified as T1 tumors

[b]Most pleural (and pericardial) effusions with lung cancer are caused by the tumor. In a few patients, however, multiple cytopathological examinations of pleural (and/or pericardial) fluid are negative for tumor cells, and the fluid is nonbloody and not an exudate. When these elements and clinical judgment dictate that the effusion is not related to the tumor, the effusion should be excluded as a staging element, and the patient should be classified as having T1, T2, T3, or T4 disease

T status is determined by the tumor size and location and the presence of invasion of adjacent structures in the thorax. The T status descriptors are described in Table 1.1.

Because of its superior spatial resolution over that of MRI and PET, CT more accurately measures the size of primary tumors and readily identifies features of tumors at advanced T stages, such as gross chest wall involvement with rib destruction and bulging chest wall abnormalities. However, CT is not as accurate in identifying more subtle chest wall involvement, such as invasion of the parietal pleura, in contrast with the tumor merely abutting this structure. In one study, CT had a sensitivity rate of 63 % in distinguishing T3–T4 tumors from T0–T2 tumors, and its specificity rate was 84 % [104]. Some CT findings that suggest invasion of the chest wall include obliteration of the extrapleural fat plane, contact of the tumor with the pleural surface more than 3 cm in length, a high ratio of tumor-pleura contact to tumor height, and formation of an obtuse angle between the tumor and the pleura [105]. Despite its superior contrast resolution compared to CT, the accuracy

Table 1.2 NSCLC stage groups and TNM subsets (International staging system for lung cancer, seventh edition

Occult carcinoma	TX	N0	M0
Stage 0	Tis	N0	M0
Stage IA	T1a, b	N0	M0
Stage IB	T2a	N0	M0
Stage IIA	T1a, b	N1	M0
	T2a	N1	M0
	T2b	N0	M0
Stage IIB	T2b	N1	M0
	T3	N0	M0
Stage IIIA	T1, T2	N2	M0
	T3	N1, N2	M0
	T4	N0, N1	M0
Stage IIIB	T4	N2	M0
	Any T	N3	M0
Stage IV	Any T	Any N	M1a, b

Used with permission from Goldstraw et al. [99]

of MRI in identifying chest wall invasion is insufficient and similar to that of CT [104, 106].

For assessment of direct mediastinal involvement of lung tumors, CT and MRI findings suggestive of microscopic invasion of the mediastinum are tumor contact along the mediastinum of more than 3 cm, an angle of contact with the aorta greater than 90°, and a lack of a preserved fat plane between the mass and mediastinal structures [107–109]. Although one study found that MRI was superior to CT in identifying mediastinal invasion by a lung tumor [104], the accuracy of both imaging methods in assessment of mediastinal involvement was disappointing, with sensitivity rates of 55 % for CT and 64 % for MRI [110].

The superb soft tissue contrast resolution and multiplanar capabilities of MRI are ideally suited for evaluation of neurovascular invasion by lung tumors. This is particularly helpful in the evaluation of superior sulcus tumors. An absolute contraindication to surgery for superior sulcus tumors, for which surgical resection in the absence of nodal disease is associated with longer survival durations [111], is invasion of the brachial plexus roots or trunks above the level of the T1 nerve root. Also, the brachial plexus can be readily assessed in the sagittal plane using MRI, but is barely detectable using CT [112]. At the time of imaging, MRI can determine whether the carotid and vertebral arteries are involved by a lung tumor, which is a relative contraindication to surgery. MRI also can determine whether the contralateral vessels are severely affected by atherosclerotic disease, in which case the patient may not be a candidate for surgery [113]. Researchers have developed MRI sequences to overcome flow artifacts and improve vascular and cardiac images in motion. MRI also is used to determine whether and, if so, to what extent a tumor directly involves the heart in the preoperative assessment of surgical candidates.

Nodal Disease (N Status)

The seventh edition of the TNM staging system is identical to the sixth edition in terms of N staging (Table 1.1).

The role of chest radiography in N staging of NSCLC is limited, as mild to modest nodal enlargement is difficult to detect radiographically. Bulky bilateral adenopathy indicates stage IIIB disease. If the patient is too ill or is unwilling to undergo treatment, chest radiography should suffice for staging. In the majority of patients, however, a more accurate staging method is needed.

CT is routinely used for noninvasive N staging of lung tumors. The sole criterion for differentiating benign and metastatic lymph nodes in cross-sectional imaging studies is size: specifically, a short axis diameter greater than 1 cm [114]. Researchers chose this threshold to create a fine balance between sensitivity and specificity in an effort to minimize false-negative results. A meta-analysis that pooled evaluations of the lymph nodes of 5,111 patients with lung cancer in 43 different studies found that the sensitivity and specificity rates for CT in detecting metastases in the mediastinal lymph node compartments according to size criteria were 51 and 86 %, respectively. Similarly, two other meta-analyses showed sensitivity rates of 61–64 % and specificity rates of 74–79 % for CT in distinguishing benign from metastatic lymph nodes [115, 116]. The accuracy of CT in detecting nodal metastases is similar to that of MRI, as the accuracy rates for CT have ranged from 56 to 82 %, whereas those for MRI have ranged from 50 to 82 % [104, 110, 117–120]. These low accuracy numbers result from the fact that normal-sized lymph nodes can harbor tumor cells and, conversely, that nodal enlargement may reflect a benign reactive process [121, 122]. Recent attempts to use MRI to identify lung cancer nodal metastases based on internal characteristics of lymph nodes, such as high signal intensity, eccentric cortical thickening, and obliterated fatty hilum, had similarly disappointing results, with accuracy rates ranging from 70 to 73 % [123, 124].

The accuracy of ^{18}FDG-PET is superior to that of CT in N staging. However, the results of ^{18}FDG-PET performed for this purpose should be interpreted with caution and in conjunction with CT assessment, as nonneoplastic inflammatory processes have increased ^{18}FDG activity. As with that of pulmonary nodules, PET is less accurate than CT in the evaluation of lymph nodes smaller than 10 mm in diameter. N staging using integrated ^{18}FDG-PET-CT is more accurate than that using ^{18}FDG-PET alone [66, 125].

In a pooled analysis of results of multiple studies evaluating a total of 2,865 patients with lung cancer, the sensitivity and specificity rates for ^{18}FDG-PET in identifying metastatic lymph nodes were 74 and 85 %, respectively [126]. In a meta-analysis of 17 studies comprising 833 patients with lung cancer, the overall sensitivity and specificity rates for ^{18}FDG-PET in detecting nodal metastases were 83 and 92 %, respectively, whereas the sensitivity and specificity rates for chest CT were 59 and 78 %, respectively [127]. In cases with enlarged lymph nodes, the specificity and accuracy of ^{18}FDG-PET and ^{18}FDG-PET-CT decrease, but their sensitivity in detecting nodal metastatic spread increases [128–132]. In one meta-analysis of patients with lung cancer who had enlarged lymph nodes, the median sensitivity and specificity rates for ^{18}FDG-PET were 100 and 78 %, respectively [116]. The lower specificity rate in the presence of enlarged lymph nodes means that almost a quarter of the patients diagnosed with metastatic lymph nodes according to CT and ^{18}FDG-PET findings actually did not have nodal metastasis, but rather had reactive or inflammatory lymphadenopathy. In patients whose mediastinal lymph nodes are smaller than 1 cm in diameter, about 20 % have false-negative PET results; in a meta-analysis of patients with lung cancer, the sensitivity and specificity rates for ^{18}FDG-PET scanning of small nodes were 82 and 93 %, respectively [116].

Because of the accuracies previously described in identifying lymph node metastases, ASCO recommends performing a confirmatory biopsy in lung cancer cases with ^{18}FDG-avid mediastinal lymph nodes so that patients with operable disease will not be denied curative surgery [65]. An ^{18}FDG-PET scan is justified even when a highly suspicious enlarged lymph node is identified on the initial chest CT scan. The ^{18}FDG-PET scan may influence the site of biopsy by identifying a previously unsuspected metastasis (which may upstage the disease), or a metastasis for which biopsy is safer than a biopsy of the initially intended mediastinal lymph node. Whereas mediastinoscopy and transbronchial lymph node biopsy are unable to sample all lymph node stations, tissue sampling remains the most accurate method of preoperative identification of occult metastatic disease in mediastinal lymph nodes smaller than 1 cm in diameter.

Distant Metastasis (M Status)

The goal of identifying of metastatic lung cancer is preventing nontherapeutic thoracotomy. The seventh edition of the TNM staging system divides metastatic disease into M1a for metastases in the thoracic cavity and M1b for extrathoracic metastases. In addition, the M1a category includes malignant pleural effusions and nodules and metastatic pulmonary nodules in the contralateral lung [99]. The common sites of distant metastatic disease in patients with NSCLC are the adrenal glands, liver, brain, and bone.

Establishing the diagnosis of a malignant pleural effusion, an M1a disease [99], is frequently difficult because fluid sampling via thoracentesis is positive for malignancy in only 66 % of patients [133]. Pleural nodules in the presence of pleural fluid are strongly indicative of malignant effusion; however, the pleura does not always exhibit nodularity on CT scans. ^{18}FDG-PET is helpful in identifying pleural metastases, but reported studies of the accuracy of ^{18}FDG-PET in establishing the diagnosis of a malignant effusion are few, with reported sensitivity rates of 92–100 %, specificity rates of 67–71 %, negative predictive values of 100 %, and positive predictive values of 63–79 % [134, 135]. ^{18}FDG-PET scanning for pleural malignancies should be interpreted with caution and in conjunction with CT scanning, as pleural inflammation following talc pleurodesis can persist for years and will exhibit increased ^{18}FDG uptake in the absence of malignant cells [136]. However, a negative PET result, that is, without increased pleural FDG uptake, can be useful in confirming the absence of metastatic pleural disease, particularly when the results of thoracentesis are also negative for metastasis.

In patients with early-stage NSCLC (stage I or II) according to their initial chest CT scans and with no clinical symptoms, additional imaging for metastatic disease has a low yield [137–139]. Some advise further extrathoracic staging of tumors in such patients whose histological type has an increased likelihood of extrathoracic metastasis at the time of presentation, such as adenocarcinoma or large cell carcinoma [19, 137, 140, 141]; however, a study of a large series of patients with early-stage lung cancer did not find this approach to be productive [139]. Nevertheless, a study in which researchers performed biopsy analysis of normal-appearing adrenal glands in patients with NSCLC staged using chest CT found that 12 % of the glands harbored metastatic disease [142]. Another study compared autopsy results with CT scans of the adrenal glands in 73 patients with NSCLC and 18 patients with SCLC within 90 days before death, which showed that CT detected only 20 % of adrenal metastases; the authors attributed this low sensitivity of CT to the absence of substantial structural changes in the glands [143].

Because of these findings, the American College of Chest Physicians [144] and ASCO [65] issued guidelines recommending ^{18}FDG-PET scanning for staging of NSCLC. Further imaging is advised depending on patient symptoms or for abnormal lesions that remain indeterminate following initial investigations using ^{18}FDG-PET and CT. Except in the brain, ^{18}FDG-PET is more sensitive and specific than CT and bone scanning in detecting metastatic disease [145–147]. For example, in a study of 303 patients, the sensitivity and specificity rates for ^{18}FDG-PET in the identification of metastatic disease were 83 and 90 %, respectively [68]. ^{18}FDG-PET also has detected unexpected distant metastases in approximately 15 % of patients with lung cancer [71] and prevented nontherapeutic thoracotomy in 20 % of patients with this disease [68, 69]. PET scanning has the benefits of imaging the entire body in one examination and assessing areas less effectively evaluated using conventional imaging, such as the skin, muscles, and pelvis, facilitating detection of unusual metastatic foci.

The adrenal glands are the most common sites of metastatic disease in patients with NSCLC [148, 149], and isolated adrenal metastasis occurs in up to 6 % of patients [150]. However, the majority of adrenal nodules, as observed at initial presentation in up to 20 % of patients, are benign [142, 148, 149, 151–159]. Adrenal nodules with a radiodensity of 10 HU or less on CT scans may confidently be diagnosed as adrenal adenomas. This criterion has 98 % sensitivity but only 71 % specificity [160], as 30 % of adenomas do not contain a sufficient amount of lipid to be measured using CT [161]. In these cases, an effective choice is MRI using chemical shift analysis to determine whether microscopic amounts of lipid are present and thus differentiate a benign adenoma from a malignant nodule [162–164]. Chemical shift analyses (MRI) and Hounsfield unit measurements (CT) can be erroneous when the adrenal nodule is small. CT and MRI features of adrenal metastasis include diameter greater than 3 cm, high signal intensity on T2-weighted MRI sequences, poorly defined margins, an irregularly enhancing rim, and invasion of adjacent structures [165].

^{18}FDG-PET can be helpful in establishing the benignity of adrenal nodules. Studies have shown that although the sensitivity and specificity rates for ^{18}FDG-PET scanning of adrenal masses are high (100 and 80–90 %, respectively), adenomas can have increased FDG uptake [146, 166]. The accuracy of identifying an adrenal metastasis is increased when an adrenal nodule has greater ^{18}FDG avidity than the liver as opposed to using a specific standardized uptake value (Fig. 1.14a–c) [167]. Because uptake can be high in adenomas, ASCO recommends biopsy analysis of an isolated adrenal mass identified on imaging studies to rule out distant metastatic disease if the cancer would otherwise be potentially resectable.

NSCLC frequently metastasizes to the liver, but the liver is rarely an isolated site of disease, particularly without evidence of metastatic disease to regional lymph nodes. One meta-analysis found that only 3 % of asymptomatic patients with NSCLC had liver metastases on CT scans. ^{18}FDG-PET can detect liver metastases with accuracy rates ranging from 92 to 100 % [147, 151, 168] and only rare false-positive findings; nevertheless, the data in those studies were limited and were not compared with results of systematic biopsies or state-of-the-art liver imaging with CT or MRI. When a liver lesion is suspected to be a metastasis according to any imaging modality, the suspicion should be confirmed using biopsy if the disease is otherwise potentially resectable [65]. In most cases, liver metastases do not significantly alter management of lung cancer because they are not isolated [169].

Routine screening for brain metastases in asymptomatic patients presenting with newly diagnosed NSCLC remains controversial and is not universally recommended by ASCO [65]. Authors reported that when brain CT was performed in asymptomatic patients undergoing NSCLC staging, the median prevalence of brain metastasis was 3 % (range, 0–21 %) [137, 170–177]. In comparison, when brain CT was performed in a combination of symptomatic and asymptomatic patients, the prevalence of brain metastases was 14 % (range, 6–32 %) [178–186]. Asymptomatic brain metastases are more common in patients with advanced intrathoracic disease than those presenting with early disease [141, 187]. Patients with stage I or II lung cancer have had a brain lesion detection rate of 4 % using CT or MRI, whereas those with stage III disease have had a detection rate of 11.4 % [177]. Although MRI can detect smaller and more numerous brain metastases than CT scan [177], evidence showing that MRI can identify more patients with NSCLC metastases than CT scan is lacking. Consequently, ASCO determined that both CT and MRI are acceptable for evaluation of brain metastases of lung cancer. One of these imaging studies should be performed in patients who have neurological signs of a brain-occupying lesion or have symptoms, as well as asymptomatic patients with stage III lung cancer who are being considered for aggressive local therapy such as thoracotomy or irradiation [65].

^{18}FDG-PET is not recommended for assessment of brain metastases of lung cancer. The sensitivity rate for ^{18}FDG-PET in detection of brain metastases has been shown to be as low as 60 % [147]. ^{18}FDG accumulates avidly in the gray matter, which is the location of most metastatic lesions, thus limiting their detectability.

Although patients with skeletal metastases from lung cancer often are symptomatic and/or have laboratory test results indicating calcium and phosphate level abnormalities [185], one study demonstrated that up to 27 % of asymptomatic patients had skeletal metastases [188]. False-positive abnormalities on technetium 99 m methylene diphosphonate bone scintigrams are numerous, owing to the frequency of degenerative and traumatic skeletal changes which also cause radiotracer accumulation. ^{18}FDG-PET is superior to bone scintigraphy in identifying skeletal metastases. Specifically, ^{18}FDG-PET is able to identify metastatic deposits in the bone marrow that typically are not detected by bone scintigraphy, and ^{18}FDG-PET yields few false-positive results. Furthermore, rates of the specificity, sensitivity, negative predictive value, positive predictive value, and accuracy of ^{18}FDG-PET scanning in the assessment of bone metastases have exceeded 90 % [145, 147, 188, 189]. Bone scintigraphy is therefore considered optional in patients who have evidence of bone metastases according to ^{18}FDG-PET unless they have symptoms suggestive of bone metastases in regions not included on PET scans. Because of the potential for false-positive uptake on both ^{18}FDG-PET scans and bone scintigrams, patients with lung cancer who are candidates for surgery are required to undergo histological confirmation or corroboration of bone metastasis using morphological imaging (radiography, CT, or MRI) of a lesion that will upstage their disease [65].

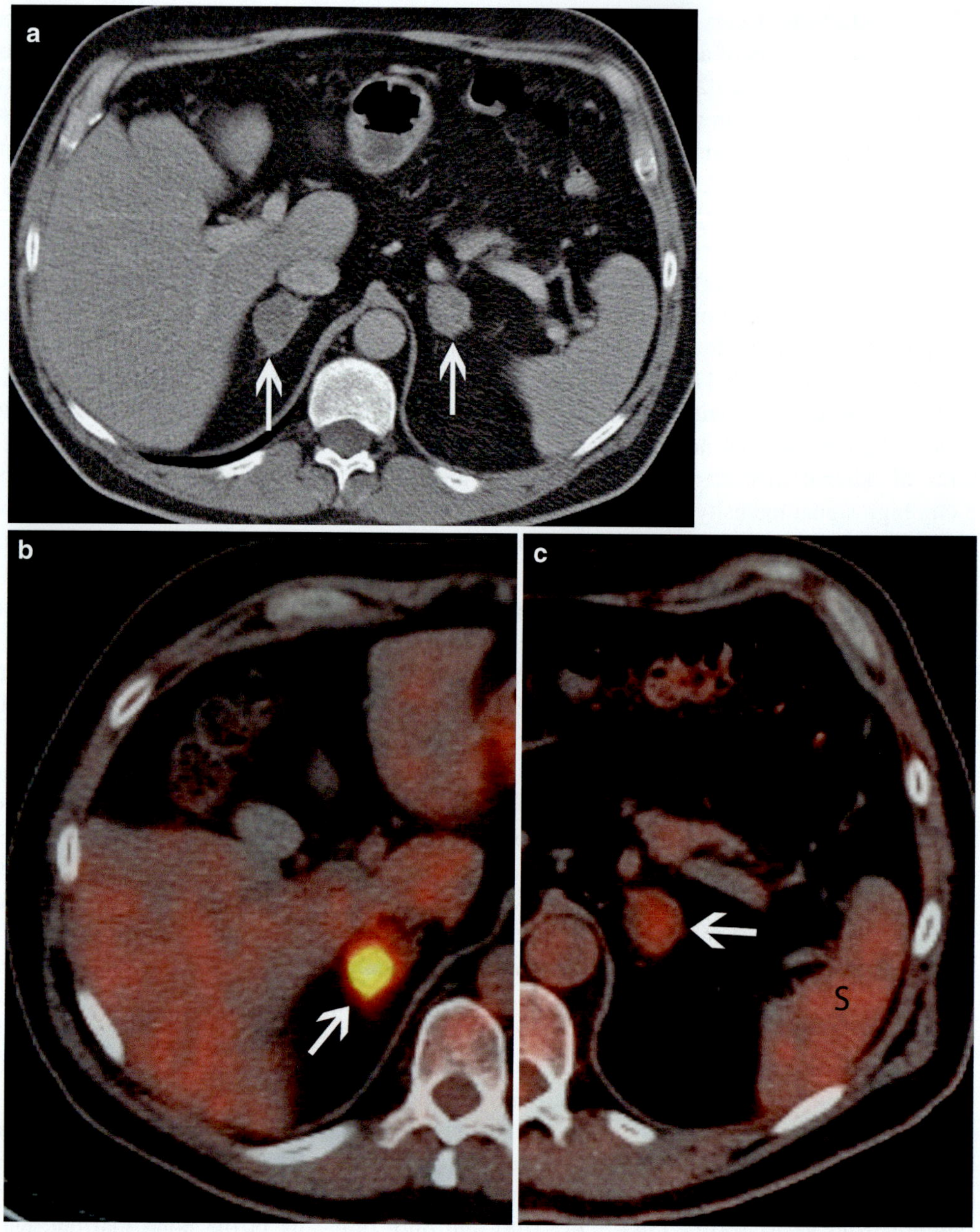

Fig 1.14 (**a**) Contrast-enhanced CT scans with abdominal window settings through the upper abdomen showing bilateral adrenal gland nodules (*arrows*) in a 58-year-old man with metastatic lung adenocarcinoma. (**b**) Fused image from subsequent PET-CT examination showing avid ^{18}FDG uptake in a right adrenal nodule (*arrow*), which was consistent with metastatic disease. (**c**) Fused image from same PET-CT showing background level activity, similar to splenic activity, in a left adrenal nodule, suggesting a benign etiology such as incidental adrenal adenoma. *S* spleen

To summarize staging of NSCLC, imaging with a chest CT scan that includes the adrenal glands and liver is routine. If the disease does not appear to be metastatic, further staging with ^{18}FDG-PET or PET-CT is recommended [65]. Additional imaging, such as brain imaging for early-stage disease or dedicated bone imaging (plain film, scintigraphy, or MRI), is performed if the patient is symptomatic or to clarify uncertain initial ^{18}FDG-PET and CT findings. Patients with locally advanced disease scheduled to receive aggressive therapy (surgery or irradiation) should undergo dedicated brain imaging (MRI or contrast-enhanced CT) even if they are asymptomatic. Biopsy analysis of nodes suspected to have metastases (i.e., those larger than 1 cm in diameter or with increased FDG activity) is required for confirmation of the presence of nodal disease. A positive imaging finding that would change the clinical management of lung cancer, such as an isolated distant metastasis in a patient whose disease is otherwise resectable, should be verified by biopsy.

SCLC

The number of studies on the best imaging methods for staging of SCLC is lower than that for NSCLC, which is probably due to the dismal prognosis of these patients. The great majority of SCLC patients undergo nonsurgical treatment. The Veterans Administration Lung Cancer Study Group developed a simplified method of dichotomous staging of

SCLC [190]. According to this method, limited SCLC includes tumors confined to the hemithorax of origin, mediastinum, and/or supraclavicular lymph nodes. Tumor spread beyond these sites constitutes extensive disease. Most patients with SCLC have disseminated disease at initial presentation [191]. The common sites of metastatic disease are the liver, bone, bone marrow, brain, and retroperitoneal lymph nodes, which can be identified on the initial staging chest CT scan.

Multiple studies, including bone marrow aspiration, brain MRI, CT scanning of the chest and abdomen, and bone scintigraphy, are commonly performed for staging of SCLC [192], but radiologists and oncologists have yet to reach a consensus regarding the routine use of imaging modalities for this purpose. Researchers have attempted to use a single imaging modality for the entire body and reduce the multiplicity of studies currently used for staging of this disease. MRI is able to fill this role, but it has not gained popularity [191]. Staging of SCLC with ^{18}FDG-PET or PET-CT is not recommended according to the second edition of the Evidence-Based Clinical Practice Guidelines of the American College of Chest Physicians [192] because of a lack of randomized prospective trials showing that ^{18}FDG-PET improves staging. Many studies of SCLC have investigated fewer than 50 patients and lacked reference standards to verify the staging accuracy of ^{18}FDG-PET [193–198]. Nevertheless, recent reports suggested that staging of SCLC using ^{18}FDG-PET resulted in a change in management in 8–16 % of patients [199, 200]. As for NSCLC, PET-CT is more accurate than chest CT alone for staging of SCLC but is less accurate than conventional imaging in detecting brain metastases [193–201].

Isolated bone and bone marrow metastases of SCLC are not common [190, 202, 203]. Therefore, evaluation for osseous metastatic disease using bone scintigraphy, bone marrow aspiration, or MRI is not performed in asymptomatic patients with limited SCLC, but rather is usually reserved for patients with extensive disease. Brain metastases, on the other hand, are common in patients with SCLC. Specifically, intracranial lesions are seen at presentation in up to 24 % of asymptomatic patients who undergo contrast-enhanced brain MRI. Therefore, dedicated brain imaging is advocated by many oncologists as part of routine staging workup [191, 204]. Liver and retroperitoneal lymph node metastases are also common at presentation in patients with SCLC but are usually asymptomatic [190, 202]. Thus, staging of SCLC should include contrast-enhanced imaging of the entire liver using either CT or MRI.

Uncommon Primary Pulmonary Malignancies

Some types of primary lung tumors are rare, but when they do occur, they often have radiological features that may suggest their diagnosis.

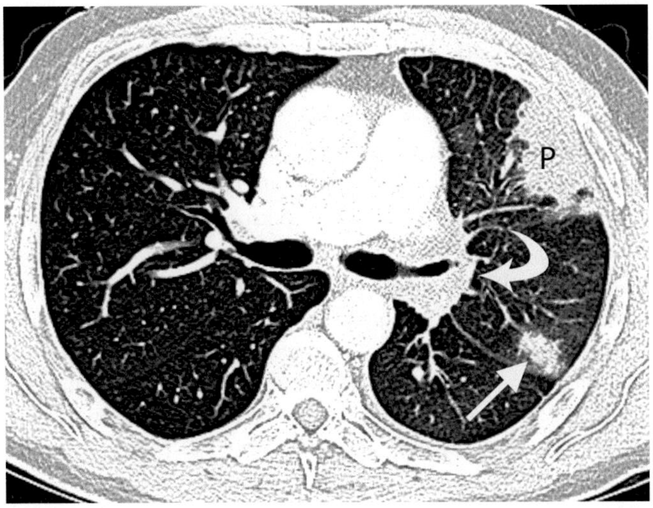

Fig. 1.15 Contrast-enhanced chest CT scan with lung window settings showing a large left upper lobe primary tumor (*P*) and left hilar lymphadenopathy (*curved arrow*) in a 74-year-old man with sarcomatoid carcinoma of the lung. A satellite metastasis (*arrow*) is shown in the same lobe

Sarcomatoid Carcinoma

Carcinomas with pleomorphic, sarcomatoid, or sarcomatous elements are uncommon. On radiological images, these neoplasms can appear either as large peripheral masses or polypoid endobronchial lesions with attendant atelectasis or postobstructive pneumonia [205–208]. Calcification and cavitation are unusual, but necrosis and hemorrhage can appear as heterogeneous attenuation on CT scans [206–208]. Also, hilar and mediastinal adenopathy are uncommon [207]. Pleural effusion can occur as a result of local invasion [209]. Metastases develop in sites similar to those in patients with lung cancer: lung, liver, bones, adrenal glands, and brain (Fig. 1.15) [208].

Pulmonary Blastoma

The typical appearance of pulmonary blastoma is a single, large (2.5–26.0 cm), well-marginated peripheral mass [210–213]. Multiplicity, cavitation, and calcification are rare [213]. Local invasion of the mediastinum and pleura occurs in 8 and 25 % of cases, respectively [211]. Hilar and mediastinal lymph node metastasis occurs in 30 % of resected cases [211]. Extrathoracic metastases are common and have distributions similar to that of primary lung cancer [211, 214].

Neoplasms of the Tracheobronchial Glands

Tracheobronchial gland neoplasms are usually located in the central airways but may occasionally manifest as peripheral pulmonary nodules. These tumors are frequently missed on chest radiographs unless they are large enough to cause obstructions and postobstructive lung parenchymal findings, such as atelectasis or pneumonia, as the tracheal air column and proximal bronchi are "blind spots" on radiographs for many radiologists. CT, which readily demonstrates the airways, is an important diagnostic tool for adult patients who present with new-onset "asthma."

Adenoid cystic carcinomas are confined to the trachea or main central bronchi in 80 % of patients, whereas 10–15 % of these tumors may manifest as peripheral pulmonary nodules [215–218]. The typical radiological appearance of an adenoid cystic carcinoma is an endotracheal or endobronchial mass, usually lobulated or polypoid, that narrows the airway lumen (Fig. 1.16). These lesions can be circumferential and may manifest as diffuse stenosis [219]. Metastatic spread of an adenoid cystic carcinoma has a distribution similar to that of metastatic spread of NSCLC [218]. Adenoid cystic carcinomas exhibit slow, progressive local growth [216] and metastasize at a late stage; consequently, patients with this cancer are usually considered candidates for surgery. CT is used for surgical planning and readily demonstrates the extratracheal extent of these tumors. However, CT can underestimate the longitudinal extent of an adenoid cystic carcinoma [220] even when it is evaluated in multiplanar reformatted reconstructions, as this tumor has a tendency to infiltrate beneath the mucosa, a microscopic phenomenon that is not identifiable on CT scans.

Mucoepidermoid carcinomas typically occur as central endobronchial masses in the main or lobar bronchi. Less common presentations include a polypoid intraluminal nodule in the trachea and pulmonary nodule or mass in the lung periphery [221–223]. Mucoepidermoid carcinomas are usually slow-growing, low-grade neoplasms with benign clinical courses, although some have more aggressive high-grade features [223–225]. These two forms, adenoid cystic and mucoepidermoid carcinomas, have similar radiological appearances and thus cannot be distinguished from each other using imaging studies alone [223].

Malignant Mesenchymal Lung Tumors

Spindle cell sarcomas (malignant fibrous histiocytoma, hemangiopericytoma, fibrosarcoma, leiomyosarcoma, and synovial sarcoma) are the most common primary pulmonary sarcomas [226–229]. They are most often located in the periphery of the lung, although central and endobronchial masses can occur [227, 228, 230–232]. Authors have reported spindle cell sarcomas as large as 25 cm in diameter; their large size at presentation probably results from their slow growth and tendency to metastasize late. These tumors are typically sharply marginated and occasionally calcified [226–228, 230, 233]. Cavitation is uncommon, although heterogeneous attenuation resulting from necrosis in the mass may be seen on CT scans [226, 233]. In particular, the rich vascularity of hemangiopericytomas in the lung can be demonstrated using CT, MRI, and ultrasound, but this tumor cannot be radiologically distinguished from other sarcomas,

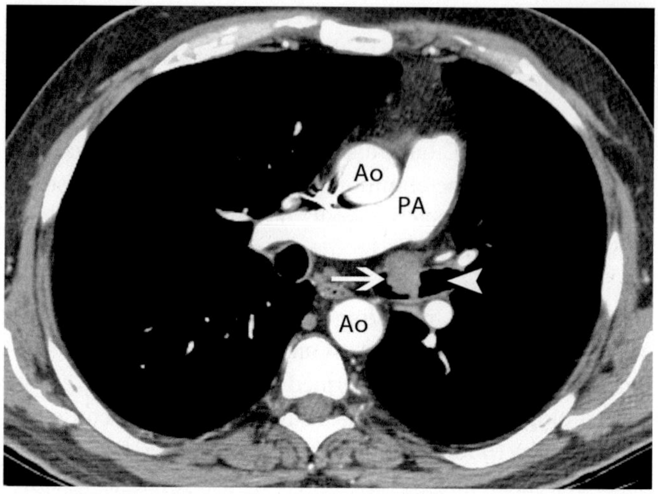

Fig 1.16 Contrast-enhanced chest CT scan with mediastinal window settings showing an irregular nodule (*arrow*) in the left main bronchus with both endobronchial and extrabronchial extension in a 51-year-old man with primary adenoid cystic carcinoma of the left bronchus. Because the tumor did not completely obstruct the airway, the distal left main bronchus (*arrowhead*) remained patent. *Ao* aorta, *PA* pulmonary artery

which can contain similar-appearing vascularity. Features of these tumors that suggest hypervascularity include feeding arteries that can be visualized directly using CT or MR angiography and indirect signs such as avid nodule enhancement on contrast-enhanced chest CT or MRI scans. Evidence of internal hemorrhaging includes high attenuation on unenhanced chest CT scans and hyperintense areas on both T1- and T2-weighted images [232, 234, 235].

Sarcomas of vascular origin (angiosarcomas and epithelioid hemangioendotheliomas) are extremely rare primary lung tumors [228, 236, 237]. Angiosarcomas of the lung are described as multiple bilateral nodules, but most probably represent metastases, and a primary tumor located outside the lung that must be excluded [228]. Pulmonary epithelioid hemangioendothelioma usually appears radiologically as multiple 1–2-cm bilateral pulmonary nodules, although about 25 % of patients have single nodules and unilateral distribution [236, 238, 239]. Authors recently described irregular thickening of the bronchovascular bundles and perilobular structures caused by lymphangitic spread and associated multiple bilateral pulmonary nodules on high-resolution CT scans [240]. Calcification is rarely detected radiologically but is frequently detected histologically [238, 239]. Although primary lung sarcomas are usually indolent, the presence of hemorrhagic pleural effusion is a sign of poor prognosis [236].

Primary Lung Lymphoma

The radiological findings for primary lymphoma of the lung may vary according to the criteria used to define this disease. The most widely accepted definition is intrathoracic monoclonal lymphoid proliferation without extrathoracic sites of disease at presentation and for at least 3 months after diagnosis. Some authors restrict the diagnosis to pulmonary parenchymal disease only, whereas others include hilar adenopathy with or without mediastinal adenopathy [241–247]. The parenchymal manifestations of lymphoma include solitary or multiple nodules or masses, focal or multifocal consolidation, reticulonodular opacities, and atelectasis (Fig. 1.17) [242, 248–252]. Hilar adenopathy is rare, and pleural effusion occurs in 7–25 % of patients [242, 249, 253].

Secondary Malignant Lung Tumors

Metastasis to the lungs occurs via multiple routes: the pulmonary and bronchial arteries, lymphatics, and airways. The four patterns of metastasis to the lung parenchyma are parenchymal nodules, interstitial thickening (lymphangitic carcinomatosis), tumor emboli with or without pulmonary hypertension or infarction, and airway obstruction by an endobronchial tumor.

Parenchymal nodules are the most common manifestations of metastatic disease in the lungs and are usually multiple and predominantly located in the lower lobes (Fig. 1.18) [254]. When multiple pulmonary nodules are present, they are usually well demarcated, although they may have irregular margins as seen with some adenocarcinomas [255]. They can vary in size from large "cannonball" metastases, as seen with sarcomas, to multiple, small 1-mm nodules distributed in a miliary pattern, as seen with thyroid cancer (Fig. 1.19a, b).

Use of multidetector spiral CT, with improved resolution and decreasing slice thickness, has led to increased sensitivity in the detection of pulmonary nodules. However, the appearance of these nodules on CT is not specific, and many of the nodules identified using CT are benign. When pulmonary nodules are new, growing, and multiple in a patient with a primary malignancy, they are most likely metastases. When an oncologist is in doubt about whether they are metastases, he or she should consider biopsy analysis of the largest nodule. Monitoring of small nodules (<4 mm in diameter) in a patient with a known malignancy is recommended for assessment of their growth, as these nodules are below the resolution of PET.

Solitary lung metastases are uncommon, as researchers have observed them in 2–10 % of patients presenting with pulmonary nodules [2, 10, 256]. Certain primary malignancies are more likely than others to metastasize to the lung in the form of a solitary nodule, including sarcoma, melanoma, and carcinoma of the colon, kidney, testicle, or breast [2, 257, 258]. Reliable radiological criteria distinguishing a primary lung tumor from a solitary pulmonary metastasis are lacking [10, 256] because their imaging features overlap.

Pulmonary metastatic nodules may have an unusual appearance. Cavitation in metastatic nodules is detected using chest radiography in approximately 4 % of patients

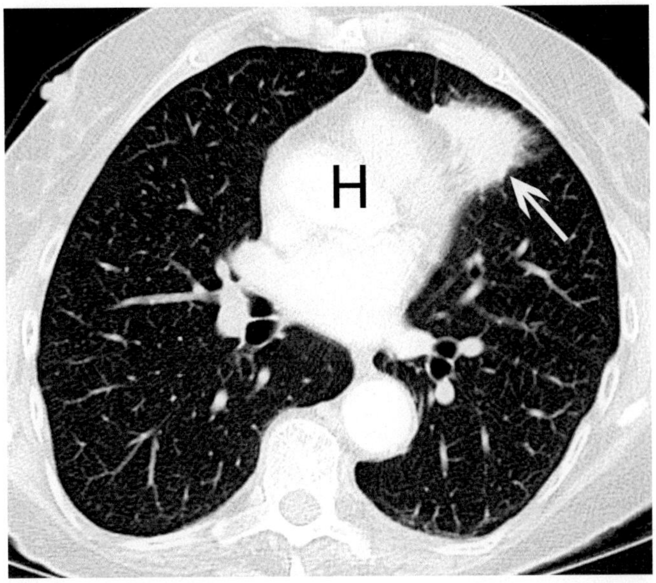

Fig. 1.17 Contrast-enhanced chest CT scan with lung window settings demonstrating an irregular consolidative mass in the lingula (*arrow*) in an 81-year-old woman with primary B-cell lymphoma of the lung. *H* heart

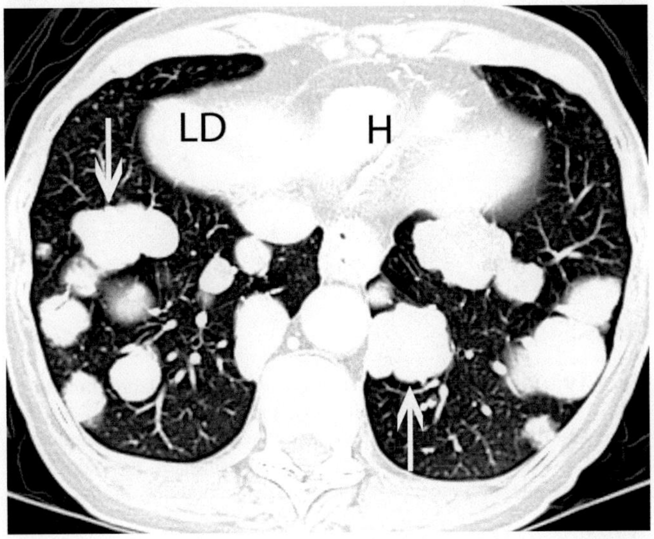

Fig. 1.18 Contrast-enhanced chest CT scan with mediastinal window settings showing a very large number of rounded, well-circumscribed bilateral pulmonary nodules (*two marked with arrows*) with a lower lobe predominance in a 68-year-old woman 3 years after treatment of an adenoid cystic carcinoma in the right neck. Biopsy analysis demonstrated a metastatic adenoid cystic carcinoma, cribriform type. *LD* liver dome, *H* heart

with metastases, most often those of squamous cell histology (Fig. 1.20a–c) [259, 260]. On CT scans, however, cavitation is seen in 9 % of metastatic nodules, with equal distribution of the adenocarcinoma and squamous cell carcinoma subtypes of NSCLC [261]. Metastatic sarcoma also can cavitate, and a pneumothorax can be the presenting feature of the disease [262, 263]. As described previously, pulmonary

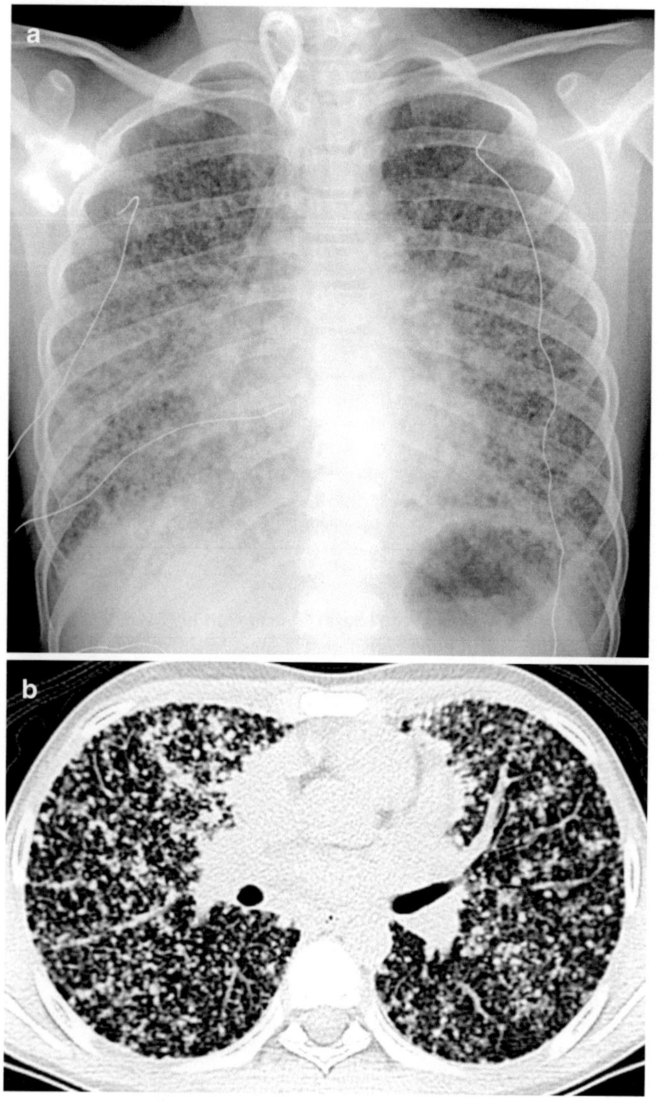

Fig. 1.19 (**a**) Chest radiograph demonstrating a very large number of diffuse bilateral nodules approximately 3 mm in size in diameter in a 13-year-old boy with metastatic papillary thyroid cancer. (**b**) Noncontrast chest CT scan with lung window settings through the mid-lungs confirming the presence of bilateral miliary nodules in a random distribution

nodules with certain calcification patterns are considered benign except in patients with primary osteosarcoma or chondrosarcoma, as calcification and ossification can occur in pulmonary metastases of these tumors [262]. Calcification in pulmonary metastases of other primary malignancies is much less common, but authors have reported it in patients with synovial sarcoma, giant cell tumors of the bone, and carcinomas of the colon, ovary, breast, and thyroid [262, 264–266]. A solid pulmonary nodule surrounded by a ground-glass halo suggests peritumoral hemorrhage (Fig. 1.21) [255] but should be distinguished from other disease processes that have this appearance, such as invasive fungal infections, AIS, and lymphoma [267–269].

Lymphangitic carcinomatosis is uncommon but can occur in patients with primary tumors in the lung, breast, stomach, pancreas, prostate, cervix, or thyroid [262, 270]. Chest radiographic findings of lymphangitic carcinomatosis may mimic those of pulmonary edema, from which it must be distinguished, and include thickened bronchovascular markings, interlobular septal thickening, and, in some cases, pleural effusion [271, 272]. Up to 50 % of patients with pathologically proven lymphangitic carcinomatosis have normal-appearing chest radiographs [273, 274]. A study showed that the use of chest CT, in addition to a chest radiograph, increased the rate of confident diagnosis of lymphangitic carcinomatosis from 54 % (by clinical examination, history, and chest radiography alone) to 92 %, whereas a lack of imaging resulted in no confident diagnoses [275]. On thin-section CT scans, lymphangitic carcinomatosis typically appears with irregular nodular thickening of the interlobular septa and peribronchovascular bundles [272, 276]. This pattern of interstitial thickening causes a CT appearance of polygonal shapes with a central dot superimposed on the normal lung architecture (Fig. 1.22). This appearance, in association with nodularity of the interlobular septa, is pathognomonic for lymphangitic carcinomatosis and distinguishes it from pulmonary edema, in which septal thickening is smooth [277]. When nodularity is not seen, the nondependent distribution and asymmetry of lymphangitic carcinomatosis may help differentiate it from edema. Approximately 30 % of patients with lymphangitic carcinomatosis also present with pleural effusion, and 40 % present with mediastinal or hilar adenopathy [272].

Tumor emboli are rarely identified using imaging despite being observed microscopically in as many as 26 % of patients with lung metastases at autopsy [278, 279]. These emboli are usually located in small or medium-sized pulmonary arteries, which make radiology-based diagnosis of them difficult [280]. On CT scans, tumor emboli appear as dilation or beading of the subsegmental arteries (Fig. 1.23a, b), which may be accompanied by peripheral wedge-shaped areas of low parenchymal attenuation owing to pulmonary infarction [281–283]. Researchers have described the tree-in-bud appearance (branching peripheral centrilobular opacities) as a manifestation of pulmonary tumor embolism [284, 285]. Tumors frequently associated with pulmonary tumor emboli are hepatomas, breast and renal cell carcinomas, gastric and prostatic cancers, and choriocarcinomas [279, 280].

Endobronchial metastasis is uncommon, and its origin is most frequently renal, colorectal, or breast carcinoma or melanoma [286–291]. Secondary chest radiography findings of endobronchial metastases are caused by bronchial obstruction and include atelectasis, postobstructive pneumonitis, and air trapping. On CT scans, endobronchial metastases appear as polypoid, sometimes branching intraluminal soft tissue masses (Fig. 1.24a, b) [292].

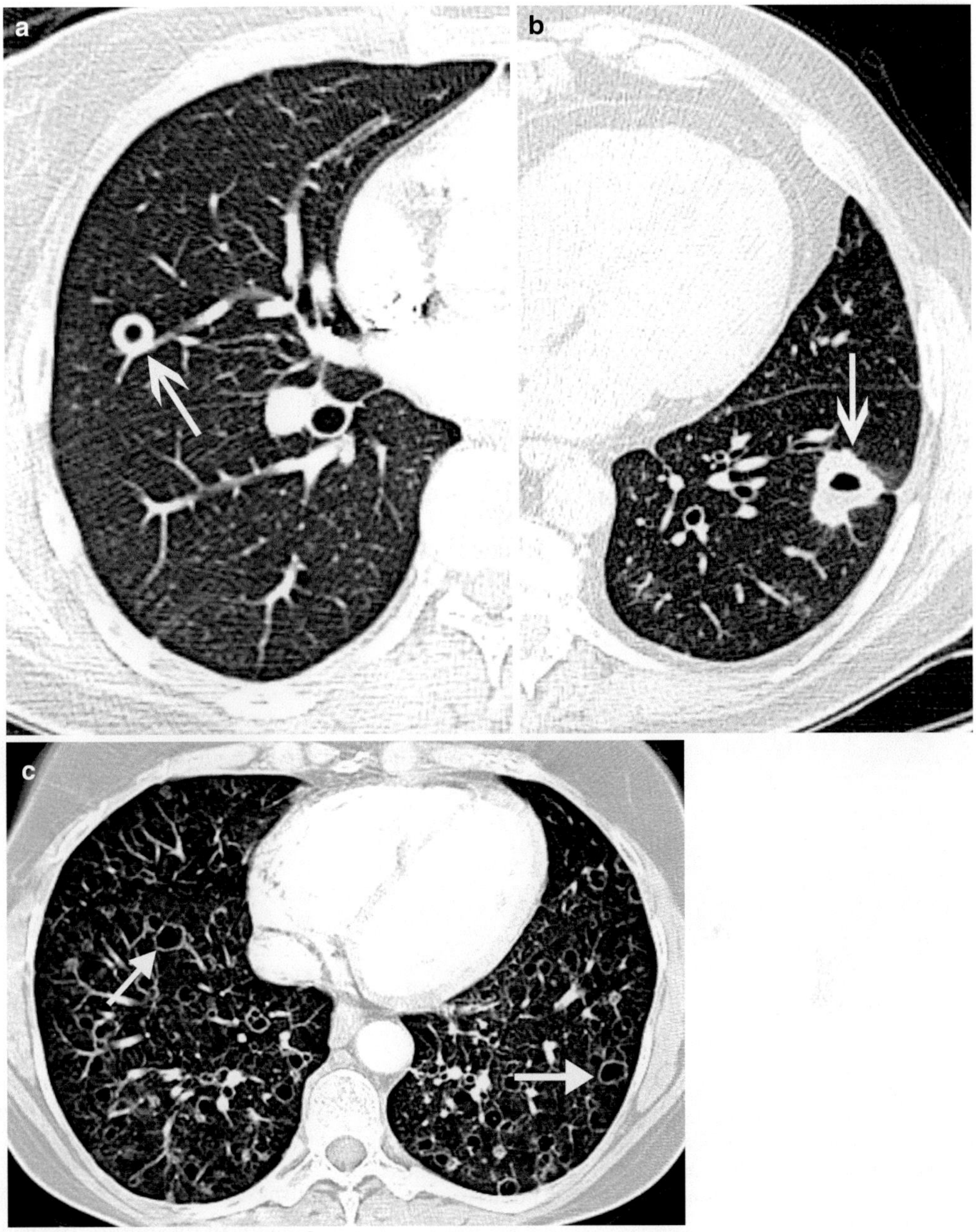

Fig. 1.20 Chest CT scans with lung window settings showing cavitary metastases in the lung. (**a**) A well-circumscribed round nodule with a central lucency (*arrow*) in a 38-year-old woman with metastatic rectal adenocarcinoma with mucinous features. (**b**) A somewhat irregular nodule with a central lucency (*arrow*) corresponding to pulmonary metastasis in a 62-year-old man with keratinizing squamous cell carcinoma of the tongue. (**c**) Bilateral small cyst-like structures (*arrows*) with thin walls in a 58-year-old woman with widely metastatic adenocarcinoma of the lung

Primary Malignant Pleural Tumors

Mesothelioma

Imaging plays an integral part in the diagnosis, staging, and treatment response assessment of mesothelioma. This disease poses challenges in imaging because of its complex three-dimensional configuration. Treatment options for mesothelioma, which range from conservative management to radical surgery, depend on staging, which requires accurate delineation of the tumor using imaging. Typically, mesothelioma manifests as a unilateral pleural mass with moderate to large pleural effusion. The subtypes of mesothelioma do not have distinct imaging features and are only identified histologically. This locally aggressive tumor rarely metastasizes to distant sites, yet most patients present with advanced disease and die within 1 year after presentation [293–300].

Imaging of Mesothelioma

Malignant pleural mesothelioma (MPM) is often detected first on chest radiographs as a unilateral pleural abnormality with moderate to large effusion [301–305]. In 45–60 % of patients, mesothelioma manifests as a smooth, lobular pleural mass that infiltrates the pleural space and fissures [301–303]. As the tumor grows, it typically encases the lung and causes an

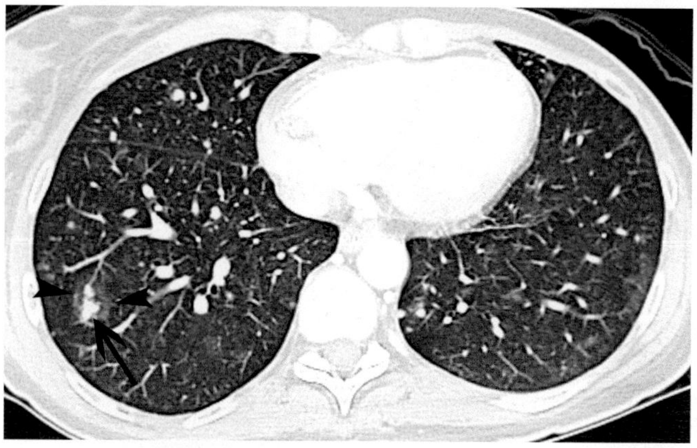

Fig. 1.21 Contrast-enhanced chest CT scan with lung window settings showing multiple small nodules with ground-glass halos in a 38-year-old woman 2 years after treatment of an angiosarcoma of the left breast. The largest nodule (*arrow*) in the right lower lobe is bilobed and measures 2.2 cm in length, including the surrounding ground-glass halo (*arrowheads*)

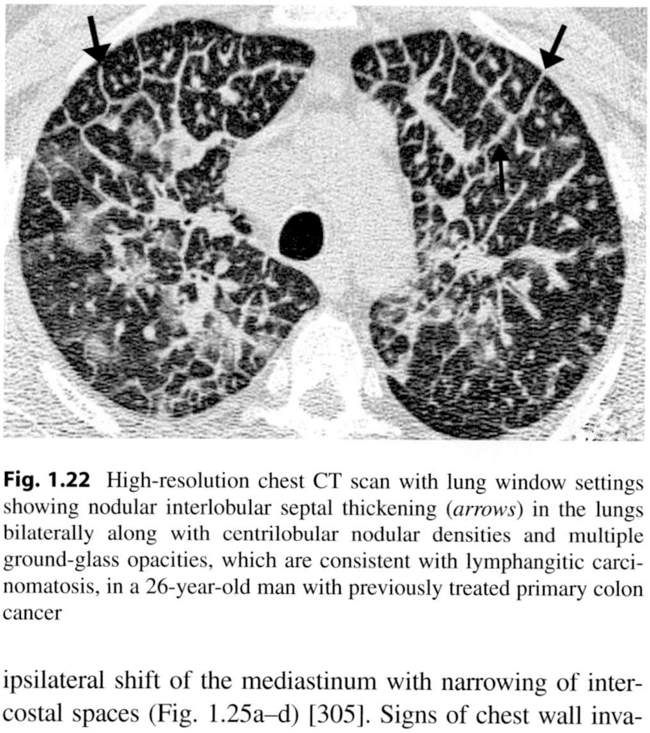

Fig. 1.22 High-resolution chest CT scan with lung window settings showing nodular interlobular septal thickening (*arrows*) in the lungs bilaterally along with centrilobular nodular densities and multiple ground-glass opacities, which are consistent with lymphangitic carcinomatosis, in a 26-year-old man with previously treated primary colon cancer

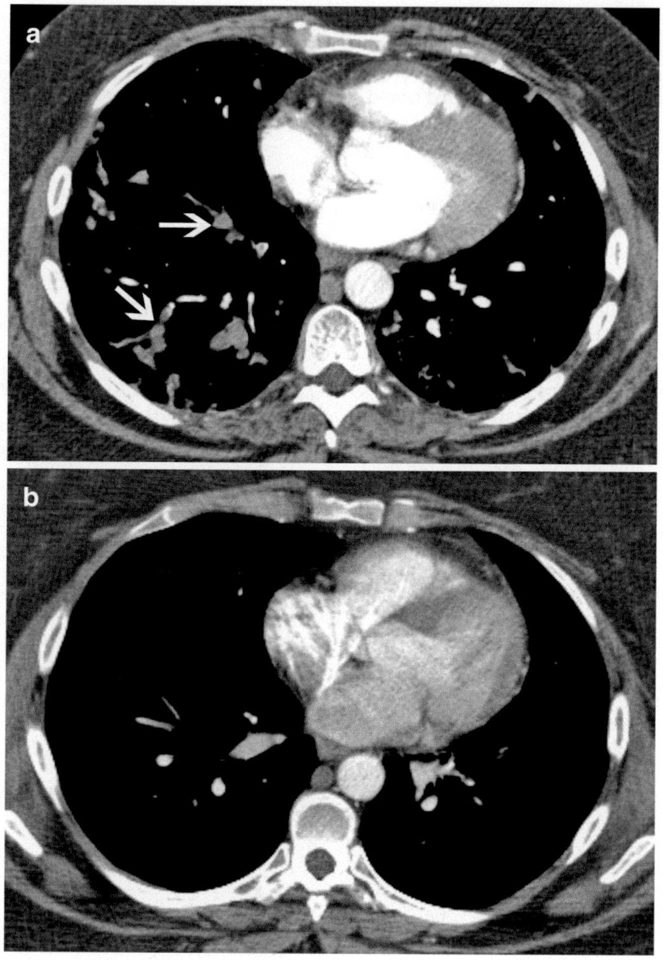

Fig. 1.23 (**a**) Contrast-enhanced chest CT scan with mediastinal window settings demonstrating beading of the pulmonary arteries (*arrows*) secondary to pulmonary arterial tumor emboli in a 41-year-old woman with chondrosarcoma of the right pelvis and sacrum after hemipelvectomy. (**b**) Contrast-enhanced chest CT scan performed 7 months before the scan in (**a**), showing no abnormalities in the pulmonary vessels

ipsilateral shift of the mediastinum with narrowing of intercostal spaces (Fig. 1.25a–d) [305]. Signs of chest wall invasion of MPM on plain chest radiographs are osseous destruction and periosteal reaction of the ribs [302, 305, 306]. Lymph node involvement is rarely assessed using chest radiography because the tumor abuts and obscures the contours of the ipsilateral mediastinum and hilum. Metastasis of MPM to the lungs may produce pulmonary nodules or thickening of the interlobular septa [305, 307, 308] but is uncommon at presentation. Contralateral pleural abnormalities are usually caused by underlying asbestos-related pleural disease, although they can be caused by pleural metastases in rare cases.

Contrast-enhanced multidetector chest CT is the examination of choice for the initial evaluation of MPM and has surpassed MRI as the primary modality for determining the T status of this tumor. To ensure that the entire pleura is evaluated, scanning must include the chest from the thoracic inlet to the level of the L3 vertebra [309]. Occasionally, more caudal imaging may be required if a bulky tumor causes deflection of the hemidiaphragm.

On CT scans, the features of MPM and other metastases to the pleura can overlap. The vast majority of patients with MPM have pleural effusion and nodular pleural thickening, usually with lower zone predominance. Whereas abnormal, nodular-enhancing pleura can be readily demonstrated using CT, this may not be the case early in MPM or following surgical intervention for pleurodesis. Biopsy analysis is required for definitive diagnosis to distinguish between MPM and pleural metastatic disease.

Late in the course of MPM, the tumor grows circumferentially around the lung (Fig. 1.25a–d) [184, 305, 310–314].

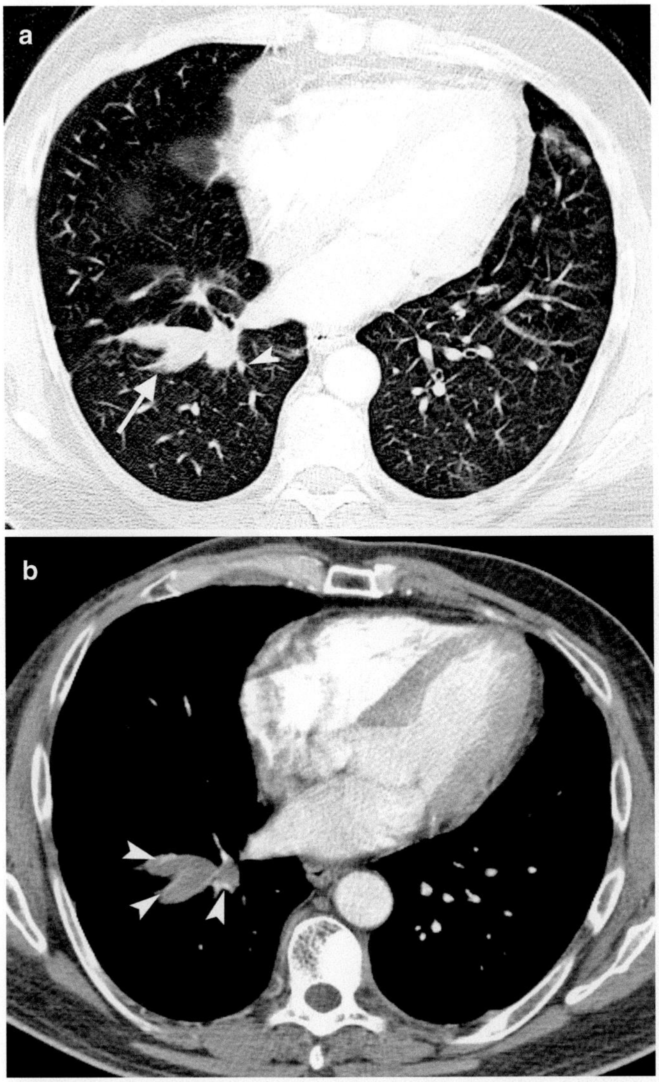

Fig. 1.24 Contrast-enhanced chest CT scan with (**a**) lung and (**b**) mediastinal window settings demonstrating three large tubular opacities appearing to branch in the right lower lobe, which are compatible with metastatic disease in the segmental right lower lobe bronchi, in a 53-year-old man with invasive ductal breast carcinoma that became metastasized. The small high-density linear structures at the periphery of these opacities (*arrowhead*) are the pulmonary vessels running adjacent to the airways

Aggressive tumors can invade local structures. Chest wall invasion obscures and infiltrates the extrapleural fat and intercostal muscles, displaces ribs, and may destroy adjacent bones [310, 313, 315]. Occasionally, CT scans demonstrate focal chest wall involvement at a site of a previous biopsy, surgical scar, or chest tube tract [308]. Direct mediastinal extension of MPM can cause infiltration of fat planes, and concomitant invasion of local mediastinal structures—the great vessels, esophagus, and trachea—may occur; tumor tissue surrounding more than 50 % of a structure strongly suggests invasion [308, 316]. Pericardial invasion of MPM is suggested by nodular pericardial thickening, which may be accompanied by pericardial effusion. Using up-to-date imaging techniques with thin-section images as well as coronal and sagittal reconstructions, radiologists can demonstrate gross diaphragmatic invasion of MPM directly rather than relying solely on indirect signs of tumor diaphragmatic invasion (Fig. 1.26). In assessment of diaphragmatic invasion, a clear fat plane between the inferior diaphragmatic surface and adjacent abdominal organs and a smooth diaphragmatic contour suggest that the tumor does not extend through the diaphragm [316].

CT is limited in the evaluation of mesothelioma. Because of the complex shape of the pleura, differentiating abnormal pleura from adjacent pleural effusion or a collapsed adjacent lung can be difficult. A complicating factor is that many patients with MPM have undergone invasive biopsy or pleurodesis, resulting in inflammatory and/or fibrotic changes that can mimic malignancy by the time of the staging CT scan.

MRI is usually reserved for patients with MPM whose disease is potentially resectable and who have equivocal findings on initial chest CT scans regarding chest wall, pericardial, or diaphragmatic invasion. Marked enhancement of MPM on MRI scans using gadolinium-based contrast agents and the multiplanar imaging capabilities of MRI are particularly useful for delineating multifocal chest wall invasion and transdiaphragmatic invasion by this tumor [317]. The signal intensity of MPM typically is equal to or slightly greater than that of the adjacent chest wall muscle on T1-weighted images and moderately greater on T2-weighted images. Administration of a contrast agent produces intense enhancement of the pleural tumor. As on CT scans, loss of normal fat planes, gross extension into mediastinal fat, and tumor tissue surrounding more than 50 % of a mediastinal structure on MRI scans all suggest tumor invasion [316].

MPM exhibits ^{18}FDG avidity on PET scans [318–323], but the poor spatial resolution of PET limits its use as the sole imaging method for MPM. However, use of integrated PET-CT has improved identification of regions of MPM involvement with increased ^{18}FDG uptake and the accuracy of staging in patients with MPM [324]. ^{18}FDG-PET does not overcome the limitations of other imaging methods in the evaluation of microscopic transdiaphragmatic invasion of MPM, though. The major strength of ^{18}FDG-PET in imaging MPM is delineation of metastatic spread that is not detected morphologically, including that in lymph nodes and at distant sites. Moreover, authors have reported that ^{18}FDG-PET can predict survival rates in patients with mesothelioma when the entire pleural disease is assessed according to total glycolytic volume but not when disease foci are assessed according to the maximal standardized uptake value [325].

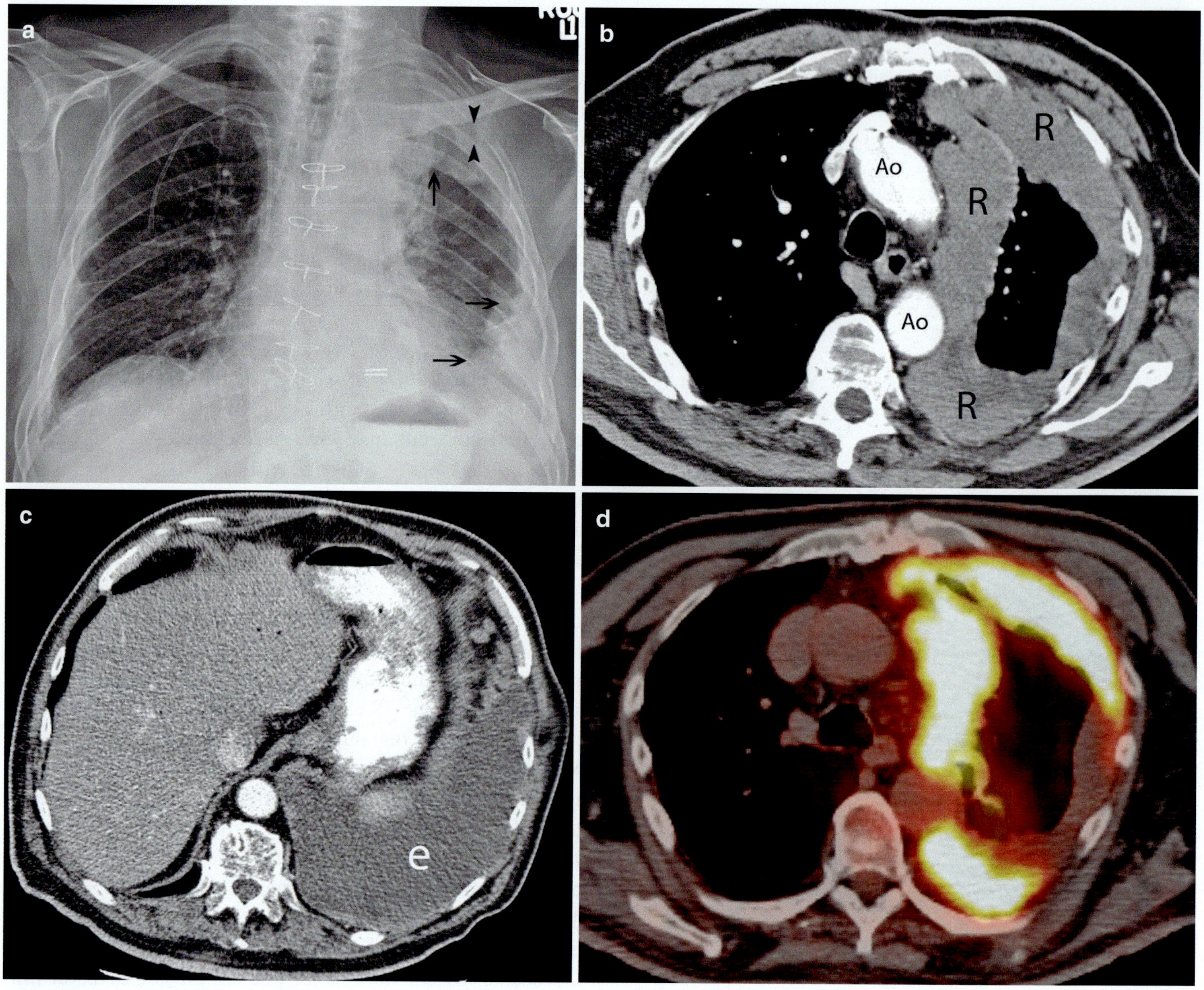

Fig. 1.25 (**a**) Chest radiograph showing an irregular thickened pleural rind (*arrows*) as well as a dependent pleural effusion in the left hemithorax in a 66-year-old man with MPM. Of note is that the left hemithorax is smaller than the right one, including narrowing of the left intercostal spaces (*arrowheads*). (**b**, **c**) Contrast-enhanced chest CT scan with mediastinal window settings demonstrating a (**b**) lobular circumferential pleural rind (*R*) enclosing the left lung and (**c**) dependent moderate pleural effusion (*e*). (**d**) Fused image from a subsequent PET-CT examination demonstrating avid ^{18}FDG uptake throughout the pleural tumor. *Ao* aorta, *T* trachea

Staging of Primary MPM

The International Mesothelioma Interest Group staging system for MPM has been gaining acceptance for differentiation of patients who would benefit from surgical resection from those needing palliative treatment only (Tables 1.3 and 1.4) [326]. The presence of an advanced locoregional primary tumor (T4); N2–N3 disease in the mediastinal, internal mammary, and/or supraclavicular lymph nodes; and M1 disease preclude surgery. Because the extent of the local tumor and regional lymph node status are factors in selecting patients for potentially curative resection of mesothelioma and because all imaging modalities are suboptimal in this evaluation, extended surgical staging is offered to surgery candidates. This staging includes mediastinal nodal biopsy analysis of sites suspicious for metastases by imaging studies, which can be performed using mediastinoscopy, transbronchial biopsy, or transthoracic needle biopsy as well as laparoscopy and peritoneal lavage for exclusion of transdiaphragmatic involvement [326].

Primary Tumor (T Status)

The T status distinguishes MPM tumors that are resectable from those that are not (T3 and T4 disease, respectively) [327]. In patients with locally advanced mesothelioma, features of potentially resectable T3 disease include a solitary

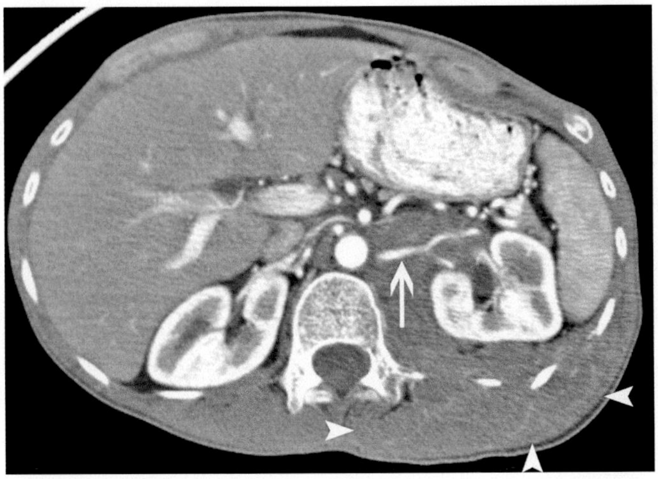

Fig. 1.26 Contrast-enhanced chest CT of the upper abdomen, mediastinal window settings, in a 48-year-old woman with recurrent pleural mesothelioma. The tumor extends below the diaphragm and into the left retroperitoneal space, where it partially encircles the left kidney and encases the left renal artery (*arrow*). The tumor also transverses the posterior intercostal spaces and invades the left abdominal wall (*arrowheads*)

focus of chest wall involvement, endothoracic fascial involvement, mediastinal fat extension, and nontransmural pericardial involvement. Unresectable T4 disease may have diffuse tumor extension or multiple invasive chest wall foci; direct extension to the mediastinal organs, spine, internal pericardial surface, or contralateral pleura; or transdiaphragmatic invasion. Many of these T-stage-differentiating factors are descriptors identified in the pathology specimen that are often minute or microscopic and thus cannot be detected using current imaging techniques.

In an early study from the 1990s, MRI and nonspiral CT had nearly equal diagnostic accuracy in overall staging of mesothelioma (~50–65 %) [317]. However, the investigators observed two significant differences in the accuracy of CT and MRI in T staging: invasion of the diaphragm (accuracy rate: 55 and 82 % for CT and MRI, respectively; $P=0.01$) and invasion of endothoracic fascia or a single chest wall focus (accuracy rate: 46 and 69 % for CT and MRI, respectively; $P=0.05$).

Because of the poor spatial resolution of PET, the sensitivity rate for ^{18}FDG-PET alone in T staging of mesothelioma is 19 % [319]. However, the accuracy of integrated modern multidetector CT and ^{18}FDG-PET was greater than that of either nonspiral CT or ^{18}FDG-PET alone in a previously published study, with a sensitivity rate in staging of T4 disease of 67 % [324].

Because of limitations in evaluating the minute and microscopic invasion that affect T status and therefore staging of mesothelioma, the goal of imaging of T4 disease is identification of visible tumor, whereas accurate staging of apparent T3 disease requires extensive surgical staging via laparoscopy. In a study assessing the value of laparoscopy in staging prior to surgical resection of MPM, 9 % (10/109) of patients had diaphragmatic invasion or peritoneal metastases at laparoscopy, but cross-sectional imaging identified only 3 % (3/109) of these patients with transdiaphragmatic extension of disease [328].

Nodal Disease (N Status)

Hilar lymph node enlargement (N1 disease) usually cannot be differentiated from the primary tumor in patients with MPM because the latter engulfs the hilar region. A more important goal for imaging is to correctly identify mediastinal and supraclavicular involvement of MPM, as survival rates are poor in patients with mediastinal, supraclavicular, or internal mammary nodal metastases [329, 330]. Patients with N2 or N3 MPM are precluded from curative resection.

Using the criterion of 1 cm as the upper limit for the short axis diameter of a benign mediastinal lymph node, the accuracy rate for both CT and MRI in determining the N status of MPM is approximately 50 % [317, 331]. In comparison, the sensitivity of ^{18}FDG-PET in detecting nodal metastatic MPM is poor: only 11 % for ^{18}FDG-PET alone and 38 % for integrated PET-CT [319, 324]. ^{18}FDG-PET therefore cannot replace invasive mediastinal lymph node staging in patients with MPM. However, ^{18}FDG-PET does play an important role in staging of mediastinal lymph nodes by guiding biopsy toward the most suspect lymph node or nodes. Aggressive biopsy, whether performed using mediastinoscopy or via transesophageal or transbronchial routes, cannot access all lymph nodes, and the pattern of lymphatic spread of MPM is less predictable than that of other intrathoracic tumors [318, 321, 322, 330]. This may explain the poorer sensitivity of mediastinoscopy-based staging (36 %) than of intraoperative staging of N2 disease in patients with MPM in one study [328]. Another study found the overall nodal staging sensitivity of mediastinoscopy in patients with MPM to be 80 % [331]. Thus, sampling of all FDG-avid lymph nodes may be necessary to improve preoperative staging of MPM in patients who are candidates for extrapleural pneumonectomy.

Metastatic Disease (M Status)

Researchers have considered distant hematogenous spread of MPM to be rare, yet distant metastasis can be the initial recurrence following extrapleural pneumonectomy [329], suggesting the presence of undetected metastatic disease prior to surgery. The increasing use of ^{18}FDG-PET-CT in staging MPM has shown that distant hematogenous disease is more common than previously thought. ^{18}FDG-PET can often detect hematogenous metastatic MPM not detected using the other routine imaging methods

Table 1.3 TNM International staging system for diffuse MPM

T (primary tumor)	
T1a	Tumor limited to ipsilateral parietal pleura, including mediastinal and diaphragmatic pleura; no involvement of visceral pleura
T1b	Tumor involving ipsilateral parietal pleura, including mediastinal and diaphragmatic pleura; scattered foci of tumor also involving visceral pleura
T2	Tumor involving each ipsilateral pleural surface with at least one of the following features: Involvement of diaphragmatic muscle Confluent visceral pleural tumor (including fissures) or extension of tumor from visceral pleura into underlying pulmonary parenchyma
T3	Locally advanced but potentially resectable tumor; tumor involving all of ipsilateral pleural surfaces with at least one of the following: Involvement of endothoracic fascia Extension into mediastinal fat Solitary, completely resectable focus of tumor extending into soft tissues of chest wall Nontransmural involvement of pericardium
T4	Locally advanced, technically unresectable tumor; tumor involving all of ipsilateral pleural surfaces with at least one of the following: Diffuse extension or multifocal masses of tumor in chest wall with or without associated rib destruction Direct transdiaphragmatic extension of tumor to peritoneum Direct extension of tumor to contralateral pleura Direct extension of tumor to one or more mediastinal organs Direct extension of tumor into spine Tumor extending through to internal surface of pericardium with or without pericardial effusion; tumor involving myocardium
N (lymph nodes)	
NX	Regional lymph nodes not assessable
N0	No regional lymph node metastases
N1	Metastases in ipsilateral bronchopulmonary or hilar lymph nodes
N2	Metastases in subcarinal or ipsilateral mediastinal lymph nodes, including ipsilateral internal mammary nodes
N3	Metastases in contralateral mediastinal, contralateral internal mammary, and ipsilateral or contralateral supraclavicular lymph nodes
M (metastases)	
MX	Distant metastases not assessable
M0	No distant metastases
M1	Distant metastases present

Used with permission from Truong et al. [326]

Table 1.4 Classification of mesothelioma stage according to TNM descriptors

Stage	Description
Ia	TIaN0M0
Ib	TIbN0M0
II	T2N0M0
IIII	Any T3M0
	Any N1M0
	Any N2M0
IV	Any T4
	Any N3
	Any M1

Used with permission from Truong et al. [326]

[319, 322, 324]. These metastases can be focal or diffuse, with involvement of the brain, lung, bone, adrenal gland, peritoneum, abdominal lymph nodes, and abdominal wall. In one study, use of ^{18}FDG-PET alone in staging of MPM identified 11 % of patients with MPM as having extrathoracic metastatic disease, obviating futile surgery [322]. In another study, ^{18}FDG-PET-CT identified extrathoracic metastases that were not detected using clinical examination and morphological imaging in 24 % of patients with MPM [324].

In summary, CT, MRI, and ^{18}FDG-PET-CT can be used for staging of mesothelioma, but because of their suboptimal accuracy in T and N staging of this cancer and the morbidity and mortality associated with extrapleural pneumonectomy, extended surgical staging is still required for MPM patients being evaluated for resection. The use of integrated PET-CT in routine staging of MPM can lead to more appropriate selection of patients for extrapleural pneumonectomy, predominantly by identifying previously unsuspected sites of extrathoracic metastatic disease.

Localized Fibrous Tumor of the Pleura

Although localized fibrous tumor of the pleura is usually benign, malignant tumors do occur. At times, histological distinction of the benign and malignant forms is difficult. However, some imaging features are seen more often with malignant than benign tumors.

Both malignant and benign fibrous tumor of the pleura can grow slowly and appear as incidental masses on routine chest radiographs. Studies of patients with localized fibrous tumors of the pleura published from 1942 to 1972 found that 72 % of patients were symptomatic at presentation, whereas studies published from 1973 to 1980 found symptoms in only 54 % of patients. This decrease in the prevalence of symptoms in patients with localized fibrous tumors of the pleura may be related to increased imaging of asymptomatic populations and resultant early detection of incidental tumors [332]. These tumors are often large at presentation and are sharply defined, smooth, or somewhat lobulated masses of homogenous density ranging in diameter from 1 to 40 cm [332–334]. In a large series in which investigators assessed localized fibrous tumors of the pleura, nearly 80 % of the tumors occupied the lower hemithorax, about 30 % (both benign and malignant forms) occupied more than a half of a hemithorax, and 91 % had at least one well-defined border [332]. In patients with small lesions, ≤4 cm in diameter, the typical imaging appearance of extraparenchymal growths can be seen, as these tumors form obtuse angles with the chest wall. In those with larger lesions, however, establishing the site of disease origin is more difficult. No features on plain radiographs distinguish benign and malignant fibrous tumor of the pleura.

Localized fibrous tumors of the pleura typically displace rather than invade thoracic organs, causing compressive atelectasis (Fig. 1.27). Features suggestive of, but not definitively indicative of, a malignant localized fibrous tumor of the pleura are ipsilateral pleural effusion, tumor diameter larger than 10 cm, and central low attenuation consistent with necrosis [332, 334]. Low-attenuation regions on CT are seen in 100 % of malignant fibrous tumor of the pleura tumors as well as 35 % of benign tumors [332]. Authors have reported calcification in 7–26 % of cases of these tumors and that it usually occurs with large lesions in association with necrosis [332, 334, 335]. These tumors avidly enhance with contrast injection. Homogenous enhancement is typically seen with benign but not malignant tumors. In comparison, researchers observed that heterogenous enhancement after intravenous contrast injection occurred in all patients with malignant fibrous tumors of the pleura and 60 % of those with benign tumors [332]. Chest wall involvement of these tumors is rare but can occur; in patients with benign tumors, it primarily manifests as rib sclerosis, while in those with malignant forms, chest wall involvement takes the form of soft tissue invasion [332].

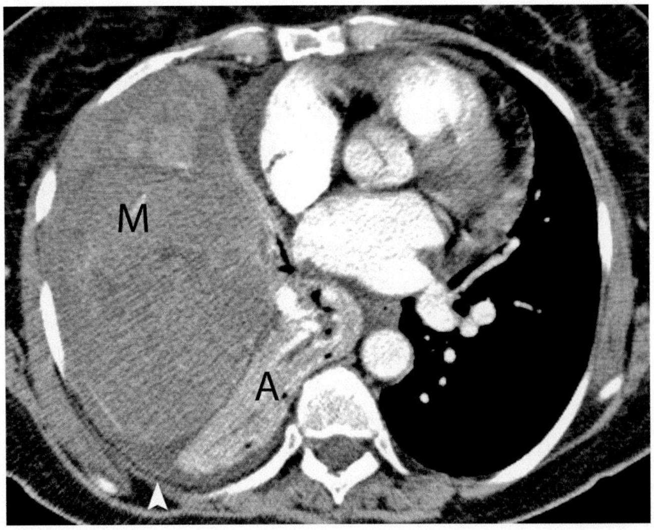

Fig. 1.27 Contrast-enhanced chest CT scan with mediastinal window settings showing a large 25-cm heterogeneous mass (*M*) occupying the majority of the right lower hemithorax in a 64-year-old woman with a localized fibrous tumor of the pleura. The mass was resected, revealing a malignant solitary fibrous tumor of the pleura. Histologically, the mass was largely homogeneous with focal areas of necrosis and 50 % hyalinization. A represents compressive atelectasis of the lung

The MRI features of localized fibrous tumors of the pleura reflect histological findings and the relative amounts of fibrous tissue, necrosis, and hemorrhaging. Typically, these tumors have predominant low or intermediate signal intensity on both T1- and T2-weighted images [332, 336–340], which reflect the tumor's fibrous collagenous tissue. In some cases, high, heterogeneous signal intensity on T2-weighted images is observed, reflecting necrosis and cystic or myxoid degeneration. Intense enhancement after intravenous injection of a gadolinium-based contrast agent is typical. Although the multiplanar imaging capabilities of MRI have been beneficial in demonstrating the relationship of a fibrous tumor of the pleura with the diaphragm for preoperative planning of these tumors, lately, thin-section multidetector CT has been replacing MRI, as the former better shows the vascular pedicle of the tumor as an aid in surgical resection [341].

Few studies, which assessed only small numbers of patients, have examined the use of ^{18}FDG-PET imaging of localized fibrous tumors of the pleura. These studies demonstrated that all of the malignant tumors assessed using PET had increased FDG activity, whereas the benign tumors did not. Further studies are needed to determine the true sensitivity and specificity of FDG-PET in discriminating malignant and benign localized fibrous tumors of the pleura [342, 343].

Secondary Malignant Pleural Tumors

Pleural metastases can appear on the different imaging modalities as pleural nodularity, which is highly suggestive of malignancy, or as nonspecific pleural effusion. The presence of a malignant pleural effusion at the time of initial staging is a poor prognostic sign (considered M1a NSCLC) and renders the disease inoperable. The major sources of pleural metastases are carcinomas of the lung, breast, ovary, and stomach, and lymphoma. Not all pleural metastases occur with pleural effusion. An autopsy series looking at 191 patients with malignancy found that 29 % of them had pleural metastases, only half of whom had accompanying pleural effusion [344]. The etiology of a pleural effusion may be a condition other than a pleural metastasis even in a patient with a known primary malignancy, such as a reactive fluid collection or infection. Cytological analysis of malignant pleural fluid has identified malignant cells in only about two-thirds of cases of NSCLC [133]. Moreover, repeat thoracentesis has yielded metastasis-positive specimens in only another 30 % of cases [345]. Biochemical analysis of pleural fluid does not accurately differentiate benign and malignant effusion [346–348]. Thoracoscopy and pleuroscopy have excellent diagnostic yields (>95 %) [349] but are invasive and require a trained surgical staff and appropriate facilities.

Chest radiographic findings of pleural effusion are variable. Malignant pleural effusion can be large (opacifying the entire hemithorax), moderate, or small. It also can be loculated or free-flowing. Determining whether a lobular contour on a chest radiograph is caused by pleural fluid loculation or soft tissue nodularity is impossible. Thus, ultrasound, CT, or MRI is required for further characterization of a pleural lobulation. CT and MRI provide a better overview of the entire pleural surface than ultrasound and are not operator dependent. However, morphological imaging, including CT and MRI, cannot be the sole imaging method used in diagnosis of malignant pleural effusion unless pleural nodularity is definitely identified, as empyemas and parapneumonic effusion can have similar imaging characteristics [350–352]. Multiple pleural nodules and nodular pleural thickening are seen almost exclusively in patients with malignant effusion. However, their absence does not exclude metastatic disease, as metastatic pleural nodules may be too small to identify using imaging [350].

The accuracy of the different imaging methods in identifying malignant pleural tumors is unknown. Studies attempting to assess imaging accuracy in this context have been limited to strictly selected groups of patients because cytological findings are not accurate and thus are suboptimal as reference standards. Studies investigating the role of CT in differentiation of benign and malignant pleural thickening in the absence of pleural fluid have found that the following features are highly specific for malignant pleural tumors: circumferential thickening (100 % specificity), pleural nodularity (94 %), parietal pleural thickening greater than 1 cm (94 %), and mediastinal pleural involvement (88 %) [311]. Also, a study of 50 patients with early-stage NSCLC who were candidates for surgery assessed the value of preoperative thoracoscopy versus CT in determining T status [350]. Thoracoscopic staging ruled out malignant pleural effusion in 7 (14 %) patients with radiologically obvious effusion, and it identified radiologically silent malignant pleural effusion in 3 (6 %) patients. In that study, errors in thoracoscopic staging did not result in any inappropriate operations. However, errors in CT staging would have resulted in the performance of operations unlikely to help the patients or inappropriately excluded patients from surgery. Thoracoscopic staging was more accurate than CT staging in this cohort of patients with NSCLC and negative mediastinoscopic findings for nodal metastases.

Studies have shown that ^{18}FDG-PET is an accurate diagnostic tool in differentiating benign and malignant pleural effusion in patients with malignant disease, with sensitivity rates ranging from 88 to 100 % and specificity rates ranging from 71 to 94 % [134, 135, 353–356]. In one of these studies, the sensitivity rate, specificity rate, positive predictive value, negative predictive value, and accuracy rate of ^{18}FDG-PET in detection of pleural involvement were 100, 71, 63, 100, and 80 %, respectively, in 92 patients with NSCLC and pleural abnormalities [135]. When the findings of a CT scan performed separately were combined with those of the ^{18}FDG-PET study, the specificity rate increased from 71 to 76 %, the positive predictive value increased from 63 to 67 %, and the accuracy rate increased from 80 to 84 %. The relatively low specificity and positive predictive value of ^{18}FDG-PET were caused by false-positive increased ^{18}FDG uptake in cases of infection.

Of note is that foci of pleural ^{18}FDG uptake require careful evaluation on corresponding CT images. In patients who have undergone talc pleurodesis, PET can show increased ^{18}FDG activity that can persist for years owing to inflammation. Talc pleurodesis has a typical CT appearance of pleural thickening with increased linear high attenuation correlating with the talc deposition. Pleural ^{18}FDG activity correlating with this classic CT pattern should be attributed to talc deposits rather than a tumor [136].

Pleural nodularity detected using any imaging modality is highly suggestive of metastatic disease. Although early studies using ^{18}FDG-PET and integrated ^{18}FDG-PET-CT showed that ^{18}FDG-PET is highly accurate in identification of malignant pleural effusion, reports of its performance in the absence of morphological abnormalities have yet to be published.

Conclusion

Lung and pleural tumors are radiologically diverse. In some cases, specific imaging features, such as macroscopic fat and certain calcification patterns, may point toward a definite diagnosis, obviating the need for biopsy. Usually, radiological findings suggestive of malignancy are complementary with pathological data in guiding treatment decisions. Good communication among the radiologist, pathologist, and clinical team is required for selection of the most advantageous imaging method for each patient. This multidisciplinary approach optimizes imaging protocols selected by the radiologist and limits the number of required imaging techniques for identification and correct staging in the most efficient, cost-effective way.

References

1. Hulka BS. Cancer screening. Degrees of proof and practical application. Cancer. 1988;62(8 Suppl):1776–80.
2. Steele JD. The solitary pulmonary nodule. Report of a cooperative study of resected asymptomatic solitary pulmonary nodules in males. J Thorac Cardiovasc Surg. 1963;46:21–39.
3. Walske BR. The solitary pulmonary nodule: a review of 217 cases. Dis Chest. 1966;49:302–4.
4. Gurney JW. Determining the likelihood of malignancy in solitary pulmonary nodules with Bayesian analysis. Part I. Theory. Radiology. 1993;186(2):405–13.
5. Yankelevitz DF, Henschke CI. Does 2-year stability imply that pulmonary nodules are benign? AJR Am J Roentgenol. 1997; 168(2):325–8.
6. Berger WG, Erly WK, Krupinski EA, Standen JR, Stern RG. The solitary pulmonary nodule on chest radiography: can we really tell if the nodule is calcified? AJR Am J Roentgenol. 2001;176(1): 201–4.
7. Black C, de Verteuil R, Walker S, Ayres J, Boland A, Bagust A, et al. Population screening for lung cancer using computed tomography, is there evidence of clinical effectiveness? A systematic review of the literature. Thorax. 2007;62(2):131–8.
8. Heitzman ER, editor. The lung: radiologic-pathologic correlations. 2nd ed. St. Louis: CV Mosby; 1984.
9. Zwirewich CV, Vedal S, Miller RR, Muller NL. Solitary pulmonary nodule: high-resolution CT and radiologic-pathologic correlation. Radiology. 1991;179(2):469–76.
10. Siegelman SS, Khouri NF, Leo FP, Fishman EK, Braverman RM, Zerhouni EA. Solitary pulmonary nodules: CT assessment. Radiology. 1986;160(2):307–12.
11. Mahoney MC, Shipley RT, Corcoran HL, Dickson BA. CT demonstration of calcification in carcinoma of the lung. AJR Am J Roentgenol. 1990;154(2):255–8.
12. Siegelman SS, Zerhouni EA, Leo FP, Khouri NF, Stitik FP. CT of the solitary pulmonary nodule. AJR Am J Roentgenol. 1980;135(1): 1–13.
13. Swensen SJ, Harms GF, Morin RL, Myers JL. CT evaluation of solitary pulmonary nodules: value of 185-H reference phantom. AJR Am J Roentgenol. 1991;156(5):925–9.
14. Siegelman SS, Khouri NF, Scott Jr WW, Leo FP, Hamper UM, Fishman EK, et al. Pulmonary hamartoma: CT findings. Radiology. 1986;160(2):313–7.
15. Kui M, Templeton PA, White CS, Cai ZL, Bai YX, Cai YQ. Evaluation of the air bronchogram sign on CT in solitary pulmonary lesions. J Comput Assist Tomogr. 1996;20(6):983–6.
16. Henschke CI, Yankelevitz DF, Mirtcheva R, McGuinness G, McCauley D, Miettinen OS. CT screening for lung cancer: frequency and significance of part-solid and nonsolid nodules. AJR Am J Roentgenol. 2002;178(5):1053–7.
17. Swensen SJ, Morin RL, Schueler BA, Brown LR, Cortese DA, Pairolero PC, et al. Solitary pulmonary nodule: CT evaluation of enhancement with iodinated contrast material – a preliminary report. Radiology. 1992;182(2):343–7.
18. Swensen SJ, Viggiano RW, Midthun DE, Muller NL, Sherrick A, Yamashita K, et al. Lung nodule enhancement at CT: multicenter study. Radiology. 2000;214(1):73–80.
19. Bankier AA, O'Donnell CR, Boiselle PM. Quality initiatives. Respiratory instructions for CT examinations of the lungs: a hands-on guide. Radiographics. 2008;28(4):919–31.
20. Hasegawa M, Sone S, Takashima S, Li F, Yang ZG, Maruyama Y, et al. Growth rate of small lung cancers detected on mass CT screening. Br J Radiol. 2000;73(876):1252–9.
21. Godoy MC, Naidich DP. Subsolid pulmonary nodules and the spectrum of peripheral adenocarcinomas of the lung: recommended interim guidelines for assessment and management. Radiology. 2009;253(3):606–22.
22. Awaya H, Matsumoto T, Honjo K, Miura G, Emoto T, Matsunaga N. A preliminary study of discrimination among the components of small pulmonary nodules by MR imaging: correlation between MR images and histologic appearance. Radiat Med. 2000;18(1):29–38.
23. Cronin P, Dwamena BA, Kelly AM, Bernstein SJ, Carlos RC. Solitary pulmonary nodules and masses: a meta-analysis of the diagnostic utility of alternative imaging tests. Eur Radiol. 2008;8(9):1840–56.
24. Schaefer JF, Vollmar J, Schick F, Vonthein R, Seemann MD, Aebert H, et al. Solitary pulmonary nodules: dynamic contrast-enhanced MR imaging–perfusion differences in malignant and benign lesions. Radiology. 2004;232(2):544–53.
25. Conti PS, Lilien DL, Hawley K, Keppler J, Grafton ST, Bading JR. PET and [18 F]-FDG in oncology: a clinical update. Nucl Med Biol. 1996;23(6):717–35.
26. Gould MK, Maclean CC, Kuschner WG, Rydzak CE, Owens DK. Accuracy of positron emission tomography for diagnosis of pulmonary nodules and mass lesions: a meta-analysis. JAMA. 2001; 285(7):914–24.
27. Gupta NC, Frank AR, Dewan NA, Redepenning LS, Rothberg ML, Mailliard JA, et al. Solitary pulmonary nodules: detection of malignancy with PET with 2-[F-18]-fluoro-2-deoxy-D-glucose. Radiology. 1992;184(2):441–4.
28. Gupta NC, Maloof J, Gunel E. Probability of malignancy in solitary pulmonary nodules using fluorine-18-FDG and PET. J Nucl Med. 1996;37(6):943–8.
29. Hubner KF, Buonocore E, Gould HR, Thie J, Smith GT, Stephens S, et al. Differentiating benign from malignant lung lesions using "quantitative" parameters of FDG PET images. Clin Nucl Med. 1996;21(12):941–9.
30. Patz Jr EF, Lowe VJ, Hoffman JM, Paine SS, Burrowes P, Coleman RE, et al. Focal pulmonary abnormalities: evaluation with F-18 fluorodeoxyglucose PET scanning. Radiology. 1993;188(2):487–90.
31. Scott WJ, Schwabe JL, Gupta NC, Dewan NA, Reeb SD, Sugimoto JT. Positron emission tomography of lung tumors and mediastinal lymph nodes using [18F]fluorodeoxyglucose. The members of the PET-Lung Tumor Study Group. Ann Thorac Surg. 1994;58(3):698–703.
32. Jeong SY, Lee KS, Shin KM, Bae YA, Kim BT, Choe BK, et al. Efficacy of PET/CT in the characterization of solid or partly solid solitary pulmonary nodules. Lung Cancer. 2008;61:186–94. Epub 2008 Feb 15

33. Kernstine KH, Grannis Jr FW, Rotter AJ. Is there a role for PET in the evaluation of subcentimeter pulmonary nodules? Semin Thorac Cardiovasc Surg. 2005;17(2):110–4.
34. Marom EM, Sarvis S, Herndon 2nd JE, Patz Jr EF. T1 lung cancers: sensitivity of diagnosis with fluorodeoxyglucose PET. Radiology. 2002;223(2):453–9.
35. Erasmus JJ, McAdams HP, Patz Jr EF, Coleman RE, Ahuja V, Goodman PC. Evaluation of primary pulmonary carcinoid tumors using FDG PET. AJR Am J Roentgenol. 1998;170(5):1369–73.
36. Higashi K, Ueda Y, Seki H, Yuasa K, Oguchi M, Noguchi T, et al. Fluorine-18-FDG PET imaging is negative in bronchioloalveolar lung carcinoma. J Nucl Med. 1998;39(6):1016–20.
37. Kim BT, Kim Y, Lee KS, Yoon SB, Cheon EM, Kwon OJ, et al. Localized form of bronchioloalveolar carcinoma: FDG PET findings. AJR Am J Roentgenol\. 1998;170(4):935–9.
38. Lowe VJ, Fletcher JW, Gobar L, Lawson M, Kirchner P, Valk P, et al. Prospective investigation of positron emission tomography in lung nodules. J Clin Oncol. 1998;16(3):1075–84.
39. Prauer HW, Weber WA, Romer W, Treumann T, Ziegler SI, Schwaiger M. Controlled prospective study of positron emission tomography using the glucose analogue [18f]fluorodeoxyglucose in the evaluation of pulmonary nodules. Br J Surg. 1998; 85(11):1506–11.
40. Pan T, Mawlawi O, Nehmeh SA, Erdi YE, Luo D, Liu HH, et al. Attenuation correction of PET images with respiration-averaged CT images in PET/CT. J Nucl Med. 2005;46(9):1481–7.
41. Dewan NA, Gupta NC, Redepenning LS, Phalen JJ, Frick MP. Diagnostic efficacy of PET-FDG imaging in solitary pulmonary nodules. Potential role in evaluation and management. Chest. 1993;104(4):997–1002.
42. Fletcher JW, Kymes SM, Gould M, Alazraki N, Coleman RE, Lowe VJ, et al. A comparison of the diagnostic accuracy of 18 F-FDG PET and CT in the characterization of solitary pulmonary nodules. J Nucl Med. 2008;49(2):179–85.
43. Kubota K, Matsuzawa T, Fujiwara T, Ito M, Hatazawa J, Ishiwata K, et al. Differential diagnosis of lung tumor with positron emission tomography: a prospective study. J Nucl Med. 1990;31(12): 1927–32.
44. Marom EM, Erasmus JJ, Patz EF. Lung cancer and positron emission tomography with fluorodeoxyglucose. Lung Cancer. 2000;28(3):187–202.
45. Quint LE, Francis IR, Wahl RL, Gross BH, Glazer GM. Preoperative staging of non-small-cell carcinoma of the lung: imaging methods. AJR Am J Roentgenol. 1995;164(6):1349–59.
46. Strauss LG, Conti PS. The applications of PET in clinical oncology. J Nucl Med. 1991;32(4):623–48; discussion 649–50.
47. Bandi V, Lunn W, Ernst A, Eberhardt R, Hoffmann H, Herth FJ. Ultrasound vs. CT in detecting chest wall invasion by tumor: a prospective study. Chest. 2008;133(4):881–6.
48. Gloeckler Ries LA, Reichman ME, Lewis DR, Hankey BF, Edwards BK. Cancer survival and incidence from the Surveillance, Epidemiology, and End Results (SEER) program. Oncologist. 2003;8(6):541–52.
49. Hayata Y, Funatsu H, Kato H, Saito Y, Sawamura K, Furose K. Results of lung cancer screening programs in Japan. Recent Results Cancer Res. 1982;82:163–73.
50. Lilienfield A, Archer PG, Burnett CH, Chamberlain EW, Davis D, Davis RL. An evaluation of radiographic and cytologic screening for early detection of lung cancer: a cooperative pilot study of the American Cancer Society and the Veterans Administration. Cancer Res. 1966;26:2083–121.
51. Nash FA, Morgan JM, Tomkins JG. South London Lung Cancer Study. Br Med J. 1968;2(607):715–21.
52. Weiss W, Boucot KR. The Philadelphia Pulmonary Neoplasm Research Project. Early roentgenographic appearance of bronchogenic carcinoma. Arch Intern Med. 1974;134(2):306–11.
53. Brett GZ. The value of lung cancer detection by six-monthly chest radiographs. Thorax. 1968;23(4):414–20.
54. Wilde J. A 10 year follow-up of semi-annual screening for early detection of lung cancer in the Erfurt County, GDR. Eur Respir J. 1989;2(7):656–62.
55. Black WC, Welch HG. Screening for disease. AJR Am J Roentgenol. 1997;168(1):3–11.
56. Flehinger BJ, Melamed MR. Current status of screening for lung cancer. Chest Surg Clin N Am. 1994;4(1):1–15.
57. Fontana RS, Sanderson DR, Taylor WF, Woolner LB, Miller WE, Muhm JR, et al. Early lung cancer detection: results of the initial (prevalence) radiologic and cytologic screening in the Mayo Clinic study. Am Rev Respir Dis. 1984;130(4):561–5.
58. Frost JK, Ball Jr WC, Levin ML, Tockman MS, Baker RR, Carter D, et al. Early lung cancer detection: results of the initial (prevalence) radiologic and cytologic screening in the Johns Hopkins study. Am Rev Respir Dis. 1984;130(4):549–54.
59. Kubik A, Polak J. Lung cancer detection. Results of a randomized prospective study in Czechoslovakia. Cancer. 1986;57(12): 2427–37.
60. Marcus PM, Bergstralh EJ, Fagerstrom RM, Williams DE, Fontana R, Taylor WF, et al. Lung cancer mortality in the Mayo Lung Project: impact of extended follow-up. J Natl Cancer Inst. 2000; 92(16):1308–16.
61. Henschke CI, Yankelevitz DF, Libby DM, Pasmantier MW, Smith JP, Miettinen OS. Survival of patients with stage I lung cancer detected on CT screening. N Engl J Med. 2006;355(17):1763–71.
62. Bach PB, Jett JR, Pastorino U, Tockman MS, Swensen SJ, Begg CB. Computed tomography screening and lung cancer outcomes. JAMA. 2007;297(9):953–61.
63. Aberle DR, Adams AM, Berg CD, Black WC, Clapp JD, Fagerstrom RM, et al. Reduced lung-cancer mortality with low-dose computed tomographic screening. N Engl J Med. 2011;365(5):395–409.
64. Field JK, Baldwin D, Brain K, Devaraj A, Eisen T, Duffy SW, et al. CT screening for lung cancer in the UK: position statement by UKLS investigators following the NLST report.Thorax. 2011; 66(8):736–7. Epub 2011 Jul 1.
65. Pfister DG, Johnson DH, Azzoli CG, Sause W, Smith TJ, Baker Jr S, et al. American Society of Clinical Oncology treatment of unresectable non-small-cell lung cancer guideline: update 2003. J Clin Oncol. 2004;22(2):330–53.
66. Lardinois D, Weder W, Hany TF, Kamel EM, Korom S, Seifert B, et al. Staging of non-small-cell lung cancer with integrated positron-emission tomography and computed tomography. N Engl J Med. 2003;348(25):2500–7.
67. Pieterman RM, van Putten JW, Meuzelaar JJ, Mooyaart EL, Vaalburg W, Koeter GH, et al. Preoperative staging of non-small-cell lung cancer with positron-emission tomography. N Engl J Med. 2000;343(4):254–61.
68. Reed CE, Harpole DH, Posther KE, Woolson SL, Downey RJ, Meyers BF, et al. Results of the American College of Surgeons Oncology Group Z0050 trial: the utility of positron emission tomography in staging potentially operable non-small cell lung cancer. J Thorac Cardiovasc Surg. 2003;126(6):1943–51.
69. van Tinteren H, Hoekstra OS, Smit EF, van den Bergh JH, Schreurs AJ, Stallaert RA, et al. Effectiveness of positron emission tomography in the preoperative assessment of patients with suspected non-small-cell lung cancer: the PLUS multicentre randomised trial. Lancet. 2002;359(9315):1388–93.
70. Vansteenkiste JF, Stroobants SG, De Leyn PR, Dupont PJ, Bogaert J, Maes A, et al. Lymph node staging in non-small-cell lung cancer with FDG-PET scan: a prospective study on 690 lymph node stations from 68 patients. J Clin Oncol. 1998;16(6):2142–9.
71. Verhagen AF, Bootsma GP, Tjan-Heijnen VC, van der Wilt GJ, Cox AL, Brouwer MH, et al. FDG-PET in staging lung cancer: how does it change the algorithm? Lung Cancer. 2004;44(2):175–81.

72. Rosado-de-Christenson ML, Templeton PA, Moran CA. Bronchogenic carcinoma: radiologic-pathologic correlation. Radiographics. 1994; 14(2):429–46; quiz 447–8.
73. Sider L. Radiographic manifestations of primary bronchogenic carcinoma. Radiol Clin North Am. 1990;28(3):583–97.
74. Theros EG. 1976 Caldwell Lecture: varying manifestation of peripheral pulmonary neoplasms: a radiologic-pathologic correlative study. AJR Am J Roentgenol. 1977;128(6):893–914.
75. Woodring JH. Unusual radiographic manifestations of lung cancer. Radiol Clin North Am. 1990;28(3):599–618.
76. Kishi K, Homma S, Kurosaki A, Motoi N, Kohno T, Nakata K, et al. Small lung tumors with the size of 1 cm or less in diameter: clinical, radiological, and histopathological characteristics. Lung Cancer. 2004;44(1):43–51.
77. Noguchi M, Morikawa A, Kawasaki M, Matsuno Y, Yamada T, Hirohashi S, et al. Small adenocarcinoma of the lung. Histologic characteristics and prognosis. Cancer. 1995;75(12):2844–52.
78. Takashima S, Li F, Maruyama Y, Hasegawa M, Takayama F, Kadoya M, et al. Discrimination of subtypes of small adenocarcinoma in the lung with thin-section CT. Lung Cancer. 2002;36(2):175–82.
79. Kondo T, Yamada K, Noda K, Nakayama H, Kameda Y. Radiologic-prognostic correlation in patients with small pulmonary adenocarcinomas. Lung Cancer. 2002;36(1):49–57.
80. Suzuki K, Kusumoto M, Watanabe S, Tsuchiya R, Asamura H. Radiologic classification of small adenocarcinoma of the lung: radiologic-pathologic correlation and its prognostic impact. Ann Thorac Surg. 2006;81(2):413–9.
81. Travis WD, Brambilla E, Noguchi M, Nicholson AG, Geisinger KR, Yatabe Y, et al. International association for the Study of Lung Cancer/American Thoracic Society/European Respiratory Society: International multidisciplinary classification of lung adenocarcinoma. J Thorac Oncol. 2011;6(2):244–85.
82. Lee KS, Kim Y, Han J, Ko EJ, Park CK, Primack SL. Bronchioloalveolar carcinoma: clinical, histopathologic, and radiologic findings. Radiographics. 1997;17(6):1345–57.
83. Strollo DC, Rosado-de-Christenson ML, Franks TJ. Reclassification of cystic bronchioloalveolar carcinomas to adenocarcinomas based on the revised World Health Organization Classification of Lung and Pleural Tumours. J Thorac Imaging. 2003;18(2):59–66.
84. Weisbrod GL, Towers MJ, Chamberlain DW, Herman SJ, Matzinger FR. Thin-walled cystic lesions in bronchioalveolar carcinoma. Radiology. 1992;185(2):401–5.
85. Okubo K, Mark EJ, Flieder D, Wain JC, Wright CD, Moncure AC, et al. Bronchoalveolar carcinoma: clinical, radiologic, and pathologic factors and survival. J Thorac Cardiovasc Surg. 1999;118(4):702–9.
86. Aquino SL, Halpern EF, Kuester LB, Fischman AJ. FDG-PET and CT features of non-small cell lung cancer based on tumor type. Int J Mol Med. 2007;19(3):495–9.
87. Tsunezuka Y, Shimizu Y, Tanaka N, Takayanagi T, Kawano M. Positron emission tomography in relation to Noguchi's classification for diagnosis of peripheral non-small-cell lung cancer 2 cm or less in size. World J Surg. 2007;31(2):314–7.
88. Byrd RB, Carr DT, Miller WE, Payne WS, Woolner LB. Radiographic abnormalities in carcinoma of the lung as related to histological cell type. Thorax. 1969;24(5):573–5.
89. Filderman AE, Shaw C, Matthay RA. Lung cancer. Part I: etiology, pathology, natural history, manifestations, and diagnostic techniques. Invest Radiol. 1986;21(1):80–90.
90. Shin MS, Jackson LK, Shelton Jr RW, Greene RE. Giant cell carcinoma of the lung. Clinical and roentgenographic manifestations. Chest. 1986;89(3):366–9.
91. Garcia-Yuste M, Matilla JM, Cueto A, Paniagua JM, Ramos G, Canizares MA, et al. Typical and atypical carcinoid tumours: analysis of the experience of the Spanish Multi-centric Study of neuroendocrine tumours of the lung. Eur J Cardiothorac Surg. 2007; 31(2):192–7.
92. Zwiebel BR, Austin JH, Grimes MM. Bronchial carcinoid tumors: assessment with CT of location and intratumoral calcification in 31 patients. Radiology. 1991;179(2):483–6.
93. McCaughan BC, Martini N, Bains MS. Bronchial carcinoids. Review of 124 cases. J Thorac Cardiovasc Surg. 1985;89(1):8–17.
94. Muller NL, Miller RR. Neuroendocrine carcinomas of the lung. Semin Roentgenol. 1990;25(1):96–104.
95. Valli M, Fabris GA, Dewar A, Hornall D, Sheppard MN. Atypical carcinoid tumour of the lung: a study of 33 cases with prognostic features. Histopathology. 1994;24(4):363–9.
96. Chong S, Lee KS, Kim BT, Choi JY, Yi CA, Chung MJ, et al. Integrated PET/CT of pulmonary neuroendocrine tumors: diagnostic and prognostic implications. AJR Am J Roentgenol. 2007; 188(5):1223–31.
97. Urschel JD. Surgical treatment of peripheral small cell lung cancer. Chest Surg Clin N Am. 1997;7(1):95–103.
98. Govindan R, Ihde DC. Practical issues in the management of the patient with small cell lung cancer. Chest Surg Clin N Am. 1997; 7(1):167–81.
99. Goldstraw P, Crowley J, Chansky K, Giroux DJ, Groome PA, Rami-Porta R, et al. The IASLC Lung Cancer Staging Project: proposals for the revision of the TNM stage groupings in the forthcoming (seventh) edition of the TNM Classification of malignant tumours. J Thorac Oncol. 2007;2(8):706–14.
100. Ahuja V, Coleman RE, Herndon J, Patz Jr EF. The prognostic significance of fluorodeoxyglucose positron emission tomography imaging for patients with nonsmall cell lung carcinoma. Cancer. 1998;83(5):918–24.
101. Berghmans T, Dusart M, Paesmans M, Hossein-Foucher C, Buvat I, Castaigne C, et al. Primary tumor standardized uptake value (SUVmax) measured on fluorodeoxyglucose positron emission tomography (FDG-PET) is of prognostic value for survival in non-small cell lung cancer (NSCLC): a systematic review and meta-analysis (MA) by the European Lung Cancer Working Party for the IASLC Lung Cancer Staging Project. J Thorac Oncol. 2008;3(1):6–12.
102. Goodgame B, Pillot GA, Yang Z, Shriki J, Meyers BF, Zoole J, et al. Prognostic value of preoperative positron emission tomography in resected stage I non-small cell lung cancer. J Thorac Oncol. 2008;3(2):130–4.
103. Hanin FX, Lonneux M, Cornet J, Noirhomme P, Coulon C, Distexhe J, et al. Prognostic value of FDG uptake in early stage non-small cell lung cancer. Eur J Cardiothorac Surg. 2008;33(5):819–23.
104. Webb WR, Gatsonis C, Zerhouni EA, Heelan RT, Glazer GM, Francis IR, et al. CT and MR imaging in staging non-small cell bronchogenic carcinoma: report of the Radiologic Diagnostic Oncology Group. Radiology. 1991;178(3):705–13.
105. Ratto GB, Piacenza G, Frola C, Musante F, Serrano I, Giua R, et al. Chest wall involvement by lung cancer: computed tomographic detection and results of operation. Ann Thorac Surg. 1991;51(2):182–8.
106. Padovani B, Mouroux J, Seksik L, Chanalet S, Sedat J, Rotomondo C, et al. Chest wall invasion by bronchogenic carcinoma: evaluation with MR imaging. Radiology. 1993;187(1):33–8.
107. Glazer HS, Kaiser LR, Anderson DJ, Molina PL, Emami B, Roper CL, et al. Indeterminate mediastinal invasion in bronchogenic carcinoma: CT evaluation. Radiology. 1989;173(1):37–42.
108. Herman SJ, Winton TL, Weisbrod GL, Towers MJ, Mentzer SJ. Mediastinal invasion by bronchogenic carcinoma: CT signs. Radiology. 1994;190(3):841–6.
109. McLoud TC. CT of bronchogenic carcinoma: indeterminate mediastinal invasion. Radiology. 1989;173(1):15–6.
110. Martini N, Heelan R, Westcott J, Bains MS, McCormack P, Caravelli J, et al. Comparative merits of conventional, computed tomographic, and magnetic resonance imaging in assessing

mediastinal involvement in surgically confirmed lung carcinoma. J Thorac Cardiovasc Surg. 1985;90(5):639–48.
111. Komaki R, Roth JA, Walsh GL, Putnam JB, Vaporciyan A, Lee JS, et al. Outcome predictors for 143 patients with superior sulcus tumors treated by multidisciplinary approach at the University of Texas MD. Anderson Cancer Center. Int J Radiat Oncol Biol Phys. 2000;48(2):347–54.
112. Bruzzi JF, Komaki R, Walsh GL, Truong MT, Gladish GW, Munden RF, et al. Imaging of non-small cell lung cancer of the superior sulcus: part 1: anatomy, clinical manifestations, and management. Radiographics. 2008;28(2):551–60; quiz 620.
113. Dartevelle P, Macchiarini P. Surgical management of superior sulcus tumors. Oncologist. 1999;4(5):398–407.
114. Glazer GM, Gross BH, Quint LE, Francis IR, Bookstein FL, Orringer MB. Normal mediastinal lymph nodes: number and size according to American Thoracic Society mapping. AJR Am J Roentgenol. 1985;144(2):261–5.
115. Dwamena BA, Sonnad SS, Angobaldo JO, Wahl RL. Metastases from non-small cell lung cancer: mediastinal staging in the 1990s–meta-analytic comparison of PET and CT. Radiology. 1999; 213(2):530–6.
116. Gould MK, Kuschner WG, Rydzak CE, Maclean CC, Demas AN, Shigemitsu H, et al. Test performance of positron emission tomography and computed tomography for mediastinal staging in patients with non-small-cell lung cancer: a meta-analysis. Ann Intern Med. 2003;139(11):879–92.
117. Klein JS, Webb WR. The radiologic staging of lung cancer. J Thorac Imaging. 1991;7(1):29–47.
118. Musset D, Grenier P, Carette MF, Frija G, Hauuy MP, Desbleds MT, et al. Primary lung cancer staging: prospective comparative study of MR imaging with CT. Radiology. 1986;160(3):607–11.
119. Staples CA, Muller NL, Miller RR, Evans KG, Nelems B. Mediastinal nodes in bronchogenic carcinoma: comparison between CT and mediastinoscopy. Radiology. 1988;167(2):367–72.
120. Webb WR. MR imaging in the evaluation and staging of lung cancer. Semin Ultrasound CT MR. 1988;9(1):53–66.
121. Gdeedo A, Van Schil P, Corthouts B, Van Mieghem F, Van Meerbeeck J, Van Marck E. Prospective evaluation of computed tomography and mediastinoscopy in mediastinal lymph node staging. Eur Respir J. 1997;10(7):1547–51.
122. McLoud TC, Bourgouin PM, Greenberg RW, Kosiuk JP, Templeton PA, Shepard JA, et al. Bronchogenic carcinoma: analysis of staging in the mediastinum with CT by correlative lymph node mapping and sampling. Radiology. 1992;182(2):319–23.
123. Kim HY, Yi CA, Lee KS, Chung MJ, Kim YK, Choi BK, et al. Nodal metastasis in non-small cell lung cancer: accuracy of 3.0-T MR imaging. Radiology. 2008;246(2):596–604.
124. Yi CA, Shin KM, Lee KS, Kim BT, Kim H, Kwon OJ, et al. Non-small cell lung cancer staging: efficacy comparison of integrated PET/CT versus 3.0-T whole-body MR imaging. Radiology. 2008;248(2):632–42.
125. Antoch G, Stattaus J, Nemat AT, Marnitz S, Beyer T, Kuehl H, et al. Non-small cell lung cancer: dual-modality PET/CT in preoperative staging. Radiology. 2003;229(2):526–33.
126. Toloza EM, Harpole L, McCrory DC. Noninvasive staging of non-small cell lung cancer: a review of the current evidence. Chest. 2003;123(1 Suppl):137S–46.
127. Birim O, Kappetein AP, Stijnen T, Bogers AJ. Meta-analysis of positron emission tomographic and computed tomographic imaging in detecting mediastinal lymph node metastases in nonsmall cell lung cancer. Ann Thorac Surg. 2005;79(1):375–82.
128. Al-Sarraf N, Gately K, Lucey J, Wilson L, McGovern E, Young V. Lymph node staging by means of positron emission tomography is less accurate in non-small cell lung cancer patients with enlarged lymph nodes: analysis of 1,145 lymph nodes. Lung Cancer. 2008;60(1):62–8.
129. de Langen AJ, Raijmakers P, Riphagen I, Paul MA, Hoekstra OS. The size of mediastinal lymph nodes and its relation with metastatic involvement: a meta-analysis. Eur J Cardiothorac Surg. 2006;29(1):26–9.
130. Dietlein M, Weber K, Gandjour A, Moka D, Theissen P, Lauterbach KW, et al. Cost-effectiveness of FDG-PET for the management of potentially operable non-small cell lung cancer: priority for a PET-based strategy after nodal-negative CT results. Eur J Nucl Med. 2000;27(11):1598–609.
131. Scott WJ, Shepherd J, Gambhir SS. Cost-effectiveness of FDG-PET for staging non-small cell lung cancer: a decision analysis. Ann Thorac Surg. 1998;66(6):1876–83; discussion 1883–5.
132. Spiro SG, Porter JC. Lung cancer – where are we today? Current advances in staging and nonsurgical treatment. Am J Respir Crit Care Med. 2002;166(9):1166–96.
133. The American Thoracic Society and The European Respiratory Society. Pretreatment evaluation of non-small-cell lung cancer. Am J Respir Crit Care Med. 1997;156(1):320–32.
134. Erasmus JJ, McAdams HP, Rossi SE, Goodman PC, Coleman RE, Patz EF. FDG PET of pleural effusions in patients with non-small cell lung cancer. AJR Am J Roentgenol. 2000;175(1):245–9.
135. Schaffler GJ, Wolf G, Schoellnast H, Groell R, Maier A, Smolle-Juttner FM, et al. Non-small cell lung cancer: evaluation of pleural abnormalities on CT scans with 18 F FDG PET. Radiology. 2004;231(3):858–65.
136. Kwek BH, Aquino SL, Fischman AJ. Fluorodeoxyglucose positron emission tomography and CT after talc pleurodesis. Chest. 2004;125(6):2356–60.
137. Grant D, Edwards D, Goldstraw P. Computed tomography of the brain, chest, and abdomen in the preoperative assessment of non-small cell lung cancer. Thorax. 1988;43(11):883–6.
138. Silvestri GA, Lenz JE, Harper SN, Morse RA, Colice GL. The relationship of clinical findings to CT scan evidence of adrenal gland metastases in the staging of bronchogenic carcinoma. Chest. 1992;102(6):1748–51.
139. Tanaka K, Kubota K, Kodama T, Nagai K, Nishiwaki Y. Extrathoracic staging is not necessary for non-small-cell lung cancer with clinical stage T1-2 N0. Ann Thorac Surg. 1999;68(3):1039–42.
140. Figlin RA, Piantadosi S, Feld R. Intracranial recurrence of carcinoma after complete surgical resection of stage I, II, and III non-small-cell lung cancer. N Engl J Med. 1988;318(20):1300–5.
141. Robnett TJ, Machtay M, Stevenson JP, Algazy KM, Hahn SM. Factors affecting the risk of brain metastases after definitive chemoradiation for locally advanced non-small-cell lung carcinoma. J Clin Oncol. 2001;19(5):1344–9.
142. Pagani JJ. Non-small cell lung carcinoma adrenal metastases. Computed tomography and percutaneous needle biopsy in their diagnosis. Cancer. 1984;53(5):1058–60.
143. Allard P, Yankaskas BC, Fletcher RH, Parker LA, Halvorsen Jr RA. Sensitivity and specificity of computed tomography for the detection of adrenal metastatic lesions among 91 autopsied lung cancer patients. Cancer. 1990;66(3):457–62.
144. Silvestri GA, Gould MK, Margolis ML, Tanoue LT, McCrory D, Toloza E, et al. Noninvasive staging of non-small cell lung cancer: ACCP evidenced-based clinical practice guidelines (2nd edition). Chest. 2007;132(3 Suppl):178S–201.
145. Bury T, Barreto A, Daenen F, Barthelemy N, Ghaye B, Rigo P. Fluorine-18 deoxyglucose positron emission tomography for the detection of bone metastases in patients with non-small cell lung cancer. Eur J Nucl Med. 1998;25(9):1244–7.
146. Erasmus JJ, Patz Jr EF, McAdams HP, Murray JG, Herndon J, Coleman RE, et al. Evaluation of adrenal masses in patients with bronchogenic carcinoma using 18 F-fluorodeoxyglucose positron emission tomography. AJR Am J Roentgenol. 1997;168(5): 1357–60.

147. Marom EM, McAdams HP, Erasmus JJ, Goodman PC, Culhane DK, Coleman RE, et al. Staging non-small cell lung cancer with whole-body PET. Radiology. 1999;212(3):803–9.
148. Englemen RM, McNamara WL. Bronchogenic carcinoma: a statistical review of two hundred twenty four autopsies. J Thorac Surg. 1954;27:227–37.
149. Mathews MJ, Kanhouwa S, Pickren J, Robinette D. Frequency of residual and metastatic tumor in patients undergoing curative surgical resection for lung cancer. Cancer Treat Red. 1973;4:63–7.
150. Postmus PE, Brambilla E, Chansky K, Crowley J, Goldstraw P, Patz Jr EF, et al. The IASLC Lung Cancer Staging Project: proposals for revision of the M descriptors in the forthcoming (seventh) edition of the TNM classification of lung cancer. J Thorac Oncol. 2007;2(8):686–93.
151. Bury T, Dowlati A, Paulus P, Corhay JL, Hustinx R, Ghaye B, et al. Whole-body 18FDG positron emission tomography in the staging of non-small cell lung cancer. Eur Respir J. 1997; 10(11):2529–34.
152. Bury T, Dowlati A, Paulus P, Hustinx R, Radermecker M, Rigo P. Staging of non-small-cell lung cancer by whole-body fluorine-18 deoxyglucose positron emission tomography. Eur J Nucl Med. 1996;23(2):204–6.
153. Erasmus JJ, Munden RF. The role of integrated computed tomography positron-emission tomography in esophageal cancer: staging and assessment of therapeutic response. Semin Radiat Oncol. 2007;17(1):29–37.
154. Ettinghausen SE, Burt ME. Prospective evaluation of unilateral adrenal masses in patients with operable non-small-cell lung cancer. J Clin Oncol. 1991;9(8):1462–6.
155. Nielsen Jr ME, Heaston DK, Dunnick NR, Korobkin M. Preoperative CT evaluation of adrenal glands in non-small cell bronchogenic carcinoma. AJR Am J Roentgenol. 1982;139(2): 317–20.
156. Oliver Jr TW, Bernardino ME, Miller JI, Mansour K, Greene D, Davis WA. Isolated adrenal masses in nonsmall-cell bronchogenic carcinoma. Radiology. 1984;153(1):217–8.
157. Pagani JJ. Normal adrenal glands in small cell lung carcinoma: CT-guided biopsy. AJR Am J Roentgenol. 1983;140(5):949–51.
158. Pagani JJ, Bernardino ME. Incidence and significance of serendipitous CT findings in the oncologic patient. J Comput Assist Tomogr. 1982;6(2):268–75.
159. Sparup J, Friis M, Brenoe J, Vejlsted H, Villumsen B, Olesen KP, et al. Computed tomography and the TNM classification of lung cancer. Scand J Thorac Cardiovasc Surg. 1990;24(3):207–11.
160. Boland GW, Lee MJ, Gazelle GS, Halpern EF, McNicholas MM, Mueller PR. Characterization of adrenal masses using unenhanced CT: an analysis of the CT literature. AJR Am J Roentgenol. 1998; 171(1):201–4.
161. Pena CS, Boland GW, Hahn PF, Lee MJ, Mueller PR. Characterization of indeterminate (lipid-poor) adrenal masses: use of washout characteristics at contrast-enhanced CT. Radiology. 2000;217(3):798–802.
162. Schwartz LH, Ginsberg MS, Burt ME, Brown KT, Getrajdman GI, Panicek DM. MRI as an alternative to CT-guided biopsy of adrenal masses in patients with lung cancer. Ann Thorac Surg. 1998;65(1):193–7.
163. Outwater EK, Siegelman ES, Huang AB, Birnbaum BA. Adrenal masses: correlation between CT attenuation value and chemical shift ratio at MR imaging with in-phase and opposed-phase sequences. Radiology. 1996;200(3):749–52.
164. Boland GW, Goldberg MA, Lee MJ, Mayo-Smith WW, Dixon J, McNicholas MM, et al. Indeterminate adrenal mass in patients with cancer: evaluation at PET with 2-[F-18]-fluoro-2-deoxy-D-glucose. Radiology. 1995;194(1):131–4.
165. Mayo-Smith WW, Boland GW, Noto RB, Lee MJ. State-of-the-art adrenal imaging. Radiographics. 2001;21(4):995–1012.
166. Yun M, Kim W, Alnafisi N, Lacorte L, Jang S, Alavi A. 1F-FDG PET in characterizing adrenal lesions detected on CT or MRI. J Nucl Med. 2001;42(12):1795–9.
167. Caoili EM, Korobkin M, Brown RK, Mackie G, Shulkin BL. Differentiating adrenal adenomas from nonadenomas using (18) F-FDG PET/CT: quantitative and qualitative evaluation. Acad Radiol. 2007;14(4):468–75.
168. Hustinx R, Paulus P, Jacquet N, Jerusalem G, Bury T, Rigo P. Clinical evaluation of whole-body 18F-fluorodeoxyglucose positron emission tomography in the detection of liver metastases. Ann Oncol. 1998;9(4):397–401.
169. Patz Jr EF, Erasmus JJ, McAdams HP, Connolly JE, Marom EM, Goodman PC, et al. Lung cancer staging and management: comparison of contrast-enhanced and nonenhanced helical CT of the thorax. Radiology. 1999;212(1):56–60.
170. Butler AR, Leo JS, Lin JP, Boyd AD, Kricheff II. The value of routine cranial computed tomography in neurologically intact patients with primary carcinoma of the lung. Radiology. 1979;131(2):399–401.
171. Cole Jr FH, Thomas JE, Wilcox AB, Halford 3rd HH. Cerebral imaging in the asymptomatic preoperative bronchogenic carcinoma patient: is it worthwhile? Ann Thorac Surg. 1994; 57(4):838–40.
172. Jacobs L, Kinkel WR, Vincent RG. 'Silent' brain metastasis from lung carcinoma determined by computerized tomography. Arch Neurol. 1977;34(11):690–3.
173. Jennings EC, Aungst CW, Yatco R. Asymptomatic patients with primary carcinomia; computerized axial tomography study. N Y State J Med. 1980;80(7 Pt 1):1096–8.
174. Kormas P, Bradshaw JR, Jeyasingham K. Preoperative computed tomography of the brain in non-small cell bronchogenic carcinoma. Thorax. 1992;47(2):106–8.
175. Osada H, Kojima K, Tsukada H, Nakajima Y, Imamura K, Matsumoto J. Cost-effectiveness associated with the diagnosis and staging of non-small-cell lung cancer. Jpn J Thorac Cardiovasc Surg. 2001;49(1):1–10.
176. Osada H, Nakajima Y, Taira Y, Yokote K, Noguchi T. The role of mediastinal and multi-organ CT scans in staging presumable surgical candidates with non-small-cell lung cancer. Jpn J Surg. 1987;17(5):362–8.
177. Yokoi K, Kamiya N, Matsuguma H, Machida S, Hirose T, Mori K, et al. Detection of brain metastasis in potentially operable non-small cell lung cancer: a comparison of CT and MRI. Chest. 1999;115(3):714–9.
178. Bilgin S, Yilmaz A, Ozdemir F, Akkaya E, Karakurt Z, Poluman A. Extrathoracic staging of non-small cell bronchogenic carcinoma: relationship of the clinical evaluation to organ scans. Respirology. 2002;7(1):57–61.
179. Crane JM, Nelson MJ, Ihde DC, Makuch RW, Glatstein E, Zabell A, et al. A comparison of computed tomography and radionuclide scanning for detection of brain metastases in small cell lung cancer. J Clin Oncol. 1984;2(9):1017–24.
180. Habets JM, van Oosterhout AG, ten Velde GP, Wilmink JT, Twijnstra A. Diagnostic value of CT in the detection of brain metastasis in small cell lung cancer patients. J Belge Radiol. 1992;75(3):179–81.
181. Hooper RG, Tenholder MF, Underwood GH, Beechler CR, Spratling L. Computed tomographic scanning of the brain in initial staging of bronchogenic carcinoma. Chest. 1984;85(6): 774–6.
182. Johnson DH, Windham WW, Allen JH, Greco FA. Limited value of CT brain scans in the staging of small cell lung cancer. AJR Am J Roentgenol. 1983;140(1):37–40.
183. Levitan N, Hong WK, Byrne RE, Gale ME, Bromer RH, Levine HL, et al. Role of computerized cranial tomography in the staging of small cell carcinoma of the lung. Cancer Treat Rep. 1984;68(11):1375–7.

184. Mintz BJ, Tuhrim S, Alexander S, Yang WC, Shanzer S. Intracranial metastases in the initial staging of bronchogenic carcinoma. Chest. 1984;86(6):850–3.
185. Salvatierra A, Baamonde C, Llamas JM, Cruz F, Lopez-Pujol J. Extrathoracic staging of bronchogenic carcinoma. Chest. 1990; 97(5):1052–8.
186. Tarver RD, Richmond BD, Klatte EC. Cerebral metastases from lung carcinoma: neurological and CT correlation. Work in progress. Radiology. 1984;153(3):689–92.
187. Earnest FT, Ryu JH, Miller GM, Luetmer PH, Forstrom LA, Burnett OL, et al. Suspected non-small cell lung cancer: incidence of occult brain and skeletal metastases and effectiveness of imaging for detection – pilot study. Radiology. 1999;211(1):137–45.
188. Schirrmeister H, Arslandemir C, Glatting G, Mayer-Steinacker R, Bommer M, Dreinhofer K, et al. Omission of bone scanning according to staging guidelines leads to futile therapy in non-small cell lung cancer. Eur J Nucl Med Mol Imaging. 2004;31(7): 964–8.
189. Hsia TC, Shen YY, Yen RF, Kao CH, Changlai SP. Comparing whole body 18 F-2-deoxyglucose positron emission tomography and technetium-99 m methylene diophosphate bone scan to detect bone metastases in patients with non-small cell lung cancer. Neoplasma. 2002;49(4):267–71.
190. Darling GE. Staging of the patient with small cell lung cancer. Chest Surg Clin N Am. 1997;7(1):81–94.
191. Jelinek JS, Redmond 3rd J, Perry JJ, Burrell LM, Benedikt RA, Geyer CA, et al. Small cell lung cancer: staging with MR imaging. Radiology. 1990;177(3):837–42.
192. Samson DJ, Seidenfeld J, Simon GR, Turrisi 3rd AT, Bonnell C, Ziegler KM, et al. Evidence for management of small cell lung cancer: ACCP evidence-based clinical practice guidelines (2nd edition). Chest. 2007;132(3 Suppl):314S–23.
193. Blum R, MacManus MP, Rischin D, Michael M, Ball D, Hicks RJ. Impact of positron emission tomography on the management of patients with small-cell lung cancer: preliminary experience. Am J Clin Oncol. 2004;27(2):164–71.
194. Bradley JD, Dehdashti F, Mintun MA, Govindan R, Trinkaus K, Siegel BA. Positron emission tomography in limited-stage small-cell lung cancer: a prospective study. J Clin Oncol. 2004; 22(16):3248–54.
195. Brink I, Schumacher T, Mix M, Ruhland S, Stoelben E, Digel W, et al. Impact of [18 F]FDG-PET on the primary staging of small-cell lung cancer. Eur J Nucl Med Mol Imaging. 2004; 31(12):1614–20.
196. Kamel EM, Zwahlen D, Wyss MT, Stumpe KD, von Schulthess GK, Steinert HC. Whole-body (18)F-FDG PET improves the management of patients with small cell lung cancer. J Nucl Med. 2003;44(12):1911–7.
197. Schumacher T, Brink I, Mix M, Reinhardt M, Herget G, Digel W, et al. FDG-PET imaging for the staging and follow-up of small cell lung cancer. Eur J Nucl Med. 2001;28(4):483–8.
198. Shen YY, Shiau YC, Wang JJ, Ho ST, Kao CH. Whole-body 18 F-2-deoxyglucose positron emission tomography in primary staging small cell lung cancer. Anticancer Res. 2002;22(2B):1257–64.
199. Niho S, Fujii H, Murakami K, Nagase S, Yoh K, Goto K, et al. Detection of unsuspected distant metastases and/or regional nodes by FDG-PET [corrected] scan in apparent limited-disease small-cell lung cancer. Lung Cancer. 2007;57(3):328–33.
200. Vinjamuri M, Craig M, Campbell-Fontaine A, Almubarak M, Gupta N, Rogers JS. Can positron emission tomography be used as a staging tool for small-cell lung cancer? Clin Lung Cancer. 2008;9(1):30–4.
201. Kut V, Spies W, Spies S, Gooding W, Argiris A. Staging and monitoring of small cell lung cancer using [18F]fluoro-2-deoxy-D-glucose-positron emission tomography (FDG-PET). Am J Clin Oncol. 2007;30(1):45–50.
202. Abrams J, Doyle LA, Aisner J. Staging, prognostic factors, and special considerations in small cell lung cancer. Semin Oncol. 1988;15(3):261–77.
203. Stahel RA, Mabry M, Skarin AT, Speak J, Bernal SD. Detection of bone marrow metastasis in small-cell lung cancer by monoclonal antibody. J Clin Oncol. 1985;3(4):455–61.
204. Hochstenbag MM, Twijnstra A, Wilmink JT, Wouters EF, ten Velde GP. Asymptomatic brain metastases (BM) in small cell lung cancer (SCLC): MR-imaging is useful at initial diagnosis. J Neurooncol. 2000;48(3):243–8.
205. Ishida T, Tateishi M, Kaneko S, Yano T, Mitsudomi T, Sugimachi K, et al. Carcinosarcoma and spindle cell carcinoma of the lung. Clinicopathologic and immunohistochemical studies. J Thorac Cardiovasc Surg. 1990;100(6):844–52.
206. Kim KI, Flint JD, Muller NL. Pulmonary carcinosarcoma: radiologic and pathologic findings in three patients. AJR Am J Roentgenol. 1997;169(3):691–4.
207. Nappi O, Glasner SD, Swanson PE, Wick MR. Biphasic and monophasic sarcomatoid carcinomas of the lung. A reappraisal of “carcinosarcomas” and “spindle-cell carcinomas”. Am J Clin Pathol. 1994;102(3):331–40.
208. Wick MR, Ritter JH, Humphrey PA. Sarcomatoid carcinomas of the lung: a clinicopathologic review. Am J Clin Pathol. 1997;108(1):40–53.
209. Kim K, Flint JDA, Muller NL. Pulmonary carcinosarcoma: radiologic and pathologic findings in three patients. Am J Roentgenol. 1997;169:691–4.
210. Boldrini R, Devito R, Diomedi-Camassei F, Francalanci P, Inserra A, Boglino C, et al. Pulmonary blastomas of childhood: histologic, immunohistochemical, ultrastructural aspects and therapeutic considerations. Ultrastruct Pathol. 2005;29(6):493–501.
211. Francis D, Jacobsen M. Pulmonary blastoma. Curr Top Pathol. 1983;73:265–94.
212. Liman ST, Altinok T, Topcu S, Tastepe AI, Uzar A, Demircan S, et al. Survival of biphasic pulmonary blastoma. Respir Med. 2006;100(7):1174–9.
213. Weisbrod GL, Chamberlain DW, Tao LC. Pulmonary blastoma, report of three cases and a review of the literature. Can Assoc Radiol J. 1988;39(2):130–6.
214. LeMense GP, Reed CE, Silvestri GA. Pulmonary blastoma: a rare lung malignancy. Lung Cancer. 1996;15(2):233–7.
215. Allen MS. Malignant tracheal tumors. Mayo Clin Proc. 1993;68(7):680–4.
216. Conlan AA, Payne WS, Woolner LB, Sanderson DR. Adenoid cystic carcinoma (cylindroma) and mucoepidermoid carcinoma of the bronchus. Factors affecting survival. J Thorac Cardiovasc Surg. 1978;76(3):369–77.
217. Dalton ML, Gatling RR. Peripheral adenoid cystic carcinoma of the lung. South Med J. 1990;83(5):577–9.
218. Gallagher CG, Stark R, Teskey J, Kryger M. Atypical manifestations of pulmonary adenoid cystic carcinoma. Br J Dis Chest. 1986;80(4):396–9.
219. McCarthy MJ, Rosado-de-Christenson ML. Tumors of the trachea. J Thorac Imaging. 1995;10(3):180–98.
220. Spizarny DL, Shepard JA, McLoud TC, Grillo HC, Dedrick CG. CT of adenoid cystic carcinoma of the trachea. AJR Am J Roentgenol. 1986;146(6):1129–32.
221. Trentini GP, Palmieri B. Mucoepidermoid tumor of the trachea. Chest. 1972;62(3):336–8.
222. Turnbull AD, Huvos AG, Goodner JT, Foote Jr FW. Mucoepidermoid tumors of bronchial glands. Cancer. 1971;28(3):539–44.
223. Yousem SA, Hochholzer L. Mucoepidermoid tumors of the lung. Cancer. 1987;60(6):1346–52.
224. Klacsmann PG, Olson JL, Eggleston JC. Mucoepidermoid carcinoma of the bronchus: an electron microscopic study of the low grade and the high grade variants. Cancer. 1979;43(5):1720–33.

225. Spencer H. Bronchial mucous gland tumours. Virchows Arch. 1979;383(1):101–15.
226. Katz DS, Lane MJ, Leung AN, Marcus FS, Sakata MK. Primary malignant pulmonary hemangiopericytoma. Clin Imaging. 1998;22(3):192–5.
227. Moran CA, Suster S, Abbondanzo SL, Koss MN. Primary leiomyosarcomas of the lung: a clinicopathologic and immunohistochemical study of 18 cases. Mod Pathol. 1997;10(2):121–8.
228. Suster S. Primary sarcomas of the lung. Semin Diagn Pathol. 1995;12(2):140–57.
229. Zeren H, Moran CA, Suster S, Fishback NF, Koss MN. Primary pulmonary sarcomas with features of monophasic synovial sarcoma: a clinicopathological, immunohistochemical, and ultrastructural study of 25 cases. Hum Pathol. 1995;26(5):474–80.
230. Attanoos RL, Appleton MA, Gibbs AR. Primary sarcomas of the lung: a clinicopathological and immunohistochemical study of 14 cases. Histopathology. 1996;29(1):29–36.
231. Janssen JP, Mulder JJ, Wagenaar SS, Elbers HR, van den Bosch JM. Primary sarcoma of the lung: a clinical study with long-term follow-up. Ann Thorac Surg. 1994;58(4):1151–5.
232. Yousem SA, Hochholzer L. Primary pulmonary hemangiopericytoma. Cancer. 1987;59(3):549–55.
233. Halle M, Blum U, Dinkel E, Brugger W. CT and MR features of primary pulmonary hemangiopericytomas. J Comput Assist Tomogr. 1993;17(1):51–5.
234. Lorigan JG, David CL, Evans HL, Wallace S. The clinical and radiologic manifestations of hemangiopericytoma. AJR Am J Roentgenol. 1989;153(2):345–9.
235. Yilmaz E, Akkoclu A, Kargi A, Sevinc C, Komus N, Catalyurek H, et al. Radiography, Doppler sonography, and MR angiography of malignant pulmonary hemangiopericytoma. AJR Am J Roentgenol. 2003;181(4):1079–81.
236. Bagan P, Hassan M, Le Pimpec Barthes F, Peyrard S, Souilamas R, Danel C, et al. Prognostic factors and surgical indications of pulmonary epithelioid hemangioendothelioma: a review of the literature. Ann Thorac Surg. 2006;82(6):2010–3.
237. Weiss SW, Ishak KG, Dail DH, Sweet DE, Enzinger FM. Epithelioid hemangioendothelioma and related lesions. Semin Diagn Pathol. 1986;3(4):259–87.
238. Dail DH, Liebow AA, Gmelich JT, Friedman PJ, Miyai K, Myer W, et al. Intravascular, bronchiolar, and alveolar tumor of the lung (IVBAT). An analysis of twenty cases of a peculiar sclerosing endothelial tumor. Cancer. 1983;51(3):452–64.
239. Ross GJ, Violi L, Friedman AC, Edmonds PR, Unger E. Intravascular bronchioloalveolar tumor: CT and pathologic correlation. J Comput Assist Tomogr. 1989;13(2):240–3.
240. Sakamoto N, Adachi S, Monzawa S, Hamanaka A, Takada Y, Hunada Y, et al. High resolution CT findings of pulmonary epithelioid hemangioendothelioma: unusual manifestations in 2 cases. J Thorac Imaging. 2005;20(3):236–8.
241. Bragg DG, Chor PJ, Murray KA, Kjeldsberg CR. Lymphoproliferative disorders of the lung: histopathology, clinical manifestations, and imaging features. AJR Am J Roentgenol. 1994;163(2):273–81.
242. Cordier JF, Chailleux E, Lauque D, Reynaud-Gaubert M, Dietemann-Molard A, Dalphin JC, et al. Primary pulmonary lymphomas. A clinical study of 70 cases in nonimmunocompromised patients. Chest. 1993;103(1):201–8.
243. Fiche M, Caprons F, Berger F, Galateau F, Cordier JF, Loire R, et al. Primary pulmonary non-Hodgkin's lymphomas. Histopathology. 1995;26(6):529–37.
244. Nicholson A, Harris N. Marginal zone B-cell lymphoma of the mucosa-associated lymphoid tissue (MALT) type. In: Travis WDBE, Muller-Hermelink HK, Harris CC, editors. World Health Organization classification of tumors: tumours of the lung, pleura, thymus and heart. Lyon, France: IARC Press; 2004. p. 88–90.
245. Ramani S, Karnad AB. Primary pulmonary non-Hodgkin's lymphoma. South Med J. 1995;88(2):243–5.
246. Saltzstein SL. Pulmonary malignant lymphomas and pseudolymphomas: classification, therapy, and prognosis. Cancer. 1963; 16:928–55.
247. Toh HC, Ang PT. Primary pulmonary lymphoma–clinical review from a single institution in Singapore. Leuk Lymphoma. 1997; 27(1–2):153–63.
248. King LJ, Padley SP, Wotherspoon AC, Nicholson AG. Pulmonary MALT lymphoma: imaging findings in 24 cases. Eur Radiol. 2000;10(12):1932–8.
249. Koss MN. Pulmonary lymphoid disorders. Semin Diagn Pathol. 1995;12(2):158–71.
250. Lee KS, Kim Y, Primack SL. Imaging of pulmonary lymphomas. AJR Am J Roentgenol. 1997;168(2):339–45.
251. Li G, Hansmann ML, Zwingers T, Lennert K. Primary lymphomas of the lung: morphological, immunohistochemical and clinical features. Histopathology. 1990;16(6):519–31.
252. O'Donnell PG, Jackson SA, Tung KT, Hassan B, Wilkins B, Mead GM. Radiological appearances of lymphomas arising from mucosa-associated lymphoid tissue (MALT) in the lung. Clin Radiol. 1998;53(4):258–63.
253. Kennedy JL, Nathwani BN, Burke JS, Hill LR, Rappaport H. Pulmonary lymphomas and other pulmonary lymphoid lesions. A clinicopathologic and immunologic study of 64 patients. Cancer. 1985;56(3):539–52.
254. Crow J, Slavin G, Kreel L. Pulmonary metastasis: a pathologic and radiologic study. Cancer. 1981;47(11):2595–602.
255. Hirakata K, Nakata H, Haratake J. Appearance of pulmonary metastases on high-resolution CT scans: comparison with histopathologic findings from autopsy specimens. AJR Am J Roentgenol. 1993;161(1):37–43.
256. Primack SL, Lee KS, Logan PM, Miller RR, Muller NL. Bronchogenic carcinoma: utility of CT in the evaluation of patients with suspected lesions. Radiology. 1994;193(3):795–800.
257. Clagett OT, Woolner LB. Surgical treatment of solitary metastatic pulmonary lesion. Med Clin North Am. 1964;48:939–43.
258. Toomes H, Delphendahl A, Manke HG, Vogt-Moykopf I. The coin lesion of the lung. A review of 955 resected coin lesions. Cancer. 1983;51(3):534–7.
259. Chaudhuri MR. Cavitary pulmonary metastases. Thorax. 1970; 25(3):375–81.
260. Dodd GD, Boyle JJ. Excavating pulmonary metastases. Am J Roentgenol Radium Ther Nucl Med. 1961;85:277–93.
261. Seo JB, Im JG, Goo JM, Chung MJ, Kim MY. Atypical pulmonary metastases: spectrum of radiologic findings. Radiographics. 2001;21(2):403–17.
262. Libshitz HI, North LB. Pulmonary metastases. Radiol Clin North Am. 1982;20(3):437–51.
263. Patel AM, Ryu JH. Angiosarcoma in the lung. Chest. 1993; 103(5):1531–5.
264. Franchi M, La Fianza A, Babilonti L, Bolis PF, Dore R, Legnani L, et al. Serous carcinoma of the ovary: value of computed tomography in detection of calcified pleural and pulmonary metastatic implants. Gynecol Oncol. 1990;39(1):85–8.
265. Hall FM, Frank HA, Cohen RB, Ezpeleta ML. Ossified pulmonary metastases from giant cell tumor of bone. AJR Am J Roentgenol. 1976;127(6):1046–7.
266. Jimenez JM, Casey SO, Citron M, Khan A. Calcified pulmonary metastases from medullary carcinoma of the thyroid. Comput Med Imaging Graph. 1995;19(4):325–8.
267. Gaeta M, Blandino A, Scribano E, Minutoli F, Volta S, Pandolfo I. Computed tomography halo sign in pulmonary nodules: frequency and diagnostic value. J Thorac Imaging. 1999;14(2):109–13.
268. Kim Y, Lee KS, Jung KJ, Han J, Kim JS, Suh JS. Halo sign on high resolution CT: findings in spectrum of pulmonary diseases

with pathologic correlation. J Comput Assist Tomogr. 1999; 23(4):622–6.
269. Primack SL, Hartman TE, Lee KS, Muller NL. Pulmonary nodules and the CT halo sign. Radiology. 1994;190(2):513–5.
270. Filderman AE, Coppage L, Shaw C, Matthay RA. Pulmonary and pleural manifestations of extrathoracic malignancies. Clin Chest Med. 1989;10(4):747–807.
271. Levin B. Subpleural interlobular lymphectasia reflecting metastatic carcinoma. Radiology. 1959;72(5):682–8.
272. Munk PL, Muller NL, Miller RR, Ostrow DN. Pulmonary lymphangitic carcinomatosis: CT and pathologic findings. Radiology. 1988;166(3):705–9.
273. Janower ML, Blennerhassett JB. Lymphangitic spread of metastatic cancer to the lung. A radiologic-pathologic classification. Radiology. 1971;101(2):267–73.
274. Sadoff L, Grossman J, Weiner H. Lymphangitic pulmonary metastases secondary to breast cancer with normal chest x-rays and abnormal perfusion lung scans. Oncology. 1975;31(3–4):164–71.
275. Grenier P, Chevret S, Beigelman C, Brauner MW, Chastang C, Valeyre D. Chronic diffuse infiltrative lung disease: determination of the diagnostic value of clinical data, chest radiography, and CT and Bayesian analysis. Radiology. 1994;191(2):383–90.
276. Stein MG, Mayo J, Muller N, Aberle DR, Webb WR, Gamsu G. Pulmonary lymphangitic spread of carcinoma: appearance on CT scans. Radiology. 1987;162(2):371–5.
277. Ren H, Hruban RH, Kuhlman JE, Fishman EK, Wheeler PS, Zerhouni EA, et al. Computed tomography of inflation-fixed lungs: the beaded septum sign of pulmonary metastases. J Comput Assist Tomogr. 1989;13(3):411–6.
278. Kane RD, Hawkins HK, Miller JA, Noce PS. Microscopic pulmonary tumor emboli associated with dyspnea. Cancer. 1975; 36(4):1473–82.
279. Winterbauer RH, Elfenbein IB, Ball Jr WC. Incidence and clinical significance of tumor embolization to the lungs. Am J Med. 1968;45(2):271–90.
280. Chan CK, Hutcheon MA, Hyland RH, Smith GJ, Patterson BJ, Matthay RA. Pulmonary tumor embolism: a critical review of clinical, imaging, and hemodynamic features. J Thorac Imaging. 1987;2(4):4–14.
281. Kang CH, Choi JA, Kim HR, Oh YH, Kim HK, Kang EY. Lung metastases manifesting as pulmonary infarction by mucin and tumor embolization: radiographic, high-resolution CT, and pathologic findings. J Comput Assist Tomogr. 1999;23(4):644–6.
282. Kim AE, Haramati LB, Janus D, Borczuk A. Pulmonary tumor embolism presenting as infarcts on computed tomography. J Thorac Imaging. 1999;14(2):135–7.
283. Shepard JA, Moore EH, Templeton PA, McLoud TC. Pulmonary intravascular tumor emboli: dilated and beaded peripheral pulmonary arteries at CT. Radiology. 1993;187(3):797–801.
284. Franquet T, Gimenez A, Prats R, Rodriguez-Arias JM, Rodriguez C. Thrombotic microangiopathy of pulmonary tumors: a vascular cause of tree-in-bud pattern on CT. AJR Am J Roentgenol. 2002;179(4):897–9.
285. Tack D, Nollevaux MC, Gevenois PA. Tree-in-bud pattern in neoplastic pulmonary emboli. AJR Am J Roentgenol. 2001;176(6):1421–2.
286. Albertini RE, Ekberg NL. Endobronchial metastasis in breast cancer. Thorax. 1980;35(6):435–40.
287. Amer E, Guy J, Vaze B. Endobronchial metastasis from renal adenocarcinoma simulating a foreign body. Thorax. 1981;36(3):183–4.
288. Braman SS, Whitcomb ME. Endobronchial metastasis. Arch Intern Med. 1975;135(4):543–7.
289. Jariwalla AG, Seaton A, McCormack RJ, Gibbs A, Campbell IA, Davies BH. Intrabronchial metastases from renal carcinoma with recurrent tumour expectoration. Thorax. 1981;36(3):179–82.
290. Sutton Jr FD, Vestal RE, Creagh CE. Varied presentations of metastatic pulmonary melanoma. Chest. 1974;65(4):415–9.
291. Zias EA, Owen RP, Borczuk A, Reichel J, Frater RW. An unusual presentation of metastatic colon cancer to the lung. Chest. 1998;113(1):244–6.
292. Marom EM, Goodman PC, McAdams HP. Focal abnormalities of the trachea and main bronchi. AJR Am J Roentgenol. 2001; 176(3):707–11.
293. Alberts AS, Falkson G, Goedhals L, Vorobiof DA, Van der Merwe CA. Malignant pleural mesothelioma: a disease unaffected by current therapeutic maneuvers. J Clin Oncol. 1988;6(3):527–35.
294. De Pangher Manzini V, Brollo A, Franceschi S, De Matthaeis M, Talamini R, Bianchi C. Prognostic factors of malignant mesothelioma of the pleura. Cancer. 1993;72(2):410–7.
295. Fusco V, Ardizzoni A, Merlo F, Cinquegrana A, Faravelli B, De Palma M, et al. Malignant pleural mesothelioma. Multivariate analysis of prognostic factors on 113 patients. Anticancer Res. 1993;13(3):683–9.
296. Herndon JE, Green MR, Chahinian AP, Corson JM, Suzuki Y, Vogelzang NJ. Factors predictive of survival among 337 patients with mesothelioma treated between 1984 and 1994 by the Cancer and Leukemia Group B. Chest. 1998;113(3):723–31.
297. Huncharek M, Kelsey K, Mark EJ, Muscat J, Choi N, Carey R, et al. Treatment and survival in diffuse malignant pleural mesothelioma; a study of 83 cases from the Massachusetts General Hospital. Anticancer Res. 1996;16(3):1265–8.
298. Ong ST, Vogelzang NJ. Chemotherapy in malignant pleural mesothelioma. A review J Clin Oncol. 1996;14(3):1007–17.
299. Tammilehto L, Maasilta P, Kostiainen S, Appelqvist P, Holsti LR, Mattson K. Diagnosis and prognostic factors in malignant pleural mesothelioma: a retrospective analysis of sixty-five patients. Respiration. 1992;59(3):129–35.
300. Yates DH, Corrin B, Stidolph PN, Browne K. Malignant mesothelioma in south east England: clinicopathological experience of 272 cases. Thorax. 1997;52(6):507–12.
301. Antman KH. Clinical presentation and natural history of benign and malignant mesothelioma. Semin Oncol. 1981;8(3):313–20.
302. Heller RM, Janower ML, Weber AL. The radiological manifestations of malignant pleural mesothelioma. Am J Roentgenol Radium Ther Nucl Med. 1970;108(1):53–9.
303. Solomon A. Radiological features of diffuse mesothelioma. Environ Res. 1970;3(4):330–8.
304. Taylor RA, Johnson LP. Mesothelioma: current perspectives. West J Med. 1981;134(5):379–83.
305. Wechsler RJ, Rao VM, Steiner RM. The radiology of thoracic malignant mesothelioma. Crit Rev Diagn Imaging. 1984;20(4): 283–310.
306. Steiner RM, Cooper MW, Brodovsky H. Rib destruction: a neglected finding in malignant mesothelioma. Clin Radiol. 1982;33(1):61–5.
307. Hillerdal G. Pleural plaques and risk for bronchial carcinoma and mesothelioma. A prospective study. Chest. 1994;105(1):144–50.
308. Miller BH, Rosado-de-Christenson ML, Mason AC, Fleming MV, White CC, Krasna MJ. From the archives of the AFIP. Malignant pleural mesothelioma: radiologic-pathologic correlation. Radiographics. 1996;16(3):613–44.
309. Benamore RE, O'Doherty MJ, Entwisle JJ. Use of imaging in the management of malignant pleural mesothelioma. Clin Radiol. 2005;60(12):1237–47.
310. Kawashima A, Libshitz HI. Malignant pleural mesothelioma: CT manifestations in 50 cases. AJR Am J Roentgenol. 1990; 155(5):965–9.
311. Leung AN, Muller NL, Miller RR. CT in differential diagnosis of diffuse pleural disease. AJR Am J Roentgenol. 1990;154(3): 487–92.
312. Mirvis S, Dutcher JP, Haney PJ, Whitley NO, Aisner J. CT of malignant pleural mesothelioma. AJR Am J Roentgenol. 1983;140(4):665–70.

313. Ng CS, Munden RF, Libshitz HI. Malignant pleural mesothelioma: the spectrum of manifestations on CT in 70 cases. Clin Radiol. 1999;54(7):415–21.
314. Rabinowitz JG, Efremidis SC, Cohen B, Dan S, Efremidis A, Chahinian AP, et al. A comparative study of mesothelioma and asbestosis using computed tomography and conventional chest radiography. Radiology. 1982;144(3):453–60.
315. Wong RJ, Lin DT, Schoder H, Patel SG, Gonen M, Wolden S, et al. Diagnostic and prognostic value of [(18)F]fluorodeoxyglucose positron emission tomography for recurrent head and neck squamous cell carcinoma. J Clin Oncol. 2002;20(20):4199–208.
316. Patz Jr EF, Shaffer K, Piwnica-Worms DR, Jochelson M, Sarin M, Sugarbaker DJ, et al. Malignant pleural mesothelioma: value of CT and MR imaging in predicting resectability. AJR Am J Roentgenol. 1992;159(5):961–6.
317. Heelan RT, Rusch VW, Begg CB, Panicek DM, Caravelli JF, Eisen C. Staging of malignant pleural mesothelioma: comparison of CT and MR imaging. AJR Am J Roentgenol. 1999;172(4):1039–47.
318. Benard F, Sterman D, Smith RJ, Kaiser LR, Albelda SM, Alavi A. Metabolic imaging of malignant pleural mesothelioma with fluorodeoxyglucose positron emission tomography. Chest. 1998;114(3):713–22.
319. Flores RM, Akhurst T, Gonen M, Larson SM, Rusch VW. Positron emission tomography defines metastatic disease but not locoregional disease in patients with malignant pleural mesothelioma. J Thorac Cardiovasc Surg. 2003;126(1):11–6.
320. Gerbaudo VH, Sugarbaker DJ, Britz-Cunningham S, Di Carli MF, Mauceri C, Treves ST. Assessment of malignant pleural mesothelioma with (18)F-FDG dual-head gamma-camera coincidence imaging: comparison with histopathology. J Nucl Med. 2002; 43(9):1144–9.
321. Nanni C, Castellucci P, Farsad M, Pinto C, Moretti A, Pettinato C, et al. Role of 18 F-FDG PET for evaluating malignant pleural mesothelioma. Cancer Biother Radiopharm. 2004;19(2):149–54.
322. Schneider DB, Clary-Macy C, Challa S, Sasse KC, Merrick SH, Hawkins R, et al. Positron emission tomography with f18-fluorodeoxyglucose in the staging and preoperative evaluation of malignant pleural mesothelioma. J Thorac Cardiovasc Surg. 2000;120(1):128–33.
323. Zubeldia J, Abou-Zied M, Nabi H. 11. Evaluation of Patients with Known Mesothelioma with 18 F-Fluorodeoxyglucose and PET Comparison with Computed Tomography. Clin Positron Imaging. 2000;3(4):165.
324. Erasmus JJ, Truong MT, Smythe WR, Munden RF, Marom EM, Rice DC, et al. Integrated computed tomography-positron emission tomography in patients with potentially resectable malignant pleural mesothelioma: staging implications. J Thorac Cardiovasc Surg. 2005;129(6):1364–70.
325. Francis RJ, Byrne MJ, van der Schaaf AA, Boucek JA, Nowak AK, Phillips M, et al. Early prediction of response to chemotherapy and survival in malignant pleural mesothelioma using a novel semiautomated 3-dimensional volume-based analysis of serial 18 F-FDG PET scans. J Nucl Med. 2007;48(9):1449–58.
326. Truong MT, Marom EM, Erasmus JJ. Preoperative evaluation of patients with malignant pleural mesothelioma: role of integrated CT-PET imaging. J Thorac Imaging. 2006;21(2):146–53.
327. Rusch VW. A proposed new international TNM staging system for malignant pleural mesothelioma from the International Mesothelioma Interest Group. Lung Cancer. 1996;14(1):1–12.
328. Rice DC, Erasmus JJ, Stevens CW, Vaporciyan AA, Wu JS, Tsao AS, et al. Extended surgical staging for potentially resectable malignant pleural mesothelioma. Ann Thorac Surg. 2005; 80(6):1988–92; discussion 92-3.
329. Rusch VW, Venkatraman E. The importance of surgical staging in the treatment of malignant pleural mesothelioma. J Thorac Cardiovasc Surg. 1996;111(4):815–25; discussion 25-6.
330. Sugarbaker DJ, Flores RM, Jaklitsch MT, Richards WG, Strauss GM, Corson JM, et al. esection margins, extrapleural nodal status, and cell type determine postoperative long-term survival in trimodality therapy of malignant pleural mesothelioma: results in 183 patients. J Thorac Cardiovasc Surg. 1999;117(1):54–63. discussion -5.
331. Schouwink JH, Kool LS, Rutgers EJ, Zoetmulder FA, van Zandwijk N, Vijver MJ, et al. The value of chest computer tomography and cervical mediastinoscopy in the preoperative assessment of patients with malignant pleural mesothelioma. Ann Thorac Surg. 2003;75(6):1715–8. discussion 8-9.
332. Rosado-de-Christenson ML, Abbott GF, McAdams HP, Franks TJ, Galvin JR. From the archives of the AFIP: localized fibrous tumor of the pleura. Radiographics. 2003;23(3):759–83.
333. Desser TS, Stark P. Pictorial essay: solitary fibrous tumor of the pleura. J Thorac Imaging. 1998;13(1):27–35.
334. Ferretti GR, Chiles C, Choplin RH, Coulomb M. Localized benign fibrous tumors of the pleura. AJR Am J Roentgenol. 1997; 169(3):683–6.
335. Sandvliet RH, Heysteeg M, Paul MA. A large thoracic mass in a 57-year-old patient. Solitary fibrous tumor of the pleura. Chest. 2000;117(3):897–900.
336. Dynes MC, White EM, Fry WA, Ghahremani GG. Imaging manifestations of pleural tumors. Radiographics. 1992;12(6): 1191–201.
337. George JC. Benign fibrous mesothelioma of the pleura: MR findings. AJR Am J Roentgenol. 1993;160(1):204–5.
338. Harris GN, Rozenshtein A, Schiff MJ. Benign fibrous mesothelioma of the pleura: MR imaging findings. AJR Am J Roentgenol. 1995;165(5):1143–4.
339. Tateishi U, Nishihara H, Morikawa T, Miyasaka K. Solitary fibrous tumor of the pleura: MR appearance and enhancement pattern. J Comput Assist Tomogr. 2002;26(2):174–9.
340. Tublin ME, Tessler FN, Rifkin MD. US case of the day. Solitary fibrous tumor of the pleura (SFTP). Radiographics. 1998; 18(2):523–5.
341. Usami N, Iwano S, Yokoi K. Solitary fibrous tumor of the pleura: evaluation of the origin with 3D CT angiography. J Thorac Oncol. 2007;2(12):1124–5.
342. Hara M, Kume M, Oshima H, Shibamoto Y, Iida A, Mori Y, et al. F-18 FDG uptake in a malignant localized fibrous tumor of the pleura. J Thorac Imaging. 2005;20(2):118–9.
343. Kohler M, Clarenbach CF, Kestenholz P, Kurrer M, Steinert HC, Russi EW, et al. Diagnosis, treatment and long-term outcome of solitary fibrous tumours of the pleura. Eur J Cardiothorac Surg. 2007;32(3):403–8.
344. Rodriguez-Panadero F, Borderas Naranjo F, Lopez Mejias J. Pleural metastatic tumours and effusions. Frequency and pathogenic mechanisms in a post-mortem series. Eur Respir J. 1989; 2(4):366–9.
345. Light RW, Erozan YS, Ball Jr WC. Cells in pleural fluid. Their value in differential diagnosis. Arch Intern Med. 1973; 132(6):854–60.
346. Burgess LJ, Maritz FJ, Taljaard JJ. Comparative analysis of the biochemical parameters used to distinguish between pleural transudates and exudates. Chest. 1995;107(6):1604–9.
347. Ceyhan BB, Demiralp E, Celikel T. Analysis of pleural effusions using flow cytometry. Respiration. 1996;63(1):17–24.
348. Metintas M, Ozdemir N, Solak M, Artan S, Ozdemir M, Basaran N, et al. Chromosome analysis in pleural effusions. Efficiency of this method in the differential diagnosis of pleural effusions. Respiration. 1994;61(6):330–5.
349. Menzies R, Charbonneau M. Thoracoscopy for the diagnosis of pleural disease. Ann Intern Med. 1991;114(4):271–6.
350. Arenas-Jimenez J, Alonso-Charterina S, Sanchez-Paya J, Fernandez-Latorre F, Gil-Sanchez S, Lloret-Llorens M. Evaluation

of CT findings for diagnosis of pleural effusions. Eur Radiol. 2000;10(4):681–90.
351. Falaschi F, Battolla L, Mascalchi M, Cioni R, Zampa V, Lencioni R, et al. Usefulness of MR signal intensity in distinguishing benign from malignant pleural disease. AJR Am J Roentgenol. 1996; 166(4):963–8.
352. Shiono T, Yoshikawa K, Takenaka E, Hisamatsu K. MR imaging of pleural and peritoneal effusion. Radiat Med. 1993;11(4): 123–6.
353. Duysinx B, Nguyen D, Louis R, Cataldo D, Belhocine T, Bartsch P, et al. Evaluation of pleural disease with 18-fluorodeoxyglucose positron emission tomography imaging. Chest. 2004;125(2):489–93.
354. Gupta NC, Rogers JS, Graeber GM, Gregory JL, Waheed U, Mullet D, et al. Clinical role of F-18 fluorodeoxyglucose positron emission tomography imaging in patients with lung cancer and suspected malignant pleural effusion. Chest. 2002;122(6):1918–24.
355. Kramer H, Pieterman RM, Slebos DJ, Timens W, Vaalburg W, Koeter GH, et al. PET for the evaluation of pleural thickening observed on CT. J Nucl Med. 2004;45(6):995–8.
356. Toaff JS, Metser U, Gottfried M, Gur O, Deeb ME, Lievshitz G, et al. Differentiation between malignant and benign pleural effusion in patients with extra-pleural primary malignancies: assessment with positron emission tomography-computed tomography. Invest Radiol. 2005;40(4):204–9.

The Staging of Lung Cancer

2

David C. Rice

Introduction

Staging is one of the most important components in the management of lung cancer. Accurate staging is important because it allows the clinician to predict prognosis and assign appropriate therapy and also provides a system that allows clinicians and researchers to stratify patients into reasonably homogenous groups so that treatment outcomes can be appropriately compared. Tumor staging is broadly broken down into clinical staging and pathologic staging. Clinical stage refers to the best prediction of lung cancer stage prior to the commencement of therapy. Pathologic stage refers to the best prediction of stage following pathologic analysis of the patient's tumor, lymph nodes, and/or metastases and is usually applied following surgical resection or exploration. The distinction between clinical and pathologic stage becomes slightly less clear, however, when patients undergo some form of histologic staging without surgical resection or exploration. Thus, a patient may undergo histologic assessment of mediastinal nodes by endobronchial ultrasound (EBUS) fine-needle aspiration (FNA) prior to surgical resection. The information thus gained is considered to contribute to the clinical not pathologic stage, which would be determined by the pathologic findings at surgery. If the same patient was found to have ipsilateral lymph node metastases at EBUS and then went on to receive nonsurgical therapy, he would be considered to have pathologic stage N2 (p-stage IIIa) disease. Ultimately, pathologic stage is determined by the highest level histologic evidence that is available. Following preoperative therapy (such as chemotherapy and radiation), subsequent pathologic staging is associated with the prefix "y". Thus a patient with ipsilateral nodal metastases might be downstaged by preoperative chemotherapy from pN2 prior to treatment to ypN0 after pathologic analysis of the post-chemotherapy surgical specimen.

In common with most other solid malignancies, lung cancer staging is defined by the local extent of the primary tumor (T), involvement of associated lymph nodes (N), and whether or not metastases (M) exist. The TNM classification for lung cancer was originally proposed by Mountain in the early 1970s based on an analysis of 2,155 surgically resected patients at the MD Anderson Cancer Center (MDACC). This staging system was adopted by the American Joint Committee on Cancer (AJCC) in 1973 and by the Union Internationale Contre le Cancer (UICC) the following year. In 1997, Mountain refined the staging system based on analysis of an expanded dataset, which included 5,319 surgically treated patients collected from the MD Anderson Cancer Center between 1975 and 1988 and the North American Lung Cancer Study Group between 1977 and 1982 [1]. The sixth iteration of the lung cancer staging system was in 1997. At the time it was clear that there were significant limitations with the staging system. First, the system was based almost exclusively on outcome analysis of patients who underwent surgical resection, a subset of patients, which represents a small proportion of the population of patients with lung cancer. Second, the stage classifications were based on analysis of a relatively small number of patients, so there were small populations of patients and whose stage assignment was frequently based on intuition rather than data-derived evidence. Third, most patients in the analysis came from a single academic institution, and all were treated at North American centers; thus, the relevance and applicability to patients with lung cancer in other geographic regions was uncertain. Acknowledging these limitations, the International Association for the Study of Lung Cancer (IASLC) convened a lung cancer staging workgroup in 1998 and collected data on a total of 100,869 patients from multiple institutions worldwide [2]. The database included lung tumor cases diagnosed between 1990 and 2000, a relatively short time interval during which staging methods have remained fairly consistent and that allowed at least 5 years of follow-up

D.C. Rice, M.D.
Minimally Invasive Surgery Program, Thoracic Surgery,
The University of Texas MD Anderson Cancer Center,
1515 Holcombe Blvd., Box 445, FC9.2012, Houston, TX 77030, USA
e-mail: drice@mdanderson.org

A. Weissferdt, C.A. Moran, *Diagnostic Pathology of Pleuropulmonary Neoplasia*,
DOI 10.1007/978-1-4419-0787-5_2,

before analysis. Ultimately, there were a total of 81,015 analyzable cases from 46 institutions in 19 countries of which 67,725 were non-small cell lung cancer, 13,290 were small cell lung cancer, and 513 were carcinoid tumors. The IASLC published their staging analyses in a series of publications in 2007 [3–6], and the data were externally validated using the population-based Surveillance, Epidemiology and End Results (SEER) cancer registry data [3]. In January 2010, the revised staging criteria for tumor (T) and metastases (M) were officially adopted by the 7th edition of the American Joint Commission on Cancer (AJCC) and the International Union Against Cancer (UICC) Staging Manual.

The Revised TNM Staging System for Non-small Cell Lung Cancer (AJCC 7th Edition)

Based on the findings of the IASLC Staging Project, a number of changes were incorporated into the previous staging system (AJCC 6th edition). These included changes in the criteria for T and M staging; however, no changes were adopted for nodal (N) staging (Table 2.1). The major differences in T-stage included changes in the stage assignment based on size. Major cutoff points that portended changes in outcome were seen for tumors at 2, 3, 5, and 7 cm. Thus, T1 tumors are now subclassified as T1a (tumor ≤2 cm) and T1b (tumor >2 and ≤3 cm), T2 tumors as T2a (tumor >3 and ≤5 cm) and T2b (tumor >5 and ≤7 cm), and T3 (tumor >7 cm), which in the previous AJCC 6th edition was included in the T2 group. Furthermore, changes in the classification of satellite nodules and ipsilateral, different-lobe nodules were made. Because of an observed improved survival over T4 tumors (by direct invasion), homo-lobar satellite nodules were reclassified as T3, and hetero-lobar, ipsilateral nodules (previously, M1) were reclassified as T4 [5]. The revisions included in the AJCC 7th edition staging system did not affect other previous anatomic determinates of tumor stage such as visceral pleural involvement, invasion of a major bronchus, post-obstructive atelectasis, and invasion of the carina, mediastinum, or other organs by direct extension. These factors retain their prognostic significance and stage assignment (Table 2.1).

The IASLC also recommended changes to the staging of metastases (M). Major results from their analysis included the finding that patients with metastases outside the thorax had worse survival than those with metastases confined to the chest. Thus, the AJCC 7th edition now divides the M1 descriptor into M1a (intrathoracic metastases) and M1b (extrathoracic metastases). In addition, patients with ipsilateral pleural effusion (T4/stage IIIb in the AJCC 6th edition) have been found to have survival similar to patients with M1a metastases and are now classified as such (stage IV) [4]. And, as described previously, patients with hetero-lobar, ipsilateral nodules (previously, M1) have been reclassified as T4 (stage IIIb instead of stage IV) to reflect prognosis superior to that of patients with metastatic disease.

The IASLC also examined nodal stage, and though significant changes in survival were noted between patients with single-zone N1 and multi-zone N1 metastases and between single-zone N2 and multi-zone N2 metastases, because these survival differences did not maintain significance independent of T-stage, no revisions in the nodal staging system were recommended (Fig. 2.1). Nonetheless, it is worthwhile noting that extent of nodal involvement within a given N class did appear to influence survival with nodal metastases to multiple zones adversely impacting survival compared to single-zone disease [6]. Patients with a single N1 nodal zone involved fared the best, whereas patients with multiple positive N2 zones had very poor survival. Interestingly, however, patients with a single N2 zone involved had similar survival to patients with multiple N1 zones.

Significance of the Revised TNM Classification System for Non-small Cell Lung Cancer (AJCC 7th Edition)

The clinical utility of the revised staging system for non-small cell lung cancer has been evaluated by several investigators [7–9]. A group of 1,154 patients who had undergone complete surgical resection for NSCLC at the University of Texas, MD Anderson Cancer Center, was retrospectively classified according to both the AJCC 6th edition and 7th edition staging systems. The AJCC 7th edition staging system was more effective at ordering and differentiating patients ($p = 0.009$) [10]. In addition, we found that the application of AJCC 7th edition to patients previously staged by AJCC 6th edition resulted in a change in overall stage assignment in 17.5 % of cases, with the most common stage shifts consisting of patients being upstaged from stage IB to IIA and downstaged from IIIB to IIIA (Table 2.2). This has implications with respect to treatment assignment, as patients with stage II NSCLC are generally treated with adjuvant chemotherapy, and surgery may be recommended for patients with stage IIIa disease but is generally contraindicated for stage IIIb tumors. In a similar manner, Suzuki and colleagues applied both AJCC 6th and the revised TNM systems to 1,623 patients who underwent lung cancer resection [11]. Better separation of stage survival curves were seen using the revised TNM system as well as an increase in the proportion of patients with stage IIA, IIB, IIIA, and IV tumors and a decrease in the numbers of patients with stage IB and IIIB disease. The largest shifts occurred in upstaging of IB to IIA and downstaging of IIIB to IIIA. Lyons and colleagues have

Table 2.1 Tumor, node, and metastases (TNM) definitions

Primary tumor (T)	
TX	Primary tumor cannot be assessed, or tumor proven by the presence of malignant cells in sputum or bronchial washings but not visualized by imaging or bronchoscopy
T0	No evidence of primary tumor
Tis	Carcinoma in situ
T1	Tumor 3 cm or less in greatest dimension, surrounded by lung or visceral pleura, without bronchoscopic evidence of invasion more proximal than the lobar bronchus (i.e., not in the main bronchus)[a]
T1a	Tumor 2 cm or less in greatest dimension
T1b	Tumor more than 2 cm but 3 cm or less in greatest dimension
T2	Tumor more than 3 cm but 7 cm or less or tumor with any of the following features (T2 tumors with these features are classified T2a if 5 cm or less): involves main bronchus, 2 cm or more distal to the carina; invades visceral pleura (PL1 or PL2); associated with atelectasis or obstructive pneumonitis that extends to the hilar region but does not involve the entire lung
T2a	Tumor more than 3 cm but 5 cm or less in greatest dimension
T2b	Tumor more than 5 cm but 7 cm or less in greatest dimension
T3	Tumor more than 7 cm or one that directly invades any of the following: parietal pleural (PL3), chest wall (including superior sulcus tumors), diaphragm, phrenic nerve, mediastinal pleura, parietal pericardium; or tumor in the main bronchus (less than 2 cm distal to the carina[a] but without involvement of the carina); or associated atelectasis or obstructive pneumonitis of the entire lung or separate tumor nodule(s) in the same lobe
T4	Tumor of any size that invades any of the following: mediastinum, heart, great vessels, trachea, recurrent laryngeal nerve, esophagus, vertebral body, carina, separate tumor nodule(s) in a different ipsilateral lobe
Regional lymph nodes (N)	
NX	Regional lymph nodes cannot be assessed
N0	No regional node metastases
N1	Metastases to ipsilateral peribronchial and/or ipsilateral hilar node(s) and intrapulmonary nodes, including involvement by direct extension
N2	Metastases to ipsilateral mediastinal and/or subcarinal lymph node(s)
N3	Metastases in contralateral mediastinal, contralateral hilar, ipsilateral or contralateral scalene, or supraclavicular node(s)
Distant metastasis (M)	
M0	No distant metastasis
M1	Distant metastasis
M1a	Separate tumor nodule(s) in a contralateral lobe tumor with pleural nodules or malignant pleural (or pericardial) effusion[b]
M1b	Distant metastasis (in extrathoracic organs)

Reprinted with permission from the *AJCC Cancer Staging Manual, 7th Edition,* 2010, American Joint Committee on Cancer

[a]The uncommon superficial spreading tumor of any size with its invasive component limited to the bronchial wall, which may extend proximally to the main bronchus, is also classified as T1a

[b]Most pleural (and pericardial) effusions with lung cancer are due to tumor. In a few patients, however, multiple cytopathologic examinations of pleural (pericardial) fluid are negative for tumor, and the fluid is nonbloody and is not an exudate. Where these elements and clinical judgment dictate that the effusion is not related to the tumor, the effusion should be excluded as a staging element and the patient should be classified as M0

reported similar results [12]. In an analysis of 414 surgical cases, 18 % of patients had a change in stage designation after application of the revised TNM staging system, with 6 % of patients downstaged (mainly from IIIB) and 12 % upstaged (mainly from stage IB).

Noninvasive Staging of Lung Cancer

Computed Tomography

Computed tomography (CT) is usually the initial imaging modality used to define the anatomic extent of lung cancer. It provides not only staging information but also provides information about anatomic relationships that are important for surgical or radiation therapy planning. CT scans for lung cancer staging should be contrast enhanced to define anatomic relationships between the tumor and the mediastinal and pulmonary vessels and also to visualize mediastinal and hilar lymph nodes [13]. CTs should be performed at a minimum of 3.75-mm collimation (slice thickness) and should extend from the supraclavicular region to below the kidneys to allow for visualization of supraclavicular lymph nodes, both adrenal glands, and the majority of the liver [14].

CT scans can provide rough information about tumor size, but at the stage-determining cut points (e.g., 3, 5 and 7 cm), it is not sufficiently sensitive to determine T-stage. However, at the extremes of tumor size, T-stage may be reliably predicted [15]. Thus, a tumor measuring 1 cm on CT will most likely be a true T1 tumor at pathology, and a 10 cm tumor will likely be a T3 tumor. For tumors that abut the surface of the lung, CT cannot reliably determine visceral

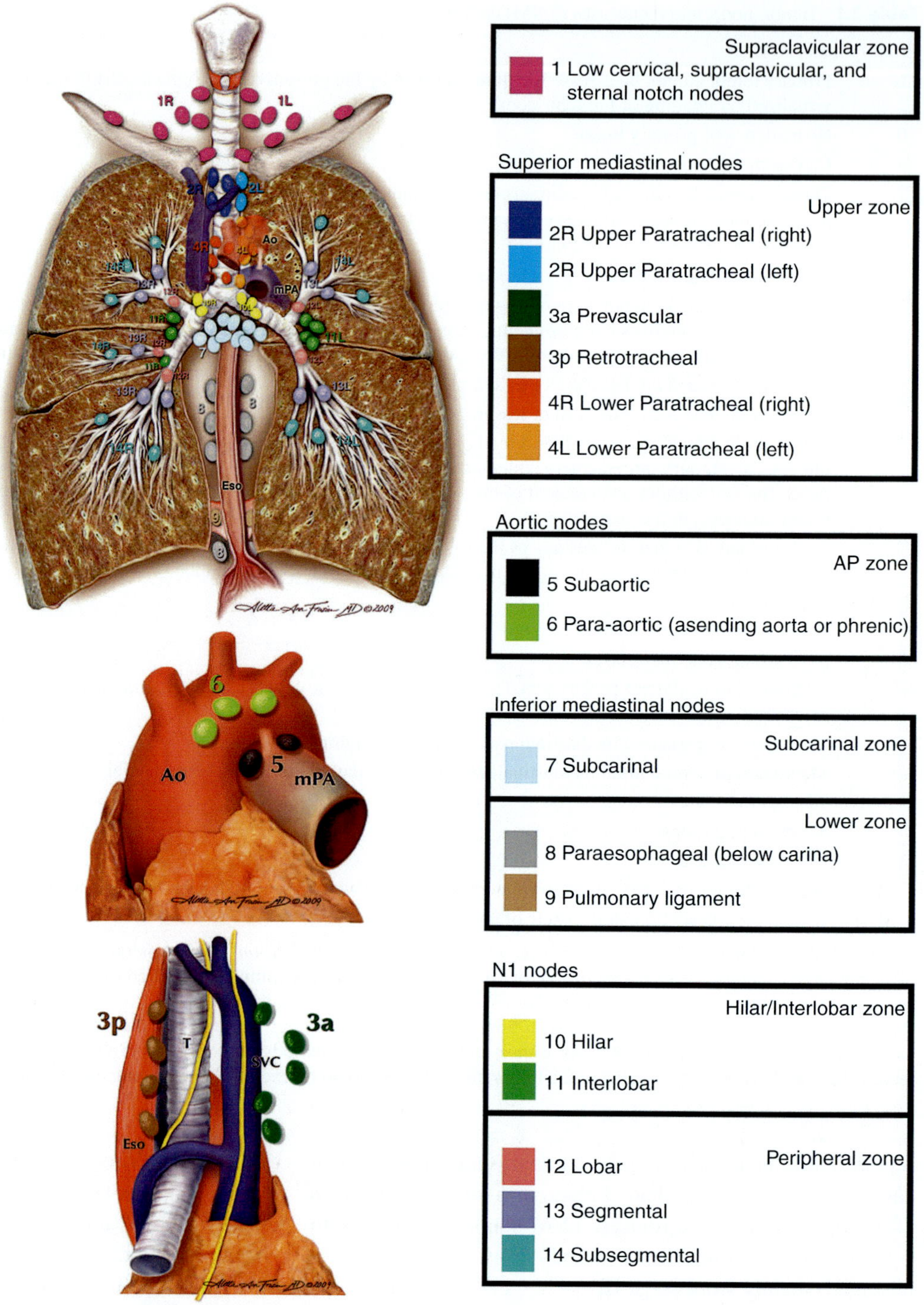

Fig. 2.1 The International Association for the Study of Lung Cancer (IASLC) lymph node map, including the proposed grouping of lymph node stations into "zones" for the purposes of prognostic analyses

pleural invasion, and so the differentiation of T1 from T2 (by visceral pleural invasion) is not possible, though pleural puckering is often suggestive of visceral pleural invasion. Chest wall invasion is often obvious on CT but may also be subtle enough to not be detected except at the time of surgery. Tumors extending into tissue outside of the chest wall or rib erosion are usually reliable predictors of chest wall invasion (T3), and the accuracy of CT for predicting chest wall invasion has been reported to be only 39–87 % [16, 17]. Invasion of mediastinal structures such as the esophagus, mediastinal fat, pericardium, and trachea can similarly be imprecise on CT unless there is extensive invasion. Generally, additional confirmatory tests will be required to establish invasion such as bronchoscopy, esophagoscopy, and esophageal (EUS) or endobronchial ultrasound (EBUS), and clinical findings such as phrenic nerve paralysis or intrascapular pain (suggestive of aortic involvement) can aid in establishing T4 status when coupled with CT findings. Invasion of the spine can often be diagnosed if bone destruction is evident; however, early

Table 2.2 TNM stage groupings

Anatomic stage/prognostic groups			
Occult carcinoma	TX	N0	M0
Stage 0	Tis	N0	M0
Stage IA	T1a	N0	M0
	T1b	N0	M0
Stage IB	T2a	N0	M0
Stage IIA	T2b	N0	M0
	T1a	N1	M0
	T1b	N1	M0
	T2a	N1	M0
Stage IIB	T2b	N1	M0
	T3	N0	M0
Stage IIIA	T1a	N2	M0
	T1b	N2	M0
	T2a	N2	M0
	T2b	N2	M0
	T3	N1	M0
	T3	N2	M0
	T4	N0	M0
	T4	N1	M0
Stage IIIB	T1a	N3	M0
	T1b	N3	M0
	T2a	N3	M0
	T2b	N3	M0
	T3	N3	M0
	T4	N2	M0
	T4	N3	M0
Stage IV	Any T	Any N	M1a
	Any T	Any N	M1b

Reprinted with permission from the *AJCC Cancer Staging Manual, 7th Edition,* 2010, American Joint Committee on Cancer

invasion may be missed. In cases of suspected spine involvement, magnetic resonance imaging (MRI) complements CT imaging in assessing vertebral invasion. In a prospective study by Webb, CT was able to discriminate between advanced-stage (T3/T4) and early stage lung cancers (T1/T2) with a sensitivity, specificity, and accuracy of 84, 70, and 78 %, respectively [17].

CT can readily identify noncalcified nodules in other lobes but does not provide pathologic diagnosis. Therefore, unless different-lobe nodules are obviously metastatic, their histology should be determined if they would change stage assignment. In the case of larger nodules (>1 cm), this can usually be easily accomplished via percutaneous CT-guided biopsy or navigational bronchoscopic biopsy. Frequently, however, the clinician is faced with multiple small nodules or ground-glass opacities (GGO) that are impossible to biopsy without video-assisted thoracoscopy (VATS) and maybe even thoracotomy. The judgment of the clinician is required to decide whether to pursue histologic sampling or not and whether their presence will influence definitive therapy.

CT and Mediastinal Nodal Staging

By convention, a cutoff point of 1 cm or greater is used to differentiate a potentially metastatically involved node from a noninvolved node. Unfortunately, the accuracy of CT for predicting metastases to the mediastinal nodes is low, the false-positive rate of CT in the diagnosis of nodal metastases is between 15 and 80 % [18], and the false-negative rate is as high as 12 % [19–21]. A recent meta-analysis by Toloza et al. included 3,438 patients from 20 studies and found that pooled sensitivity and specificity of CT scanning was 57 and 82 %, respectively, with a positive predictive value of only 56 % [22]. An inherent limitation of CT prediction of nodal metastases is that lymph node size is not a reliable indicator of nodal metastatic disease. In a recent analysis of 256 patients (2,891 nodes), Prenzel and colleagues reported that at least 77 % of patients without nodal metastases had at least one lymph node greater than 1 cm in diameter. Furthermore, 12 % of patients with N2 metastases had no enlarged nodes on CT scanning [23].

Positron Emission Tomography (PET)

A major advance in the preoperative staging of lung cancer has been the development of positron emission tomography (PET). PET works by taking advantage of the fact that cancer cells and cells with high metabolic activity have increased cellular uptake of glucose and increased rates of glycolysis. Radiolabeled fluorodeoxyglucose (FDG), a glucose analog, undergoes uptake by cancer cells but following phosphorylation is unable to undergo further metabolization and is retained intracellularly. The intensity of FDG uptake can be quantified (standardized uptake value or SUV) and is considered abnormal if greater than 2.5 or if it is above the normal background uptake in the mediastinum [24]. PET provides information about the metabolic activity of a lesion, but its spatial resolution is poor compared to the precise anatomic information that CT can provide [24, 25]. The development of integrated PET/CT scanners where 2D axial CT images are co-localized with colorized PET data has enabled more accurate assessment of location of metabolic activity than either modality when performed separately [26]. It should be noted that the CT component of most integrated PET/CT scans is performed without intravenous contrast, making detailed information about the relationships of pulmonary vasculature to tumors or mediastinal and hilar nodes not possible. Furthermore, as the CT is performed without breath holding, the lung parenchyma is underinflated and subject to motion artifact which obscures detail. This is particularly relevant when evaluating small (<5 mm) intraparenchymal nodules.

PET/CT rarely provides additional information regarding T-stage over what is available from a contrast-enhanced CT, though there is some evidence to suggest that the level of FDG uptake may offer prognostic information regarding survival [24]. Its main role in the staging and pretreatment assessment of lung cancer lies in its ability to predict mediastinal nodal and distant metastases.

PET/CT and Mediastinal Staging

PET/CT has significantly improved our ability to predict the presence of metastatic disease in mediastinal nodes. CT is limited by the fact that patients can have enlarged mediastinal nodes without metastatic involvement, and conversely, cancer can involve nodes without necessarily causing their enlargement (defined as >1 cm in short axis dimension). PET, however, relies on metabolic activity of tissue rather than on anatomic size criteria and thus has an advantage over CT in this regard. Standardized quantitative criteria for an abnormal PET scan finding in the mediastinum have not been defined; however, an SUV > 2.5 or uptake greater than the background activity of lung or liver is frequently used [27]. False positivity may occur with inflammatory tissue. Thus, patients with granulomatous inflammation or infection may have nodes with increased FDG uptake leading to falsely positive scans. Furthermore, there must be a critical mass of FDG-avid tissue to allow its detection, thus nodes with only microscopic involvement with metastases will not appear FDG avid. The spatial resolution with current generation PET scanners is about 7 mm. Accordingly, an FDG-avid node smaller than this is generally highly suspicious for metastatic involvement, whereas a non-avid node may still harbor tumor. A recent analysis of 2,865 patients with lung cancer demonstrated a pooled sensitivity and specificity of 74 and 85 %, respectively [28]. Most studies have reported negative predictive values of 90 % or greater, and in general, a patient with a negative PET scan and a peripheral lung cancer may proceed to definitive therapy without further evaluation of the mediastinum. The American College of Surgeons Oncology Group (ACOSOG) ZD0050 trial prospectively evaluated the use of PET (not integrated PET/CT) in the preoperative staging and work-up of patients with proven lung cancer [29]; 303 patients were enrolled in the study, of which 76 % were clinical stage I prior to PET scanning. PET identified unsuspected metastatic disease in 6 %; however, PET overdiagnosed metastatic disease in 7 % of patients who were subsequently found to be without metastases. PET identified 82 of 302 (27 %) patients as having N2/3 disease; however, only 46/82 (56 %) were true positives (positive predictive value = 56 %, negative predictive value = 87 %). Overall, PET identified 61 (20 %) patients in whom nontherapeutic thoracotomy could potentially be avoided. There was a relatively high rate of false positives in this study (44 %), which strongly argues in favor of histologic confirmation of PET-positive mediastinal nodes. Indeed, both the American College of Chest Physicians and the European Society of Thoracic Surgeons recommend mediastinal nodal sampling to confirm PET-positive mediastinal nodes.

Patients with small peripheral lung cancers that have negative nodes by PET and CT criteria may safely undergo either surgical resection or ablative therapy as their physiologic performance allows. The incidence of occult N2 metastases in this group of patients is between 5 and 11 % [30–32]. Patients with central tumors, however, are at significantly higher risk for occult N2 disease. In a study by Lee et al., patients with peripheral tumors smaller than 2 cm and a radiologically negative mediastinum had a 3 % incidence of occult N2 nodal metastases but increased to 22 % if the tumor was centrally located [33]. The incidence of occult N2 disease increased substantially for tumors that were greater than 2 cm and centrally located and approached 30 %. Thus, even patients who have negative mediastinal nodes by PET and CT should be considered for histologic assessment of the mediastinal nodes if they have central tumors that are greater than 2 cm in size. The same applies to cases where the risks of surgery are great and the marginal benefit of an operative approach would be greatly offset by the presence of occult nodal disease, examples might include patients who require pneumonectomy, resection of Pancoast tumors, and patients with severe comorbidities or of extremely advanced age.

Invasive Staging for Lung Cancer

Invasive surgical staging is generally performed either with surgery (mediastinoscopy, anterior mediastinotomy [Chamberlain procedure], or VATS lymph node sampling) or via endoscopy (transbronchial needle aspiration, with or without endobronchial ultrasound [EBUS] guidance, and esophageal ultrasound [EUS] fine-needle aspiration). Occasionally transthoracic CT-guided biopsy may be performed to sample nodes not immediately adjacent to the tracheobronchial or esophageal structures and therefore inaccessible to mediastinoscopy or endoscopic methods.

Cervical Mediastinoscopy

Cervical mediastinoscopy (CM) was first described by Carlens at the Karolinska Institute, Sweden in 1959 [34]. It has remained the gold standard method of histologic sampling of mediastinal nodes since then but will likely be replaced by less invasive endoscopic methods, as a growing

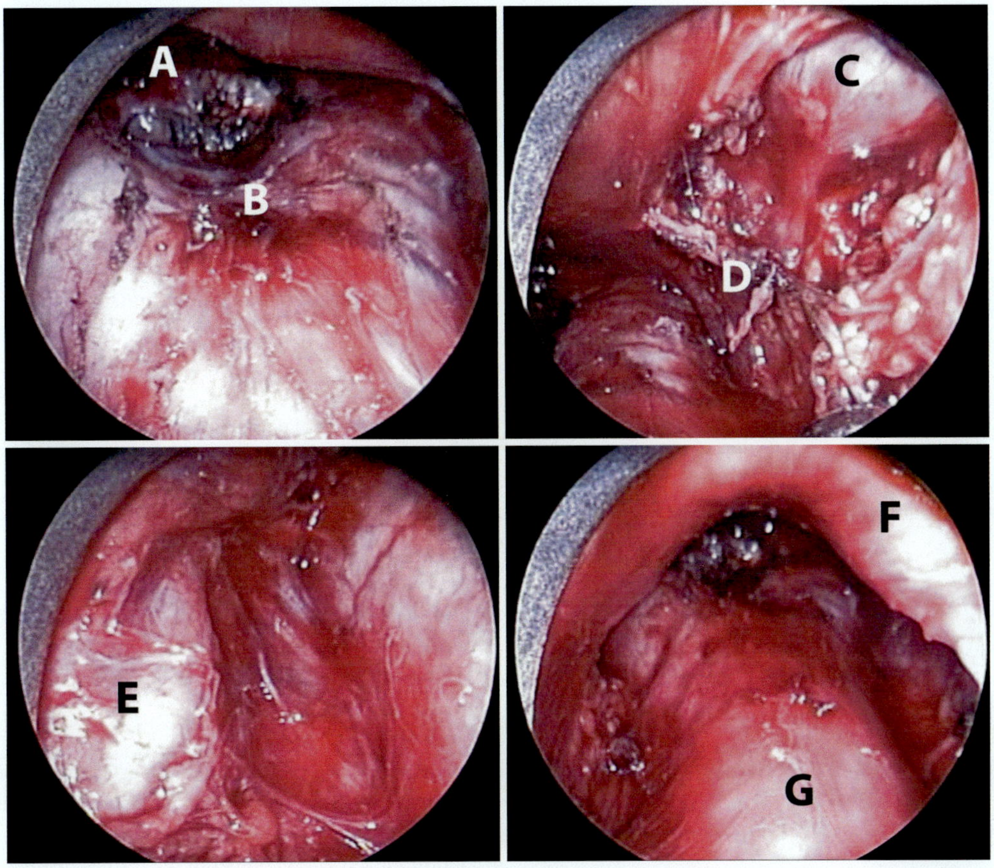

Fig. 2.2 Videomediastinoscopy. The following mediastinal structures are visible: *A* – subcarinal lymph node with right main pulmonary artery overlying; *B* – carina; *C* – superior vena cava; *D* – azygos vein; *E* – left recurrent laryngeal nerve; *F* – innominate artery; *G* – distal trachea

body of literature suggests similar efficacy of EBUS and EUS [35]. Mediastinoscopy is performed as an outpatient surgery under general anesthesia and is now more commonly performed with a videomediastinoscope, which greatly improves visualization [36]. The patient is placed in a supine position, and a 2-cm transverse incision is placed 1 cm above the suprasternal notch. The platysma is divided and the strap muscles separated in the midline, exposing the underlying anterior surface of the trachea. Incision of a thin layer of investing fascia allows entry into the avascular pretracheal space. The mediastinoscope is then directed into this space under direct vision. Further dissection is performed bluntly with the aid of a suction/cautery device. The development of the videomediastinoscope significantly enhanced visualization and now allows for extremely accurate dissection and nodal sampling (Fig. 2.2). The mediastinoscope can readily access stations 2R, 2L, 4R, 4L, and 7, and attempts to sample nodes from these stations should be made. It is extremely unusual not to be able to sample nodal tissue from the 4R, 4L, and 7 stations in nearly every patient. Nodes in the 2L region are not infrequently absent or diminutive. Furthermore, excessive dissection in the left paratracheal region does place the left recurrent laryngeal nerve at potential risk for traction injury, so judgment is required whether to persist in the pursuit of small, high left paratracheal nodes. With extensive dissection distally, nodes in the 10L and 10R stations may be occasionally accessed, though this is not routinely performed (Table 2.3).

Mediastinoscopy has been shown to be highly accurate for detecting N2 and N3 metastases. In a large single-institution series from Duke Medical Center, Lemaire and colleagues reported a sensitivity of 86 % and a negative predictive value (NPV) of 95 % [37]. A meta-analysis of 5,687 patients found similar results with a sensitivity and NPV of 81 and 93 %, respectively [38]. However, these results may reflect outcomes at specialized centers. Little and colleagues reported results from a large American College of Surgeons database that recorded patterns of surgical care among more than 11,000 patients with lung cancer. Mediastinoscopy was performed in only 27 % of cases, and among these, nodal tissue was present in the final pathological report in only 47 % of cases. This suggests that in practice mediastinoscopy is not only infrequently performed but inadequate for staging more than half of the time. A visual inspection of the peritracheal soft tissue is insufficient for staging purposes, and nodal tissue must be obtained from the paratracheal and subcarinal regions in all cases.

Structures at risk for injury during mediastinoscopy include the ascending aorta, superior vena cava, azygos vein, trachea, bronchi, left recurrent laryngeal nerve, right main

Table 2.3 IASLC definition of intrathoracic nodal stations

Nodal station	Description	Definition
Level 1 (left/right)	Low cervical, supraclavicular, sternal notch	*Upper border*: lower margin of cricoid cartilage *Lower border*: clavicles bilaterally, in the midline, the upper border of the manubrium
Level 2 (left/right)	Upper paratracheal nodes	2R: *Upper border*: apex of the lung and pleural space, midline, the upper border of the manubrium *Lower border*: intersection of the caudal margin of innominate vein with the trachea 2L: *Upper border*: apex of the lung and pleural space, midline, the upper border of the manubrium *Lower border*: superior border of the aortic arch
Level 3	Prevascular and retrotracheal nodes	3a: Prevascular *On the right* *Upper border*: apex of chest *Lower border*: level of carina *Anterior border*: posterior sternum *Posterior border*: anterior to superior vena cava *On the left* *Upper border*: apex of chest *Lower border*: level of carina *Anterior border*: posterior sternum *Posterior border*: left carotid artery 3p: Retrotracheal *Upper border*: apex of chest *Lower border*: level of carina
Level 4	Lower paratracheal nodes	4R: paratracheal and pretracheal nodes extending to the left lateral border of the trachea *Upper border*: intersection of caudal margin of innominate vein with the trachea *Lower border*: lower border of azygos vein 4L: left of the left lateral border of the trachea, medial to the ligamentum arteriosum *Upper border*: upper margin of the aortic arch *Lower border*: upper rim of the left main pulmonary artery
Level 5	Subaortic/aortopulmonary nodes	Subaortic nodes lateral to the ligamentum arteriosum *Upper border:* the lower border of the aortic arch *Lower border*: upper rim of the left main pulmonary artery
Level 6	Para-aortic nodes (ascending aorta or phrenic)	Nodes anterior and lateral the ascending aorta and aortic arch *Upper border*: tangential line to the upper aspect of the aortic arch *Lower border*: the lower border of the aortic arch
Level 7	Subcarinal	*Upper border*: the carina *Lower border*: Left: the upper aspect of the lower lobe bronchus on the left Right: the lower border of the bronchus intermedius
Level 8 (left/right)	Paraesophageal nodes (below the carina)	Nodes adjacent to the wall of the esophagus and to the right or left of the midline excluding subcarinal nodes *Upper border*: Left: the upper border of the lower lobe bronchus Right: lower border of the bronchus intermedius on the right *Lower border*: the diaphragm
Level 9 (left/right)	Pulmonary ligament nodes	Nodes within the pulmonary ligament *Upper border*: the inferior pulmonary vein *Lower border*: the diaphragm
Level 10 (left/right)	Hilar nodes	Nodes immediately adjacent to the main stem bronchus and hilar vessels including proximal portion of the pulmonary vein and the main pulmonary artery *Upper border*: Right: the lower aspect of the azygos vein Left: the upper aspect of the pulmonary artery *Lower border*: Interlobar region bilaterally

Table 2.3 (continued)

Level 11 (left/right)	Interlobar nodes	Between the origin of the lobar bronchi
Level 12	Lobar nodes	Adjacent to the lobar bronchi
Level 13	Segmental nodes	Adjacent to the segmental bronchi
Level 14	Subsegmental nodes	Adjacent to the subsegmental bronchi

pulmonary artery, innominate artery, right pleura, and esophagus. Despite this, the procedure is extremely safe with a reported risk of death as low as 0.05 % in specialized centers. Reported rates of morbidity include recurrent laryngeal nerve paresis (0.55 %), hemorrhage (0.32 %), tracheal injury (0.09 %), and pneumothorax (0.09 %) [37].

Extended Mediastinoscopy

The prevascular and subaortic regions are inaccessible to conventional mediastinoscopy but may be accessed by what is termed "extended mediastinoscopy" (ECM) [39]. Using the standard cervical incision for CM, blunt dissection is performed anterior to the arch of the aorta between the innominate artery on the right and the left carotid artery on the left. A mediastinoscope can be passed into the preaortic area to biopsy nodes at the level 5 and 6 stations. Sensitivity and negative predictive values as high as 75 and 94 %, respectively, have been reported with selective use of ECM.

Anterior Mediastinotomy

The main indication to perform anterior mediastinotomy (also known as a Chamberlain procedure) is to access nodes or tumor in the prevascular regions (station 3a on the right and 5 and 6 on the left), areas that are beyond the reach of conventional mediastinoscopy [40]. The technique involves either a left- or right-sided transverse parasternal incision (usually 4–5 cm in length) with either resection of the second costal cartilage or an incision in the second or third intercostal space. The parietal pleura is swept laterally using blunt dissection. Occasionally, the internal mammary artery is encountered and must be ligated, though it is preferable to avoid it altogether. For this reason, prior use of an ipsilateral mammary artery for coronary artery bypass grafting is a relative contraindication for anterior mediastinotomy. Sensitivity of the procedure is approximately 80–90 % with a false-negative rate of about 10 %.

Video-Assisted Thoracoscopy

Video-assisted thoracoscopy (VATS) has been championed by several authors as being useful for evaluation of aortopulmonary window nodes. It has the advantage of providing excellent visualization and being able to resect essentially all tissue in the aortopulmonary window, thus providing a highly accurate way of assessing nodal involvement. In addition to paratracheal and subcarinal nodes, VATS can sample nodes in the inferior pulmonary ligament and paraesophageal regions that are beyond the scope of CM. Furthermore, visualization of the entire pleural cavity is useful for identification of occult pleural metastases. Landreneau and colleagues reported a sensitivity and specificity of 100 % in a small series of patients with enlarged aortopulmonary window, peri-azygos, and subcarinal nodes [41]. Cerfolio and colleagues found that left-sided VATS was more accurate than either EUS or anterior mediastinotomy for suspected nodes in the aortopulmonary window [42]. The chief disadvantage of the procedure is that it requires single-lung ventilation and usually an overnight hospitalization.

Transbronchial Needle Aspiration

Transbronchial needle aspiration (TBNA) can be useful for biopsying mediastinal nodes (especially the subcarinal station) at the time of bronchoscopy. The procedure requires a therapeutic bronchoscope with a working channel large enough to pass a flexible 19- or 22-gauge needle and its sheath [43, 44]. Nodes in the subcarinal region can be easily biopsied, but because the technique is blind, relying on an estimation of the site of nodes from CT imaging, it is much less reliable for paratracheal nodes unless they are quite enlarged. The technique has been shown to be highly operator dependent with reported sensitivity rates ranging from 37 to 89 %. Because of these technical limitations, a recent American College of Chest Physicians practice survey reported that the technique was routinely used by only 12 % of pulmonologists [45]. In an effort to improve the sensitivity of TBNA, Herth and colleagues investigated the use of concomitant radial probe ultrasound for localization of lymph nodes at the time of TBNA to improve accuracy [46]. In 200 patients with enlarged mediastinal nodes and proven or suspected lung cancer, use of radial probe ultrasound immediately prior to TBNA improved sampling sensitivity for paratracheal nodes from 58 to 84 % ($p<0.001$) but not for nodes in the subcarinal region (74 % vs 86 %, p=NS) [47]. The improved sensitivity achieved by coupling ultrasound imaging with TBNA led to the development of the integrated linear endobronchial ultrasound bronchoscope, which has now radically changed how we currently stage the mediastinum.

Endobronchial Ultrasound Transbronchial Needle Aspiration

Over the last decade endobronchial ultrasound transbronchial needle aspiration (EBUS-TBNA) has rapidly gained acceptance as a method of histologically sampling the mediastinal lymph nodes in patients with lung cancer or other causes of mediastinal adenopathy. The technique is performed using a modified bronchoscope with a linear ultrasound array at its working end and a flexible 22-gauge needle and sheath that exits the working channel of the bronchoscope at 30° to the scope axis (Fig. 2.3). The ultrasound array provides real-time 2D image guidance so that both peritracheal and peribronchial nodes may be biopsied (Figs. 2.4 and 2.5). The procedure is usually performed (for staging purposes) under general anesthesia although it may also be done with sedation and topical anesthesia, particularly if biopsy of only a single nodal station is anticipated. EBUS-TBNA can sample paratracheal nodes (stations 2 and 4), subcarinal nodes (station 7), and hilar nodes (stations 10 and 11), the latter which are usually beyond the reach of cervical mediastinoscopy. Its clinical utility for staging lung cancer was initially described by Yasafuku in 2004 [48]: 102 patients with proven or suspected lung cancer underwent staging with CT, PET, and EBUS. EBUS identified 24 patients with N2 metastases and with only 2 false negatives and had higher sensitivity and negative predictive value than PET scanning (92 % vs 80 %, 97 % vs 92 %, respectively) [49]. Numerous studies have since confirmed the accuracy of EBUS, and two recent meta-analyses have shown pooled sensitivity rates of between 88 and 93 % [50, 51]. Even in patients with a negative mediastinum on 2D and metabolic imaging, PET has shown benefit in detecting occult mediastinal nodes. Herth and colleagues performed EBUS on 97 patients with lung cancer who had a negative mediastinum by PET and CT scanning [52]. EBUS identified occult N2 disease in five patients and unsuspected N3 disease in one patient. An additional two patients were found to have occult N1 nodes. Altogether EBUS upstaged 8 % of patients. Three studies have compared the accuracy of EBUS to that of mediastinoscopy (CM) for staging the mediastinum in lung cancer. Ernst and colleagues performed EBUS-TBNA followed by CM on 66 patients with lung cancer and mediastinal adenopathy [53]. The diagnostic yield of EBUS was higher than CM (91 % vs 78 %, $p=0.007$), and the main difference was in a better ability of EBUS to obtain diagnostic tissue from the subcarinal station. However, on a per patient basis, there was no statistical difference between EBUS and CM in defining the true N-stage. A Dutch study performed a randomized trial comparing up-front CM to EBUS plus EUS (esophageal ultrasound) staging followed by CM only if endoscopic staging was negative. In this study that included 241 patients, endoscopic staging and CM had similar false-negative rates (8 and 9 %, respectively) and similar sensitivity and negative predictive values (85 % vs 80 % and 84 % vs 86 %, respectively; $p=\text{NS}$); however, the combination of endoscopic staging and selective use of CM had a sensitivity of 94 %, significantly higher than either CM or endoscopic staging alone [54]. Lastly, a recently published prospective case–control study by Yasafuku and colleagues compared EBUS-TBNA to CM in 153 patients [55]. Though CM examined more nodes per patient compared to EBUS-TBNA (4 vs 3) and more nodes overall (573 vs 426), there were no significant differences in sensitivity rates (79 % vs 81 %) and negative predictive values (90 % vs 91 %). We may conclude, therefore, that EBUS-TBNA appears to be as accurate as CM at staging the mediastinum in patients with lung cancer.

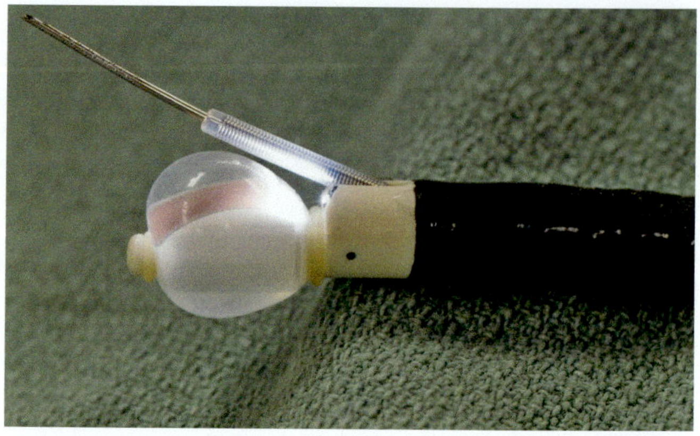

Fig. 2.3 The linear endobronchial ultrasound scope (Olympus Corp, BF-UC180F). The curvilinear ultrasound probe is covered with a saline-filled balloon to aid acoustic coupling with the tracheal wall. A 22-gauge needle and sheath exits the bronchoscope at 30° off-axis

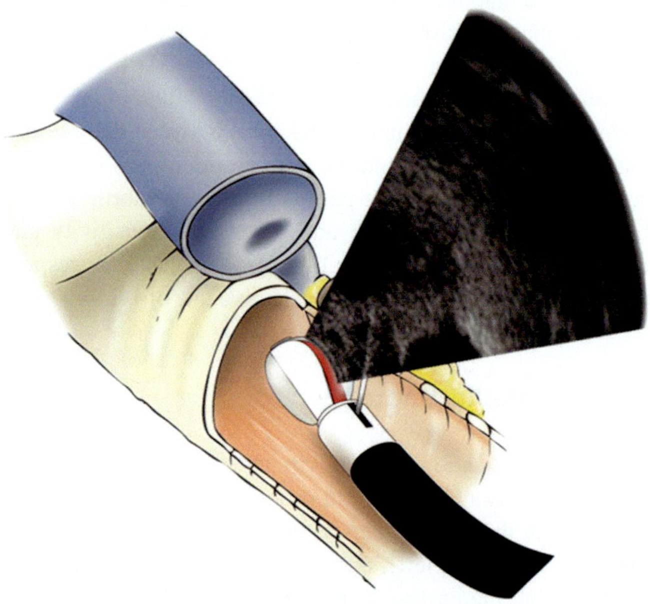

Fig. 2.4 The EBUS scope is passed perorally into the trachea. The node of interest is visualized with ultrasound, and a needle is placed into the node under real-time image guidance

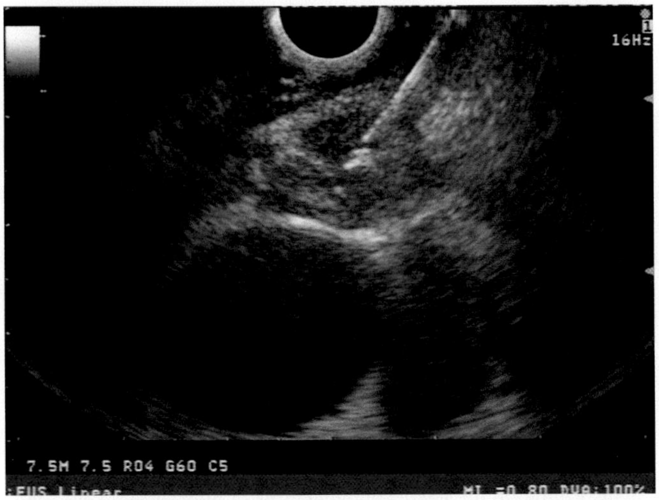

Fig. 2.5 EBUS-TBNA showing the needle inside a left paratracheal node. The round, hypoechoic structure at the bottom of the picture is the left main pulmonary artery

Esophageal Ultrasound (EUS)

Endoscopic esophageal ultrasound (EUS) offers the ability to sample lymph nodes that are not contiguous with the tracheobronchial tree and therefore offers an attractive complement to EBUS to allow "total" endoscopic staging of the mediastinum. EUS can access lymph nodes in the left paratracheal (station 4L), subcarinal (station 7), paraesophageal (station 8), and inferior pulmonary ligament (station 9) regions [56]. Occasionally, nodes in the aortopulmonary window (stations 5/6) may also be sampled. Several comparative studies have shown that EUS has similar sensitivity as EBUS-TBNA in assessment of mediastinal nodes [57, 58]; however, the combination of EBUS and EUS appears to be more accurate than either procedure alone. In a prospective study of 33 patients with lung cancer, Villman and colleagues performed EBUS and EUS and showed an accuracy of 89 and 86 %, respectively [59]. However, the combined accuracy of both procedures was 100 %. Similarly, Wallace et al. performed EBUS and EUS in 138 consecutive patients with lung cancer [60]. The sensitivity and negative predictive value for both procedures was identical – 69 and 88 %, respectively. Combined sensitivity and NPV were 93 and 97 %.

References

1. Mountain CF. Revisions in the international system for staging lung cancer. Chest. 1997;111(6):1710–7.
2. Goldstraw P, Crowley J, Chansky K, Giroux DJ, Groome PA, Rami-Porta R, et al. The IASLC Lung Cancer Staging Project: proposals for the revision of the TNM stage groupings in the forthcoming (seventh) edition of the TNM classification of malignant tumours. J Thorac Oncol. 2007;2(8):706–14.
3. Groome PA, Bolejack V, Crowley JJ, Kennedy C, Krasnik M, Sobin LH, et al. The IASLC Lung Cancer Staging Project: validation of the proposals for revision of the T, N, and M descriptors and consequent stage groupings in the forthcoming (seventh) edition of the TNM classification of malignant tumours. J Thorac Oncol. 2007; 2(8):694–705.
4. Postmus PE, Brambilla E, Chansky K, Crowley J, Goldstraw P, Patz Jr EF, et al. The IASLC Lung Cancer Staging Project: proposals for revision of the M descriptors in the forthcoming (seventh) edition of the TNM classification of lung cancer. J Thorac Oncol. 2007; 2(8):686–93.
5. Rami-Porta R, Ball D, Crowley J, Giroux DJ, Jett J, Travis WD, et al. The IASLC Lung Cancer Staging Project: proposals for the revision of the T descriptors in the forthcoming (seventh) edition of the TNM classification for lung cancer. J Thorac Oncol. 2007; 2(7):593–602.
6. Rusch VW, Crowley J, Giroux DJ, Goldstraw P, Im JG, Tsuboi M, et al. The IASLC Lung Cancer Staging Project: proposals for the revision of the N descriptors in the forthcoming seventh edition of the TNM classification for lung cancer. J Thorac Oncol. 2007; 2(7):603–12.
7. Detterbeck FC, Boffa DJ, Tanoue LT. The new lung cancer staging system. Chest. 2009;136(1):260–71.
8. Boffa DJ, Detterbeck FC, Smith EJ, Rami-Porta R, Crowley J, Zelterman D, et al. Should the 7th edition of the lung cancer stage classification system change treatment algorithms in non-small cell lung cancer? J Thorac Oncol. 2010;5(11):1779–83.
9. Kameyama K, Takahashi M, Ohata K, Igai H, Yamashina A, Matsuoka T, et al. Evaluation of the new TNM staging system proposed by the International Association for the Study of Lung Cancer at a single institution. J Thorac Cardiovasc Surg. 2009;137(5):1180–4.
10. Kassis ES, Vaporciyan AA, Swisher SG, Correa AM, Bekele BN, Erasmus JJ, et al. Application of the revised lung cancer staging system (IASLC Staging Project) to a cancer center population. J Thorac Cardiovasc Surg. 2009;138(2):412–8.e1–2.
11. Suzuki M, Yoshida S, Tamura H, Wada H, Moriya Y, Hoshino H, et al. Applicability of the revised International Association for the Study of Lung Cancer staging system to operable non-small-cell lung cancers. Eur J Cardiothorac Surg. 2009;36(6):1031–6.
12. Lyons G, Quadrelli S, Jordan P, Colt H, Chimondeguy D. Clinical impact of the use of the revised International Association for the Study of Lung Cancer staging system to operable non-small-cell lung cancers. Lung Cancer. 2011;74(2):244–7.
13. Truong MT, Munden RF, Movsas B. Imaging to optimally stage lung cancer: conventional modalities and PET/CT. J Am Coll Radiol. 2004;1(12):957–64.
14. Gross BH, Brown RK, Kalemkerian GP. Optimal anatomic coverage for CT in staging lung cancer: lessons from PET-CT correlation. Lung Cancer. 2011;73(1):59–62.
15. Gdeedo A, Van Schil P, Corthouts B, Van Mieghem F, Van Meerbeeck J, Van Marck E. Comparison of imaging TNM [(i) TNM] and pathological TNM [pTNM] in staging of bronchogenic carcinoma. Eur J Cardiothorac Surg. 1997;12(2):224–7.
16. Glazer HS, Duncan-Meyer J, Aronberg DJ, Moran JF, Levitt RG, Sagel SS. Pleural and chest wall invasion in bronchogenic carcinoma: CT evaluation. Radiology. 1985;157(1):191–4.
17. Webb WR, Gatsonis C, Zerhouni EA, Heelan RT, Glazer GM, Francis IR, et al. CT and MR imaging in staging non-small cell bronchogenic carcinoma: report of the Radiologic Diagnostic Oncology Group. Radiology. 1991;178(3):705–13.
18. Eggeling S, Martin T, Bottger J, Beinert T, Gellert K. Invasive staging of non-small cell lung cancer – a prospective study. Eur J Cardiothorac Surg. 2002;22(5):679–84.
19. Daly BD, Mueller JD, Faling LJ, Diehl JT, Bankoff MS, Karp DD, et al. N2 lung cancer: outcome in patients with false-negative computed tomographic scans of the chest. J Thorac Cardiovasc Surg. 1993;105(5):904–10; discussion 10–1.
20. McLoud TC, Bourgouin PM, Greenberg RW, Kosiuk JP, Templeton PA, Shepard JA, et al. Bronchogenic carcinoma: analysis of staging

in the mediastinum with CT by correlative lymph node mapping and sampling. Radiology. 1992;182(2):319–23.
21. Kerr KM, Lamb D, Wathen CG, Walker WS, Douglas NJ. Pathological assessment of mediastinal lymph nodes in lung cancer: implications for non-invasive mediastinal staging. Thorax. 1992;47(5):337–41.
22. Toloza EM, Harpole L, McCrory DC. Noninvasive staging of non-small cell lung cancer: a review of the current evidence. Chest. 2003;123(1 Suppl):137S–46.
23. Prenzel KL, Monig SP, Sinning JM, Baldus SE, Brochhagen HG, Schneider PM, et al. Lymph node size and metastatic infiltration in non-small cell lung cancer. Chest. 2003;123(2):463–7.
24. Berghmans T, Dusart M, Paesmans M, Hossein-Foucher C, Buvat I, Castaigne C, et al. Primary tumor standardized uptake value (SUVmax) measured on fluorodeoxyglucose positron emission tomography (FDG-PET) is of prognostic value for survival in non-small cell lung cancer (NSCLC): a systematic review and meta-analysis (MA) by the European Lung Cancer Working Party for the IASLC Lung Cancer Staging Project. J Thorac Oncol. 2008; 3(1):6–12.
25. Marom EM, McAdams HP, Erasmus JJ, Goodman PC, Culhane DK, Coleman RE, et al. Staging non-small cell lung cancer with whole-body PET. Radiology. 1999;212(3):803–9.
26. Lardinois D, Weder W, Hany TF, Kamel EM, Korom S, Seifert B, et al. Staging of non-small-cell lung cancer with integrated positron-emission tomography and computed tomography. N Engl J Med. 2003;348(25):2500–7.
27. Cerfolio RJ, Bryant AS. Ratio of the maximum standardized uptake value on FDG-PET of the mediastinal (N2) lymph nodes to the primary tumor may be a universal predictor of nodal malignancy in patients with nonsmall-cell lung cancer. Ann Thorac Surg. 2007;83(5):1826–9; discussion 9–30.
28. Silvestri GA, Gould MK, Margolis ML, Tanoue LT, McCrory D, Toloza E, et al. Noninvasive staging of non-small cell lung cancer: ACCP evidenced-based clinical practice guidelines (2nd edition). Chest. 2007;132(3 Suppl):178S–201.
29. Reed CE, Harpole DH, Posther KE, Woolson SL, Downey RJ, Meyers BF, et al. Results of the American College of Surgeons Oncology Group Z0050 trial: the utility of positron emission tomography in staging potentially operable non-small cell lung cancer. J Thorac Cardiovasc Surg. 2003;126(6):1943–51.
30. Cerfolio RJ, Bryant AS. Survival of patients with unsuspected N2 (stage IIIA) nonsmall-cell lung cancer. Ann Thorac Surg. 2008;86(2):362–6; discussion 6–7.
31. Veeramachaneni NK, Battafarano RJ, Meyers BF, Zoole JB, Patterson GA. Risk factors for occult nodal metastasis in clinical T1N0 lung cancer: a negative impact on survival. Eur J Cardiothorac Surg. 2008;33(3):466–9.
32. Park HK, Jeon K, Koh WJ, Suh GY, Kim H, Kwon OJ, et al. Occult nodal metastasis in patients with non-small cell lung cancer at clinical stage IA by PET/CT. Respirology. 2010;15(8):1179–84.
33. Lee PC, Port JL, Korst RJ, Liss Y, Meherally DN, Altorki NK. Risk factors for occult mediastinal metastases in clinical stage I non-small cell lung cancer. Ann Thorac Surg. 2007;84(1):177–81.
34. Carlens E. Mediastinoscopy: a method for inspection and tissue biopsy in the superior mediastinum. Dis Chest. 1959;36:343–52.
35. Ginsberg RJ. Evaluation of the mediastinum by invasive techniques. Surg Clin North Am. 1987;67(5):1025–35.
36. Sortini A, Navarra G, Santini M, Occhionorelli S, Sartori A, Bresadola V, et al.]Video-assisted mediastinoscopy. A new application of television technology in surgery]. Minerva Chir. 1994;49(9):803–5.
37. Lemaire A, Nikolic I, Petersen T, Haney JC, Toloza EM, Harpole Jr DH, et al. Nine-year single center experience with cervical mediastinoscopy: complications and false negative rate. Ann Thorac Surg. 2006;82(4):1185–9; discussion 9–90.
38. Toloza EM, Harpole L, Detterbeck F, McCrory DC. Invasive staging of non-small cell lung cancer: a review of the current evidence. Chest. 2003;123(1 Suppl):157S–66.
39. Ginsberg RJ, Rice TW, Goldberg M, Waters PF, Schmocker BJ. Extended cervical mediastinoscopy. A single staging procedure for bronchogenic carcinoma of the left upper lobe. J Thorac Cardiovasc Surg. 1987;94(5):673–8.
40. McNeill TM, Chamberlain JM. Diagnostic anterior mediastinotomy. Ann Thorac Surg. 1966;2(4):532–9.
41. Landreneau RJ, Hazelrigg SR, Mack MJ, Fitzgibbon LD, Dowling RD, Acuff TE, et al. Thoracoscopic mediastinal lymph node sampling: useful for mediastinal lymph node stations inaccessible by cervical mediastinoscopy. J Thorac Cardiovasc Surg. 1993; 106(3):554–8.
42. Cerfolio RJ, Bryant AS, Eloubeidi MA. Accessing the aortopulmonary window (#5) and the paraaortic (#6) lymph nodes in patients with non-small cell lung cancer. Ann Thorac Surg. 2007;84(3):940–5.
43. Wang KP. Transbronchial needle aspiration and percutaneous needle aspiration for staging and diagnosis of lung cancer. Clin Chest Med. 1995;16(3):535–52.
44. Harrow EM, Abi-Saleh W, Blum J, Harkin T, Gasparini S, Addrizzo-Harris DJ, et al. The utility of transbronchial needle aspiration in the staging of bronchogenic carcinoma. Am J Respir Crit Care Med. 2000;161(2 Pt 1):601–7.
45. Dasgupta A, Mehta AC. Transbronchial needle aspiration. An underused diagnostic technique. Clin Chest Med. 1999;20(1): 39–51.
46. Herth FJ, Becker HD, Ernst A. Ultrasound-guided transbronchial needle aspiration: an experience in 242 patients. Chest. 2003; 123(2):604–7.
47. Herth F, Becker HD, Ernst A. Conventional vs endobronchial ultrasound-guided transbronchial needle aspiration: a randomized trial. Chest. 2004;125(1):322–5.
48. Yasufuku K, Chiyo M, Sekine Y, Chhajed PN, Shibuya K, Iizasa T, et al. Real-time endobronchial ultrasound-guided transbronchial needle aspiration of mediastinal and hilar lymph nodes. Chest. 2004;126(1):122–8.
49. Yasufuku K, Nakajima T, Motoori K, Sekine Y, Shibuya K, Hiroshima K, et al. Comparison of endobronchial ultrasound, positron emission tomography, and CT for lymph node staging of lung cancer. Chest. 2006;130(3):710–8.
50. Adams K, Shah PL, Edmonds L, Lim E. Test performance of endobronchial ultrasound and transbronchial needle aspiration biopsy for mediastinal staging in patients with lung cancer: systematic review and meta-analysis. Thorax. 2009;64(9):757–62. Epub 2009 May 18. Review.
51. Gu P, Zhao YZ, Jiang LY, Zhang W, Xin Y, Han BH. Endobronchial ultrasound-guided transbronchial needle aspiration for staging of lung cancer: a systematic review and meta-analysis. Eur J Cancer. 2009;45(8):1389–96. Epub 2009 Jan 3. Review.
52. Herth FJ, Eberhardt R, Krasnik M, Ernst A. Endobronchial ultrasound-guided transbronchial needle aspiration of lymph nodes in the radiologically and positron emission tomography-normal mediastinum in patients with lung cancer. Chest. 2008;133(4):887–91.
53. Ernst A, Anantham D, Eberhardt R, Krasnik M, Herth FJ. Diagnosis of mediastinal adenopathy-real-time endobronchial ultrasound guided needle aspiration versus mediastinoscopy. J Thorac Oncol. 2008;3(6):577–82.
54. Annema JT, van Meerbeeck JP, Rintoul RC, Dooms C, Deschepper E, Dekkers OM, et al. Mediastinoscopy vs endosonography for mediastinal nodal staging of lung cancer: a randomized trial. JAMA. 2010;304(20):2245–52.
55. Yasufuku K, Pierre A, Darling G, de Perrot M, Waddell T, Johnston M, et al. A prospective controlled trial of endobronchial ultrasound-guided transbronchial needle aspiration compared with mediastinoscopy for

mediastinal lymph node staging of lung cancer. J Thorac Cardiovasc Surg. 2011;142(6):1393–400.e1.

56. Gress FG, Savides TJ, Sandler A, Kesler K, Conces D, Cummings O, et al. Endoscopic ultrasonography, fine-needle aspiration biopsy guided by endoscopic ultrasonography, and computed tomography in the preoperative staging of non-small-cell lung cancer: a comparison study. Ann Intern Med. 1997;127(8 Pt 1):604–12.
57. Eloubeidi MA, Cerfolio RJ, Chen VK, Desmond R, Syed S, Ojha B. Endoscopic ultrasound-guided fine needle aspiration of mediastinal lymph node in patients with suspected lung cancer after positron emission tomography and computed tomography scans. Ann Thorac Surg. 2005;79(1):263–8.
58. Savides TJ, Perricone A. Impact of EUS-guided FNA of enlarged mediastinal lymph nodes on subsequent thoracic surgery rates. Gastrointest Endosc. 2004;60(3):340–6.
59. Vilmann P, Krasnik M, Larsen SS, Jacobsen GK, Clementsen P. Transesophageal endoscopic ultrasound-guided fine-needle aspiration (EUS-FNA) and endobronchial ultrasound-guided transbronchial needle aspiration (EBUS-TBNA) biopsy: a combined approach in the evaluation of mediastinal lesions. Endoscopy. 2005;37(9):833–9.
60. Wallace MB, Pascual JM, Raimondo M, Woodward TA, McComb BL, Crook JE, et al. Minimally invasive endoscopic staging of suspected lung cancer. JAMA. 2008;299(5):540–6.

3 Non-Small Cell Carcinomas

Introduction

Lung cancer is the leading cause of death in the USA in comparison to other types of malignancies. In 2007, it was estimated that more than 203,000 people in the USA were diagnosed with lung carcinoma, including approximately 110,000 men and 93,000 women. On the other hand, in general terms, approximately 158,000 people died due to this malignancy at a similar rate between men and women—about 88,000 men and 70,000 women. Interestingly, when one compares different ethnic groups, one may observe that black men have the highest incidence of lung cancer followed by white men; however, the contrary occurs for women, in which white women appear to be more commonly affected than black women. Despite the alarming numbers, lung cancer has decreased by about 1.8 % among white men and 2.7 % among black men from previous years (1996–2006). Unfortunately, an increase of 0.2 % has been observed among white women while it has remained the same for black women from previous years (1991–2006) [1]. According to the Surveillance Epidemiology and End Results (SEER), from 2004 to 2008, the median age at diagnosis was 71 years of age. The age group most commonly affected is for those between 55 and 74 years of age with approximately 60 % of cases. The incidence of lung cancer in patients under 44 years appears to be less than 2 % with approximately 9 % in those between the ages of 45 and 54 years. Also interesting to note is the SEER estimate for the 5-year relative survival (survival of cancer patients compared to the general population) of lung cancer patients, which is estimated at 15.6 %. On the other hand, the prevalence of patients with lung cancer up to 2008 in the USA was estimated to be more than 373,000 men and women [2]. Also in the same report, it was estimated that the lifetime risk of being diagnosed with lung cancer is at about 1 in 14 men and women.

Several factors have been mentioned in the pathogenesis of lung cancer, including smoking and second-hand smoke; exposure to chemical compounds such as asbestos, radon, arsenic, silica, chromium, dietary habits, and familial history and genetics. Most of these factors may be closely linked to the different occupational hazards or environmental conditions which an individual may be exposed to. One may also argue that the occurrence of lung cancer may in many cases be multifactorial.

In general terms, the largely denominated non-small cell carcinomas are by far the most common primary tumors in the lung. Even though the histopathological growth patterns of these tumors are vast, most tumors can be grouped into the two main categories of adenocarcinoma and squamous cell carcinoma. Currently, it appears that adenocarcinoma is the more common histological type, while squamous cell carcinoma has been linked more frequently with the use of tobacco [3–9]. In a recent retrospective histological study of the 1980s on the frequency of these two variants of carcinoma, Wahbah et al. [10] encountered about 29 % of tumors that were diagnosed as adenocarcinomas while squamous cell carcinoma accounted for 39 % of the cases. However, by 2003, it appears that the frequency between those two variants changed as adenocarcinomas came to represent 40 % of the tumors diagnosed while squamous cell carcinomas decreased to 29 %.

Based on current statistics on non-small cell carcinoma, it is obvious that more work is needed not only to detect early cases of these tumors but also to develop new strategies leading to improve the survival and treatment in patients with advanced disease. Even though the slight decrease that has been appreciated in the general numbers of lung carcinoma may appear very low, it is encouraging that at least the number of cases has not increased. It is likely that in the future with the new advances in chemotherapy and with better educational campaigns, the survival rate of these patients will improve just as the total number of cases may decrease.

A. Weissferdt, C.A. Moran, *Diagnostic Pathology of Pleuropulmonary Neoplasia*,
DOI 10.1007/978-1-4419-0787-5_3, © Springer Science+Business Media New York 2013

Clinical Aspects

Non-small cell carcinomas are by far the most common malignant tumors in the lung. As mentioned, most of the cases are diagnosed in patients above 55 years. However, some authors have stated that the average diagnosis age for men and women is about 59 years [10]. The symptomatology elicited by patients with lung carcinoma will largely depend on several issues, which include anatomic location of the tumor; size of the tumor, which can also be viewed as clinical stage at the time of diagnosis; and possible secretion of hormones by the tumor, which provide a different set of signs and symptoms. For instance, in patients whose tumors are located in the main stem bronchus or the so-called central tumors, the patients likely will present with symptoms of obstruction that may include wheezing, coughing, dyspnea, hemoptysis, and possibly obstructive pneumonia. On the other hand, for tumors that are located in the periphery of the lung, the patients may be asymptomatic, and the tumor may become apparent during a routine chest radiographic study. However, when peripheral tumors reach a larger size, patients may present with symptoms of chest pain, shortness of breath, and other nonspecific symptomatology. In some cases, the presence of productive cough with expectoration of large amounts of mucoid material (bronchorrea) has been associated with mucinous tumors of the lung, more specifically with the so-called bronchioloalveolar carcinoma. In addition, some pulmonary carcinomas may also present with symptoms associated with the inappropriate secretion of hormones that may lead to clinical conditions such as Cushing's syndrome, acromegaly, inappropriate secretion of antidiuretic hormone, or other paraneoplastic syndromes. Another association that has been documented in patients with non-small cell carcinoma is the association with some infectious conditions such as tuberculosis, fibrotic interstitial lung disease, and bronchiectasis. In some cases, patients may present with acute symptoms leading to superior vena cava syndrome, pleuritic pain, or Pancoast syndrome [11–16]. However, regardless of the clinical presentation, diagnostic imaging plays an important role in the diagnosis of these tumors, and ultimately tissue diagnosis is still the gold standard for the diagnosis of lung carcinoma.

Table 3.1 Histopathological approach to the diagnosis of adenocarcinoma

Bronchioloalveolar carcinoma (Fig. 3.7)
Single nodule
In situ adenocarcinoma
Minimally invasive adenocarcinoma
Multinodular
Pneumonic type
Well-differentiated (Fig. 3.10)
Moderately differentiated (Fig. 3.11)
Poorly differentiated (Fig. 3.12)
Variants (Figs. 3.15, 3.16, 3.17, 3.18, 3.19, 3.20, 3.21, 3.22, 3.23, 3.24, 3.25, 3.26, 3.27, and 3.28)
Colloid
Papillary—micropapillary—with morular component
Signet ring cell
Secretory endometrioid-like
Hepatoid
Oncocytic
Adenomatoid
Cribriform
Intestinal-like
Choriocarcinoma-like
Warthin-like

Classification

Table 3.1 depicts the current evolution toward the diagnosis and approach to the classification of non-small cell carcinomas, namely, adenocarcinomas with the different histopathological variants. Traditionally, the histopathological classification of non-small cell carcinomas has been rather straightforward and simple to the point that in the past terms such as non-small cell carcinoma were commonly used in the diagnostic line in the majority of cases without any specific designation to whether the tumor was adenocarcinoma or squamous cell carcinoma. This specific designation was essentially construed to designate tumors as small or non-small cell carcinomas. However, more recently, due to new developments in molecular biology and consequently in new therapeutic modalities, it has become imperative to become more specific, and pathologists are frequently asked to refine their diagnosis as to more specific subtypes. It is also important to highlight that due to this necessity to provide a more specific diagnosis, pathologists are more often required to perform a battery of immunohistochemical stains in biopsies in which the histology is not clear enough to make the distinction between adenocarcinoma and a different type of carcinoma. On the other hand, more recently, a different approach to the histopathological classification of non-small cell carcinoma, namely, adenocarcinoma, has been presented [17], which, although novel, has its own shortcomings.

Classification of Adenocarcinoma

Traditionally, the histopathological classification of adenocarcinoma has been simple and straightforward, as tumors are classified depending on their glandular differentiation into well-, moderately, and poorly differentiated adenocarcinomas. Even though a special reference has been made for "bronchioloalveolar carcinoma" (BAC) in most pathologists' minds, BAC represents a well-differentiated adenocarcinoma. This classification of adenocarcinomas is widely used and proven to work for the most part very well in the diagnosis of these tumors. More recently, Travis et al. [17] presented a study on the classification of adenocarcinoma. It is important to highlight some issues regarding this schema:

- The authors did not present a study based on actual cases; on the contrary, the authors limited themselves to study what they described as more than 11,000 citations from which they selected 312 articles that according to the authors met "specified eligibility".
- It is obvious that the authors' intention was to rid the literature from the term "BAC", as the authors state that the term is no longer used. However, if the authors' contention is correct and that the term "bronchioloalveolar carcinoma" is no longer used, the citations that they provide speak very much against their thesis.
- The authors, without any actual number of cases of their own, present a classification introducing two new categories for the diagnosis of adenocarcinoma:
  - Adenocarcinoma in situ—a localized small (≤3 cm) adenocarcinoma with lepidic growth; no stromal, vascular or pleural invasion; non-mucinous or mucinous variants.
  - Minimally invasive adenocarcinoma—solitary small (≤3 cm) adenocarcinoma with predominant lepidic growth; ≤5 mm invasion in greatest dimension in one focus.
- The authors concluded under "validation" that this "new" proposal is based on the best available evidence and that because of the lack of universal diagnostic criteria in the literature, there is a need for future validation. It is important to highlight here that the authors of this "new" classification have presented a schema based on review of the literature, not reviewing actual cases of adenocarcinoma that fit their definitions, and at the end state that this "new classification" still needs validation.

Based on those definitions, it is obvious that such tumors not only cannot be diagnosed on small biopsy material but also they cannot be diagnosed unless the entire tumor is submitted for histopathological evaluation and proper staging has also been performed. In the citations relevant to their point of the creation of this "new" classification, the authors make special mention of about a dozen articles out of the 312 that they claimed to have reviewed. It is important at this point to carefully evaluate those references.

In 2001, Yamamoto et al. [18] reported their experience with what the authors called BAC. The authors reported 42 patients with small peripheral tumors of no more than 2 cm in diameter. All the patients had wedge resection or segmentectomy and were followed for a period of 30 months, in which time all were alive without recurrence. Further details gathered from this report show that the initial diagnosis in 39 of the 42 patients was adenocarcinoma and that lymph node sampling at the time of surgery, obviously for staging purposes, was performed in all the patients. According to the measurements provided for these tumors, the authors cite that the tumors varied from 4 to 25 mm. Interestingly, the current criteria state that tumors under 5 mm are best classified as atypical adenomatous hyperplasia (AAH). Unfortunately, in Yamamoto's report, it is not stated how many of the patients reported had tumors under 5 mm.

In 2002, Watanabe et al. [19] presented their experience by describing 17 patients as BAC with pure ground-glass attenuation, and in whom after a follow-up of 32 months, none of the patients showed any evidence of recurrence or metastatic disease. Interestingly, in the description of the tumors, the authors state that the diameter of the tumors varied from 5 mm to 1.2 cm, but more importantly, the authors state that 16 of the 17 patients had tumors of 1 cm or less. Once again, the specifics about how many were 5 mm are not presented. Such information is crucial as the diagnosis of AAH becomes an important differential diagnosis.

Also, Suzuki et al. [20] presented their experience with a retrospective study in which the authors evaluated 1,540 cases of lung adenocarcinoma. The authors found that 69 cases showed a large ground-glass opacity component. Histologically, 47 of these cases were coded as BAC and 22 as adenocarcinomas. Interestingly, in 16 of these patients, lymph nodes were not available for review, and in 2 cases, vascular invasion was present while in 2 patients pleural invasion was also observed. One important aspect in this study is the fact that the exact size of each of the tumors is not presented; the authors state that the dimensions ranged from 6 to 41 mm but there were no specifics regarding each particular tumor.

In 2004, Sakurai et al. [21] reported a retrospective analysis of 108 patients in whom 25 (23 %) were labeled as BAC. Even though the authors state that they follow the World Health Organization (WHO) definition of these tumors, when they described the size of these tumors, they were limited to state that these tumors ranged from 0.5 to 3.0 cm with a mean of 1.9. Once again, it is very difficult to clearly identify whether the majority of tumors were under 1 cm or even how many of these cases were 0.5 cm, which is the cutoff for AAH.

Interestingly, in a different report, Yamada and Kohno [22] presented their experience with 39 pure ground-glass opacity tumors of less than 2 cm in diameter. The authors described that single lesions were present in 30 patients, while in 9 patients multiple lesions were observed. Even though, the authors state that 29 patients had BAC without active fibroblastic proliferation and 8 patients had AAH. In the table produced by the authors under AAH, the size in 12 cases was described as under 12 mm and in 4 cases from 10 to 20 mm; this description is rather confusing as it is known that the diagnosis of AAH is made on lesions under 5 mm.

More interesting is the observation that in 32 cases of what the authors called localized BAC, the tumors measured less than 1 cm. Once again, the specific sizes of each one of the tumors described is absent.

Similarly, Yoshida et al. [23] reported their experience with 50 patients with tumors that according to the authors varied in size from 2 to 21 mm. Interestingly, in the table providing the sizes of the tumors resected, one encounters that the size used for the diagnosis of AAH ranged from 5 to 14 mm while in the cases classified as BAC types A and B, which are the ones supposed to represent in situ adenocarcinoma, the sizes of the tumors varied ranging from 9 to 10 mm and 6 to 21 mm, respectively. This definition by sizes clearly shows a conflict as there is an obvious overlap between the size of AAH and BAC types A and B. One could argue that the authors of this study decided to ignore the WHO definition of AAH as a lesion of 5 mm or less in diameter; however, the upper range in their cases of AAH (14 mm) is bigger than the type A and middle way from the type B BAC.

Koike et al. [24] also presented a similar experience with 46 patients with what the authors referred to as "noninvasive BAC". Even though the authors state that the median size of the tumor by imaging was 1.6 cm and by gross inspection 1.5, the range provided was for tumors between 0.8 and 3 cm and 0.7 and 4.5 cm, respectively. Two important issues arise from this information: one, that there are tumors above 3 cm that fulfill the criteria for noninvasive lesions, and two, that based on the information provided, one cannot specify how many tumors were under 1 cm or 2 cm or even 3 cm. Therefore, meaningful and unequivocal conclusions cannot be drawn from this study regarding the size of tumors.

A more detailed analysis of similar tumors was presented by Vasquez et al. [25] with their experience of 279 cases from 1993 to 2007. In this study, the authors documented 20 cases of a BAC (7 %) and 207 cases of adenocarcinoma with a BAC component, which the authors further stratified into three categories depending on the proportion of the BAC component into 1–50 %, 50–90 %, and 90–99 %. Based on the survival curves presented by the authors, one can see tumors categorized as BAC and adenocarcinoma with BAC component fare better in comparison to other types of adenocarcinoma with a survival of 100 and 95 % for BAC tumors and adenocarcinomas with BAC component, respectively when compared to other types of adenocarcinoma that showed 75% survival at 10 years. However, it is of interest to highlight that only one case of the 20 tumors coded as BAC was larger than 2 cm, while 11 were under 1 cm and 8 under 2 cm. That clearly points in favor of the importance of a small type of tumor. Also in the cases classified as adenocarcinoma with BAC component, the great majority of cases was composed of tumors less than 2 cm (179/207) with only 28 cases under 3 cm. However, it is also important to mention that the authors did not provide further analysis whether the separation between 1 and 90 % provides meaningful statistically significant differences in survival. At this point, it is also important to mention that the authors did not address the issue of whether the entire tumor was evaluated, mainly in those cases prior to the WHO publication of 2004.

Lastly, Yoshizawa et al. [26] recently reported their experience with 514 cases from the files of Memorial Sloan-Kettering Cancer Center. Two important issues arise from this publication: (1) the information provided completely lacks materials and methods, and (2) the authors failed to clearly specify if the tumors that they described—mainly those under the designation of in situ or minimally invasive adenocarcinomas—were completely evaluated by histological means. Taken the size of the tumors described, it is likely that the tumors were gathered from several years prior to the publication of this "new" classification, thus raising serious consideration as to whether the entire lesion was completely evaluated in order to properly interpret the lesion as in situ or minimally invasive adenocarcinoma. However, more importantly is the fact that only one case of in situ adenocarcinoma and seven of minimally invasive adenocarcinoma were found in this study, basing the entire report on only eight tumors representing approximately 1.5 % of the lesions reported. This clearly speaks volumes in favor of, at the very least, being very cautious with this "new" classification system.

On the other hand, the literature cited by Travis et al. [17] in favor of a minimally invasive adenocarcinoma technically consists of three reports. Sakurai et al. [27] reported a study of 380 cases of peripheral adenocarcinoma of 2 cm or less. The authors essentially separated these tumors into four categories: grade 0 for tumors that had pure BAC growth pattern and grades 1–3 for similar tumors but with different types of stromal invasion. Interestingly, the authors stated that vascular invasion was not present in those tumors graded 0, but it was present in some lesions of grades 1 and 2, and it was present in 68 % in those of grade 3. In the table presented by the authors under grade 0 with their respective sizes, one can note that the size of these tumors ranged from 0.4 to 2 cm. However, specifics about the total number of cases that were 0.4 or even 0.5 are missing. In addition, two tumors graded 1 and 2 had lymphatic invasion, which according to the latest WHO definition of BAC is a feature not acceptable in order to classify a tumor as BAC. Yim et al. [28] also reported a study of 141 patients with clinical stage I or II adenocarcinoma. The cases were classified depending on the extent of BAC into 4 groups. Groups 1 and 2 belong to either pure BAC or the so-called minimally invasive adenocarcinoma with a <5 mm invasive component. A few important features need to be highlighted about this study. It is not clear whether the material available for microscopic evaluation in the cases of in situ or minimally invasive adenocarcinoma consisted of representative sections or whether the entire tumor was evaluated. The authors also acknowledge that most of the discrepancies occurred regarding whether invasion was present or absent. In addition, according to this report, only 8 patients were in group 1, while 21 patients were in group II, which represented approximately 21 % of the total number of cases presented. More interesting is the fact that once again the specific size of the tumors for group I are not provided and they are designated as 1.1 cm ± 0.45, which raises the possibility that some of these lesions may have been at least borderline AAH. Also, when one looks into the tumor size of group II (minimally invasive adenocarcinoma), one encounters that the size is 1.85 ± 1.61, also raising the possibility that some of these lesions may have fallen under the designation of AAH. Lastly, Borczuk et al. [29] presented a series of 178 adenocarcinomas from a period of 3 years (1997–2000) in which the author claimed that the size of the invasiveness in adenocarcinoma is an independent predictor of survival. The authors stated that lymph node metastases were not present in adenocarcinomas with less than 0.6 cm invasion and concluded that these tumors had a more indolent clinical outcome after resection. What is not clear from this report is whether the authors examined the tumor entirely or only representative sections. In addition, one other factor that is not mentioned in the cases designated as minimally invasive adenocarcinoma is whether deeper sections of the "scar" were evaluated. It is common to see cases in which deeper sections of scar areas may contain a more solid tumor proliferation. Unfortunately, those latter features remain unanswered and potentially may play a role in the final interpretation of these tumors. Nevertheless, according to the authors, they encountered only 8 cases out of 178 that belong to the BAC category and 24 to the minimally invasive category, which in essence correspond to a minority of cases. Interestingly, some clinicians have noticed that the provided new classification schema may lead to misguided treatment and diagnosis. Witt [30] in a letter to the editor raised concerns about the questionable inclusion of this so-called minimally invasive adenocarcinoma and added that terms such as in situ adenocarcinoma and minimally invasive adenocarcinoma have the potential of misguidance, especially due to their limitation on resection. However, more important is the issue raised that the basis for diagnosis in the majority of cases relies on biopsy material.

On the other hand, if one compares the proposed "new" classification schema against large series of pulmonary carcinoma, one finds that perhaps the answer is not in providing new and questionable classification schemas but rather that survival rate is more closely determined by early detection. Sawabata et al. [31] in a report from the Japanese lung cancer registry studying more than 11,000 cases of adenocarcinoma clearly demonstrated that those tumors in early stages will fare much better than those in late stages of the disease, clearly emphasizing early detection and diagnosis. In addition, it has been documented that small peripheral tumors may have metastatic disease to lymph nodes without showing pleural invasion and without being clinically apparent. Takizawa et al. [32] reported a study of 157 patients who underwent lobectomy and complete hilar/mediastinal lymphadenectomy for small peripheral adenocarcinomas between the sizes of 1.1 and 2.0 cm. The authors found that 17 % of the patients had metastatic disease in lymph nodes and more specifically 8 % of these patients with "well-differentiated adenocarcinoma" had lymph node metastasis. The authors concluded that due to the fact that lymph node metastasis was not noticed during surgery, the intraoperative assessment is not reliable for identifying lymph node metastasis. Also, Konaka et al. [33] reported their experience with 171 patients, 136 of whom had peripheral adenocarcinomas with a tumor size less than 2 cm. A 22 % incidence of lymph node metastasis was identified in tumors between 1.5 and 2.0 cm; however, no lymph node metastasis was observed in tumors under 1.0 cm. Thus, the authors concluded that systematic mediastinal and hilar lymph node dissection is necessary even for patients with tumors of less than 2.0 cm; however, for patients with tumors under 1.0 cm, the patients may be good candidates for video-assisted lobectomy. Interestingly, Warren and Faber [34] reported their experience with 173 cases of non-small cell carcinoma in stage I. The authors did not find any statistically significant difference between lobectomy and segmentectomy in patients with tumors under 3.0 cm. In the results provided in this study, although not very clear as to the different histologies and tumor size, one can summarize that at least 44 of these tumors were adenocarcinomas and under 2.0 cm.

Based on current data available, it is likely that the outcome of patients with peripheral tumors relates more to the stage of the patient at the time of diagnosis. Changes in nomenclature should be carefully investigated before changes in treatment are seriously considered. In addition, the current schema provided under "new classification" based on review of the literature and not on actual cases has the potential to be misleading not only with regard to the diagnosis but also the treatment of these tumors.

At this point, it is important to turn our attention to the issue, which appears to be the center not only of the latest WHO report from 2004 but also of its authors' latest attempt to classify adenocarcinoma. The concept of BAC dates back more than a 100 years [35]. First described by Malassez in 1876 as a primary pulmonary neoplasm with an unusual alveolar pattern of growth, in his description [35], the tumor appeared to be multinodular, which is the reason the author chose the name of "Cancer Encephaloide of the Lung (Epithelioma)". Twenty-seven years later, Musser [36] described a similar tumor under the designation of "Primary Cancer of the Lung". Both of those descriptions are essentially similar in terms of histopathological description;

however, the most important aspect in which they differ is in terms of gross description. In Malassez's case, the gross description is that of multinodular tumor replacing lung parenchyma, while in Musser's case, the description is that of a diffuse process similar to an infectious process such as bronchopneumonia. These two particular descriptions have provided us with the current knowledge about the two main patterns of growth of this particular pulmonary neoplasm. One important aspect that needs to be emphasized is the fact that metastatic disease was present in both of those descriptions.

During the next 50 years, a sizable number of cases with similar histopathological and macroscopic characteristics were presented in the literature [37–45]. The cases were either of the multinodular or diffuse type, while histopathologically, the tumors either showed the alveolar lining replaced by a columnar or by a low cuboidal type of cellular proliferation. Numerous terms have been used to coin this type of unusual neoplasm, including alveolar cell cancer, primary multiple carcinoma, multiple nodular carcinoma, diffuse lung carcinoma, alveolar carcinoma, carcinosis, carcinomatoides alveogenica multicentrica, alveolar cell tumor, and pulmonary alveolar adenomatosis. However, the discussion of these cases revolved around the existence of or lack of alveolar epithelium. Nevertheless, the concept of a tumor growing along alveolar structures did not change, nor did the fact that in almost all the cases described up to the first half of the twentieth century, the tumors were not limited to the lung parenchyma. In the majority of cases, tumor seeding the pleura, peribronchial lymph nodes, or tumor outside of the thoracic cavity was documented. Interestingly, despite the discussion around alveolar epithelium, some authors suggested the possibility of an infectious origin for these types of tumors and made an analogy to similar tumors seen in animals, namely, sheep, the so-called Jaagsiekte. Because of the lack of agreement on the etiology of these tumors regarding the true nature as originating from alveolar epithelium or from finer terminal bronchioles, the setting for the term BAC was born.

The definition of BAC has somewhat changed over the years. In 1960, Liebow [46] coined the term BAC and provided a definition to diagnose this particular neoplasm. Liebow's definition of BAC was that of a well-differentiated adenocarcinoma and added that the distinction between this type of tumor and the "ordinary" adenocarcinoma as far as cell of origin was not clear. In addition, Liebow reinforced the concept that there are three main forms for this neoplasm: (1) single nodular, (2) disseminated nodular, and (3) diffuse forms. Also, Liebow stated that this particular neoplasm is capable of invading lymph nodes, pleura, and extrathoracic organs. This latter feature may be seen in over 50 % of the cases at death [46]. In Liebow's opinion, the tumor may have a long dormancy or slow growth, particularly those presenting as isolated nodules. He also alluded to the fact that 50 % of patients present with bilateral disease. In 1980, in the fascicle of tumors of the lower respiratory tract by the Armed Forces Institute of Pathology [47], the definition offered was that of "a lesion with relatively bland cytological features that arises in the periphery of the lung and spreads on the walls of the distal air spaces". In the 1995 fascicle of tumors of the lower respiratory tract, second series of the Armed Forces Institute of Pathology [48], the definition is that of a subset of adenocarcinoma distinctive enough to warrant separation from the other subtypes. In the two most recent publications of the World Health Organization [49, 50], the tumor is defined as an adenocarcinoma with bronchioloalveolar pattern and no evidence of stromal, vascular, or pleural invasion, essentially the definition is of an in situ tumor. However, like with any diagnosis of an in situ malignancy, it is imperative to properly exclude an invasive tumor. In that particular setting, this can be accomplished only by complete histological evaluation of the tumor, a feature that has been largely ignored by the proponents of this interpretation.

However, it is important to consider previous literature regarding tumors that have been coded as BAC. Overholt et al. [51] presented a study of 15 patients treated surgically, 11 of whom were well without evidence of metastasis at follow-up. However, they also documented one patient who developed metastatic disease to the brain and two who developed ipsilateral disease. Belgrad et al. [52] and Munnel et al. [53] also made a similar claim in a study of patients with localized disease. The patients were treated surgically, and according to the authors, surgery may have eradicated the tumor. However, the authors [52] also acknowledge that in those tumors in which there was diffuse involvement of a lobe, the prognosis may not be the same. On the other hand, Watson and Farpour [54] studied 265 patients in whom the clinical behavior of the tumor in some patients was more aggressive. In this particular study, 82 cases were autopsied showing metastatic disease, while 16 of 82 patients who were treated with excisional surgery survived more than 5 years.

However, other authors have questioned the validity of this entity stating that BAC represents a pattern rather than a specific entity based on the fact that many tumors from extrathoracic origin can metastasize to the lung in a manner indistinguishable from pulmonary BAC [55, 56]. Bennett and Sasser [56] in a study of 30 cases of BAC concluded that there is no morphological, histogenetical, or clinical basis to separate BAC from adenocarcinoma of the lung. Contrary to that opinion, Delarue et al. [57] presented their views in a reappraisal of BAC insisting on considering this tumor a specific clinicopathological entity. The authors outlined their criteria for the diagnosis of this tumor as (1) absence of primary adenocarcinoma elsewhere, (2) absence of intrinsic tumor of bronchogenic origin, (3) peripheral location involving alveolar ducts and sacs, and (4) unaffected interstitium. However, the authors noted that metastatic adenopathies and malignant pleural effusions might occur. The overall survival rate of the 74 patients studied was of 34 % at 3 years. Marco and Galy [58] presented their experience of BAC in 29 patients, whom the authors separated into three main groups depending on the extent of the disease. Group 3 in this particular study was composed of patients with pleural and lymph node involvement. Over the years, different opinions contrasting and differentiating BAC from conventional adenocarcinoma have been presented while others have attempted to further divide BAC [59] . Singh et al. [60–61] have considered that in addition to the peripheral lesion recognized as BAC, two other subtypes may also occur in these tumors, Clara cell and type II pneumocyte subtypes of BAC. Other authors have also supported such an opinion and have stated that BAC and peripheral bronchogenic adenocarcinoma are derived from secretory cells that resemble bronchiolar Clara cells, and thus, are different from conventional bronchogenic adenocarcinoma [62]. Other authors have also attempted to correlate histopathological features of BAC with survival; for instance Manning et al. [63] stated in a study of 34 cases of BAC, in which BAC was separated into type 1 and type 2, that type 1 is associated with mucus production and is most likely to be multicentric, while type 2 does not show much mucus production and is most likely to be solitary. The authors observed a 5-year survival of 72 % in the non-mucinous type (type 2), while the mucinous type (type 1) had a survival of 25 %. Clayton [64] arrived at a somewhat different conclusion in a study of 45 cases of BAC. In this study, the author found that 24 of 36 non-mucinous tumors had aerogenous spread and that those patients were either dead of disease or alive with metastasis, while for 12 non-mucinous tumors without aerogenous spread, the 5-year survival rate was 61 %. The author also stated that smaller tumors have a better prognosis and that the presence of alveolar spread rather than cell type was the most important feature to predict prognosis. Thomas et al. [65] in a 21-year retrospective study concluded that BAC is a valid term but that it represents a heterogeneous population of tumors and further stated that BAC should be retained as a term describing a growth pattern. In the authors' experience, BAC has a bad prognosis, which may be attributed to the fact that many patients are asymptomatic until the disease is advanced and inoperable. In a large study between the years 1968 and 1986, Elson et al. [66] accumulated 193 cases of BAC; of those cases, only 39 cases were selected as pure BAC. However, in this study, it is not clear what type of material was available for review, and it is likely that it was derived from cytology, biopsy, and surgical resection material. Thus, it is difficult to determine the validity of the "pure BAC". In 1991, from the Mayo Clinic, Daly et al. [67] presented a study of 134 patients with BAC, ten of the patients described (7.5 %) had lymph node metastasis, and although the great majority were stage I, there were several cases in stages II, IIIA, and IIIB. The survival in this particular study for patients with T1N0M0 tumors at 5 years was of 90 % in contrast to patients with T2N0M0 disease in whom it was 55 %. The authors concluded that BAC has a unique natural history that is more influenced by a local neoplastic process than by lymph node metastases. Interestingly from the same institution, Feldman et al. [68] presented a study of 25 patients with metastatic BAC in which the authors compared the response to chemotherapy to that of conventional adenocarcinoma. The authors concluded that the chemotherapeutic response and the median times of progression of disease were similar in both groups and further stated that metastatic BAC is an aggressive disease that is associated with poor prognosis, similar to metastatic conventional adenocarcinoma of the lung. Similar experience was also reported by Breathnach et al. [69] in their report of 28 BAC in stages IIIB and IV. The authors in this particular report stated that patients with advanced BAC are more likely to have bilateral disease but are less likely to develop brain metastasis. In a different study from Taiwan, in which the authors collected 50 cases of BAC, the authors included patients in different stages of disease and concluded that BAC frequently presents with lymphatic spread or systemic metastasis at diagnosis and that most localized BAC fare better than the diffuse type of BAC [70]. Also, Fujimoto et al. [71] presented a study based in Japan in which the authors collected 53 cases of BAC and found no difference in survival between surgically resected patients with BAC and those with non-BAC tumors. However, the authors stated that patients with stage IV BAC have a better response to chemotherapy than those with non-BAC tumors. It is of interest to note that BAC has been perceived as a tumor of increased frequency in younger individuals, females, and nonsmokers [72, 73], with a reported incidence of as high as 14 %, depending on the source cited. Read et al. [74] presented an epidemiological study of BAC over a decade (1979–1989) by analyzing the SEER database and concluded that even though there appears to be an increase in BAC, this tumor represents less than 4 % of all primary non-small cell carcinomas of the lung. In a different analysis of the SEER database, Raz encountered that BAC is not associated with younger mean age and that the tumor is not associated with an age less than 50 years at diagnosis [75]. It has also been suggested by some authors that BAC may have an environmental etiology other than tobacco use [73]. In addition, the tumor is believed to behave better in children although the tumor is rare in the pediatric age group [76].

The more recent literature on BAC using the latest definition by the WHO has also provided conflicting information regarding BAC. For instance, Breathnach et al. [77] in a study focusing on the survival and recurrences of BAC stage I disease found that when stage I BAC and adenocarcinoma of the conventional type were compared, the 5-year survival rate for BAC is 83 % and 63 % for other types of adenocarcinoma. Rena et al. [78] also reported similar findings in a study of 28 patients of stage I BAC in which the authors found a 5-year disease-free rate of 81 % and a long-term survival rate of 86 % against 51 and 71 % of adenocarcinoma of the conventional type, respectively. Interestingly, even as the authors state that the WHO criteria were followed in these cases, 20 patients were diagnosed by fine-needle aspiration biopsy, which very much goes against the current existing criteria by the WHO. Gaeta et al. [79] in a study of 20 cases of BAC focusing on pattern of recurrence after surgical resection concluded that diffuse BAC may develop from prior focal carcinoma and that the mucinous type is the one most likely to become diffuse. Interestingly in this study, the authors included three different types of BAC—mucinous, non-mucinous, and mixed adenocarcinomas with prominent bronchioloalveolar pattern. However, a study by Ebright et al. [80] concluded that the most important predictors of survival in BAC are clinical pattern and pathological stage rather than degree of invasion on histological examination.

Similar to the new claim about the classification of adenocarcinoma, Travis et al. [81] have provided their views in a symposium on BAC in which the authors defended the relevance of the WHO pathological criteria for the diagnosis of BAC. In their results the authors stated that there is existing evidence that indicates that patients with solitary, small, peripheral BAC have a 100 % survival at 5 years. The authors stated that the basis for the newly proposed classification of BAC comes from a study by Noguchi et al. [82] on the histological characteristics and prognosis of small adenocarcinomas of the lung. In this study [82] 236 cases of resected peripheral adenocarcinomas of the lung were reviewed, which was limited to lesions no more than 2 cm in greatest diameter. The authors separated different tumor types into categories ranging from A to F, and the ones belonging to types A and B were classified as localized BAC. The difference between these two groups is the presence of foci of structural collapse of alveoli in type B; both groups together amounted to 28 cases, 14 of each category. Closer analysis of the data presented showed that although general information is provided for the 236 cases studied, the authors did not provide a specific tumor size for types A and B, and the authors were limited to state that "they are usually larger than 1 cm", thus leaving the possibility that some of these lesions may have been smaller than 1 cm. In addition, even though the authors stated that no lymph node metastasis was present in any of the 28 cases, they stated that 3 of 34 (not the 28 cases specified) showed pleural involvement, while 2 of 34 (again not the initial 28 cases) showed vascular involvement. Also previously quoted by Travis et al. [81], as an indication for the clinical impact of the WHO criteria over the diagnosis of BAC is a study conducted by Zell et al. [83]. In this study, the authors presented a retrospective analysis from a population-based Cancer Surveillance Program of three Southern California counties from 1995 to 2003, in which the authors analyzed cases diagnosed as BAC before and after May 1999, the time in which the new criteria for the diagnosis of BAC were published by the WHO. The authors stated that the overall survival for BAC patients diagnosed after 1999 is 53 months in contrast to 32 months before May 1999. Interestingly, the authors stated that at time of presentation, 48 % of the patients had localized disease, 26 % had regional spread, and 24 % had metastatic disease. Furthermore, the authors stated that BAC was found to have a "significantly" prolonged median overall survival (42 months), 1-year survival of 69 %, 2-year survival of 58 %, and 5-year survival of 41 %. When patients were stratified, the overall median survival rate for patients with localized disease was 98 months. Interestingly, the authors stated that the incidence of BAC before 1999 was 5 % and after 1999 was 5.5 %, raising the possibility that even with the new restrictions on the criteria for the diagnosis of BAC, the incidence did not change, and as a matter of fact, increased. In addition, the authors further stated that from January 1995 to May 1999 (before the latest version of the WHO), the 1-year survival rate was 66.5 % and the 2-year survival rate was 54 %. On the other hand, after June 1999 to December 2003 (after the latest version of the WHO), the 1-year survival rate was 72.5 % and the 2-year survival rate was 63.3 %. Essentially, it is this 6–9 % difference that the proponents of the WHO criteria use to support the current criteria for the diagnosis of BAC. Interestingly, the same authors, Zell et al. [84] identified 1,909 patients from the California Cancer Registry between 1999 and 2003 with histologically confirmed diagnosis of BAC and complete tumor-nodes-metastasis (TNM) staging. Of these 1,909 patients, 627 patients (very likely the same group of patients used in the previous publication), or 33 %, were stage I, and 572, or 30 %, were stage II. The authors stated that their analysis was essentially based on current criteria established by the WHO. Data from this study show that BAC stage 1 has a 1-year survival rate of 94 % and a 5-year survival rate of 65 %, while BAC stage II has a 1-year survival rate of 89 % with a 5-year survival rate of 45 %. These data having the benefit of a larger population are in no way closer to the 100 % survival rate quoted in the study of Noguchi et al. [83]. Furthermore, Zell et al. [84] found that there is better survival improvement in patients in late stages of disease. However, that is in direct contradiction with the WHO current criteria, which limit the diagnosis of BAC to tumors that do not show pleural, lymphatic, and interstitial involvement.

On the other hand, it is of great interest to review the stated survival rates in prior publications on BAC before the current WHO criteria took place. For instance, Grover et al. [85] collected the experience of the Lung Cancer Study

Group by collecting a large series of 235 cases diagnosed as pure BAC between the years 1977 and 1988. The authors concluded that the mortality rate for patients with BAC stage I (T1N0MO) was that of 7 %/year, thus, in other words, a survival rate of about 65 % at 5 years, similar to the findings by Zell et al. [84] after using the "new" criteria and in no way similar to that of Noguchi with their study of 28 cases.

More recently, Garfield et al. [86] raised concerns about the current definition of BAC, mainly in cases with multifocal involvement, and stated that the current definition is inapplicable for patients with stages IIIB and IV. Similar concerns were also raised by Damhuis et al. [87], who found an unfavorable prognosis of stage I BAC with a 5-year survival rate of 24 %. Although the authors provided possible explanations for this rather poor outcome for these patients, they concluded that by the current definition it is difficult to establish a diagnosis of BAC before surgery and question whether the diagnosis of "BAC with invasive component" should be maintained.

The dissatisfaction with the WHO criteria for the diagnosis of BAC has been made clear by different authors [88, 89]. Sidhu et al. [88] in an ultrastructural analysis of 155 cases of BAC stated that the unique characteristic of BAC is its cell type and that the extent of lepidic growth, degree of differentiation, and degree of stromal desmoplasia cannot be used as definitional requirements. The authors further characterized the current definition of the WHO as a form of in situ *adenocarcinoma*, in which BAC is defined as a pattern and not as an entity, and when it is accepted as an entity, then only if the lesion is not invasive. Thus, the current criteria negate that BAC has the potential to spread and make the staging of these tumors impractical. Thus, with this current definition, BAC may become an extremely rare entity if it exists at all [88]. Hajdu [89] went even further in his opinion about the current WHO definition of BAC by stating "a group of pathologists changed the definition of BAC, it was de facto implied that BAC is a carcinoma in situ and that invasive BAC does not exist."

Based on the past and present literature, [17, 49, 82], it is clear that the type of references provided clearly contradicts the authors' claims about the "new" classification schema. Indeed, it is likely that smaller tumors may behave in a more favorable fashion as has been amply demonstrated by several series of cases. However, that in itself does not warrant a change in name for any entity and more importantly serious thought has to be given to the treatment for patients with small adenocarcinomas. Still staging appears to be the most solid prognostic factor, and by all means early diagnosis appears to be the goal in the treatment of these tumors. Special care should be given to the possibility of misinterpretation of "in situ adenocarcinoma" in biopsy material as it may lead to improper choice of treatment. This is an area in which more work will emerge in the future and hopefully more comprehensive studies will shed more light on this difficult topic.

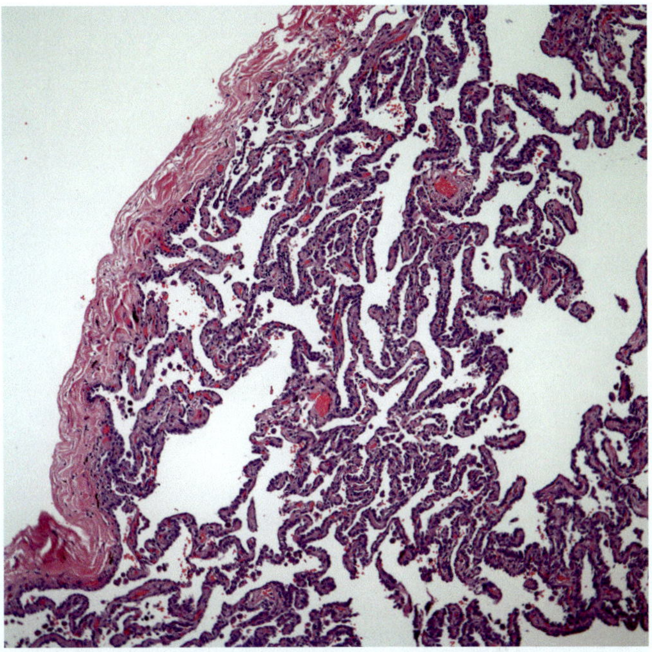

Fig. 3.1 Peripheral tumor showing a lepidic growth pattern in situ adenocarcinoma

Because traditionally BAC has been described as presenting in three different macroscopic forms, it is important to properly address those features:

1. The localized form of the disease in which there is a peripheral mass in the lung parenchyma (Figs. 3.1, 3.2, 3.3, and 3.4). This type of presentation is the one classified by the WHO as in situ adenocarcinoma and which may be the one presenting as a ground-glass opacity by imaging. Usually, these tumors are under 3 cm in greatest diameter and do not show areas of necrosis and/or hemorrhage. They are well-defined but not encapsulated tumors. The cut surface appears homogenous and tan in color.
2. The multinodular pattern in which the tumor involves extensive areas of the lung parenchyma in a milliary fashion almost mimicking metastatic disease, the nodules are of varying sizes but they are usually under 1 cm in greatest diameter, and this type of presentation may involve a lobe or the entire lung parenchyma (Figs. 3.5a,b and 3.6a,b).
3. The diffuse form in which the appearance is that of a pneumonic process (Fig. 3.7a–d). In this pattern, the tumor also involves extensive areas of lung parenchyma that may involve one lobe or the entire lung parenchyma, no tumor masses or nodules are identified in this presentation, and the appearance is that of a nonneoplastic process.

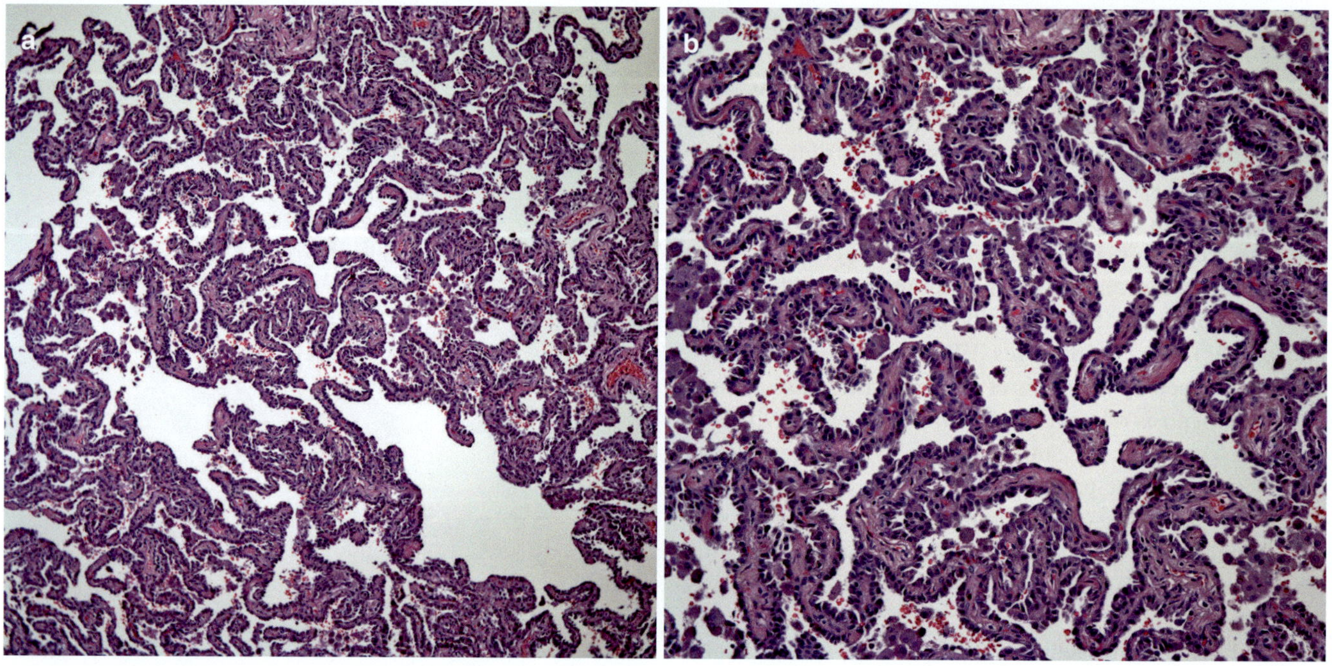

Fig. 3.2 (**a**) Prominent lepidic growth pattern. (**b**) The neoplastic cells do not involve the interstitium

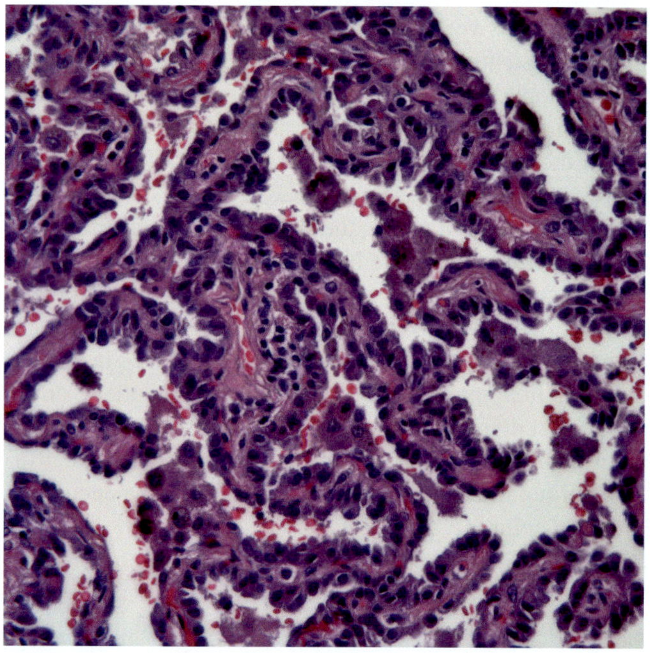

Fig. 3.3 Higher magnification showing a rather bland cellular proliferation with very mild nuclear atypia

However, even though the growth pattern is essentially similar for this tumor, the WHO and the new schema for adenocarcinoma [17] consider in situ disease only the single nodular presentation. What is more interesting about the WHO criteria and those more recently presented is that a tumor is defined by the size that it may attain, which is essentially 3 cm or less, without explanation that similar histology may be seen in tumors larger than 3 cm; obviously, one is left with the diagnosis of adenocarcinoma for similar lesions beyond 3 cm in largest dimension.

The histopathological features of BAC recapitulate those of their gross appearance:

1. The nodular form of the tumor shows the presence of an almost intact normal lung parenchyma; however, closer inspection shows areas in which the alveolar walls are being replaced by either a low cuboidal or cylindrical type of epithelium that lines the alveolar walls either entirely or partially and that follows very much the outlines of the normal alveolar walls. The tumor does not show increased mitotic activity and/or cellular pleomorphism with nuclear atypia. The proliferation is rather bland but distinct from the normal alveolar lining.
2. The multinodular pattern resembles a metastatic tumor in terms of the extensive areas of normal lung parenchyma separating the tumor nodules. These nodules appear to be discretely affecting extensive areas of the lung parenchyma, not in a continuous form but rather in a nodular pattern. Either low cuboidal and/or columnar type of mucinous epithelium lines the alveoli; in some areas, it is possible to identify normal alveoli that are filled with an acellular mucinous material. Mitotic figures and cellular pleomorphism with nuclear atypia are not common. Necrosis and/or hemorrhage is not common in this pattern.
3. The diffuse pattern of BAC is almost invariably of the mucinous type; in this pattern, two important features may be easily identifiable, one is the presence of extensive areas in which the alveoli are filled with mucinous material

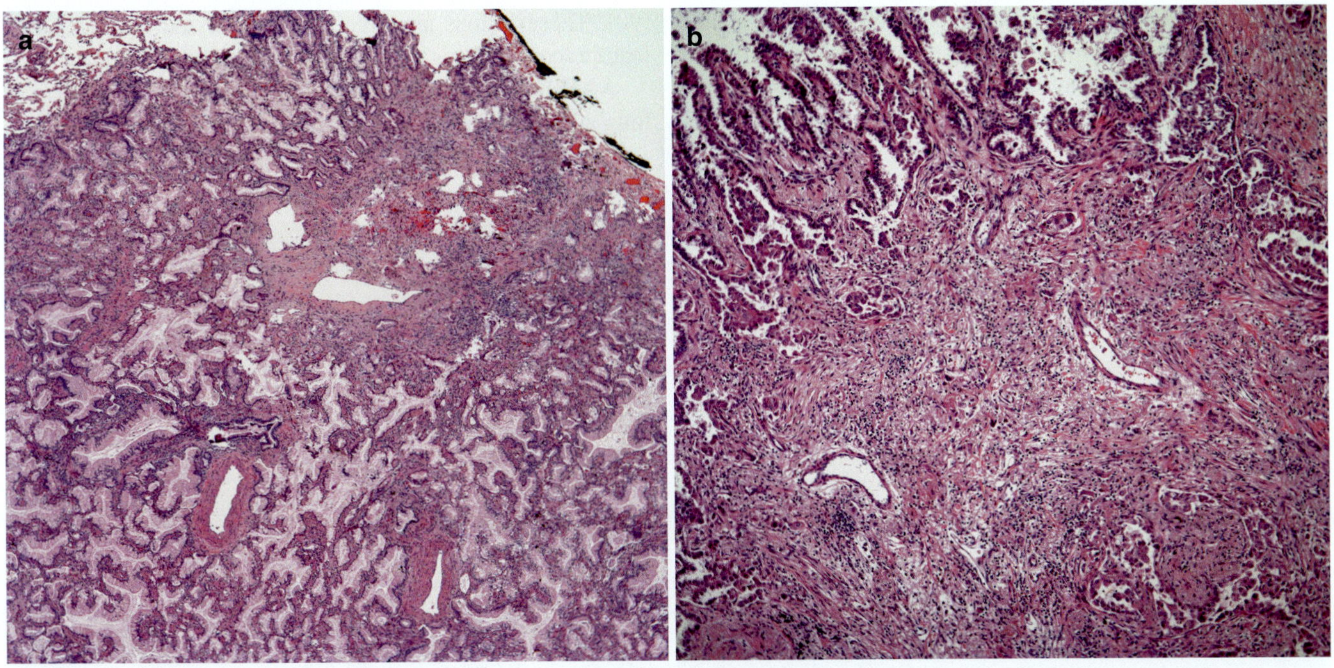

Fig. 3.4 (**a**) Peripheral tumor with lepidic growth pattern and central scar; minimally invasive adenocarcinoma (**b**) Closer magnification showing tumor in the periphery and a central scar

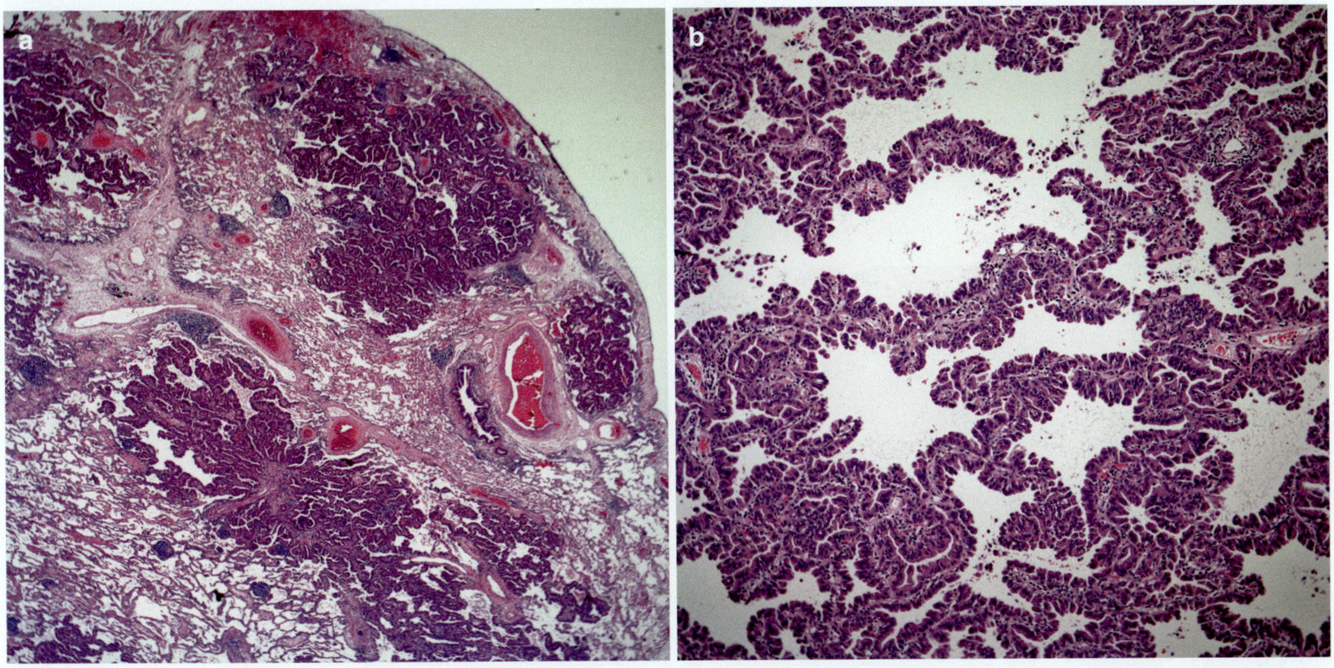

Fig. 3.5 (**a**) Multinodular tumor with similar lepidic growth pattern, note the interspersed normal lung parenchyma. (**b**) Higher magnification showing similar cellular characteristics as the so-called in situ adenocarcinoma. This tumor can occupy extensive areas of the lung parenchyma

containing mucinophages and two, the presence of alveoli that are being replaced by a columnar mucinous type of epithelium. The low-power magnification of this type can be easily misread as some type of pneumonic process. Thus, this type of pattern has been called pneumonic type.

The most important differential diagnosis is separating BAC from AAH. The histopathological characteristics of these two lesions are very similar, and in many occasions, the only way to separate them is strictly by size. AAH is defined as a lesion of no more than 0.5 cm in greatest diameter. However, in small core needle biopsies, the distinction between these two conditions on histological grounds may prove to be very difficult. One other lesion that may be important to include in the differential diagnosis is papillary adenoma of type 2 pneumocytes [90]. These lesions are exceedingly rare, and one important feature to consider is that they occur in a central location.

AAH has been observed to be frequently associated with lung adenocarcinoma with a bronchioloalveolar component,

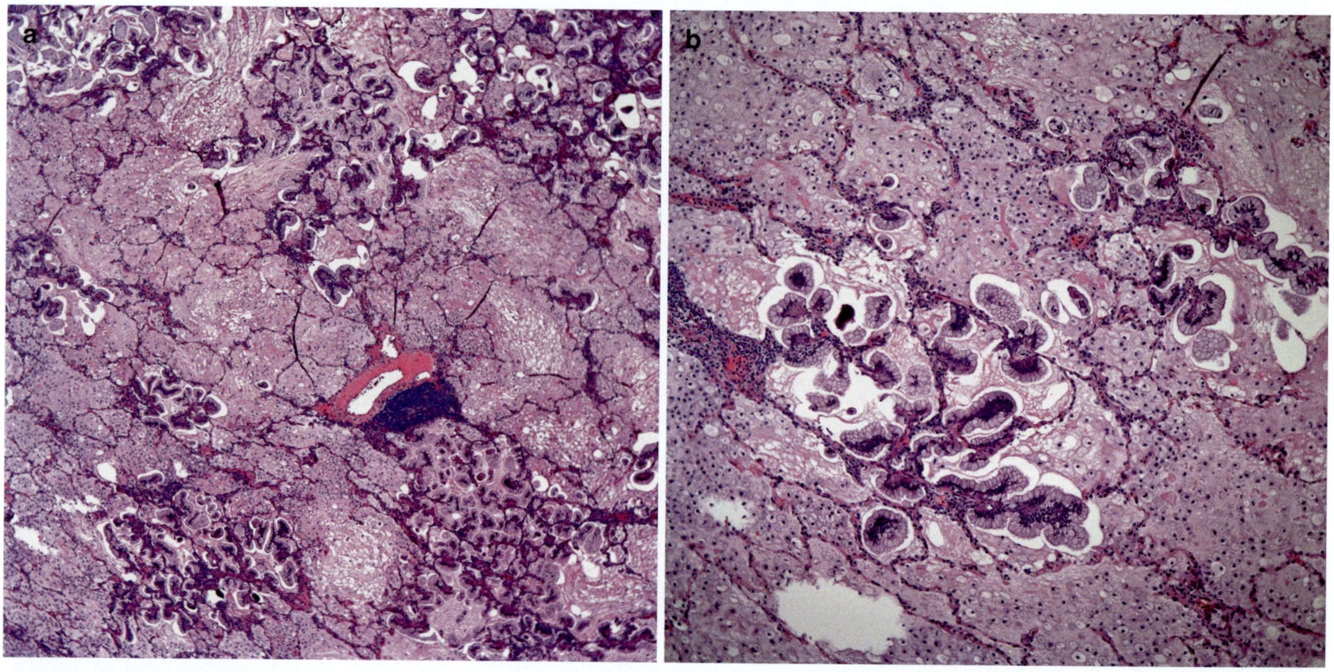

Fig. 3.6 (**a**) Multinodular tumor showing a prominent mucinous component. (**b**) Closer magnification of two separate nodules in pools of mucoid material

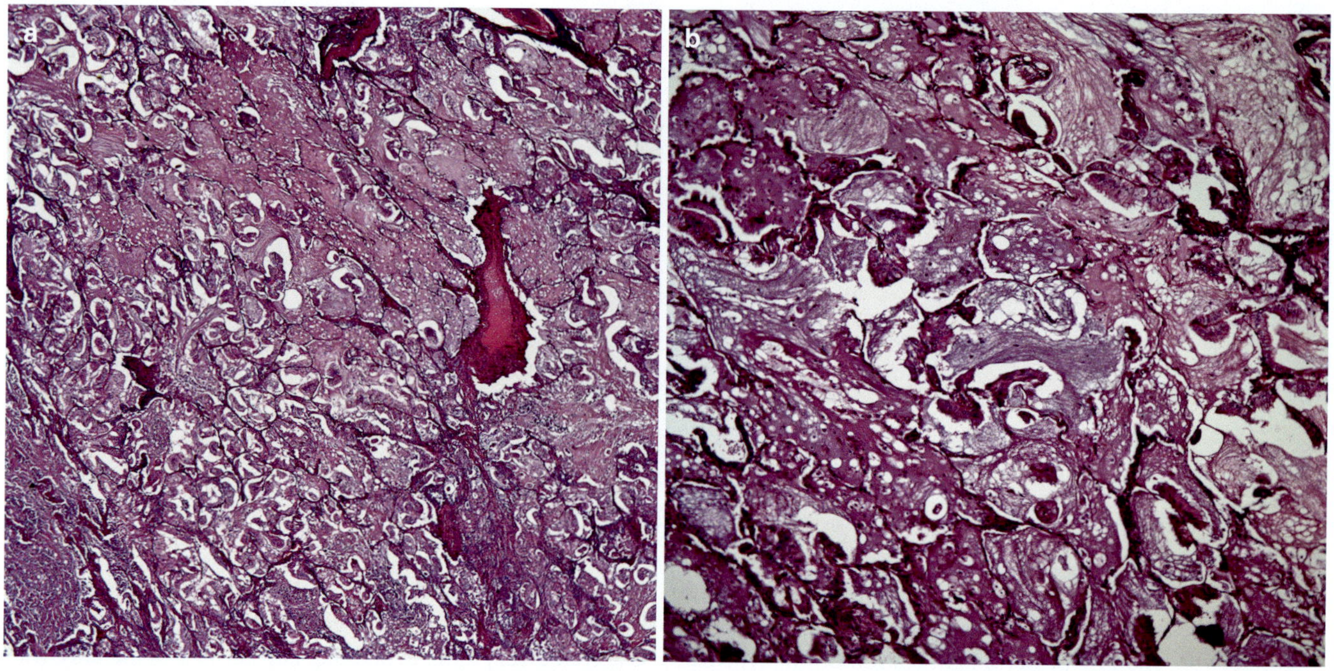

Fig. 3.7 (**a**) Low power of a BAC pneumonic type (mucinous adenocarcinoma) in which the alveolar spaces are filled with edematous fluid. (**b**) The outlines of the alveolar walls are still preserved. (**c**) Other areas with prominent edematous fluid filling alveolar spaces. (**d**) Higher magnification showing alveolar walls lined by mucinous epithelium

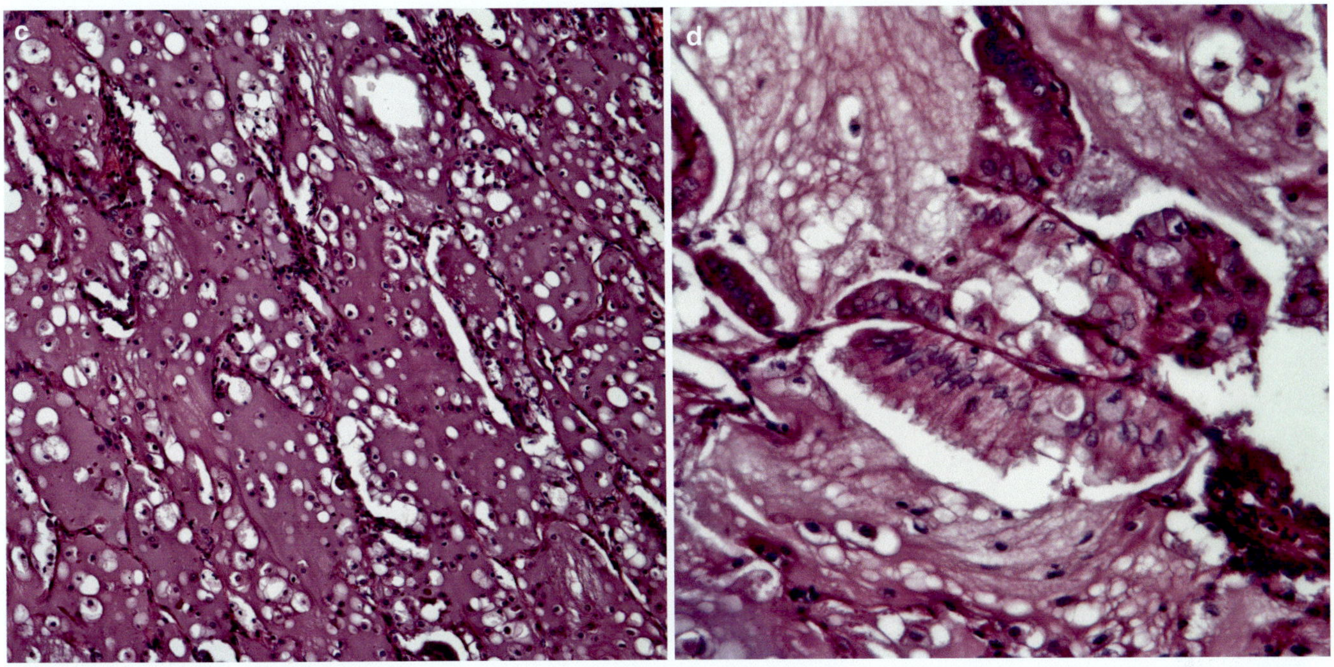

Fig. 3.7 (continued)

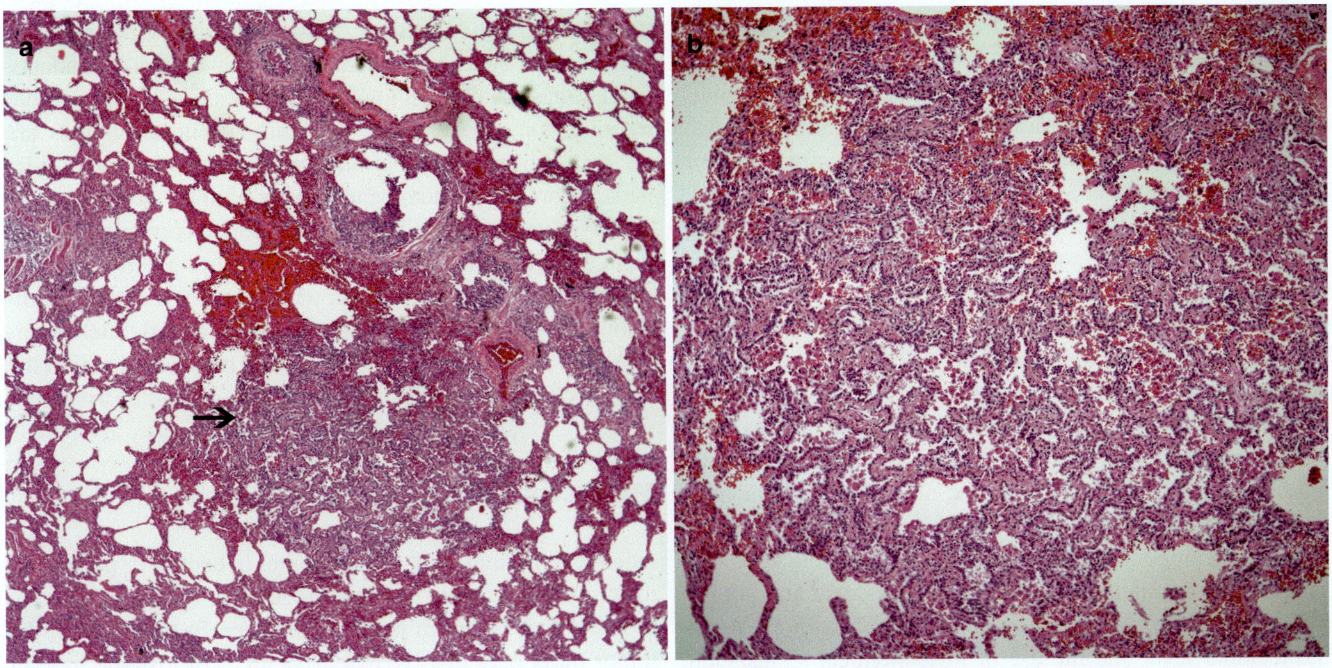

Fig. 3.8 (**a**) Well-demarcated tumor nodules under 0.5 cm (see *arrow*) surrounded by normal lung parenchyma. (**b**) Close magnification showing a lepidic growth pattern similar to that seen in BAC

and histologically, AAH may be indistinguishable from BAC [91, 92]. Koga et al. [91] in a study of 3641 resections for lung adenocarcinoma found that AAH was present in 57 % of these tumors and proposed that these lesions may be precursors of lung adenocarcinoma, specifically BAC. Interestingly, Morandi et al. [93] attempted to correlate the genetic relationship among AAH, BAC, and adenocarcinoma, concluding that their results suggest that AAH and the associated cancer are genetically independent and that less frequently AAH foci could represent an early spread of cells from the main tumor, rather than a precursor tumor (Figs. 3.8a,b and 3.9a,b).

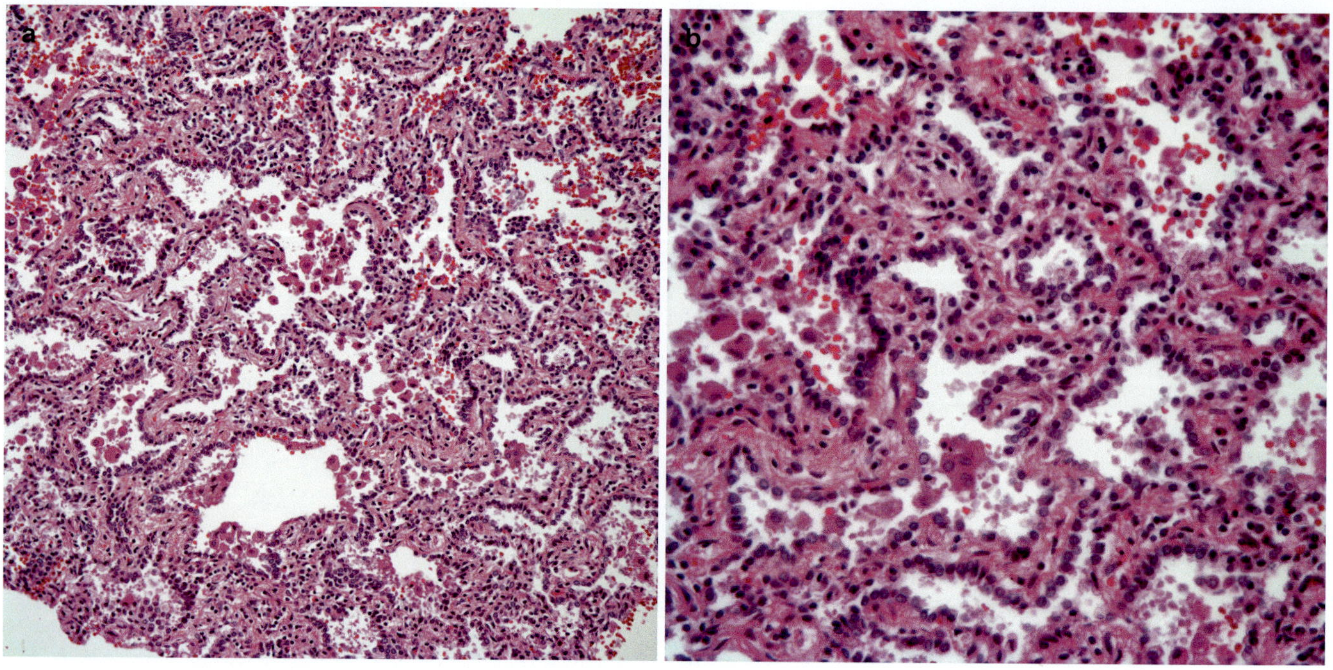

Fig. 3.9 (**a**) AAH showing a prominent lepidic growth pattern. (**b**) Higher magnification showing very mild nuclear atypia

Traditional Classification of Adenocarcinoma

Essentially, the diagnosis and further grading of adenocarcinomas is rather straightforward. For practical purposes, we have traditionally graded adenocarcinomas depending on their differentiation into well, moderate, and poorly differentiated. Four main patterns of growth have been recognized including acinar, solid, papillary, and the previously described bronchioloalveolar. Even though it is a matter of debate whether any of these particular growth patterns should be associated with clinical behavior, recently Solis et al. [94] presented a study of adenocarcinomas in which the presence of a solid component imparts a more aggressive behavior to adenocarcinomas.

Depending on the degree of differentiation, the intracellular mucin or the intraglandular mucinous content may vary. In tumors that are better differentiated, the glandular malignant component may show intraluminal collections of mucinous material, while in the solid component and poorly differentiated tumors, the presence of mucin is more at the intracellular level and the use of histochemical stains such as mucicarmine and diastase periodic acid-Schiff (DPAS) may prove to be beneficial in properly identifying the mucinous content. Also important to mention is the occurrence of Clara cell granules in peripheral lung adenocarcinomas by ultrastructural studies. Ogata and Endo [95] suggested that irrespective of the histological growth pattern, peripheral adenocarcinomas could show Clara cell differentiation. Regarding specific types of adenocarcinomas associated with particular groups, Hirata et al. [96] suggested that bronchial gland cell-type adenocarcinoma occurs more commonly in younger patients (mean age: 50 years) than in older patients. On the other hand, some authors [97] have separated adenocarcinomas not by histological differentiation but by cellular morphology and anatomic site; thus, adenocarcinomas are divided into parenchymal adenocarcinomas, bronchial adenocarcinomas, and adenocarcinomas of uncertain origin.

To some extent, the patterns mentioned correlate with the degree of differentiation of a particular tumor. However, it is common to observe tumors in which the degree of differentiation ranges from well to poorly differentiated. Such determination may not be possible in small biopsies in which the full spectrum of histological variability cannot be assessed.

Macroscopic Features

Adenocarcinomas may present either in central or peripheral location. The tumor size may range from more than 0.6 cm to more than 10 cm in greatest diameter. In many cases, the tumor mass may involve extensive areas of a single lobe or extensive areas of the entire lung. The tumors may be well demarcated but not encapsulated, grayish to light brown. Areas of hemorrhage and/or necrosis may be present. When the tumors are in a central location, the tumor may appear as compressing airway structures or in some cases actually obstructing the airway. On the other hand, peripheral tumors, although they may share the same macroscopic characteristics as the central tumors, may appear to be in a subpleural location. In some instances, puckering or retraction of the pleura may be present. In this setting, it is important to carefully evaluate the possibility of gross pleural invasion due to the fact that tumors under 3 cm with pleural invasion will be placed in a different clinical stage. Thus, the identification of pleural invasion in small tumors becomes crucial. We recommend the inking of the pleural surface in order to properly evaluate such features under light microscopic examination. The use of histochemical stains to determine pleural invasion can be helpful; however, in many circumstances, a good morphological evaluation of the conventional hematoxylin-eosin section is sufficient. Although in most instances, lung carcinomas present as a solitary lung tumor, Miller et al. [98] reported a study of 50 consecutive adenocarcinomas, documenting that 12 % of the cases studied presented as multiple tumors. Important to highlight in this setting is the size of the adjacent nodules—if those lesions are under 0.5 cm in diameter and with the proper histology, these lesions may fall under the category of AAH. On the contrary, if these nodules are larger than 0.5 cm with the proper histology, then the possibility of multifocal adenocarcinoma must be considered.

Morphological Features

Well-Differentiated Adenocarcinoma

The low-power magnification of well-differentiated adenocarcinoma is of a glandular proliferation replacing normal lung parenchyma. The tumors appear to be well defined but not encapsulated. The glandular appearance of the tumor is easily identified, and the malignant glands are composed of columnar or mucinous epithelium with round to oval cells, ample cytoplasm, round nuclei, and prominent nucleoli (Fig. 3.10a–d). In some well-differentiated tumors, the cytological features of the neoplastic glandular proliferation are bland with virtual absence of mitotic activity. However, in some cases, mitotic figures are present and areas of hemorrhage and necrosis may be conspicuous. In some cases, the glandular proliferation may be embedded in dense areas of fibrocollagenous tissue. The acinar and the papillary growth patterns are commonly seen in well-differentiated adenocarcinomas.

Moderately Differentiated Adenocarcinoma

A glandular proliferation is apparent in moderately differentiated adenocarcinoma just as in the well-differentiated counterpart. However, one can observe the formation or partial formation of glandular structures of variable size. The cellular component may exhibit more nuclear atypia, and mitotic figures are more easily identifiable (Fig. 3.11a–d). Areas of necrosis and/or hemorrhage can be present as well as areas of an inflammatory reaction. Similarly to the well-differentiated adenocarcinomas, the acinar and papillary growth patterns are also most commonly seen in this type of adenocarcinoma.

Poorly Differentiating Adenocarcinoma

These tumors are characterized by the presence of sheets of neoplastic cells with only focal areas of glandular

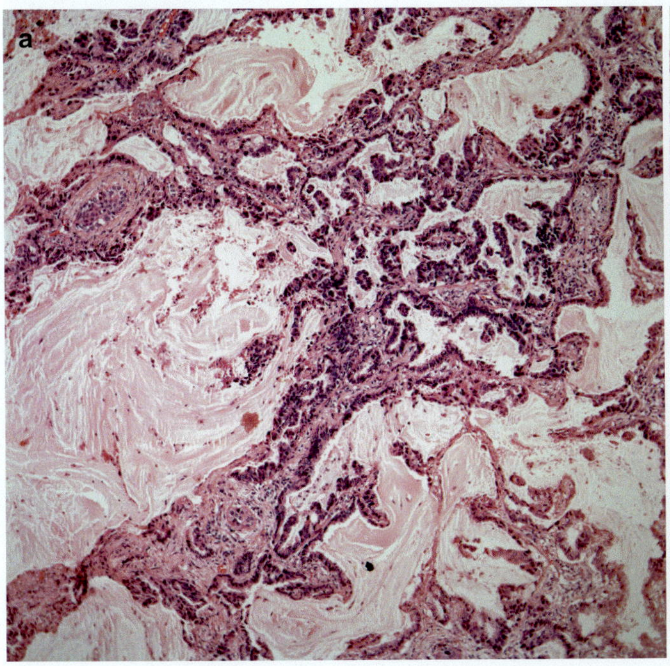

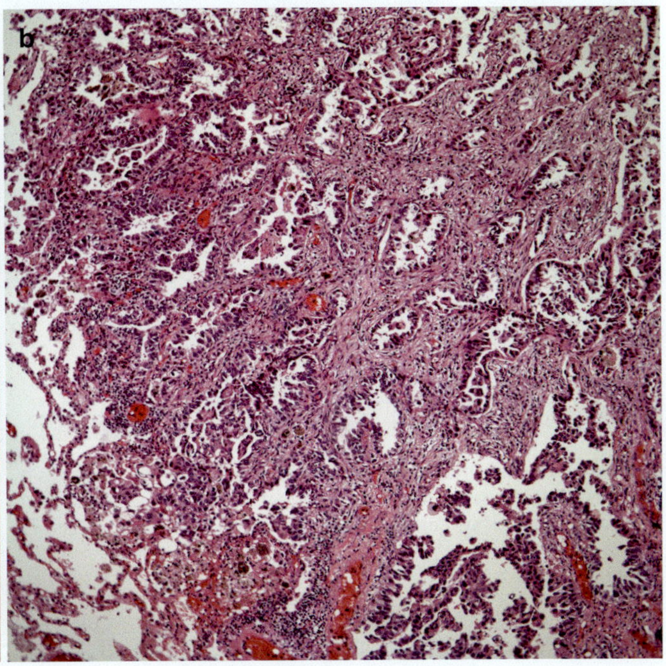

Fig. 3.10 (**a**) Well-differentiated adenocarcinoma showing glandular proliferation replacing lung parenchyma with areas of mucin deposition. (**b**) Glandular proliferation in a more fibrotic background. (**c**) Glandular proliferation composed of glands of different sizes. (**d**) Higher magnification showing glands with mild nuclear atypia and low mitotic activity

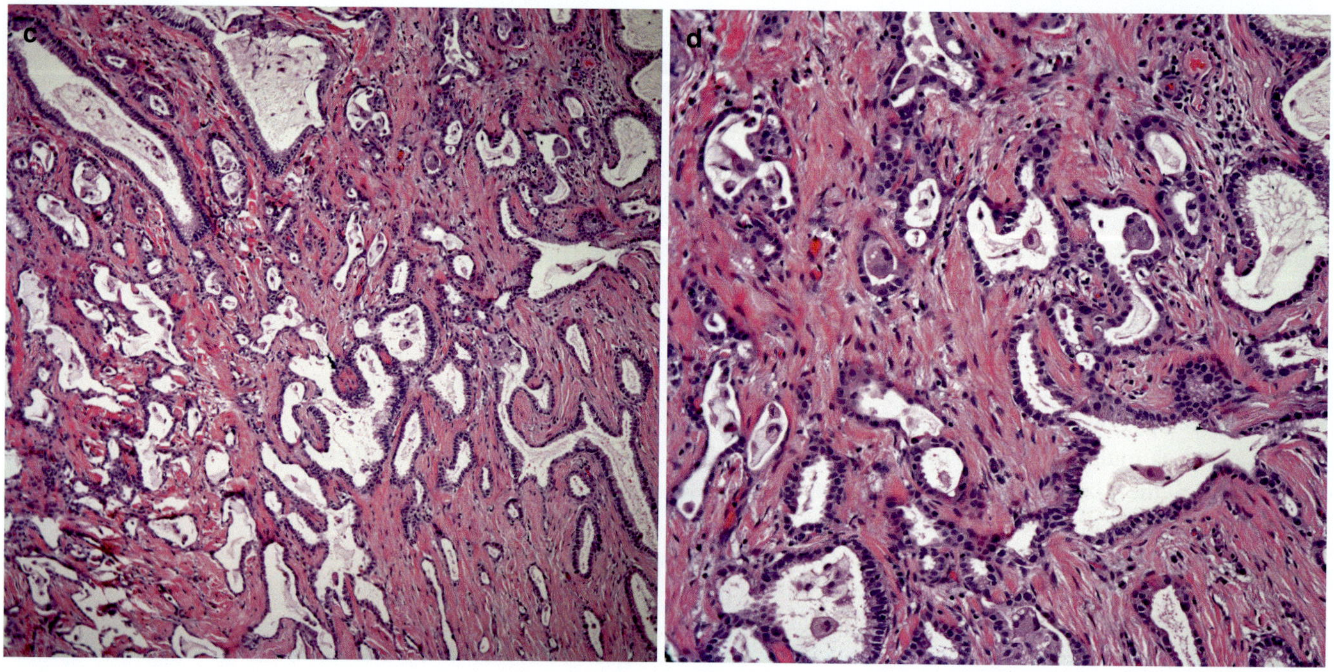

Fig. 3.10 (continued)

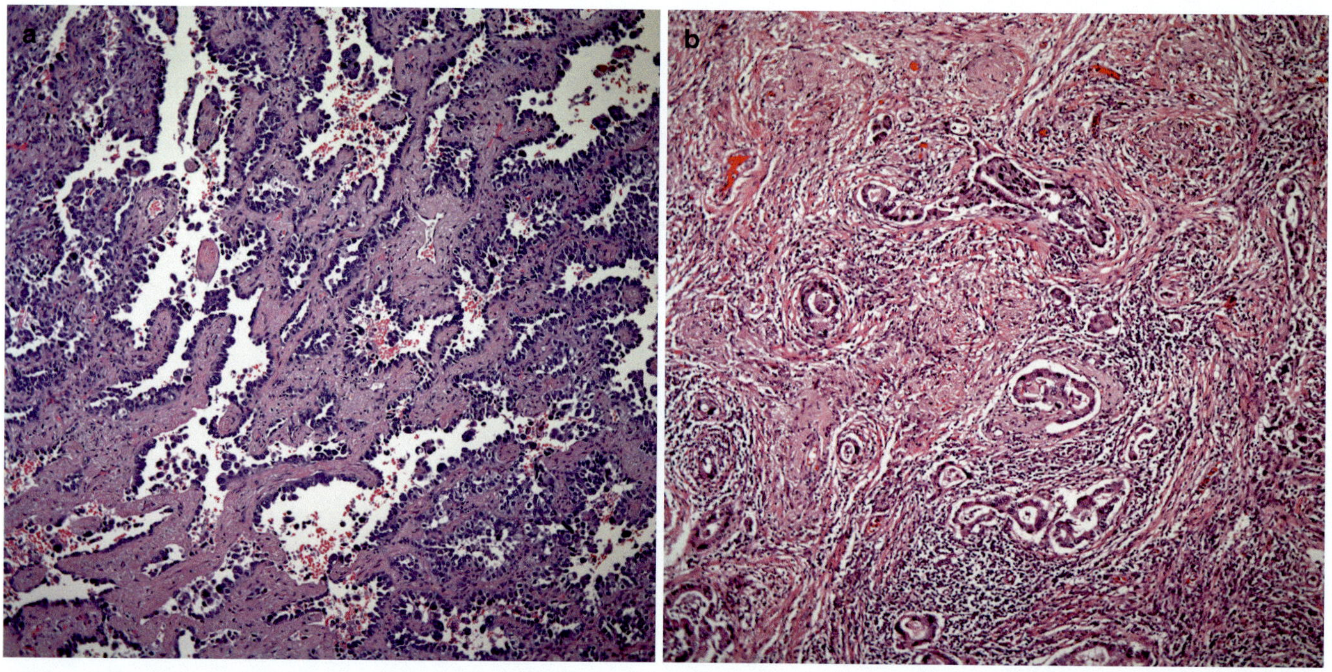

Fig. 3.11 (**a**) Moderately differentiated adenocarcinoma showing a glandular proliferation replacing normal lung parenchyma. (**b**) Malignant glands are embedded in a fibrotic and inflammatory background. (**c**) Acinar proliferation of malignant glands replacing lung parenchyma. (**d**) Higher magnification showing moderate nuclear atypia and mitotic activity

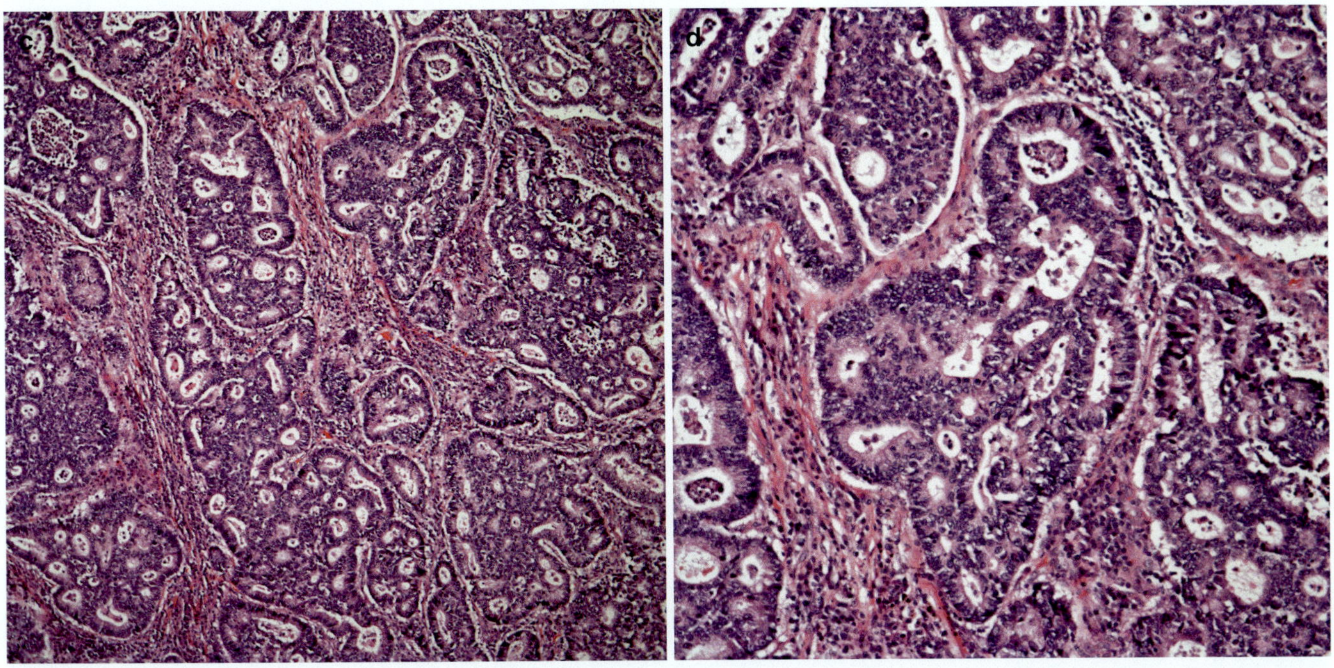

Fig. 3.11 (continued)

differentiation. One of the most common patterns of growth for the poorly differentiated adenocarcinomas is the solid growth pattern in which focal areas of abortive glandular formation may still be remaining. High-power magnification of the malignant cellular component may display cells with ample cytoplasm, round to oval nuclei, and prominent nucleoli. At the cytoplasmic level, the cells may show vacuolization, which may be helpful to pursue histochemical studies such as mucicarmine or DPAS to demonstrate the presence of intracellular mucin. In addition, one may find more conventional areas of glandular differentiation, which will be an important clue in the classification of these tumors as adenocarcinomas (Fig. 3.12a–f).

It is important to emphasize that the most important pieces of information that are crucial in the staging of lung carcinomas are the size of the tumor, the presence of pleural involvement, and the involvement of lymph nodes. Even though modern radiographic techniques provide very important and valid information regarding the size of tumors, it is still the responsibility of the pathologist to determine the size of the tumor by gross examination. Regarding pleural involvement, the gross evaluation is crucial as in many instances it can determine whether pleural involvement is present or not. Also important for proper staging is the dissection of all possible lymph nodes in cases of lobectomies or pneumonectomies. Ideally, dissecting lymph nodes and providing the level in which they are situated may help in providing an additional tool in the treatment of these patients.

Immunohistochemical Features

In the current practice of thoracic pathology, it is becoming of increasing importance to properly address the issue of adenocarcinoma or other type of non-small cell carcinoma. Even though in a majority of cases such distinction is easily demonstrated by light microscopic features, there are some cases, mainly in small biopsy material, in which such distinction is not easily recognized. Therefore, the use of immunohistochemical markers has become more popular in establishing such a separation between adenocarcinoma and other non-small cell carcinoma (see Table 3.2). Numerous immunohistochemical markers have been traditionally used as markers of adenocarcinoma. Positive staining for many carcinomatous epitopes including carcinoembryonic antigen (CEA), B72.3, CD15 (Leu M1), BER-EP4, broad-spectrum keratin, low molecular weight keratin (CAM 5.2), keratin 7, keratin 20, CDX2, surfactant protein, and PE-10 has been used with some success. However, the use of these markers will have more meaning depending on the setting in which they may be used. In addition, Dabbs et al. [99] in a study of estrogen and progesterone receptors in lung adenocarcinomas, using estrogen receptor clones 6 F11 and 1D5, found that 56 % of BAC and 80 % of adenocarcinomas with no special type show positive nuclear staining with the 6 F11 clone, while no staining was seen with the 1D5 clone. In addition, the authors report no staining for progesterone receptors.

Regarding the separation of primary lung non-small cell carcinoma, it is our experience that the use of TTF-1, Napsin A, p63, and keratin 5/6 can help with proper classification of a particular non-small cell carcinoma. For instance, adenocarcinoma will commonly express positive staining for TTF-1 and Napsin A (Figs. 3.13 and 3.14) but negative staining for keratin 5/6. The use of p63 although important has to be carefully evaluated when tumors show positive staining in addition to negative staining for TTF-1, Napsin A, and keratin 5/6. This particular immunoprofile can be seen in adenocarcinomas as in our experience, p63 may stain about 30 % of adenocarcinoma. On the other hand, positive staining for TTF-1 may not necessarily indicate primary lung adenocarcinoma, as positive staining for TTF-1 has been described in endometrial adenocarcinomas [100] and adenocarcinomas of the sinonasal cavity. Also important to note is the fact that CDX2 staining is commonly seen in adenocarci-

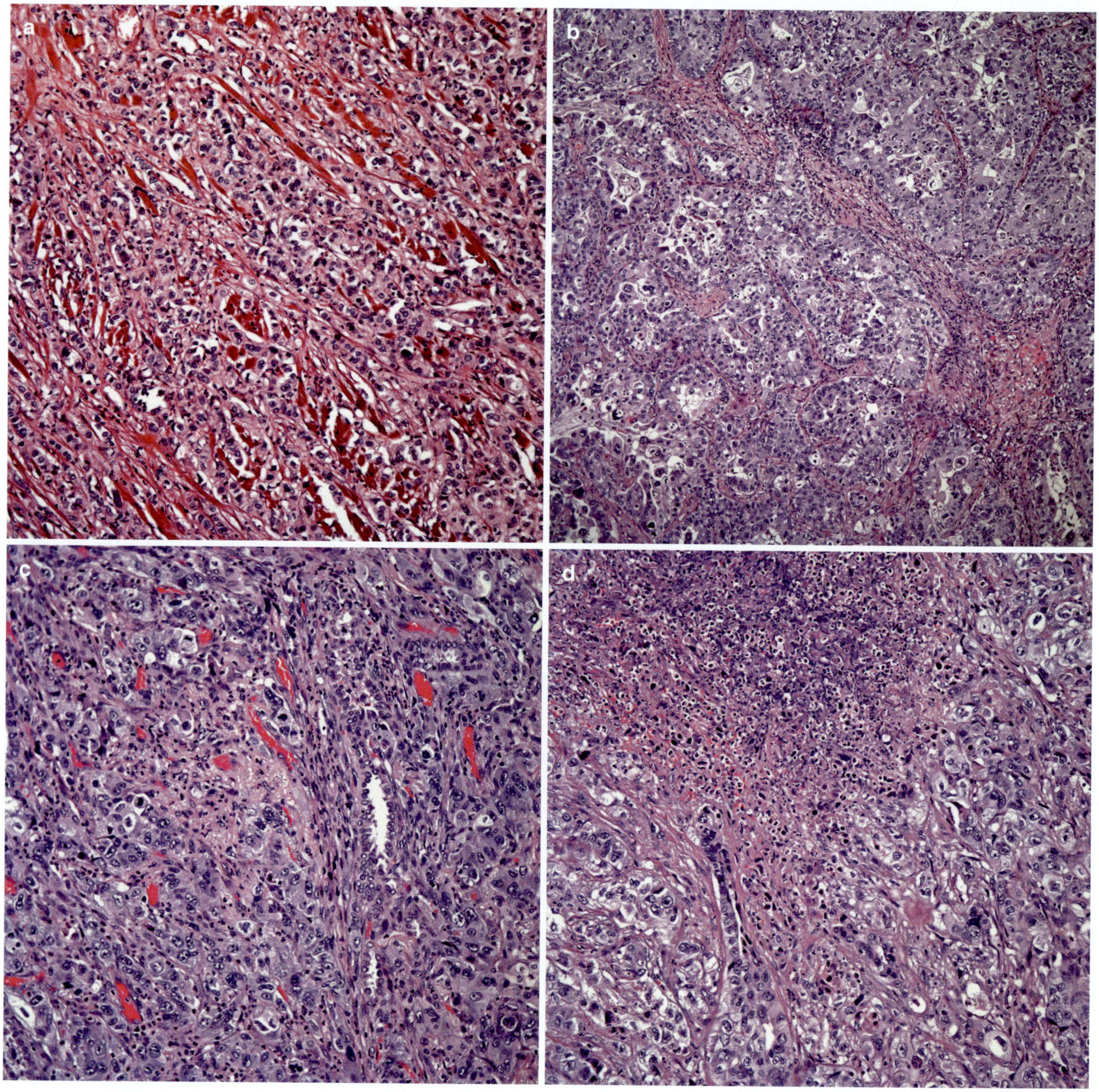

Fig. 3.12 (**a**) Poorly differentiated adenocarcinoma showing cords of neoplastic cells dissecting fibroconnective tissue. (**b**) In some areas, a glandular proliferation is still present. (**c**) Solid areas with only focal glandular changes. (**d**) Prominent nuclear atypia with poorly formed glands and areas of necrosis. (**e**) Prominent solid component of malignancy. (**f**) In focal areas, the presence of clear cells may be observed

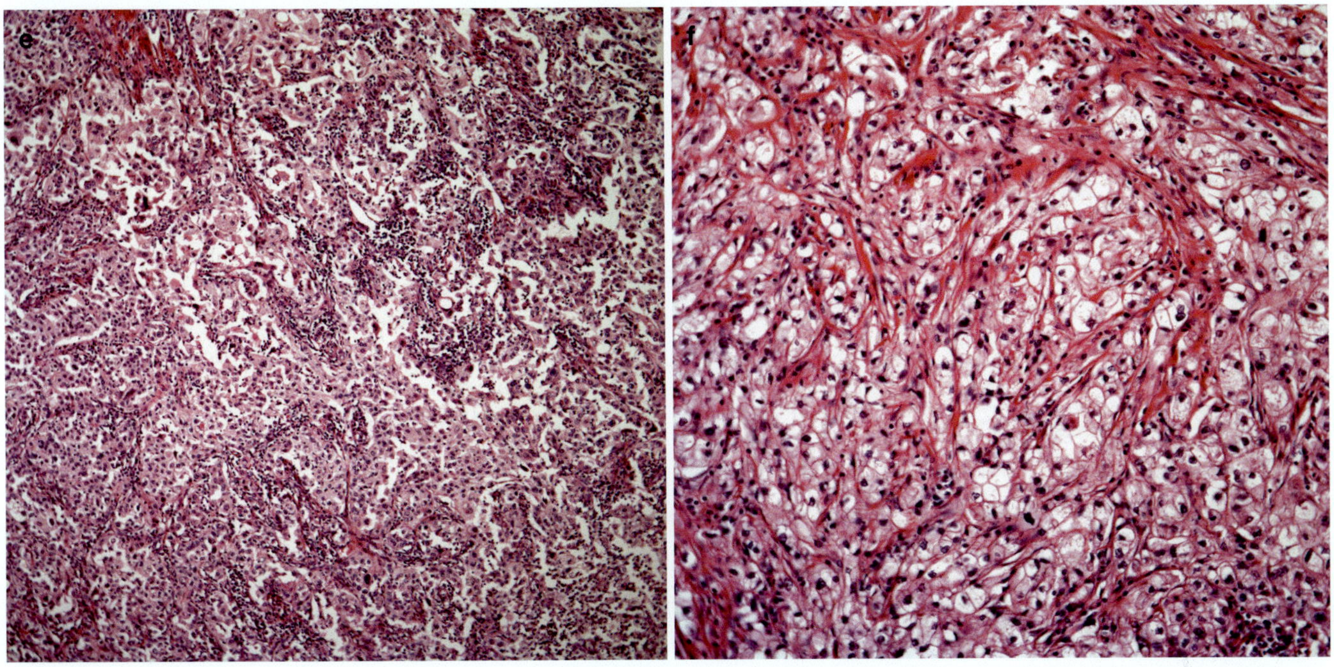

Fig. 3.12 (continued)

Table 3.2 Commonly used immunohistochemical stains in the diagnosis of non-small cell carcinoma

Tumor	Stains	Expected result
Adenocarcinoma	TTF-1	Positive
	Napsin A	Positive
	p63	Negative—positive in 30 % of cases
	Keratin 5/6	Negative—positive in unusual rare cases
	Keratin 7	Positive
	Keratin 20	Negative—positive in some cases
	CDX2	Negative—positive in mucinous tumors
	PAX-8	Negative
Squamous cell carcinoma	TTF-1	Negative
	Napsin A	Negative
	p63	Positive
	Keratin 5/6	Positive
	Keratin 7	Negative—positive in some cases
	Keratin 20	Negative
	CDX-2	Negative
	PAX8	Negative[a]

[a]PAX8 is positive in thymic squamous cell carcinomas

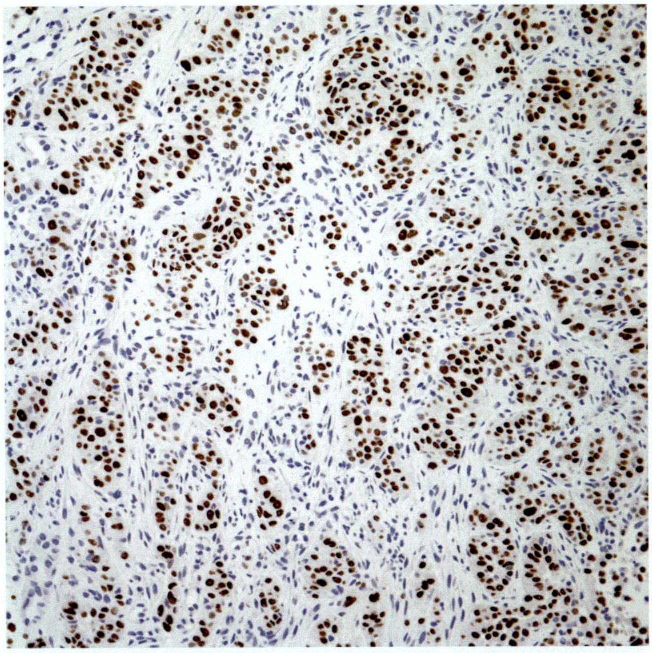

Fig. 3.13 Immunohistochemical stain for TTF-1 showing strong nuclear staining

nomas of the gastrointestinal tract; however, similar positive staining may also be seen in mucinous adenocarcinomas primary of the lung. The same applies for the use of keratin 20 that commonly is associated with adenocarcinomas of the gastrointestinal tract; however, positive staining can also be seen in some primary lung adenocarcinomas.

Histological Variants

Although traditionally adenocarcinomas are conceptualized as tumors with glandular proliferation, adenocarcinomas may display a wide diversity of cellular components that in many instances may pose problems with proper classification,

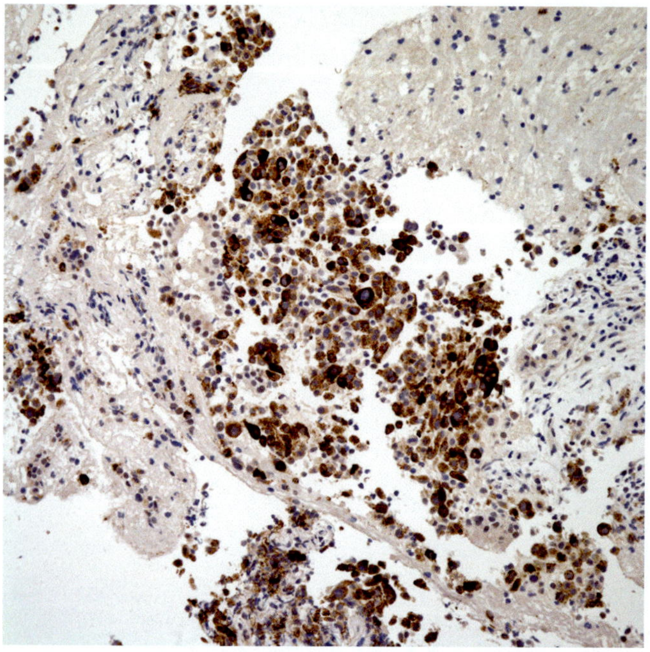

Fig. 3.14 Immunohistochemical stain for Napsin A showing strong positive staining in tumor cells

namely, when one is confronted with limited material for evaluation. Because of those different growth patterns, many adenocarcinomas carry specific histopathological descriptive terms.

Mucinous (So-Called Colloid) Carcinoma

Over the last two decades, this particular variant of adenocarcinoma has evolved from initial descriptions of a benign tumor—to borderline tumor—to what is now known as adenocarcinoma. Currently, most of those entities have been grouped under the term mucin-rich adenocarcinoma [101]. However, one point in which most descriptions of these tumors have agreed is that this tumor may behave as a low-grade adenocarcinoma. Interestingly, the authors of the "new" classification of adenocarcinoma [17] have stated that this tumor has an aggressive behavior, which is contrary to every single manuscript that has been published on that topic. Also controversial has been the designation by the latest WHO publication [50] of tumors resembling colloid carcinoma under the designation of mucinous cystadenoma, a lesion that has been described as a case report and most likely represents colloid carcinoma. One important issue that needs not to be confused is the fact that colloid carcinoma must be separated from the mucinous variant of BAC. Colloid carcinoma more often presents as a single subpleural and intrapulmonary tumor amenable to complete surgical resection, while the mucinous variant of BAC is a tumor of diffuse distribution along the pulmonary parenchyma often involving an entire lung, complete lobe, very often being multicentric. These tumors need not to be confused as the survival of these patients has been clearly defined in the literature. In order to shed more light in this topic, let us review previous publications:

Mucinous Cystadenoma. This represents one of the earliest designations provided for these tumors. Such nomenclature was introduced by Kragel et al. [102] in 1990 by describing two patients, a man and a woman, both 62 years of age, who were found to have a solitary lung tumor on radiographic examination. Both tumors were located in the right middle lobe, and surgical resection of the tumors was performed. Grossly both tumors were described as cystic, while microscopically, they were described as having abundant mucin production with the presence of columnar epithelium.

On the other hand, Traub [103] contested that the same tumors have already been described under the designation of *multilocular cystic carcinoma*. Nevertheless, Kragel et al. [102] argued that the tumors described by Traub belong to the mucinous variant of BAC. Interestingly, this particular entity is separated in the latest version of World Health Organization (WHO) [50] as a specific tumor; most other authors consider it to be part of the spectrum of mucinous-rich (colloid) carcinomas of the lung.

Pulmonary Mucinous Cystic Tumor. This term was introduced by Dixon et al. [104] in a case report of a 59-year-old man who apparently had had a pulmonary mass for 11 years prior to resection. Surgical resection of the tumor was performed, and the tumor mass was described as cystic. Histologically, the description of the tumor is essentially similar to that of Kragel et al. and Traub [102, 103]. However, important to note is that in Dixon's case, the authors mention the presence of an atypical glandular component. Nonetheless, the authors avoided the term "carcinoma" and regarded their neoplasm as an indolent lesion with favorable prognosis based on the negative clinical follow-up of 5 years.

Higashima et al. [105] also described similar cases as that described by Dixon [104] with a different interpretation. The cases described by Higashima show similar gross and microscopic features but were named "cystic mucinous adenocarcinoma of the lung" and believed that they were a variant of mucus-producing adenocarcinoma of the lung different from previous tumors described as mucinous tumors, specifically mucinous cystadenoma.

Davison et al. [106] described a similar case in a 69-year-old woman with a peripheral lung nodule incidentally found during a routine physical examination. In this particular case, the gross and microscopic features described are essentially the same as those previously reported under the terms cystadenoma, mucinous tumor, and cystic mucinous adenocarcinoma. Further, the author described a solid focus of well-differentiated adenocarcinoma; thus, the authors opted for the designation of adenocarcinoma arising in a mucinous cystadenoma of the lung. These reports raise the idea that first there is a benign mucinous cystadenoma, which can undergo malignancy. Such an idea, although interesting, has no foundation, as likely the only description of a mucinous cystadenoma most likely represents colloid carcinoma.

Pulmonary Mucinous Cystic Tumors of Borderline Malignancy. Graeme-Cook and Mark [107] in 1991 introduced this new term based on a study of 11 cases of primary mucinous cystic tumors of the lung. The descriptions of these tumors again reflected the cystic and mucinous nature of these tumors, which in some cases showed a "solid epithelial proliferation". The follow-up provided, which ranged from 1 to 9 years, appears to be of an "indolent" tumor. However, despite the fact that the authors considered this tumor "neoplastic," the term carcinoma was avoided in favor of that of a borderline tumor.

Mucinous (So-Called Colloid) Carcinoma. This represents the latest designation for the family of mucin-rich neoplasms and attempts to include all previous designations for these tumors. The term was introduced in 1992 [108] based on a study of 24 cases. Clinically, grossly, and microscopically, the tumors described showed an overlap of features with previous cases. Also, areas with a solid epithelial glandular proliferation were observed in some of the cases. The most important contrasting feature present in this series is that the follow-up, ranging from 2 to 192 months, identified some patients with metastatic lesions to bone and brain. Recurrences of the tumors were also recorded while in some other patients, the follow-up was uneventful.

Based on all those previous descriptions, it is likely that all those descriptions referred to a single pathological entity. Clinically, grossly, and histologically, there are only minor differences in all these tumors. If one accepts the concept of benign and malignant tumors, it is difficult to find exact criteria how to separate those tumors, a situation that becomes crucial as one evaluates small biopsy specimens. On the other hand, if one is to approach these tumors as low-grade carcinomas with metastatic potential, it becomes crucial that the tumor requires complete surgical resection with close follow-up. It appears that at least in one of the reported series of these cases, such an argument can be easily accepted as some of the patients presented went on to develop metastatic disease. Thus, some authors have advocated to classify these tumors as carcinomas of low-grade malignant potential. Important to note is that in some cases in which the tumor is solitary and amenable to complete surgical resection, that may be the only treatment required. However, for those patients who present with widespread pulmonary involvement and in advance clinical staging, the prognosis may be dismal.

Gross Features

Mucinous tumors of the lung are characterized by a soft mucoid consistency. In addition, these tumors may show easily identifiable cystic structures. In some cases, the tumor although mucoid in consistency may appear as a more solid tumor mass; however, closer inspection may show the presence of microcystic structures. The size of these tumors may vary from 1 cm to widely disseminated tumors in the lung parenchyma.

Microscopic Features

Characteristically, the low-power view of mucinous tumors of the lung is the overwhelming presence of extensive areas of mucoid material destroying normal lung parenchyma. These areas may only contain small clusters of atypical cells or single cells with atypical features. In some cases, the low-power view may be of a cystic tumor, while in other cases, the tumor may show microcystic structures filled with mucoid material. One of the most important features of these tumors is the presence of residual alveolar wall lined by mucinous-producing epithelium resembling intestinal type of epithelium. The presence of mucinous type of epithelium may be focal, and careful search for these areas may be necessary in cases in which such a finding is not readily visible (Fig. 3.15a–f). In a minority of cases, one may find the presence of focal solid areas of adenocarcinoma, which may appear as a conventional adenocarcinoma, or adenocarcinoma with papillary features. It is important to properly sample these tumors as the most characteristic findings may be present only focally, while other areas may show only extensive mucoid material distributed haphazardly in the lung parenchyma destroying normal architecture.

Immunohistochemical Features

Just like any other primary lung adenocarcinoma, the use of TTF-1 and keratin 7 may help in decorating the epithelial component of the tumor. However, it is important to use an immunohistochemical panel that may aid in ruling out tumors with similar histology but different origin. Thus, the use of keratin 20, CDX2, CD10, and gross cystic disease fluid protein may help in ruling out tumors from gastrointestinal, genitourinary, and breast origin. Nevertheless, in practice, colloid carcinomas often are negative for TTF-1 and Napsin A, while the tumor may show positive staining for CDX2.

Clinical Behavior

As one can draw from the different publications on these tumors, the clinical behavior of these tumors may follow an indolent course in which patients are treated with complete surgical resection, while in other patients, the behavior is that of an aggressive tumor with widespread metastatic disease. The most important feature to predict prognosis is the staging at the time of diagnosis. For those tumors that are small and amenable to complete surgical resection, the course may be more innocuous while those tumors that are large or have spread outside the lung parenchyma or even outside of the thoracic cavity the prognosis may be more guarded. However, as mentioned earlier, it is highly important not to confuse or group colloid carcinoma with the mucinous variant of BAC

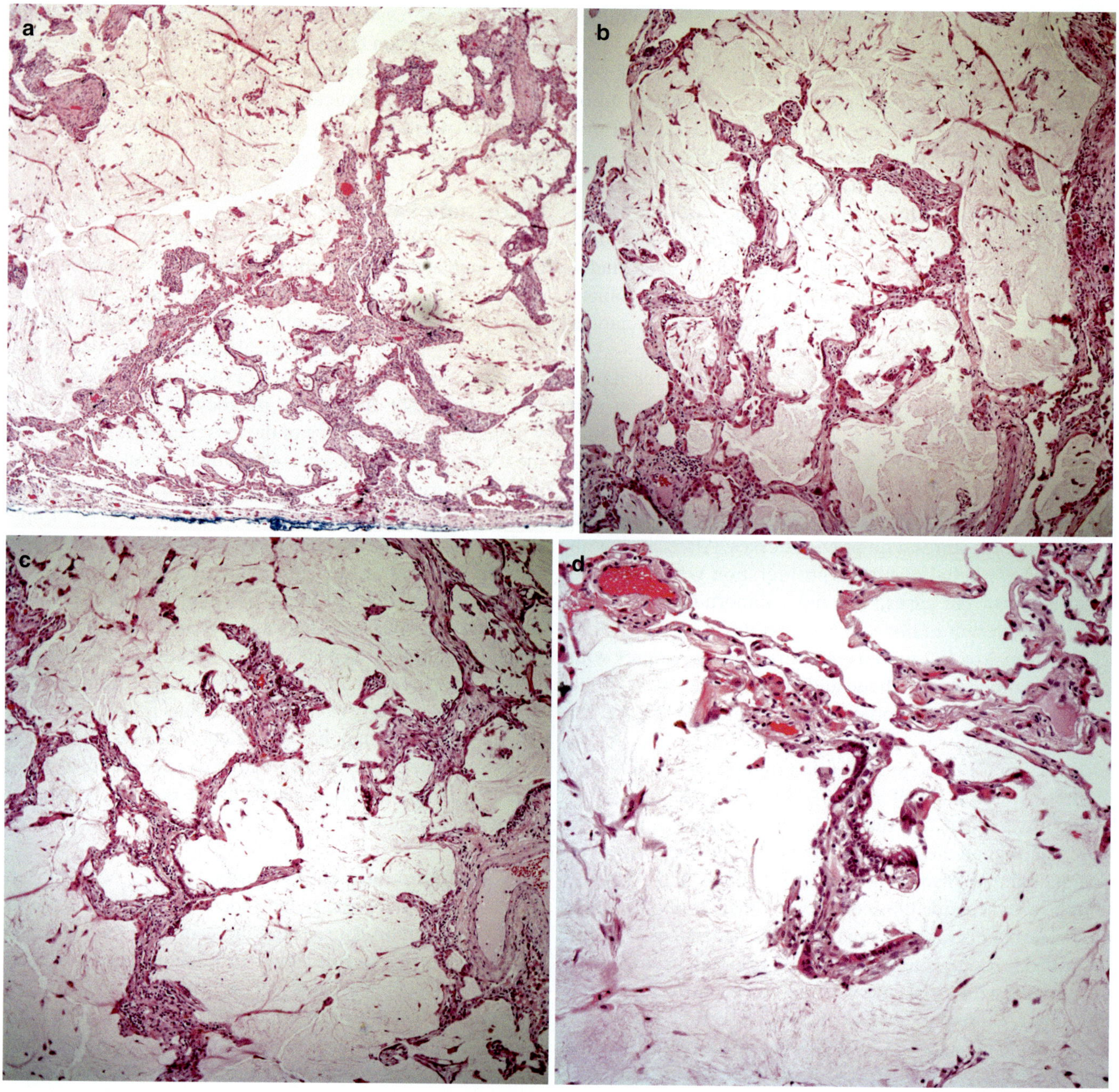

Fig. 3.15 (**a**) Low-power view of a colloid carcinoma of the lung showing extensive pools of mucoid material. (**b**) Some lung parenchyma is still preserved but distended by pools of mucin. (**c**) In focal areas, there is lining of the alveolar wall by mucinous epithelium. (**d**) Closer view of the mucinous epithelium lining alveolar walls. (**e**) Cystically dilated areas filled with mucious material. Note the mucinous epithelium lining the cystic wall. (**f**) Closer view at the mucinous epithelium lining cystic walls

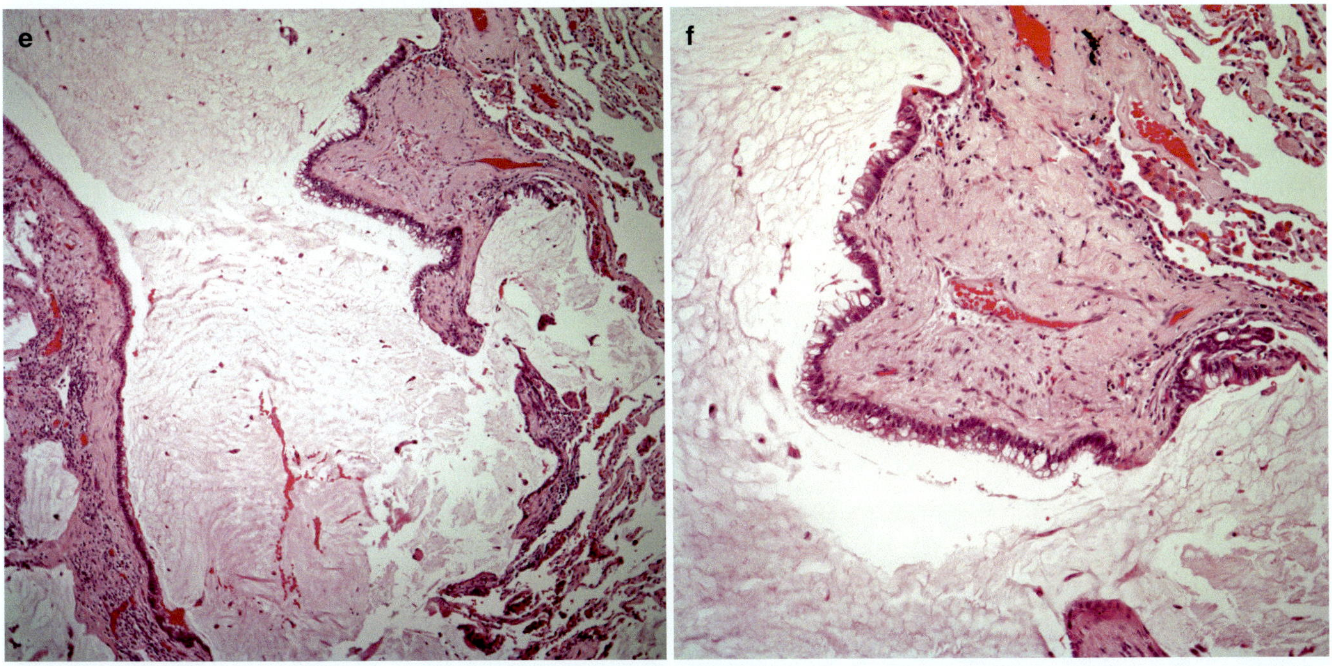

Fig. 3.15 (continued)

which likely has wide distribution within the lung parenchyma, while colloid carcinoma often presents as a subpleural solitary tumor.

Papillary Carcinoma

Although there has been an acknowledgment of carcinomas with papillary features, those cases had been grouped under other designations including variants of BAC. Several studies of this type of growth pattern have calculated that it represents approximately 10 % of all adenocarcinomas of the lung.

Silver and Askin [109] in 1997 introduced the term "true" papillary carcinomas of the lung as a separate entity. The authors described 31 patients with primary papillary carcinomas and set the parameters for the diagnosis of such tumors. In their report, Silver and Askin [109] concluded that tumors with this morphology should have at least 75 % of papillary features in order to qualify for this designation. The tumor appears to affect men and women equally, although in some reports, a slight predominance in women have been reported [110]. No particular lung or pulmonary segments for its occurrence have been identified. The tumor is more common in adult individuals with a mean age of 64 years. The great majority of these patients will present with a single solitary pulmonary tumor although in a few cases the tumor may be multifocal. Only a few studies of this variant of carcinoma have been presented in the literature [109–111], and these studies appear to support that it represents a separate clinicopathological entity that appears to be more aggressive than conventional adenocarcinoma.

Gross Features

The tumors may present as a central or peripheral tumor. The tumor mass may vary in size from 1 to more than 10 cm in greatest dimension. The tumors appear to be well delimited and light brown, and at cut surface, they may show a homogenous surface. In a few cases, the tumor may show necrosis and/or hemorrhage.

Histological Features

The low-power magnification is that of a papillary neoplasm destroying normal lung parenchyma. The papillary pattern in some areas may acquire a more complex configuration with papillary cores of different sizes and length. Closer examination of these papillary cores shows that they contain delicate fibrovascular cores. The papillary cores are lined by neoplastic cells in which the nuclei are displaced toward the periphery of the cells; the nuclei may show grooves and intranuclear inclusions. Mitotic figures are not common; however, the tumor may show the presence of psammoma bodies haphazardly distributed in tumoral areas (Fig. 3.16a–h). In some cases, although the pattern is that of a papillary carcinoma, the cytological features are those of an oncocytic papillary carcinoma.

Immunohistochemical Features

Because of the predominant papillary growth pattern and the possibility of metastatic lesions to the lung with similar histology, the use of immunohistochemical studies including keratin 7, TTF-1, Napsin A, thyroglobulin and Pax8 is an important aid in the diagnosis of these tumors.

Molecular Biology

Despite the relatively low frequency of this type of adenocarcinoma of the lung, molecular biology studies have been performed in order to determine whether this type of tumor deserves to be separated as a real clinicopathological entity and also to determine differences with other types of lung carcinoma, mainly BAC. In that regard, it has been determined that papillary carcinomas show loss of heterozygosity (LOH) on chromosome 3p in approximately 80 % of cases in contrast to 14 % in BAC [110].

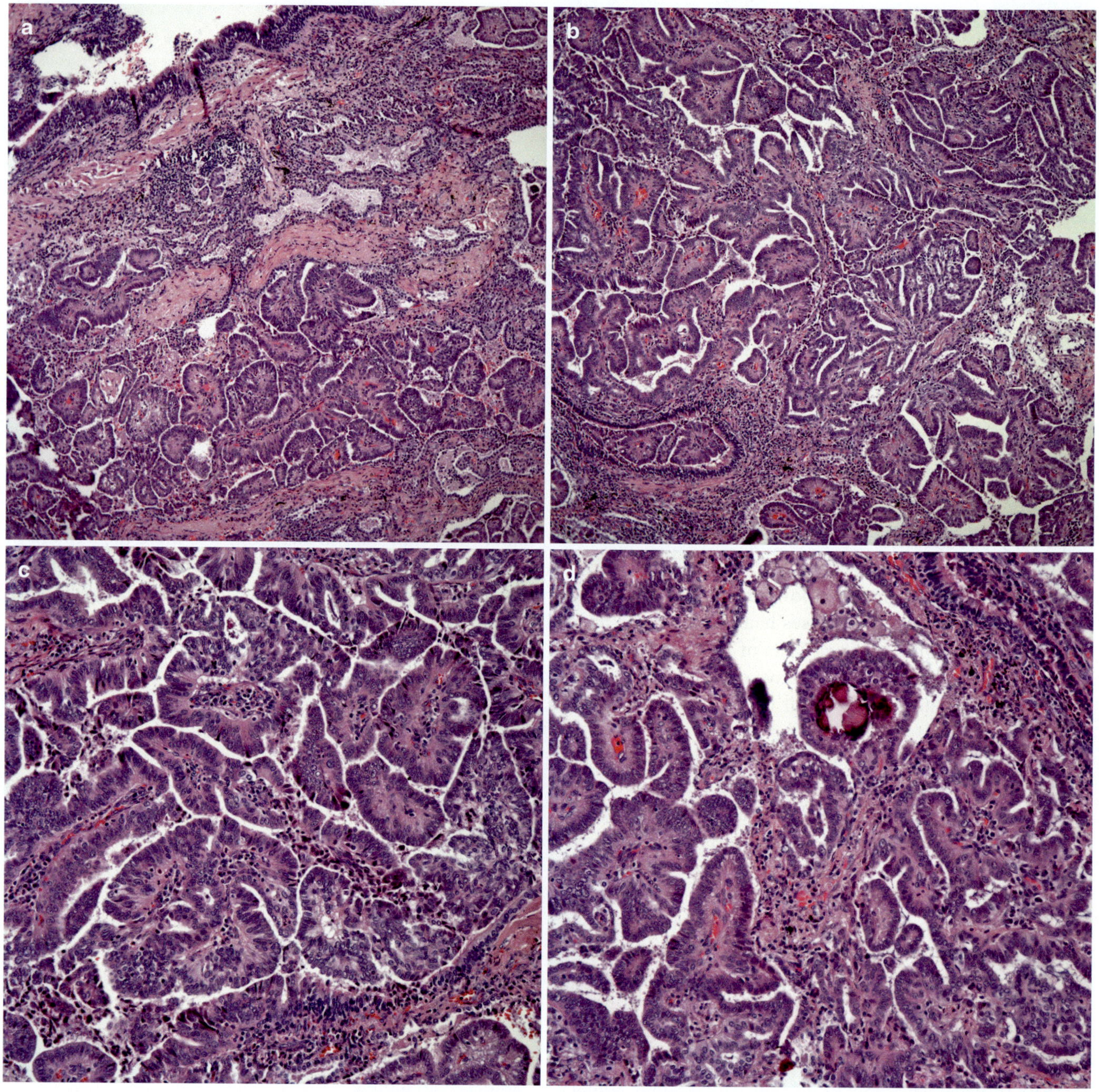

Fig. 3.16 (**a**) Low-power view of a papillary carcinoma of the lung. (**b**) Papillary fronds replacing normal lung architecture. (**c**) Closer view at the papillary proliferation showing thin fibrovascular cords in some of the papillations. (**d**) The presence of psammoma bodies may be subtle. (**e**) Extensive areas of psammoma bodies are uncommon. (**f**) Breakdown of papillary structures floating in edematous fluid. (**g**) In focal areas, papillary structures are floating in pools of mucin. (**h**) Higher magnification of the papillary structures showing cells with clear nuclei

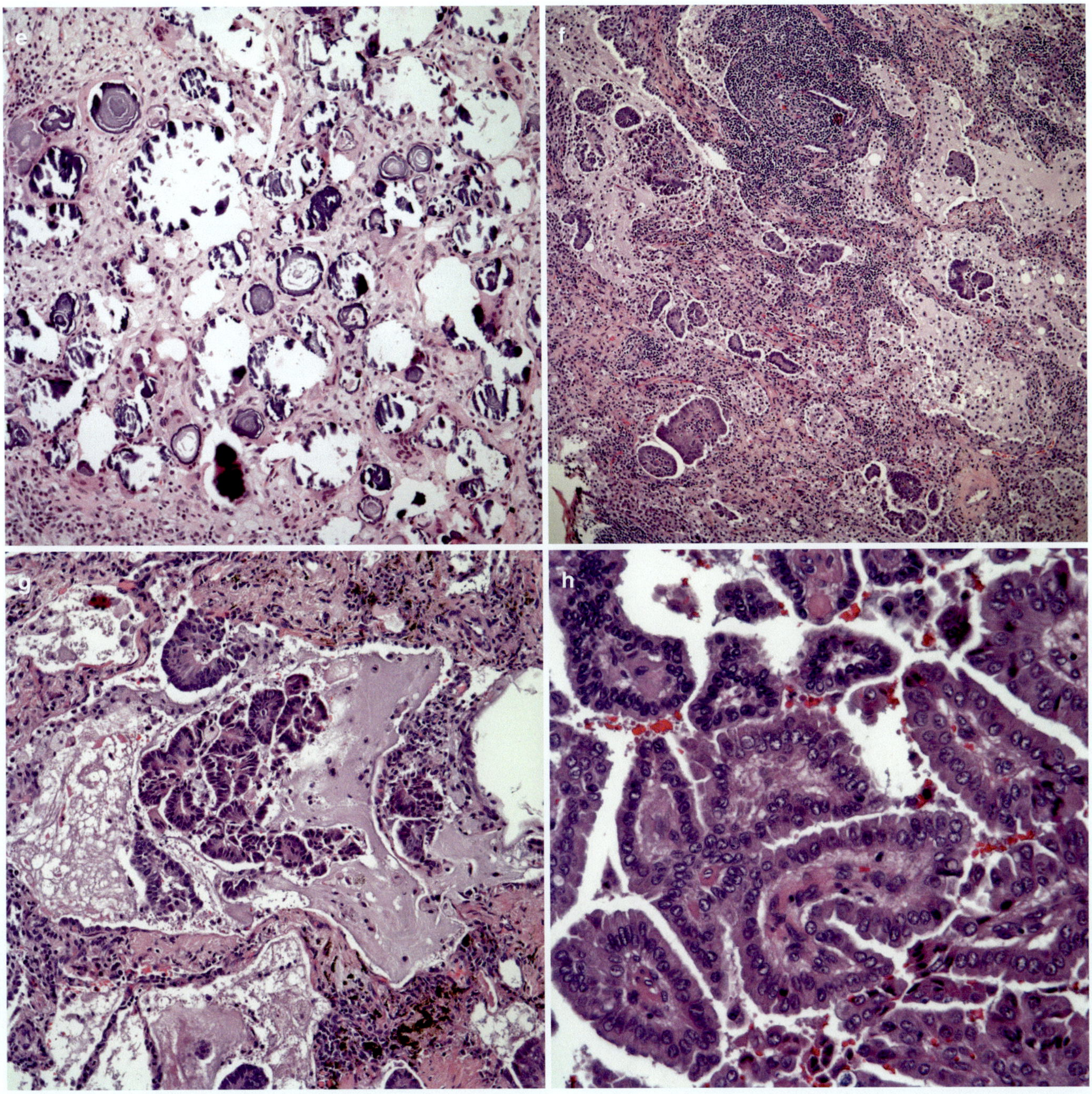

Fig. 3.16 (continued)

Clinical Behavior

The prognosis and survival rate for patients with papillary carcinoma appears to be linked to the clinical staging. In the series presented by Silver and Askin [109], 75 % of the patients studied had recurrence or metastatic disease. However, when analyzed by stage, patients in early stages fare better. In the study by Silver and Askin [109], with a mean follow up of 3.4 years over 50 % of the patients in stage I were alive, while only 25 % in stage II were alive.

Papillary Carcinoma with Prominent Morular Component

This variant or papillary carcinoma has been recently described [112]. Three cases of this unusual growth pattern were described in adult patients between the ages of 25 and 68 years. Clinically, these patients presented with similar symptoms as those seen in any lung carcinoma, namely, cough, dyspnea, and chest pain. No lung or lung segment appears to have predilection for this tumor.

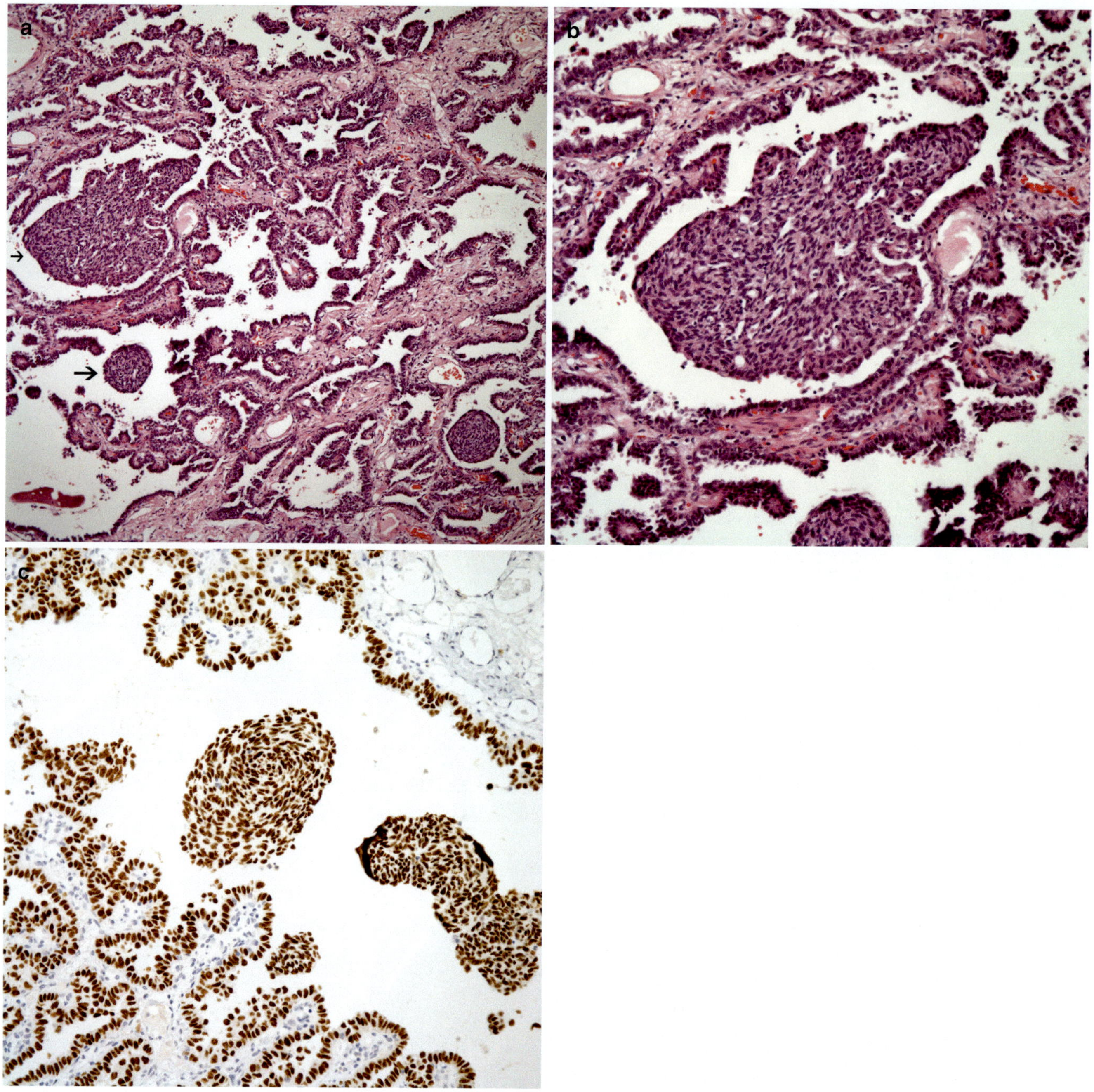

Fig. 3.17 (**a**) Papillary carcinoma with morular component (see *arrows*). (**b**) Close magnification at the morular component showing spindling of the cells. (**c**) Immunohistochemical stain for TTF-1 showing strong positive staining in the cells lining the papillary structures and in the morular component

Gross Features

The tumors described varied in size from 2.5 to 3.5 cm in greatest dimension and were well-defined tumor masses, soft, white to tan, and with no evidence of necrosis or hemorrhage.

Microscopic Features

These tumors share similar features as true papillary carcinomas in the sense of a predominantly papillary architecture. However, within the papillary structures, one can identify the presence of small cellular aggregates in the form of "morules." These "morules" are distributed among papillary structures in a haphazard fashion and without attachment to papillary structures (Fig. 3.17a–c). In all the cases described, areas of conventional adenocarcinoma were also present.

Immunohistochemical Studies

The tumor characteristically shows positive staining for keratin, carcinoembryonic antigen (CEA), Napsin A, and TTF-1 while thyroglobulin is negative. Interestingly, TTF-1 is also positive in the morular component of the tumor.

Clinical Behavior

All patients underwent surgical resection. However, the follow-up provided is too short to determine a more definitive clinical behavior. However, it is possible that their behavior may be similar to the classical true papillary carcinoma.

Micropapillary Carcinoma

Only a few series of micropapillary carcinoma have been presented in the literature [113–117], as this variant of adenocarcinoma represents a relatively new entity. Nevertheless, it appears to be a unanimous agreement that tumors with these histopathological features behave more aggressively. In the reported series, the finding of metastatic disease was observed in more than 25 % of cases. Therefore, it has been stated that this growth pattern needs to be carefully evaluated in adenocarcinomas, and its presence should alert of the possible aggressive behavior of this tumor. It is important to mention that the presence of a micropapillary growth pattern may vary from case to case. In some cases, it has been reported to be rather focal while in other cases, it may be more extensive. Also, important to recognize is that micropapillary features may be associated with any type of adenocarcinoma and not only the conventional true papillary carcinoma of the lung. In addition, the presence of micropapillary features in a tumor is not associated with the size of the tumor.

The first to recognize this type of pattern and making an analogy with similar tumors in the breast and bladder was Amin et al. [113] with the description of 35 cases. In this series of cases, most patients were in late stages of disease (stages III and IV). However, those patients in stage I went on to develop metastatic disease in a relatively short period of time, thus emphasizing the concept that tumors with this type of growth pattern may show a more aggressive behavior.

Microscopic Features

The most important feature distinguishing papillary from micropapillary growth pattern is that in the former the papillary structures show the presence of fibrovascular cores while in the latter such cores are absent. Therefore, tumors with this type of pattern may show the presence of clusters of cells filling alveolar spaces detached from the lining of the alveolar wall resembling free-floating cells (Fig. 3.18a–d). These clusters of cells may vary in size from a few cells to sizable clusters of malignant cells. This growth pattern has predilection for invading vascular spaces mimicking metastatic disease to the lung. Closer view of the malignant cells shows cells with mild to moderate amounts of amphophilic cytoplasm, round to oval nuclei with inconspicuous nucleoli. Mitotic figures are present but not in large numbers. Although areas of necrosis and hemorrhage may be present, they are not very common.

Immunohistochemical Features

In the series of cases reported by Amin et al. [113], the authors studied 15 cases by immunohistochemical means using antibodies for keratin 7, keratin 20, and TTF-1. Of the 15 cases studied, 14 cases showed positive staining for keratin 7, and 12 cases showed positive staining for TTF-1. Interestingly, two cases also showed positive staining for keratin 20. Based on this study, it is important to note that not all of these tumors may show positive staining for TTF-1 or keratin 7, thus leaving a small percentage of cases in which good clinical correlation needs to be made in order to address the possibility of metastatic lesions to the lung, mainly from tumors of breast and bladder origin. Thus, it may be important to widen this panel of immunohistochemical studies depending on the particular setting in which one may find this tumor.

Clinical Behavior

As previously stated and based on the reported series of these tumors, micropapillary carcinoma has a tendency to present in late stages of disease with metastatic disease to lymph nodes and pleura, or metastasis outside of the thoracic cavity. In the reported series, the majority of cases have been in stages III and IV. Thus, it is important to note that the clinical outcome of these patients is also related to staging at the time of diagnosis.

Signet Ring Cell Carcinoma

Signet ring cell carcinoma represents another unusual variant of adenocarcinoma, which has been reported seldom and for which there are only a few series of cases documenting this unusual growth pattern [118–121]. There does not appear to be any gender predisposition or a predisposition for any lung or lung segment. The ages of the patients described have varied from 30 to 75 years of age. In Hayashi's study [120], the authors concluded that signet ring cell adenocarcinomas are closely related to bronchial gland cell-type adenocarcinoma. Although signet ring cells may occasionally be seen in otherwise conventional adenocarcinomas, in the cases reported, the signet ring cell component has been a predominant feature. In addition, in the series of cases presented by Castro et al. [121], the authors included cases in which signet ring cell features composed at least 75 % of the tumor. The tumors may appear in a central or peripheral location, and symptoms may be related to tumor size and anatomic location. The tumors have been described as soft, gray, and with or without areas of hemorrhage and/or necrosis. The tumor size may also vary from 1 cm to more than 5 cm in greatest diameter.

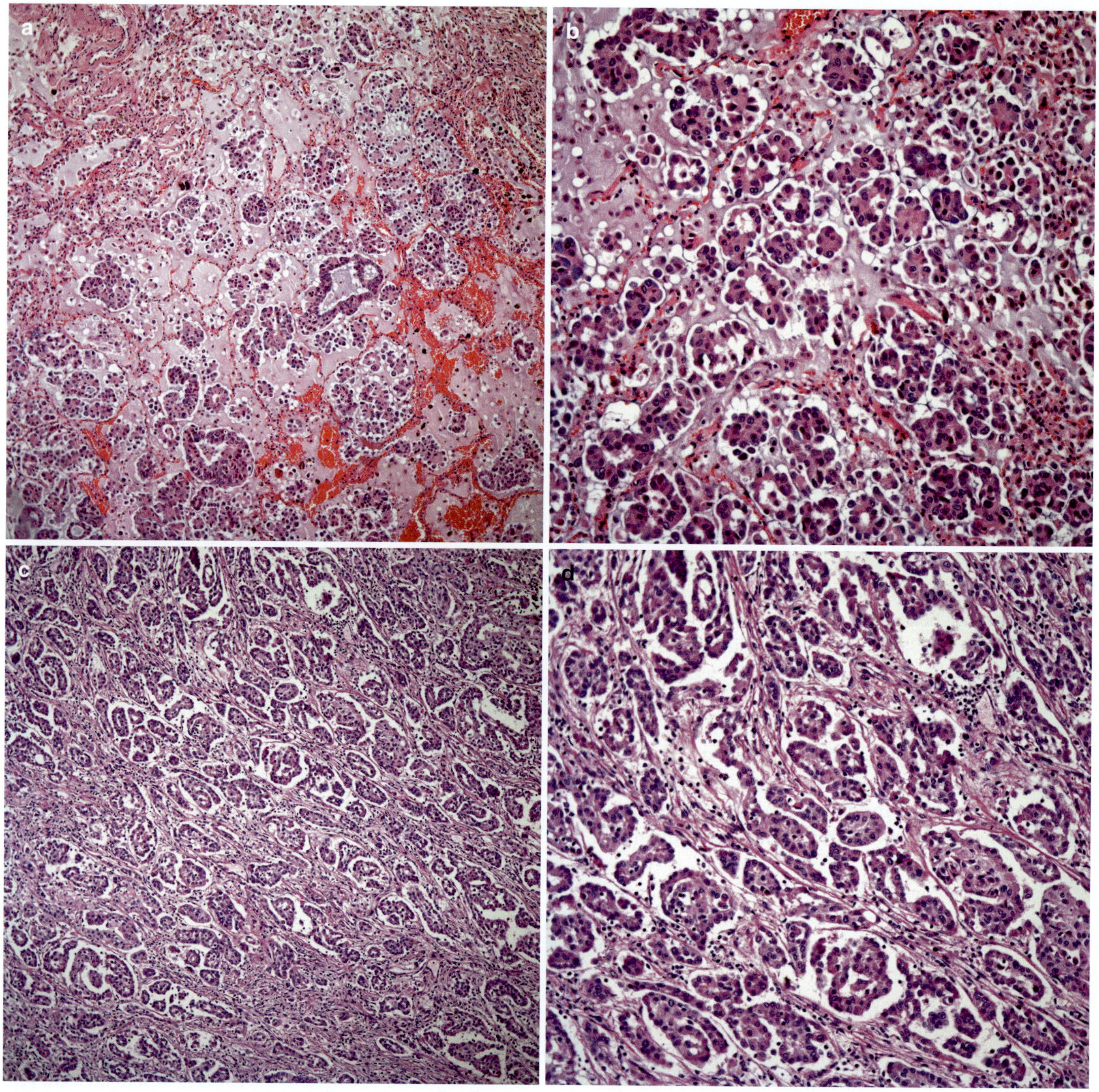

Fig. 3.18 (**a**) Lung parenchyma with micropapillae floating in alveolar spaces. (**b**) Micropapillae floating in alveolar spaces, note the absence of fibrovascular cords. (**c**) In other areas, the micropapillae appear to destroy normal lung parenchyma. (**d**) The cellular proliferation does not show increased mitotic activity or nuclear atypia

Microscopic Features

Two histopathological growth patterns have been described for signet ring cell adenocarcinoma: acinar and diffuse. In the acinar pattern, the tumor cells are distributed in small nests of tumor cells separated by thin bands of fibroconnective tissue, which may contain an inflammatory infiltrate. On higher magnification, these nests of tumor cells are composed of medium-size cells with clear cytoplasm and nuclei displaced toward the periphery imparting the so-called signet ring cell appearance. High nuclear atypia and/or mitotic figures are not common. In some areas, the tumoral cells appear to be filling alveolar spaces. In the diffuse pattern, sheets of malignant cells arranged in cords or distributed haphazardly appear to dissect, infiltrate, and destroy areas of normal lung parenchyma. The cytological features in the growth pattern are similar to that seen in the acinar growth pattern (Fig. 3.19a–e). Histochemical studies for PAS with and without diastase and mucicarmine (Fig. 3.20) show strong positive cytoplasmic staining for mucin.

Immunohistochemical Features

Although the number of cases reported has emphasized the histopathological growth pattern of signet ring cells, immunohistochemical studies have been limited. Hayashi et al. [120] reported that signet ring cell adenocarcinomas of the lung are positive for MUC-1 and negative for MUC-2, while the opposite is true for tumors of gastrointestinal origin. In the series of cases reported by Castro et al. [121], the authors performed a limited immunohistochemical study on a few of the cases reported and observed that keratin 7 was positive in 50 % of the cases studied and TTF-1 and CEA showed positive staining in

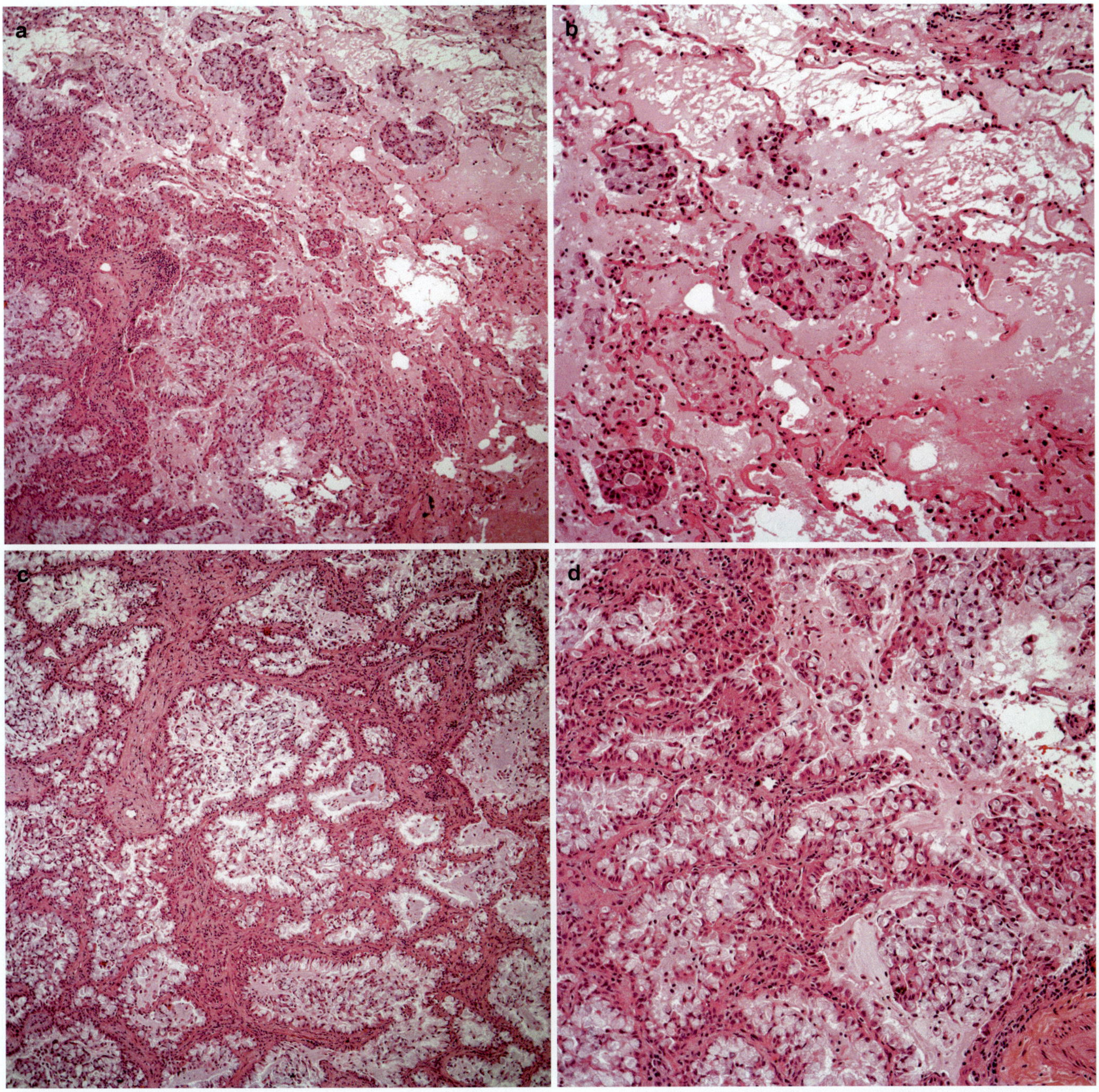

Fig. 3.19 (**a**) Low-power view of a signet ring cell carcinoma of the lung. Note the presence of cluster of malignant cells and edematous fluid filling alveolar spaces. (**b**) Closer view at the neoplastic cells filling alveolar spaces and admixed with edematous fluid. (**c**) Acinar growth pattern of signet ring cell carcinoma. (**d**) Delicate bands of fibroconnective separate areas of tumor cells. (**e**) Closer view showing the classic cytological features of signet ring cells

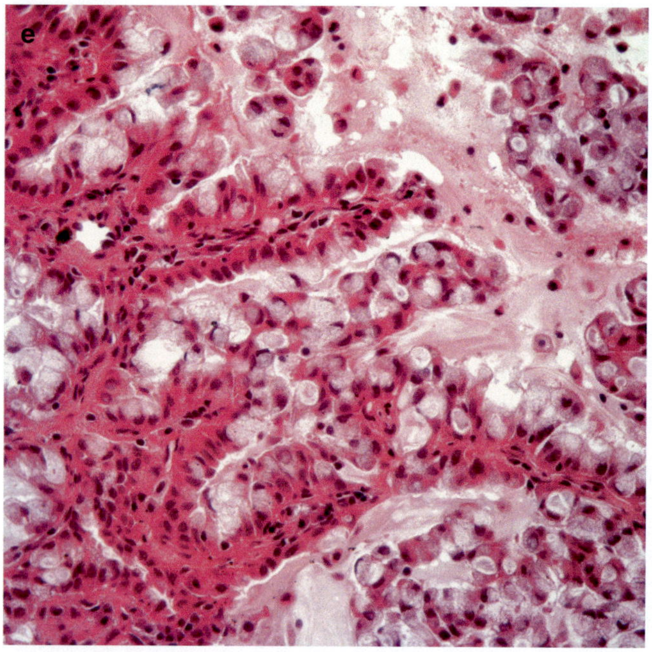

Fig. 3.19 (continued)

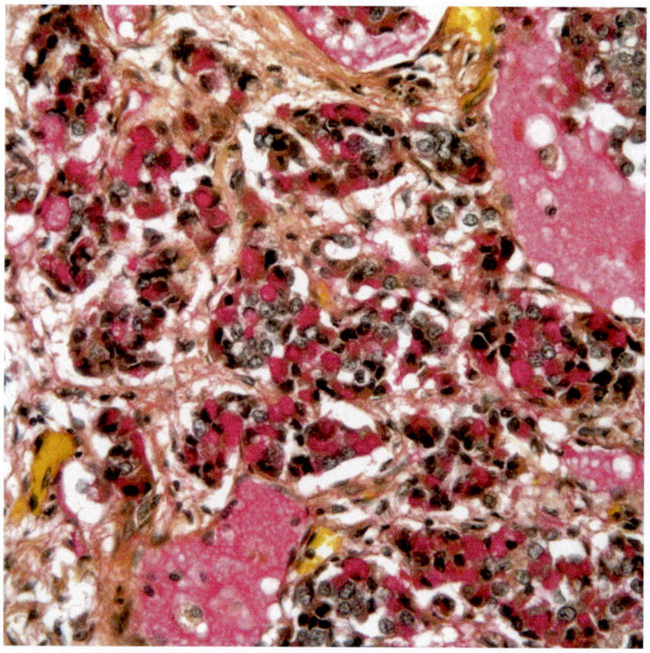

Fig. 3.20 Mucicarmine histochemical stain showing strong positive reaction (intracellular mucin) in tumor cells

all the cases studied. Keratin 20 was negative in all the cases studied. A practical approach to this type of histopathological growth pattern should include keratins 7 and 20 but also TTF-1 and CDX2 as well as gross cystic disease fluid protein and mammaglobin to rule out the possibility of a gastrointestinal or breast carcinoma.

From the molecular point of view, mucinous tumors just like carcinomas with signet ring cell features have been observed to have the echinoderm microtubule-associated protein-like 4 gene-anaplastic lymphoma kinase (EML4-ALK) translocation therefore raising the possibility that these tumors may be amenable to treatment with ALK inhibitors.

Clinical Behavior

Similar to signet ring cell carcinomas of the gastrointestinal tract, their lung counterparts also follow an aggressive behavior. In the series reported by Castro et al. [121], 50 % of the patients in whom follow-up was obtained have died within 12 months. Thus, it appears important to separate these tumors from other adenocarcinomas with more favorable histology.

"Secretory Endometrioid-Like" Adenocarcinoma

This growth pattern for adenocarcinoma has been recognized recently [121]. Although only a few cases have been reported in the literature, the authors have been able to evaluate many other cases with similar features. The most important aspect of recognizing these tumors as a specific growth pattern of adenocarcinoma is to emphasize and separate these tumors from fetal adenocarcinoma (pulmonary blastoma, monophasic type). Separating these two tumors may have important therapeutic considerations. The patients described so far are adult men and women between the ages of 52 and 81 years. There appears no predilection for any lung or lung segment. The tumors may be central or peripheral lung masses, and the patients may also present with symptoms depending on the anatomic location of the tumor.

Microscopic Features

The low-power view is that of a complex glandular proliferation destroying normal lung parenchyma. This complex glandular architecture is composed of branching tubules and papillae with a variable dense desmoplastic stroma. Higher magnification shows that the glands are composed of a monolayer of medium to large cuboidal to columnar cells lining the tubules and papillae. Cytoplasmic clearing reminiscent of secretory type of endometrium is the most striking feature. Areas of necrosis and/or hemorrhage may also alternate in some cases. High mitotic activity and/or prominent nuclear atypia is not common (Fig. 3.21a–e).

Immunohistochemical Features

In the cases reported by Steinhauer et al. [122], the tumors were positive for keratin 7 and TTF-1, while tumor cells were negative for keratin 20, WT-1, chromogranin, and progesterone and estrogen receptors.

Clinical Behavior

The clinical behavior for these tumors may be closely related to the clinical staging at the time of diagnosis.

Hepatoid Adenocarcinoma

This type of histopathological growth pattern is extremely unusual, and only a few cases have been reported in the literature [123–129]. All the reported cases have been in adult men between the ages of 35 and 82 years. The size of the tumors has varied from 3 cm to more than 10 cm in greatest dimension. The most important characteristic of this particular tumor is the production of alpha-fetoprotein.

Microscopic Features

The tumor characteristically shows the presence of a neoplastic cellular proliferation arranged in cords or sheets of

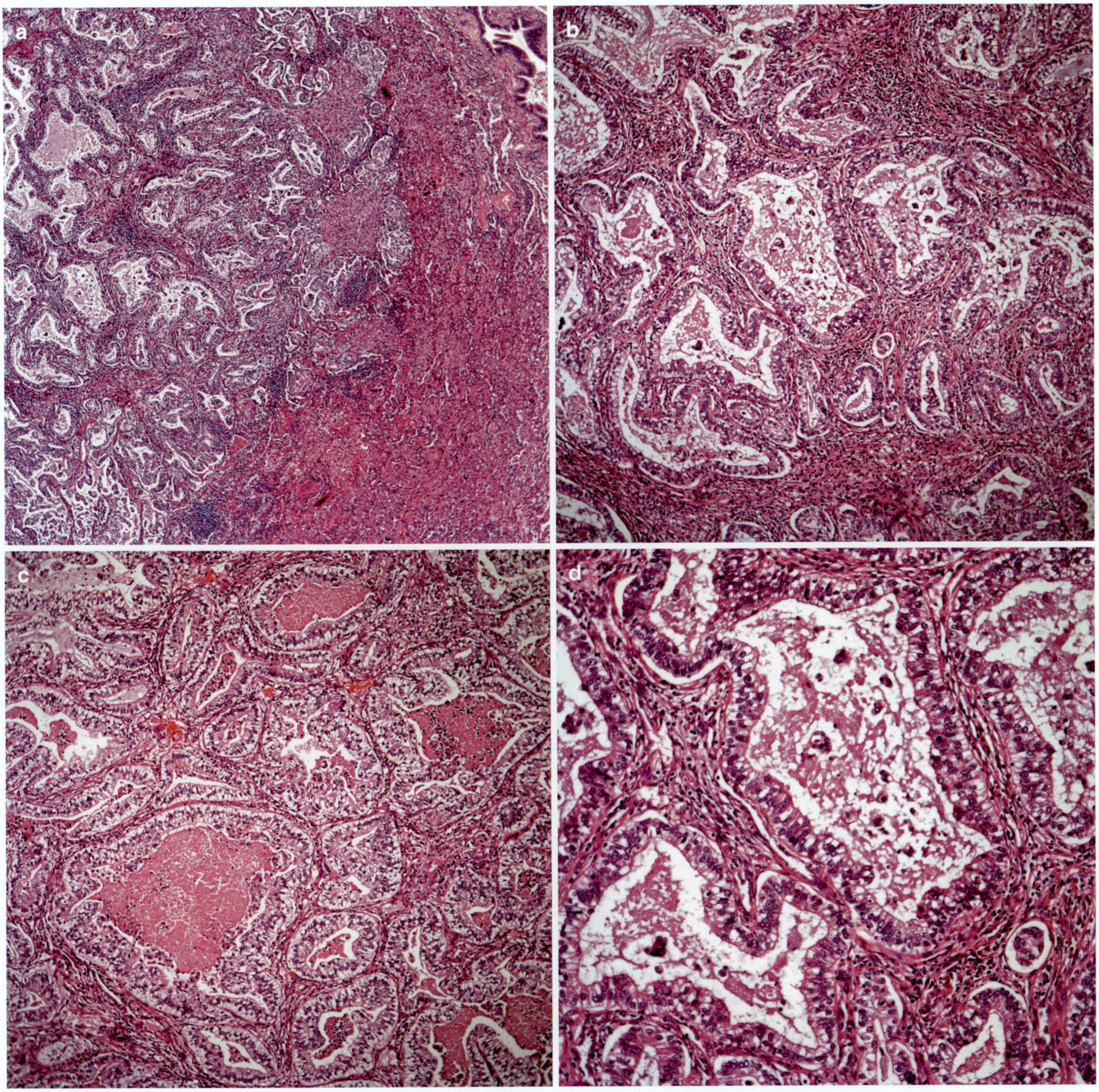

Fig. 3.21 (**a**) Low-power view of a secretory endometrioid-like adenocarcinoma of the lung. Note the compressed lung parenchyma. (**b**) Atypical glandular proliferation replacing normal lung parenchyma. (**c**) Neoplastic glands with comedo-like necrosis. (**d**) Malignant glands in a back-to-back arrangement. (**e**) Higher magnification showing malignant glands with features similar to those seen in secretory endometrium

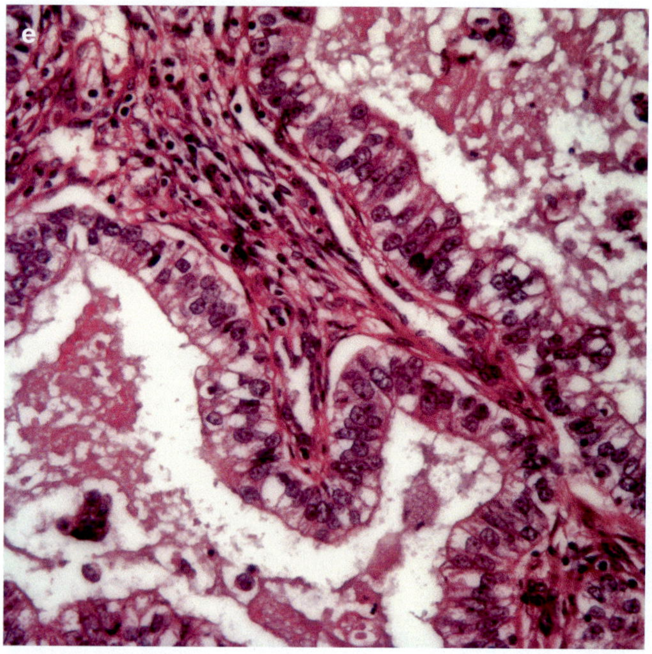

Fig. 3.21 (continued)

tumor cells. Higher magnification shows a neoplastic cellular proliferation of medium-size cells with ample eosinophilic cytoplasm and round to oval nuclei, some of them showing prominent nucleoli (Fig. 3.22a–d). This cellular proliferation mimics the normal architecture of the liver parenchyma. In some cells, it is possible to identify the presence of hyaline globules, which can be more apparent with histochemical stains for PAS. Necrosis, hemorrhage, and/or increased mitotic activity is not common in these tumors.

Immunohistochemical Features

The most important immunohistochemical features are the presence of positive staining for alpha-fetoprotein. However, due the rarity of these neoplasms, there does not exist a more extensive immunohistochemical study of these cases.

Clinical Behavior

Of the few cases reported, the majority of patients have died within 2 years after initial diagnosis. However, there are a couple of cases in which the clinical course has been less aggressive with survival of more than 3 years.

Oncocytic Adenocarcinoma

This is a relatively newly described growth pattern of adenocarcinoma. Solis et al. [130] described 16 patients with primary oncocytic lung carcinomas. The patients were adult individuals between the ages of 47 and 81 (median: 75 years), who complained of symptoms of cough, chest pain, and shortness of breath. Interestingly, 88 % of the patients were in stage I while the remaining 12 % were in stages II and III. The tumor size ranged from 1.2 to 4.9 cm in greatest dimension. In addition, it was noted that only two of the patients were non smokers, while the rest of the patients were either current or former smokers. Nevertheless, the main histological characteristic of these neoplasms was the presence of prominent oncocytic cytoplasmic features.

Histological Features

The tumors as they were described belong to the conventional types of well, moderately, and poorly differentiated adenocarcinomas. The growth patterns described were acinar, solid, papillary, and bronchioloalveolar, which were present in different proportions. Cytologically, the tumors were composed of medium-size cells with ample eosinophilic cytoplasm, round nuclei, and prominent nucleoli (Fig. 3.23a–g). Scattered larger cells were present resembling "oncoblasts." Necrosis was observed in seven cases that represented 10–50 % of the tumors. Mitotic activity was present in all the tumors and ranged from 1 to 8 mitotic figures/10 HPF.

Immunohistochemical and Molecular Features

Keratin 7 and TTF-1 showed positive staining in the tumors studied, while thyroglobulin was negative and cytokeratin 20 was focally positive in two cases. Mitochondrial antigen showed variable staining. In addition, DC-LAMP and PE-10 immunohistochemical stains were performed to document the presence of Clara cell differentiation; however, variable positive staining was obtained in a few cases. From a molecular point of view, three cases (20 %) harbored EGFR mutations while three cases showed K-ras mutations.

Clinical Behavior

The overall survival was 88 % while the recurrence-free survival was of 75 % at 2 years. In general terms, five patients had recurrence (ranged 3–32 months) while two patients died of tumor (7–47 months). We consider that similar to other types of adenocarcinoma, clinical staging at the time of diagnosis is the most reliable parameter to evaluate prognosis.

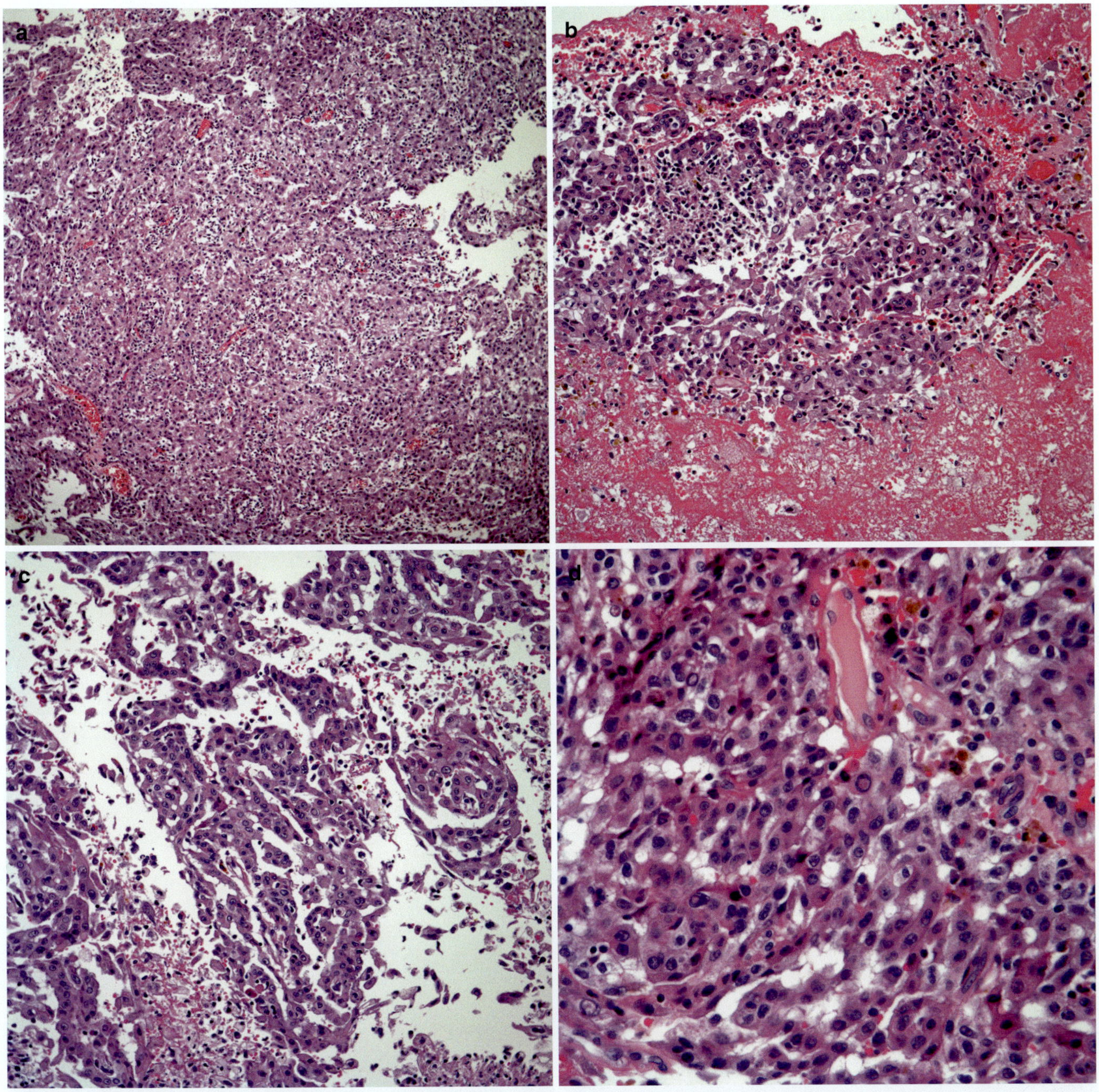

Fig. 3.22 (**a**) Hepatoid adenocarcinoma of the lung showing sheets of neoplastic cells. (**b**) The neoplastic cells are embedded in fibrinoid exudates. (**c**) Neoplastic cells arranged in cords mimicking "liver plates". (**d**) Higher magnification showing medium-size cells with round nuclei, some showing nucleoli while others show intranuclear inclusions

Miscellaneous Features

As it is expected, the growth patterns of adenocarcinoma are not limited to those that have been described in the literature. In some cases, different growth patterns may be seen as a small or large component of these tumors to a point of making the diagnosis of a primary lung tumor more challenging. Some of those growth patterns may include a cribriform pattern (Fig. 3.24a,b) that may be easily confused with metastatic breast carcinoma or an intestinal pattern in which the tumor acquires features similar to those seen in colorectal adenocarcinomas (Fig. 3.25a,b). Adenomatoid adenocarcinoma shows features in which the tumor resembles true adenomatoid tumors (Fig. 3.26a,b). Two other unusual growth patterns include adenocarcinomas with prominent syncytial giant cells, which can mimic choriocarcinomas (Fig. 3.27a–e). As a matter of fact, in some cases of these tumors, it is possible to detect increase of human chorionic gonadotropin in their serum. Also, adenocarcinomas

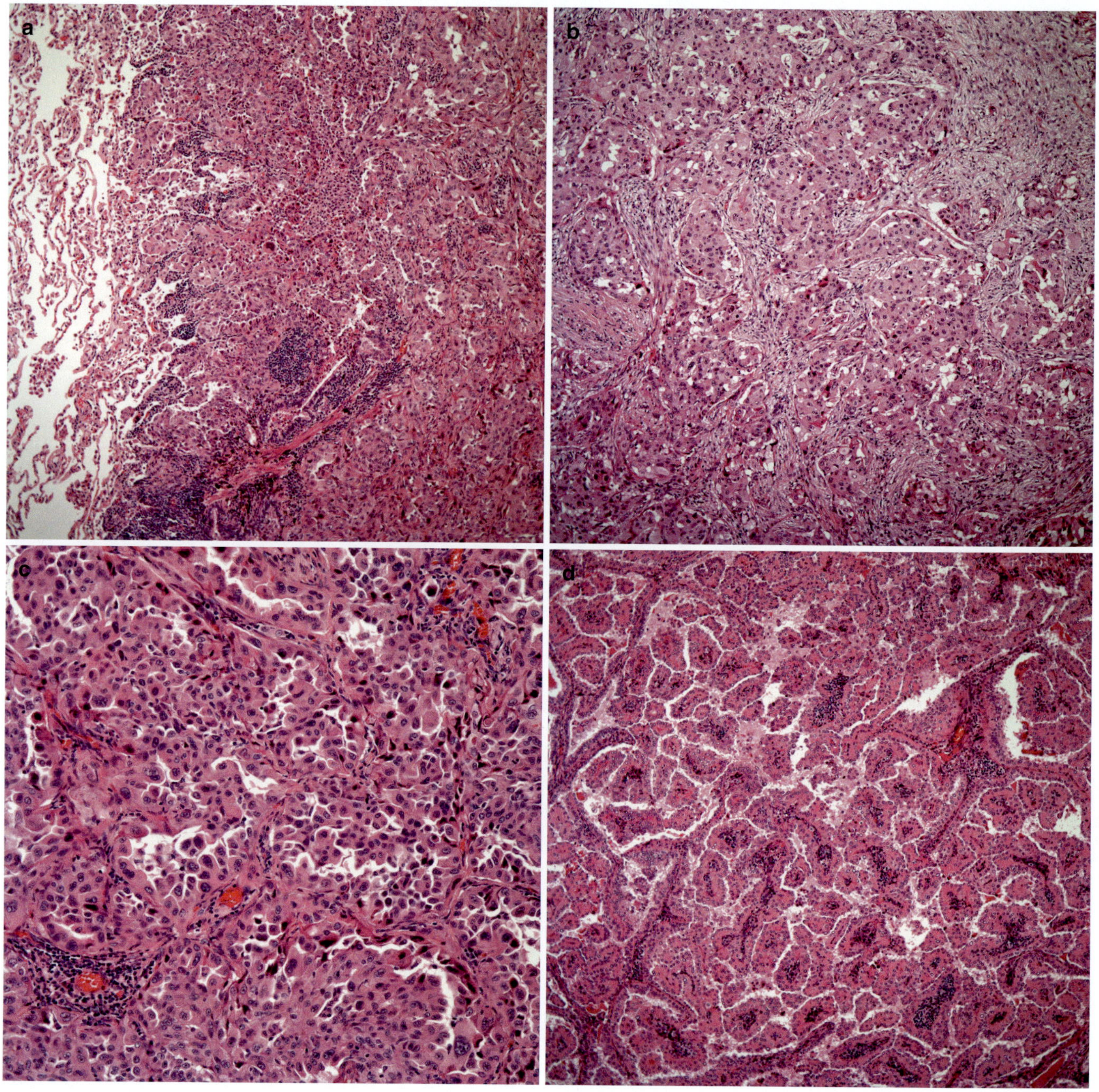

Fig. 3.23 (**a**) Oncocytic adenocarcinoma of the lung showing neoplastic cells destroying normal lung architecture. (**b**) Nests of neoplastic cells replacing lung parenchyma. (**c**) More conventional glandular proliferation. Note the marked oncocytic changes. (**d**) Prominent papillary growth pattern. (**e**) Papillary fronds admixed with inflammatory cells. (**f**) Papillary proliferation with focal glandular areas containing "colloid-like" material. (**g**) Higher magnification showing cells with ample oncocytic cytoplasm. Note the absence of marked nuclear atypia or mitotic activity

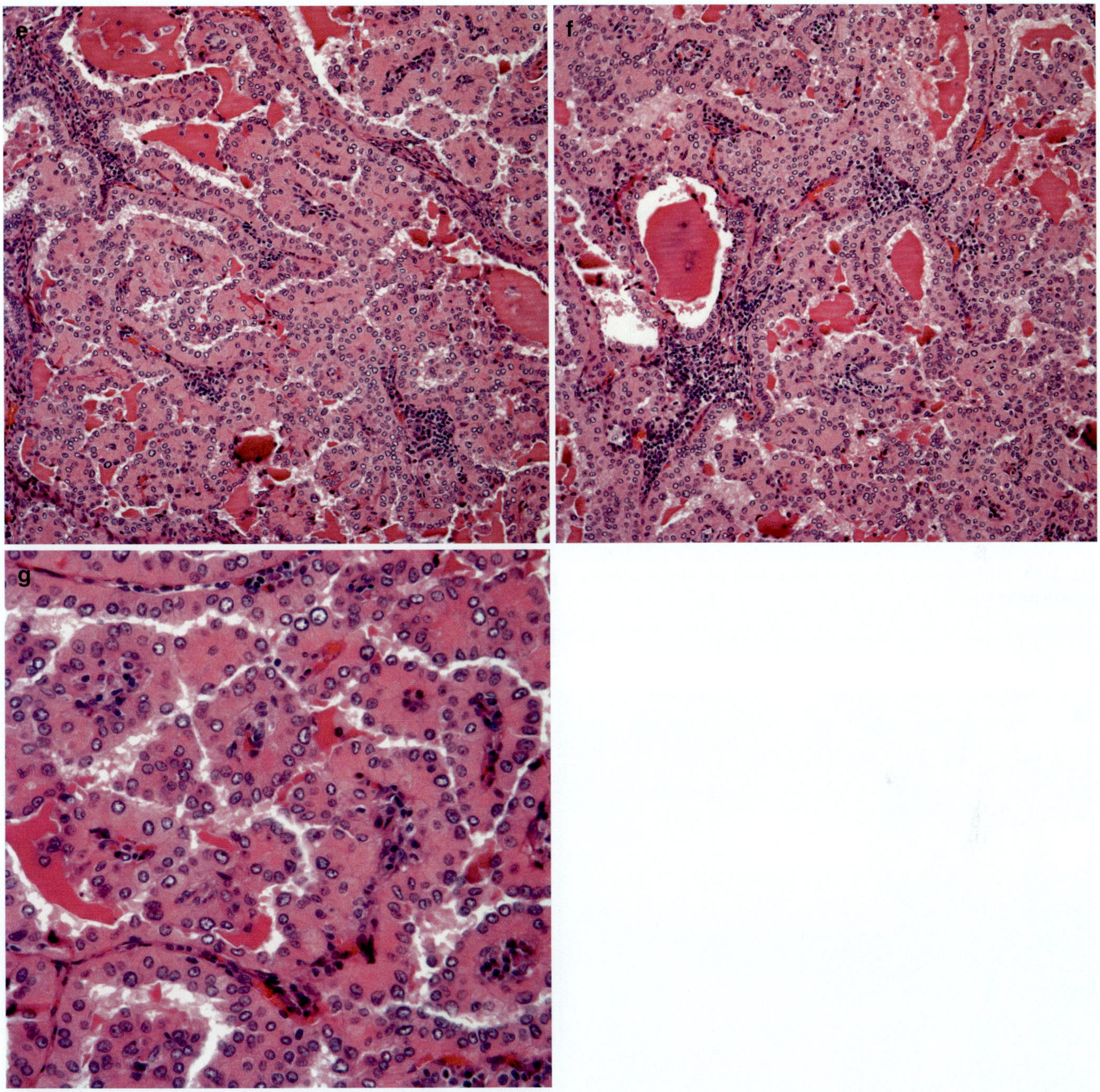

Fig. 3.23 (continued)

showing features similar to those described for Warthin tumors can occasionally be seen (Fig. 3.28a,b).

In addition, it is important to mention that some adenocarcinoma may also show unusual cytological features such as the presence of malignant glands, which are lined by ciliated epithelium. This feature may pose a problem in interpretation as the presence of ciliated epithelium is often associated with a benign glandular proliferation. Also important to mention is the association of some adenocarcinomas with prominent granulomatous changes (Fig. 3.29a,b). In such instances, it is worth pursuing these cases with special stains to rule out the possibility of a concurrent infectious process.

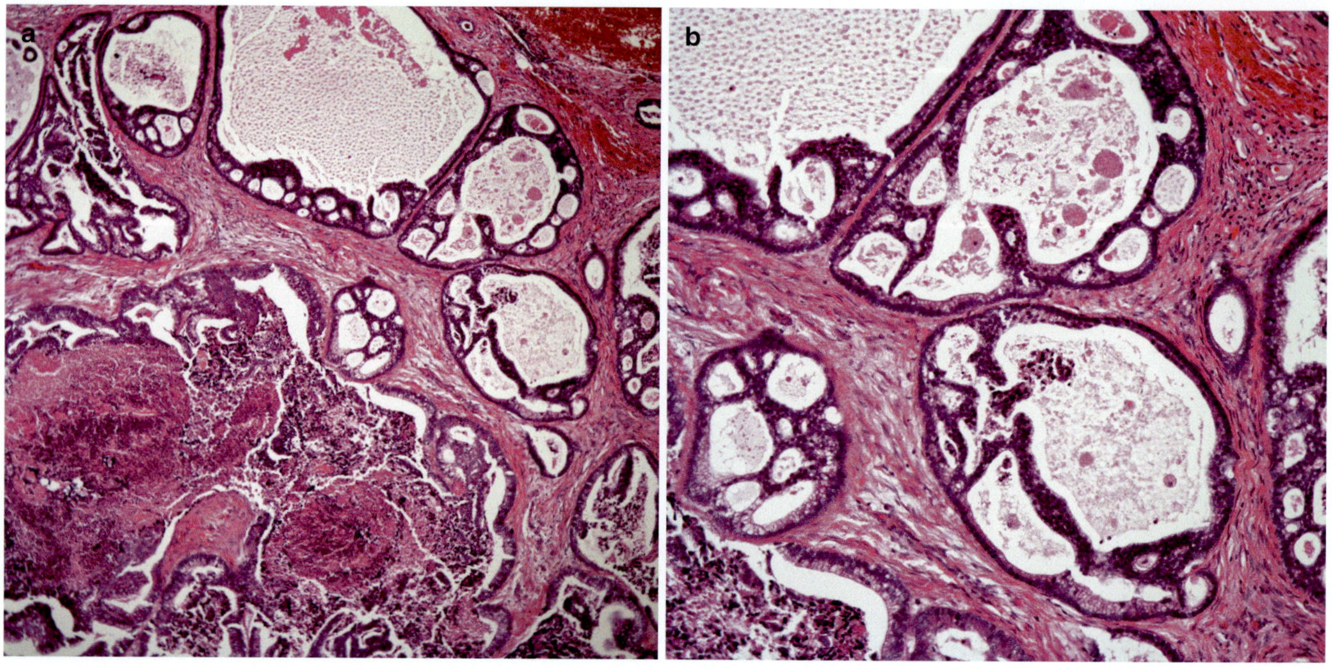

Fig. 3.24 (**a**) Pulmonary adenocarcinoma with prominent cribriform pattern. (**b**) Higher magnification showing so-called Roman bridge-like growth pattern

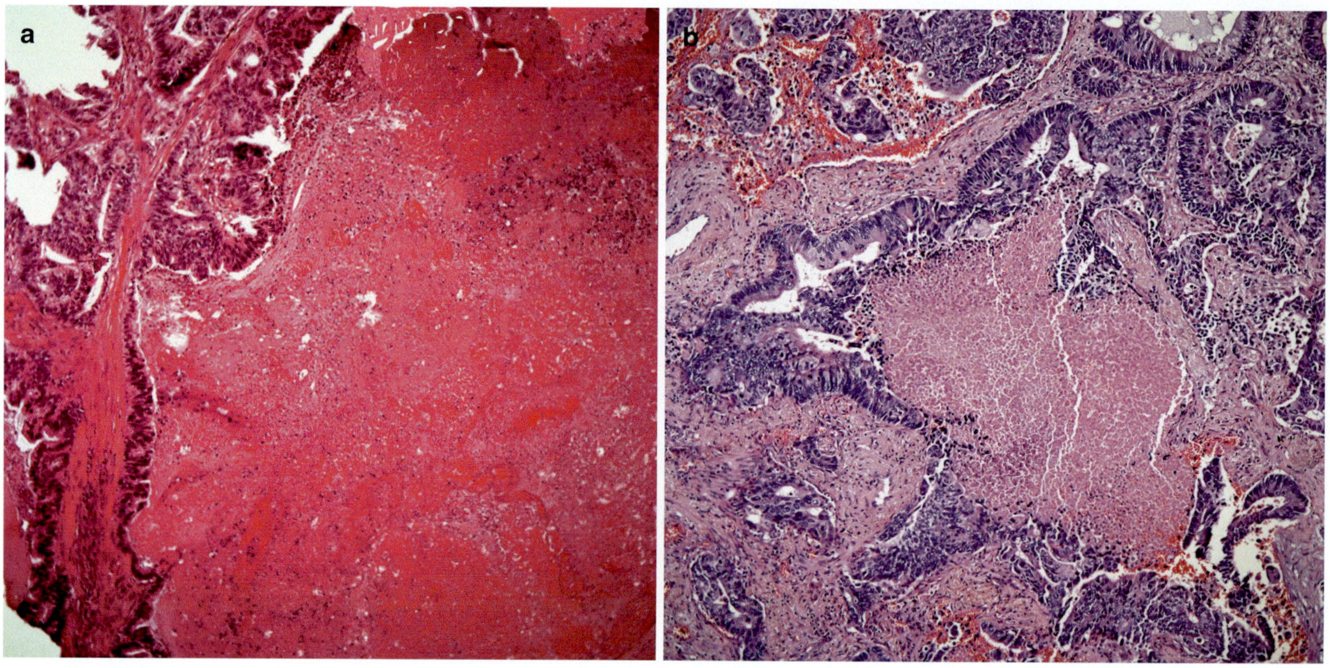

Fig. 3.25 (**a**) Intestinal-type adenocarcinoma of the lung showing extensive areas of hemorrhage and necrosis. (**b**) More glandular appearance with extensive necrosis

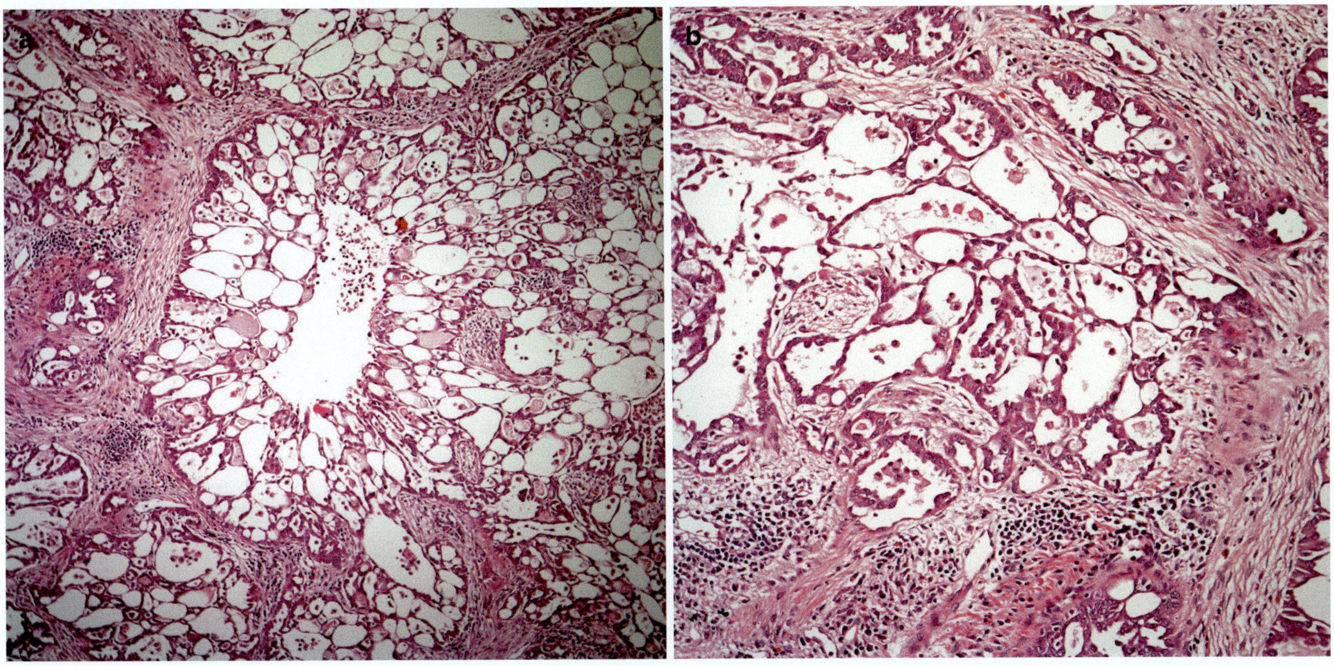

Fig. 3.26 (**a**) Lung adenocarcinoma with prominent adenomatoid growth pattern. (**b**) Higher magnification of adenomatoid adenocarcinoma. Note the absence of marked nuclear atypia or mitotic activity

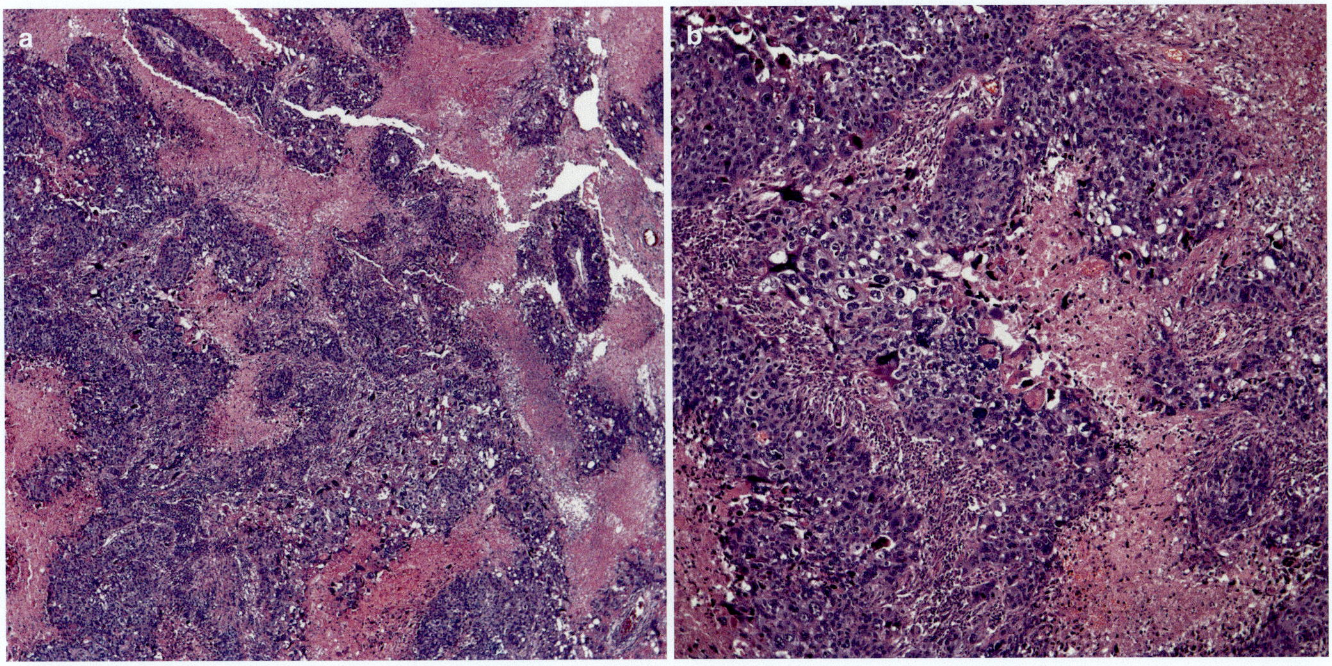

Fig. 3.27 (**a**) Low-power view of a pulmonary adenocarcinoma mimicking choriocarcinoma. (**b**) High-grade neoplastic cellular proliferation with extensive necrosis. (**c**) Dual neoplastic cellular proliferation with presence of multinucleated giant cells. (**d**) In some areas, more conventional glandular component is present. (**e**) Immunohistochemical stain for human chorionic gonadotropin showing positive staining in tumor cells

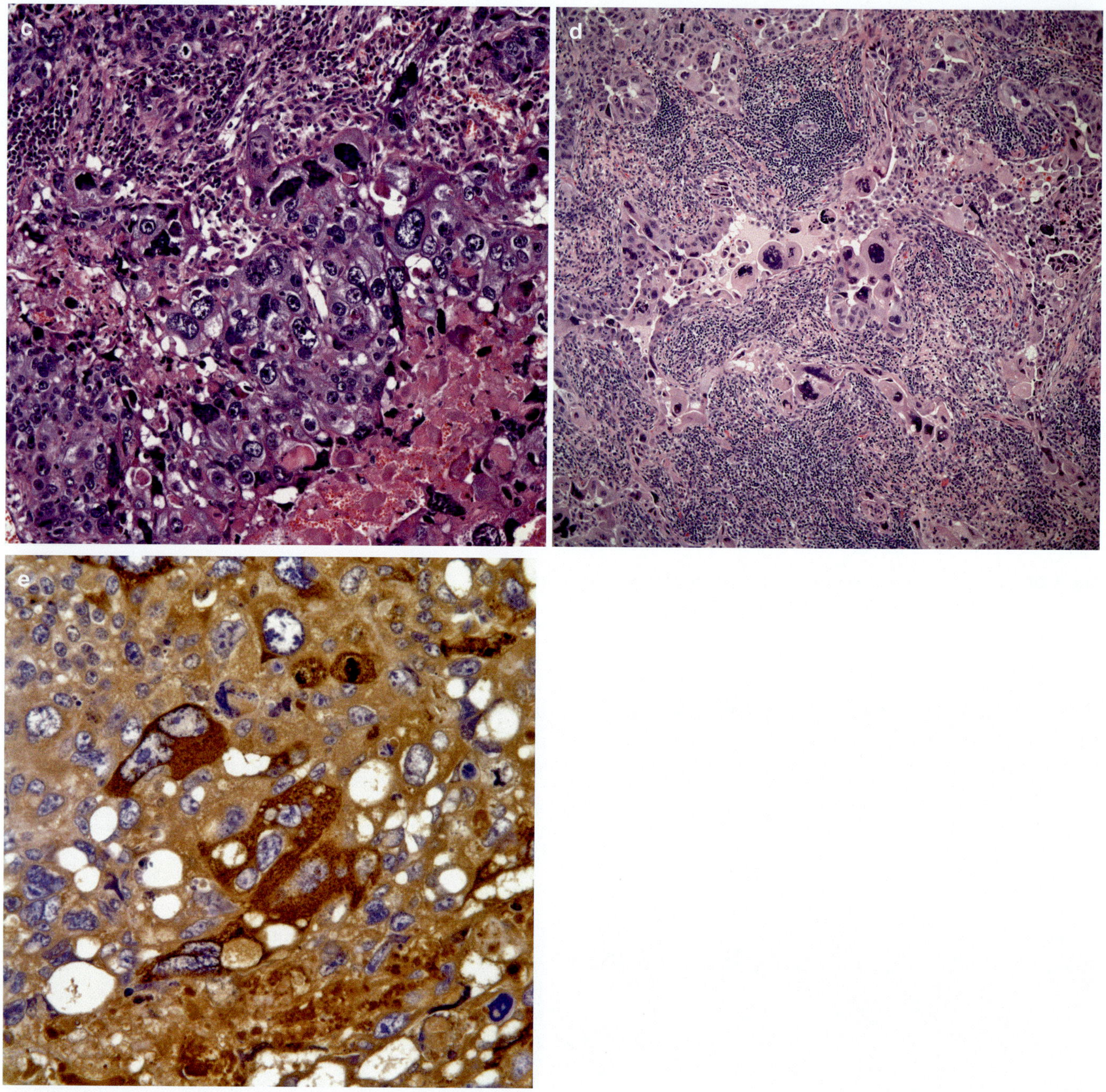

Fig. 3.27 (continued)

Squamous Cell Carcinoma

Even though squamous cell carcinoma is statistically less common than adenocarcinoma, it is a major component of the non-small cell category of tumors. Just like the other variants of non-small cell carcinoma, the overall survival of patients with squamous cell carcinoma depends on the clinical stage at the time of diagnosis. Worth mentioning is also the fact that squamous cell carcinomas are commonly associated with tobacco use. In this type of tumor one can often observe the different evolutional changes of the disease, represented by the presence of mild, moderate, and severe dysplasia that may eventually progress to in situ and/or invasive squamous cell carcinoma.

At this point, it is important to address the features of the different forms of noninvasive neoplasia, characterized by the different dysplasias and carcinoma in situ:

- *Mild dysplasia*: This diagnosis is made when one encounters cellular atypia at the basal or just above the basal cell

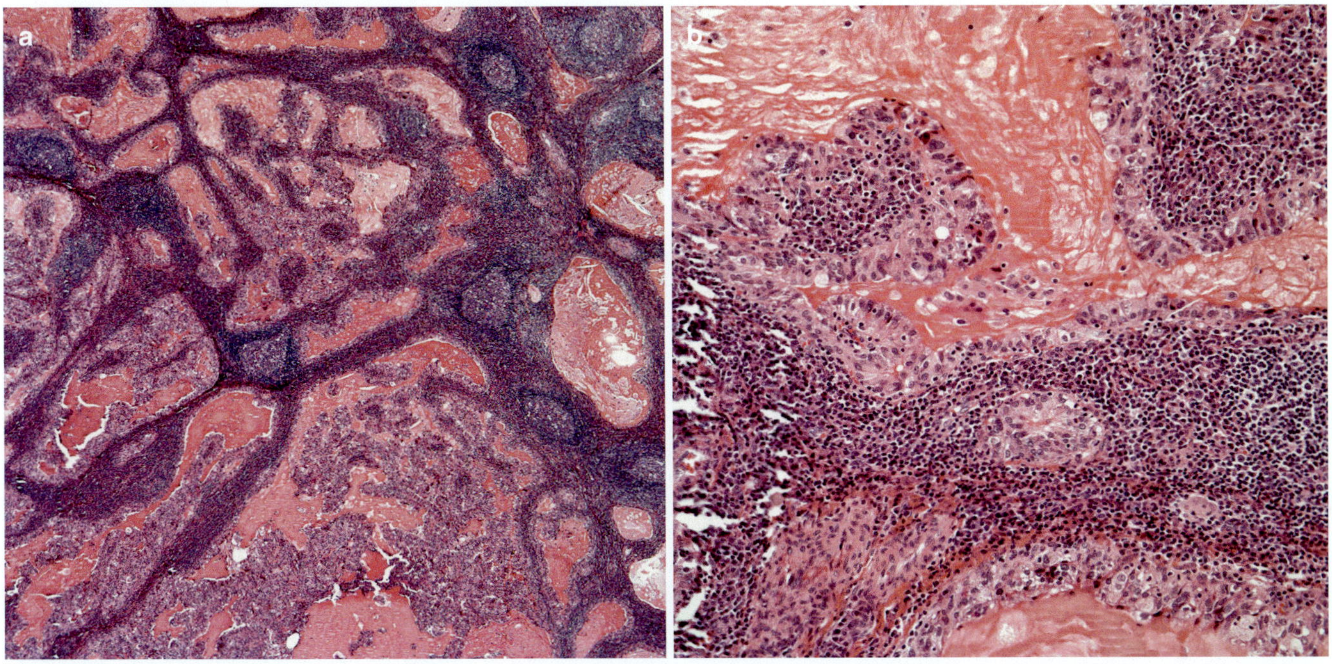

Fig. 3.28 (**a**) Pulmonary adenocarcinoma with Warthin-like growth pattern. (**b**) Higher magnification showing glandular with inflammatory component

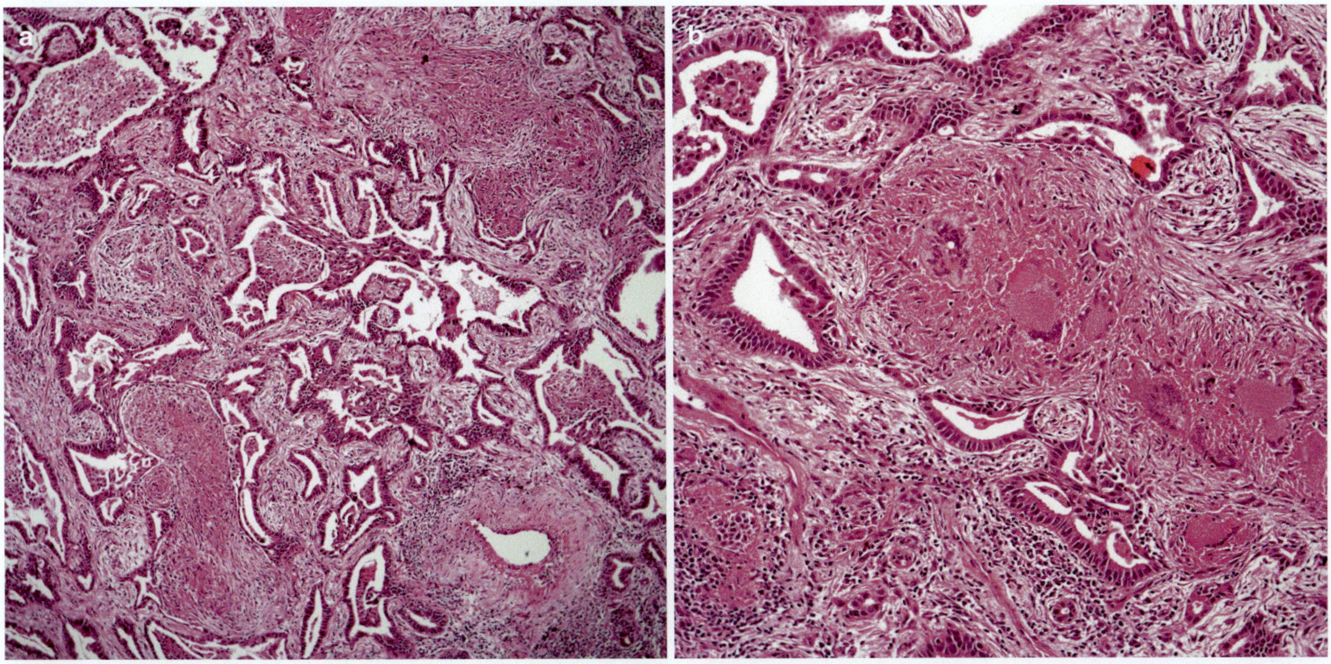

Fig. 3.29 (**a**) Pulmonary adenocarcinoma with associated granulomatous reaction. (**b**) Closer view of the granulomatous inflammatory reaction. Note the presence of giant cells

layer. The nuclei may be more hyperchromatic, and mitotic figures may be seen. However, no mitotic figures or cellular atypia is seen in the midportion of the mucosa, which shows normal maturation.

- *Moderate dysplasia*: Essentially similar to the findings in mild dysplasia, however, the cellular atypia and mitotic activity are not limited to the lower portion of the mucosa. In addition, the cellular atypia may be more pronounced, and mitotic figures may be seen in the midportion of the mucosa. However, one is still able to identify maturation of the upper portion of the mucosa.

- *Severe dysplasia/carcinoma in situ*: Both of those conditions are intrinsically associated and represent the same pathological process. Histologically, the mucosa shows full thickness cellular atypia and mitotic figures occupy the entire mucosa, while maturation is essentially absent. Atypical mitotic figures may be seen at any level, and cellular atypia is much more pronounced (Figs. 3.30a,b and 3.31a,b). In some cases, the process may extend into endobronchial glands, without however being invasive. Careful attention must be placed to that feature and careful evaluation is needed in cases in which there is marked chronic inflammation, which may either obscure the true nature of the process or mimic an invasive neoplasm. In some unusual cases of in situ squamous cell carcinoma, it is possible to observe the presence of changes in the epithelium, which histologically are similar to the changes seen in Paget's disease. Although this pagetoid change may be extensive, one is still able to find areas of more conventional squamous cell differentiation.

Invasive Squamous Cell Carcinoma

Traditionally, squamous cell carcinomas of the lung just like their counterparts in other anatomic areas have been divided into well, moderately, and poorly differentiated types. Most of the factors influencing such differentiation refer to either the presence of keratinization or presence of intercellular bridges. Thus, the closer the tumor mimics normal squamous epithelium, the better will be the grade of differentiation.

Clinical Features

Similar to other non-small cell carcinomas, patients may complain of cough, dyspnea, hemoptysis, and/or thoracic pain. These symptoms are generally associated with the anatomic location of the tumor. Those tumors that are centrally located are more likely to produce symptoms associated with obstruction, while those tumors that are in the periphery of the lung are more likely to produce thoracic pain due to the large size that some tumors may reach.

Macroscopic Features

Squamous cell carcinomas may present as polypoid tumors obstructing the lumen of the airway. On the other hand, they may be seen extrinsically pushing into airway structures as the tumors reach a larger size. Also, squamous cell carcinomas may be seen in the periphery of the lung in a subpleural location or infiltrating the pleura with direct invasion into the soft tissues of the chest wall.

The tumors may range in size from under 1 cm to tumor masses larger than 10 cm in greatest dimension. They are white tan and well demarcated but not encapsulated. The cut surface of these tumors may be homogeneous or show

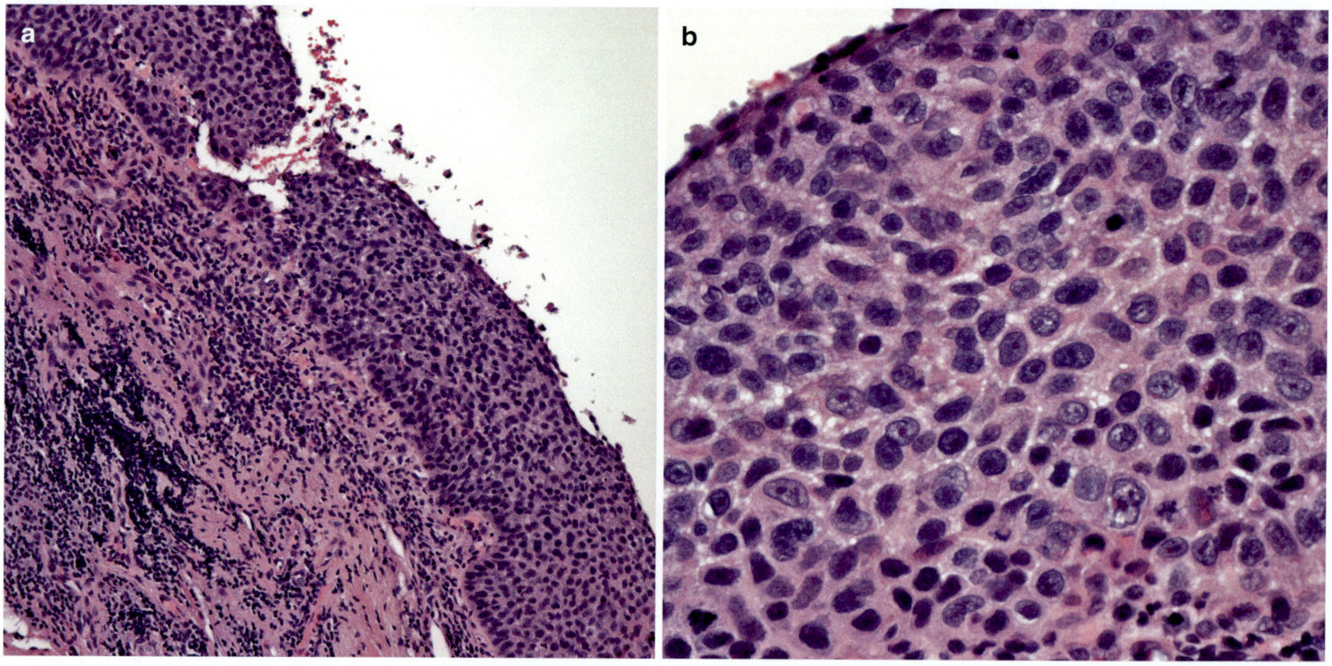

Fig. 3.30 (**a**) Squamous epithelium showing squamous cell carcinoma in situ. (**b**) Higher magnification showing full thickness dysplasia. Note the presence of mitotic figures

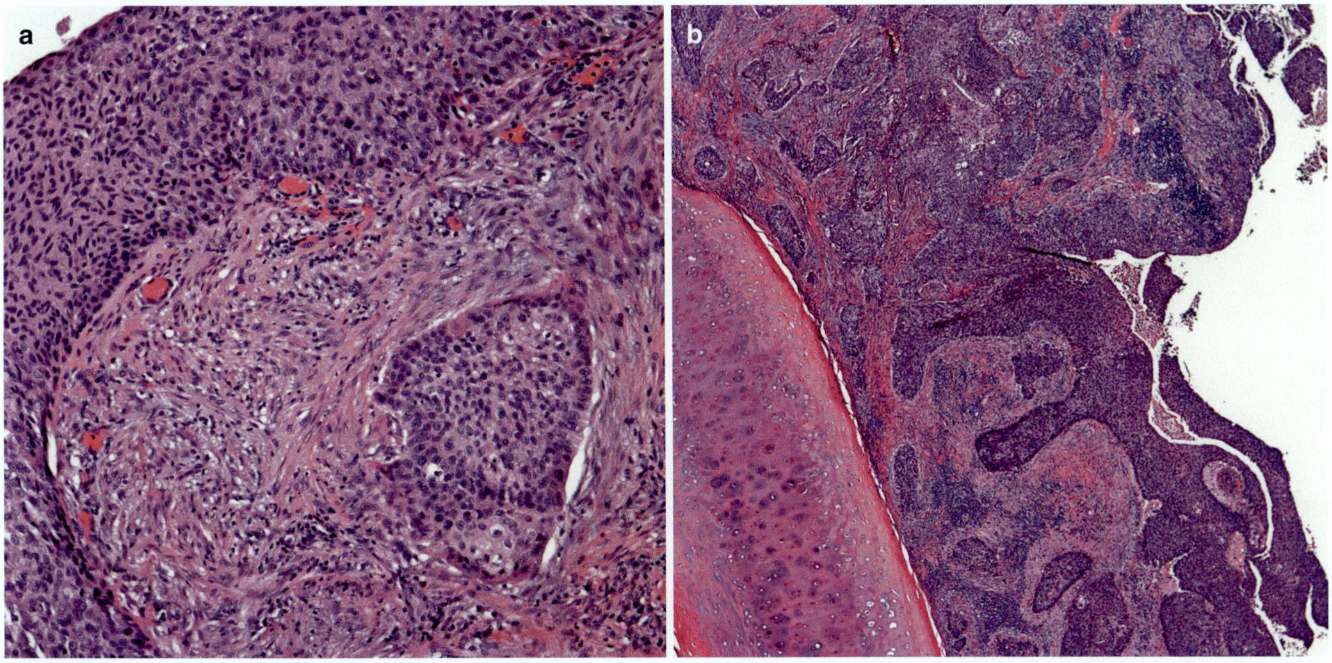

Fig. 3.31 (**a**) Squamous cell carcinoma predominantly in situ with only a focal microscopic focus of microinvasion. (**b**) Invasive squamous cell carcinoma with overlying in situ component

extensive areas of necrosis and/or hemorrhage. In some cases, the tumor is characterized by a cavitary tumor mass.

Histological Features

As stated previously, conventionally squamous cell carcinomas have been graded as well-, moderately, and poorly differentiated tumors. Their features are as follows:

- *Well-differentiated squamous cell carcinoma*: These tumors appear to show areas of keratinization and easily identifiable intercellular bridges. The tumor may grow in sheets or ribbons destroying normal lung parenchyma. The neoplastic cells are oval with moderate amounts of eosinophilic cytoplasm, small nuclei, and inconspicuous nucleoli. Mitotic figures are present and can be numerous (Fig. 3.32a–d). Areas of necrosis and/or hemorrhage are usually absent or may be only focally present.
- *Moderately differentiated squamous cell carcinoma*: The tumor may still show areas in which one can identify either keratinization or intercellular bridges. However, the tumor may show more extensive areas of hemorrhage and necrosis, which may obscure the true nature of the neoplasm. Mitotic figures and cellular pleomorphism are more prominent (Fig. 3.33a–c).
- *Poorly differentiated squamous cell carcinoma*: The tumor has a tendency to grow in sheets in which the tumor may not show definitive evidence of squamous differentiation. Extensive necrosis and hemorrhage may be present. The presence of cellular pleomorphism and mitotic activity is marked. However, in focal areas, one may still be able to find areas unequivocally showing squamous cell differentiation (Fig. 3.34a–f).

Histological Variants

Squamous cell carcinoma may show a variety of different growth patterns that can pose a problem in the diagnosis of these tumors. When the tumors show extensive areas of keratinization, the diagnosis is rather straightforward; however, when the tumor does not display this feature or belong to the unusual growth pattern associated with this subtype, then the diagnosis may not be so easily made, one may even have to apply immunohistochemical studies to properly determine the exact nature of the tumor. Some of the unusual features that may be present in squamous cell carcinoma include the following.

Exophytic Squamous Cell Carcinoma

This is an unusual variant of squamous cell carcinoma also known to some as "Sherwin tumor" in honor of one of the earliest. Sherwin et al. [131] documented the existence of

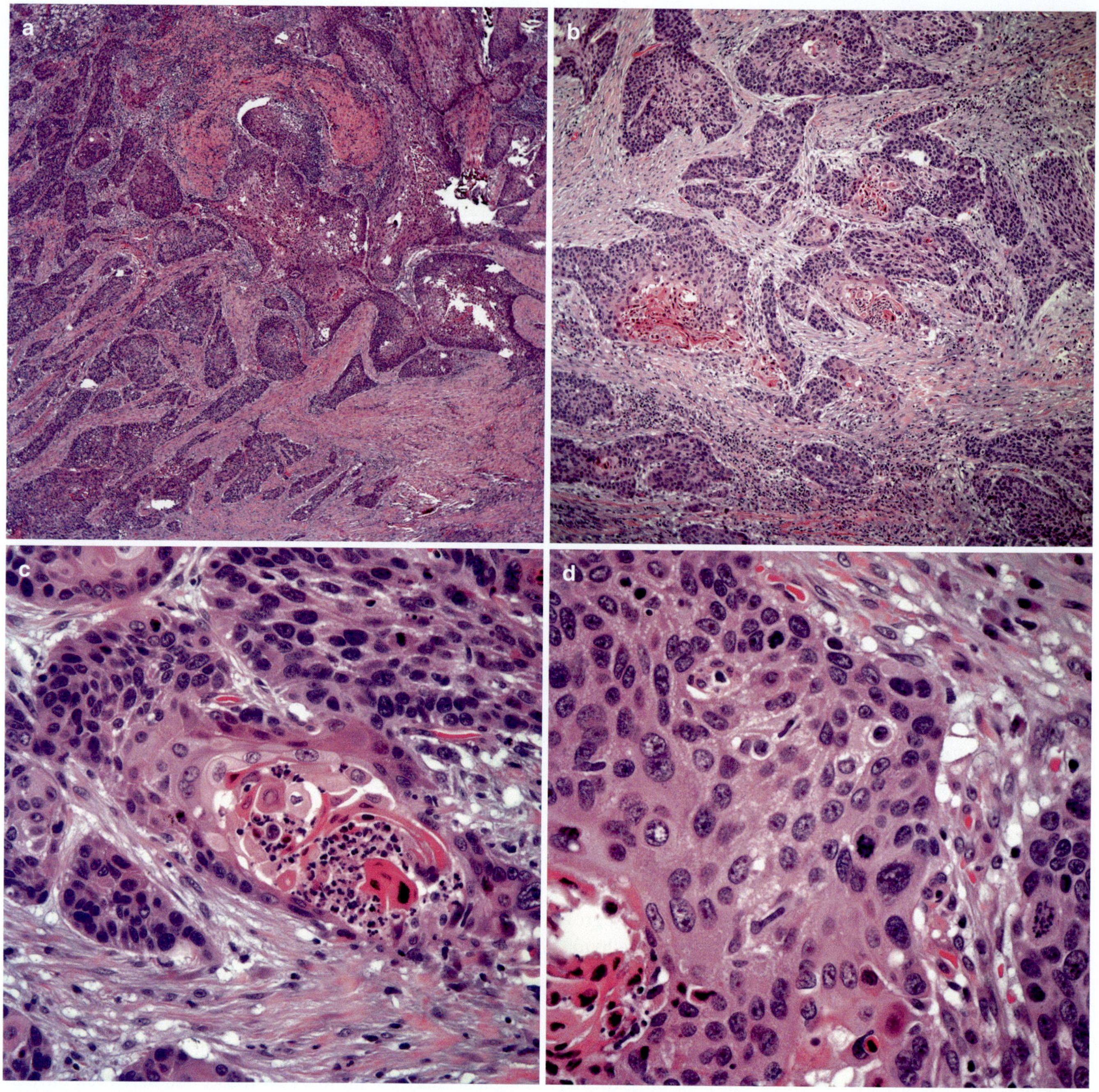

Fig. 3.32 (**a**) Well-differentiated squamous cell carcinoma showing keratinizing atypical squamous epithelium. (**b**) Haphazard tumor growth. Note the presence of keratinization. (**c**) Higher magnification showing keratin pearls. (**d**) Single-cell keratinization and cells showing intercellular bridges

this neoplasm after reviewing 85 patients diagnosed with squamous cell carcinoma. The author isolated nine patients in whom the tumor had the characteristic of an exophytic neoplasm. The patients were between the ages of 50 and 74 years and have undergone resection of the tumor. Some of the patients had lobectomy while others had pneumonectomy. The authors found that those patients with pneumonectomy had a more favorable outcome than those who were treated with lobectomy. Microscopically, the tumors, as the name implies, grew in an exophytic manner obstructing the airway. The tumors were of the well-differentiated type, and none of the patients had metastasis to lymph nodes. The authors noted that this type of squamous cell carcinoma might have a more favorable outcome than other more

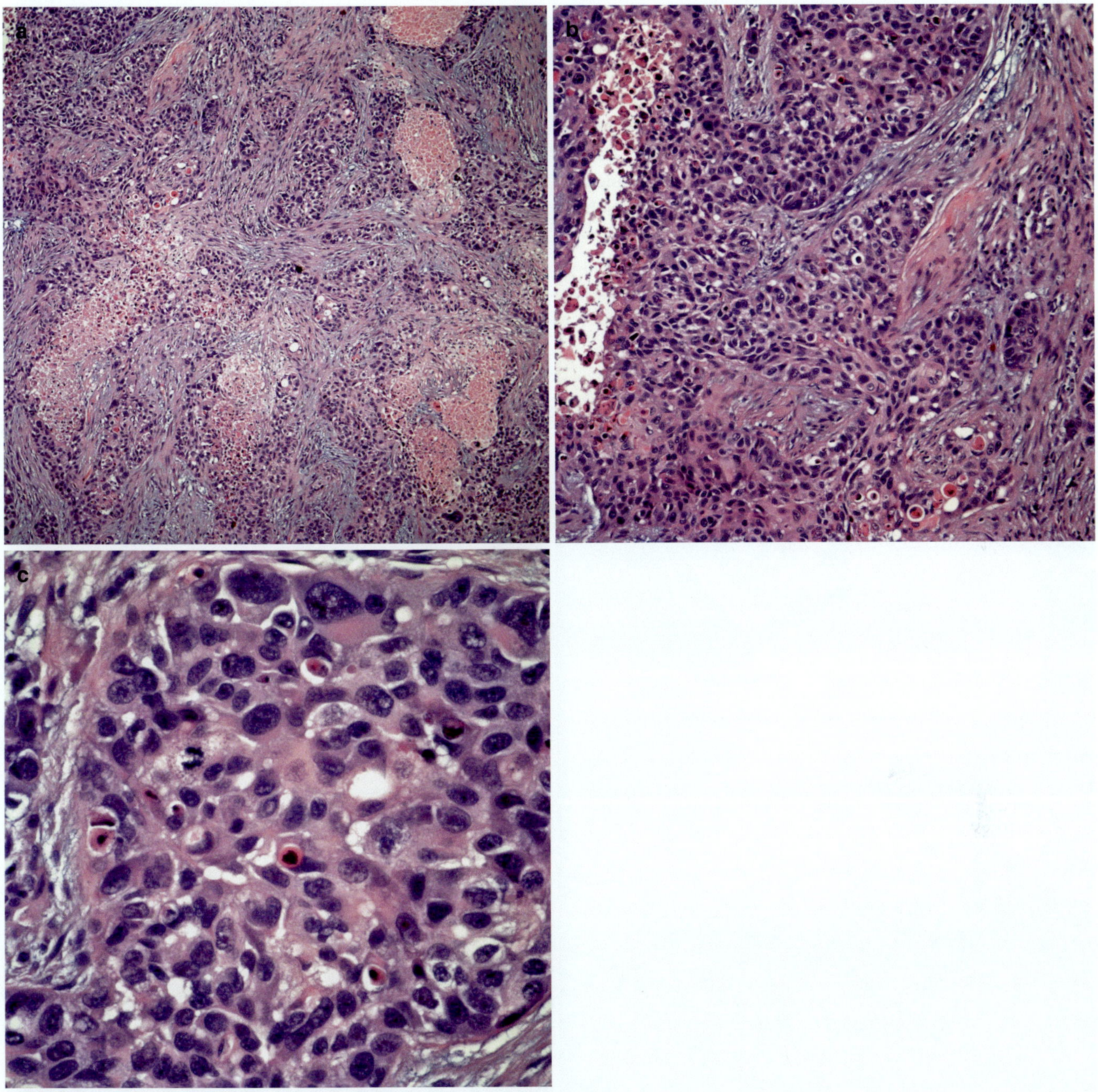

Fig. 3.33 (**a**) Moderately differentiated squamous cell carcinoma showing areas of necrosis. (**b**) Squamous carcinoma replacing lung parenchyma. (**c**) Higher magnification showing nuclear atypia and single cell keratinization

infiltrative tumors. Dulmet-Brender et al. [132] also presented their experience of 34 cases collected over 35 years and concluded that these tumors are almost always T1N0MO stage. However, the authors noted that the prognosis was not any better than that for any other non-small cell carcinoma of the same stage. The authors concluded that these tumors represent a special variant of squamous cell carcinoma rather than a tumor that is detected at an earlier stage. More recently, Cooper et al. [133] documented a similar occurrence in a 75-year-old woman in whom the initial chest radiographic studies were unremarkable, but the endobronchial tumor became evident on computed tomography (CT) scan. Resection of the mass was performed showing a papillary endobronchial neoplasm that did not extend into the adjacent lung parenchyma. Microscopically, all these lesions appear to have the same characteristics, namely, an exophytic tumor with squamous appearance, in some cases with extensive keratinization (Fig. 3.35a,b). Some tumors may acquire a papillary growth pattern in which the papillary projections show only a thin line of fibroconnective tissue with no evidence of invasion. The most important histological characteristic is the limitation of the tumor to extend exophytically into the bronchial lumen without invasion into the bronchial wall. On rare occasions, tumor extension into endobronchial glands may be seen but that is not common, and one should not see the presence of bronchial wall invasion. The papillary fronds of exophytic squamous cell carcinoma show cellular atypia, nuclear pleomorphism, and mitotic activity with some atypical mitoses.

Although the diagnosis of these tumors should not pose a problem from the histological point of view, there are some other lesions that may present in similar fashion and that may

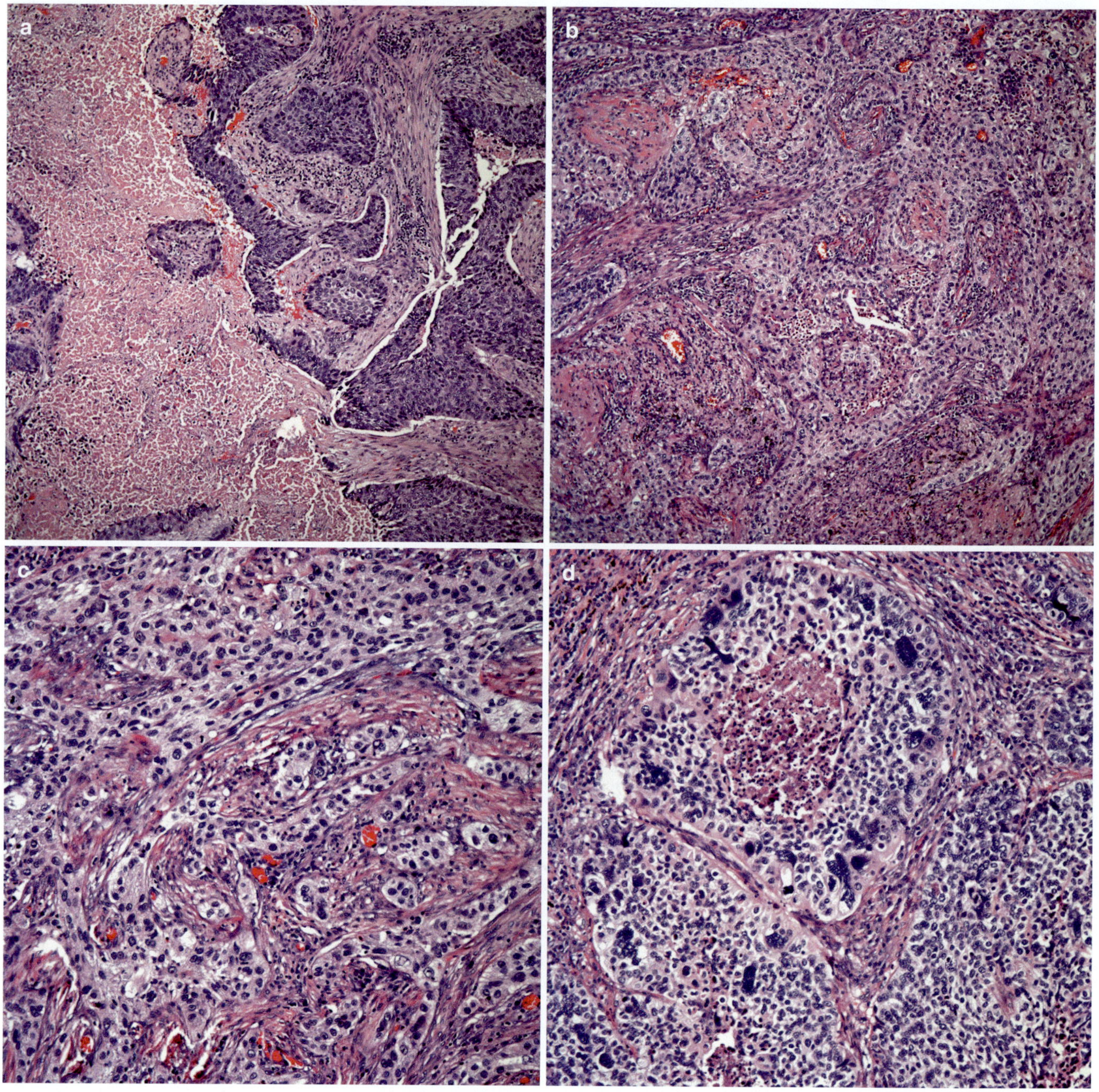

Fig. 3.34 (**a**) Low-power view of a poorly differentiated squamous cell carcinoma with necrosis. (**b**) Islands of neoplastic cells replacing lung parenchyma. (**c**) The tumors can grow in sheets of non-keratinizing epithelium. (**d**) Prominent nuclear atypia. (**e**) Nests of neoplastic cells resembling a neuroendocrine growth pattern. (**f**) Higher magnification showing islands of tumor cells with prominent nuclear pleomorphism and focal areas of keratinization

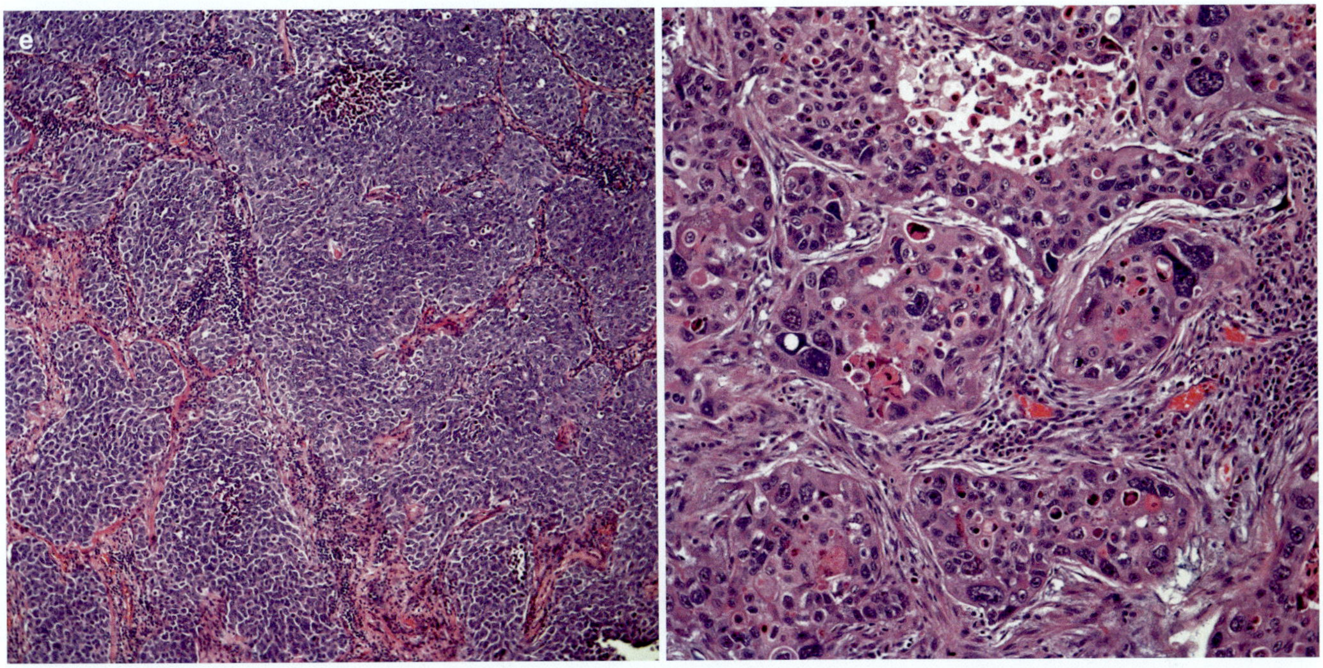

Fig. 3.34 (continued)

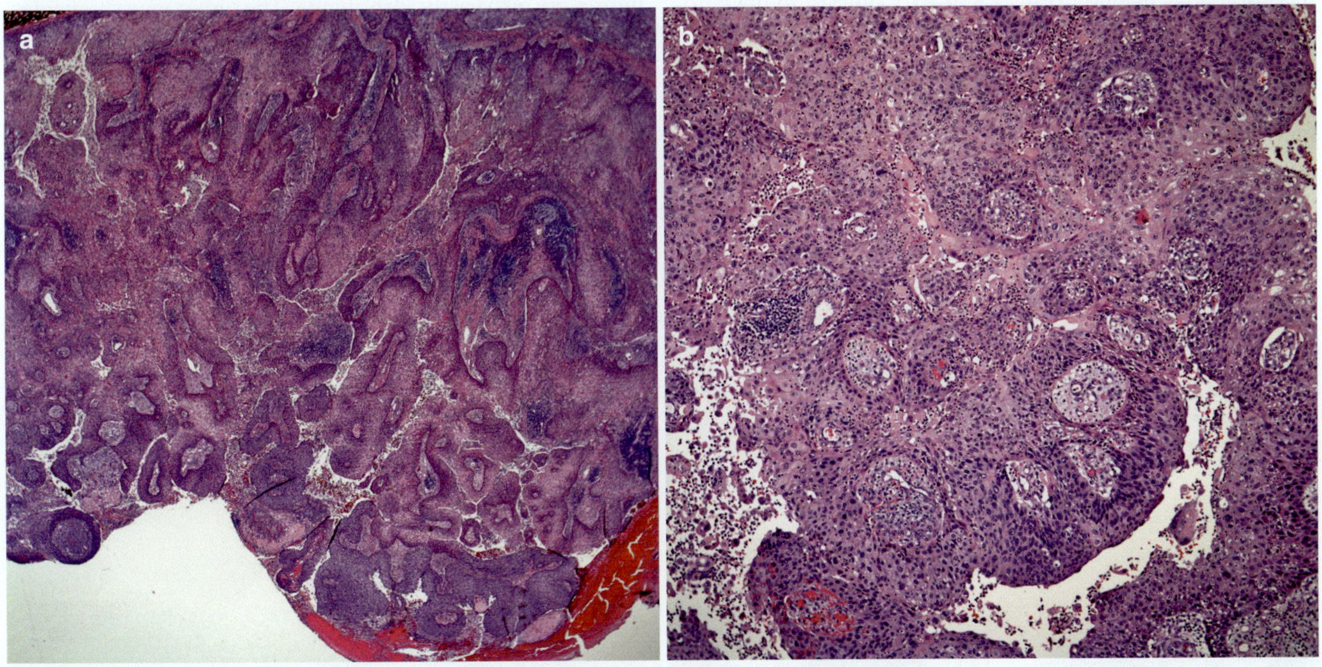

Fig. 3.35 (**a**) Exophytic squamous cell carcinoma. Note the keratoacanthomatous-like growth pattern. (**b**) Extensive areas of keratinization are common in this tumor

enter in the differential diagnoses. Laubscher [134] in 1969 described a tumor under the name of solitary squamous cell papilloma; histologically, the tumor was a keratinizing, noninvasive squamous cell neoplasm that based on the illustrations provided shares some features with the cases described by Sherwin et al. [131]. Nevertheless, the existence of noninvasive papillary neoplasms, such as solitary condylomatous papillomas and lower respiratory tract papillomatosis, is well known in the literature. Those cases show squamous epithelium in which there is still evidence of some maturation and in which focal areas may show areas of transition between squamous and non-squamous epithelium [134–137].

Cystic Squamous Cell Carcinoma

This variant of squamous cell carcinoma is based on the gross appearance of the tumor. These tumors are characterized by prominent cystically dilated spaces, which may be filled with necrotic or inflammatory debris. However, in the periphery of the tumor, one usually encounters otherwise conventional strands of squamous cell carcinoma that may be present in the form of squamous cell buds or ribbons of squamous cell carcinoma. Usually, these tumors are of the well-differentiated type that have undergone cystic and necrotic changes (Fig. 3.36a,b).

Small Cell Squamous Cell Carcinoma

This growth pattern is likely the most unusual and represents a very small percentage of these tumors. Interestingly, there is not a single series of cases reported, and in the great majority there are only single anecdotal cases that have been presented in textbooks [138]. Microscopically, the tumor shows a proliferation of rather small cells with oval nuclei and inconspicuous nucleoli (Fig. 3.37a–e). Contrary to the chromatin pattern in true small cell carcinomas, the one of the small cell variant of squamous cell carcinoma is not the typical "salt-and-pepper" type. Rather, the tumor cells possess a more smooth type of scant cytoplasm. In an endobronchial biopsy, one important clue to the diagnosis is the finding of adjacent squamous cell carcinoma in situ. On the other hand, in cases in which squamous cell carcinoma in situ is absent, one needs to identify areas in which the tumor may show focal keratinization or other clues of squamous cell differentiation. In more complicated cases, the use of immunohistochemical studies including neuroendocrine markers and keratin 5/6 and p63 may be helpful as the small cell variant of squamous cell carcinoma may show positive staining for keratin 5/6 and p63 with negative staining for neuroendocrine markers. However, one needs to be fully aware that some squamous cell carcinomas may show focal positive staining for some of the neuroendocrine markers, namely, synaptophysin.

Spindle Cell Squamous Cell Carcinoma

This is an unusual type of squamous cell carcinoma that can be confused with other spindle cell neoplasms, namely, sarcomas. The growth pattern is characterized by fascicles of fusiform cells with elongated nuclei and inconspicuous nucleoli, mitotic figures are increased, and atypical mitotic figures are also easily identifiable. The tumor may show interlacing fascicles or a subtle storiform growth pattern mimicking spindle cell sarcomas (Fig. 3.38a,b). However, in focal areas, the tumors may show areas of keratinization in the form of keratin pearls, single-cell keratinization, or frank foci of keratinization. The use of immunohistochemical studies

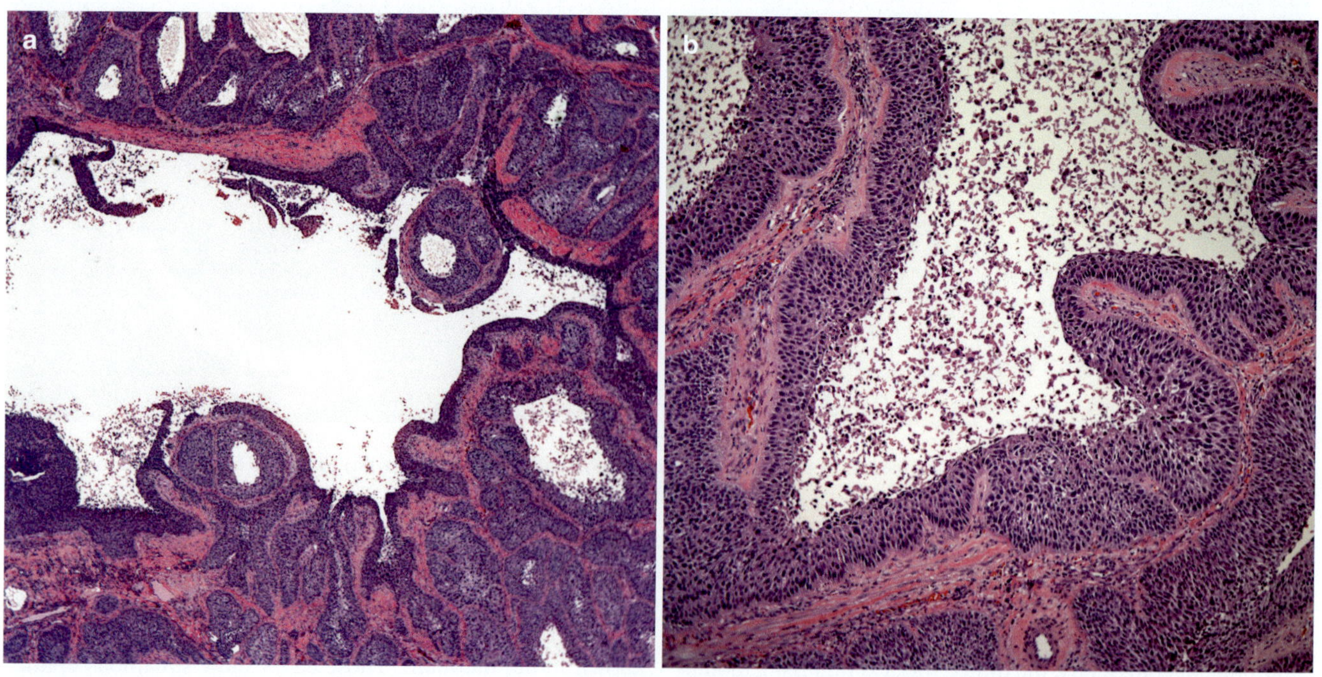

Fig. 3.36 (**a**) Cystic squamous cell carcinoma characterized by dilated cystic structures. (**b**) Higher magnification showing the cystic structures lined by squamous carcinoma

including epithelial markers such as broad spectrum keratin low molecular weight keratin, keratin 5/6, or p63 may help in separating these tumors from primary pulmonary sarcomas. Also, the use of electron microscopic studies may also be helpful as spindle cell carcinomas may show epithelial differentiation characterized by the presence of intercellular junctions and tonofilaments [139].

Basaloid Squamous Cell Carcinoma

This is an unusual variant of squamous cell carcinoma in which the growth pattern resembles that seen in basal cell carcinomas of the skin. The cells are arranged in islands of tumor cells with palisading of the nuclei. Mitotic figures are numerous, and nuclear atypia is prominent (Fig. 3.39a–c).

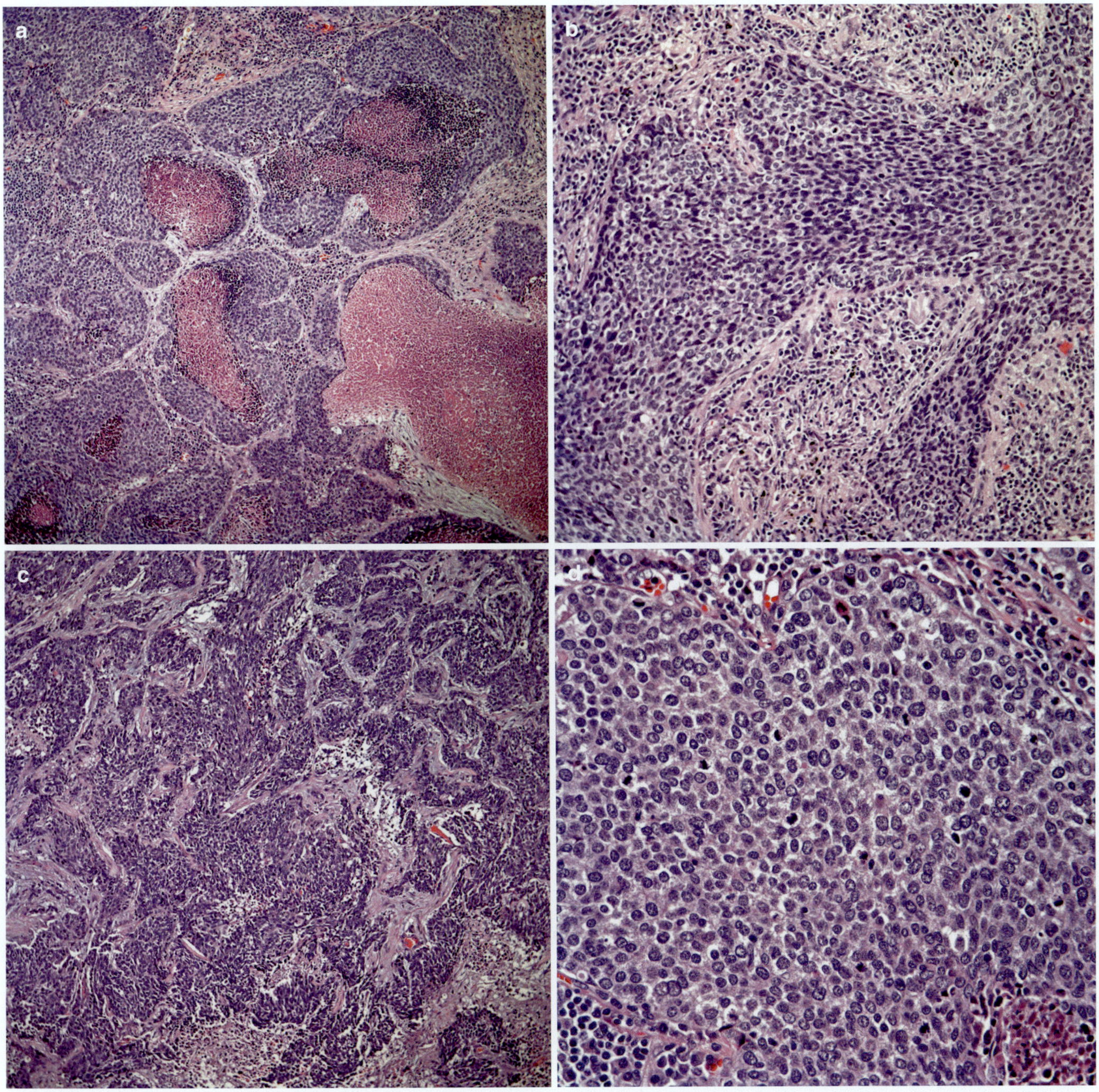

Fig. 3.37 (**a**) Small cell variant of squamous carcinoma showing comedo-like necrosis. (**b**) In other areas, the growth pattern is more in keeping with squamous carcinoma. (**c**) Haphazard arrangement of neoplastic cells replacing normal lung parenchyma. (**d**) Higher magnification showing cells with inconspicuous nucleoli, resembling small cell carcinoma. (**e**) In other areas, cells with more conspicuous nucleoli are seen

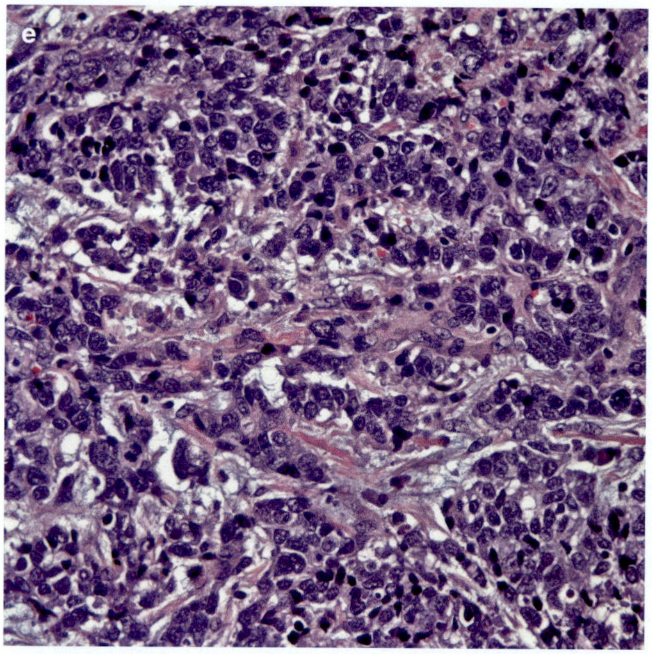

Fig. 3.37 (continued)

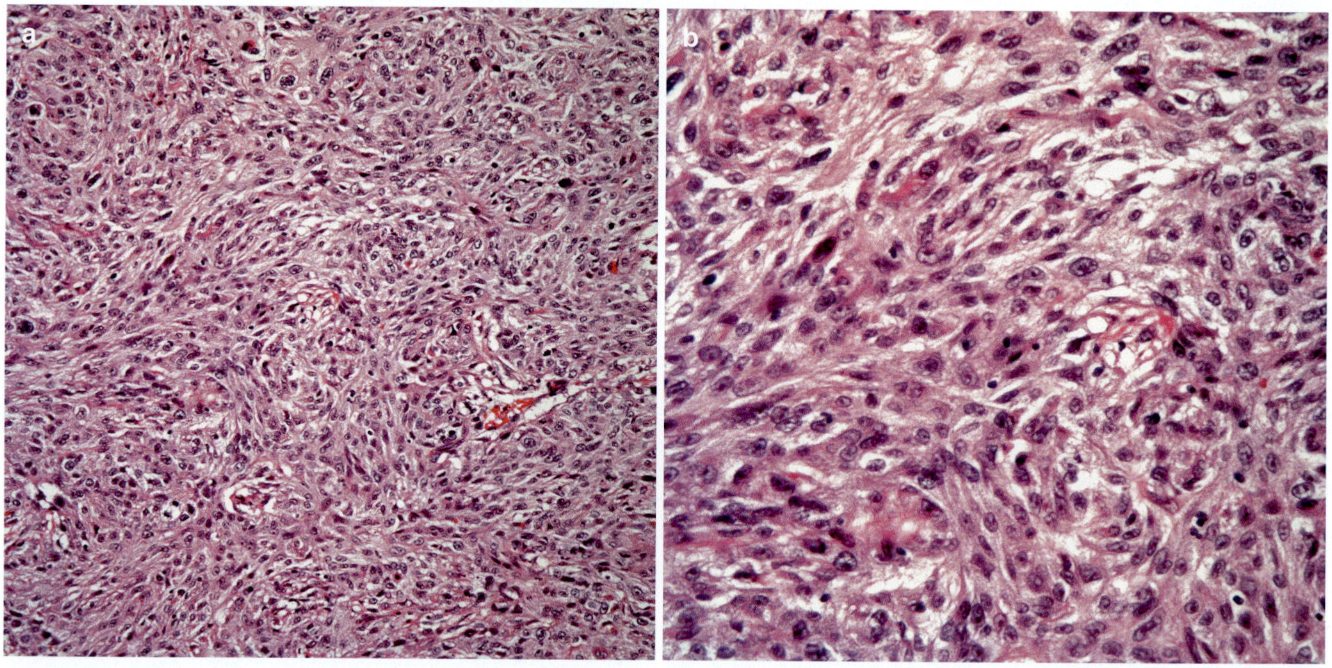

Fig. 3.38 (**a**) Spindle cell squamous carcinoma showing a prominent spindle cell proliferation mimicking a mesenchymal neoplasm. (**b**) Higher magnification showing prominent nuclear pleomorphism

The cells may acquire a fusiform appearance with elongated nuclei and inconspicuous nucleoli. In some cases, areas of keratinization are present, while in other cases, the squamous cell differentiation may be more subtle. However, because a basaloid pattern may be present in other tumors, namely, neuroendocrine carcinomas or the so-called basaloid carcinomas of the lung, it is important to make sure that the tumor in question really represents a true basaloid squamous cell carcinoma. Once again, the use of immunohistochemical markers, namely, keratin 5/6 and/or p63, may be of help.

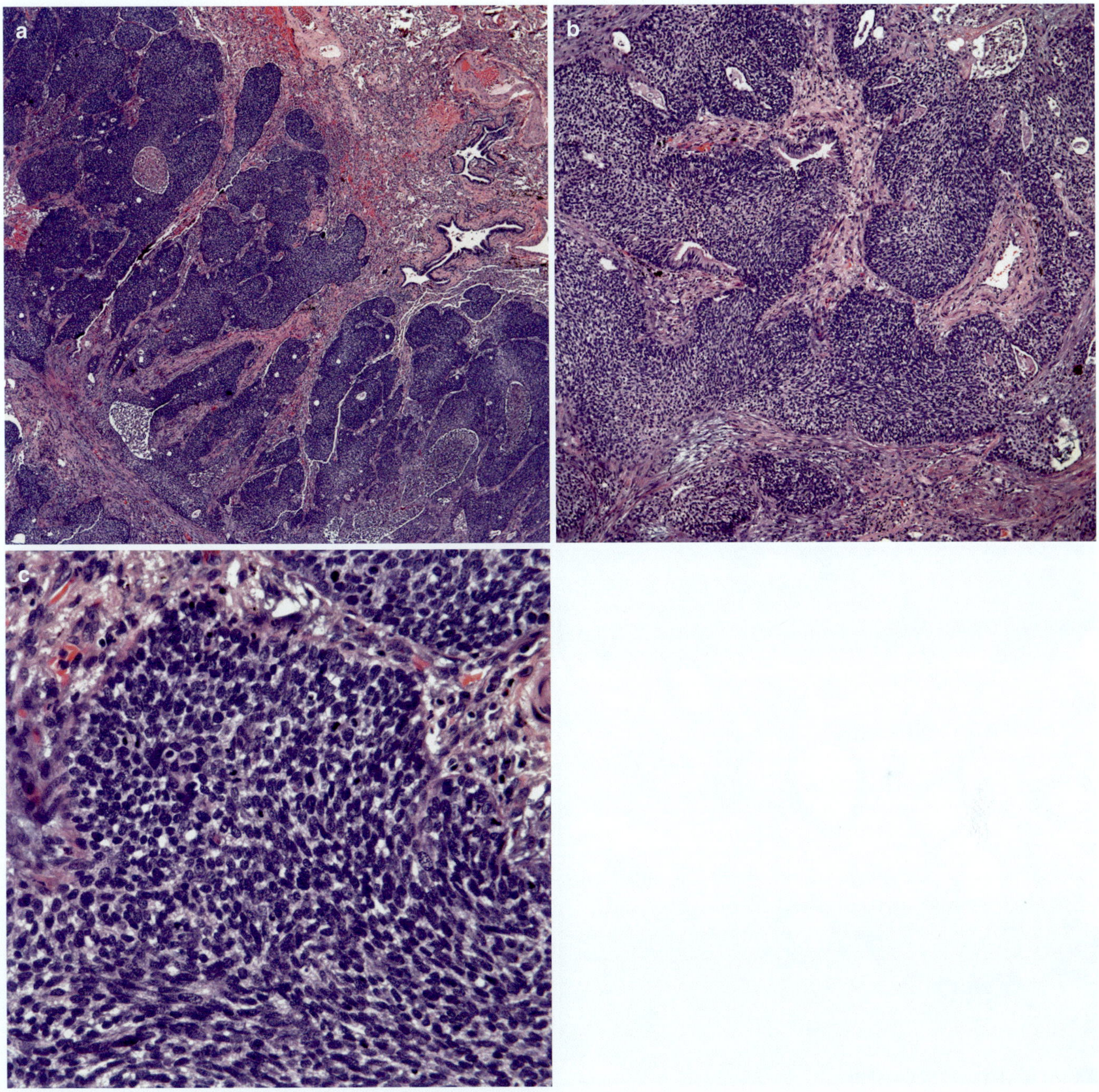

Fig. 3.39 (**a**) Basaloid squamous carcinoma of the lung. Note the similarity with the cutaneous tumor. (**b**) Islands of tumor cells with classical basaloid features. (**c**) Higher magnification showing increased mitotic activity

Microcystic Squamous Cell Carcinoma

This growth pattern of squamous cell carcinoma represents a recently described entity in which the authors [140] described three cases with features reminiscent to certain cutaneous adnexal neoplasms. The three patients were adult individuals between 72 and 83 years of age who presented with the usual symptoms of cough, chest pain, and hemoptysis. Follow-up information for two of these patients showed one patient alive after 76 months, while another patient had died 38 months after initial diagnosis.

Histologically, the tumors were described as peripheral tumors with an infiltrative growth pattern into the surrounding lung parenchyma. The tumors were characterized by

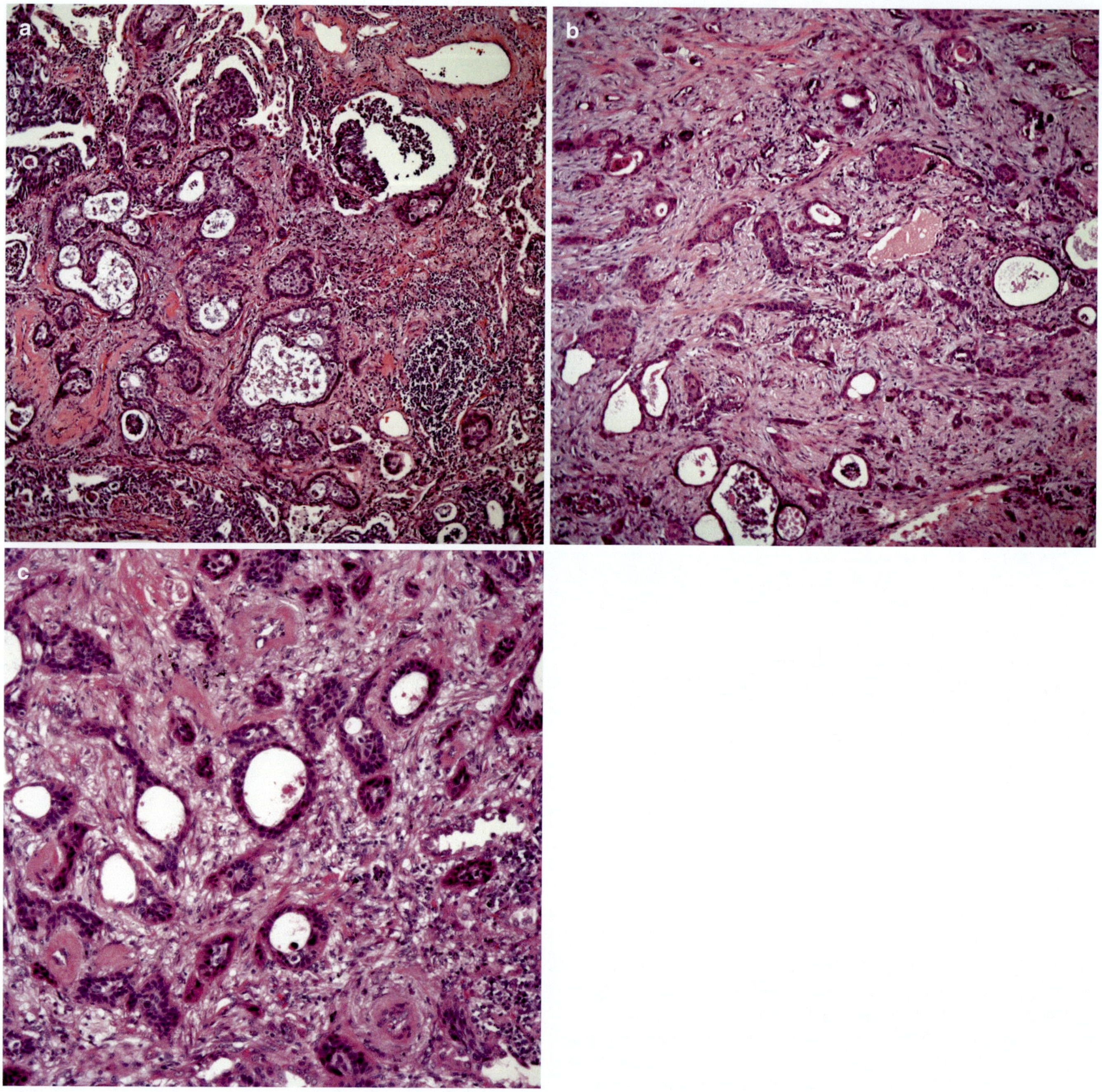

Fig. 3.40 (**a**) Microcystic carcinoma of the lung showing features similar to those seen in dermal tumors. (**b**) Areas of keratinization with microcysts are present. (**c**) Prominent syringomatous features may also be present

irregular islands, nests, and strands of mild to moderately pleomorphic keratinocytes. Cystic changes imparting a glandular appearance were noted in these cases. The neoplastic cells were embedded in a desmoplastic stroma, which appeared to compress some of the tumor nests into thin, slender strands of neoplastic cells (Fig. 3.40a–c). Mitotic activity was present and ranged from 4 to 19 mitotic figures/10 HPF. Even though focal areas of comedo-like necrosis were present in one case, extensive areas of necrosis were not identified. In general, the authors stated that the overall features of these tumors were reminiscent to those described for microcystic adnexal carcinoma of the skin. In view of that similarity, it is important, before rendering a final diagnosis of primary microcystic squamous cell carcinoma of the lung, to properly determine that the patient does not have any prior history of adnexal squamous cell carcinoma.

Miscellaneous Growth Patterns

The versatility of squamous cell carcinomas of the lung mirrors that of adenocarcinomas in terms of a wide variety of growth patterns that may be confused with another tumor. Squamous cell carcinomas of the lung may also in addition to the conventional growth pattern show prominent ameloblastic-like areas resembling ameloblastomas of the jaw, which could raise the possibility of metastatic carcinoma to the lung (Fig. 3.41a,b). In more unusual cases, squamous cell carcinomas may display areas with a prominent granular appearance (Fig. 3.42a–c). This pattern is rather unusual, and in most of the cases, is associated with more conventional areas of squamous cell carcinoma. In addition, some cases of squamous cell carcinomas may also show adenoid cystic-like features strongly resembling primary adenoid cystic carcinomas (Fig. 3.43a,b). Lastly, some squamous cell carcinomas of the lung, appear to have an interstitial growth pattern with entrapped alveoli (Fig. 3.44a,b) or respiratory epithelium mimicking a glandular neoplasm or an even adenosquamous carcinoma.

Immunohistochemical and Molecular Features

Currently, there are numerous immunohistochemical markers that have been described as useful in separating squamous cell carcinomas from other types of non-small cell carcinomas. Keratin 5/6 (Fig. 3.45) and p63 (Fig. 3.46) are a couple of those markers that may help in separating squamous cell carcinomas from other non-small cell carcinomas in cases in which such separation may be required [141, 142]. The main use of those stains is owed to the trend toward making a more specific diagnosis than non-small cell carcinomas. In addition, in cases in which the patient has a history of squamous cell carcinoma of extrathoracic origin and the lung biopsy shows a non-small cell carcinoma, the use of keratin 5/6, p63, and TTF-1 may be helpful to differentiate between a second primary tumor or metastatic process. Also, these stains may be helpful in cases in which the patients have a previous history of lung tumor and the question arises whether the new tumor represents another primary lesion or recurrence of their prior tumor. There are other immunohistochemical stains that have shown positive staining in squamous cell carcinomas including CD117; however, the relevance of such staining remains unclear at present [142]. On the other hand, at the molecular level, Yoshino et al. [143] studied 22 cases of squamous cell carcinomas of the lung and encountered that LOH was more frequently observed in squamous cell carcinomas than in adenocarcinomas of the lung and that LOH tends to be associated with smoking status. Also Chujo et al. [144], in a comparative genomic hybridization analysis, encountered overrepresentation of chromosome 3q in squamous cell carcinomas of the lung and concluded that an increase copy number at 3q may contribute to the development of these tumors.

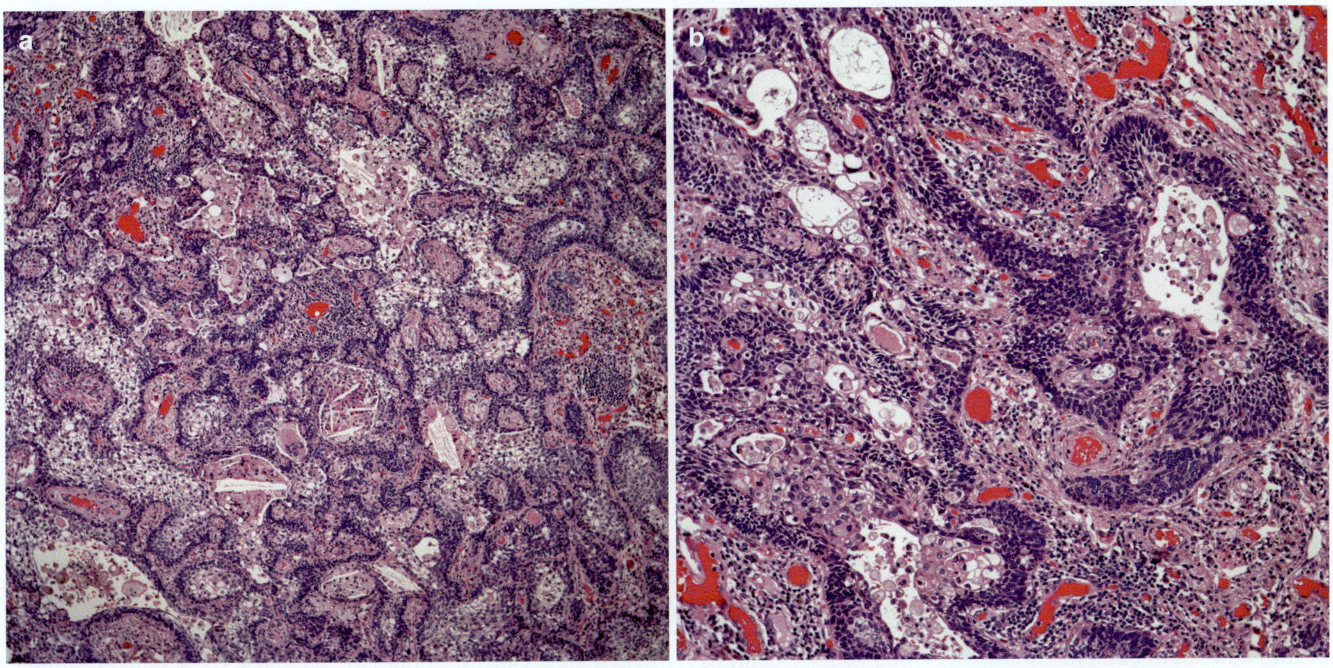

Fig. 3.41 (**a**) Squamous cell carcinoma with prominent ameloblastic-like growth pattern. (**b**) Higher magnification showing focal basaloid and keratinizing squamous cell carcinoma

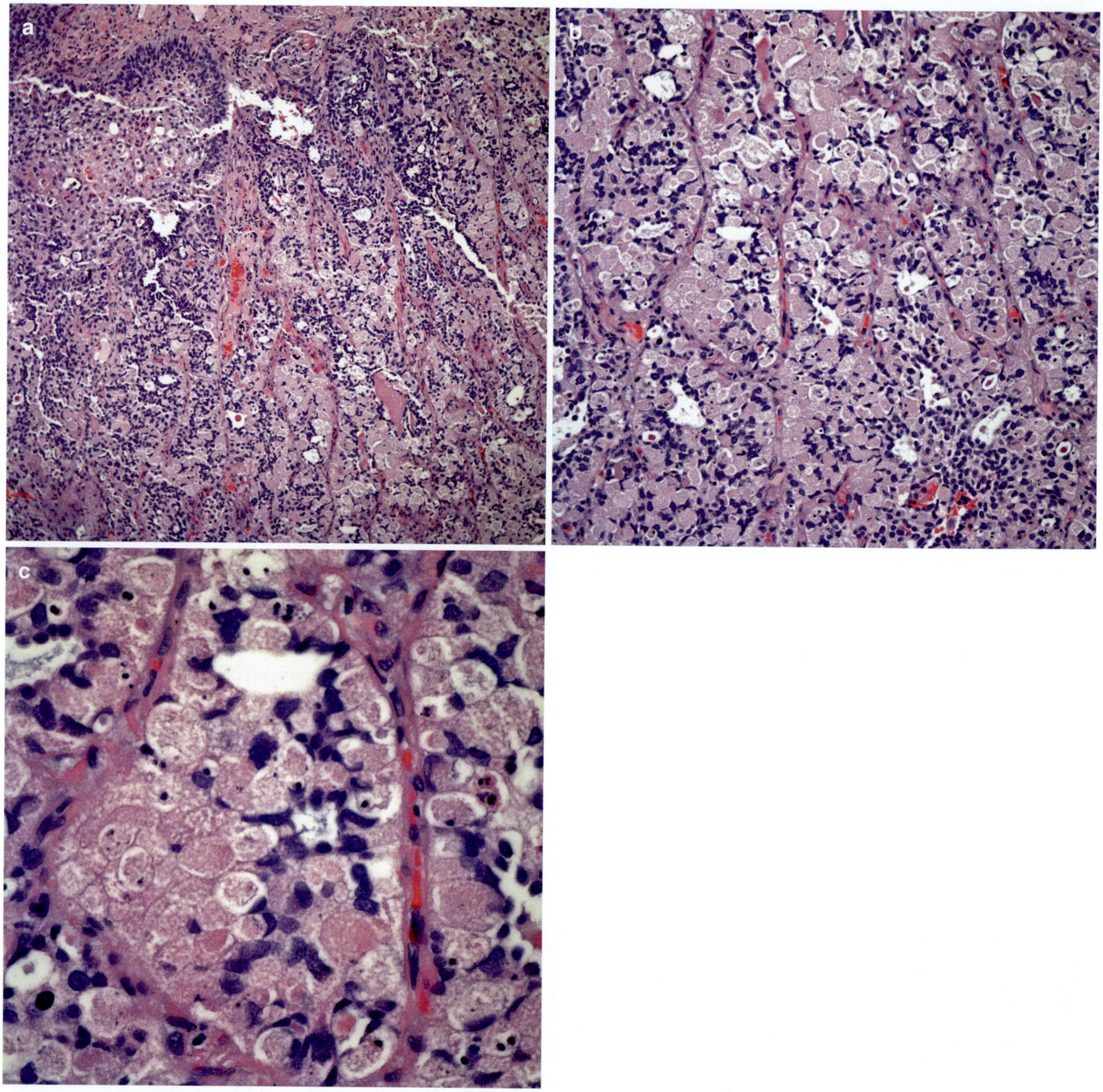

Fig. 3.42 (**a**) Squamous cell carcinoma with areas of granular-like growth pattern. (**b**) Closer view at the granular-like pattern showing cells with nuclei displaced to the periphery and granular cytoplasm. (**c**) Higher magnification showing the granular content of the cells

Large Cell Carcinoma

Large cell carcinoma is a carcinoma that does not show adenocarcinomatous or squamous cell differentiation. In the general context, one is required to exercise care when diagnosing non-small cell carcinoma since this generic designation does not automatically mean that a tumor is of large cell type nor is making the diagnosis of large cell carcinoma an appropriate way to classify a tumor as not being a small cell carcinoma. Currently, the use of immunohistochemical studies including TTF-1, p63, Napsin A, and keratin 5/6 may reduce the percentage of cases that are classified as large cell carcinomas. For practical purposes large cell carcinoma may be an entity that should be reserved for resected tumors in which one can be certain of the lack of adenocarcinoma, squamous cell carcinoma, or any other tumor type. In past publications [145–147], it has been estimated that large cell carcinomas may represent somewhere between 6 and 20 %

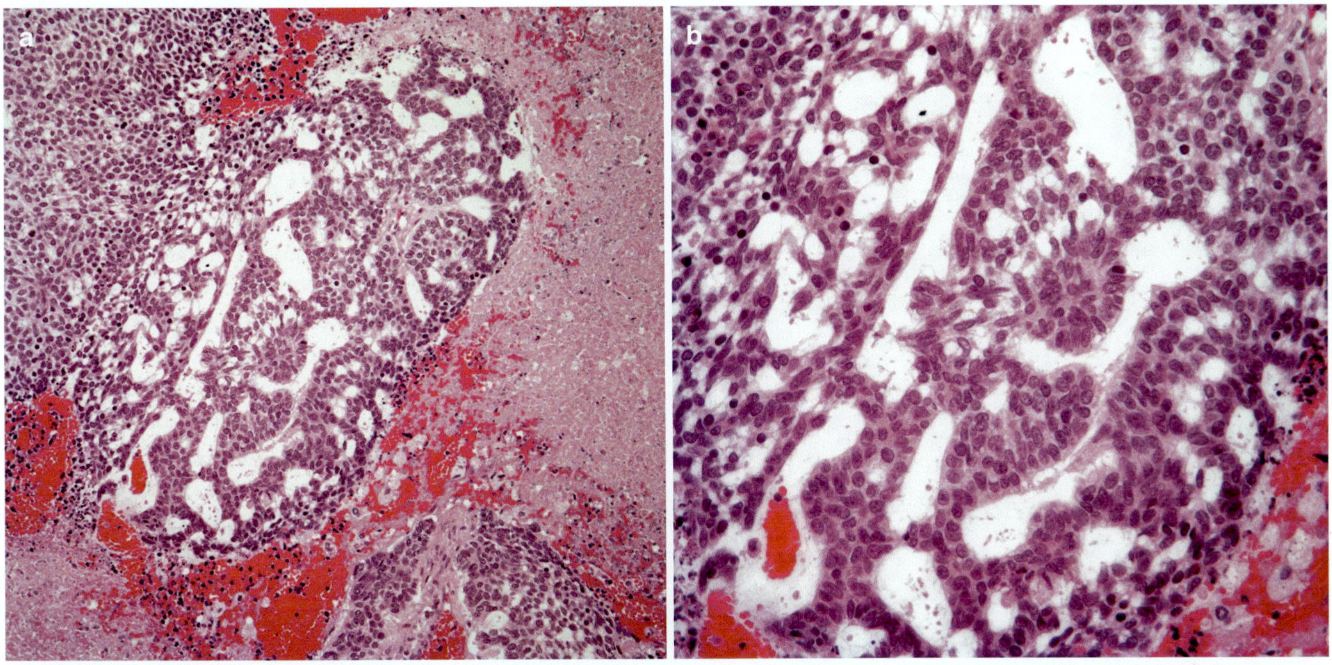

Fig. 3.43 (**a**) Adenoid cystic-like areas may be seen in some squamous carcinomas. (**b**) The cellular proliferation is arranged in cords with subtle cystic features

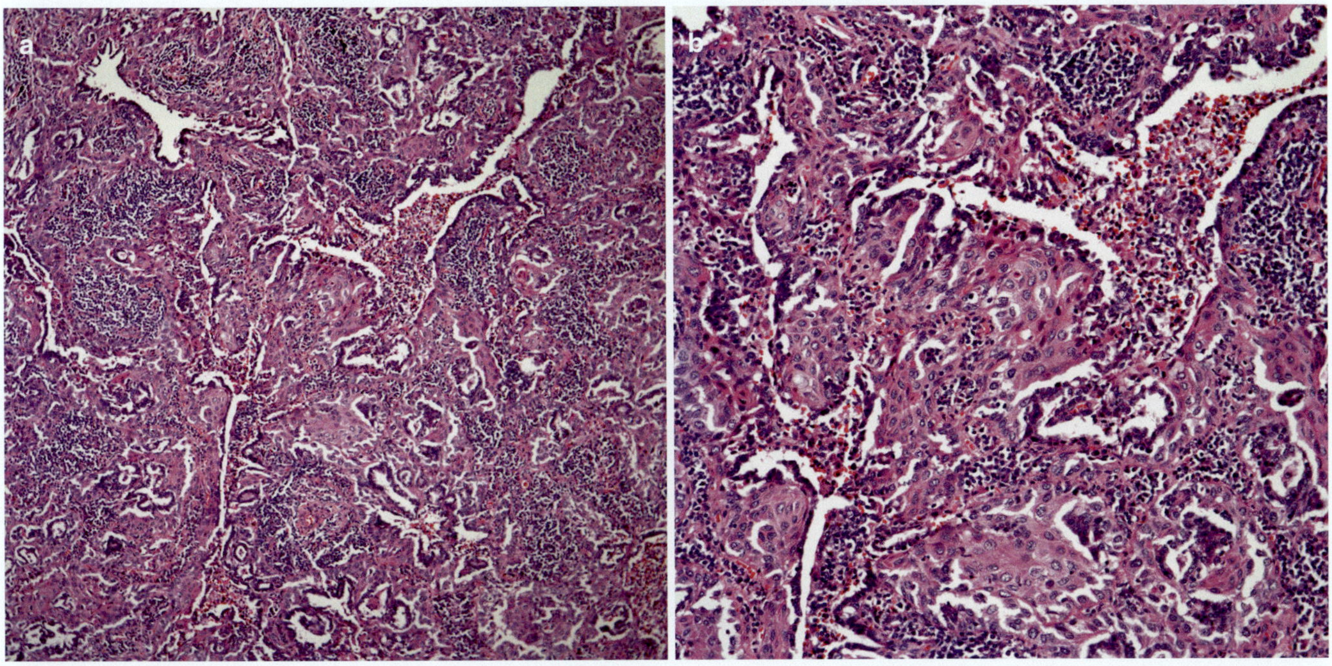

Fig. 3.44 (**a**) Squamous carcinoma with interstitial growth pattern. Note the entrapment of alveolar and airway structures. (**b**) Closer magnification showing squamous carcinoma

of all lung carcinomas. However, this percentage may be affected by the use of ancillary studies currently used in diagnostic surgical pathology. It is also important to separate this type of tumors from the so-called large cell neuroendocrine carcinoma, which is a tumor that must have a neuroendocrine growth pattern in addition to positive neuroendocrine markers. One also has to appreciate the fact that a percentage of "non-small cell carcinomas" may show positive staining for neuroendocrine markers. Thus, care must be exercised to properly classify a carcinoma as large cell carcinoma.

In the past, some authors have been opposed to this type of denomination, arguing that "large cell undifferentiated

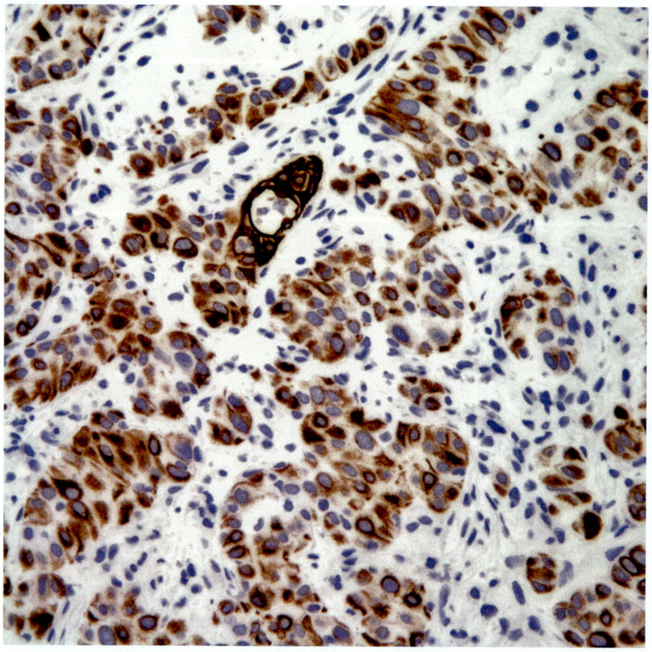

Fig. 3.45 Immunohistochemical stain for keratin 5/6 showing positive staining in tumor cells

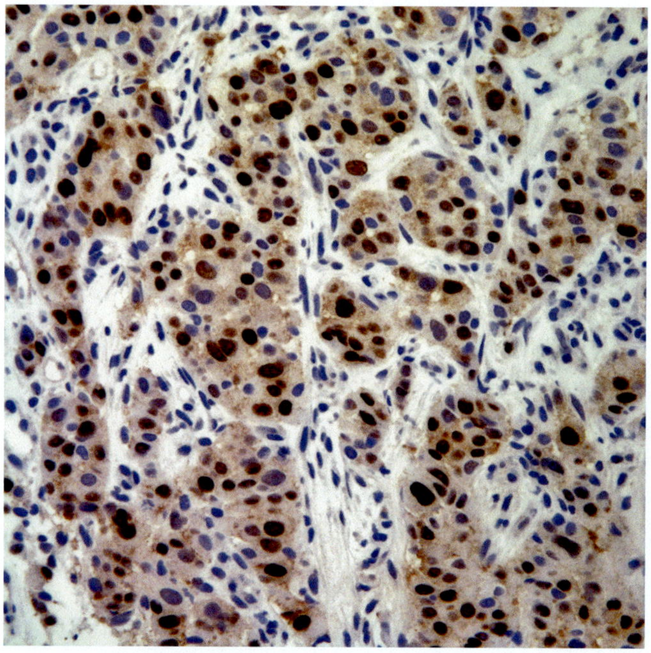

Fig. 3.46 Immunohistochemical stain for p63 showing nuclear positive staining in tumor cells

carcinoma of the lung" may represent either poorly differentiated adenocarcinoma or squamous cell carcinoma. Churg [145] provided such a conclusion after an ultrastructural analysis of 7 cases of "large cell carcinoma". Yesner [146] considers that the biology of large cell carcinoma is similar to that of adenocarcinoma characterized by their peripheral location in about 72 % of the cases, and similar metastatic pattern. Thus, large cell carcinoma is basically defined as a diagnosis of exclusion. Contrary to that, Albain et al. [147] in a study of large cell carcinoma of the lung found that these tumors can be either central or peripheral lesions that may be more common in female patients. Albain et al. [147] were able to group cases in which ultrastructurally, there was differentiation toward adenocarcinoma or squamous cell carcinoma. However, they observed that in about one-third of the cases studied (48 cases), no such differentiation was encountered. Kodama et al. [148] also reported similar findings in an ultrastructural study of 18 cases of large cell carcinomas in which the authors were also able to find adenocarcinoma, squamous cell carcinoma, and neuroendocrine differentiation in 14 cases. Only 4 of the 18 cases studied did not show any type of differentiation. These studies raise the possibility that large cell carcinoma of the lung is a rare entity after utilization of all the diagnostic tools available for proper identification of any particular differentiation.

Clinical Features

Similar to other pulmonary carcinomas, patients with large cell carcinoma may show symptoms depending on the anatomic location of the tumor. Patients with central tumors are more likely to present with symptoms of obstruction, hemoptysis, cough, and dyspnea; while those patients with peripheral tumors may have larger tumors whose size may elicit symptoms of chest pain, obstructive pneumonia, weight loss, etc.

Gross Features

The tumors may have a central or peripheral location and present as large tumor masses compressing airway structures. The tumors are bulky, and at cut surface, they may show a tan-light color with areas of necrosis or hemorrhage. The tumors are well defined but not encapsulated, and they may exceed more than 10 cm in greatest dimension with involvement of extensive areas of lung parenchyma.

Histological Features

Low-power magnification of this tumor is characterized by the presence of sheets of cells without any particular arrangement. The sheets are composed of a discohesive neoplastic cellular proliferation composed of larger cells with moderate amounts of light eosinophilic cytoplasm, round to oval nuclei, and prominent nucleoli (Fig. 3.47a–d). Mitotic figures and atypical mitoses are commonly seen as well as extensive areas of necrosis or inflammatory exudates. In some cases, the presence of osteoclast-like giant cells has been described [149]. Also, cases in which the tumor shows ectopic gonadotropin production by tumor cells have been identified [150].

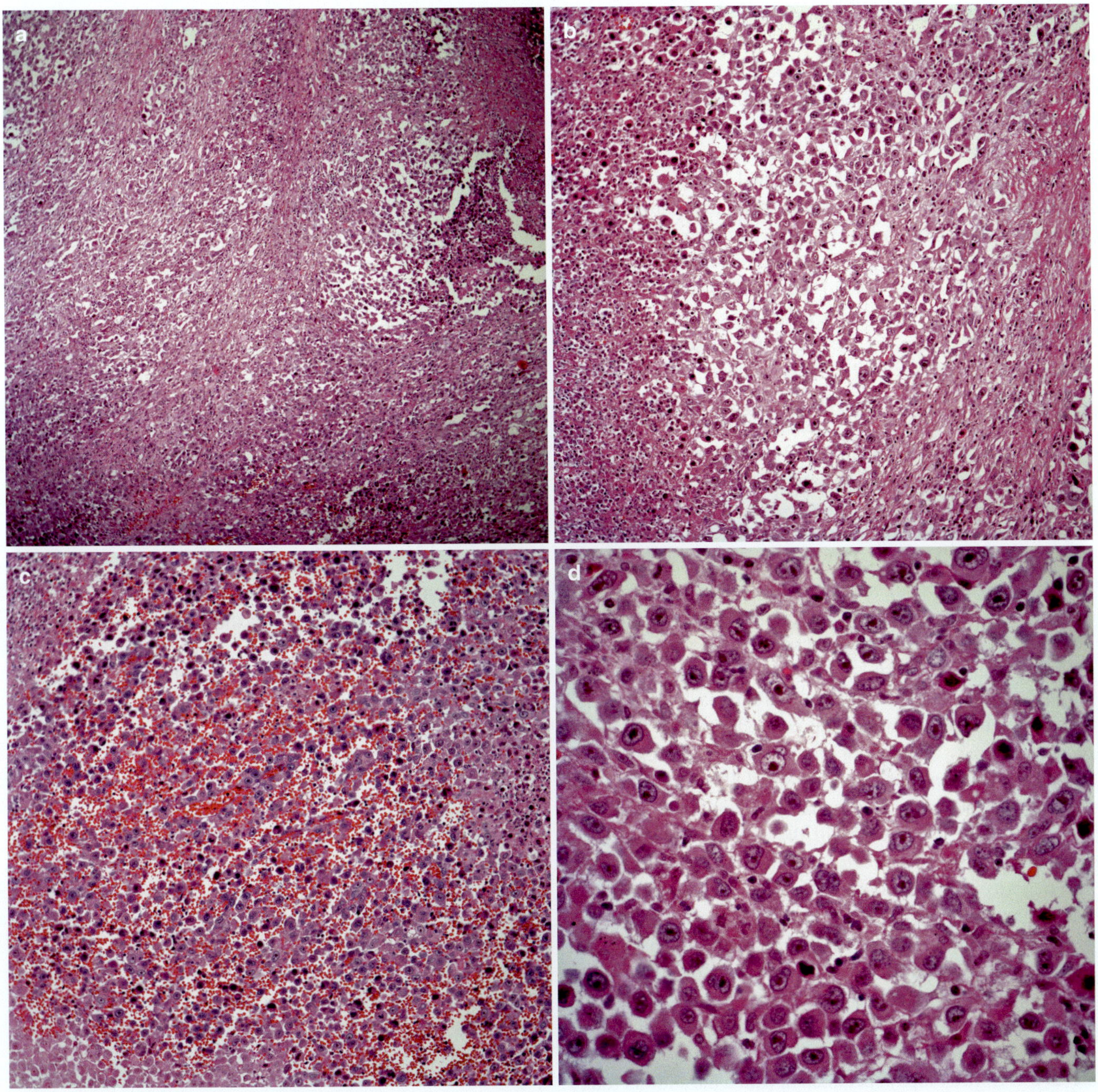

Fig. 3.47 (**a**) Large cell carcinoma showing areas of necrosis. (**b**) Closer view at the neoplastic cellular proliferation with any particular differentiation. (**c**) Large cell with discohesive growth pattern. (**d**) Higher magnification showing large cells with ample cytoplasm, round nuclei, and prominent nucleoli

In those cases, it is believed that the tumor cells are responsible for the elaboration and secretion of the hormone.

Immunohistochemical and Molecular Biology Features

Large cell carcinomas are positive for broad spectrum keratin, low molecular weight keratin, keratin 7, and epithelial membrane antigen (EMA). However, they may not show positive staining for TTF-1, p63, and keratin 5/6. Other carcinomatous epitopes that may be useful in this particular setting include CEA and CD15, as these makers may be useful in separating carcinoma from other types of malignancy.

More recently, Zhong et al. [151] identified LKB1 mutation in large cell carcinoma of the lung and stated that acquired loss of function of LKB1 may be involved in the pathogenesis of large cell carcinoma.

Adenosquamous Carcinoma

As its name implies, this tumor should contain areas that by themselves are diagnosed as either squamous cell carcinoma or adenocarcinoma by light microscopy. It is likely that in the past many cases that had been classified under this designation may have represented unusual variants of either squamous cell carcinoma with a glandular pattern, solid areas of adenocarcinoma, or tumors that were classified as adenosquamous carcinoma based on the presence of mucin by mucicarmine stains in solid areas of poorly differentiated squamous cell carcinomas. Therefore, it is difficult to define a specific percentage for the incidence of adenosquamous carcinoma. Nevertheless, the tumor has been recognized for quite some time and represents a specific neoplasm with a reported more aggressive behavior than conventional squamous or adenocarcinoma [152–163]. The proportion of either component is debatable and varies according to various authors from 5 to 10 %. However, in practice, it is likely that 5 % of either component is the threshold for making such a diagnosis. However, in a small biopsy, the presence of both of these components may not be obvious; therefore, the diagnosis of adenosquamous carcinoma is more appropriately left for complete surgical resections.

Fitzgibbons and Kern [152] in 1985 reported a study of seven cases of adenosquamous cell carcinoma of the lung and determined that these tumors represented less than 1 % of all lung carcinomas. The authors reviewed 1,125 cases of lung carcinoma between the years 1968 and 1984 and identified 21 cases diagnosed as adenosquamous carcinoma; however, only 7 of those 21 cases fulfill the criteria of unequivocal areas of either squamous cell carcinoma or adenocarcinoma. The majority of the tumors were peripheral, and in most, the predominant tumor was squamous cell carcinoma, either well or moderately differentiated. The lowest percentage recorded in this series of cases for either tumor component was 10 %. Interestingly, although the great majority of cases represented surgical resections in the form of wedge resection, lobectomy, and pneumonectomy, one of the cases included in this series was from a biopsy specimen in which the authors found equal proportions of both components. Also, the majority of patients had larger tumors (>3 cm). Naunheim et al. [153] using similar criteria as the ones applied by Fitzgibbons and Kern [152] reported a study of 20 cases of adenosquamous carcinoma after a review of 873 cases of lung carcinoma between the years of 1974 and 1985 and estimated a 2.3 % for the incidence of this tumor. However, only 12 cases in this series were derived from surgical resection material. In 8 of the cases described, only biopsy material was available. In two separate studies on adenosquamous carcinoma, probably using the same patient population, Sridhar et al. [154, 155] encountered 103 and 127 patients diagnosed with adenosquamous carcinoma between the years 1977 and 1986 and estimated an incidence of 8 % for this tumor. However, there are important differences between the study by Sridhar [155] and the one of Fitzgibbons [150] in terms of case selection. For instance, in the study by Sridhar et al. [155], the authors included essentially biopsy material (91 cases) and cytology specimens (12 cases); also, the authors did not specify criteria for the diagnosis of these tumors for the cases included in this study. Therefore, it is likely that a sizable percentage of the cases included may not have been true adenosquamous carcinomas. One of the largest series of adenosquamous carcinomas of the lung is the one by Takamori et al. [156] in which the authors identified 56 cases diagnosed out of 2,160 surgical resections for lung carcinoma. The authors estimated a 2.6 % incidence and histologically included cases with a minimum of 5 % of each component in order to be designated as adenosquamous carcinoma. The authors analyzed adenosquamous carcinoma in relation to squamous cell carcinoma and/or adenocarcinoma and determined that adenosquamous carcinoma follows a more aggressive behavior, particularly those in stages I and II.

Clinical Features

Adenosquamous carcinoma, just the same as other types of non-small cell carcinomas of the lung, may present with similar symptoms that may include cough, dyspnea, hemoptysis, pneumonia, chest pain, and weight loss. There is not a particular clinical setting that is specific for adenosquamous cell carcinoma.

Gross Features

Similar to other more common non-small cell carcinomas such as adenocarcinoma or squamous cell carcinoma, adenosquamous carcinoma may present as a peripheral or central tumor, which may range in size from 1 cm to more than 10 cm in greatest dimension. In some reports of adenosquamous carcinoma, a more common peripheral location has been noted. However, these tumors may be peripheral or central. There are no specific gross features that distinguish adenosquamous carcinoma from other non-small cell carcinomas.

Histological Features

As previously stated, the tumor is characterized by the presence of unequivocal areas of squamous cell carcinoma and adenocarcinoma (Fig. 3.48a–d) that by themselves can be diagnosed as such. The proportion of either of those components should be at least 5 %. The squamous cell carcinoma is more likely to be of the well or moderately differentiated type in which areas of keratinization and intercellular bridges are still possible to identify. Similarly, the adenocarcinomatous component will often show areas of glandular or tubular differentiation. These two components may merge with only a subtle transition between them but without any abrupt change. Two distinct tumor nodules are identified, one show-

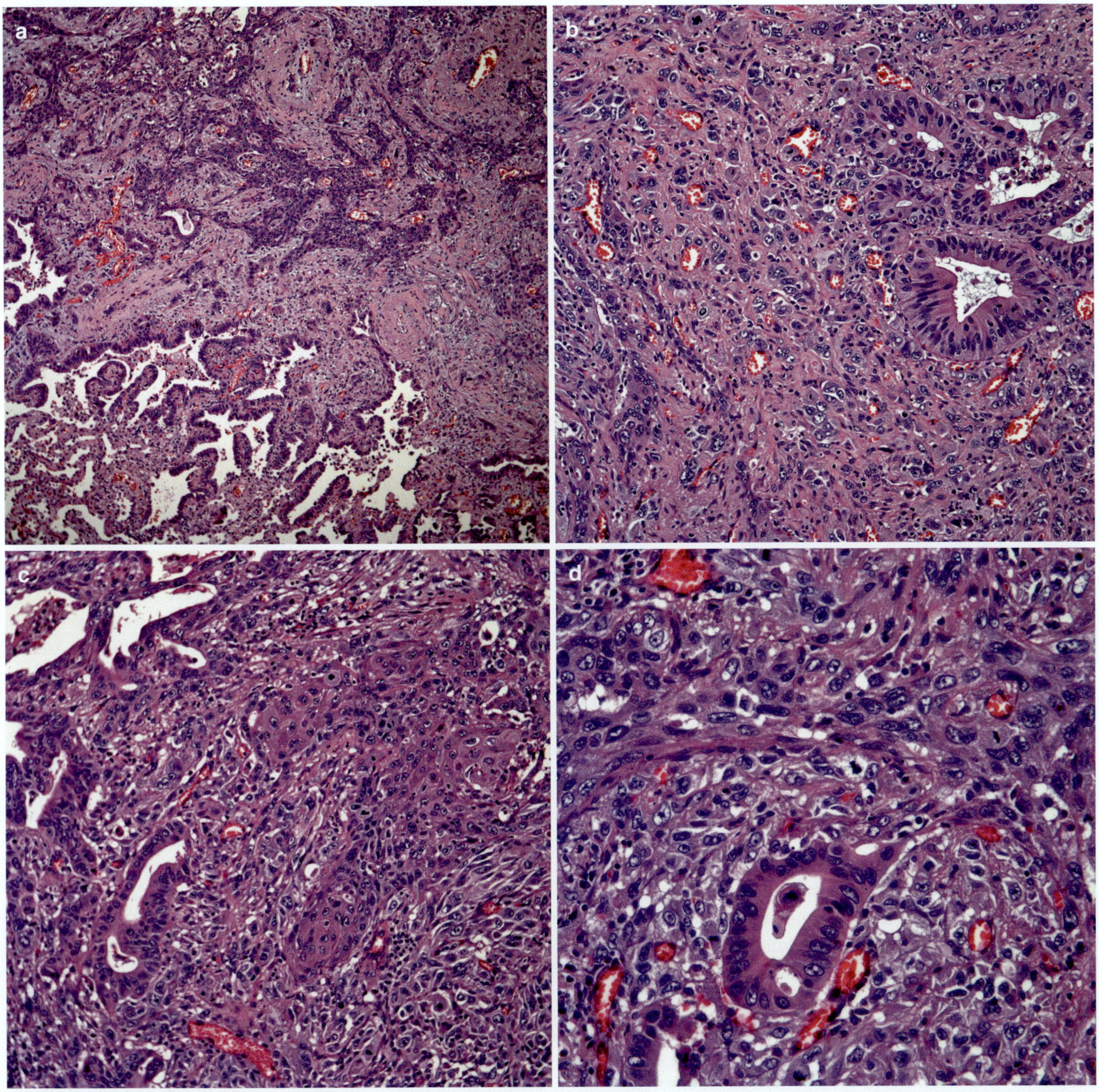

Fig. 3.48 (**a**) Low-power view of an adenosquamous carcinoma showing both tumor components. (**b**) Solid proliferation of poorly differentiated squamous carcinoma admixed with adenocarcinoma. (**c**) More conventional areas of both squamous and adenocarcinoma. (**d**) Higher magnification showing adenocarcinoma and squamous cell carcinoma

ing squamous cell carcinoma and the other adenocarcinoma, such occurrence should raise the possibility of two separate tumors.

Immunohistochemical and Molecular Biology Features

From the immunohistochemical point of view, the tumor may show positive staining for markers that are more commonly seen with any of these two particular tumors. For instance, p63 and keratin 5/6 for in the squamous cell component while TTF-1 and Napsin A are positive in the adenocarcinomatous component. In addition, CD44, CD44v6, and CD44v7-8 have also been seen to decorate the squamous cell component of adenosquamous carcinoma. However, these antibodies are not reliable in cases in which the differentiation of the tumor is poor [164].

Kanazawa et al. [165] compared the genetic alterations of p53 and K-ras chromosomal abnormalities at 9p21 and

9q31–32. The author found p53 overexpression and mutation both components of the tumors and suggested a monoclonal transition from squamous cell carcinoma to adenocarcinoma. Kang et al. [166] studied the mutation status of EGFR kinase domain from exon 18 to 21 in 25 cases of adenosquamous carcinoma and found identical EGFR mutations in both components. Thus, the authors suggested the possibility of monoclonality in the histogenesis of adenosquamous carcinoma. On the other hand, Liang et al. [167] found that trisomy 12 correlates with elevated expression of p21ras in a single case of adenosquamous carcinoma. These molecular alterations may in due course play an important role in the treatment of patients with adenosquamous carcinoma.

Sarcomatoid Carcinoma and Pleomorphic Carcinoma

These two entities are presented together due to the similarity in their histopathological characteristics as well as the controversy that exists whether these tumors are two separate entities or part of a spectrum of differentiation of the same tumor. However, it is important to separate these tumors, at least for the purpose of this text, from similar tumors that may have heterologous elements in the form of cartilage, osteoid, or other mesenchymal components; such tumors are discussed under the term carcinosarcoma. Therefore, by definition, the terms sarcomatoid carcinoma and pleomorphic carcinoma are reserved for those tumors that almost exclusively show a malignant epithelial spindle cell component. However, we will make an attempt to separate sarcomatoid carcinoma from pleomorphic carcinoma as much as it is possible. Other names that have been used to designate these tumors include spindle cell carcinoma, carcinoma with pseudosarcomatous stroma, and metaplastic carcinoma; on the other hand, terms that have been used to describe pleomorphic carcinomas include giant cell carcinoma, sarcomatoid carcinoma, carcinoma with pseudosarcomatous stroma, and pseudosarcomatous carcinoma.

In 1988, Humphrey et al. [168] reported a study of eight pulmonary tumors that the authors described as pulmonary carcinomas with a sarcomatoid component. In this study, the authors, although expressing the fact that spindle cell squamous cell carcinoma is less controversial, proposed that pulmonary carcinomas exhibiting evidence of epithelial differentiation in a spindle cell component be termed "spindle cell carcinomas," while those in which one can identify the presence of malignant cartilage, bone, or muscle be termed carcinosarcomas. Matsui et al. [169] reported three cases of spindle cell carcinoma of the lung two of which were termed "monophasic" spindle cell carcinomas and one of which was called adenosquamous carcinoma with a spindle cell component. These tumors expressed keratin and vimentin in different degrees. The authors concluded that the spindle cell component displays a spectrum of phenotypes originating from squamous cell carcinoma, while the term "monophasic" spindle cell carcinoma is an extreme phenotype of squamous cell carcinoma pretending mesenchymal differentiation. In a different study on sarcomatoid carcinomas of the lung, Ro et al. [170] analyzed 14 cases in which the authors provided more specific criteria for inclusion: (1) the concurrent presence of malignant epithelial and sarcomatoid spindle cell components and (2) positive immunoreactivity for antikeratin antibodies or ultrastructural demonstration of epithelial differentiation in sarcomatoid tumors in which the epithelial component was inconspicuous. The patients were between the ages of 43 and 78 years, and 12 of the 14 patients were men. Histologically, the most common growth pattern in the sarcomatoid component of these tumors was that of malignant fibrous histiocytoma in ten cases; two additional cases showed a fibrosarcomatous pattern while in two additional cases, the term unclassified sarcomatous component was used. The majority of patients were in late stages of disease (11 patients in stages III and IV). Based on those features, the authors concluded that primary tumors of the lung showing extensive "sarcomatoid" components should be carefully evaluated for epithelial differentiation using immunohistochemical and/or electron microscopic studies. Also, the authors stated that sarcomatoid carcinomas of the lung are aggressive neoplasms that usually present in late stages.

On the other hand, the term pleomorphic carcinoma was introduced by Fishback et al. [171] in order to group all those cases that in the past have been designated as spindle cell carcinomas or giant cell carcinomas [171–180]. The authors presented a study of 78 cases, corresponding to 57 men and 21 women between the ages of 35 and 83 years (mean: 62 years). Clinically, the patients presented with variable symptomatology including chest pain, cough, and hemoptysis. A small percentage of patients (14 %) were asymptomatic. Almost half of the patients were in stages I and II (41 % were stage I and 6 % were stage II) while 39 % were in stage III and 12 % in stage IV. Histologically, only 22 % of the cases studied showed only a spindle and/or giant cell component, while the remaining tumors show foci of adenocarcinoma (45 %), large cell carcinoma (25 %), and squamous cell carcinoma (8 %). The authors found that 53 out of 69 patients in whom clinical follow-up was available died within 6 years (mean: 23 months, median: 10 months). In addition, there was a significant shortening of survival for patients with tumor size greater than 5 cm, clinical stage greater than I, and lymph node involvement. This latter feature was the single most important prognostic factor, whereas the presence of adenocarcinoma or squamous cell carcinoma did not influence the prognosis. Interestingly, this report shows that the presence of spindle and/or giant cell carcinoma may be seen in association with other types of histology besides squamous cell carcinoma. It has also been stated that pleomorphic carcinoma may represent a genetically distinct entity separate from adenocarcinoma or squamous cell carcinoma. Przygodzki et al. [181] performed a comparative DNA sequence and immunohistochemical analysis on 22 cases of pleomorphic carcinoma, 42 cases of squamous cell carcinoma, and 97 cases of adenocarcinoma. The authors found that pleomorphic carcinoma shows that p53 mutations were more common in exon 7, while p53 mutations in adenocarcinoma and squamous cell carcinoma were more common in exon 8. In addition, K-ras-2 mutations are present in only a few cases of pleomorphic carcinoma (9 %—2/22 cases studied), while they are more common in adenocarcinoma (36 %—35/97 cases studied), and they were not present in squamous cell carcinoma.

Gross Features

There are not any specific gross features that distinguish sarcomatoid/pleomorphic carcinoma from other types of non-small cell carcinomas. However, these tumors can attain a large size, and in many cases, the patients are in late stages of disease. They can occupy large portions of the lung parenchyma as they can reach more than 10 cm in greatest dimension. At cut surface, they may show a tan color with a homogenous surface with or without areas of necrosis or hemorrhage. They can be either in a central or peripheral location.

Histological Features

This most salient histopathological feature in these tumors is the presence of a spindle cellular proliferation that can be arranged in a fascicular pattern mimicking any of the conventional sarcomas of the soft tissues. The cells are elongated, some with a "cigar shaped" type of nucleus and inconspicuous nucleoli. Mitotic figures are easily identifiable and atypical forms are common. Areas of necrosis and hemorrhage are not uncommon. In cases that have been reported under the rubric of pleomorphic carcinoma, the tumors essentially show the same histological characteristics as those described for sarcomatoid carcinomas except for the additional presence of multinucleated malignant giant cells that can be bi-, tri-, or multinucleated (Fig. 3.49a–e). However, no heterologous component should be present in this type of tumors.

Immunohistochemical and Ultrastructural Features

The use of immunohistochemical studies should help in separating these tumors mainly from true sarcomas. Epithelial markers such as keratins and EMA are reported positive in these tumors. In addition, we have seen some cases in which actin is positive as well as vimentin. However, desmin, myoglobin, caldesmon, and CD31 should be negative in the tumor cells. In addition, ultrastructurally, the tumor cells may display the presence of epithelial differentiation by showing tonofilaments and/or desmosomes.

Rhabdoid Carcinoma

Primary lung carcinomas that resemble tumors of the kidney known as malignant rhabdoid tumors have been well documented in the literature [182–192]. Malignant rhabdoid tumors appear to occur in a ubiquitous distribution, and those occurring outside the kidney have also been called extrarenal rhabdoid tumors or pseudo-rhabdoid tumors. Whether this particular tumor represents a specific clinicopathological entity or a growth pattern is beyond the scope of this chapter. Here, we will limit ourselves to discuss only those tumors occurring in the lung. In general, these tumors are rare as primary lung neoplasms, and although there is controversy as to how to properly designate these tumors, herein they will be regarded as "rhabdoid carcinomas" rather than the ambiguous term of "rhabdoid phenotype" or "dedifferentiated carcinoma". We consider that these tumors represent a specific growth pattern of a heterogeneous group of tumors which in the lung may include adenocarcinoma, large cell carcinoma, or neuroendocrine carcinomas. However, as has been stated clearly by Wick et al. [192], the setting in which one makes this particular diagnosis may dictate a particular interpretation. Rhabdoid carcinomas occurring in the lung will show areas with of "rhabdoid" features in a proportion of no less than 10 % of the tumor, while by immunohistochemistry, the tumor cells may show, at least focally, positive staining for epithelial markers (keratin and EMA). Ultrastructural studies, show cytoplasmic accumulation of intermediate filaments or mitochondria. However, in the majority of pulmonary rhabdoid tumors, a component of the conventional type of non-small cell carcinoma is usually present, thus leading to the concept that the "rhabdoid" component is a growth pattern rather than a specific clinicopathological entity.

The credit for the first description of "rhabdoid tumor" in the lung is awarded to Rubenchik et al. [182] who described an intrapulmonary tumor in a 74-year-old man. The tumor was characterized by the presence of rhabdoid features, which by electron microscopy show the presence of cytoplasmic intermediate filaments that are characteristic of malignant rhabdoid tumors of the kidney. However, as the tumor became better known and more cases have been documented in the lung, many of these tumors - event those showing extensive rhabdoid changes -contain areas of more conventional non-small cell carcinoma, which can be either in the form of adenocarcinoma, large cell carcinoma, or sarcomatoid carcinoma. Because of the association of rhabdoid features with more conventional carcinoma, some authors have proposed the term "dedifferentiated phenotype" for these tumors [187]. Although some authors have reported a "good" prognosis for these tumors, we believe that staging at the time of diagnosis may play a more significant role in the outcome of patients with this particular carcinoma.

Histological Features

As the name implies, the tumor resembles the so-called malignant rhabdoid tumor of the kidney. The low-power magnification is that of a tumor that destroys normal lung

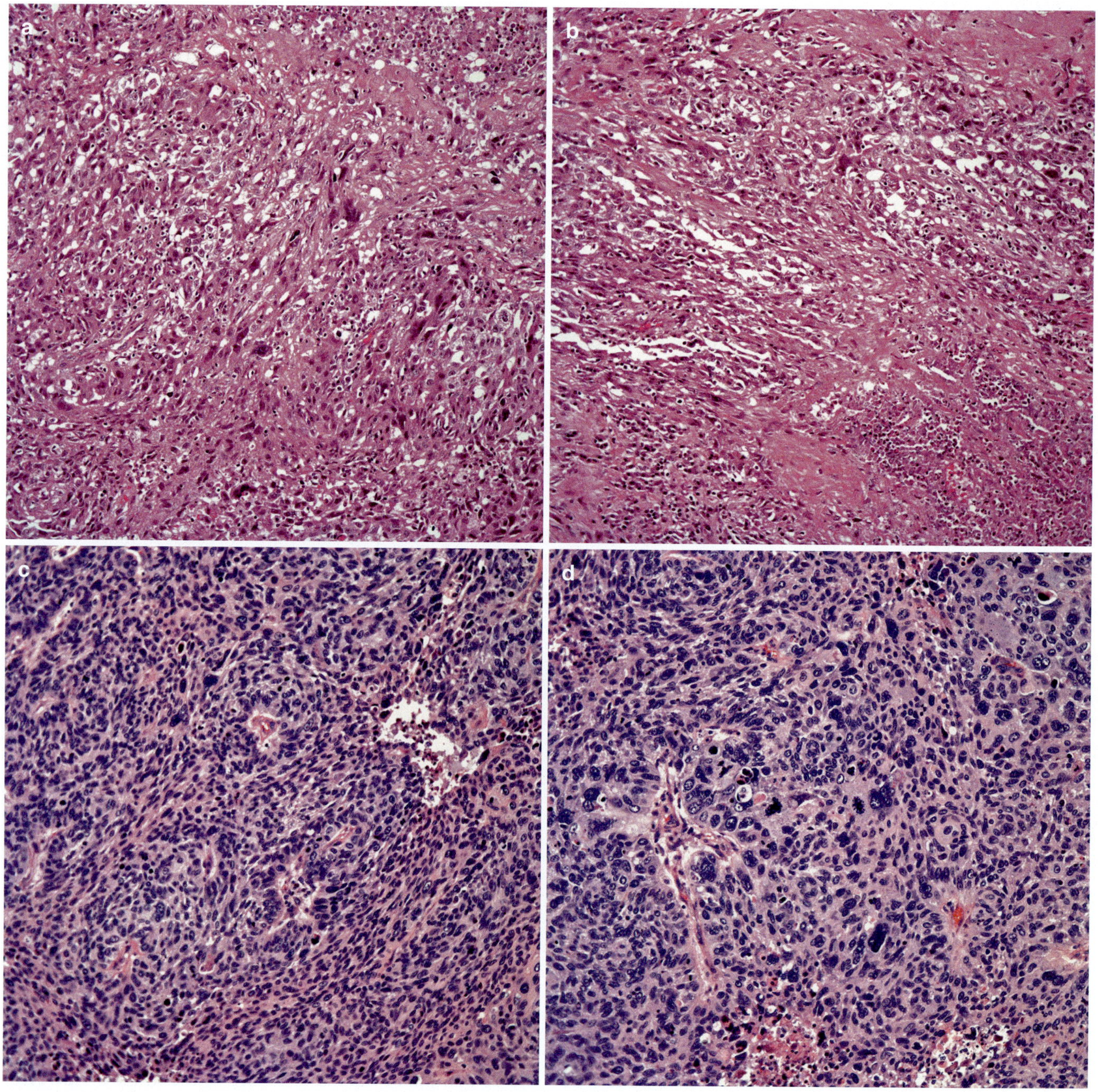

Fig. 3.49 (**a**) Pleomorphic carcinoma showing areas of spindle cells admixed with giant cells. (**b**) Predominantly spindle cell proliferation with areas of necrosis. (**c**) Spindle cell proliferation mimicking a mesenchymal neoplasm. (**d**) Scattered multinucleated giant cells in a predominantly spindle cell proliferation. (**e**) Highly pleomorphic multinucleated giant cells

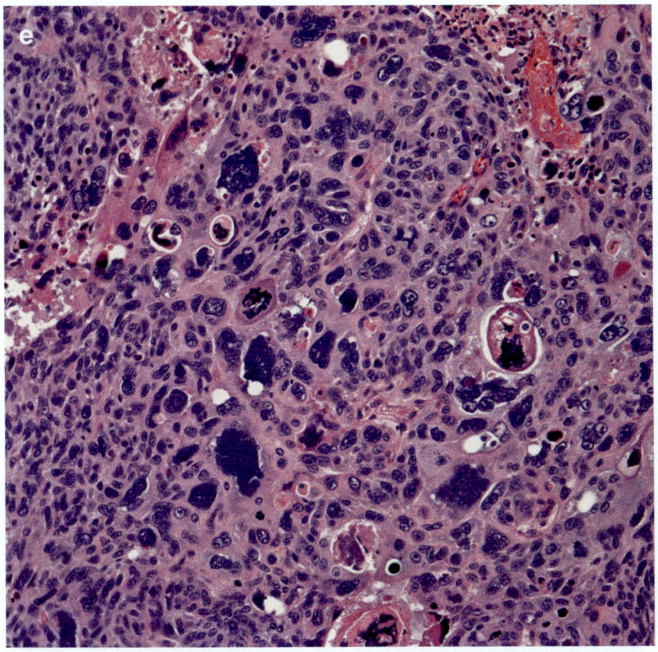

Fig. 3.49 (continued)

parenchyma; it appears well demarcated but not encapsulated. The tumor has a tendency to grow in sheets of tumor cells with some discohesion or in a vaguely nested pattern. At high-power magnification, the neoplastic cells are composed of larger cells with abundant eosinophilic cytoplasm, the nuclei are round to oval, and in some cells, they are displaced towards the periphery of the cells, while in others, it is more centrally located and contains prominent nucleoli (Fig. 3.50a–c). Other unusual features include the presence of a spindle cell (sarcomatous) component or multinucleated giant cells. In some cases of rhabdoid carcinoma, it is possible to identify areas of more conventional non-small cell carcinoma, even though this latter feature may be only focal. Although the diagnosis of rhabdoid carcinoma can be accomplished in a small biopsy, a resected specimen will provide the advantage of studying more tissue to determine the possibility of areas of more conventional carcinoma.

Immunohistochemical Features

In the majority of cases reported and in the ones that we have been able to examine, the use of epithelial markers (keratins and EMA) has proven to provide positive results. However, the positive staining for epithelial markers may be only focal. Other immunohistochemical markers that may also show positive staining in tumor cells include CD34, CD56, actin, vimentin, and rarely desmin. However, myoglobin has not been reported positive in these tumors.

Differential Diagnosis

Since the lung is a common site for metastatic tumors, it is important to properly address such possibility in tumors showing rhabdoid changes. In this setting, malignant melanoma or sarcomas are tumors that may metastasize to the lung and show similar cytologic features. Thus, the use of immunohistochemical studies including S-100 protein, HMB45, Melan A, myoglobin, caldesmon, and SOX2 would be important to rule out such possibility. As always, a good clinical history will be important in a context in which the possibility of metastatic disease is considered.

Lymphoepithelioma-Like Carcinoma (LELC)

LELC appear to be the counterpart of similar tumors that commonly occur in the head and neck area and are also referred to as undifferentiated carcinoma or Schmincke tumor. This particular tumor has also been described in several other areas within the thoracic cavity (thymus) or outside of the thoracic cavity.

The real incidence of this tumor as primary lung carcinoma is difficult to assess due to its rarity as well as the demographic distribution of this tumor.

LELC of the lung has been described predominantly in Asian individuals. Most of what is reported in the literature represents individual case reports with only a few small series of cases [193–208]. Begin et al. [193] are credited for the first description of this type of tumor in the lung after the authors described a 40-year-old female, nonsmoker of Asian background, with a lung tumor that histologically resembled LELC of the nasopharynx. The authors also suggested that the immunological profile was suggestive of Ebstein-Barr virus (EBV) infection. Han et al. [194] reported one of the largest series of LELC of the lung in 32 patients and compared them to conventional non-small cell carcinomas of the lung. In Han's series, there were more tumors in men than in women and the age ranged from 39 to 73 years, with the majority of patients in early stages of disease (stages I and II). The authors concluded that LELC has a better prognosis when compared to conventional non-small cell carcinomas, even in late stages of the disease. Tumor necrosis (>5 %) and tumor recurrence were associated with poor prognosis. Chan et al. [195] in a series of 11 cases of LELC also arrived to similar conclusions, as their patient demographics were similar to the series of Han et al. [194], and stated that LELC of the lung may have a variable behavior with the possibility of cases behaving aggressively. Butler et al. [196] reported a small series of four cases in adults of which three were women and one a man. Interestingly, three of the patients were Caucasians and one of Asian background. The authors of this report also found a more favorable outcome in the cases described. Although the great majority of cases described occur in adult individuals, LELC has also been described in the pediatric age group. Curcio et al. [202] described a case of LELC in an 8-year-old child

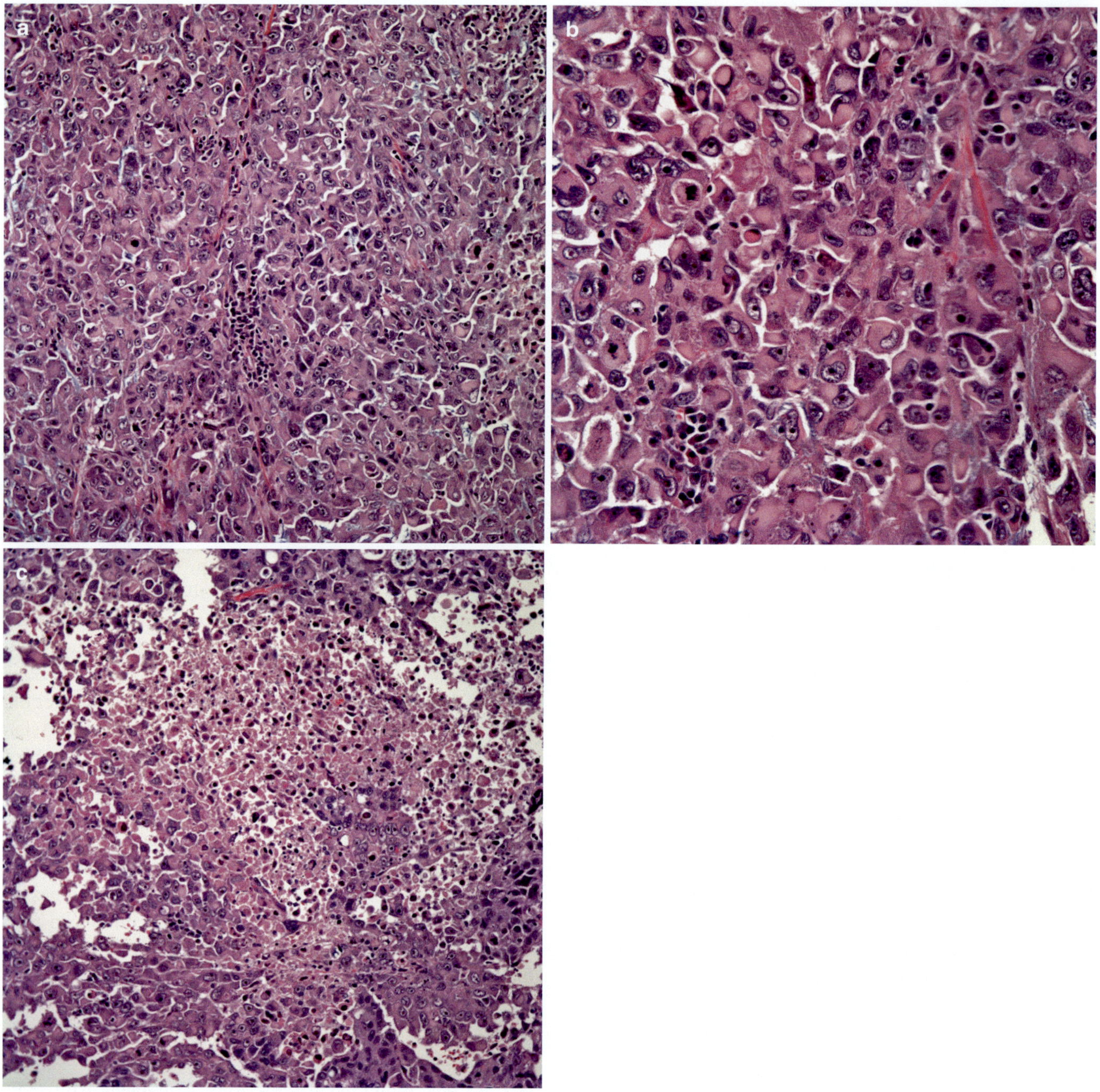

Fig. 3.50 (**a**) Rhabdoid carcinoma showing sheets of neoplastic cells. (**b**) Neoplastic cells showing abundant eosinophilic cytoplasm and nuclei displaced towards the periphery. (**c**) Rhabdoid cells admixed with necrosis

of Asian background, who underwent pneumonectomy and chemotherapy for a primary LELC of the lung. In situ hybridization studies demonstrated nuclear positivity for EBER-1 in tumor cells while the adjacent lymphocytes were negative. Other reports on LELC of the lung have been more focused in the identification of EBV [203–208]. There appears to be a strong association of EBV and the development of this tumor in the lung. However, in most of the cases in which EBV has been found in association with LELC, the patients were predominantly of Asian background. In addition, the tumor does not appear to be related to tobacco use. In 1991, Gal et al. [203] described a single case of LELC of the lung and identified the presence of EBV in the carcinoma cells but not in the lymphoid stroma. Thus, the authors suggested a possible oncogenic relationship between EBV and LELC of the lung. Chen et al. [206] performed a study of 127 cases of non-small cell carcinomas of the lung including LELC (5 cases) and encountered EBER-1 positivity in other non-small cell carcinomas of the lung besides LELC. Although the intensity of staining was recorded as stronger in LELC, squamous cell carcinomas also show positive nuclear staining for EBER-1, and in general, the authors estimated that about 8 % of non-small cell carcinomas may show such a reaction. The authors concluded that EBV infection might play a different role in the tumorigenesis of primary LELC of the lung than in the conventional variants of non-small cell carcinoma. Castro et al. [207] analyzed the relationship between EBV and LELC of the lung in 6 Caucasian patients by in situ hybridization studies and found that all the cases were negative for EBV. Thus, the authors suggested that there is no relationship between EBV and LELC of the lung in Western patients. More recently, Chang et al. [208] analyzed 23 cases of pulmonary LELC and documented an association between serum levels of EBV and tumor size. The authors also documented that nearly all cases had Bcl-2-oncoprotein expression and that latent membrane protein-1, p53, and c-erb B-2 expression was low.

Clinical Features

Like with any other non-small cell carcinoma, there is not a specific type of symptomatology associated with this type of neoplasm. Patients may present with cough, dyspnea, hemoptysis, or be completely asymptomatic, and the tumor is detected by chest radiological examination during routine examination. In most of the cases described, it appears that at least 50 % of the patients are in early stage of disease (stages I and II).

Histological Features

The hallmark of this neoplasm is the presence of a lymphocytic background that at low power may mimic an inflammatory reaction. The inflammatory stroma is predominantly composed of mature lymphocytes, but in some cases, plasma cells may be also be present. Admixed with this lymphocytic or lymphoplasmacytic stroma, are sheets of cells growing in ribbons or small islands. The neoplastic cellular proliferation is composed of medium-size cells, round to oval in shape and with indistinct cellular borders and moderate amounts of cytoplasm. The nucleus is round, and vesiculation of the nuclei may be seen with many cells displaying prominent nucleoli (Fig. 3.51a–c). Mitotic figures are easily encountered. Although in the great majority of cases, necrosis and/or hemorrhage are uncommon, these features can be seen in a small proportion of cases. In many cases, the neoplastic cellular proliferation appears to be haphazardly distributed in the lymphoid stroma without any particular pattern.

Differential Diagnosis

The most important differential diagnosis is the exclusion of a metastatic LELC from the head and neck area. Because all

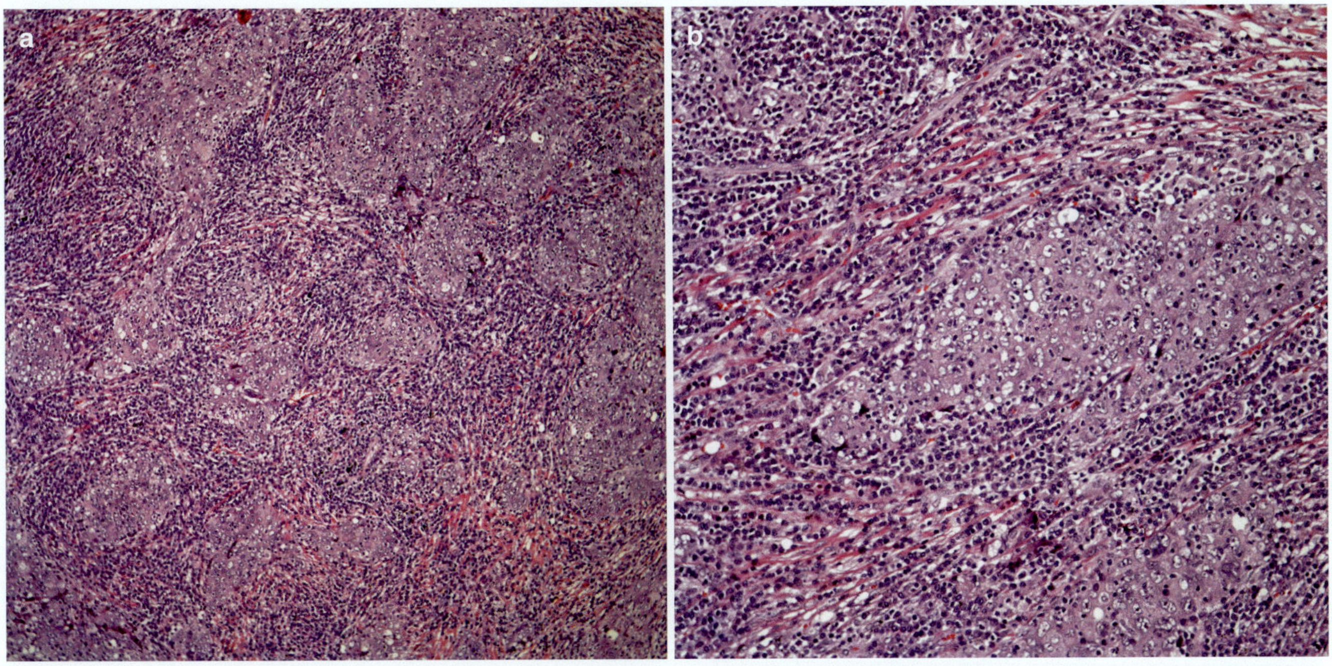

Fig. 3.51 (**a**) Lymphoepithelioma-like carcinoma showing neoplastic cells admixed with heavy inflammation. (**b**) The neoplastic cells are arranged in small islands embedded in an inflammatory background. (**c**) Closer magnification showing neoplastic cells admixed with inflammatory cells

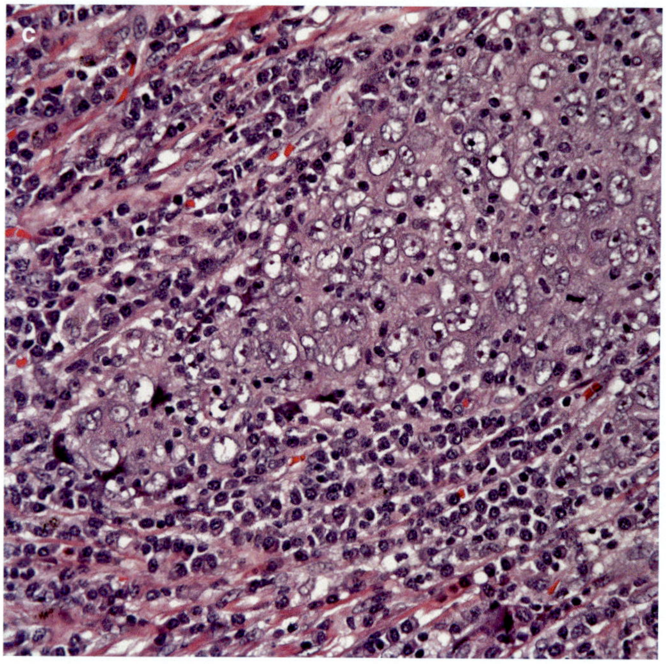

Fig. 3.51 (continued)

these tumors share similar histology, a complete clinical history should be of great help. However, due to the presence of a marked lymphocytic stroma, another lesion that may enter the differential diagnosis is lymphoma. The use of markers for epithelial differentiation should lead to proper interpretation.

Immunohistochemical Features

As has been reported by different authors, the use of epithelial markers including keratins and EMA may be of help in the diagnosis of this type of tumor. However, this tumor also shows positive staining for lymphoid markers including leukocyte common antigen (LCA) and Bcl-2 in the lymphoid component. Perhaps the most important study to perform in these tumors, although not for diagnostic purposes, would be in situ hybridization for EBV, mainly in a patients of Asian background.

References

1. http://www.cdc.gov/cancer/lung/statistics/index.html. Accessed on 1 June 2011.
2. http://seer.cancer.gov/csr/1975_2008/ Accessed on 1 June 2011.
3. Stanley K, Stjernsward J. Lung cancer: a worldwide health problem. Chest. 1989;96 Suppl 1:1S–5S.
4. Garfikel L, Silverberg E. Lung cancer and smoking trends in the United States over the past 25 years. CA Cancer J Clin. 1991;41:137–45.
5. Rubin SA. Lung cancer: past, present, and future. J Thorac Imaging. 1991;7:1–8.
6. Aronchik JM. Clinical aspects of lung cancer. Semin Roentgenol. 1990;25:5–11.
7. Gritz ER. Lung cancer: now, more than ever, a feminist issue. CA Cancer J Clin. 1993;43:197–9.
8. Devesa SS, Shaw GL, Blot WJ. Changing patterns of lung carcinoma. Cancer Epidemiol Biomarkers Prev. 1991;1:29–34.
9. Rosado-de-Christenson ML, Templeton PA, Moran CA. Bronchogenic carcinoma: radiologic/pathologic correlation. Radiographics. 1994;14:429–46.
10. Wahbah M, Boroumand N, Castro Y, et al. Changing trends in the distribution of the histologic types of lung cancer: a review of 4,439 cases. Ann Diagn Pathol. 2007;11:89–96.
11. Pietra GG. The pathology of carcinoma of the lung. Semin Roentgenol. 1990;25:25–33.
12. Haque AK. Pathology of carcinoma of the lung: an update on current concepts. J Thorac Imaging. 1991;7:9–20.
13. Boyards MC. Clinical manifestations of carcinoma of the lung. J Thorac Imaging. 1991;7:21–8.
14. Grippi MA. Clinical aspects of lung cancer. Semin Roentgenol. 1990;25:12–24.
15. Frazer RG, Pare JAP, Frazer RS, Genereux GP. Neoplastic diseases of the lung. In: Frazer RG et al., editors. Diagnosis of diseases of the chest. 3rd ed. Philadelphia: Saunders; 1989. p. 1327–99.
16. Morita T. A statistical study of lung cancer in the annual of pathological autopsy cases in Japan from 1958–1997, with reference to time trends of lung cancer in the world. Jpn J Cancer Res. 2002;93:15–23.
17. Travis WD, Brambilla E, Noguchi M, et al. International association for the study of lung cancer/American Thoracic Society/European Respiratory Society International Multidisciplinary Classification of Lung Adenocarcinoma. J Thorac Oncol. 2011;6:244–85.
18. Yamamoto Y, Tsuchida M, Watanabe T, et al. Early resection of a prospective study of limited resection for bronchioloalveolar adenocarcinoma of the lung. Ann Thorac Surg. 2001;71:971–4.
19. Watanabe S, Watanabe T, Arai K, et al. Results of wedge resection for focal bronchioloalveolar carcinoma showing pure ground-glass attenuation on computed tomography. Ann Thorac Surg. 2002;73:1071–5.
20. Suzuki K, Asamura H, Kusumoto M, et al. "Early" peripheral lung cancer: prognostic significance of ground glass opacity on thin-section computed tomography scan. Ann Thorac Surg. 2002;74:1635–9.
21. Sakurai H, Dobashi Y, Mizutani E, et al. Bronchioloalveolar carcinoma of the lung 3 centimeters of less in diameter: a retrospective assessment. Ann Thorac Surg. 2004;78:1728–33.
22. Yamada S, Kohno T. Video-assisted thoracic surgery for pure ground-glass opacities 2 cm or less in diameter. Ann Thorac Surg. 2004;77:1911–5.
23. Yoshida J, Nagai K, Yokose T, et al. Limited resection trial for pulmonary ground-glass opacity nodules: fifty-case experience. J Thorac Cardiovasc Surg. 2004;129:991–6.
24. Koike T, Togashi K, Shirato T, et al. Limited resection for non-invasive bronchioloalveolar carcinoma diagnosed by intraoperative pathologic examination. Ann Thorac Surg. 2009;88:1106–11.
25. Vasques M, Carter D, Brambilla E, et al. Solitary and multiple resected adenocarcinomas after CT screening for lung cancer: Histopathologic features and their prognostic implications. Lung Cancer. 2009;64:148–54.
26. Yoshizawa A, Motoi N, Riely GJ, et al. Impact of proposed IASLC/ATS/ERS classification of lung adenocarcinoma: prognostic subgroups and implications for further revision of staging based on analysis of 514 stage I cases. Mod Pathol. 2011;24:653–64.
27. Sakurai H, Maeshima A, Watanabe S, et al. Grade of stromal invasion in small adenocarcinomas of the lung. Am J Clin Pathol. 2004;28:198–206.
28. Yim J, Zhu LC, Chiriboga L, et al. Histological features are important prognostic indicators in early stages lung adenocarcinoma. Mod Pathol. 2007;20:233–41.

29. Borczuk AC, Qian F, Kazeros A, et al. Invasive size is an independent predictor of survival in pulmonary adenocarcinoma. Am J Surg Pathol. 2009;33:462–9.
30. Witt R. Letter to the Editor. J Thorac Oncol. 2011;6:1451.
31. Sawabata N, Miyaoka E, Asamura H, et al. Japanese lung cancer registry study of 11,663 surgical cases in 2004: demographic and prognosis changes over decade. J Thorac Oncol. 2011;6:1229–35.
32. Takizawa T, Terashima M, Koike T, et al. Lymph node metastasis in small peripheral adenocarcinoma of the lung. J Thorac Cardiovasc Surg. 1998;116:276–80.
33. Konaka C, Ikeda N, Hiyoshi T, et al. Peripheral non-small lung cancers 2.0 cm or less in diameter: proposed criteria for limited pulmonary resection based upon clinicopathological presentation. Lung Cancer. 1998;21:185–91.
34. Warren W, Faber LP. Segmentectomy versus lobectomy in patients with stage I pulmonary carcinoma: five-year survival and patterns of intrathoracic recurrence. J Thorac Cardiovasc Surg. 1994;107: 1087–94.
35. Malassez L. Examen histologique d'un cas de cancer encephaloide du poumon (Epithelioma). Arch Physiol Norm Pathol. 1876;3:352–72.
36. Musser JH. Primary cancer of the lung. Univ Penn Bull. 1903;16:289–96.
37. Sweany HC. A so-called alveolar cell cancer of the lung. Arch Pathol. 1935;19:203–7.
38. Casilli AR, White HJ. Rare forms of primary malignant lung tumors. Am J Clin Pathol. 1940;10:623–41.
39. Geever KT. Alveolar cell tumor of the human lung. Arch Pathol. 1942;33:551–69.
40. Herbut PA. Bronchiolar origin of "alveolar cell tumor" of the lung. Am J Pathol. 1944;20:911–29.
41. Wood DA, Pierson PH. Pulmonary alveolar adenomatosis in man. Am Rev Tuberc. 1945;51:205–23.
42. Ikeda K. Alveolar cell carcinoma of the lung. Am J Clin Pathol. 1945;15:50–63.
43. Osserman KE, Neuhof H. Mucocellular papillary adenocarcinoma of the lung. J Thorac Surg. 1946;15:272–8.
44. Drymalski GW, Thompson R, Sweany HC. Pulmonary adenomatosis. Am J Pathol. 1948;20:1083–93.
45. Dela Rue NC, Graham EA. Alveolar cell carcinoma of the lung (pulmonary adenomatosis, jaagsiekte?). J Thorac Surg. 1948;18:237–51.
46. Liebow AA. Bronchiolo-alveolar carcinoma. Adv Intern Med. 1960;10:329–58.
47. Carter D, Eggleston JC, editors. Tumors of the lower respiratory tract, Fascicle 17, Second series. Bethesda: Armed Forces Institute of Pathology; 1980. p. 127
48. Colby TV, Koss MN, Travis WD, editors. Tumors of the lower respiratory tract. Atlas of tumor pathology, Fascicle #13. Washington, D.C.: Armed Forces Institute of Pathology; 1995. p. 203.
49. Travis WD, Colby TV, Corrin B, et al. Histological typing of lung and pleural tumours. World Health Organization, 3rd ed. Berlin/ New York: Springer; 1999. p. 36
50. Travis WD, Brambilla E, Muller-Hermelink K, Harris CC, editors. Pathology and genetics of the tumours of the lung, pleura, thymus, and heart. World Health Organization classification of tumors. Lyon: IARC Press; 2004. p.38
51. Overholt RH, Meissner WA, Delmonico E. Favorable bronchiolar carcinoma. Chest. 1955;27:403–13.
52. Belgrad R, Good A, Woolner LB. Alveolar-cell carcinoma (terminal bronchiolar carcinoma): a study of surgically excised tumors with special emphasis on localized lesions. Radiology. 1962;79:789–98.
53. Munell ER, Lawson RC, Keller DF. Solitary bronchiolar (alveolar cell) carcinoma of the lung. J Thorac Cardiovasc Surg. 1966;52:261–70.
54. Watson I, Farpour A. Terminal bronchiolar or "alveolar cell" cancer of the lung: two hundred sixty-five cases. Cancer. 1966;19: 776–80.
55. Rosenblatt MB, Lisa JR, Collier F. Primary and metastatic bronchiolo-alveolar carcinoma. Chest. 1967;52:147–52.
56. Bennett DE, Sasser WF. Bronchiolar carcinoma: a valid clinicopathologic entity? A study of 30 cases. Cancer. 1969;24:876–87.
57. Delarue NC, Anderson W, Sanders D, Starr J. Bronchiolo-alveolar carcinoma: a reappraisal after 24 years. Cancer. 1972;29:90–7.
58. Marco M, Galy P. Bronchioloalveolar carcinoma: clinicopathologic relationships, natural history, and prognosis in 29 cases. Am Rev Respir Dis. 1973;107:621–9.
59. Schraunagel D, Peloquin A, Pare JAP, Wang NS. Differentiating bronchioloalveolar carcinoma from adenocarcinoma. Am Rev Respir Dis. 1982;125:74–9.
60. Singh G, Katyal SL. Bronchioloalveolar carcinomas: a heterogeneous group. Am Rev Respir Dis. 1982;125:183.
61. Singh G, Katyal SL, Torikata C. Carcinoma of type II pneumocytes: immunodiagnosis of a subtype of "bronchioloalveolar carcinomas". Am J Pathol. 1981;102:195–208.
62. Dermer GB. Origin of bronchioloalveolar carcinoma and peripheral bronchial adenocarcinoma. Cancer. 1982;49:881–7.
63. Manning JT, Spjut HJ, Tsechen JA. Bronchioloalveolar carcinoma: the significance of two histopathologic types. Cancer. 1984;54:525–34.
64. Clayton F. Bronchiloalveolar carcinomas. Cell types, patterns of growth, and prognostic correlates. Cancer. 1986;57:1555–64.
65. Thomas JJ, Tullett WM, Stack BHR. Bronchioloalveolar cell carcinoma: a 21-year retrospective study of cases at the Western Infirmary, Glasgow. Br J Dis Chest. 1985;79:132–40.
66. Elson CE, Moore SP, Johnston WW. Morphologic and immunohistochemical studies of bronchioloalveolar carcinoma at Duke University Medical Center, 1968–1986. Anal Quant Cytol Histol. 1989;11:261–74.
67. Daly RC, Trastek VF, Pairolero PC, et al. Bronchoalveolar carcinoma: factors affecting survival. Ann Thorac Surg. 1991;51: 368–77.
68. Feldman ER, Eagan RT, Schaid DJ. Metastatic bronchioloalveolar carcinoma and metastatic adenocarcinoma of the lung: comparison of clinical manifestations, chemotherapeutic responses, and prognosis. Mayo Clin Proc. 1992;67:27–32.
69. Breathnach OS, Ishibe N, Williams J, et al. Clinical features of patients with stage IIIb and IV bronchioloalveolar carcinoma of the lung. Cancer. 1999;86:1165–73.
70. Hsu CP, Chen CY, Hsu NY. Bronchioloalveolar carcinoma. J Thorac Cardiovasc Surg. 1995;110:374–81.
71. Fujimoto N, Segawa Y, Takigawa N, et al. Clinical investigation of bronchioloalveolar carcinoma: a retrospective analysis of 53 patients in a single institution. Anticancer Res. 1999;19:1369–74.
72. Barkley JE, Green MR. Bronchioloalveolar carcinoma. J Clin Oncol. 1996;14:2377–86.
73. Goodwin LO, Mason JM, Hajdu SI. Gene expression patterns of paired bronchioloalveolar carcinoma and benign lung tissue. Ann Clin Lab Sci. 2001;31:369–75.
74. Read WL, Page NC, Tierney RM, et al. The epidemiology of bronchioloalveolar carcinoma over the last two decades: analysis of the SEER database. Lung Cancer. 2004;45:137–42.
75. Raz DJ, Jablons DM. Bronchioloalveolar carcinoma is not associated with younger age at diagnosis: an analysis of the SEER database. J Thorac Oncol. 2006;1:339–43.
76. Ohye RG, Cohen DM, Caldwell S, Qualman SJ. Pediatric bronchioloalveolar carcinoma: a favorable pediatric malignancy? J Pediatr Surg. 1998;33:730–2.
77. Breathnach OS, Kwiatowski DJ, Finkelstein DM, et al. Bronchioloalveolar carcinoma of the lung: recurrences and survival in patients with stage I disease. J Thorac Cardiovasc Surg. 2001;121:42–7.
78. Rena O, Papalia E, Ruffini E, et al. Stage I pure bronchioloalveolar carcinoma: recurrences, survival and comparison with adenocarcinoma. Eur J Cardiothorac Surg. 2003;23:409–14.

79. Gaeta M, Blandino A, Pergolizzi S, et al. Patterns of recurrence of bronchioloalveolar cell carcinoma after surgical resection: a radiological, histological, and immunohistochemical study. Lung Cancer. 2003;42:319–26.
80. Ebright MI, Zakoski MF, Martin J, et al. Clinical pattern and pathologic stage but not histologic features predict outcome for bronchioloalveolar carcinoma. Ann Thorac Surg. 2002;74:1640–7.
81. Travis WD, Garg K, Franklin WA, et al. Bronchioloalveolar carcinoma and lung adenocarcinoma: the clinical importance and research relevance of the 2004 World Health Organization pathologic criteria. J Thorac Oncol. 2006;1:S13–9.
82. Noguchi M, Morikawa A, Kawasaki M, et al. Small adenocarcinoma of the lung: histologic characteristics and prognosis. Cancer. 1995;75:2844–52.
83. Zell JA, Ou SHI, Ziogas A, Culver HA. Epidemiology of bronchioloalveolar carcinoma: improvement in survival after release of the 1999 WHO classification of lung tumors. J Clin Oncol. 2005;23:8396–405.
84. Zell JA, Ou SHI, Ziogas A, Culver HA. Validation of the proposed international association for the study of lung cancer non-small cell lung cancer staging system revisions for advanced bronchioloalveolar carcinoma using data from the California Cancer Registry. J Thorac Oncol. 2007;2:1078–85.
85. Grover FL, Piantadosi S. Recurrence and survival following resection of bronchioloalveolar carcinoma of the lung – The Lung Cancer Study Group experience. Ann Surg. 1989;209:779–90.
86. Garfield DH, Cadranel JL, Wislez M, et al. The bronchioloalveolar carcinoma and peripheral adenocarcinoma spectrum of diseases. J Thorac Oncol. 2006;1:344–59.
87. Damhuis RAM, Schutte PR, Varin OCM, et al. Poor results after surgery for bronchioloalveolar carcinoma. Eur J Surg Oncol. 2006;32:573–6.
88. Sidhu SG, Wieczorek R, Cassai ND, Zhu CC. The concept of bronchioloalveolar cell adenocarcinoma: redefinition, a critique of the 1999 WHO classification, and an ultrastructural analysis of 155 cases. Int J Surg Pathol. 2003;11:89–99.
89. Hajdu SI. A note from history: the story of bronchioloalveolar carcinoma. Ann Clin Lab Sci. 2005;35:336–8.
90. Noguchi M, Kodama T, Shimosato Y, et al. Papillary adenoma of type 2 pneumocytes. Am J Surg Pathol. 1986;10:134–9.
91. Koga T, Hashimoto S, Sugio K, et al. Lung adenocarcinoma with bronchioloalveolar component is frequently associated with foci of high-grade atypical adenomatous hyperplasia. Am J Clin Pathol. 2002;117:464–70.
92. Travis WD, Linnoila RI, Horowitz M, et al. Pulmonary nodules resembling bronchioloalveolar carcinoma in adolescent cancer patients. Mod Pathol. 1988;1:372–7.
93. Morandi L, Asioli S, Cavazza A, et al. Genetic relationship among atypical adenomatous hyperplasia, bronchioloalveolar carcinoma, and adenocarcinoma of the lung. Lung Cancer. 2007;56:35–42.
94. Solis LM, Behrens C, Raso MG, Lin HY, Kadara H, Yuan P, et al. Histologic patterns and molecular characteristics of lung adenocarcinoma associated with clinical outcome. Cancer. 2011;118:2889–99. doi:10.1002/cncr.26584.
95. Ogata T, Endo K. Clara cell granules of peripheral lung cancers. Cancer. 1984;54:1635–44.
96. Hirata H, Noguchi M, Shimosato Y, et al. Clinicopathologic and immunohistochemical characteristics of bronchial gland cell type adenocarcinoma of the lung. Am J Clin Pathol. 1990;93:20–5.
97. Edwards CW. Pulmonary adenocarcinoma: review of 106 cases and proposed new classification. J Clin Pathol. 1987;40:125–35.
98. Miller RA, Nelems B, Evans KG, et al. Glandular neoplasia of the lung: a proposed analogy to colonic tumors. Cancer. 1988;61:1009–14.
99. Dabbs DJ, Landreneau RJ, Liu Y, et al. Detection of estrogen receptors by immunohistochemistry in pulmonary adenocarcinoma. Ann Thorac Surg. 2002;73:403–6.
100. Siami K, McCluggage G, Ordonez NG, et al. Thyroid transcription factor-1 expression in endometrial and endocervical adenocarcinomas. Am J Surg Pathol. 2007;31:1759–63.
101. Moran CA. Mucin-rich tumors of the lung. Adv Anat Pathol. 1995;2:299–305.
102. Kragel PJ, Devaney KO, Meth BM, Linnoila I, Frierson HF, Travis WD. Mucinous cystadenoma of the lung: a report of two cases with immunohistochemical and ultrastructural analysis. Arch Pathol Lab Med. 1990;114:1053–6.
103. Traub B. Mucinous cystadenoma of the lung [letter]. Arch Pathol Lab Med. 1991;115:740.
104. Dixon AY, Moran JF, Wesselius LJ, McGregor DH. Pulmonary mucinous cystic tumor: case report with review of the literature. Am J Surg Pathol. 1993;17:722–8.
105. Higashima M, Doi O, Kodama K, Yokouchi H, Tateishi R. Cystic mucinous adenocarcinoma of the lung: two cases of cystic variant of mucinous-producing lug adenocarcinoma. Chest. 1992;101:763–6.
106. Davison AM, Lowe JW, Da Costa P. Adenocarcinoma arising in a mucinous cystadenoma of the lung. Thorax. 1992;47:129–30.
107. Graeme-Cook F, Mark EJ. Pulmonary mucinous cystic tumors of borderline malignancy. Hum Pathol. 1991;22:185–90.
108. Moran CA, Hochholzer L, Fishback N, Koss MN. Mucinous (so-called colloid) carcinoma of the lung. Mod Pathol. 1992;5:634–8.
109. Silver S, Askin FB. True papillary carcinoma of the lung. A distinct clinicopathologic entity. Am J Surg Pathol. 1997;21:43–51.
110. Zhang J, Tomizawa Y, Yanagitani N, et al. Papillary adenocarcinoma of the lung is a more advanced adenocarcinoma than bronchioloalveolar carcinoma that is composed of two distinct histological subtypes. Pathol Int. 2005;55:619–25.
111. Aida S, Shimazaki H, Sato K, et al. Prognostic analysis of pulmonary adenocarcinoma subclassification with special consideration of papillary and bronchioloalveolar types. Histopathology. 2004;45:466–76.
112. Moran CA, Jagirdar J, Suster S. Papillary lung adenocarcinoma with prominent "morular" component. Am J Clin Pathol. 2004;122:106–9.
113. Amin M, Tamboli P, Merchant SH, et al. Micropapillary component in lung adenocarcinoma: a distinctive histologic feature with possible prognostic significance. Am J Surg Pathol. 2002;26:358–64.
114. Makimoto Y, Nabeshima K, Iwasaki H, et al. Micropapillary pattern: a distinctive pathological marker to subclassify tumours with significantly poor prognosis within small peripheral lung adenocarcinoma (< 20 mm) with mixed bronchioloalveolar and invasive subtypes (Noguchi's type C tumours). Histopathology. 2005;46:677–84.
115. Kuroda N, Hamaguchi N, Takeuchi E, et al. Lung adenocarcinoma with micropapillary pattern: a clinicopathological study of 25 cases. Acta Pathol Microbiol Immunol Scand Suppl. 2006;114:381–5.
116. Miyoshi T, Satoh Y, Okumura S, et al. Early-stage lung adenocarcinomas with micropapillary pattern, a distinct pathologic marker for a significantly poor prognosis. Am J Surg Pathol. 2003;27:101–9.
117. Hoshi R, Tsuzuku M, Horai T, et al. Micropapillary clusters in early-stage lung adenocarcinoma. A distinct cytologic sign of significantly poor prognosis. Cancer Cytopathol. 2004;102:81–6.
118. Kish JK, Ro JY, Ayala AG, McMurtrey MJ. Primary mucinous adenocarcinoma of the lung with signet-ring cells: a histochemical comparison with signet ring cell carcinomas of other sites. Hum Pathol. 1989;20:1097–102.

119. Sarma EP. Primary signet-ring cell carcinoma of the lung [letter to the editor]. Hum Pathol. 1990;21:459–60.
120. Hayashi H, Kitamura H, Nakatani Y, et al. Primary signet ring cell carcinoma of the lung: histochemical and immunohistochemical characterization. Hum Pathol. 1999;30:378–83.
121. Castro CY, Moran CA, Flieder DG, Suster S. Primary signet ring cell adenocarcinoma of the lung: a clinicopathological study of 15 cases. Histopathology. 2001;39:397–401.
122. Steinhauer JR, Moran CA, Suster S. Secretory endometrioid-like adenocarcinoma of the lung. Histopathology. 2005;47:219–20.
123. Ishikura H, Kanda M, Ito M, et al. Hepatoid adenocarcinoma: a distinctive histological subtype of alpha-fetoprotein-producing lung carcinoma. Virchows Arch A Pathol Anat Histopathol. 1990;417:73–80.
124. Arnould L, Drouot F, Fargeot P, et al. Hepatoid adenocarcinoma of the lung. Am J Surg Pathol. 1997;43:654–61.
125. Nasu M, Soma T, Fukushima H, et al. Hepatoid carcinoma of the lung with production of a-fetoprotein and abnormal prothrombin: an autopsy case report. Mod Pathol. 1997;10:1054–8.
126. Carlinfante G, Pia-Foshini M, Pasquinelli G, et al. Hepatoid carcinoma of the lung: a case report with immunohistochemical, ultrastructural and in situ hybridization findings. Histopathology. 2000;37:88–9.
127. Yasunami R, Hashimoto Z, Ogura T, et al. Primary lung cancer producing alpha-fetoprotein: a case report. Cancer. 1981;47:926–9.
128. Miyake M, Ito M, Taki T, et al. A case report of two patients with pulmonary lung cancer secreting AFP. Nippon Kyobu Geka Gakkai Zasshi. 1986;34:914–9.
129. Hayashi Y, Takanashi Y, Ohsawa H, et al. Hepatoid adenocarcinoma of the lung. Lung Cancer. 2002;38:211–4.
130. Solis LM, Raso GM, Behrens C, et al. Primary oncocytic adenocarcinoma of the lung: a clinicopathologic, immunohistochemical, and molecular biologic analysis of 16 cases. Am J Clin Pathol. 2010;133:133–40.
131. Sherwin RP, Laforret EG, Strieder JW. Exophytic endobronchial carcinoma. J Thorac Cardiovasc Surg. 1962;43:716–30.
132. Dulmet-Brender E, Jaubert F, Huchon G. Exophytic endobronchial epidermoid carcinoma. Cancer. 1986;57:1358–64.
133. Cooper L, Hagenschneider JK, Banky S, Rosado-de-Christenson ML, Suster S. Papillary endobronchial squamous cell carcinoma. Ann Diagn Pathol. 2005;9:284–8.
134. Laubscher F. Solitary squamous cell papilloma of bronchial origin. Am J Clin Pathol. 1969;52:599–603.
135. Spencer H, Dail DH, Arneaud J. Non-invasive bronchial epithelial papillary tumors. Cancer. 1980;45:1486–97.
136. Trillo A, Guha A. Solitary condylomatous papilloma of the bronchus. Arch Pathol Lab Med. 1988;112:731–3.
137. Al-Saleem T, Peale AR, Norris CM. Multiple papillomatosis of the lower respiratory tract: clinical and pathologic study of eleven cases. Cancer. 1968;6:1173–84.
138. Suster S, Huszar M, Herczeg E. Spindle cell squamous carcinoma of the lung: immunohistochemical and ultrastructural study of a case. Histopathology. 1987;11:871–8.
139. Wang BY, Gill J, Kaufman D, et al. P63 in primary pulmonary epithelium, pulmonary squamous neoplasms, and other pulmonary tumors. Hum Pathol. 2002;33:921–6.
140. Weissferdt A, Moran CA. Microscystic squamous cell carcinoma: a clinicopathological correlation of 3 cases. Am J Clin Pathol. 2011;136:436–41.
141. Pelosi G, Pasini F, Stenholm CO, et al. P63 immunoreactivity in lung cancer: yet another player in the development of squamous cell carcinomas? J Pathol. 2002;198:100–9.
142. Pelosi G, Barisella M, Pasini F, et al. CD117 immunoreactivity in stage I adenocarcinoma and squamous cell carcinoma of the lung: relevance to prognosis in a subset of adenocarcinoma patients. Mod Pathol. 2004;17:711–21.
143. Yoshino I, Osoegawa A, Yohena T, et al. Loss of heterozygosity (LOH) in non-small cell lung cancer: difference between adenocarcinoma and squamous cell carcinoma. Respir Med. 2005;99:308–12.
144. Chujo M, Noguchi T, Miura T, et al. Comparative genomic hybridization analysis detected frequent overrepresentation of chromosome 3q in squamous cell carcinoma of the lung. Lung Cancer. 2002;38:23–9.
145. Churg A. The fine structure of large cell undifferentiated carcinoma of the lung. Hum Pathol. 1978;9(2):143–56.
146. Yesner R. Large cell carcinoma of the lung. Semin Diagn Pathol. 1985;2(4):255–69.
147. Albain KS, Ture LD, Golomb HM, et al. Large cell carcinoma of the lung: ultrastructural differentiation and clinicopathologic correlations. Cancer. 1985;56:1618–23.
148. Kodama T, Shimosato Y, Koide T, et al. Large cell carcinoma of the lung – ultrastructural and immunohistochemical studies. Jpn J Clin Oncol. 1985;15:431–41.
149. Leung CS, Morava-Protzner I. Large cell carcinoma of the lung with osteoclast-like giant cells. Histopathology. 1998;32:482–4.
150. Masse SR, Dawson DT, Khaliq A. Ectopic gonadotropin in a case of anaplastic large-cell carcinoma of the lung. CMAJ. 1974;111:253–5.
151. Zhong D, Guo L, Aguirre I, et al. LKB1 mutation in large cell carcinoma of the lung. Lung Cancer. 2006;53:285–94.
152. Fitzgibbons PL, Kern WH. Adenosquamous carcinoma of the lung: a clinical and pathologic study of seven cases. Hum Pathol. 1985;16:463–6.
153. Naunheim KS, Taylor JR, Skosey C, et al. Adenosquamous lung carcinoma: clinical characteristics, treatment, and prognosis. Ann Thorac Surg. 1987;44:462–6.
154. Sridhar KS, Raub WA, Duncan RC, Hilsenbeck S. The increasing recognition of adenosquamous lung carcinoma (1977–1986). Am J Clin Oncol. 1992;15:356–62.
155. Sridhar KS, Bounassi MJ, Raub W, Richman SP. Clinical features of adenosquamous lung carcinoma in 127 patients. Am Rev Respir Dis. 1990;142:19–23.
156. Takamori S, Noguchi M, Morinaga S, et al. Clinicopathologic characteristics of adenosquamous carcinoma of the lung. Cancer. 1991;67:649–54.
157. Teruyoshi I, Kaneko S, Yokoyama H, et al. Adenosquamous carcinoma of the lung: clinicopathologic and immunohistochemical features. Am J Clin Pathol. 1992;97:678–85.
158. Mnaymneh LG, Raub WA, Sridhar KS, et al. The accuracy of the histological classification of lung carcinoma and its reproducibility: a study of 75 archival cases of adenosquamous carcinoma. Cancer Invest. 1993;11:641–51.
159. Hofmann HS, Knolle J, Neef H. The adenosquamous lung carcinoma: clinical and pathological characteristics. J Cardiovasc Surg. 1994;35:543–7.
160. Shimizu J, Oda M, Hayashi Y, et al. A clinicopathologic study of resected cases of adenosquamous carcinoma of the lung. Chest. 1996;109:989–94.
161. Hsia JY, Chen CY, Hsu CP, et al. Adenosquamous carcinoma of the lung: surgical results compared with squamous cell and adenocarcinoma. Scand Cardiovasc J. 1998;33:29–32.
162. Nakagawa K, Yasumitu T, Fukuhara K, et al. Poor prognosis after lung resection for patients with adenosquamous carcinoma of the lung. Ann Thorac Surg. 2003;75:1740–4.
163. Gawrychowski J, Brulinski K, Malinowski E, Papla B. Prognosis and survival after radical resection of primary adenosquamous lung carcinoma. Eur J Cardiothorac Surg. 2005;27:686–92.
164. Ylagan LR, Scholes J, Demopoulos R. CD44: a marker of squamous differentiation in adenosquamous neoplasms. Arch Pathol Lab Med. 2000;124:212–5.

165. Kanazawa H, Ebina M, Ino-Oka N, et al. Transition from squamous cell carcinoma to adenocarcinoma in adenosquamous carcinoma of the lung. Am J Pathol. 2000;156:1289–98.
166. Kang SM, Kang HJ, Shin JH, et al. Identical epidermal growth factor receptor mutations in adenocarcinomatous and squamous cell carcinomatous components of adenosquamous carcinoma of the lung. Cancer. 2007;109:581–7.
167. Liang JC, Kurzrock R, Gutterman JU, Gallick GE. Trisomy 12 correlates with elevated expression of p21ras in a human adenosquamous carcinoma of the lung. Cancer Genet Cytogenet. 1986;23:183–8.
168. Humphrey P, Scroggs MW, Roggli V, Shelburne JD. Pulmonary carcinomas with sarcomatoid element: an immunohistochemical and ultrastructural analysis. Hum Pathol. 1988;19:155–65.
169. Matsui K, Kitagawa M. Spindle cell carcinoma of the lung: a clinicopathologic study of three cases. Cancer. 1991;67:2361–7.
170. Ro JY, Chen JL, Lee JS, et al. Sarcomatoid carcinoma of the lung: immunohistochemical and ultrastructural studies of 14 cases. Cancer. 1992;69:376–86.
171. Fishback NF, Travis WD, Moran CA, et al. Pleomorphic (spindle/giant cell) carcinoma of the lung: a clinicopathologic correlation of 78 cases. Cancer. 1994;73:2936–45.
172. Razzuk MA, Urschel HC, Albers JE, et al. Pulmonary giant cell carcinoma. Ann Thorac Surg. 1976;21:540–5.
173. Wang NS, Seemayer TA, Ahmed MN, Knaack J. Giant cell carcinoma of the lung: a light and electron microscopic study. Hum Pathol. 1976;7:3–16.
174. Bendel WL, Ishak KG. Giant cell carcinoma of the lung: report of two cases. Am J Clin Pathol. 1961;35:435–40.
175. Nash AD, Stout AP. Giant cell carcinoma of the lung: report of 5 cases. Cancer. 1958;11:369–76.
176. Herman DL, Bullock WK, Waken JK. Giant cell adenocarcinoma of the lug. Cancer. 1966;19:1337–46.
177. Hellstrom HR, Fisher ER. Giant cell carcinoma of the lung. Cancer. 1963;16:1080–8.
178. Shin M, Jackson LK, Shelton RW, Greene RE. Giant cell carcinoma of the lung: clinical and roentgenographic manifestations. Chest. 1986;89:366–9.
179. Ginsberg SS, Buzaid AC, Stern H, Carter D. Giant cell carcinoma of the lung. Cancer. 1992;70:606–10.
180. Addis BJ, Dewar A, Thurlow NP. Giant cell carcinoma of the lung – immunohistochemical and ultrastructural evidence of dedifferentiation. J Pathol. 1988;155:231–40.
181. Przygodzki RM, Koss MN, Moran CA, et al. Pleomorphic (giant and spindle cell) carcinoma is genetically distinct from adenocarcinoma and squamous cell carcinoma by K-ras-2 and p53 analysis. Am J Clin Pathol. 1996;106:487–92.
182. Rubenchik I, Dardick I, Auger M. Cytopathology and ultrastructure of primary rhabdoid tumor of the lung. Ultrastruct Pathol. 1996;20:355–60.
183. Cavazza A, Colby TV, Tsokos M, et al. Lung tumors with rhabdoid phenotype. Am J Clin Pathol. 1996;105:182–8.
184. Chetty R, Bhana B, Batitang S, Govender D. Lung carcinomas composed of rhabdoid cells. Eur J Surg Oncol. 1997;23:432–4.
185. Miyagi I, Tsuhako K, Kinjo T, et al. Rhabdoid tumour of the lung is a dedifferentiated phenotype of pulmonary adenocarcinoma. Histopathology. 2000;37:37–44.
186. Shimazaki H, Aida S, Sato M, et al. Lung carcinoma with rhabdoid cells: a clinicopathological study and survival analysis of 14 cases. Histopathology. 2001;38:425–34.
187. Kaneko T, Honda T, Fukushima M, et al. Large cell carcinoma of the lung with rhabdoid phenotype. Pathol Int. 2002;52:643–7.
188. Hiroshima K, Shibuya K, Shimamura F, et al. Pulmonary large cell carcinoma with rhabdoid phenotype. Ultrastruct Pathol. 2003;27:55–9.
189. Tamboli P, Tropani TH, Amin MB, et al. Carcinoma of lung with rhabdoid features. Hum Pathol. 2004;35:8–13.
190. Yilmazbayhan D, Ates LE, Dilege S, et al. Pulmonary large cell carcinoma with rhabdoid phenotype. Ann Diag Pathol. 2005;9:223–6.
191. Falconieri G, Moran CA, Pizzolitto S, et al. Intrathoracic rhabdoid carcinoma: a clinicopathological immunohistochemical, and ultrastructural study of 6 cases. Ann Diagn Pathol. 2005;9:279–83.
192. Wick MR, Ritter JH, Dehner LP. Malignant rhabdoid tumors: a clinicopathologic review and conceptual discussion. Semin Diagn Pathol. 1995;12:233–48.
193. Begin LR, Eskandari J, Joncas J, Panasci L. Epstein-Barr virus related lymphoepithelioma-like carcinoma of the lung. J Surg Oncol. 1987;36:280–3.
194. Han A, Xiong M, Gu Y, et al. Lymphoepithelioma-like carcinoma of the lung with a better prognosis: a clinicopathologic study of 32 cases. Am J Clin Pathol. 2001;115:841–50.
195. Chan JKC, Hui PK, Tsang WYW, et al. Primary lymphoepithelioma-like carcinoma of the lung: a clinicopathologic study of 11 cases. Cancer. 1995;76:413–22.
196. Butler AE, Colby TV, Weiss L, Lombard C. Lymphoepithelioma-like carcinoma of the lung. Am J Surg Pathol. 1989;13:632–9.
197. Ho JC, Wong MP, Wong MK, et al. Lymphoepithelioma-like carcinoma of the lung: experience with ten cases. Int J Tuberc Lung Dis. 2004;8:890–5.
198. Guerrero A, Laflamme M, Agoff SN, et al. Primary lymphoepithelioma-like carcinoma of the lung. Can Respir J. 2001;8:431–3.
199. Frank MW, Shields TW, Joob AW, et al. Lymphoepithelioma-like carcinoma of the lung. Ann Thorac Surg. 1997;64:1162–4.
200. Wockel W, Hofler HH, Popper HH, Morresi A. Lymphoepithelioma-like carcinoma of the lung. Pathol Res Pract. 1995;191:1170–4.
201. Miller B, Montgomery C, Watne A, et al. Lymphoepithelioma-like carcinoma of the lung. J Surg Oncol. 1991;48:62–8.
202. Curcio LD, Cohen JS, Grannis FW, et al. Primary lymphoepithelioma-like carcinoma of the lung in a child: report of an Epstein-Barr virus-related neoplasm. Chest. 1997;111:250–1.
203. Gal AA, Unger ER, Koss MN, Yen BST. Detection of Epstein-Barr virus in lymphoepithelioma-like carcinoma of the lung. Mod Pathol. 1991;4:264–8.
204. Pittaluga S, Wong MP, Chung LP, Loke SL. Clonal Epstein-Bar virus in lymphoepithelioma-like carcinoma of the lung. Am J Surg Pathol. 1993;17:678–82.
205. Higashiyama M, Doi O, Kodama K, et al. Lymphoepithelioma-like carcinoma of the lung: analysis of two cases for Epstein-Barr virus infection. Hum Pathol. 1995;26:1278–82.
206. Chen FF, Yan JJ, Lai WW, et al. Epstein-Barr virus-associated nonsmall cell lung carcinoma: undifferentiated "lymphoepithelioma-like" carcinoma as a distinct entity with better prognosis. Cancer. 1998;82:2334–42.
207. Castro CY, Ostrowski ML, Barrios R, et al. Relationship between Epstein-Barr virus and lymphoepithelioma-like carcinoma of the lung: a clinicopathologic study of 6 cases and review of the literature. Hum Pathol. 2001;32:863–72.
208. Chang YL, Wu CT, Shih JY, Lee YC. New aspects in clinicopathologic and oncogene studies of 23 pulmonary lymphoepithelioma-like carcinomas. Am J Surg Pathol. 2002;26:715–23.

Neuroendocrine Carcinomas

4

Introduction

Neuroendocrine neoplasms occurring primary in the lung account for approximately 15% of this family of tumors. Unfortunately, the bulk of neuroendocrine tumors are made up by small cell lung carcinoma. In recent statistics, it has been estimated that small cell carcinomas of the lung may account for approximately 30,000 new cases on a yearly basis. Paradoxically, a disease that previously was observed predominantly in older men, now appears to affect men and women almost equally. However, it is important to keep in mind that although the gamut of primary lung tumors that may show neuroendocrine differentiation is rather complex, involving tumors not only of epithelial but also of mesenchymal or neural origin, this chapter will be limited to the most conventional epithelial carcinomas that range from the low- to the high-grade types. Another important aspect in this chapter will be the discussion with another neuroendocrine tumor that, even though not considered carcinoma, may pose a significant problem in the differential diagnosis: intrapulmonary paraganglioma.

Neuroendocrine neoplasms are ubiquitous tumors that have been the subject of much investigation for over a century. Although the low-grade tumors (carcinoid tumor) were initially described as a form of neoplasms that behave better than conventional carcinoma different studies of these tumors have focused on the concept of a family of neoplasms that may expand from the indolent and insignificant small lesion (so-called tumorlet)—more often encountered by chance—to low-, intermediate-, and high-grade malignancies. In order to provide a better understanding in terms of clinical course, behavior, and possible histogenesis, different studies including morphological, immunohistochemical, and molecular studies have attempted to shed some light on this family of neoplasms. However, a universal agreement has not been reached. Some reviews on the subject [1] are either priort to the most recent classification of lung tumors by the World Health Organization (WHO) [2] or have separated these tumors in the conventional three-way category system [3]. Although other studies have followed the WHO classification, those studies have stated the difficulty that exists in making these diagnoses on surgical biopsy specimens [4]. One of the biggest problems in achieving full agreement across all anatomic areas is the fact that the designation given to some of these tumors depends largely on the anatomic site in which they may occur. To illustrate this fact, one only has to review the WHO classification for tumors of the pleura, lung, thymus, and heart [2] in which tumors in the thymus are separated into low- and high-grade malignancies while those in the lung are separated into a four-way category system, demonstrating the inconsistency in the classification of these tumors, even in the same anatomic area—the thorax.

Siegfried Oberndorfer [5] is credited for coining the term "carcinoid tumor" in 1907. However, Bunting [6] from Johns Hopkins in 1904 had described a case under the designation of "multiple primary carcinomata" and made reference to other possible descriptions that dated back to the eighteenth century. Thus, it appears that this tumor may have been recognized well over a century ago. In 1914, Gossett and Masson [7] described similar tumors in the appendix and made an analogy to the previous description by Oberndorfer [5]. Contrary to the knowledge generated for these tumors in the gastrointestinal system, similar tumors in the respiratory tract, essentially those occurring in the bronchial wall, were being coded as bronchial adenomas [8, 9]. Gmelich et al. [10] identified the presence of Kultschitzky cells in bronchioles and established the relationship of these cells and the occurrence of these neoplasms in the lung. Interestingly, Hausman and Weimann [11] described a case with lymph node metastasis under the designation of "pulmonary tumorlet." The authors alluded to the fact that these tumors have a low malignant potential. As per their description of

A. Weissferdt, C.A. Moran, *Diagnostic Pathology of Pleuropulmonary Neoplasia*,
DOI 10.1007/978-1-4419-0787-5_4, © Springer Science+Business Media New York 2013

the case, the tumor measured 1.5 cm, and it had spindle cell morphology with lymph node metastasis. On the other hand, Azzopardi [12] in a study of 100 cases of what he called "oat cell carcinoma," based on 16 surgical cases and 84 cases from autopsy material, stated that oat cell carcinoma has positive structural features that identify this tumor including streams, ribbons, rosettes, and ductules. Judging by this definition and at least one of the illustrations presented in this review, it is possible that some of the cases presented in this study may not represent oat cell carcinoma as it is defined today. Thus, it is possible that some of the cases presented by Azzopardi [12] may correspond to intermediate-grade neuroendocrine carcinomas of today. Similar experience may be drawn from the 138 cases of oat cell carcinoma presented by Yukato et al. [13] where some of those tumors, although neuroendocrine in nature, may not necessarily be of the oat cell type, as it is defined today.

In order to shed light onto this difficult subject, many authors have employed different terms to explain the origin of these tumors. Terms such as histogenesis, differentiation, multidirectional differentiation, and/or divergent differentiation have been used, unfortunately not with the intended goal, as they have introduced more confusion into this field. Gould et al. [14] introduced the term "multidirectional differentiation" after observing the presence of neuroendocrine, mucosubstance-producing, and squamous cells in pulmonary carcinomas. In addition, Gould et al. [14] made observations that certain tumors may share similar patterns of differentiation. Interestingly, Gould et al. [14] also described cases, which by electron microscopy showed predominant features of squamous differentiation, thus designating those tumors as neuroendocrine carcinomas with squamous differentiation. The authors also alluded to the fact that some squamous and adenocarcinomas of the lung may show membrane-bound and dense-core granules by electron microscopy. However, Gould [15] also warned about the possibility of having cell populations with similar or identical patterns of differentiation, which may not necessarily share identical or even closely related embryogenesis. To that extent other authors had documented earlier the presence of neoplasms of the non-small cell type, which histologically may look like squamous cell carcinomas or adenocarcinomas and in which electron microscopic studies may show the presence of neurosecretory granules. Earlier denominations for those tumors have been atypical endocrine tumors. Such descriptions have raised high concerns about the true significance of the many classification systems available for neuroendocrine tumors [16]. In addition, tumor differentiation raises even higher issues such as the fact that some small cell carcinomas may lack the presence of immunohistochemical differentiation for neuroendocrine markers and/or the presence of neurosecretory granules by ultrastructural studies, at the same time showing the presence of ultrastructural features of epithelial tumors. A fact that is worth mentioning is that regardless of the histological subtype, all lung tumors are capable of showing neuroendocrine differentiation by immunohistochemistry or electron microscopy.

Recently, other authors [17] arguing that the current revised classification of tumors by the World Health Organization [2] clearly defines each one of the neuroendocrine tumors of the lung have introduced the term "divergent differentiation." The authors state that divergent differentiation applies to a subset of non-small cell carcinomas that are not considered neuroendocrine on morphological grounds but that show neuroendocrine differentiation with immunohistochemical markers (so-called non-small cell carcinoma with neuroendocrine differentiation). In addition, Brambilla et al. [17] state that the so-called tumorlets do not differ in the cellular composition from the so-called typical carcinoid and that these tumorlets also display divergent differentiation. Although there are reports of "metastatic tumorlets"[11], those early reports are incorrect and represent the current so-called typical carcinoid. However, the authors have personally seen a few cases in which the neuroendocrine tumor in question has measured under 0.5 cm and yet metastatic disease to the lymph nodes has been observed. These cases are highly unusual and by no means represent the more likely biological behavior of the so-called tumorlet, which in the vast majority of cases shows indolent clinical behavior.

Classification Schemas

Neuroendocrine lung neoplasms have been a subject of numerous classification approaches, many of them, although logical, fail to provide a practical approach while others, although practical, fail to properly define this complex group of tumors. Herein we evaluate the most important past and present classification systems with their respective salient features and at the same time attempt to highlight their practical use or the lack of it. Table 4.1 depicts three of the most common approaches to the classification of these tumors.

In 1977, Gould [18] introduced the terms "neuroendocrinomas" and "neuroendocrine carcinomas" by drawing an analogy of these tumors with the APUD (amine precursor uptake and decarboxylation) cell system neoplasms and their aberrant secretory activities. Gould emphasized the numerous neoplasms that may belong to this APUD system, which is not limited to the respiratory tract or to a particular group of tumors, i.e., carcinoid tumor. Gould also elaborated on abandoning traditional terms such as "bronchial adenoma"—a term that does not convey the true nature of these neoplasms and that at the same time is used to encompass a diverse group of tumoral conditions. A few important issues may be highlighted from this study: first, the preferred term of

Table 4.1 Three common approaches to the diagnosis of neuroendocrine carcinomas

Conventional	WHO	Practical
Tumorlet	Tumorlet	Carcinoid tumorlet
Size: <0.5 cm	Size: <0.5 cm	Size: <0.5 cm
Carcinoid tumor	Typical carcinoid	WDNECa
Size: >0.5 cm	Size: >0.5 cm	Size: >0.5 cm
Mitosis: <5 × 10 hpf	Mitosis: 0–1 × 10 hpf	Mitosis: 0–3 × 10 hpf
Necrosis: absent	Necrosis: absent	Necrosis: absent or focal punctuate
Atypical carcinoid	Atypical carcinoid	MDNECa
Size: >0.5 cm	Size: >0.5 cm	Size: >0.5 cm
Mitosis: 5–10 × 10 hpf	Mitosis: 2–10 × 10 hpf	Mitosis: 4–10 × 10 hpf
Necrosis: present	Necrosis: present	Necrosis: present—extensive or comedo-like
Small cell carcinoma	Small cell carcinoma	PDNECa
	Mitosis: >10 × 10 hpf	Small cell type
		Mitosis: >10 × 10 hpf
	Large cell NECa	
	Mitosis: >10 × 10 hpf	Large cell type
	NE morphology	Mitosis: >10 × 10 hpf
	NE markers: +	NE morphology
		NE markers: +/–

WDNECa=well differentiated neuroendocrine carcinoma, *MDNECa*=moderately differentiated neuroendocrine carcinoma, *PDNECa*=poorly differentiated neuroendocrine carcinoma, *NECa*=neuroendocrine carcinoma, *NE*=neuroendocrine

bronchopulmonary neuroendocrine tumor as opposed to bronchopulmonary carcinoid; second, the concept that "oat cell" carcinomas represent the malignant counterpart of carcinoid tumor; and third, the continuous use of the term undifferentiated "oat cell" carcinoma. In 1983, Gould et al. [19] presented a new classification system for neuroendocrine pulmonary neoplasms. Novel to this classification system was the introduction of a four-way classification system instead of the conventional three-way split. Gould's schema is as follows:

- *Bronchopulmonary carcinoid*—Typical histology, locally invasive, potential for recurrence, and distant metastasis. Bronchopulmonary carcinoid is separated from neuroendocrine carcinoma (see below). The cases depicted showed penetration of the bronchial wall and mediastinal soft tissue. In addition, six cases showed direct invasion into lymph nodes at the time of initial presentation.
- *Well-differentiated neuroendocrine carcinoma*—Even though it was stated that it may not represent an entirely satisfactory designation, this designation is for tumors that retain a clearly organoid pattern, moderate cellular pleomorphism, mitosis, and "true" lymph node metastasis.
- *Neuroendocrine carcinoma of intermediate-size cells*—Represents a variant of small cell neuroendocrine carcinoma; the cells are twice the size of "small cell" counterparts with prominent nucleoli and abundant mitotic figures. Interestingly, the authors state that 7 of the 11 cases presented showed features of glandular or squamous differentiation.
- *Neuroendocrine carcinoma of small cell type*—Typical "oat" cell carcinoma, abundant mitoses, and inconspicuous nucleoli. The authors comment that not all tumors in this category are neuroendocrine and recommend the systematic use of immunohistochemistry to separate those tumors that are neuroendocrine from those which are not.

In 1985, Warren et al. [20] presented a study of 81 cases of pulmonary neuroendocrine neoplasms assessing Gould's classification systems and determined their usefulness for the proper classification and treatment of patients with those neoplasms.

At the same time, Paladugu [21] presented a new classification system under the designation of bronchopulmonary Kultschitzky cell carcinomas (KCC) and reverted to the three-way category of neuroendocrine neoplasms. The authors used the designation of KCC-1, KCC-II, and KCC-III for the typical carcinoid, atypical carcinoid, and small cell carcinoma, respectively. The author provided a mortality rate of 1.7% for KCC-I and 27% for KCC-II. Histologically, the tumors coded under KCC-II showed a mitotic activity of 1 mitotic figure per high-power field (hpf). The authors concluded that their nomenclature is preferred to that of Gould given the fact that they consider the K-cell as the origin of these tumors and in addition, it is simpler and less confusing.

However, it was Arrigoni et al. [22] who in 1972 laid the basis for the concept of "atypical carcinoid" by separating those tumors based on cellular atypia and mitotic activity with an average of one mitotic figure per one or two high-power fields, thus leaving a window of 5–10 mitotic figures per 10 hpf. It is of importance to note that in either Arrigoni et al. [22], Gould et al. [19], and Paladugu's [21] classification systems, the number of mitotic figures per 10 hpf is left to some extent to interpretation, as all these authors were not dogmatic in presenting a specific number of mitotic figures to separate conventional from atypical "carcinoid tumor". Interestingly, in 1982, Mills et al. [23] presented a study of 17 cases of atypical carcinoid tumors of the lung in which the mitotic count in those tumors varied from 2 to 28 mitotic figures (mean: 14, median: 13). Also Valli et al. [24] presented a study of 33 cases of atypical carcinoid tumors of the lung in which the mitotic activity varied from 4 to 80/1.52 mm^2. In other studies [25], the reported criteria are those of increased mitotic activity, greater than one per one or two hpf. Based on those reports, one can only assume that the criteria to separate carcinoid from atypical carcinoid have been less than ideal when it comes to the issue of mitotic activity. In 1995, Capella et al. [26] revised the classification of neuroendocrine tumors of the lung, pancreas, and gut, stating the following schema:

- *Benign or low-grade malignant nonfunctioning well-differentiated tumor* as the equivalent for conventional carcinoid
- *Low-grade malignant nonfunctioning well-differentiated carcinoma* as equivalent for atypical carcinoid
- *High-grade malignant functioning or nonfunctioning poorly differentiated carcinoma* for the large cell type and the small cell or intermediate type

The mitotic count to separate typical from atypical carcinoid was established at no more than 3 mitotic figures ×10 hpf. The authors added that if metastasis or gross invasion is present, tumors should be called low-grade neuroendocrine carcinoma.

In 1991, Travis et al. [27] presented a study of 35 cases of neuroendocrine carcinomas of the lung in which criteria were presented for large cell neuroendocrine carcinoma. In this study, previous criteria for other neuroendocrine carcinomas were followed, and the large cell carcinoma was presented as a tumor with a "neuroendocrine pattern, high mitotic activity with an average of 66×10 hpf, and prominent nucleoli." The authors stated that the prognosis of large cell neuroendocrine carcinoma lies between atypical carcinoid and small cell carcinoma. However in 1998, Travis et al. [28] presented a new study of neuroendocrine neoplasms in which the authors' goal was to provide clear definitions for the four neuroendocrine tumors, in addition to modify the criteria for the diagnosis of carcinoid and atypical carcinoid. The "new" classification schema placed large cell neuroendocrine carcinoma in the high-grade category of tumors contrary to the previous study [27]. This new approach is as follows:

- Conventional carcinoid tumor is now restricted to no more than 2 mitoses×10 hpf.
- Atypical carcinoid: 2–10 mitoses×10 hpf, or necrosis (often punctuate).
- Large cell neuroendocrine carcinoma: tumors with "neuroendocrine morphology", >10 mitoses×10 hpf, cytologic features of large cell carcinoma, and positive immunohistochemical staining for neuroendocrine markers.
- Small cell carcinoma is a tumor with the cytology of small cell tumor cells (absent nucleoli), mitotic figures of >10 × 10 hpf, and frequent necrosis.

This classification system is essentially repeated in the last version of the WHO publication for the classification of tumors of the lung, pleura, thymus, and heart [2]. However, it is important to note that this represents a classification for resected specimens. It is of interest to note that in a separate study on the reproducibility of the proposed classification of neuroendocrine lung tumors conducted by Travis et al. [29], in which 5 experienced pulmonary pathologists participated in the evaluation of 40 surgical resections of neuroendocrine tumors, a unanimous agreement was reached in only 55% of the cases. The most common disagreements were between large cell neuroendocrine carcinoma and small cell carcinoma. Lastly, in 2002, Huang et al. [30] presented the latest attempt to classify neuroendocrine tumors of the lung. The authors presented a study of 234 cases and classified them into five different categories. This system essentially follows Travis' criteria [28] for the separation of carcinoid and atypical carcinoid, now named well- and moderately differentiated neuroendocrine carcinoma; the terms large cell neuroendocrine carcinoma and small cell carcinoma are kept with the prefix of "undifferentiated" with mitotic counts of more than 30×10 hpf. A new category is what the authors call "poorly differentiated neuroendocrine carcinoma," which is conceptualized as an atypical carcinoid with an increase mitotic activity of more than 10×10 hpf.

Clinical Features

The clinical presentation of neuroendocrine tumors of the lung is varied. For instance, small cell carcinoma of the lung usually presents as a large hilar mass with bulky mediastinal lymphadenopathy. In many cases, patients may present with widespread metastatic disease at the time of diagnosis. Nevertheless, in a few instances, small cell carcinomas may present with a solitary peripheral nodule. Paraneoplastic syndromes including Cushing's syndrome, inappropriate secretion of antidiuretic hormone, and carcinoid syndrome have also been reported in association with neuroendocrine carcinomas; carcinoid syndrome are associated with approximately 10% of the cases of well-differentiated histology. Other conditions that have also been associated with these tumors include Lambert-Eaton myasthenic syndrome and paraneoplastic encephalomyelitis and sensory neuropathy. In addition, depending on the location of the tumor, those in the central location may also show symptoms of pulmonary obstruction, dyspnea, cough, and/or chest pain. Patients with tumors in the periphery of the lung may be asymptomatic until the tumor reaches a larger size. Although neuroendocrine carcinomas may occur at any age, the tumors are more commonly encountered in the fifth to seventh decade of life. No gender predilection has been noted.

Macroscopic Features

Those tumors occurring in the central location may present as polypoid tumors obstructing the lumen of the airway. The tumors may measure from 1 cm to more than 10 cm in diameter. They are light brown and at cut surface appear homogenous. The presence of areas of necrosis or hemorrhage should alert for a higher grade tumor. In high-grade neuroendocrine carcinomas, it is common to encounter invasion into mediastinal structures at the time of diagnosis.

Microscopic Features

Tumorlet

The histopathological features present in the so-called tumorlet are essentially the same as those that one would find in otherwise well-differentiated neuroendocrine carcinoma (Fig. 4.1a,b). As a matter of fact, this so-called tumorlet may represent the true carcinoid tumor of the lung. However, the diagnosis of tumorlets is restricted to lesions of no more than 0.5 cm size in greatest diameter. Although this lesion is more often found incidentally in lung biopsies, nowadays with the use of more sophisticated radiological techniques, "tumorlets" are becoming more common. Even though the great majority of cases are likely to be encountered as an incidental finding in cases in which resection has taken place for other reasons, we have observed a few cases in which there has been an incidental "tumorlet carcinoid" in the lung, fulfilling all the required histopathological characteristics, but yet the tumor had metastasized to a lymph node. This occurrence should be taken into consideration when encountered with the finding of metastatic disease to the lymph node from an unknown source of disease.

Well- and Moderately Differentiated Neuroendocrine Carcinomas (Carcinoid and Atypical Carcinoid)

The current designation provided by the WHO [2] defines these tumors as having neuroendocrine morphology, namely, organoid, trabecular, insular, palisading, ribbon, and rosette-like features (Figs. 4.2a–c and 4.3a–c). However, the separation of well- and moderately differentiated neuroendocrine carcinoma according to the WHO is that the former has fewer than two mitotic figures per 10 hpf while the latter has 3–10 mitotic figures per 10 hpf. Clinically, both tumors may be associated with carcinoid syndrome [31] and show a spectrum of cell differentiation that includes spindle cells, oncocytic, and melanocytic features, among others [32–37]. Although the WHO still maintains the nomenclature of carcinoid and atypical carcinoid, some authors believe that the most accurate designation for these neoplasms is that of neuroendocrine carcinoma, which conveys the true nature of these tumors, and is the one followed in this section [22, 38]. In addition, the issue of one mitosis to separate well- from moderately differentiated tumors may be an artificial designation that in practice may not hold true. Therefore, we recommend that such criteria should be used with care as in some cases the diagnosis of moderately differentiated neuroendocrine carcinoma (atypical carcinoid) may imply the use of chemotherapy. Careful communication with the oncologist is of utmost importance to

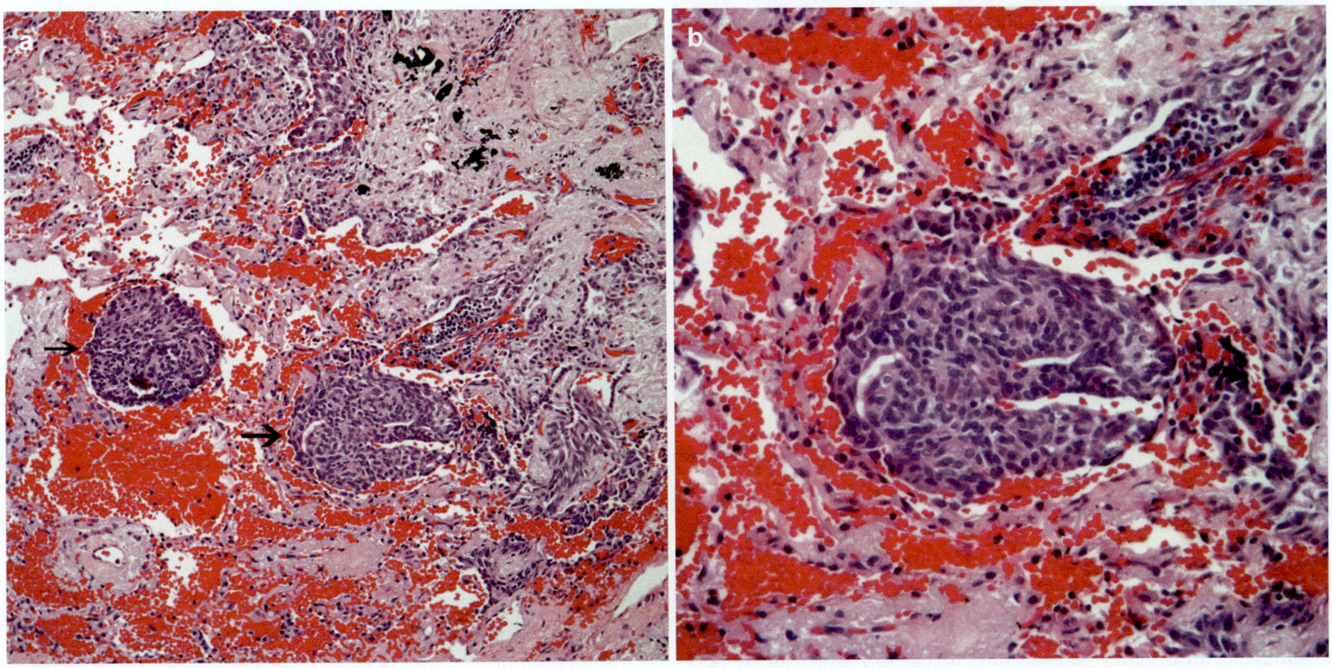

Fig. 4.1 (**a**) Carcinoid tumorlet (see *arrows*) with similar cellular characteristics of a well-differentiated neuroendocrine carcinoma, except that these lesions are under 0.5 cm in diameter. (**b**) Higher magnification showing a homogeneous cellular proliferation without mitotic activity

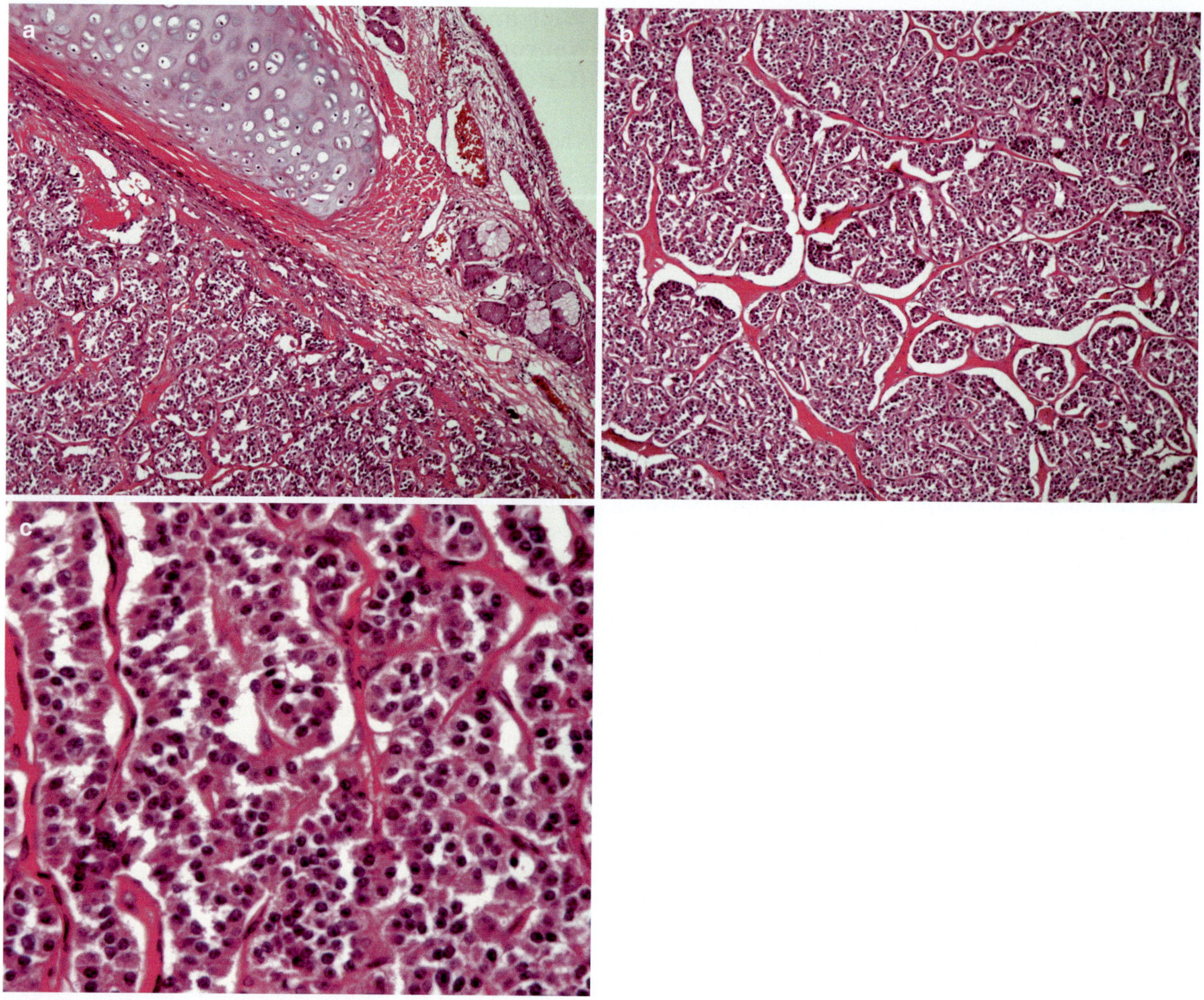

Fig. 4.2 (**a**) Well-differentiated neuroendocrine carcinoma showing a classical nested growth pattern, note the presence of bronchial epithelium and cartilage. (**b**) In other areas, the nested growth pattern is preserved with a homogeneous cellular proliferation. (**c**) Higher magnification showing absence of nuclear atypia and mitotic activity

convey such information. Recently, we evaluated 80 cases of low- and intermediate-grade neuroendocrine tumors using three different methods to count mitosis and encountered that the overall mean number of mitoses correlated with the recurrence-free survival [39]. Interestingly, the overall survival (OS) of patients when mitotic activity was counted in random fields was not dramatically different if the tumor showed fewer than 2 or between 2 and 10 mitotic figures per 10 high-power fields as the OS was 100 and 97%, respectively. An almost similar situation occurred when the mitotic figures were counted in mitotically active fields as the OS was that of 100 and 96%, respectively. Based on those results, it is possible that mitotic count may not be as reliable a parameter as it has been considered. On the contrary, the presence of necrosis may offer a better clue for clinical outcome.

At low magnification, the tumor displays an organized growth pattern, which may show nesting, solid, pseudoglandular, and/or trabecular arrangements composed of a rather homogeneous cellular proliferation characterized by small- to medium-size cells with moderate amounts of eosinophilic cytoplasm, round to oval nuclei; nucleoli may be identified in some cells. Rosette formation may be easily identifiable. The presence of necrosis in the form of comedo-like necrosis and/or hemorrhage is an important criterium for the diagnosis of moderately differentiated neuroendocrine carcinoma.

Several histological variants have been described [40–42] for both well- and moderately differentiated neuroendocrine carcinomas including:

- *Spindle cell type*: In this variant, although one may find an organoid pattern, the cell morphology is that of fusiform

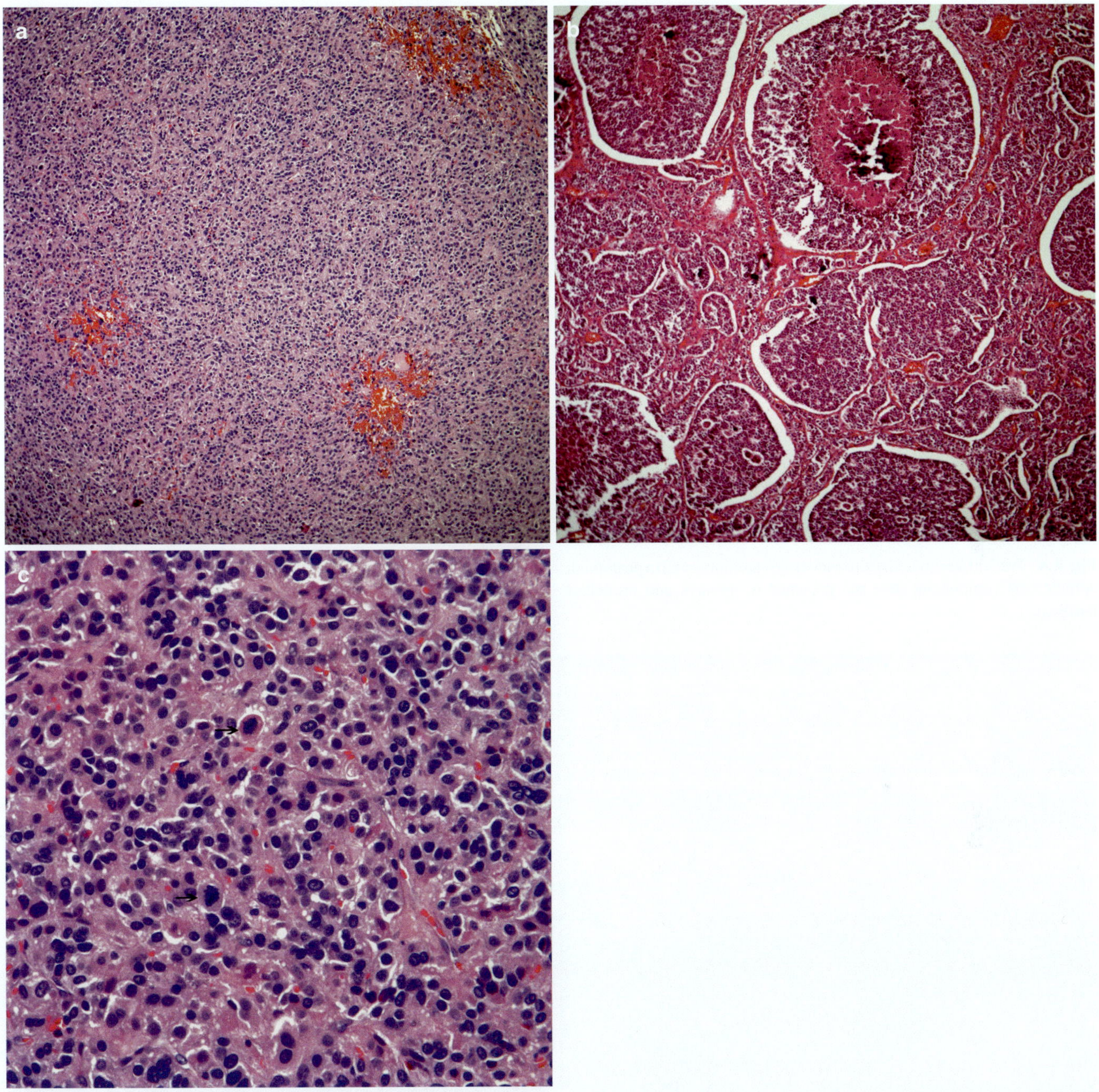

Fig. 4.3 (**a**) Moderately differentiated neuroendocrine carcinoma showing a diffuse growth pattern composed of medium-size cells. (**b**) In other areas, a nested growth pattern is present; however, note the presence of comedo-like necrosis. (**c**) High-power magnification shows the presence of mitotic activity (see *arrows*)

cells with inconspicuous nuclei and finely disperse chromatin (Figs. 4.4, 4.5, 4.6, 4.7, and 4.8). In some cases, the spindle cell proliferation may be associated with dilated blood vessels imparting a hemangiopericytic pattern. However, this variant may also display nuclear atypia and mitotic activity.

- *Oncocytic type*: The growth pattern of this neoplasm is essentially similar as those of the conventional cell type. The tumors may have a diffuse growth or a glandular appearance. Cytologically, the cells are of medium size with ample eosinophilic cytoplasm, round to oval nuclei, and in some cells prominent nucleoli are seen (Figs. 4.9, 4.10, 4.11, and 4.12). In some cases, clusters of oncocytic cells are present among tumor cells—so-called oncoblasts. This variant may also display features of moderately differentiated neuroendocrine carcinoma by displaying increased mitotic activity. However, one needs to be careful in assessing the presence of mitotic activity

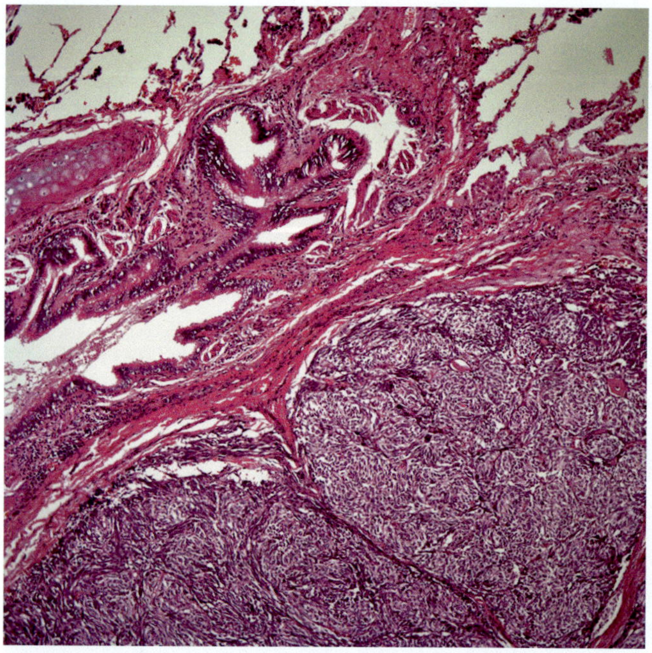

Fig. 4.4 Well differentiated neuroendocrine carcinoma with a prominent spindle cell component; note the presence of airways and bronchial cartilage

since oncocytic tumors may display areas of nuclear atypia without mitotic activity.

- *Mucinous type*: This is a rare occurrence in primary neuroendocrine carcinomas of the lung. The presence of mucus material may be limited to the intraluminal component in some cases of glandular arrangement, or more rare the mucinous component may be intermixed with the neoplastic cellular proliferation (Fig. 4.13a,b).
- *Melanocytic type*: The growth pattern is similar as those of the conventional type; however, melanin pigment may be present in cells (Fig. 4.14a,b) or distributed along the fibroconnective tissue.
- *Clear cell type*: In this variant, the neoplastic cells are characterized by the presence of clear cytoplasm (Fig. 4.15a,b). This cytoplasmic feature may be seen in either spindle cell or conventional morphology.
- *Angiectatic type*: This variant is characterized by the presence of large dilated spaces filled with blood mimicking a vascular neoplasm (Fig. 4.16). However, closer inspection of the tumor cells reveals the presence of more conventional areas of neuroendocrine morphology.

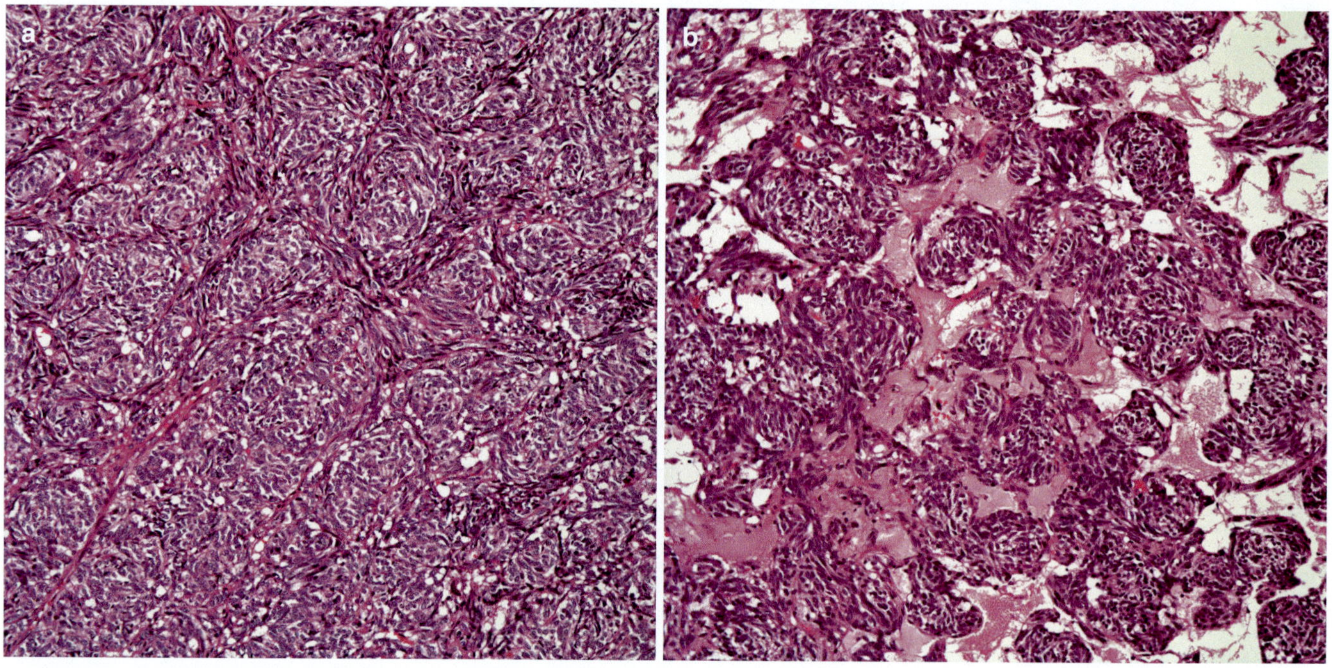

Fig. 4.5 (**a**) The cellular proliferation may show tightly packed nests of spindle cells. (**b**) Loosely arranged nests of spindle cells separated by fibroconnective tissue

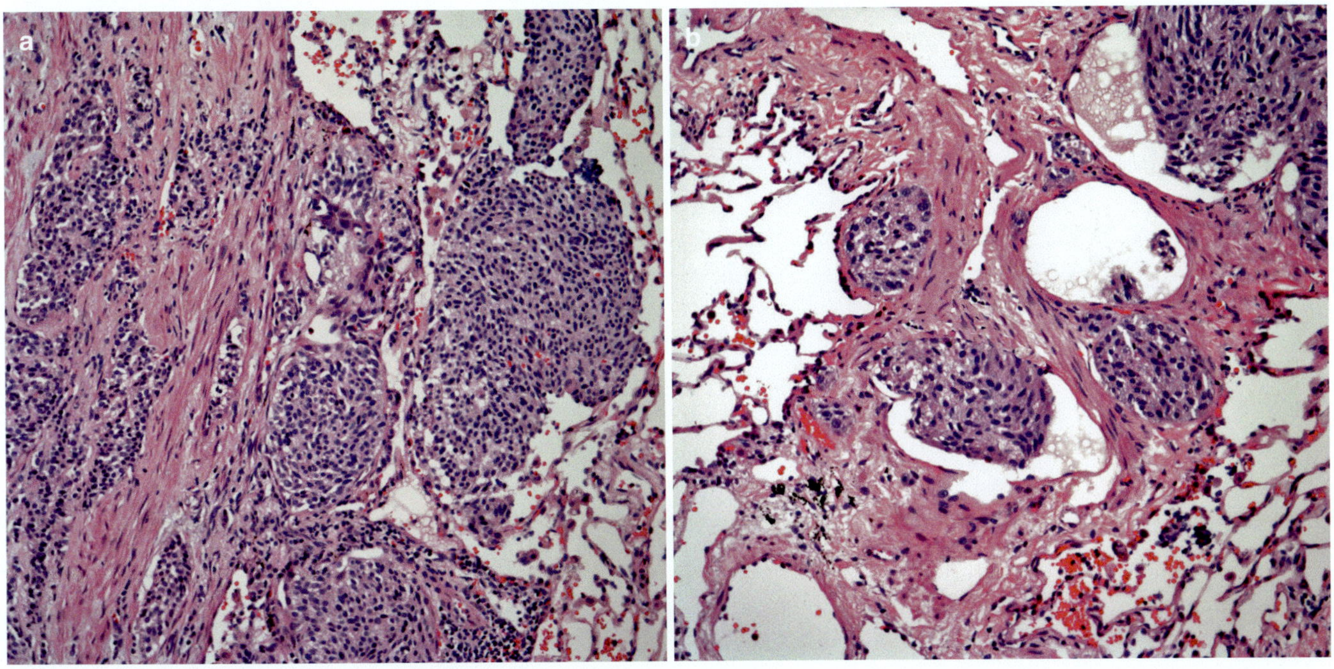

Fig. 4.6 (**a**) The tumor may spread into alveolar spaces. (**b**) The tumor may also show vascular permeation

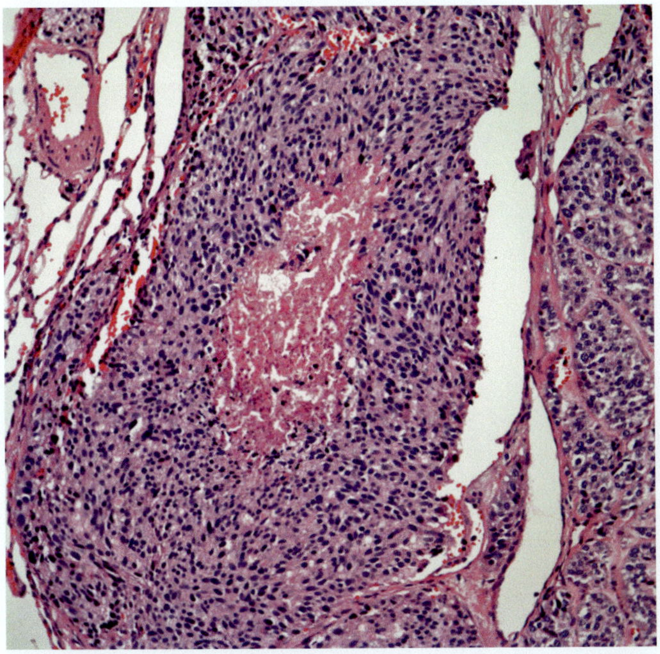

Fig. 4.7 Moderately differentiated neuroendocrine carcinoma, spindle cell type with comedo-like necrosis

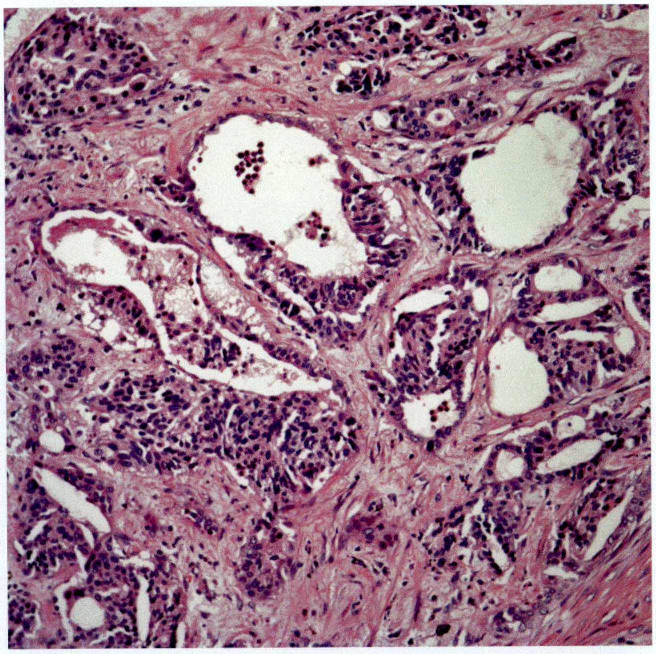

Fig. 4.8 Areas of pseudoglandular appearance may also be present

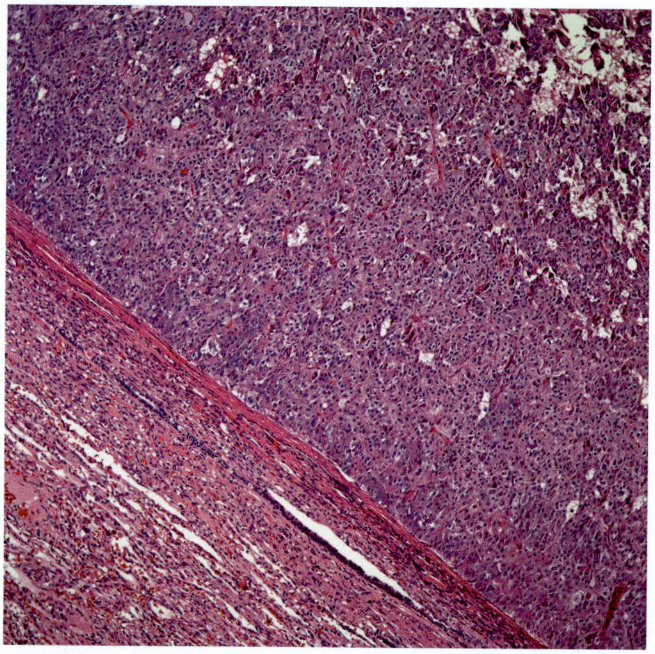

Fig. 4.9 Peripheral oncocytic neuroendocrine carcinoma showing a well-demarcated tumor

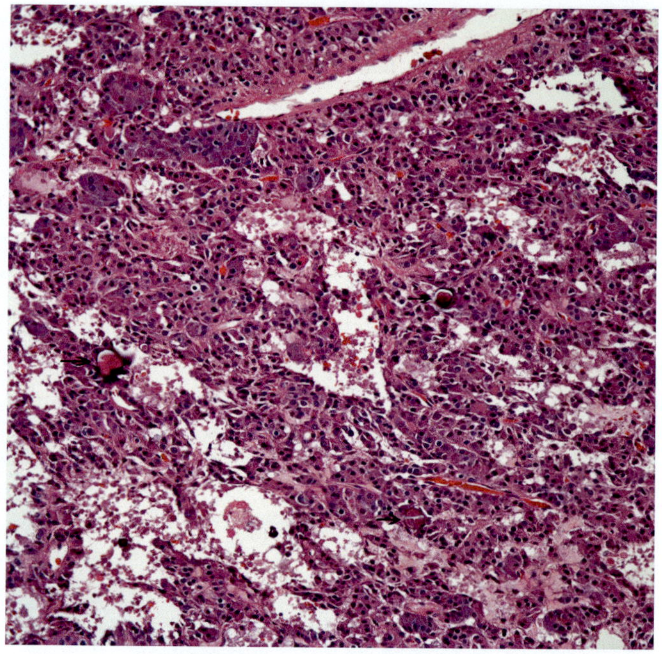

Fig. 4.11 The tumor may show numerous calcifications of "psammoma-like" type (see *arrows*)

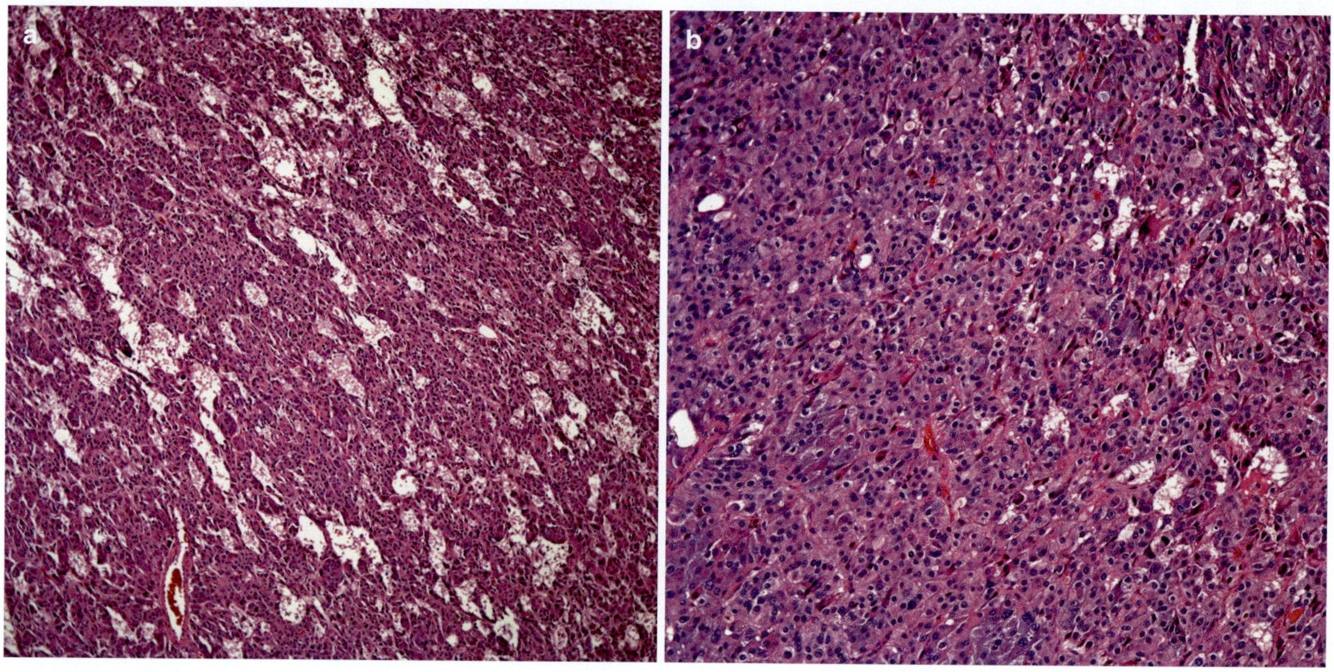

Fig. 4.10 (**a**) The tumor may be formed by cords of neoplastic cells. (**b**) The tumors may show a prominent solid growth pattern

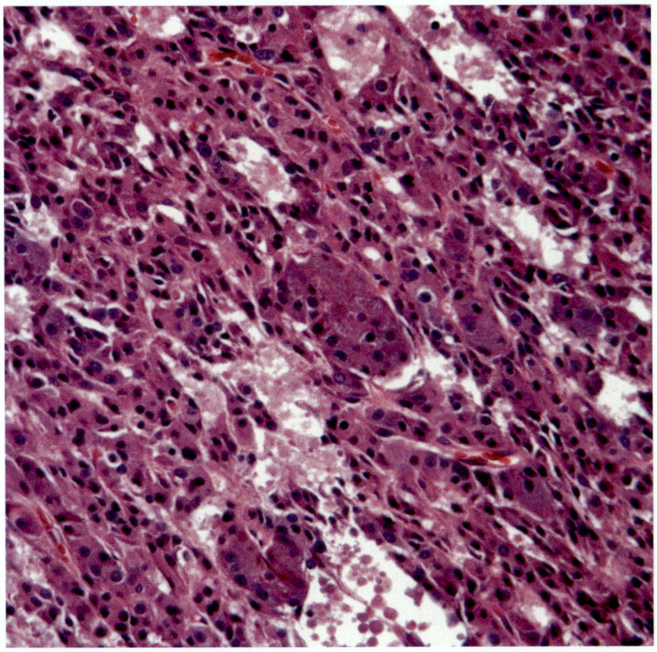

Fig. 4.12 Higher magnification showing tumor cells with ample eosinophilic cytoplasm, round nuclei, and prominent nucleoli

- *Amyloid-like type*: The morphology of these tumors is essentially the same as conventional neuroendocrine carcinoma. However, the tumor cells are admixed with areas of hyalinization imparting an amyloid-like matrix (Fig. 4.17).
- *Sclerotic type*: In these cases, the tumor cells may not be readily identifiable due to the extent of collagenization of the sclerosing changes. This type of neuroendocrine carcinoma may pose a challenge when dealing with small biopsies. However, in all the cases described, clusters of neuroendocrine cells have been present enough to make a diagnosis. Nevertheless, the sclerotic changes should not be considered any type of special feature in order to upgrade the tumor to a higher grade as such changes may be seen in low- as well as intermediate-grade tumors (Fig. 4.18a–c).
- *Metaplastic bone formation*: The growth pattern is of conventional neuroendocrine carcinoma in which the presence of well-formed bone (Fig. 4.19) is admixed with the neoplastic cellular proliferation.

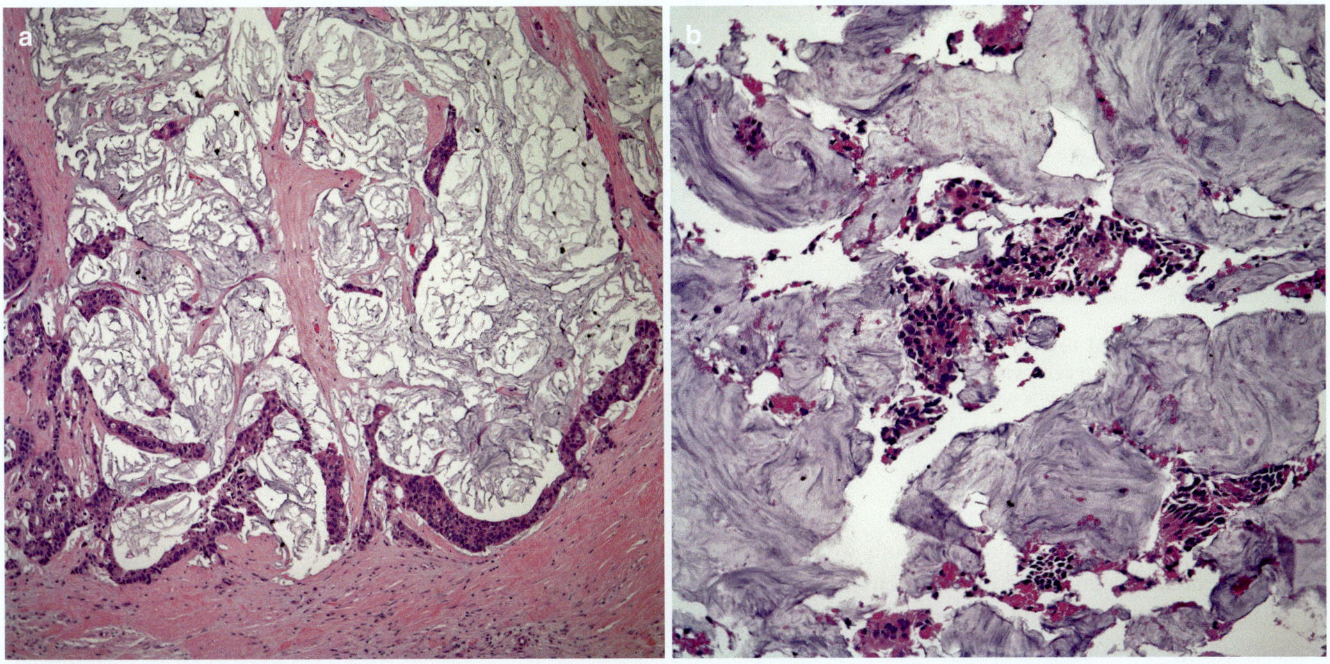

Fig. 4.13 (**a**) Mucinous neuroendocrine carcinoma showing pools of mucoid material. (**b**) In some areas, the neoplastic cells may be embedded in pools of mucoid material

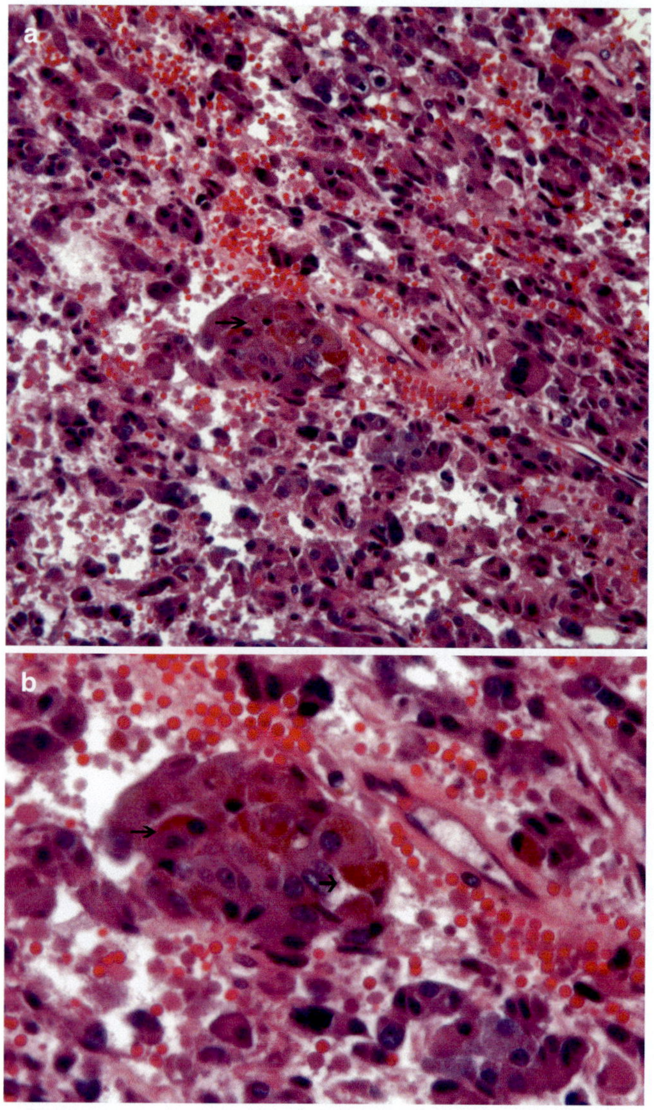

Fig. 4.14 (**a**) Pigmented neuroendocrine carcinoma with oncocytic changes. Note the cluster of cells with melanin pigment (see *arrow*). (**b**) Closer view of the cluster of cells with melanin pigment

Immunohistochemical Features

The immunohistochemical features of both well- or moderately differentiated neuroendocrine carcinomas (carcinoid and atypical carcinoid) are similar in terms of sharing positive staining using the conventional neuroendocrine markers, namely, chromogranin, synaptophysin, and CD56. In addition, the use of thyroid transcription factor-1 has also been shown to be helpful in the evaluation of neuroendocrine neoplasms of the lung [43]. More recently, Tsuta et al. [44] conducted a study of neuroendocrine carcinomas of the lung in which the tumors were stained with Sox10 for sustentacular cells. The authors stated that Sox10-positive sustentacular cells were observed in well-differentiated tumors (carcinoid tumors) but not in high-grade neuroendocrine carcinomas. On the other hand, the use of proliferation markers such as KI-67 in the separation of conventional and atypical carcinoid has found that a 4% cutoff provides significant differences for the 4-year overall survival rate [45]. In this particular study, the methodology that was followed for the classification of neuroendocrine neoplasms was the one presented by Arrigoni [22] and Warren [20], and the study was performed on resected specimens. This study raises an important issue, and that is that the complete interpretation of these tumors rests on surgical resections and not on biopsy specimens, where labeling of proliferation markers may be deceiving. Since most of the initial approach to the classification of neuroendocrine tumors is performed on a biopsy specimen, it is possible that using specific mitotic markers may be of aid in difficult cases in which there is doubt about the possibility of mitotic activity. In that regard, Tsuta et al. [46], using a mitosis specific marker—the anti-phosphohistone H3 (PHH3)—to assess mitosis in neuroendocrine carcinomas of the lung, concluded that PHH3 may be a reliable aid in determining mitotic activity.

Molecular Features

Well- and moderately differentiated tumors have also been the subject of more modern techniques such as chromosomal studies in which 11q deletions appear to be shared by both tumors [47]. Losses of 10q and 13q may also be responsible for a possible aggressive behavior shown by some of these tumors.

Clinical Behavior

Due to the lack of real comparisons between previous and current schemas for the classification of these tumors, the survival rates of patients with low- and intermediate- grade neuroendocrine carcinomas are difficult to assess and address meaningfully. Wilkins et al. [48] in 1984, obviously using a different schema (most likely Arrigoni's criteria), presented a study of 111 patients who underwent surgical resection for "bronchopulmonary carcinoid"; 11 of these patients had atypical carcinoid, and 45% of them died in a period of 33 months. Those who were still alive had been followed for 16–48 months. However, even though the authors provided a survival rate of 82% for a 10-year period, close examination of the data provided is rather limited, and no clear-cut survival rate is provided for the conventional carcinoid. A better-defined publication on "typical carcinoid" is the one presented by Schreurs [49] in a study of 93 patients and a period of 25 years. Once again, the likely criteria for classification in this study were those formulated by Arrigoni. The authors provided an important survival rate of 100% for 86 patients at 5, 10, and years (according to the authors, seven patients died of unrelated causes) for surgically treated patients.

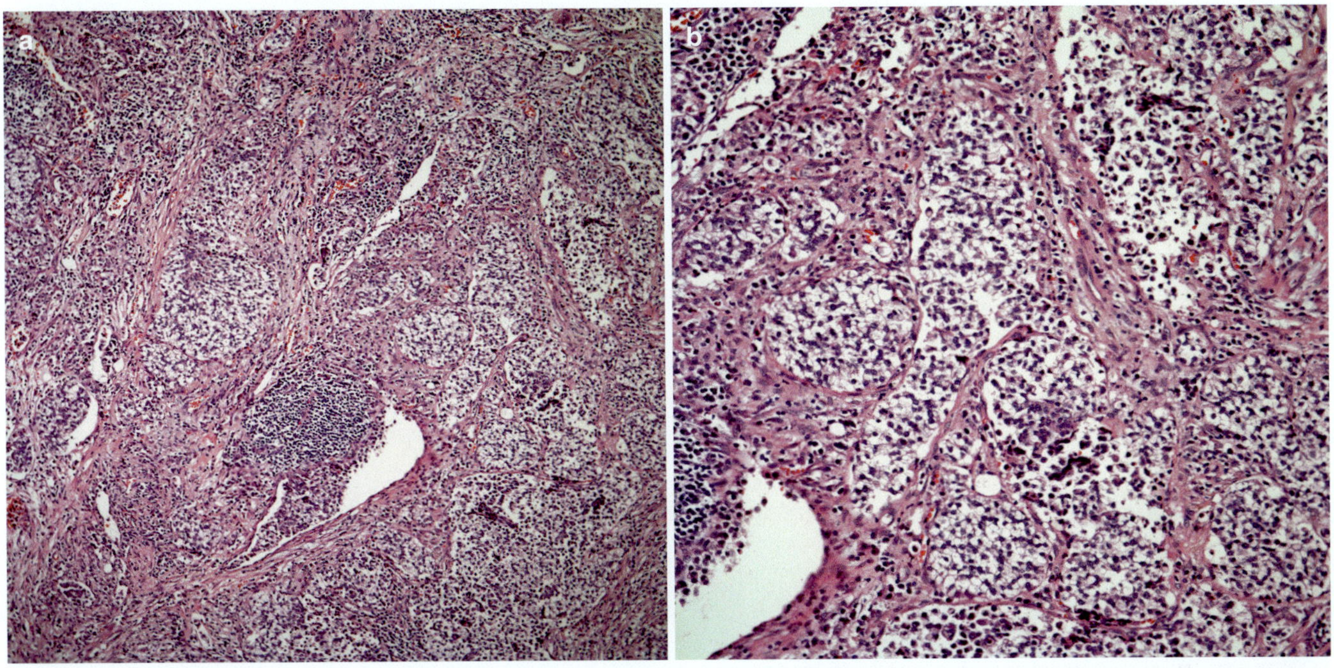

Fig. 4.15 (**a**) Neuroendocrine carcinoma showing a classical nested pattern and composed of cells with clear cytoplasm. (**b**) Higher magnification showing prominent clear cell changes

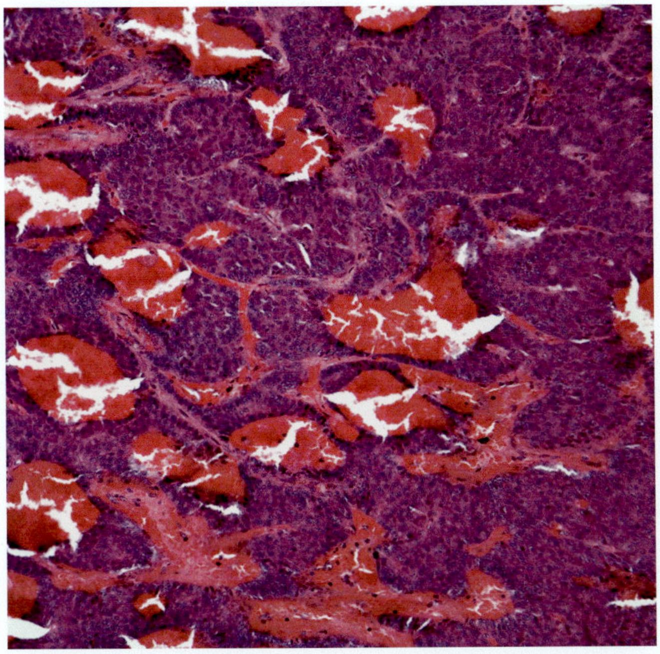

Fig. 4.16 Neuroendocrine carcinoma with presence of ectatic spaces filled with blood imparting a pseudo-vascular appearance

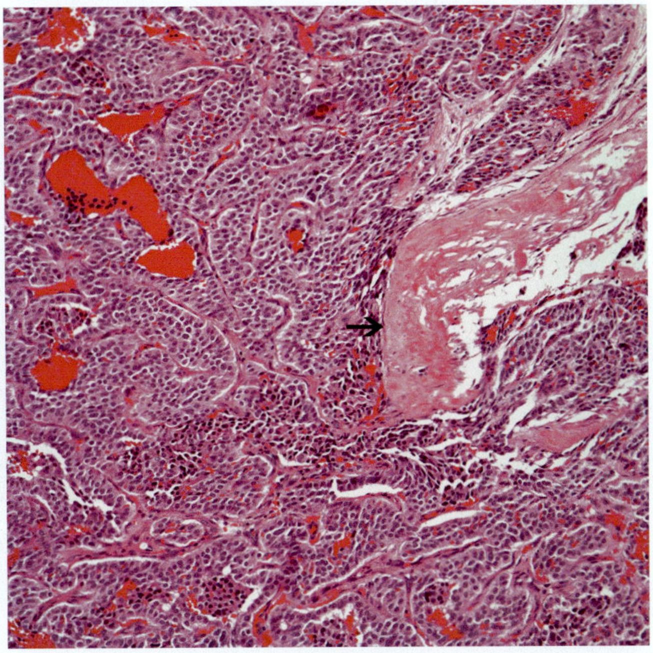

Fig. 4.17 Conventional neuroendocrine carcinoma with areas of dense hyalinization (see *arrow*) mimicking amyloid

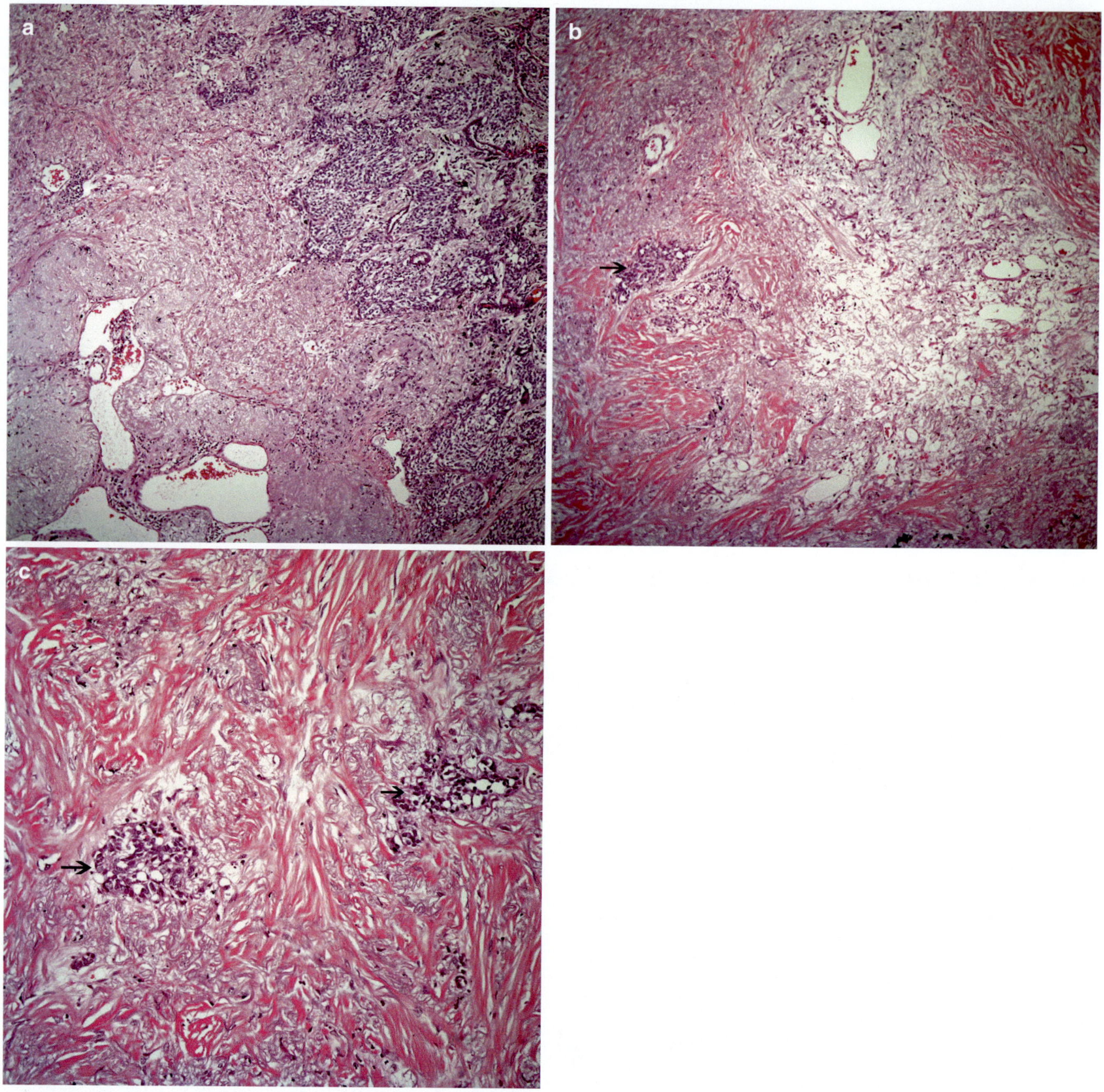

Fig. 4.18 (**a**) Neuroendocrine carcinoma with extensive areas of hyalinization in transition with tumoral areas. (**b**) Extensive hyalinization with only clusters of neuroendocrine cells (*arrow*). (**c**) Higher magnification showing the neuroendocrine cellular proliferation (*arrows*)

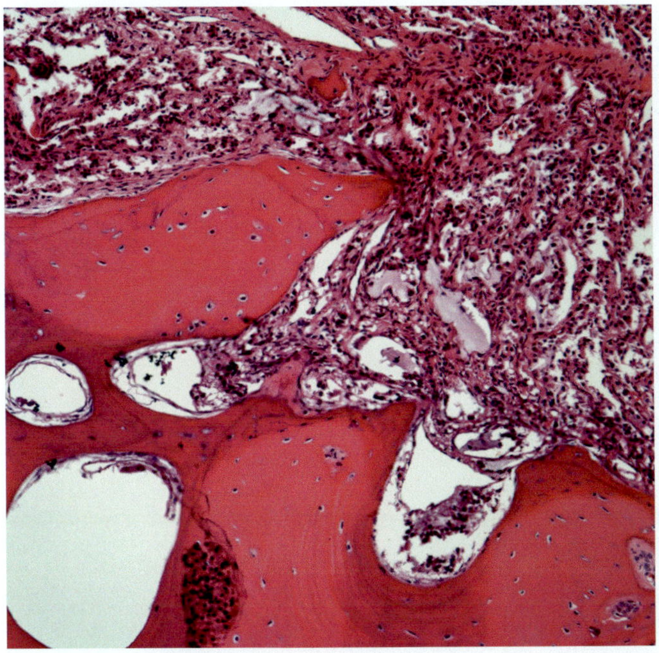

Fig. 4.19 Neuroendocrine carcinoma with metaplastic bone formation

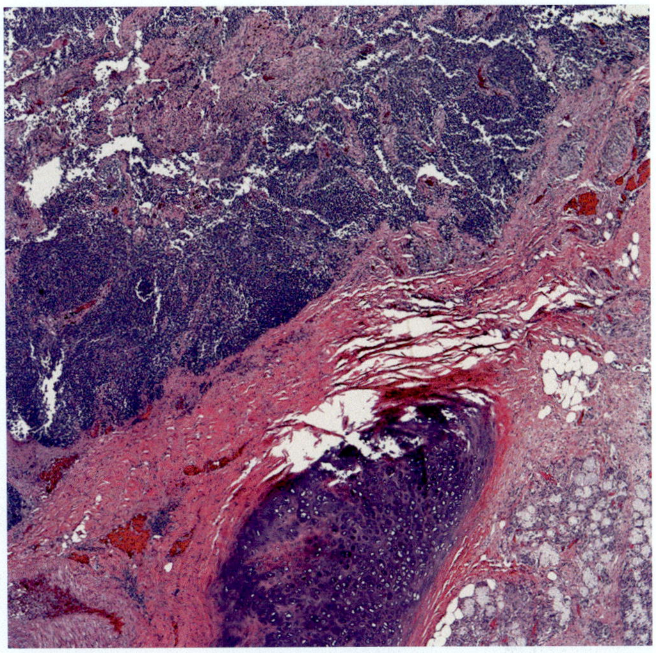

Fig. 4.20 Small cell carcinoma showing the typical cellular proliferation. Note the presence of residual normal endobronchial glands and bronchial cartilage

However, the selection process for this study excluded patients with distant metastasis. Thus, raising the issue that staging of the neoplasm at the time of diagnosis also plays an important role in this group of tumors and impacts heavily in the survival rate.

Small Cell Carcinoma

The latest version of the WHO [2] defines this tumor as a malignant tumor with cells with scant cytoplasm and absent or inconspicuous nucleoli; necrosis is extensive and mitotic count is high. The mitotic count provided is of 60 mitoses/2 mm^2. It is obvious from this definition that the authors of the WHO are far from the real practice of surgical pathology as such criteria apply only when there is a resected specimen, which rarely happens in daily practice. Nevertheless, in a study of 100 cases of small cell carcinoma [50], the authors clearly state that in over 90% of the cases, the diagnosis of small cell carcinoma can be established on small biopsy. Needless to say, an important fact that must be emphasized is that most patients with small cell carcinoma are beyond a stage that makes them amenable for surgical resection of the tumor, as has been noted in the literature [51], thus leaving the surgical pathologist confronted with a small biopsy in order to provide a definitive diagnosis.

The topic of small cell carcinoma has not been exempted from controversy. In 1985, Vollmer et al. [52] presented a study in which the authors analyzed the issue of subclassification of small cell carcinoma into oat cell or intermediate types. However, in 1988, the Pathology Committee of the International Association for the Study of Lung Cancer recommended the use of small cell carcinoma and that such designation would include tumors previously denominated as oat cell and intermediate subtypes [53]. Even terms such as small cell neuroendocrine carcinoma [54] may fall under scrutiny, as a proportion of these tumors may not show positive reaction with antibodies against neuroendocrine markers.

Macroscopic Features

As stated before, small cell carcinomas often present in late stages of the disease. The tumors are commonly centrally located, of large size and with variable proportions of necrosis.

Microscopic Features

The tumor shows a non-cohesive cellular distribution composed of small cells with scant cytoplasm, round nucleus, and inconspicuous nucleoli. Single cell necrosis or extensive areas of necrosis are common. In addition, the presence of the so-called Azzopardi phenomenon is commonly observed in these tumors. The mitotic count in resected specimens or in open lung biopsies is more than 10×10 hpf. In some areas, the morphology is that of spindle cells, with oval nuclei and inconspicuous nucleoli. Mitotic activity is

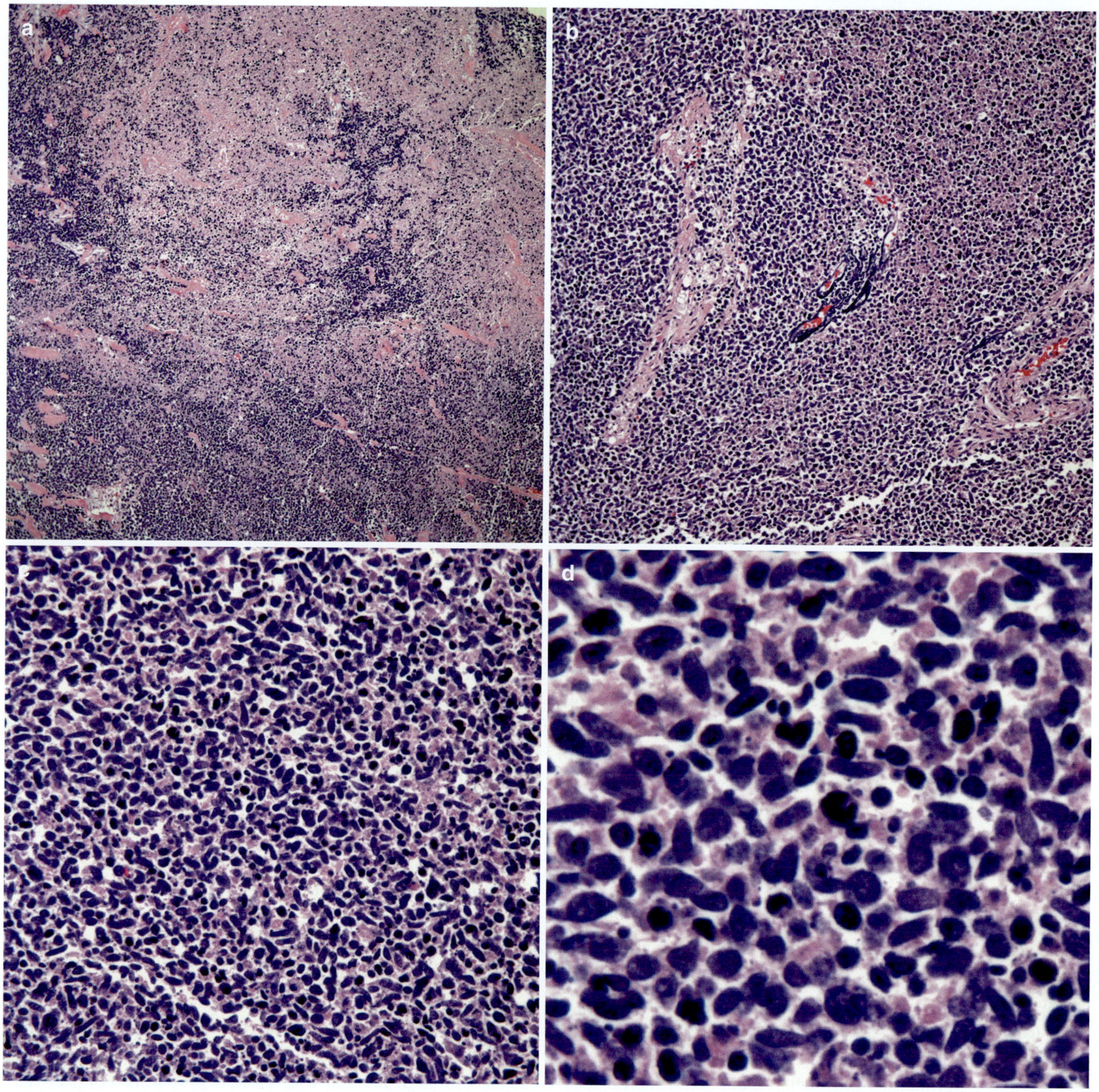

Fig. 4.21 (**a**) Small cell carcinoma with extensive necrosis. (**b**) The so-called Azzopardi phenomenon is classic in small cell carcinomas. (**c**) Closer view at the neoplastic cellular proliferation showing high mitotic activity. (**d**) Higher magnification showing small cells with absence of nucleoli

high (Figs. 4.20 and 4.21a–d). However, it is important to recognize that most of these features may be absent in a small transbronchial biopsy and that the established criteria for diagnosis of small cell carcinoma may not be met in such material. Small biopsies are characterized by the presence of crush artifact and little viable cells with only occasional mitotic figures.

Immunohistochemical Features

There are no comprehensive studies on the immunohistochemistry of small cell carcinoma. In a rather limited immunohistochemical study of small cell carcinoma [55], the authors found that neuroendocrine markers such as chromogranin were positive in 60% of open lung biopsies but only in 47% of transbronchial biopsies, while synaptophysin showed 5 and 19% positivity, respectively. Nevertheless, most authors concur that small cell carcinoma represents the end of the spectrum of neuroendocrine carcinomas of the lung. One additional factor that must be carefully analyzed is that in small, poorly preserved biopsies in which the intensity of neuroendocrine markers is marked, one must carefully exclude the possibility of a lower-grade neuroendocrine carcinoma as an alternative for small cell carcinoma [56].

The implications of a diagnosis of small cell carcinoma cannot be overemphasized, as the patients may undergo chemotherapy, radiation therapy, or both. In addition, large studies have estimated, that the long term survival of patients with small cell carcinoma is approximately 10% at 2 years [57]. However, even though there is little mention about staging for small cell carcinoma, the Veterans Administration Lung Group stages small cell carcinoma in a two-tier schema: (1) limited-stage disease, in which the tumor is confined to the ipsilateral hemithorax, and (2) extensive-stage disease, in which the tumor has grown beyond the ipsilateral hemithorax. However, more recently a TNM system has been presented, which appears to provide prognostic significance [58].

Large Cell Neuroendocrine Carcinoma, Large Cell Carcinoma with Neuroendocrine Morphology, and Large Cell Carcinoma with Neuroendocrine Differentiation

By definition, these tumors are poorly differentiated non-small cell carcinomas. According to the WHO [2], the main distinguishing features of large cell neuroendocrine carcinoma and small cell carcinoma are the presence of prominent nucleoli.

Macroscopic Features

Large cell neuroendocrine carcinomas (LCNEC) are large neoplasms usually in advance clinical stages at the time of diagnosis. The tumor may be in a central location, and it may present as well-demarcated, solid, grayish, with or without apparent necrosis.

Microscopic Features

Large cell neuroendocrine carcinomas will display a neuroendocrine morphology, namely, the presence of ribbons, rosettes, or nesting patterns combined with large zones of necrosis and a mitotic count higher than 11 mitotic figures/2 mm^2 (average 75) of viable tumor (Figs. 4.22, 4.23, 4.24, 4.25, and 4.26). This latter definition clearly applies only to resected tumors; thus, such diagnoses can hardly be accomplished on small biopsies in which one may not get enough viable tumor to evaluate the so-called neuroendocrine pattern or evaluate the mitotic count of more than 11 mitotic figures.

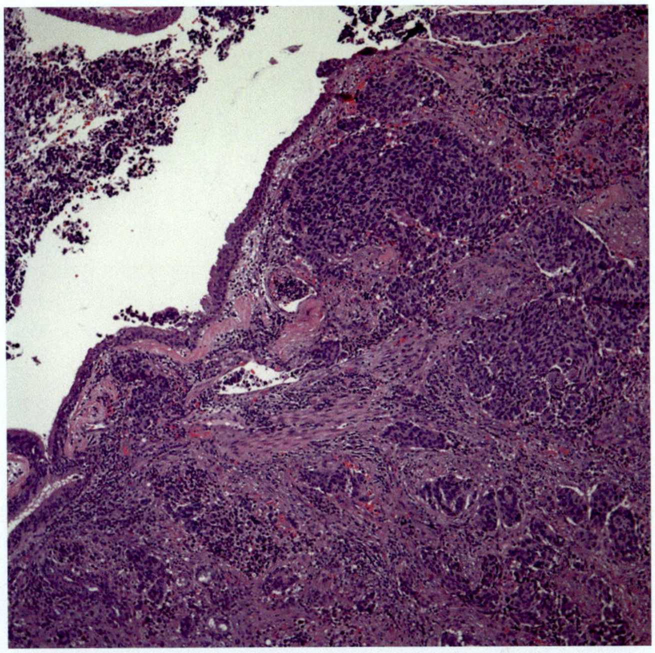

Fig. 4.22 Large cell neuroendocrine carcinoma adjacent to an airway. Note the nested neuroendocrine growth pattern of the tumor

Mooi et al. [59] described 11 primary lung carcinomas under the rubric of non-small cell carcinoma with neuroendocrine features. These tumors had been diagnosed either as large cell carcinoma or squamous cell carcinoma, but all the tumors had similarities to bronchial carcinoid and small cell carcinoma. Six of seven cases in which electron microscopy studies were available showed dense-core granules, while all cases showed positive staining for neuron-specific enolase (NSE) (most of the antibodies that are available today may not have been available in 1988). The authors also stated that neuroendocrine features may be suspected by light microscopy. Judging by some of the illustrations provided, one can assume that some of those tumors, if not all, are similar to today's designation of large cell neuroendocrine carcinoma. Dresler et al. [60] in 1997 analyzed 40 cases of large cell neuroendocrine carcinoma and concluded that large cell neuroendocrine carcinomas identified by histological examination have poor prognosis. The authors also suggested that lesions previously categorized as large cell carcinoma with neuroendocrine features should be regarded as "large cell carcinoma with occult neuroendocrine differentiation." This latter suggestion specifically addresses an issue that goes to the core of these types of tumors, which is

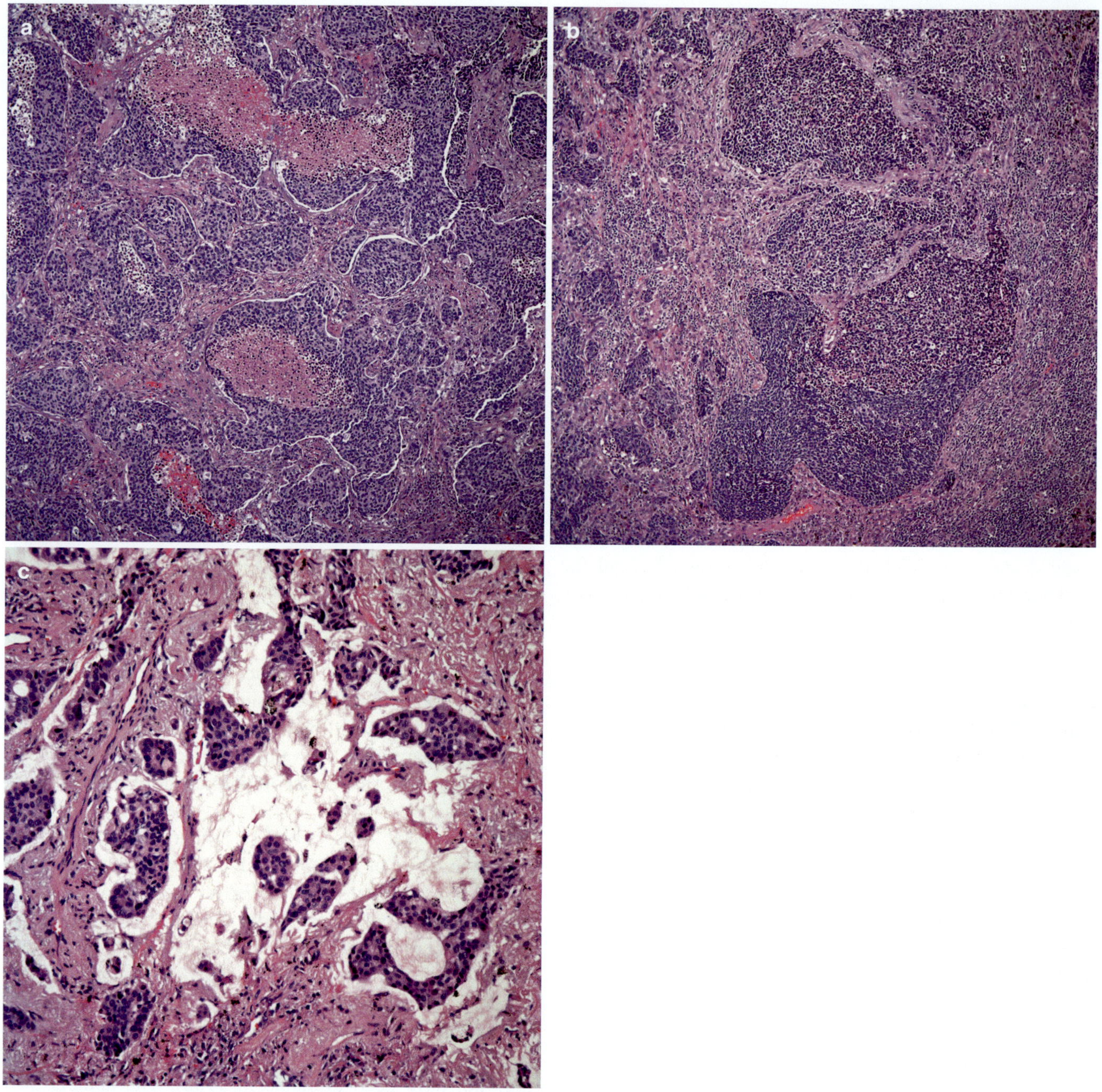

Fig. 4.23 (**a**) Areas of necrosis are commonly seen, and in some cases comedo-like necrosis is common. (**b**) In other areas, the tumor may show a basaloid component. (**c**) In more unusual tumors, areas of mucinous pools may be seen

how to group tumors that have a "neuroendocrine pattern" but yet fail to show immunoreactivity for neuroendocrine markers. As the criteria are currently presented, in order to make the diagnosis of "large cell neuroendocrine carcinoma," the tumor must have "neuroendocrine morphology" and positive staining for at least one neuroendocrine marker [2]. This issue has become even more confusing by the use of terms such as *small cell-like large cell neuroendocrine carcinoma* in some cytologic studies [61]. In addition, following the presence of nucleoli to separate small from non-small cell carcinoma may prove difficult just as using cell size for their differentiation. Marchevsky et al. [62] evaluated, by morphometric means, 28 surgically resected high-grade pulmonary neuroendocrine carcinomas (16 small cell carcinomas and 12 large cell neuroendocrine carcinomas). The authors concluded that there is considerable nuclear overlap between these entities, which helped the author to separate only 9 of 28 cases studied, and suggested the use of more generic

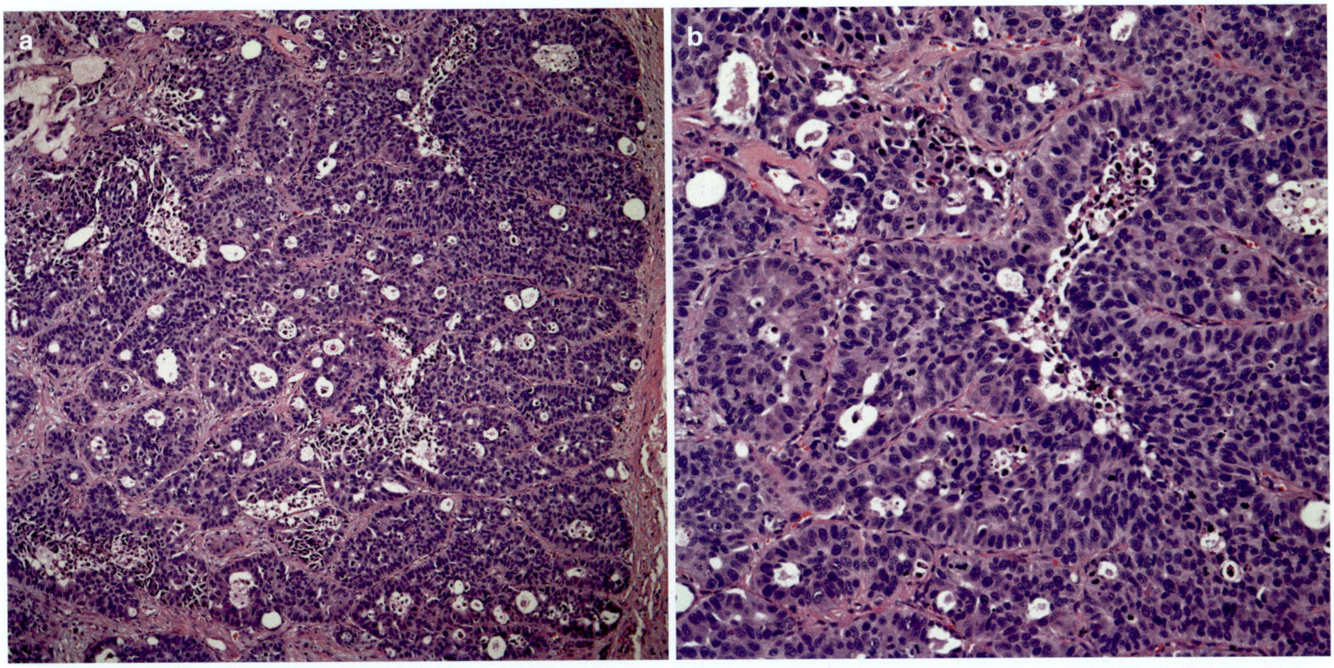

Fig. 4.24 (**a**) Important in the diagnosis of large cell neuroendocrine carcinoma is the identification of areas with neuroendocrine growth pattern. (**b**) Closer view at the neuroendocrine growth pattern showing cells larger cells with round nuclei and presence of nucleoli

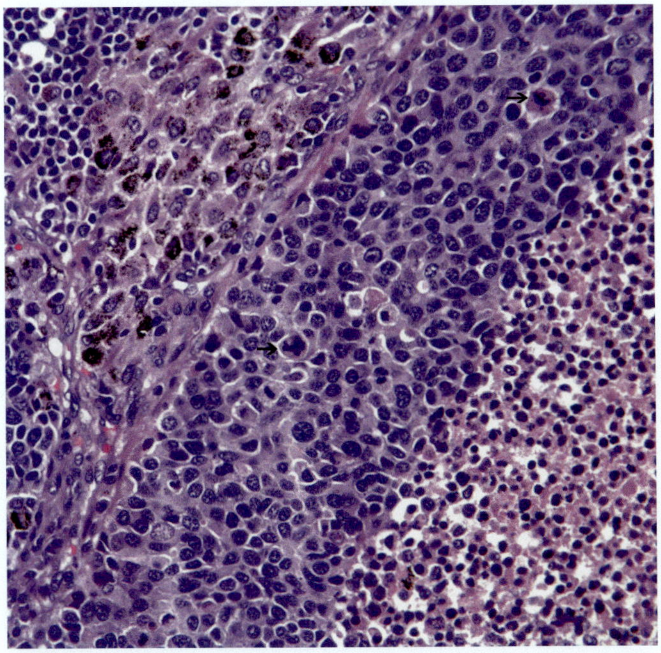

Fig. 4.25 Closer view at the neoplastic cells showing larger cells with presence of nucleoli and increased mitotic activity (see *arrows*)

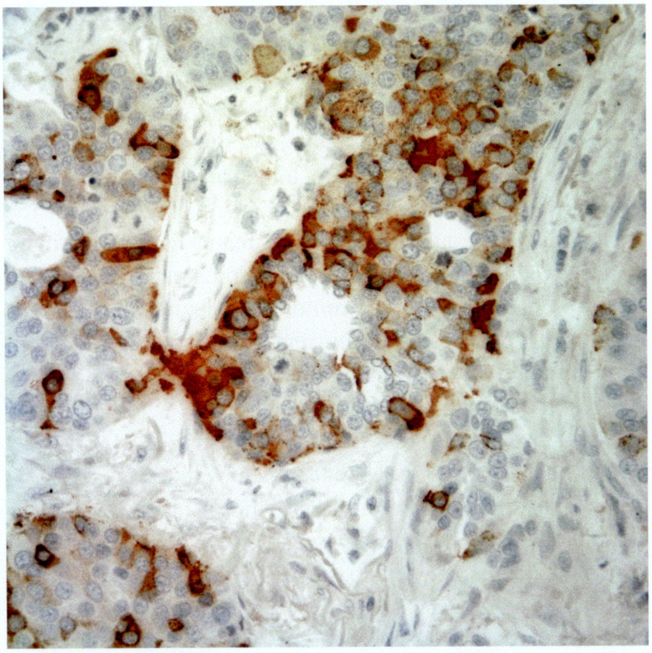

Fig. 4.26 Chromogranin showing positive staining in tumor cells

terminology such as high-grade neuroendocrine carcinoma or grade III neuroendocrine carcinoma. The entire topic of "large cell neuroendocrine carcinoma" has generated a myriad of publications in order to bring light to this confusing topic. For instance, Iyoda et al. [63], in a study of 2,070 cases of large cell carcinomas, divided such tumors into four different categories: large cell neuroendocrine carcinoma, large cell carcinoma with neuroendocrine differentiation, large cell carcinoma with neuroendocrine morphology, and "classic" large cell carcinoma. In a multivariable analysis, the authors grouped the three former entities into a single entity, which the authors denominated as large cell carcinoma with neuroendocrine features separate from the "classic" large cell carcinoma, and concluded that those tumors are more aggressive. What is interesting and important in this study is the fact that tumors in which the authors did not find morphologic evidence of neuroendocrine change were grouped as large cell carcinomas with neuroendocrine morphology. Yet on multivariable analysis, the authors found that these tumors – just the same as those grouped as large cell neuroendocrine carcinoma and large cell carcinoma with neuroendocrine differentiation – behave more aggressively compared to the "classic" large cell carcinoma. Nevertheless, their point raises another issue and that is whether it is important to determine neuroendocrine "differentiation" by immunohistochemical means and whether a specific diagnosis is warranted for those tumors. Some other publications on this topic have lumped large cell neuroendocrine carcinomas and large cell carcinoma with neuroendocrine morphology under the same designation [64]. Unfortunately, in many recent publications on the subject, even as the authors claimed that they have used rigorous application of the WHO criteria [2], the emphasis has been on those tumors that fit the criteria of morphology and immunohistochemistry, leaving unanswered the question of how to handle tumors that may show the morphology but not the immunohistochemistry of a neuroendocrine carcinoma [65–75]. In other reports, it is very difficult to discern which cases were accounted for as large cell neuroendocrine carcinoma, since the terminology used appears to be ambiguous [76–79]. More recently Glisson and Moran [80] addressed the difficulties and controversies in the diagnosis and treatment of large cell neuroendocrine carcinoma and stated that because of the rarity of this tumor and vagaries in diagnosis because of the complexity of current pathologic classification, current treatment recommendations must be based on retrospective data, which are imperfect at best.

Chromosomal and loss of heterozygosity (LOH) analyses have been undertaken to separate tumors with features of large cell neuroendocrine carcinoma [81], while in others the nomenclature used is not the one assigned by the WHO classification system [82]. In some reports, these tumors have been correlated with pathologic stage, raising the issue of staging, since these tumors may present in different pathological stages [83]. In some recent publications [84, 85], an emphasis has been made to separate large cell neuroendocrine carcinoma from small cell carcinoma by using immunohistochemistry and molecular studies. If one is to apply WHO criteria or any of the other schemas presented, such distinction should not be a difficult task, since one is small cell and the other is non-small cell carcinoma with prominent nucleoli. Furthermore, the problem of separating small from non-small cell carcinoma should not require immunohistochemistry or molecular studies.

Important to note is that some reports have concentrated on non-small cell carcinomas with neuroendocrine differentiation or neuroendocrine morphology [79, 86–91]. In a study by Howe et al. [86], the authors studied 439 cases of non-small cell carcinoma, which were evaluated using immunohistochemical stains for neuroendocrine markers. The authors reported that 36% of these tumors showed at least positive staining for one neuroendocrine marker and concluded that the presence of neuroendocrine differentiation in non-small cell carcinoma is of no prognostic significance, as has also been reported by other authors [88]. More recently, Ionescu et al. [91] arrived at a similar conclusion after reviewing 609 cases of non-small cell carcinoma. Important to mention is the fact that some adenocarcinomas may show neuroendocrine differentiation, which has been suggested as an important prognostic feature [92] while others have had a more circumspect approach about this particular issue [93].

Critical review of the literature raises some important questions:

1. The diagnosis of large cell neuroendocrine carcinoma in most of the series presented has been a diagnosis in retrospect after analysis of all large cell carcinomas.
2. The cases included in a good number of publications, despite the "rigorous" application of the WHO criteria, suggest that some of the tumors included may not exactly belong into that designation.
3. The fact that resections have been evaluated speaks volumes to the fact that these tumors have already been initially treated as non-small cell carcinomas.
4. Although all authors believe that these tumors are of high grade, there is not unanimous agreement regarding the best method of treatment for patients diagnosed with large cell neuroendocrine carcinomas. In this regard, some authors have advocated that large cell neuroendocrine carcinoma is potentially treatable with surgery [71] while others advocate additional medical treatment [94].
5. There is some confusion regarding the use of adjectives such as "neuroendocrine differentiation" and "neuroendocrine morphology."
6. Staging may still represent an important independent factor in the prognosis of these tumors. The entire issue of neuroendocrine morphology or differentiation can be summarized as follows:

- *Large cell neuroendocrine carcinoma*: tumors with neuroendocrine pattern and positive staining for neuroendocrine markers, i.e. chromogranin, synaptophysin, or CD56.
- *Large cell carcinoma with neuroendocrine features or morphology*: tumors with neuroendocrine pattern but negative staining for neuroendocrine markers.
- *Large cell carcinoma with neuroendocrine differentiation*: positive staining for neuroendocrine markers but absent neuroendocrine morphology.

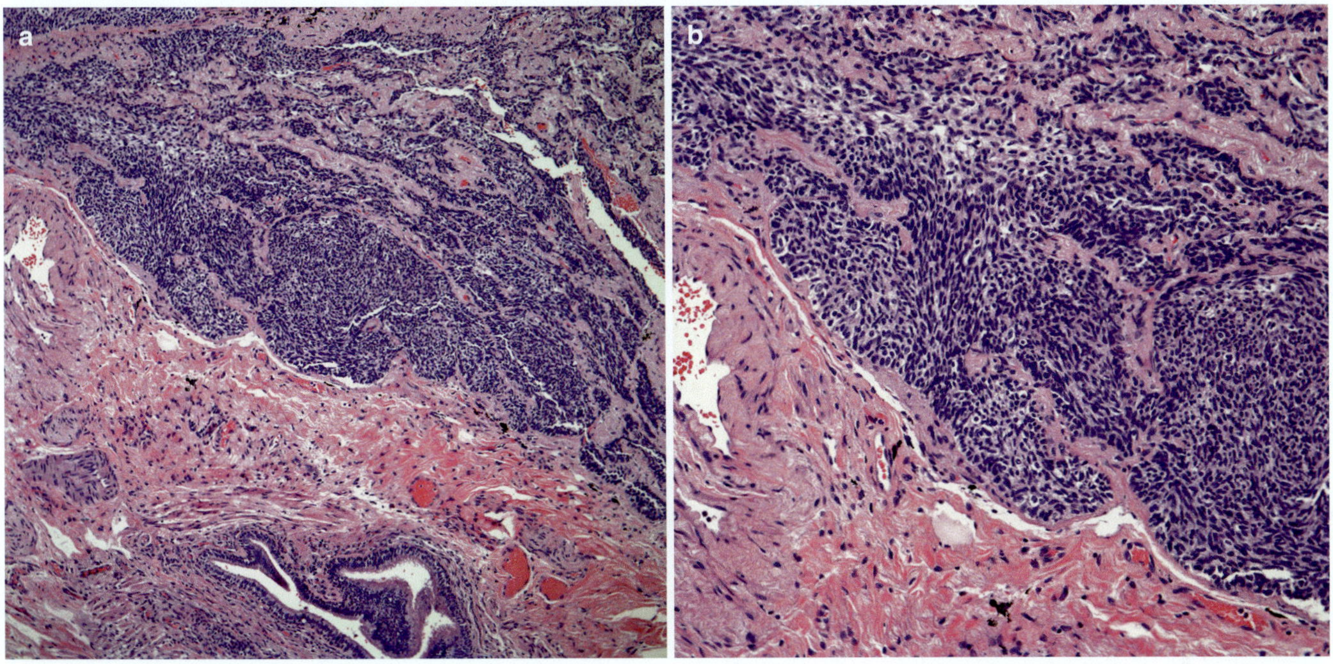

Fig. 4.27 (**a**) Basaloid carcinoma showing classic appearance with peripheral palisading of the nuclei. (**b**) Higher magnification showing a subtle spindling of the neoplastic cells

Although one would expect that the issue of large cell carcinoma may be restricted to the issue of neuroendocrine morphology or neuroendocrine differentiation, the WHO separated yet another tumor that may provide even more confusion to the current classification, the so-called basaloid carcinoma of the lung [95].

Basaloid Carcinoma

This particular neoplasm was initially described as a new morphological and phenotypical entity. However, close analysis of their histopathological description shows that 19 of the 38 cases described showed areas of squamous cell carcinoma, adenocarcinoma, and large cell carcinoma, raising the possibility that at least half of the tumors described may be grouped into one of those more specific categories. On the other hand, the WHO classification [2] recognized that the distinction between large cell neuroendocrine carcinoma and basaloid carcinoma is difficult and often requires immunohistochemical studies. Also, the WHO acknowledges that in 10% of cases of basaloid carcinoma, a neuroendocrine marker may be positive, thus raising the possibility that "basaloid carcinoma" may represent a growth pattern rather than a specific pathological entity. Other studies on basaloid carcinoma have stressed the use of immunohistochemical studies, namely, cytokeratins 1, 5, 10, and 14 (34βE12) to differentiate such tumor from large cell neuroendocrine carcinoma. However, Lyda and Weiss [96] reported an incidence of 5% positive staining for 34βE12 in neuroendocrine carcinomas. Thus, separating these tumors by immunohistochemistry may not be as straightforward as thought, if indeed they represent different neoplasms.

Microscopic Features

These tumors appear to be well defined masses destroying lung parenchyma. As the name implies, the low-power shows islands of tumor cells arranged in ribbons and forming rosettes with palisading of the nuclei. High-power magnification shows oval to spindle cells with elongated nuclei, and in some cells prominent nucleoli may be observed (Fig. 4.27a,b). The mitotic count in these tumors is high and in resected specimens is well beyond 10×10 hpf.

Carcinomas with Mixed Histologies

It is well known that pulmonary carcinomas in a small but well-represented number of cases may show combined histologies (Fig. 4.28a,b), namely, of the small cell/non-small cell categories [97–101]. It appears that the general consensus with these types of tumors is that the behavior is more aggressive than in pure small cell carcinomas, leading to a shorter survival rate. However, an important issue that needs further investigation is the possible association of small cell

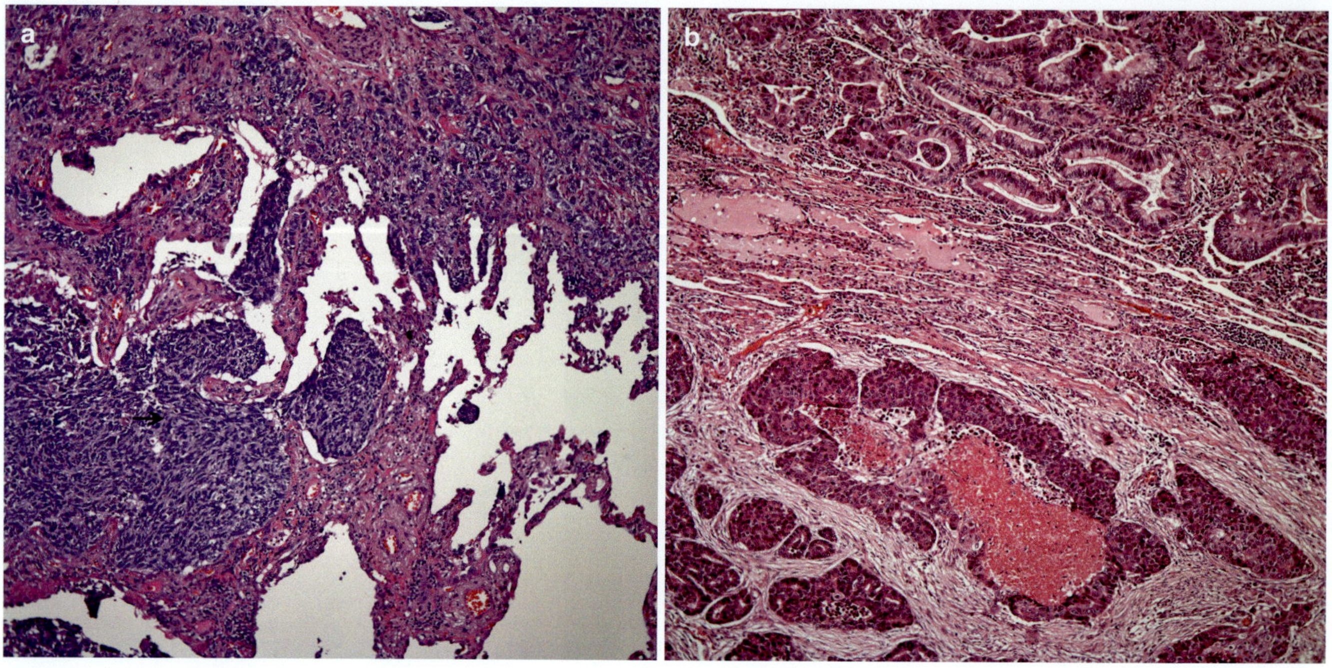

Fig. 4.28 (**a**) Combined small cell carcinoma (see *arrow*) and non-small cell carcinoma. (**b**) Combined large cell neuroendocrine carcinoma and conventional adenocarcinoma

carcinoma and large cell neuroendocrine carcinoma or large cell carcinoma with neuroendocrine differentiation. Whether that distinction has a practical value in the treatment of these patients may be just an academic exercise since both of those tumors belong to the high-grade category and may be treated with chemotherapeutic regimens for high-grade neuroendocrine carcinomas.

Molecular Biology

Genetic studies have been performed showing a gain of 3q in about 66% of small cell carcinoma while deletions of 10q, 16q, and 17p were less frequent in large cell neuroendocrine carcinoma than in small cell carcinoma [102]. Other studies have shown that gene expression profiling has failed to distinguish small cell from large cell neuroendocrine carcinomas and has led some authors to suggest that both entities should be grouped under the designation of high-grade neuroendocrine tumors [103]. Other studies have placed more emphasis on the issue of the spectrum of differentiation of neuroendocrine tumors and have found through studies of expression of gene products that there is no evidence linking carcinoids and small cell carcinoma [104]. Similar findings have been encountered by other authors [105], leading to the suggestion that small cell carcinomas are derived from epithelial cells and that bronchial carcinoids are related to neural crest-derived tumors. It also appears that human p19ARF protein encoded by the beta transcript of the $p16^{INK4a}$ gene is more commonly lost in high-grade neuroendocrine carcinomas than in conventional non-small cell carcinomas [106].

Analysis of p53, K-ras-2, and C-raf-1 by some authors has led to the suggestion that typical and atypical carcinoids are genetically distinct from high-grade neuroendocrine carcinomas [107]. Regarding atypical carcinoids, it has been documented that loss of heterozygosity at 3p14.2–p21.3 is significantly more extensive in atypical carcinoids, while typical carcinoids are strongly positive for the cytoplasmic Fhit protein, similar to normal lung epithelia [108]. Interestingly, studies on the expression of Bcl-2 have concluded that the expression of Bcl-2 is involved in the pathogenesis of small cell carcinoma and carcinoid tumors of the lung [109]. The expression of retinoblastoma (RB) protein in neuroendocrine tumors has disclosed its presence in carcinoids and atypical carcinoids, while it is absent in small cell and large cell neuroendocrine carcinoma [110, 111]. It has also been suggested that hASH-1 (human homologue of Mas1) is involved in the neuroendocrine differentiation of small and non-small cell carcinomas [112].

Conceptual Practical Approach to the Diagnosis of Neuroendocrine Carcinomas

Based on current concepts and approaches, a practical approach to the diagnosis of neuroendocrine carcinomas may be conceptualized as follows:

Surgical Resections

- Carcinoid tumorlet (neuroendocrine lesions under 0.5 cm in size)
- Well differentiated neuroendocrine carcinoma (typical carcinoid tumor): 0–3 mitotic figures × 10hpf, only focal punctuate necrosis
- Moderately differentiated neuroendocrine carcinoma (atypical carcinoid tumor): 4–10 mitotic figures × 10 hpf, and necrosis
- High-grade neuroendocrine carcinoma:
  - Small cell carcinoma: with or without positive neuroendocrine markers, tumors with >10 mitotic figures × 10 hpf, and necrosis
  - Large cell neuroendocrine carcinoma: large cell carcinoma with positive neuroendocrine morphology and positive neuroendocrine markers and large cell carcinoma with positive morphology and negative staining for neuroendocrine markers, large tumor cells with nucleoli, >10 mitotic figures × 10 hpf, and necrosis

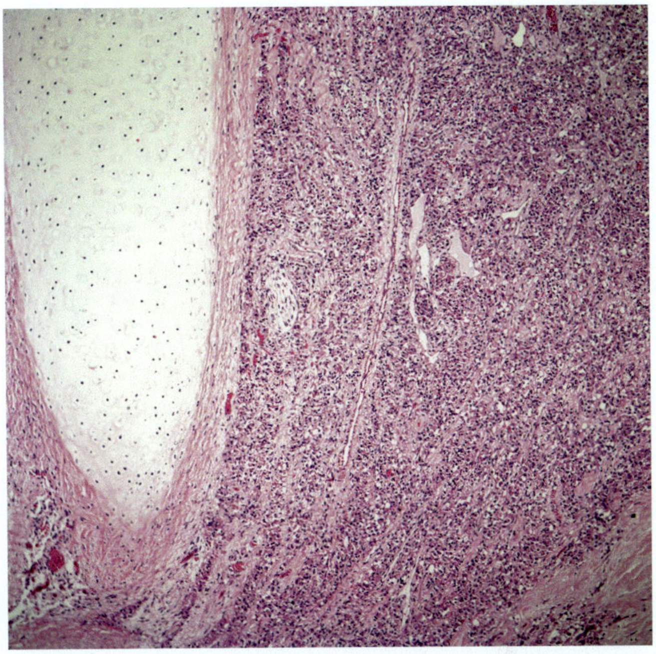

Fig. 4.29 Primary pulmonary paraganglioma showing the conventional nested growth pattern. Note the presence of bronchial cartilage

Biopsy Specimens

- Neuroendocrine carcinoma—if the tumor is in the spectrum of well- or moderately differentiated neuroendocrine carcinoma (carcinoid or atypical carcinoid) and the tumor radiologically is >0.5 cm in greatest diameter (specify the possibilities)
- Small cell carcinoma
- Squamous cell carcinoma
- Adenocarcinoma
- Large cell carcinoma

Pulmonary Paraganglioma

Pulmonary paragangliomas will be discussed in this chapter as part of the spectrum of neuroendocrine tumors; however, their clinical behavior is distinct to that of the conventional neuroendocrine carcinoma. Also, important to note is the fact that intrapulmonary paragangliomas are rare tumors in this location and every effort has to be made in order to determine the possibility of a metastatic lesion to the lung. In general, these tumors are exceedingly rare, and only a few well-described cases are reported in the literature. The tumors appear to occur in adult individuals, who clinically may present with hypertension, increase serum norepinephrine, or Cushing's syndrome [113–117].

Macroscopic Features

These tumors vary in size from under 1 cm to more than 3 cm in greatest dimension. The tumors are endobronchial and may obstruct the bronchial lumen producing symptoms of cough, wheezing, and dyspnea. Macroscopically, they cannot be separated from low- or intermediate-grade neuroendocrine carcinomas.

Microscopic Features

Low-power magnification shows that the tumor may appear as a polypoid mass filling the bronchial lumen. The classic low-power appearance of paragangliomas is the so-called Zellballen pattern. The cells are arranged in a nesting pattern in which the nests are separated by thin fibroconnective tissue and ectatic blood vessels. The tumor may also show oncocytic changes with a homogeneous cellular proliferation (Figs. 4.29, 4.30, 4.31, and 4.32). At high-power magnification, it is common to identify the presence of cells with macronuclei or bizarre nuclei but no associated mitotic activity [113–117]. Also common is the presence of large dilated vessels or the presence of extensive areas of hyalinization. In some cases, ganglion cells, represented by larger cells with eosinophilic cytoplasm, and prominent nucleoli accompany the cellular proliferation. In other cases, the tumor may show spindle cell morphology. In a few cases, lymph node involvement has been reported.

Immunohistochemical Features

The same as neuroendocrine carcinomas, paragangliomas react positively with neuroendocrine markers such as chromogranin, synaptophysin, and/or CD56. However,

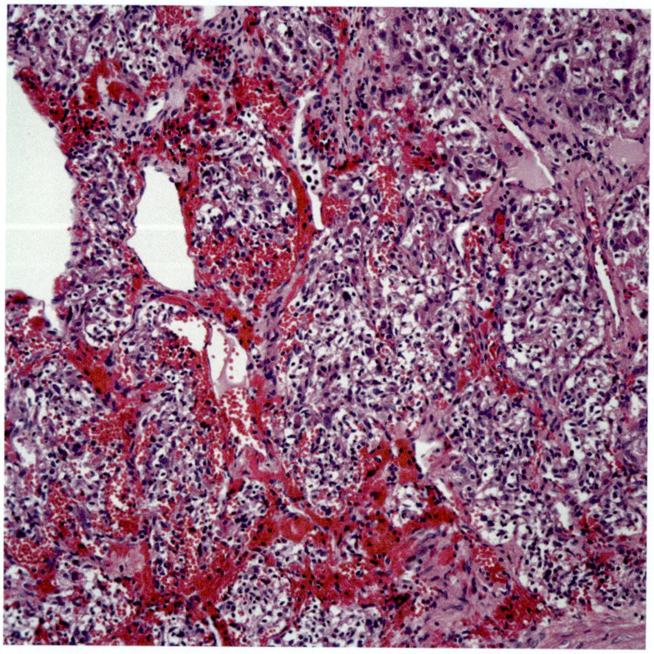

Fig. 4.30 Pulmonary paraganglioma showing a nested growth pattern composed of a homogenous cellular proliferation

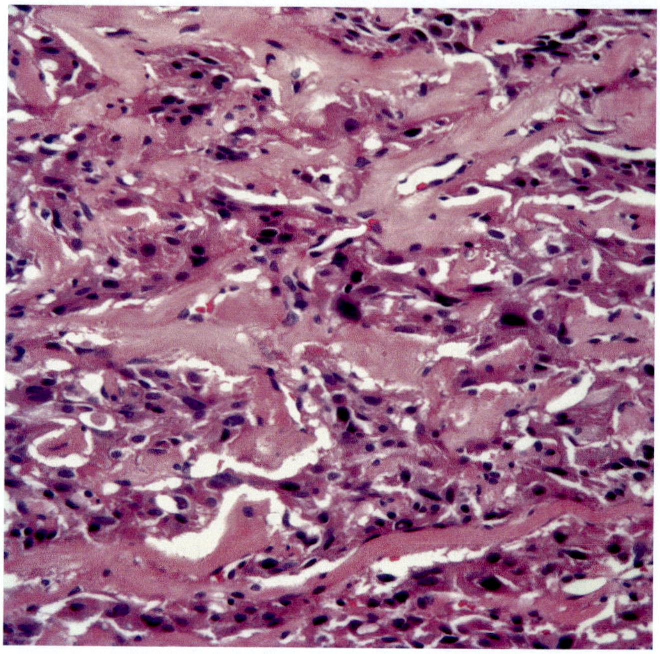

Fig. 4.32 Higher magnification of a pulmonary paraganglioma showing large nuclei but absence of mitotic activity

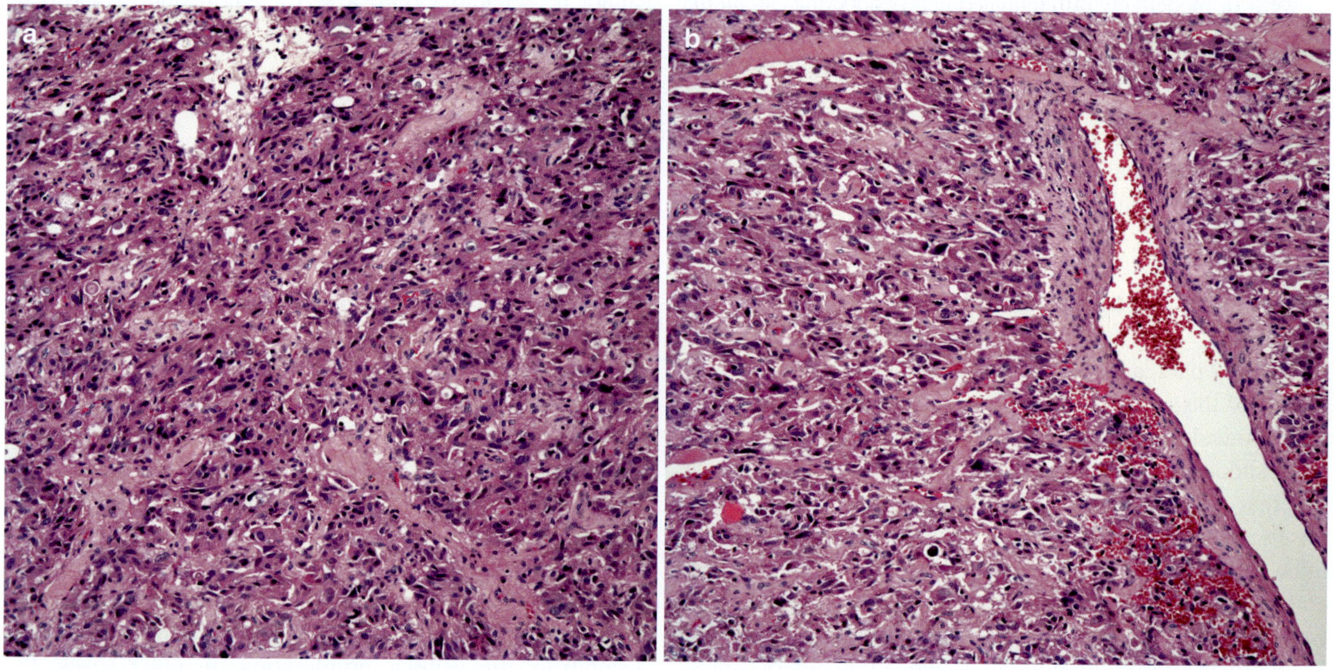

Fig. 4.31 (**a**) Cords of neuroendocrine cells separated by areas of fibrocollagen. (**b**) Dilated vascular structures are commonly seen. Note the presence of the neoplastic cells around the vessel

keratin is negative in paragangliomas, while positive in neuroendocrine carcinomas. S-100 protein is positive in the sustentacular cells of paragangliomas.

Clinical Behavior

Surgical treatment appears to be the treatment of choice and in the majority of cases is the only treatment accompanied by close follow-up. However, due to the rarity of these tumors in an intrapulmonary location, it is difficult to meaningfully determine the clinical behavior of these tumors especially when these tumors can involve lymph nodes.

References

1. Muller NL, MIller RR. Neuroendocrine carcinomas of the lung. Semin Roentgenol. 1990;XXV(1):96–104.
2. Beasley MB, Thunnissen FB, Hasleton PS, et al. Tumours of the lung, pleura, thymus and heart. Lyon: IARC Press; 2004.
3. Cerilli LA, Ritter J, Mills SE, Wick MR. Neuroendocrine neoplasms of the lung. Am J Clin Pathol. 2001;116 Suppl 1:S65–96.
4. Flieder DB. Neuroendocrine tumors of the lung: recent developments in histopathology. Curr Opin Pulm Med. 2002;8:275–80.
5. Oberndorfer S. Karzinoide Tumoren des Dunndarms. Frankfurter Zeischrift fur Pathologie. 1907;1:425–32.
6. Bunting CH. Multiple primary carcinomata of the ileum. Johns Hopkins Hosp Bull. 1904;165(December):389–94.
7. Gosset A, Masson P. Tumeurs endocrines de l'appendice. La Presse Medicale. 1914;25:237–40.
8. Kinney FJ, Kovarik JL. Bone formation in bronchial adenoma. Am J Clin Pathol. 1965;44(1):52–6.
9. Heimburger IL, Kilman JW, Battersby JS. Peripheral bronchial adenomas. J Thorac Cardiovasc Surg. 1966;52(4):542–9.
10. Gmelich JT, Bensch KG, Liebow AA. Cells of Kultschitzky type in bronchioles and their relation to the origin of peripheral carcinoid tumor. Lab Invest. 1967;17(1):88–98.
11. Hausman DH, Weimann R. Pulmonary tumorlet with hilar lymph node metastasis. Cancer. 1967;20(9):1515–9.
12. Azzopardi JG. Oat cell carcinoma of the bronchus. J Pathol Bacteriol. 1959;78(2):513–9.
13. Yutaka K, Ferguson TB, Bennett DE, Burford TH. Oat cell carcinoma of the lung. Cancer. 1969;23(3):517–24.
14. Gould VE, Memoli VA, Dardi LE. Multidirectional differentiation in human epithelial cancers. J Submicrosc Cytol. 1981;13(1):97–115.
15. Gould VE. Histogenesis and differentiation: a re-evaluation of these concepts as criteria for the classification of tumors. Hum Pathol. 1986;17(3):212–5.
16. Sheppard MN. Neuroendocrine differentiation in lung tumours. Thorax. 1991;46:843–50.
17. Brambilla E, Lantuejoul S, Sturm N. Divergent differentiation in neuroendocrine tumors. Semin Diagn Pathol. 2000;17(2):138–48.
18. Gould VE. Neuroendocrinomas and neuroendocrine carcinomas: APUD cell system neoplasms and their aberrant secretory activities. Pathol Annu. 1977;12:33–62.
19. Gould VE, Linnoila RI, Memoli VA, Warren WH. Neuroendocrine cells and neuroendocrine neoplasms of the lung. Pathol Annu 1983;18:287–330.
20. Warren WH, Gould VE, Faber LP, Kittle CF, Memoli VA. Neuroendocrine neoplasms of the bronchopulmonary tract. J Thorac Cardiovasc Surg. 1985;89(6):819–25.
21. Paladugu RR, Benfield JR, Pak HY, Ross RK, Teplitz RL. Bronchopulmonary Kultschitzky cell carcinomas: a new classification scheme for typical and atypical carcinoids. Cancer. 1985;55(6):1303–11.
22. Arrigoni MG, Woolner LB, Bernatz PE. Atypical carcinoid tumors of the lung. J Thorac Cardiovasc Surg. 1972;64(3):4113–421.
23. Mills SE, Cooper PH, Walker AN, Kron IL. Atypical carcinoid tumor of the lung. Am J Surg Pathol. 1982;6(7):643–54.
24. Valli M, Fabris GA, Dewar A, Hornall D, Sheppard MN. Atypical carcinoid tumour of the lung: a study of 33 cases with prognostic features. Histopathology. 1994;24:363–9.
25. Grote TH, Macon WR, Davis B, Greco FA, Johnson DH. Atypical carcinoid of the lung: a distinct clinicopathologic entity. Chest. 1988;93(2):370–5.
26. Capella C, Heitz PU, Hofler H, Solcia E, Kloppel G. Revised classification of neuroendocrine tumours of the lung, pancreas and gut. Virchows Arch. 1994;425:547–60.
27. Travis WD, Linnoila RI, Tsokos MG, et al. Neuroendocrine tumors of the lung with proposed criteria for large-cell neuroendocrine carcinoma An ultrastructural, immunohistochemical, and flow cytometric study of 35 cases. Am J Surg Pathol. 1991;15(6):529–53.
28. Travis WD, Rush W, Flieder DB, et al. Survival analysis of 200 pulmonary neuroendocrine tumors with clarification of criteria for atypical carcinoid and its separation from typical carcinoid. Am J Surg Pathol. 1998;22(8):934–44.
29. Travis WD, Gal AA, Colby TV, Klimstra DS, Falk R, Koss MN. Reproducibility of neuroendocrine lung tumor classification. Hum Pathol. 1998;29:272–9.
30. Huang Q, Muzitansky A, Mark EJ. Pulmonary neuroendocrine carcinomas: a review of 234 cases and statistical analysis of 50 cases treated at one institution using a simple clinicopathologic classification. Arch Pathol Lab Med. 2002;126:545–53.
31. Ricci C, Patrassi N, Massa R, Mineo C, Benedetti-Valentini F. Carcinoid syndrome in bronchial adenoma. Am J Surg. 1973;126(11):671–7.
32. Sklar JL, Churg A, Bensch KG. Oncocytic carcinoid tumor of the lung. Am J Surg Pathol. 1980;4(3):287–92.
33. Cebelin MS. Melanocytic bronchial carcinoid tumor. Cancer. 1980;46(8):1843–8.
34. Wise WS, Bonder D, Aikawa M, Hsieh CL. Carcinoid tumor of lung with varied histology. Am J Surg Pathol. 1982;6(3):261–7.
35. Grazer R, Jacobs SB, Lucas P. Melanin-containing peripheral carcinoid of the lung. Am J Surg Pathol. 1982;6(1):73–8.
36. Gal AA, Koss MN, Hochholzer L, DeRose PB, Cohen C. Pigmented pulmonary carcinoid tumor. Arch Pathol Lab Med. 1993;117:832–6.
37. Tsutsumi Y, Yazaki K. Atypical carcinoid tumor of the lung, associated with giant-cell transformation in bone metastasis. Acta Pathol Jpn. 1990;40(8):609–15.
38. Memoli VA. Well-differentiated neuroendocrine carcinoma: a designation comes of age. Chest. 1991;10:892.
39. Tsuta K, Raso MG, Kalhor N, Liu DD, Wistuba I, Moran CA. Histologic features of low-grade and intermediate grade neuroendocrine carcinoma (typical and atypical carcinoid tumors) of the lung. Lung Cancer. 2011;71:34–41.
40. Tsuta K, Kalhor N, Raso MG, Wistuba I, Moran CA. Oncocytic neuroendocrine tumors of the lung: histologic spectrum and immunohistochemical analysis of 15 cases. Hum Pathol. 2011;42:578–85.
41. Tsuta K, Kalhor N, Wistuba I, Moran CA. Clinicopathological and immunohistochemical analysis of spindle cell carcinoid tumour of the lung. Histopathology. 2011;59:526–36.
42. Kalhor N, Suster S, Moran CA. Primary sclerosing neuroendocrine carcinomas of the lung: a clinicopathologic and immunohistochemical study of 10 cases. Am J Clin Pathol. 2010;133:618–22.
43. Sturm N, Rossi G, Lantuejoul S, et al. Expression of thyroid transcription factor-1 in the spectrum of neuroendocrine cell lung proliferations with special interest in carcinoids. Hum Pathol. 2002;33:175–82.

44. Tsuta K, Raso MG, Kalhor N, Liu DC, Wistuba II, Moran CA. Sox10-positive sustentacular cells in neuroendocrine carcinoma of the lung. Histopathology. 2011;58:276–85.
45. Costes V, Marty-Ane C, Picot MC, et al. Typical and atypical bronchopulmonary carcinoid tumors: a clinicopathologic and Ki-67-labeling study. Hum Pathol. 1995;26(7):740–5.
46. Tsuta K, Liu DC, Kalhor N, Wistuba II, Moran CA. Using the mitosis-specific marker anti-phosphohistone H3 to assess mitosis in pulmonary neuroendocrine carcinomas. Am J Clin Pathol. 2011;136:252–9.
47. Walch AK, Zitzelsberger HF, Bauchinger M, et al. Typical and atypical carcinoid tumors of the lung are characterized by 11q deletions as detected by comparative genomic hybridization. Am J Pathol. 1998;153:1089–98.
48. Wilkins EW, Grillo HC, Moncure AC, Scannell JG. Changing times in surgical management of bronchopulmonary carcinoid tumor. Ann Thorac Surg. 1984;38(4):339–44.
49. Schreurs JM, Westermann JJ, Bosch JMM, Vanderschueren RGJRA, Riviere AB, Knaepen PJ. A twenty-five-year follow-up of ninety-three resected typical carcinoid tumors of the lung. J Thorac Cardiovasc Surg. 1992;104(5):1470–5.
50. Nicholson S, Beasley MB, Brambilla E, et al. Small cell carcinomas (SCLC): a clinicopathologic study of 100 cases with surgical specimens. Am J Surg Pathol. 2002;26(9):1184–97.
51. Zakowski MF. Pathology of small cell carcinoma of the lung. Semin Oncol. 2003;30(1):3–8.
52. Vollmer RT, Birch R, Ogden L, Crissman JD. Subclassification of small cell cancer of the lung: the southern cancer study group experience. Hum Pathol. 1985;16(3):247–52.
53. Hirsch FR, Matthews MJ, Aisner S, et al. Histopathologic classification of small cell lung cancer: changing concepts and terminology. Cancer. 1988;62(5):973–7.
54. Warren WH, Memoli VA, Jordan AG, Gould VE. Reevaluation of pulmonary neoplasms resected as small cell carcinomas. Cancer. 1990;65:1003–10.
55. Guinee DG, Fishback NF, Koss MN, Abbondanzo SL, Travis WD. The spectrum of immunohistochemical staining of small-cell lung carcinoma in specimens from transbronchial and open lung biopsies. Cancer. 1994;102(4):406–14.
56. Warren WH, Gould VE. Differential diagnosis of small cell neuroendocrine carcinoma of the lung. Chest Surg Clin N Am. 1997; 7(1):49–63.
57. Spiegelman D, Maurer LH, Ware JH, et al. Prognostic factors in small cell carcinoma of the lung: an analysis of 1,521 patients. J Clin Oncol. 1989;7(3):344–54.
58. Kalemkerian GP, Akerley W, Bogner P, et al. Small cell lung cancer: clinical practice guidelines in oncology. J Natl Compr Canc Netw. 2011;9(10):1086–110.
59. Mooi WJ, Dewar A, Springall D, Polak JM, Addis BJ. Non-small cell lung carcinomas with neuroendocrine features. A light microscopic, immunohistochemical and ultrastructural study of 11 cases. Histopathology. 1988;13:329–37.
60. Dresler CM, Ritter JH, Patterson GA, Ross E, Bailey MS, Wick MR. Clinical-pathological analysis of 40 patients with large cell neuroendocrine carcinoma of the lung. Ann Thorac Surg. 1997;63:180–5.
61. Yang YJ, Steele CT, Ou XL, Snyder KP, Kochman LJ. Diagnosis of high-grade pulmonary neuroendocrine carcinoma by fine-needle aspiration biopsy: non-small-cell or small-cell type? Diagn Cytopathol. 2001;25:292–300.
62. Marchevsky AM, Gal AA, Shah S, Koss MN. Morphometry confirms the presence of considerable nuclear size overlap between "small cells" and "large cells" in high-grade pulmonary neuroendocrine neoplasms. Am J Clin Pathol. 2001;116:466–72.
63. Iyoda A, Hiroshima K, Toyozaki T, Haga Y, Fujisawa T, Ohwada H. Clinical characterization of pulmonary large cell neuroendocrine carcinoma and large cell carcinoma with neuroendocrine morphology. Cancer. 2001;91:1992–2000.
64. Zacharias J, Nicholson AG, Ladas GP, Goldstraw P. Large cell neuroendocrine carcinoma and large cell carcinomas with neuroendocrine morphology of the lung: prognosis after complete resection and systematic nodal dissection. Ann Thorac Surg. 2003;75:348–52.
65. Takei H, Asamura H, Maeshima A, et al. Large cell neuroendocrine carcinoma of the lung: a clinicopathologic study of eighty-seven cases. J Thorac Cardiovasc Surg. 2002;124(2):285–92.
66. Mazieres J, Daste G, Molinier L, et al. Large cell neuroendocrine carcinoma of the lung: pathological study and clinical outcome of 18 resected cases. Lung Cancer. 2002;37:287–92.
67. Jung K-J, Lee KS, Han J, et al. Large cell neuroendocrine carcinoma of the lung: clinical, CT, and pathological findings in 11 patients. J Thorac Imaging. 2001;16:156–62.
68. Filosso PL, Ruffini E, Oliaro A, et al. Large cell neuroendocrine carcinoma of the lung: a clinicopathologic study of eighteen cases and the efficacy of adjuvant treatment with octreotide. J Thorac Cardiovasc Surg. 2005;129(4):819–24.
69. Hage R, Seldenrijk K, Bruin PD, Swieten HV, Bosch JVD. Pulmonary large cell neuroendocrine carcinoma (LCNEC). Eur J Cardiothorac Surg. 2003;23:457–60.
70. Yamanishi M, Takeuchi S, Kurashina R, et al. High survival rate of 6 cases of pulmonary large cell neuroendocrine carcinoma formerly classified as small cell carcinoma. J Nippon Med Sch. 2001;68:335–9.
71. Doddoli C, Barlesi F, Chetaille B, et al. Large cell neuroendocrine carcinoma of the lung: an aggressive disease potentially treatable with surgery. Ann Thorac Surg. 2004;77:1168–72.
72. Paci M, Cavazza A, Annessi V, et al. Large cell neuroendocrine carcinoma of the lung: a 10-year clinicopathologic retrospective study. Ann Thorac Surg. 2004;77:1163–7.
73. Jiang S-X, Kameya T, Shoji M, Dobashi Y, Shinada J, Yoshimura H. Neuroendocrine carcinoma of the lung: a histologic and immunohistochemical study of 22 cases. Am J Surg Pathol. 1998;22(5):526–37.
74. Skuladottir H, Hirsch FR, Hansen HH, Olsen JH. Pulmonary neuroendocrine tumors: incidence and prognosis of histological subtypes. A population-based study in Denmark. Lung Cancer. 2002;37:127–35.
75. Cooper WA, Thourani VH, Gal AA, Lee RB, Mansour KA, Miller JI. The surgical spectrum of pulmonary neuroendocrine neoplasms. Chest. 2001;119:14–8.
76. Veronesi G, Morandi U, Alloisio M, et al. Large cell neuroendocrine carcinoma of the lung: a retrospective analysis of 144 surgical cases. Lung Cancer. 2006;53:111–5.
77. Masuya D, Liu D, Ishikawa S, Yamamoto Y, Huang C-l, Yokomise H. Large cell carcinoma with neuroendocrine morphology of the lung. Jpn J Thorac Cardiovasc Surg. 2006;54:31–4.
78. Battafarano RJ, Fernandez FG, Ritter J, et al. Large cell neuroendocrine carcinoma: an aggressive form of non-small cell lung cancer. J Thorac Cardiovasc Surg. 2005;130:166–72.
79. Iyoda A, Hiroshima K, Baba M, Saitoh Y, Ohwada H, Fujisawa T. Pulmonary large cell carcinoma with neuroendocrine features are high-grade neuroendocrine tumors. Ann Thorac Surg. 2002;73: 1049–54.
80. Glisson BS, Moran CA. Large cell neuroendocrine carcinoma: controversies in diagnosis and treatment. J Natl Compr Canc Netw. 2011;9(10):1122–9.
81. Peng W-X, Sano T, Oyama T, Kawashima O, Nakajima T. Large cell neuroendocrine carcinoma of the lung: a comparison with large cell carcinoma with neuroendocrine morphology and small cell carcinoma. Lung Cancer. 2005;47:225–33.
82. Garcia-Yuste M, Matilla JM, Alvarez-Gago T, et al. Prognostic factors in neuroendocrine lung tumors: a Spanish multicenter study. Ann Thorac Surg. 2000;70:258–63.

83. Iyoda A, Hiroshima K, Moriya Y, et al. Prognostic impact of large cell neuroendocrine histology in patients with pathologic stage Ia pulmonary non-small cell carcinoma. J Thorac Cardiovasc Surg. 2006;132:312–5.
84. Hiroshima K, Iyoda A, Shida T, et al. Distinction of pulmonary large cell neuroendocrine carcinoma from small cell lung carcinoma: a morphological, immunohistochemical, and molecular analysis. Mod Pathol. 2006;19:1358–68.
85. Nitadori JI, Ishii G, Tsuta K, et al. Immunohistochemical differential diagnosis between large cell neuroendocrine carcinoma and small cell carcinoma by tissue microarray analysis with a large antibody panel. Am J Clin Pathol. 2006;125:682–92.
86. Howe MC, Chapman A, Kerr K, Dougal M, Anderson H, Hasleton PS. Neuroendocrine differentiation in non-small cell lung cancer and its relation to prognosis and therapy. Histopathology. 2004;46:195–201.
87. Carey FA, Save VE. Neuroendocrine differentiation in lung cancer. J Pathol. 1997;182:9–10.
88. Wertzel H, Grahmann PR, Bansbach S, Lange W, Hasse J, Bohm N. Results after surgery in undifferentiated large cell carcinoma of the lung: the role of neuroendocrine expression. Eur J Cardiothorac Surg. 1997;12:698–702.
89. Jensen SM, Gazdar AF, Cuttitta F, Russell EK, Linnoila I. A comparison of synaptophysin, chromogranin, and L-Dopa decarboxylase as markers for neuroendocrine differentiation in lung cancer cell lines. Cancer Res. 1990;50:6068–74.
90. Burnett HE, Zakhour HD, Walker C. Neuroendocrine and epithelial markers in diagnostic bronchial lung cancer biopsy specimens. Eur J Cancer. 1992;28A(4/5):853–5.
91. Ionescu D, Treaba D, Gilks CB, et al. Nonsmall cell lung carcinoma with neuroendocrine differentiation - an entity of no clinical or prognostic significance. Am J Surg Pathol. 2007;31(1):26–32.
92. Hiroshima K, Iyoda A, Shibuya K, et al. Prognostic significance of neuroendocrine differentiation in adenocarcinoma of the lung. Ann Thorac Surg. 2002;73:1732–5.
93. Souhami RL. Neuroendocrine phenotype, chemosensitivity and prognosis in adenocarcinoma of the lung. Ann Oncol. 1991;2:323–4.
94. Iyoda A, Hiroshima K, Toyozaki T, et al. Adjuvant chemotherapy for large cell carcinoma with neuroendocrine features. Cancer. 2001;92:1108–12.
95. Brambilla E, Moro D, Veale D, et al. Basal cell (Basaloid) carcinoma of the lung: a new morphologic and phenotypic entity with separate prognostic significance. Hum Pathol. 1992;23(9):993–1003.
96. Lyda MH, Weiss LM. Immunoreactivity for epithelial and neuroendocrine antibodies are useful in the differential diagnosis of lung carcinomas. Hum Pathol. 2000;331:980–7.
97. McDowell EM, Trump BF. Pulmonary small cell carcinoma showing tripartite differentiation in individual cells. Hum Pathol. 1981;12(3):286–94.
98. Tsubota YT, Kawaguchi T, Hoso T, Nishino E, Travis WD. A combined small cell and spindle cell carcinoma of the lung: report of a unique case with immunohistochemical and ultrastructural studies. Am J Surg Pathol. 1992;16(11):1008–115.
99. Adelstein DJ, Tomashefski JF, Snow NJ, Horrigan TP, Hines JD. Mixed small cell and non-small cell lung cancer. Chest. 1986;89(5):699–704.
100. Radice PA, Matthews MJ, Ihde DC, et al. The clinical behavior of "mixed" small cell/large cell bronchogenic carcinoma compared to "pure" small cell subtypes. Cancer. 1982;50(12):2894–902.
101. Ruffini E, Rena O, Oliaro A, et al. Lung tumors with mixed histologic pattern. Clinico-pathologic characteristics and prognostic significance. Eur J Cardiothorac Surg. 2002;22:701–7.
102. Ullmann R, Petzmann S, Sharma A, Cagle PT, Popper HH. Chromosomal aberrations in a series of large-cell neuroendocrine carcinomas: unexpected divergence from small-cell carcinoma of the lung. Hum Pathol. 2001;32:1059–63.
103. Jones MH, Virtanen C, Honjoh D, et al. Two prognostically significant subtypes of high-grade lung neuroendocrine tumours independent of small cell and large cell neuroendocrine carcinomas identified by gene expression profiles. Lancet. 2004;363: 775–81.
104. Sampietro G, Tomasic G, Collini P, et al. Gene product immunophenotyping of neuroendocrine lung tumors. Appl Immunohistochem Mol Morphol. 2000;8(1):49–56.
105. Anbazhagan R, Tihan T, Bornman DM, et al. Classification of small cell lung cancer and pulmonary carcinoid by gene expression profiles. Cancer Res. 1999;59(10):5119–22.
106. Gazzeri S, Valle VD, Chaussade L, Brambilla C, Larsen CJ, Brambilla E. The human p19ARF protein encoded by the beta transcript of the p16INK4a gene is frequently lost in small cell lung cancer. Cancer Res. 1998;58(17):3926–31.
107. Przygodzki RM, Finkelstein SD, Langer JC, et al. Analysis of p53, K-ras-2, and C-raf-1 in pulmonary neuroendocrine tumors: correlation with histological tumors. Am J Pathol. 1996;148(5): 1531–41.
108. Kovatich A, Friedland DM, Druck T, et al. Molecular alterations to human chromosome 3p loci in neuroendocrine lung tumors. Cancer. 1998;83:1109–17.
109. Wang DG, Johnston CF, Sloan JM, Buchanan KD. Expression of Bcl-2 in lung neuroendocrine tumours: comparison with p53. J Pathol. 1998;184:247–51.
110. Cagle PT, Naggar AK, Xu HJ, Xu SX, Benedict WF. Differential retinoblastoma protein expression in neuroendocrine tumors of the lung. Potential diagnostic implications. Am J Pathol. 1997;150:393–400.
111. Rusch VW, Klimstra DS, Venkatraman ES. Molecular markers help characterized neuroendocrine lung tumors. Ann Thorac Surg. 1996;62:798–810.
112. Ito T, Udaka N, Okudela K, Yazawa T, Kitamura H. Mechanisms of neuroendocrine differentiation in pulmonary neuroendocrine cells and small cell carcinoma. Endocr Pathol. 2003;14(2): 133–9.
113. Shibara J, Goto A, Niki T, et al. Primary pulmonary paraganglioma: report of a functioning case with immunohistochemical and ultrastructural study. Am J Surg Pathol. 2004;28(6):825–9.
114. Kee AR, Forrest CH, Brennan BA, Papadimitriou JM, Glancy RJ. Gangliocytic paraganglioma of the bronchus: a case report with follow-up and ultrastructural assessment. Am J Surg Pathol. 2003;27:1380–5.
115. Palau MA, Merino MJ, Quezado M. Corticotropin-producing pulmonary gangliocytic paraganglioma associated with Cushing's syndrome. Hum Pathol. 2006;37:623–6.
116. Aubertine CL, Flieder DB. Primary paraganglioma of the lung. Ann Diagn Pathol. 2004;8:237–41.
117. Dahir KM, Gonzales A, Revelo MP, et al. Ectopic adrenocorticotropin hormone hypertension due to a primary pulmonary paraganglioma. Endocr Pract. 2004;10:424–8.

5 Biphasic Tumors of the Lungs

Introduction

Biphasic tumors are a group of tumors that are composed of two elements: malignant epithelial and mesenchymal components. These tumors only rarely arise in the lungs and overall represent less than 2 % of all primary lung neoplasms. In the bronchopulmonary system, the tumors belonging to this group include pulmonary blastoma, pleuropulmonary blastoma, and carcinosarcoma. Pulmonary blastomas and carcinosarcomas in particular have caused great contention in the literature with regard to their histogenesis, nomenclature, and classification; and to date no universally accepted concept exists as to whether these tumors represent independent clinicopathological entities or rather constitute subtypes of other neoplasms. However, based on their distinct morphological features and the results of the latest molecular investigations indicating tumor autonomy, these neoplasms warrant inclusion as independent entities. The pertinent characteristics of the three neoplasms are summarized in Table 5.1.

Pulmonary Blastoma

History, Histopathogenesis, and Definition

Pulmonary blastomas are biphasic tumors composed of mixed epithelial and mesenchymal elements in which both components have the appearance of embryonal structures. Pulmonary blastoma was first described by Barnard in 1952 [1] reporting on a peculiar lung tumor with the features of mixed carcinomatous and sarcomatous elements resembling the developing lung of an embryo. He termed this tumor "embryoma of the lung." Three more of these cases were studied by Spencer in 1961 [2] who coined the term "pulmonary blastoma" because of their morphologic similarity to nephroblastomas of the kidney. He proposed that both epithelium and stroma derived from primitive mesenchymal tissue similar to the development of nephroblastoma in the kidney. This view was disputed in subsequent reports that, based on morphological and ultrastructural investigations, suggested that the epithelial and mesenchymal elements were distinct enough to warrant classification as a form of carcinosarcoma [3–6]. More recent immunohistochemical and molecular investigations have demonstrated similar antigen expression and gene mutations in both elements of pulmonary blastoma and confirmed that this tumor very likely is derived from a totipotential stem cell and should therefore be regarded as a distinct clinicopathological entity [7–13].

A monophasic variant of pulmonary blastoma was described by Kradin in 1982 [14] who reported a lung tumor resembling pulmonary blastoma but without the sarcomatous element, the so-called pulmonary endodermal tumor resembling fetal lung. Similar tumors were subsequently referred to as "well differentiated adenocarcinoma simulating fetal lung tubules" and "adenocarcinoma of the fetal lung type" [15–17]. It soon emerged that this monophasic type of pulmonary blastoma, although histogenetically apparently linked to the biphasic type, is more prevalent in women and has a better prognosis compared to the biphasic tumor [10, 12, 14–17]. For this reason, monophasic pulmonary blastoma, or "fetal adenocarcinoma," is listed as a variant of adenocarcinoma by the current WHO classification of lung tumors, whereas only the biphasic type is classified as a true pulmonary blastoma [18]. We regard both the monophasic and biphasic variants as pulmonary blastomas based on their distinct morphology resembling the developing lung.

A. Weissferdt, C.A. Moran, *Diagnostic Pathology of Pleuropulmonary Neoplasia*,
DOI 10.1007/978-1-4419-0787-5_5, © Springer Science+Business Media New York 2013

Table 5.1 Clinical and histological characteristics of biphasic lung tumors

	Monophasic pulmonary blastoma	Biphasic pulmonary blastoma	Pleuropulmonary blastoma	Carcinosarcoma
Median age at diagnosis	37 years	35 years	3 years	seventh decade
Sex	F	F	M=F	M
Smoking history	Yes	Yes	No	Yes
Malignant glandular component	Yes	Yes	No	Variable
Sarcomatous component	No	Yes	Yes	Yes
Morules	Yes	Yes	No	No
Cystic component	No	No	Yes	No
Associated diseases	No	No	Cystic nephroma, thyroid neoplasms, germ cell tumors, other sarcomas	Migratory polyarthritis, polyneuropathy, hypertrophic pulmonary osteoarthropathy
Prognosis	Better	Poor	Poor	Poor

M male, *F* female

Clinical Features

Pulmonary blastomas comprise only 0.25–0.5 % of all primary lung malignancies [19, 20], and to date only approximately 200 cases have been described in the literature [21]. Although initially thought to be equally common among men and women, a slight female preponderance has recently emerged [21, 22]. Pulmonary blastomas are largely tumors of adulthood with a mean age of 35 years [19], but rare cases have also been described in neonates and children or the elderly [23, 24]. Patients present with cough, chest pain, fever, or hemoptysis, but up to 40 % of cases remain entirely asymptomatic [19, 25]. Up to 80 % of cases have been shown to be related to smoking [19].

A recent Japanese series of 25 cases of the monophasic variant revealed similar clinical findings to those of the biphasic tumor with a male-to-female ratio of 2:3 and a mean age of 37 years at diagnosis [26]. Similar to biphasic pulmonary blastoma, the monophasic variant has sporadically been reported in children [27]. All pulmonary blastomas usually present as solitary parenchymal masses on computed tomography (CT) or rarely as multiple nodules [21, 28]. The radiological features are rather nonspecific and often mimic an abscess, bronchogenic cyst, or a benign neoplasm [21, 28]. If endobronchially located, carcinoid tumors often enter the differential diagnosis [21, 28].

Gross Features

Pulmonary blastomas are well-demarcated, unencapsulated tumors that are usually found in the peripheral portion of the lungs, although up to one-fourth can be found in an endobronchial location [19, 25]. The tumors are typically solitary but may on occasion show smaller satellite lesions [19]. A particular predilection for a specific lobe has not emerged [25]. Blastomas are large tumors ranging in size from 1 to 28 cm with a mean diameter of 6 cm; the monophasic variant is often slightly smaller [19]. The tumors may show variation in color ranging from white to tan or brown and have a bulging cut surface with a fish-flesh appearance [19]. As many as 50 % of blastomas can show central necrosis, and cystic breakdown is also commonly observed [19, 25].

Histological Features

Monophasic Pulmonary Blastoma

Monophasic pulmonary blastomas comprise roughly half of all pulmonary blastomas [29]. In contrast to biphasic pulmonary blastomas, the monophasic variant is composed entirely of an epithelial component [30]. Characteristically, this epithelium forms complex branching tubules lined by non-ciliated columnar cells (Figs. 5.1, 5.2, 5.3, and 5.4). These cells have clear to eosinophilic cytoplasm, uniform round to oval nuclei, and characteristic subnuclear or supranuclear cytoplasmic vacuoles reminiscent of those typically seen in endometrial glands (Figs. 5.5 and 5.6). The glands can have various growth patterns with solid or cribriform areas, cords, ribbons, or rosette-like structures (Figs. 5.7, 5.8, and 5.9). Overall, the appearance of the epithelial component in pulmonary blastomas has a striking resemblance to the developing lung during weeks 11–18 [19, 25]. In addition to the glands, the tumor cells can form peculiar round squamoid structures, so-called morules, which are composed of solid nests of cells with eosinophilic cytoplasm and optically clear nuclei [19, 25] (Figs. 5.10, 5.11, 5.12, and 5.13). Interestingly, neuroendocrine differentiation is often identified in these structures [19, 25]. Morules can be found in as many as 86–100 % of monophasic pulmonary blastomas and are a

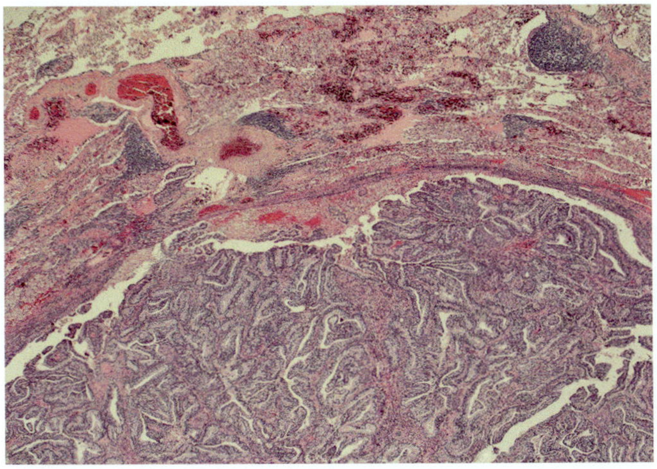

Fig. 5.1 Low-power view of monophasic pulmonary blastoma and surrounding lung parenchyma

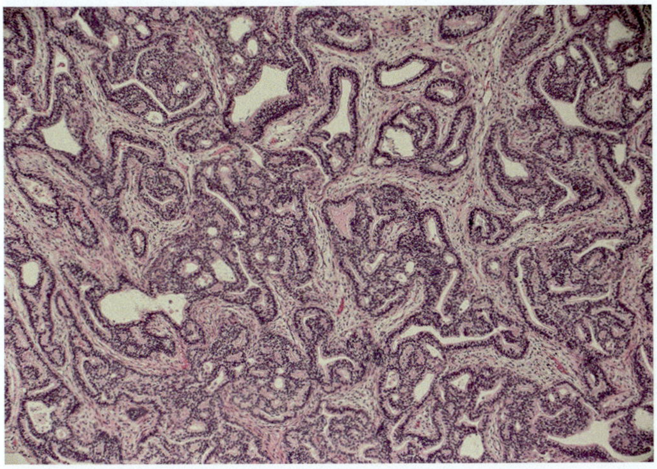

Fig. 5.2 Monophasic pulmonary blastoma demonstrating a glandular pattern of growth

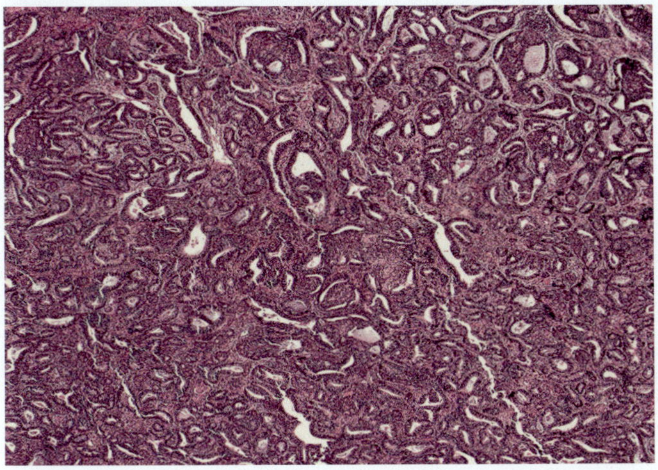

Fig. 5.3 Glands of different shape and size in monophasic pulmonary blastoma

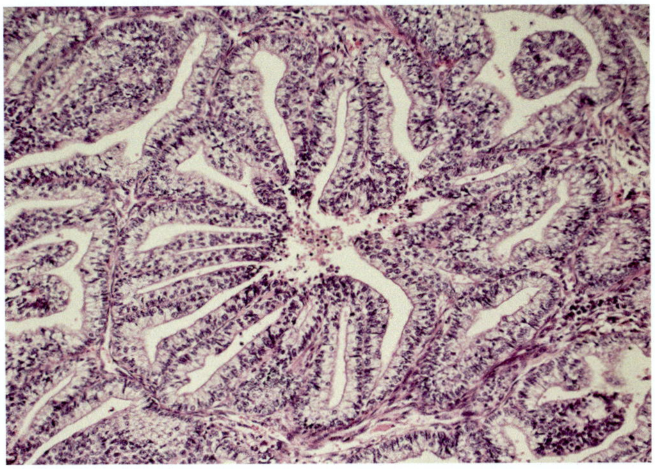

Fig. 5.4 Epithelium in monophasic pulmonary blastoma forming complex branching tubules

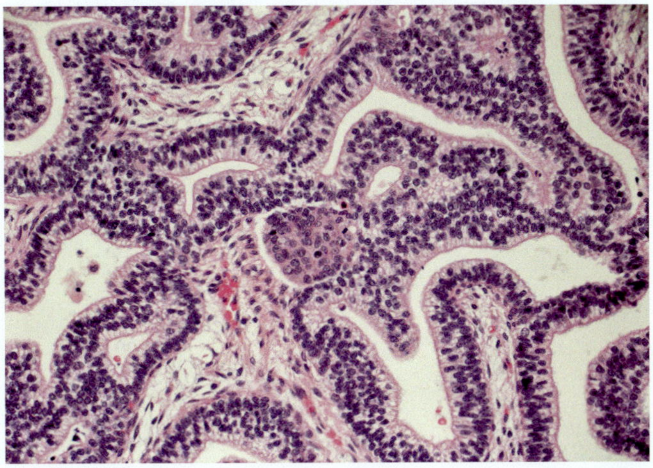

Fig. 5.5 High-power view of monophasic pulmonary blastoma with uniform round nuclei

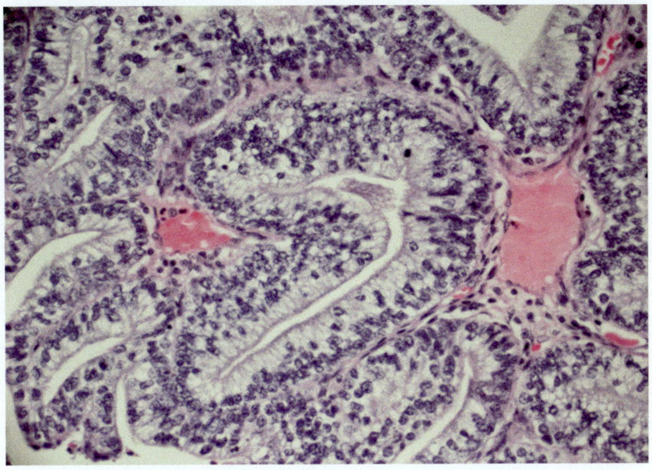

Fig. 5.6 Monophasic pulmonary blastoma with characteristic supranuclear clearing

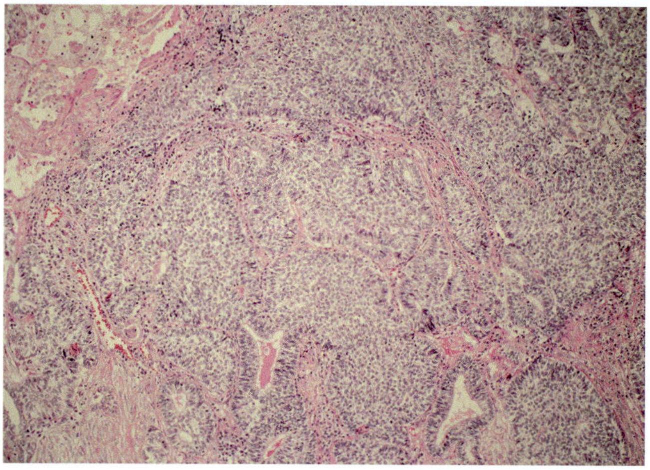

Fig. 5.7 More solid growth pattern in monophasic pulmonary blastoma

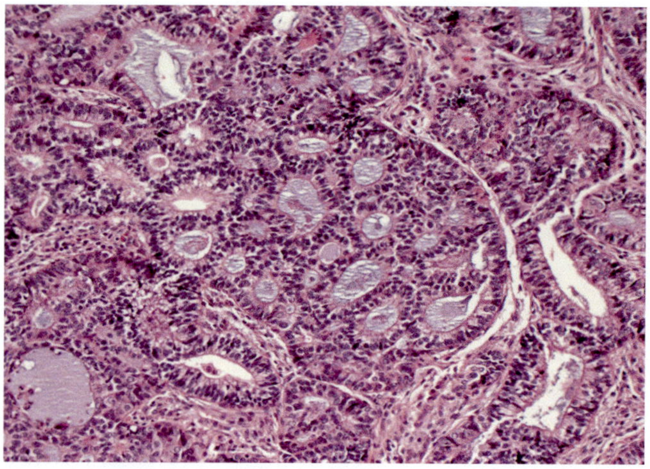

Fig. 5.8 Monophasic pulmonary blastoma with rosette-like architecture

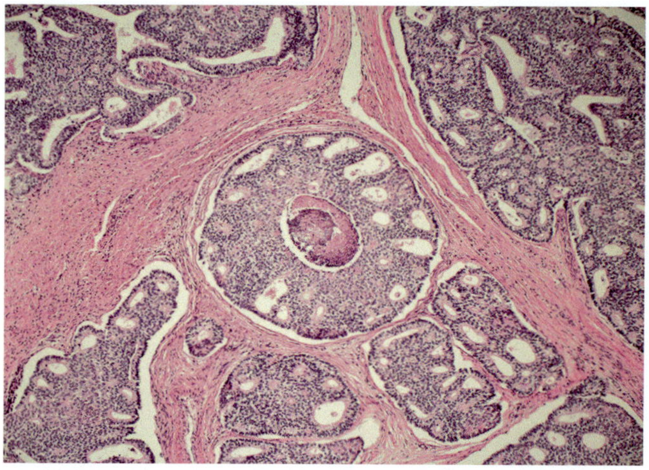

Fig. 5.9 Cribriform growth pattern in monophasic pulmonary blastoma

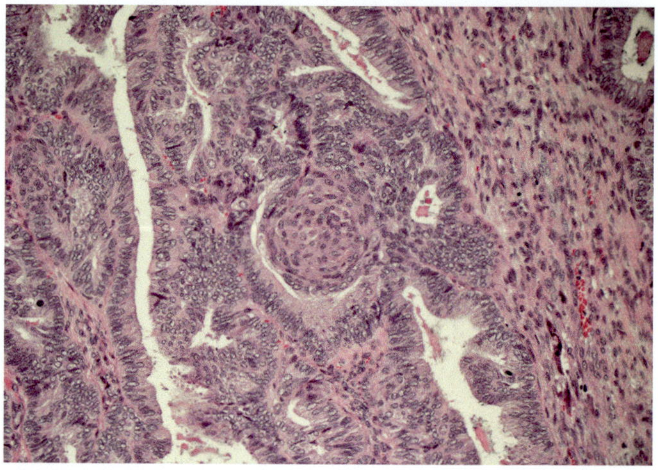

Fig. 5.10 Characteristic morule in monophasic pulmonary blastoma

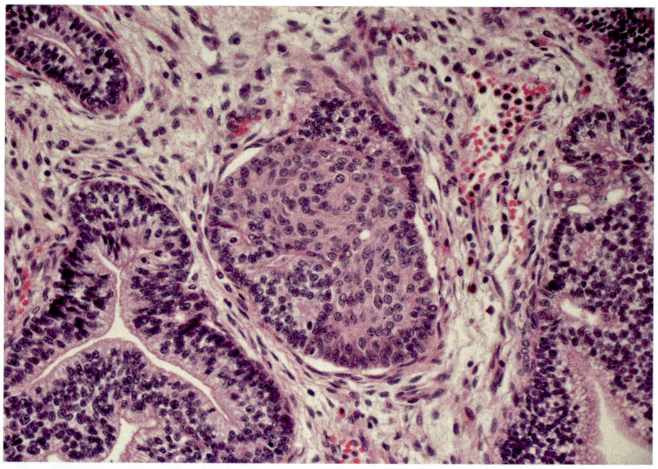

Fig. 5.11 High-power view of morule in monophasic pulmonary blastoma displaying a squamoid appearance

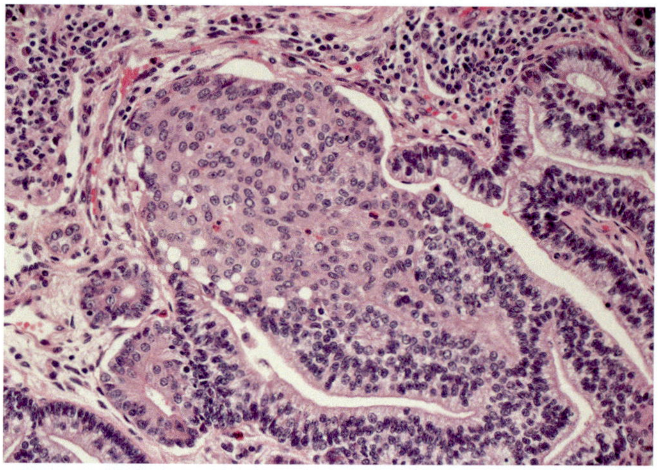

Fig. 5.12 Large morule in monophasic pulmonary blastoma filling the glandular lumen

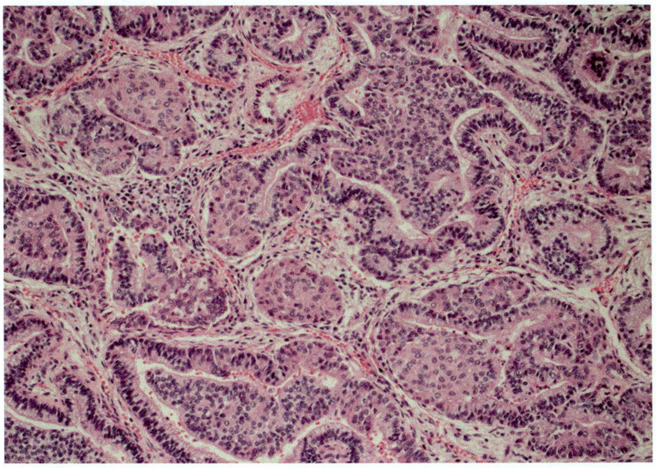

Fig. 5.13 Multiple morules in monophasic pulmonary blastoma

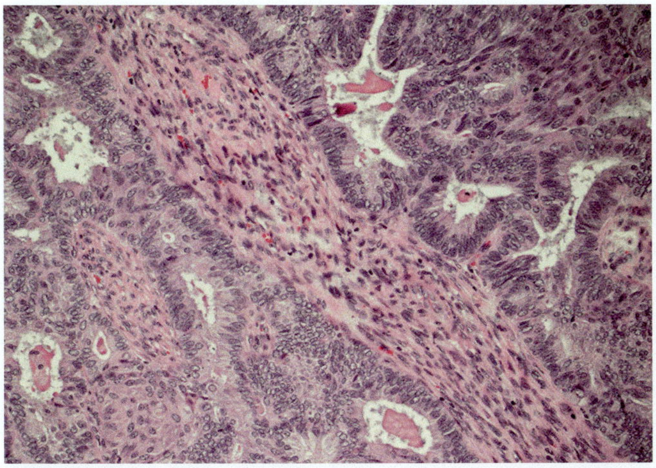

Fig. 5.14 Benign fibrous stroma separating the glands in monophasic pulmonary blastoma

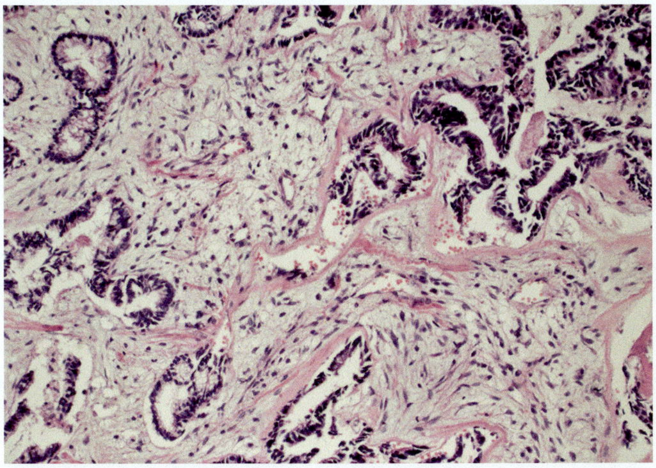

Fig. 5.15 Loose fibromyxoid stroma in monophasic pulmonary blastoma

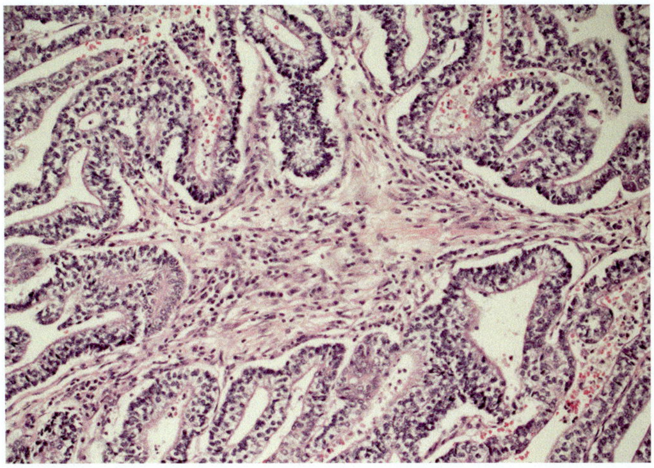

Fig. 5.16 Stroma in monophasic pulmonary blastoma showing no significant atypia or mitotic activity

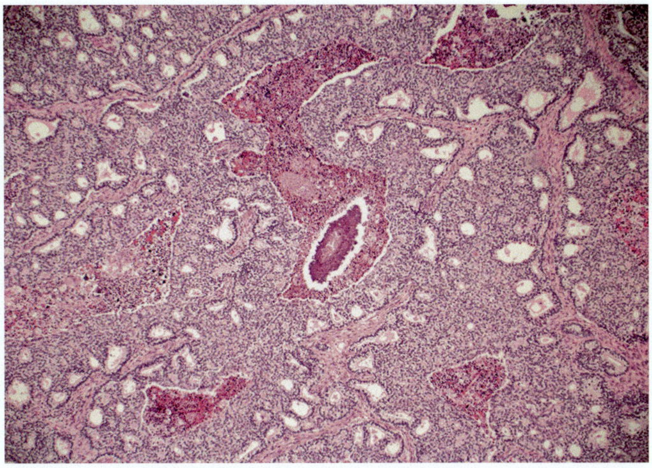

Fig. 5.17 Comedo-type necrosis in monophasic pulmonary blastoma

characteristic finding in these tumors. A scant and benign stroma separates the closely packed glands in monophasic blastoma, which is composed of bland myofibroblastic cells (Figs. 5.14 and 5.15). Low mitotic activity and focal necrosis may be present, but high mitotic activity and extensive necrosis are uncommon findings (Figs. 5.16 and 5.17). Importantly, mucin may be identified in the lumina of the glandular structures but should not be present in the cytoplasm of the epithelial cells.

Biphasic Pulmonary Blastoma

In addition to the glandular component as described previously, biphasic pulmonary blastoma is characterized by a malignant stroma with an embryonic or blastematous appearance (Figs. 5.18, 5.19, 5.20, 5.21, and 5.22). This stroma can show striking condensation around the glandular component and exhibit prominent nuclear pleomorphism

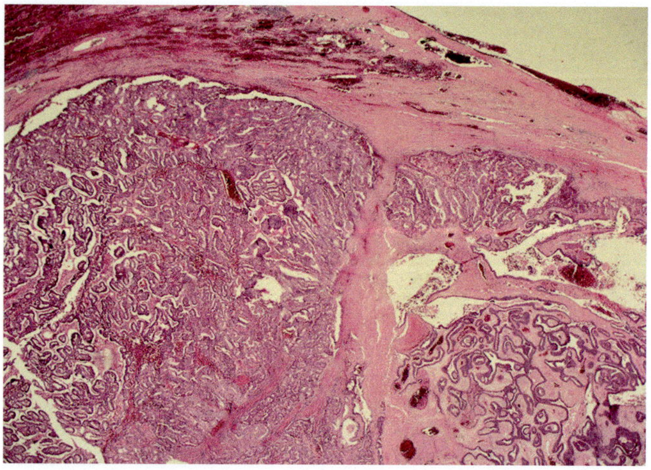

Fig. 5.18 Low-power view of biphasic pulmonary blastoma showing a well-demarcated lesion in the lung parenchyma

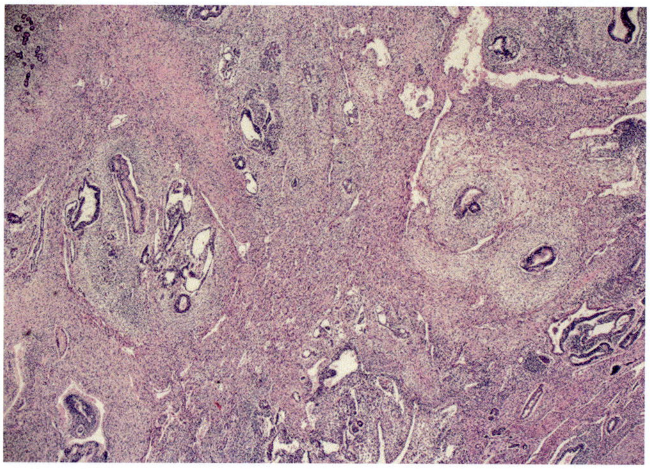

Fig. 5.19 Low-power view of biphasic pulmonary blastoma showing a mix of epithelial and mesenchymal elements

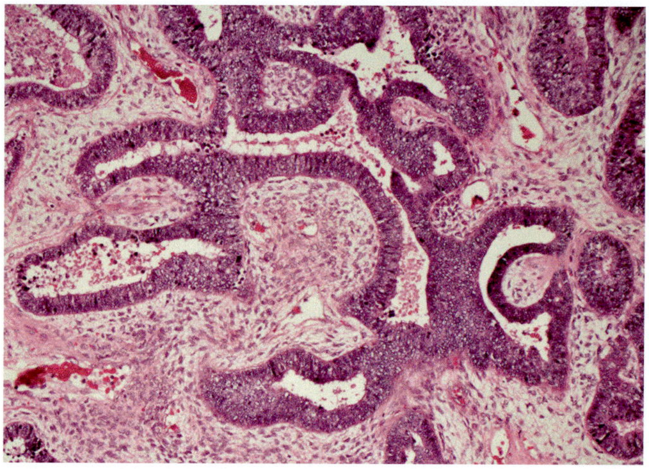

Fig. 5.20 Biphasic pulmonary blastoma containing an immature mesenchymal component in addition to the glandular structures

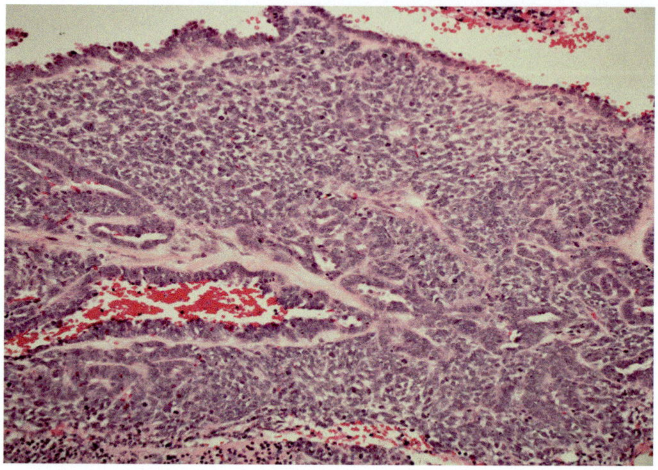

Fig. 5.21 Blastemal stroma in biphasic pulmonary blastoma

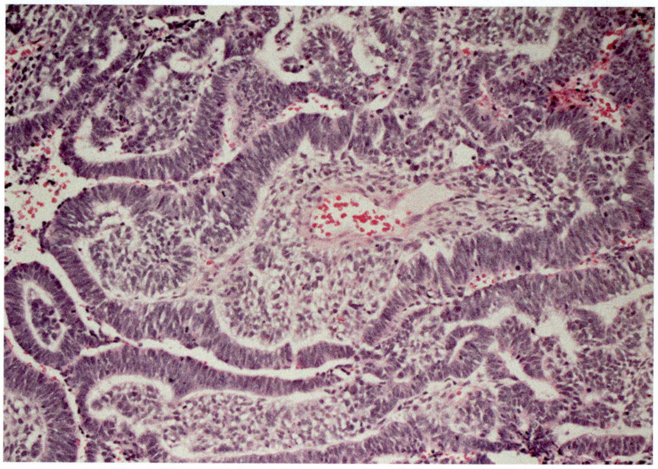

Fig. 5.22 Biphasic pulmonary blastoma with loose high-grade mesenchymal component

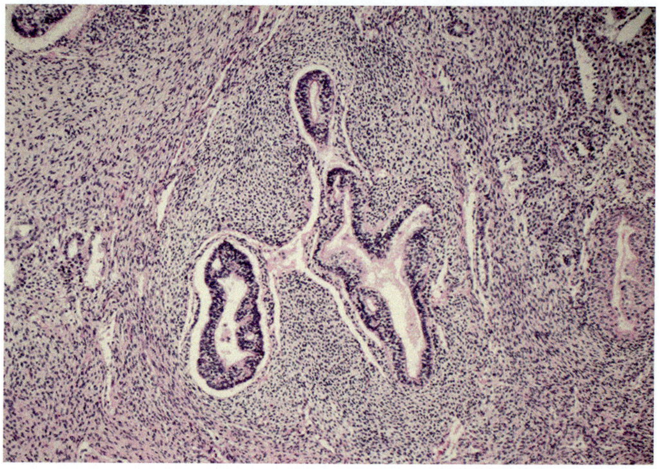

Fig. 5.23 Prominent condensation of stroma around glandular component in biphasic pulmonary blastoma

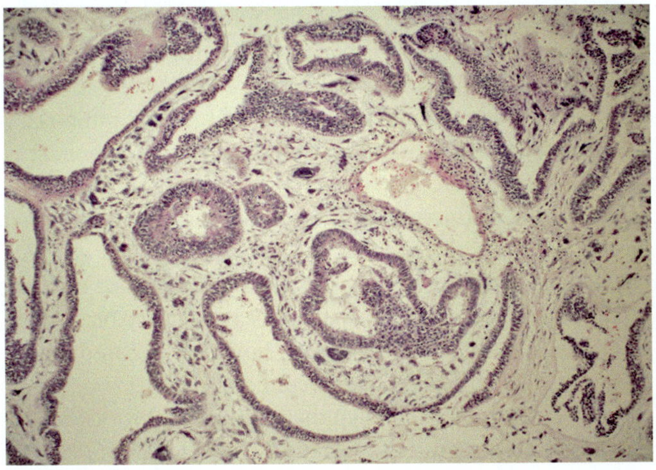

Fig. 5.24 Striking nuclear pleomorphism in the stroma of biphasic pulmonary blastoma

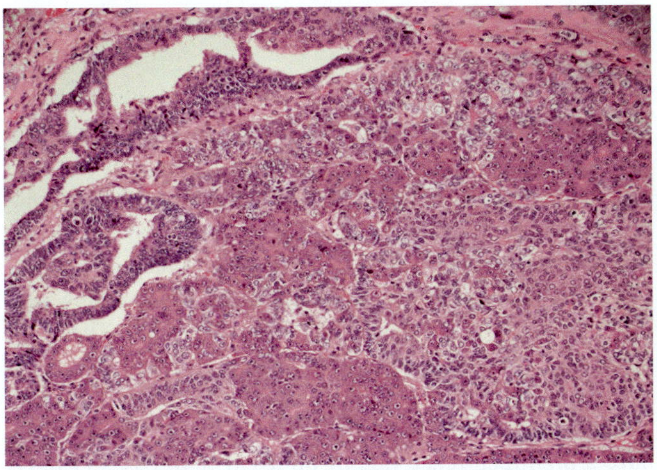

Fig. 5.25 An unusual association of pulmonary blastoma with hepatocelullar differentiation

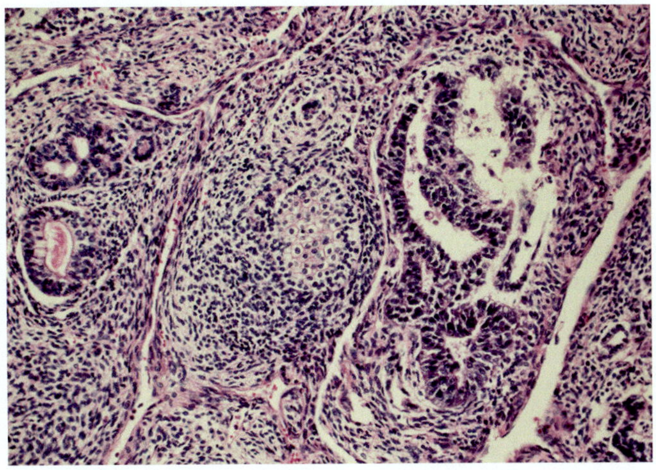

Fig. 5.26 Biphasic pulmonary blastoma with chondroid differentiation

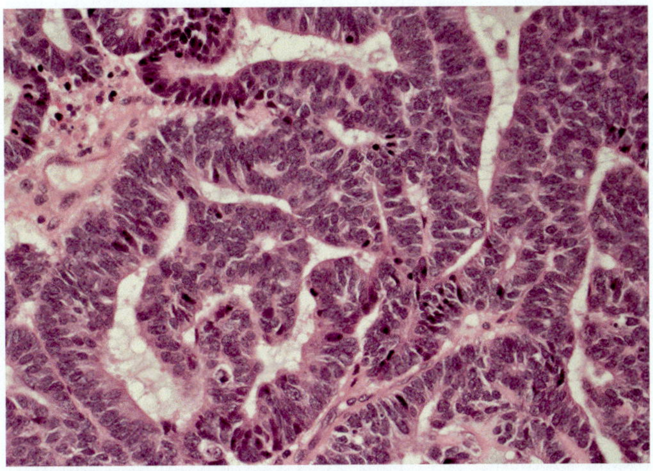

Fig. 5.27 Nuclear crowding and high mitotic activity in glandular component of biphasic pulmonary blastoma

(Figs. 5.23 and 5.24). Importantly, it can contain immature striated muscle, cartilage, osseous differentiation, smooth muscle, yolk sac-like areas, or melanocytic differentiation [19, 25, 31–34] (Figs. 5.25 and 5.26). Interestingly, morules are less frequently seen (24 % of cases) than in monophasic blastomas [19, 25]. Although nuclear pleomorphism is not a striking feature of the glands in biphasic blastoma, the mitotic activity can be as high as 24 mitoses/10 high-power fields (hpf) [25] (Fig. 5.27).

Electron Microscopy

Ultrastructural investigations of pulmonary blastomas have revealed that the epithelial cells have distinct basal lamina, apical junctional complexes, and microvilli on the apical surface. Glycogen granules and electron-dense granules may be found, but cilia or basal bodies are usually absent. The stroma shows the typical features of myofibroblastic cells: a well-developed rough endoplasmic reticulum, peripheral cytoplasmic filaments forming dense bodies, pinocytotic vesicles, and an investing basal lamina. Basement membrane-like material and occasional cell junctions may sometimes also be found. Of interest, the morules contain lamellar inclusions reminiscent of developing alveolar buds, and the characteristically optically clear nuclei have been shown to consist of intranuclear aggregates of fine filaments and fibrils [19, 25].

Immunohistochemical and Molecular Features

Pulmonary blastomas can show very heterogenous immunohistochemical staining patterns depending on the components present in the tumors. The epithelial elements display positive staining for pancytokeratin (CK), carcinoembryonic antigen (CEA), epithelial membrane antigen (EMA), thyroid transcription factor-1 (TTF-1), cytokeratin 7 (CK7), cytokeratin 5/6 (CK5/6), and surfactant protein alpha [11, 19, 25, 35, 36]. The stromal component generally shows reactivity for vimentin and depending on more differentiated elements may show positive staining for desmin, muscle-specific actin, myoglobin, or S100 protein [11, 19, 25, 35, 36]. Neuroendocrine markers like chromogranin and synaptophysin have been shown to stain the morules of pulmonary blastomas in addition to surfactant protein alpha, biotin, and CD10 [19, 25, 37].

Several investigators have tried to determine the molecular characteristics of pulmonary blastomas. Two of these studies found p53 gene mutations and p53 overexpression in the epithelial and mesenchymal components in a subset of biphasic pulmonary blastomas but no such findings in the monophasic variant [8, 9]. They concluded that both elements of biphasic pulmonary blastomas likely derived from a single totipotential stem cell. Further studies showed that β(beta)-catenin mutations were present in monophasic and biphasic pulmonary blastomas, suggesting a histogenetic linkage of the tumors [10, 12]. Single nucleotide polymorphism array and mutational analysis for p53, β(beta)-catenin, epidermal growth factor receptor (EGFR), and K-ras on a single biphasic tumor and its metastatic brain deposit showed common genetic alterations in the form of allelic imbalance on chromosomes 17p11-p13 and 14q24-q32 as well as β(beta)-catenin mutations in both elements of the primary tumor and the metastasis implying a monoclonal origin of the neoplasm [13]. The same study also described chromosomal differences between the epithelial and mesenchymal components (6p24-p25 and 6q14-q27 alterations for the epithelial element; 3p11-p14, 9p21-p24 alterations; and p53 gene mutation in the mesenchymal element) and concluded that the biphasic nature of the tumor was due to differences in accumulated genetic alterations of the epithelial and mesenchymal tumor components.

Differential Diagnosis

Monophasic pulmonary blastomas may mimic conventional gland-forming adenocarcinoma and especially primary secretory endometrial-like or metastatic endometrioid adenocarcinoma. Blastomas may be distinguished from conventional adenocarcinoma by the presence of morules and the typical embryonic appearance of the epithelium characterized by prominent subnuclear or supranuclear cytoplasmic vacuoles. In addition, blastomas lack the intracellular mucin often found in conventional adenocarcinoma, and histochemical mucin stains may prove useful to differentiate the two tumors. Secretory endometrial-like and endometrioid adenocarcinoma can be more difficult to distinguish due to a similar morphology of the glandular component and the occasional presence of squamous morules closely resembling the morules seen in blastoma. In this case, thorough clinical and radiological correlation is required, especially if the patient is a female. In those cases of biphasic pulmonary blastomas, where an additional mesenchymal component is present, carcinosarcoma enters the differential diagnosis. However, the distinctive embryonal morphology of blastoma has not been described in carcinosarcomas, nor have morules been identified in these tumors. Lastly, malignant salivary gland-like tumors can be mistaken for pulmonary blastomas. The biphasic nature of the former, however, is based on the presence of epithelial and myoepithelial elements and will display a prominent myoepithelial immunohistochemical phenotype characterized by reactivity for cytokeratin, vimentin, and actin. Such a staining pattern has not been described in pulmonary blastomas [25].

Treatment and Prognosis

Although most studies agree that complete surgical excision is the treatment of choice for pulmonary blastomas, the role of adjuvant radiation therapy and chemotherapy is not well established. Nevertheless, chemotherapy using a combination of platinum- and non-platinum-based cytotoxic agents is used in the adjuvant setting, and radiation therapy with or without chemotherapy may be used for downstaging purposes or in cases of unresectable disease [19, 38]. The prognosis of pulmonary blastomas largely depends on the histological subtype. Biphasic blastomas are generally highly aggressive tumors with an ominous outcome. These tumors have a high recurrence rate of up to 50 % of cases [19, 39] and may metastasize to the brain, mediastinum, pleura, liver, diaphragm, heart, or soft tissues [25, 39, 40]. In about half of the cases, the metastatic deposits have a monotypic appearance, whereas the other half shows a biphasic pattern [41]. Biphasic pulmonary blastomas have been shown to have a poor survival rate with two-thirds of patients dying within 2 years and 5- and 10-year survival rates of 16 and 8 %, respectively [19]. Another more recent series reported a better overall outcome with an average survival of 49.7 months and 2- and 5-year survival rates of 85.7 and 71.4 %, respectively [21]. This study, however, incorporated both biphasic and monophasic blastomas in their survival data, and all of their tumors presented at an early stage. The authors deducted that early tumor stage improves survival, supporting the results of earlier studies [30]. Other factors influencing survival were found to be small tumor size (<5 cm) and an absence of tumor recurrence and metastasis [30].

The prognosis for monophasic pulmonary blastomas is strikingly better, and some authors believe these tumors should be regarded as a low-grade malignancy [16]. Although monophasic blastomas can have a recurrence rate as high as

30 %, most of the recurrences happen in the lung rather than in distant sites, and the tumor-associated mortality is only 10–14 % (median follow-up 95 months). Negative predictive factors of survival for the monophasic variant include the presence of thoracic lymphadenopathy, metastatic disease at presentation, tumor recurrence, and tumor stage; however, contrary to the biphasic variant, tumor size does not appear to influence the clinical course [30]. It has been suggested that this improved survival compared to biphasic blastoma is due to lower biological aggressiveness and a higher tendency of monophasic blastomas to recur within the lungs thereby facilitating surgical resection [19].

Pleuropulmonary Blastoma

History, Histopathogenesis, and Definition

Pleuropulmonary blastoma is a rare neoplasm that is virtually restricted to the pediatric age group. Despite its similarity in nomenclature with the pulmonary blastoma of adulthood, pleuropulmonary blastoma is a different clinicopathological entity that needs to be differentiated from pulmonary blastoma and other biphasic tumors more commonly seen in the older age group. Before 1988, these tumors were published in the literature under various terms including "pulmonary blastoma," "pulmonary sarcoma arising in mesenchymal cystic hamartoma," "embryonal sarcoma," and "pulmonary rhabdomyosarcoma arising in congenital adenomatoid malformation or in bronchogenic cyst" [42–50]. The term "pleuropulmonary blastoma" was first used by Manivel and coworkers [51] describing 11 unique pediatric tumors involving the lungs, pleura, or mediastinum. These tumors were composed of an embryonal-like blastemal element, an uncommitted stroma with focal rhabdomyosarcomatous, chondrosarcomatous, or liposarcomatous differentiation and variable cyst formation. Although histologic similarities to the adult-type pulmonary blastoma exist, the defining feature of pleuropulmonary blastoma is a striking absence of any malignant epithelial component thereby separating pleuropulmonary blastoma from the other biphasic lung neoplasms. The authors believed that pleuropulmonary blastoma may represent the expression of the thoracic splanchnopleural or somatopleural mesoderm, which would explain the absence of a malignant epithelial component, the pluripotentiality for the various lines of mesenchymal differentiation, and the varied anatomic sites of origin in the thoracic cavity [51]. More recently, pleuropulmonary blastoma have been subdivided into three different types depending on the degree of cystic change. In addition, it could be shown that this subdivision also correlates with age at presentation and prognosis [52]. To date, however, the initial description by Manivel et al. [51] defines the entity of pleuropulmonary blastoma.

Clinical Features

Pleuropulmonary blastomas are tumors of childhood with an average age at presentation of 3 years [51, 53]. Children older than 12 years are only uncommonly affected, and rare case reports even describe the occurrence of pleuropulmonary blastoma in adults [51, 54–56]. In a more recent study, it has emerged that the median age at presentation is different for the three tumor subtypes: 10 months for type 1, 36 months for type 2, and 44 months for type 3 [57]. A distinct sex predilection has not been observed [51, 58, 59]. Patients are symptomatic with cough, fever, chest pain, respiratory distress, lethargy, weight loss, abdominal pain, or anorexia [51, 53, 54]. Pleuropulmonary blastomas commonly arise in the periphery of the lungs and less often in the pleura or mediastinum [51–53]. Although mostly an isolated lesion, pleuropulmonary blastoma rarely presents as multiple tumors [60]. Interesting findings are a striking predilection for the right hemithorax [51, 61] and a supposed limitation of type 1 pleuropulmonary blastoma to the lung parenchyma [62]. Radiologically, pleuropulmonary blastomas present as air-filled cysts or homogenous masses with partial or complete obliteration of the hemithorax and/or pleural- and mediastinal-based masses [51, 52]. Based on these findings, cystic lung disease is often suspected clinically, and the correct diagnosis is often only rendered after surgical resection [59]. A very typical imaging finding of pleuropulmonary blastoma is its peripheral location and a striking absence of any chest wall invasion [61, 63]. Pleuropulmonary blastoma is often seen in association with cystic lung diseases like bronchogenic cysts or cystic adenomatoid pulmonary malformation (CPAM) [51, 53, 58]. More importantly, pleuropulmonary blastoma is a strong marker of predisposition to develop other childhood neoplasms either affecting the same patient or a close family member [51, 64–66]. These childhood neoplasms include cystic nephroma, thyroid carcinoma, germ cell tumors, or other sarcomas [51, 64, 66]. Close surveillance of the patients and their family members are thus indicated when a diagnosis of pleuropulmonary blastoma is rendered.

Gross Features

Pleuropulmonary blastomas are large tumors that may reach up to 28 cm in size [51]. They are often multilobulated masses with a glistening surface involving mainly the lower lobes of the lungs. Frequently, the pleura is involved at presentation, and widespread tumor is encountered at resection [58]. Depending on the histological subtype, the macroscopic features range from thin-walled cystic structures (type 1) to solid firm and rubbery masses (type 3). Type 2 pleuropulmonary blastoma shows a mixture of cystic and solid areas with nodular and plaque-like thickenings or solid polypoid structures projecting into the cystic spaces [51, 58]. Areas of necrosis, hemorrhage, gelatinous, or mucoid change may be seen in all types. Rarely, intrabronchial extension can be identified [67].

Histological Features

Pleuropulmonary blastoma has been subdivided into three different types based on the degree of cystic differentiation [52, 58]. Type 1 pleuropulmonary blastoma is a multicystic lesion separated by thin fibrovascular septa lined by benign ciliated respiratory-type epithelium (Figs. 5.28 and 5.29). The stroma is composed of small round to spindle-shaped cells that may condense to form a continuous layer beneath the benign epithelium resembling the cambium layer in embryonal rhabdomyosarcoma (sarcoma botryoides) (Fig. 5.30). These stromal cells are often accompanied by cells displaying rhabdomyoblastic differentiation (Figs. 5.31 and 5.32). In addition to the cystic component, pleuropulmonary blastoma type 2 contains a solid component, whereas type 3 pleuropulmonary blastoma is entirely solid (Figs. 5.33, 5.34, and 5.35). This solid component usually shows mixed blastematous and sarcomatous features: The blastomatous element is composed of small primitive cells with little cytoplasm and increased mitotic activity; the sarcomatous component displays spindle cells in a fascicular arrangement. These components merge with a loose stroma of short fusiform cells set in a pale background. Rhabdomyoblasts, cartilaginous differentiation, anaplastic cells, and tumor giant cells are often identified in type 2 and 3 pleuropulmonary blastomas. Foci of necrosis and pseudocyst formation are also often identified in the higher-grade tumors. Recurrent or metastatic tumor shows similar histologic features to those seen in the primary lesion; however, an increased tendency of rhabdomyoblastic or

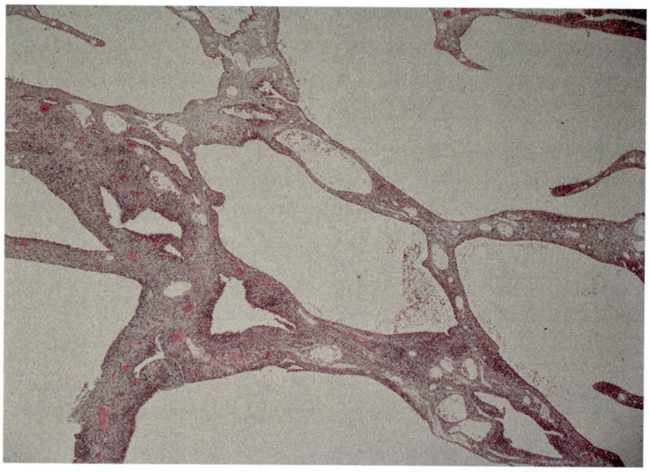

Fig. 5.28 Low-power view of type 1 pulmonary pleuropulmonary blastoma

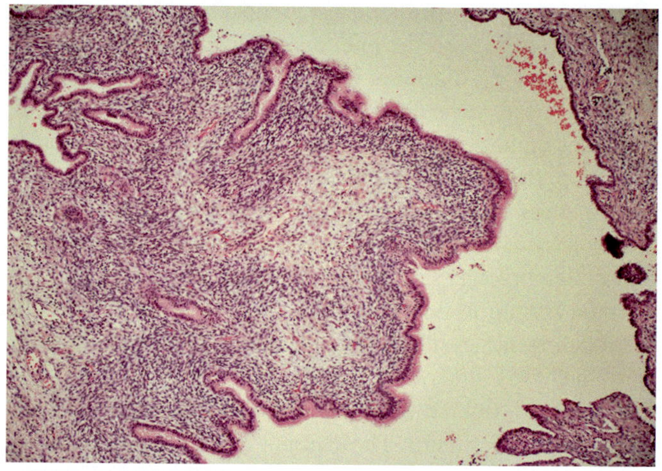

Fig. 5.30 Stromal condensation underneath the epithelium of pleuropulmonary blastoma

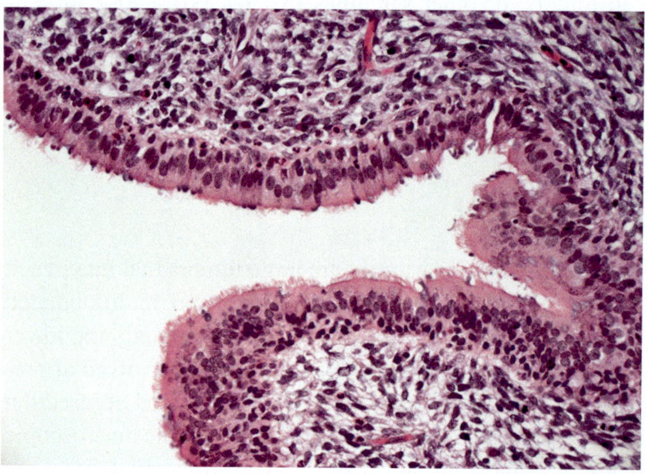

Fig. 5.29 Benign ciliated epithelium lining the septa in pleuropulmonary blastoma

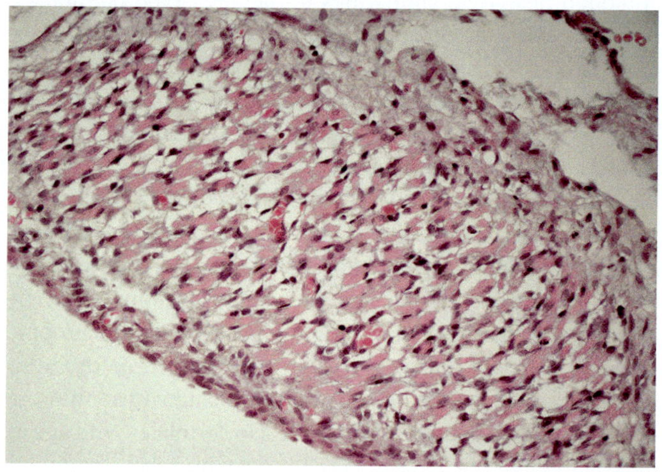

Fig. 5.31 Stromal cells in pleuropulmonary blastoma showing rhabdomyoblastic differentiation

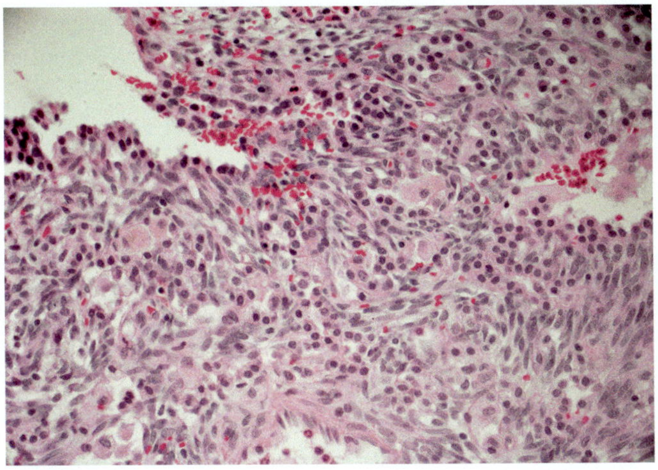

Fig. 5.32 Type 3 pleuropulmonary blastoma with focal rhabdoid differentiation

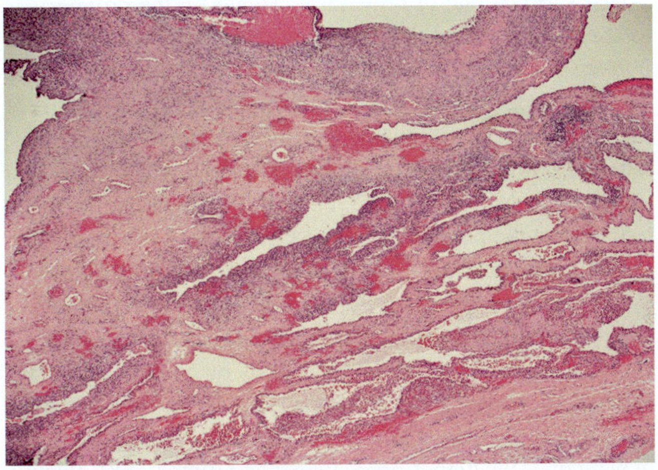

Fig. 5.33 Type 2 pleuropulmonary blastoma showing equal proportions of solid and cystic areas

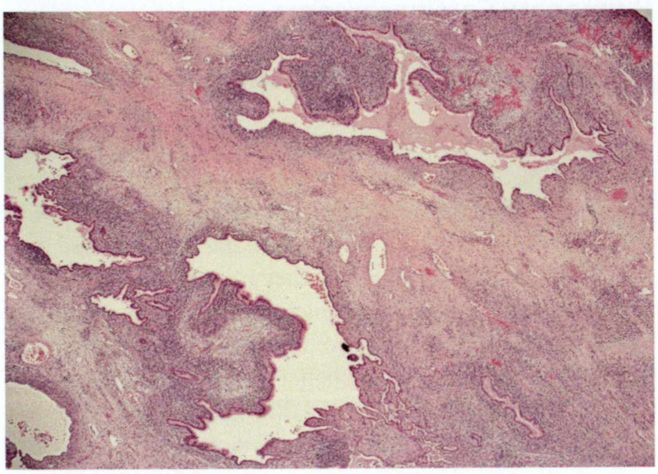

Fig. 5.34 Cystic spaces in type 2 pleuropulmonary blastoma

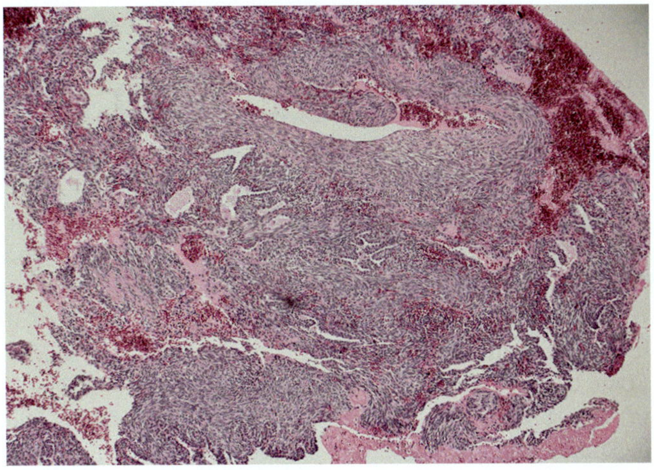

Fig. 5.35 Type 3 pleuropulmonary blastoma with predominantly solid growth pattern

spindle cell overgrowth can sometimes be seen in these deposits [52, 58].

Electron Microscopy

Electron microscopy of the blastemal elements shows undifferentiated cells with a high nuclear-cytoplasmic ratio, rounded nuclei with smooth contours, and a sparse cytoplasm with few organelles like mitochondria, ribosomes, and disorganized cristae. Occasional electron-dense intramatrical material may be found along with scattered glycogen rosettes and sparse cytoplasmic microfilaments. Intercellular junctions are only primitively developed [51, 54]. The spindle-shaped stromal cells show the features of elongated fibroblast-like cells with a well-developed rough endoplasmic reticulum and cytoplasmic lipid vacuoles. Thin cytoplasmic processes may be identified together with long intercellular junctions and sublemmal aggregates of microfilaments. Basement membranes are generally not seen [51, 54]. The rhabdomyoblasts possess thin and thick filaments in sarcomeric organization and abortive Z-band formation [51, 54]. Chondroid cells, if present, are set in a loosely granular matrix and have scalloped cell membranes and dilated rough endoplasmic reticulum with finely granular material. These cells contain abundant intermediate filaments and may also contain scattered glycogen particles and mitochondria [51, 54].

Immunohistochemical and Molecular Features

Although the diagnosis of pleuropulmonary blastoma remains largely a histological one, immunohistochemical studies may aid in the correct identification of the sarcomatous component. The most common sarcomatous element, rhabdomyosarcoma, may be confirmed with markers like desmin, myoglobin, muscle-specific actin, myogenin, and myoD1, while cartilaginous differentiation will show reactivity for S100 protein [51, 54, 58, 68, 69]. Vimentin and histiocytic markers, such as α(alpha)-1-antitrypsin, α(alpha)-1-antichymotrypsin, and CD68, have been reported to be positive in the blastematous component [51, 54, 68]. The benign epithelium is generally immunoreactive for CK and EMA [51, 54, 68].

A recurrent finding of molecular studies is the presence of trisomies 2 and 8 in pleuropulmonary blastoma [69–73]. Some of these authors noted that similar genetic abnormalities can also be seen in embryonal rhabdomyosarcoma and hepatoblastoma, suggesting a common genetic pathway in the origin of these tumors. In addition to this, Kusafuka et al. [74] described p53 mutations in two out of three pleuropulmonary blastomas, further supporting a genetic link with rhabdomyosarcoma that may show similar findings. More recently, DICER1 mutations were found in familial cases of pleuropulmonary blastoma [75]. Loss of DICER1 is thought to induce changes resembling the early stages of pleuropulmonary blastoma in the lungs of mice, and the authors speculated that the development of pleuropulmonary blastoma in humans may arise through a similar mechanism.

Differential Diagnosis

The most important differential diagnosis of pleuropulmonary blastoma includes pulmonary blastoma, rhabdomyosarcoma, and congenital cystic adenomatoid malformation (C-CAM). Pulmonary blastoma usually affects adults, arises in the lung parenchyma, and has a mostly solid growth pattern. Histologically, it is composed of malignant blastemal, stromal, and epithelial elements. Pleuropulmonary blastoma is a pediatric tumor that may arise anywhere in the thoracic cavity and typically lacks a malignant epithelial component facilitating separation from pulmonary blastoma [51]. Primary rhabdomyosarcomas of the lung are extremely rare neoplasms that show monodirectional differentiation toward skeletal muscle cells and lack the blastematous component of pleuropulmonary blastoma [51, 54]. C-CAM may be difficult to distinguish from pleuropulmonary blastoma type 1; C-CAM encompasses a spectrum of cystic lung diseases and has been subdivided into five subtypes. Especially, type 1 ("large cyst C-CAM") and type 4 ("peripheral type C-CAM") can easily be mistaken for pleuropulmonary blastoma. Due to overlapping morphological features, pleuropulmonary blastoma is best distinguished from benign cystic lung disease based on its characteristic multiloculated cystic architecture, well-developed border to the normal lung parenchyma, and, most importantly, the presence of collections of small primitive cells in the septa [76]. Careful search of the cyst walls for evidence of stromal hypercellularity is indicated in all cases of cystic lung disease in order not to miss a malignant process [77].

Treatment and Prognosis

The treatment of pleuropulmonary blastoma generally consists of complete surgical resection followed by adjuvant chemotherapy [51, 53, 58]. Although no specific cytotoxic regimens exist for these tumors, frontline chemotherapy agents include vincristine, doxorubicin, cisplatin, dactinomycin, cyclophosphamide, etoposide, or ifosfamide [53, 78]. Neoadjuvant chemotherapy followed by resection and adjuvant chemoradiation may produce long-term survival in locally advanced cases [79]. In a clinicopathological study of 50 cases of pleuropulmonary blastoma, Priest et al. [58] reported a generally aggressive behavior with an overall 5-year survival rate of only 45 %. However, the prognosis is to some degree dependent on tumor subtype with an overall 2-year survival of 80 % for type 1 lesions, 73 % for type 2, and 48 % for type 3 tumors [58]. Factors that influence treatment failure and prognosis include unresectable tumor at diagnosis, tumor recurrence, mediastinal or pleural involvement, and type 2 or 3 histology [52, 53, 58, 80]. Pleuropulmonary blastomas have the potential to metastasize and do so most often to the central nervous system, bone, liver, and soft tissues; in fact, cerebral metastasis is more common in pleuropulmonary blastoma than in any other childhood sarcoma. The cumulative risk of developing brain metastasis by 5 years after diagnosis is 11 % for type 2 tumors and 54 % for type 3 lesions [57]. Since it is known that type 1 pleuropulmonary blastoma may recur as the higher-grade type 2 or 3 tumors [58], elective surgery of all cystic lung lesions in young children is advised even if these are asymptomatic [59, 81, 82].

Pulmonary Carcinosarcoma

History, Histopathogenesis, and Definition

Since its earliest description by Kika in 1908 [83], controversy has surrounded the histogenesis and definition of carcinosarcoma. Saphir and Vass in 1938 [84] reviewed 153 cases of "carcinosarcoma" reported in the literature and proposed that, in the few cases that they regarded as truly carcinosarcomatous, the mesenchymal component of carcinosarcoma was a reactive response induced by paracrine secretion from the epithelial component. This theory was reinforced by studies of Addis and Corrin [85] and Humphrey et al. [86] who believed that the mesenchymal component derived from metaplasia of undifferentiated stem cells or carcinoma cells, respectively. Later, this theory was refuted, primarily by the fact that the mesenchymal component had malignant morphologic features and metastatic potential. This led to the biclonal theory proposing a collision between histogenetically independent neoplasms derived from separate progenitor cells (so-called collision tumors) [87, 88]. This hypothesis contrasts with the monoclonal theory put forward by Thompson et al. in 1996 [89] stating that a single totipotential stem cell can differentiate into diverse cell lines during tumorigenesis. The latter proposition has recently been supported by the results of various molecular investigations: These studies described similar genetic alterations in the epithelial and mesenchymal components of carcinosarcoma, suggesting a monoclonal origin of both elements [90, 91]. Today, the monoclonal theory appears to be the most widely accepted one.

Similar contention involves the definition of carcinosarcoma and its separation from sarcomatoid carcinoma. Both lesions may share certain morphological characteristics making separation on pure histological grounds difficult. The earlier definitions of carcinosarcoma did not require the presence of specialized mesenchymal tumor elements for diagnosis but regarded even nonspecific spindle cells as representation of the "mesenchymal" component [92, 93]. However, later other authors were able to demonstrate epithelial differentiation within both elements of such tumors by using adjunct techniques such as electron microscopy and immunohistochemistry, thereby reclassifying these lesions as sarcomatoid carcinomas [94, 95]. The same authors proposed that sarcomatoid carcinomas be divided into biphasic tumors (those demonstrating the presence of a divergent cell line) and monophasic tumors (those with a nonspecialized spindle cell component) [95]. A number of other investigators, including the recommendations by the latest WHO publication on lung tumors, however, advocate the term carcinosarcoma for those tumors that in addition to an epithelial malignancy contain unequivocal heterologous mesenchymal elements in the form of osteorsarcoma, chondrosarcoma, rhabdomyosarcoma, or liposarcoma [18, 25, 86]. Due to these controversies, opinions are still divided as to whether carcinosarcoma is best regarded as a separate clinicopathological entity or rather forms part of a spectrum with other tumors displaying sarcomatoid features. This controversy is reflected in the inclusion of carcinosarcomas as a subtype of sarcomatoid carcinoma in the most recent WHO classification [18].

Clinical Features

Carcinosarcomas belong to the rarest primary tumors of the lungs with an estimated incidence of only 0.2–0.4 % of all pulmonary neoplasms [96–98]. Carcinosarcomas predominantly affect men with a male-to-female ratio of 7:1 [96, 99, 100]. The age at presentation ranges from 29 to 81 years with a peak in the seventh decade. Tobacco use appears to be a common etiologic factor [96, 99, 101]. Carcinosarcomas may present as central lesions with an endobronchial component or arise peripherally in the lung parenchyma [92, 101–103]. Isolated cases may also present as entirely pleural-based lesions [104]. Endobronchial tumors may produce cough, dyspnea, hemoptysis, and shortness of breath, whereas peripheral lesions are more likely to induce chest pain, recurrent pneumonic episodes, weight loss, and fever [92, 96, 99, 101, 102]. Up to one-third of patients may be entirely asymptomatic [99].

Radiologically, endobronchial carcinosarcomas show features of obstructive pneumonitis or atelectasis, whereas peripheral lesions are characterized by large round parenchymal masses. The latter shows heterogeneous enhancement in the periphery and decreased attenuation centrally on CT scanning. Local invasion into the chest wall, pericardium, or pulmonary vein may be present [105].

Carcinosarcomas may be associated with paraneoplastic syndromes such as migratory polyarthritis and polyneuropathy or hypertrophic pulmonary osteoarthropathy [106–108].

Gross Features

Pulmonary carcinosarcomas are large tumors affecting primarily the upper lobes [96, 99]. Tumor sizes range from 1.5 to 16 cm with a mean size of 7 cm [96, 99]. They are usually single, well-circumscribed masses of either peripheral or central location [92]. Although single lesions are by far more common, occasionally carcinosarcomas can also present as multiple nodules [99]. If situated centrally, the tumors may have endobronchial, extrabronchial, or intrabronchial components and may show the appearance of bronchial polyps [92, 99, 103]. Extensive pleural involvement mimicking malignant mesothelioma has been described in one case [109]. Whereas the epithelial component often displays a soft and friable consistency with or without areas of necrosis and cavitation, the sarcomatous component is commonly firm, fleshy, and rubbery on gross examination [96, 99].

Histological Features

The histological features of carcinosarcoma are characterized by an admixture of carcinomatous and sarcomatous elements (Figs. 5.36 and 5.37). These may be distributed in equal proportions or show predominantly epithelial or mesenchymal differentiation [96] (Figs. 5.38 and 5.39). The most common carcinomatous component is squamous cell carcinoma, and this is particularly true for endobronchial tumors [99, 102] (Fig. 5.40). Squamous cell carcinoma is

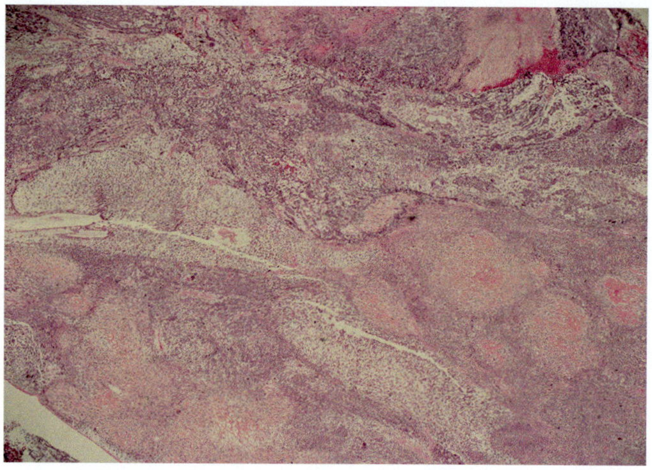

Fig. 5.36 Low-power view demonstrating the biphasic nature of carcinosarcoma

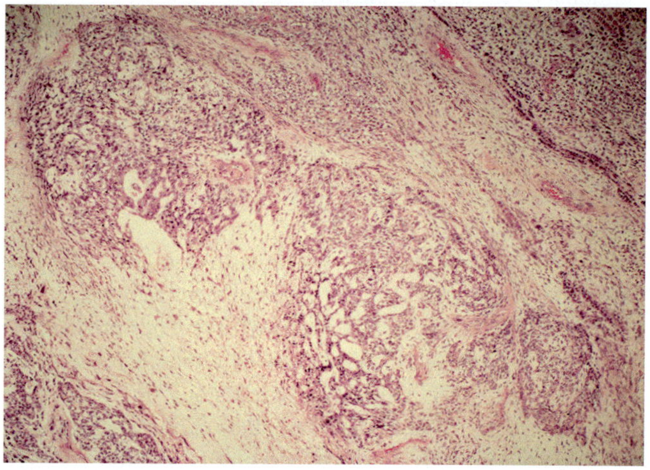

Fig. 5.37 Mixture of carcinomatous and sarcomatous elements in carcinosarcoma

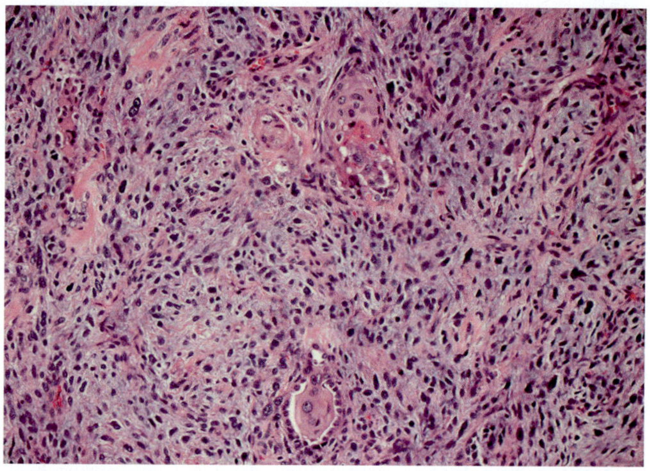

Fig. 5.38 Subtle squamous cell carcinoma component in carcinosarcoma

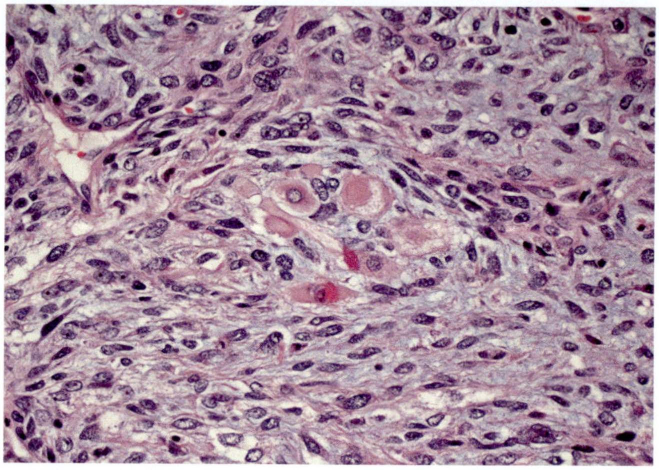

Fig. 5.39 Subtle rhabdomyoblastic cells in the mesenchymal component of a carcinosarcoma

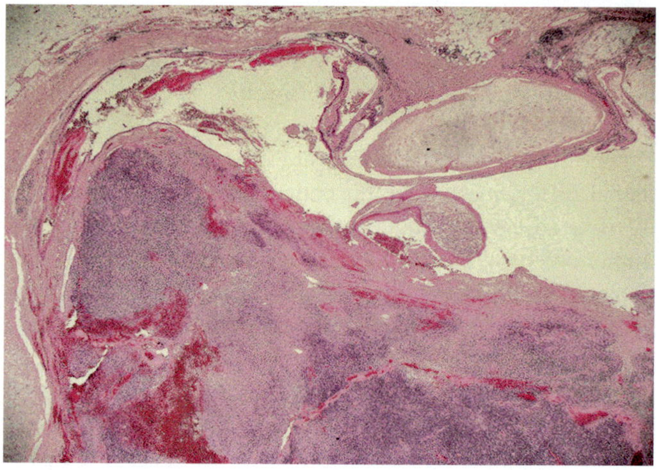

Fig. 5.40 Endobronchial carcinosarcoma growing into the bronchial lumen

followed in frequency by adenocarcinoma, adenosquamous carcinoma, and large cell carcinoma [99] (Figs. 5.41, 5.42, 5.43, 5.44, and 5.45). Among the stromal elements, rhabdomyosarcoma, osteosarcoma, and chondrosarcoma are most commonly identified, while leiomyosarcoma, liposarcoma, undifferentiated sarcoma, or osteoclast-like giant cells are less often found [92, 99, 110] (Figs. 5.46, 5.47, 5.48, 5.49, 5.50, 5.51, 5.52, 5.53, 5.54, and 5.55). Both the epithelial and mesenchymal components histologically resemble their counterparts in other organ systems and may show all stages of differentiation. Isolated case reports also comment on the presence of neuroendocrine carcinoma and salivary gland-type epithelium as part of the epithelial component in these tumors [25, 111–114]. While the majority of carcinosarcomas show permeative growth into adjacent tissues, peripheral lesions often have a pushing interface with the

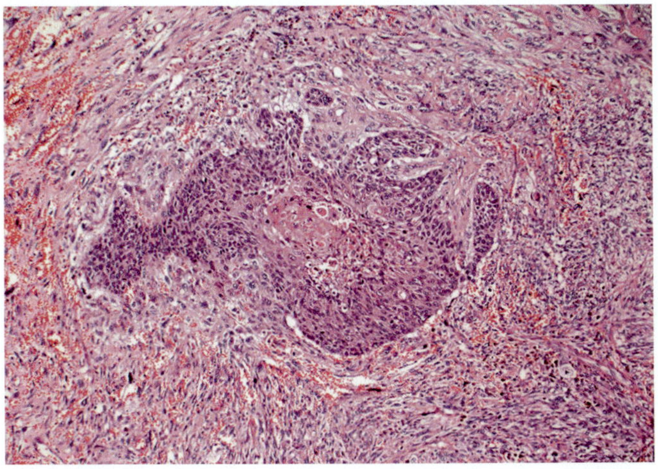

Fig. 5.41 Squamous cell carcinoma embedded in malignant mesenchymal stroma

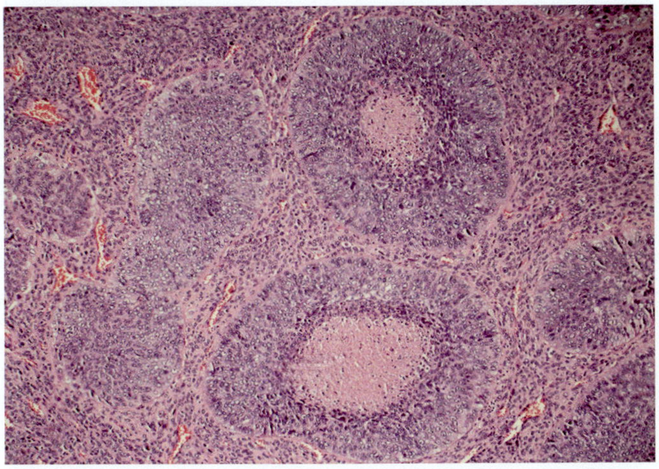

Fig. 5.42 Squamous cell carcinoma with basaloid features as part of a carcinosarcoma

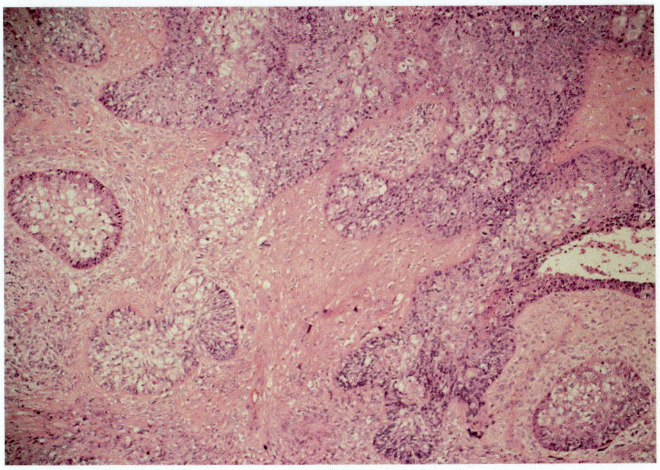

Fig. 5.43 Carcinosarcoma with clear cell changes in the squamous cell carcinoma component

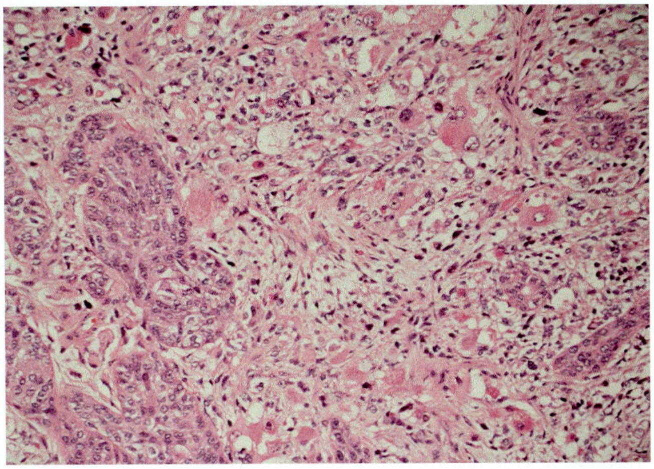

Fig. 5.44 Squamous cell carcinoma adjacent to areas of rhabdomyosarcoma in carcinosarcoma

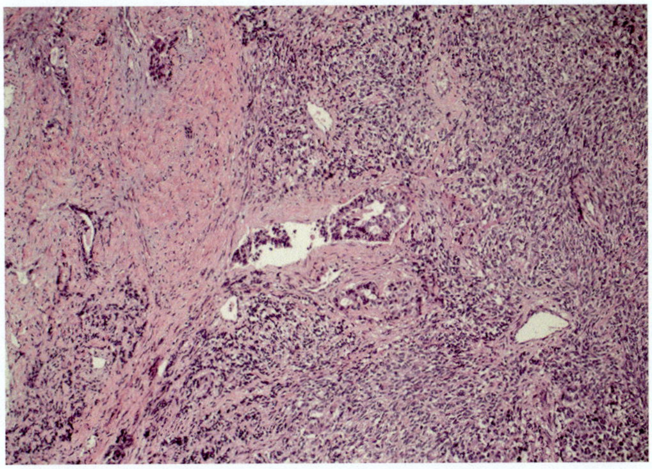

Fig. 5.45 Adenocarcinoma as part of a carcinosarcoma

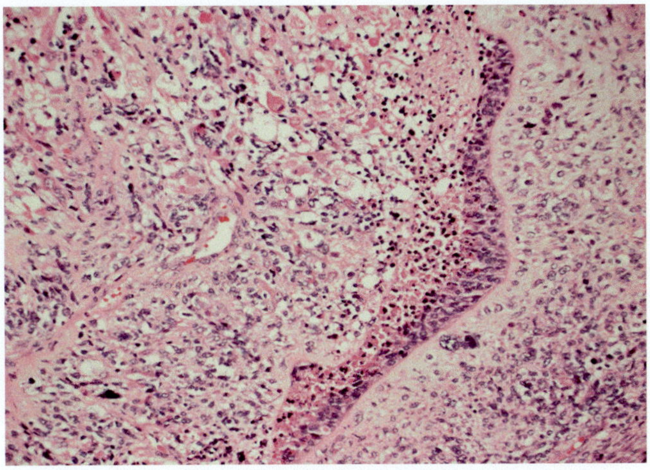

Fig. 5.46 Carcinosarcoma with rhabdomyoblastic differentiation

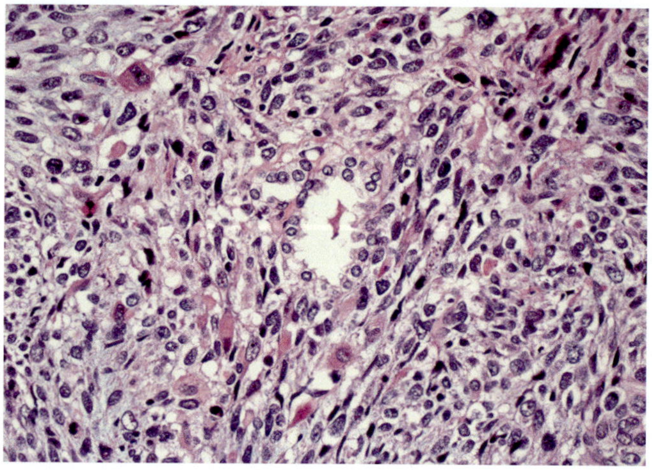

Fig. 5.47 Rhabdomyoblastic cells in a carcinosarcoma

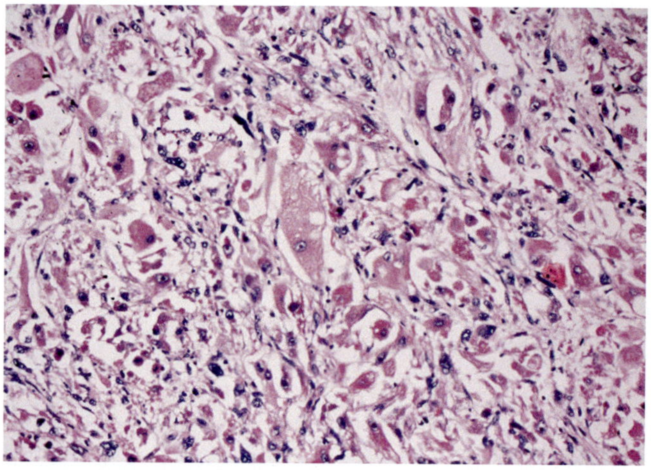

Fig. 5.48 Extensive rhabdomyoblastic differentiation in carcinosarcoma

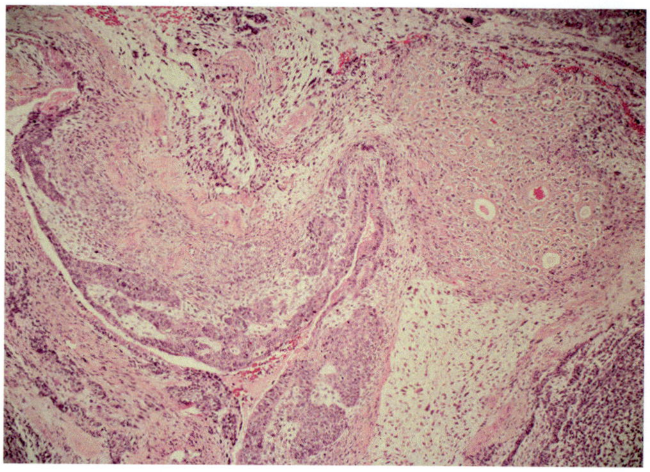

Fig. 5.49 Low-power view of a carcinosarcoma with osteosarcoma component

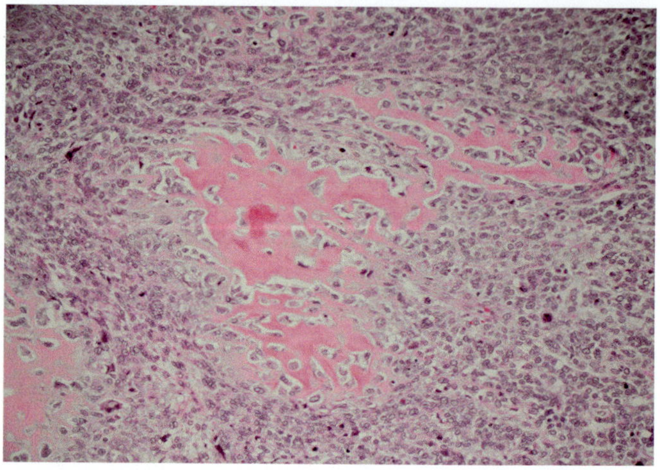

Fig. 5.50 High-power view showing malignant osteoid in a carcinosarcoma

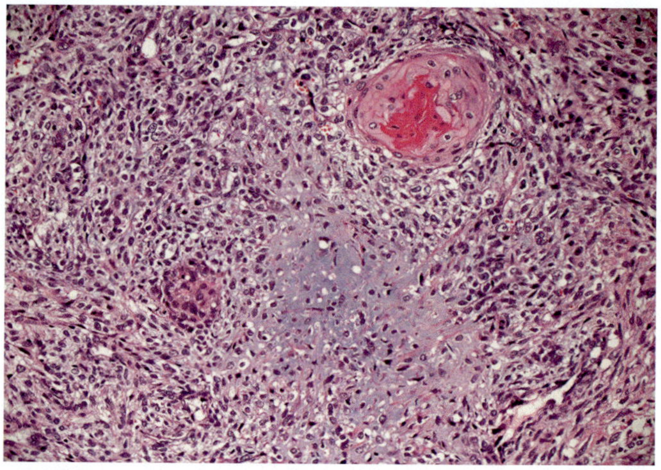

Fig. 5.51 Carcinosarcoma with squamous cell carcinoma and cartilaginous differentiation

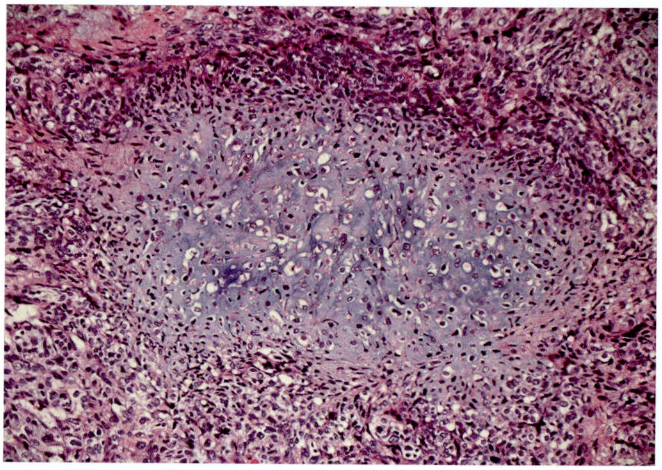

Fig. 5.52 Higher-power view of malignant cartilage in carcinosarcoma

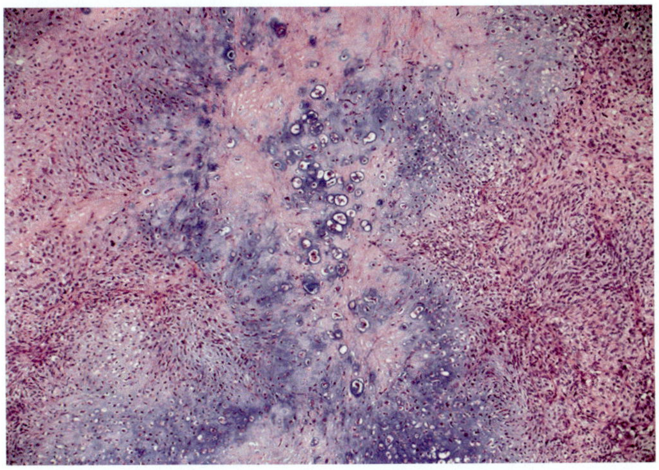

Fig. 5.53 Extensive chondrosarcoma component showing high-grade cytological atypia in carcinosarcoma

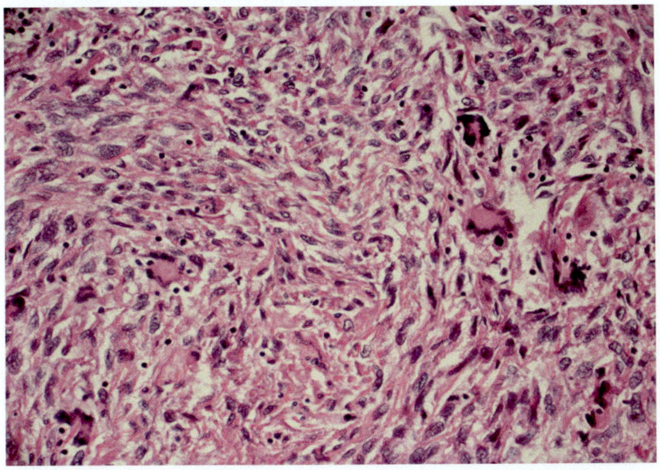

Fig. 5.54 Giant cell change in sarcomatous areas of carcinosarcoma

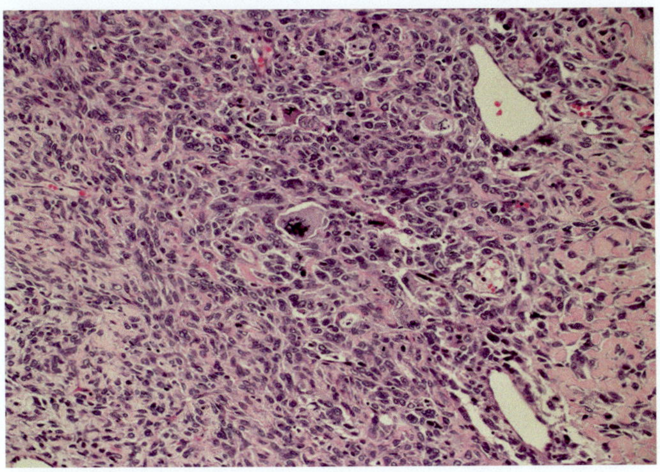

Fig. 5.55 High-grade undifferentiated sarcoma component in carcinosarcoma

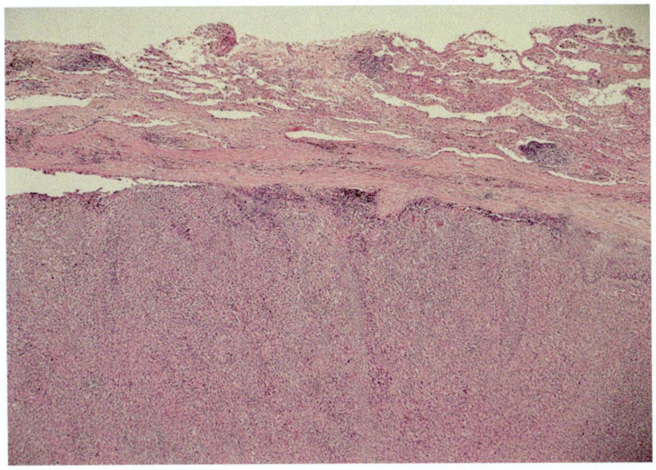

Fig. 5.56 Carcinosarcoma showing a pushing interface with the adjacent lung parenchyma

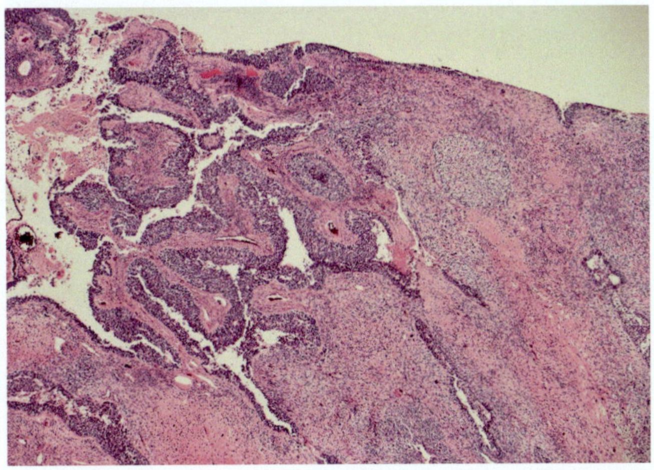

Fig. 5.57 Cystic change in carcinosarcoma lined by squamous cell carcinoma

surrounding parenchyma [101] (Fig. 5.56). Hemorrhage, necrosis, and pseudocyst formation are frequently seen [101] (Figs. 5.57, 5.58, and 5.59). Metastatic deposits of carcinosarcoma may show features of only one of the components or a mixture of both [99].

Electron Microscopy

Detailed ultrastructural investigations of carcinosarcoma have revealed that the carcinomatous component shows the typical features of epithelial cells: The cells contain tonofilaments and are widely connected by junctional complexes in the form of desmosomes. The mesenchymal cells are generally characterized by an absence of these structures

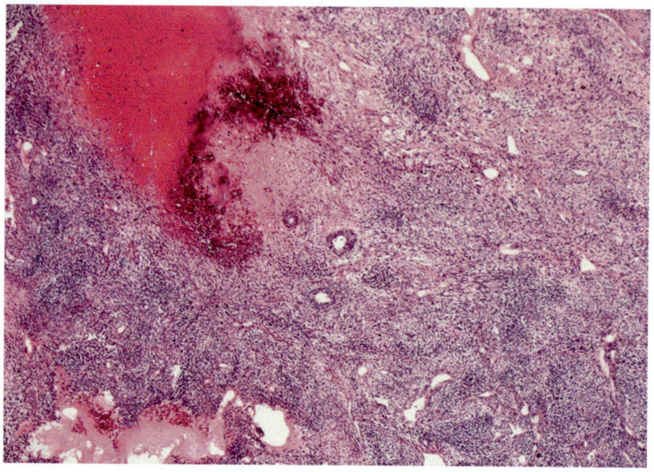

Fig. 5.58 Areas of hemorrhage in carcinosarcoma

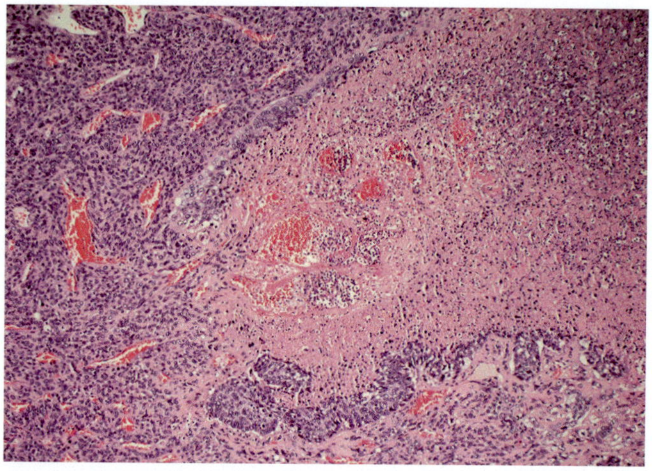

Fig. 5.59 Extensive necrosis in carcinosarcoma

and are set in a loose myxomatous matrix [109, 115]. An interesting observation was made by Yamazaki et al. [116] who described cell to cell interactions between the two components, suggesting that the different tumor cells interact with each other as well as with the matrix and that this interaction may influence the development and migration of the neoplastic cells.

Immunohistochemical and Molecular Features

Although the diagnosis of carcinosarcoma is often a histological one, immunohistochemical studies may be helpful in determining less well-differentiated tumor components. The carcinomatous elements will show reactivity for CAM5.2 and CK stains; more specifically, CK5/6 and p63 can be used to identify squamous cell carcinoma, and CK7, TTF-1, and napsin may be used in the diagnosis of adenocarcinoma. Rhabdomyoblastic differentiation can be confirmed with muscle-specific markers like desmin, myoglobin, or myogenin. S100 protein may aid to identify liposarcomatous or chondrosarcomatous areas, whereas, for practical purposes, the detection of osteosarcoma-like areas is restricted to the typical morphological appearance. Finally, if neuroendocrine differentiation is suspected, synaptophysin, chromogranin, and CD56 are the most useful markers to confirm the diagnosis.

Recent genetic studies have contributed significantly to confirm the histogenetic development of carcinosarcomas. Dacic et al. [90] have been able to detect the same allelic losses involving chromosomes 3q, 5q, and 17p in the epithelial and mesenchymal components of carcinosarcoma, strongly suggesting a monoclonal origin of this tumor and supporting the totipotential stem cell theory of tumorigenesis. Furthermore, they found fractional allelic loss to be more often present in the mesenchymal component and interpreted this to reflect transition from carcinoma to sarcoma in the process of tumor development. These findings were supported by Pardo et al. in 2008 [91] who found many common alterations between carcinomatous and sarcomatous areas characterized by gains in chromosomes 1q, 3q, 5p, 8q, and 12p. Furthermore, some studies documented an absence of K-ras and β(beta)-catenin mutations in carcinosarcoma, the latter indicative that this tumor is distinct from pulmonary blastoma, a neoplasm that has consistently shown the presence of such genetic change [9, 10, 12].

Differential Diagnosis

Carcinosarcomas may be difficult to diagnose on small endobronchial or transthoracic needle core biopsies, which will often only include one of the tumor components, and definitive diagnosis will be delayed until the tumor is formally resected. However, even on resected material, diagnostic difficulties may arise, and carcinosarcomas can be mistaken for tumors displaying similar features. One of the most controversial issues is the separation from sarcomatoid carcinoma. Whereas some authors believe that carcinosarcomas as a whole represent a subtype of sarcomatoid carcinomas [18, 101], other investigators believe that they form a specific clinicopathologic entity [25, 99]. The latter groups define carcinosarcomas as those tumors showing epithelial and specialized mesenchymal differentiation such as osteosarcoma, chondrosarcoma, or rhabdomyosarcoma. In their opinion, only tumors in which the mesenchymal component is represented by an undifferentiated spindle cell proliferation (with or without immunohistochemical cytokeratin reactivity) are classified as a sarcomatoid carcinoma.

Carcinosarcomas in which the carcinomatous element is adenocarcinoma may be confused with pulmonary blastomas. Pulmonary blastomas, however, are biphasic tumors where the stromal component is composed of an undifferentiated embryonal mesenchyma and the epithelial part resembles the tubules and acini of the fetal lung, thereby distinguishing the two tumors [117]. Teratomas displaying malignant transformation have a potential to be confused with carcinosarcoma due to the presence of malignant epithelial or mesenchymal components. However, this tumor is derived from all three germ cell layers and will most often show mature cartilage, adipose, or neural tissue in combination with a malignant epithelial element. Other tumors to consider in the differential diagnosis are malignant salivary gland-like tumors and primary mesenchymal neoplasms of the lung. Malignant salivary gland-like tumors will have a striking myoepithelial component, and the malignancy will be primarily epithelial in nature [25]. Primary mesenchymal neoplasms of the lung like rhabdomyosarcoma, leiomyosarcoma, or osteosarcoma are exceedingly rare and will not contain any carcinomatous elements.

Treatment and Prognosis

Since a large proportion of carcinosarcomas is resectable at the time of diagnosis, complete surgical resection is the treatment of choice and potentially curative if disease is localized [99, 118]. Chemotherapy and/or radiation may be indicated in cases that are not amenable to surgery or in cases of metastatic dissemination. Metastatic disease is most frequently found in lymph nodes, kidney, bone, thorax, liver, spleen, adrenal gland, and brain and can present in the form of the carcinomatous or sarcomatous component or both [99, 101]. Information on cytotoxic regimens effective in carcinosarcoma is sparse, and no universal chemotherapy recommendation exists. Some workers suggested the use of doxorubicin-based chemotherapies, believing that the sarcomatous component is the one predicting prognosis therefore modeling treatment after that of soft tissue sarcomas [114]. Other studies reported treatment responses to combination chemotherapy with doxorubicin, cisplatin, and cyclophosphamide, thereby targeting both tumor components [96, 119]. Despite all treatment modalities, the prognosis for patients with carcinosarcoma is poor. In the two largest series investigating pulmonary carcinosarcomas, the survival ranged from a median survival of 1-year to a 5-year survival rate of 21.3 % [96, 99]. A later series of 15 resected tumors reported an overall cumulative 5-year survival of 49.4 %, a rate similar to patients with primary pulmonary sarcoma [118]. Koss et al. [99] noted in their study of 66 patients that neither endobronchial location nor tumor stage had an impact on survival and that the only relevant parameter was tumor size with a cutoff at 6 cm. The eventual cause of death in patients with pulmonary carcinosarcoma is most often related to tumor recurrence and distant metastasis [114].

References

1. Barnard WG. Embryoma of lungs. Thorax. 1952;7:299–301.
2. Spencer H. Pulmonary blastomas. J Pathol Bacteriol. 1961;82:161–5.
3. Souza RC, Peasley ED, Takaro T. Pulmonary blastomas: a distinctive group of carcinosarcomas of the lung. Ann Thorac Surg. 1965;122: 259–68.
4. Bauermeister DE, Jennings ER, Beland AH, Judson HA. Pulmonary blastoma, a form of carcinosarcoma. Report of a case of 24 years' duration without treatment. Am J Clin Pathol. 1966;46:322–9.
5. McCann MP, Fu YS, Kay S. Pulmonary blastoma: a light and electron microscopic study. Cancer. 1976;38:789–97.
6. Roth JA, Elguezabal A. Pulmonary blastoma evolving into carcinosarcoma. A case study. Am J Surg Pathol. 1978;2:407–13.
7. Pacinda SJ, Ledet SC, Gondo MM, et al. p53 and MDM2 immunostaining in pulmonary blastomas and bronchogenic carcinomas. Hum Pathol. 1996;27:542–6.
8. Bodner SM, Koss MN. Mutations in the p53 gene in pulmonary blastomas: immunohistochemical and molecular studies. Hum Pathol. 1996;27:1117–23.
9. Holst VA, Finkelstein S, Colby TV, Myers JL, Yousem SA. p53 and K-ras mutational genotyping in pulmonary carcinosarcoma, spindle cell carcinoma, and pulmonary blastoma: implications for histogenesis. Am J Surg Pathol. 1997;21:801–11.
10. Sekine S, Shibata T, Matsuno Y, et al. Beta-catenin mutations in pulmonary blastomas: association with morule formation. J Pathol. 2003;200:214–21.
11. Hansen T, Bittinger F, Kortsik C, Wagner B, Kirkpatrick CJ. Expression of KIT (CD117) in biphasic pulmonary blastoma. Novel data on histogenesis. Lung. 2003;181:193–200.
12. Nakatani Y, Miyagi Y, Takemura T, et al. Aberrant nuclear/cytoplasmic localization and gene mutation of beta-catenin in classic pulmonary blastoma: beta-catenin immunostaining is useful for distinguishing between classic pulmonary blastoma and a blastomatoid variant of carcinosarcoma. Am J Surg Pathol. 2004;28:921–7.
13. Takahashi K, Kohno T, Matsumoto S, et al. Clonality and heterogeneity of pulmonary blastoma from the viewpoint of genetic alterations: a case report. Lung Cancer. 2007;57:103–8.
14. Kradin RL, Young RH, Dickersin GR, Kirkham SE, Mark EJ. Pulmonary blastoma with argyrophil cells and lacking sarcomatous features (pulmonary endodermal tumor resembling fetal lung). Am J Surg Pathol. 1982;6:165–72.
15. Kodama T, Shimosato Y, Watanabe S, Koide T, Naruke T, Shimase J. Six cases of well-differentiated adenocarcinoma simulating fetal lung tubules in pseudoglandular stage. Comparison with pulmonary blastoma. Am J Surg Pathol. 1984;8:735–44.
16. Nakatani Y, Dickersin GR, Mark EJ. Pulmonary endodermal tumor resembling fetal lung: a clinicopathologic study of five cases with immunohistochemical and ultrastructural characterization. Hum Pathol. 1990;21:1097–107.
17. Nakatani Y, Kitamura H, Inayama Y, et al. Pulmonary adenocarcinomas of the fetal lung type: a clinicopathologic study indicating differences in histology, epidemiology, and natural history of low-grade and high-grade forms. Am J Surg Pathol. 1998;22:399–411.
18. Travis WD, Brambilla E, Müller-Hermelink HK, Harris CC, editors. Pathology and geneticsof tumours of the lung, pleura, thymus and heart. World Health Organization (WHO) classification of tumors. Lyon: IARC Press; 2004. p. 40–56.
19. Koss MN. Pulmonary blastomas. Cancer Treat Res 1995;72:349–62.
20. Zaidi A, Zamvar V, Macbeth F, Gibbs AR, Kulatilake N, Butchart EG. Pulmonary blastoma: medium-term results from a regional center. Ann Thorac Surg. 2002;73:1572–5.
21. Adluri RK, Boddu SR, Martin-Ucar A, Duffy JP, Beggs FD, Morgan WE. Pulmonary blastoma – a rare tumor with variable presentation. Eur J Cardiothorac Surg. 2006;29:236–9.

22. Robert J, Pache JC, Seium Y, de Perrot M, Spiliopoulos A. Pulmonary blastoma: report of five cases and identification of clinical features suggestive of the disease. Eur J Cardiothorac Surg. 2002;22:708–11.
23. Majid OA, Rajendran U, Baker LT. Pulmonary blastoma. Ann Thorac Cardiovasc Surg. 1998;4:47–52.
24. Reichman M, Kovanlikaya A, Mathew S, Beneck D, Brill PW. Pulmonary blastoma in a neonate: a lesion distinct from pleuropulmonary blastoma with unique cytogenetic features. Pediatr Radiol. 2010;40:366–70.
25. Berho M, Moran CA, Suster S. Malignant mixed epithelial/mesenchymal neoplasms of the lung. Semin Diagn Pathol. 1995;12:123–39.
26. Sato S, Koike T, Yamato Y, Yoshiya K, Honma K, Tsukada H. Resected well-differentiated fetal pulmonary adenocarcinoma and summary of 25 cases reported in Japan. Jpn J Thorac Cardiovasc Surg. 2006;54:539–42.
27. DiFurio MJ, Auerbach A, Kaplan KJ. Well-differentiated fetal adenocarcinoma: rare tumor in the pediatric population. Pediatr Dev Pathol. 2003;6:564–7.
28. Lee HJ, Goo JM, Kim KW, Im JG, Kim JH. Pulmonary blastoma: radiologic findings in five patients. Clin Imaging. 2004;28:113–8.
29. Francis D, Jacobsen M. Pulmonary blastoma. Curr Top Pathol. 1983;73:265–94.
30. Koss MN, Hochholzer L, O'Leary T. Pulmonary blastomas. Cancer. 1991;67:2368–81.
31. Cohen RE, Weaver MG, Montenegro HD, Abdul-Karim FW. Pulmonary blastoma with malignant melanoma component. Arch Pathol Lab Med. 1990;114:1076–8.
32. Siegel RJ, Bueso-Ramos C, Cohen C, Koss M. Pulmonary blastoma with germ cell (yolk sac) differentiation: report of two cases. Mod Pathol. 1991;4:566–70.
33. Oshika Y, Matsukuma S, Hashimoto H, Takeo H, Sato K, Tanaka Y. Biphasic pulmonary blastoma with a lesion of yolk sac tumor. Gen Thorac Cardiovasc Surg. 2007;55:243–7.
34. Archie PH, Beasley MB, Ross HJ. Biphasic pulmonary blastoma with germ cell differentiation in a 36-year-old man. J Thorac Oncol. 2008;3:1185–7.
35. Rossi G, Cavazza A, Sturm N, et al. Pulmonary carcinomas with pleomorphic, sarcomatoid, or sarcomatous elements: a clinicopathologic and immunohistochemical study of 75 cases. Am J Surg Pathol. 2003;27:311–24.
36. García-Escudero A, González-Cámpora R, Villar-Rodríguez JL, Lag-Asturiano E. Thyroid transcription factor-1 expression in pulmonary blastoma. Histopathology. 2004;44:507–8.
37. Cameselle-Teijeiro J, Alberte-Lista L, Chiarelli S, et al. CD10 is a characteristic marker of tumours forming morules with biotin-rich, optically clear nuclei that occur in different organs. Histopathology. 2008;52:389–92.
38. Zagar TM, Blackwell S, Crawford J, et al. Preoperative radiation therapy and chemotherapy for pulmonary blastoma: a case report. J Thorac Oncol. 2010;5:282–3.
39. Novotny JE, Huiras CM. Resection and adjuvant chemotherapy of pulmonary blastoma: a case report. Cancer. 1995;76:1537–9.
40. Kouvaris JR, Gogou PV, Papacharalampous XN, Kostara HJ, Balafouta MJ, Vlahos LJ. Solitary brain metastasis from classic biphasic pulmonary blastoma: a case report and review of the literature. Onkologie. 2006;29:568–70.
41. Nissen MH, Jacobsen M, Vindeløv L, Olsen J, Rørth M. Pulmonary blastoma: remission with chemotherapy. Eur J Respir Dis. 1984;65:377–9.
42. Chitambar IA, Gujral JS, Aikat BK. Embryonal sarcoma of the lung. A case report with a discussion regarding its morphogenesis. J Thorac Cardiovasc Surg. 1969;57:657–62.
43. Fallon G, Schiller M, Kilman JW. Primary rhabdomyosarcoma of the bronchus. Ann Thorac Surg. 1971;12:650–4.
44. Valderrama E, Saluja G, Shende A, Lanzkowsky P, Berkman J. Pulmonary blastoma. Report of two cases in children. Am J Surg Pathol. 1978;2:415–22.
45. Weinberg AG, Currarino G, Moore GC, Votteler TP. Mesenchymal neoplasia and congenital pulmonary cysts. Pediatr Radiol. 1980;9:179–82.
46. Krous HF, Sexauer CL. Embryonal rhabdomyosarcoma arising within a congenital bronchogenic cyst in a child. J Pediatr Surg. 1981;16:506–8.
47. Weinblatt ME, Siegel SE, Isaacs H. Pulmonary blastoma associated with cystic lung disease. Cancer. 1982;49:669–71.
48. Ashworth TG. Pulmonary blastoma, a true congenital neoplasm. Histopathology. 1983;7:585–94.
49. Becroft DMO, Jagusch MF. Pulmonary sarcomas arising in mesenchymal cystic hamartomas. Pediatr Pathol. 1987;7:478.
50. Allan BT, Day DL, Dehner LP. Primary pulmonary rhabdomyosarcoma of the lung in children. Report of two cases presenting with spontaneous pneumothorax. Cancer. 1987;59:1005–11.
51. Manivel JC, Priest JR, Watterson J, et al. Pleuropulmonary blastoma. The so-called pulmonary blastoma of childhood. Cancer. 1988;62:1516–26.
52. Dehner LP. Pleuropulmonary blastoma is THE pulmonary blastoma of childhood. Semin Diagn Pathol. 1994;11:144–51.
53. Indolfi P, Casale F, Carli M, et al. Pleuropulmonary blastoma: management and prognosis of 11 cases. Cancer. 2000;89:1396–401.
54. Hachitanda Y, Aoyama C, Sato JK, Shimada H. Pleuropulmonary blastoma in childhood. A tumor of divergent differentiation. Am J Surg Pathol. 1993;17:382–91.
55. Hill DA, Sadeghi S, Schultz MZ, Burr JS, Dehner LP. Pleuropulmonary blastoma in an adult: an initial case report. Cancer. 1999;85:2368–74.
56. Zuker NB, Dietl CA, Kenna S, Fischer EG, Gardner D. Unusual survival of an adult with pleuropulmonary blastoma and neurofibromatosis. J Thorac Cardiovasc Surg. 2007;134:541–2.
57. Priest JR, Magnuson J, Williams GM, et al. Cerebral metastasis and other central nervous system complications of pleuropulmonary blastoma. Pediatr Blood Cancer. 2007;49:266–73.
58. Priest JR, McDermott MB, Bhatia S, Watterson J, Manivel JC, Dehner LP. Pleuropulmonary blastoma: a clinicopathologic study of 50 cases. Cancer. 1997;80:147–61.
59. Miniati DN, Chintagumpala M, Langston C, et al. Prenatal presentation and outcome of children with pleuropulmonary blastoma. J Pediatr Surg. 2006;41:66–71.
60. Picaud JC, Levrey H, Bouvier R, et al. Bilateral cystic pleuropulmonary blastoma in early infancy. J Pediatr. 2000;136:834–6.
61. Naffaa LN, Donnelly LF. Imaging findings in pleuropulmonary blastoma. Pediatr Radiol. 2005;35:387–91.
62. Priest JR, Hill DA, Williams GM, et al. Type I pleuropulmonary blastoma: a report from the International Pleuropulmonary Blastoma Registry. J Clin Oncol. 2006;24:4492–8.
63. Papaioannou G, Sebire NJ, McHugh K. Imaging of the unusual pediatric 'blastomas'. Cancer Imaging. 2009;9:1–11.
64. Priest JR, Watterson J, Strong L, et al. Pleuropulmonary blastoma: a marker for familial disease. J Pediatr. 1996;128:220–4.
65. Boman F, Hill DA, Williams GM, et al. Familial association of pleuropulmonary blastoma with cystic nephroma and other renal tumors: a report from the International Pleuropulmonary Blastoma Registry. J Pediatr. 2006;149:850–4.
66. Priest JR, Williams GM, Hill DA, Dehner LP, Jaffé A. Pulmonary cysts in early childhood and the risk of malignancy. Pediatr Pulmonol. 2009;44:14–30.
67. Goel P, Panda S, Srinivas M, et al. Pleuropulmonary blastoma with intrabronchial extension. Pediatr Blood Cancer. 2010;54:1026–8.
68. Cohen M, Emms M, Kaschula RO. Childhood pulmonary blastoma: a pleuropulmonary variant of the adult-type pulmonary blastoma. Pediatr Pathol. 1991;11:737–49.

69. de Krijger RR, Claessen SM, van der Ham F, et al. Gain of chromosome 8q is a frequent finding in pleuropulmonary blastoma. Mod Pathol. 2007;20:1191–9.
70. Sciot R, DalCin P, Brock P, et al. Pleuropulmonary blastoma (pulmonary blastoma of childhood): genetic link with other embryonal malignancies? Histopathology. 1994;24:559–63.
71. Novak R, Dasu S, Agamanolis D, Herold W, Malone J, Waterson J. Trisomy 8 is a characteristic finding in pleuropulmonary blastoma. Pediatr Pathol Lab Med. 1997;17:99–103.
72. Sebire NJ, Rampling D, Malone M, Ramsay A, Sheppard M. Gains of chromosome 8 in pleuropulmonary blastomas of childhood. Pediatr Dev Pathol. 2002;5:221–2.
73. Roque L, Rodrigues R, Martins C, et al. Comparative genomic hybridization analysis of a pleuropulmonary blastoma. Cancer Genet Cytogenet. 2004;149:58–62.
74. Kusafuka T, Kuroda S, Inoue M, et al. P53 gene mutations in pleuropulmonary blastomas. Pediatr Hematol Oncol. 2002;19:117–28.
75. Hill DA, Ivanovich J, Priest JR, et al. DICER1 mutations in familial pleuropulmonary blastoma. Science. 2009;325:965.
76. Hill DA, Jarzembowski JA, Priest JR, Williams G, Schoettler P, Dehner LP. Type I pleuropulmonary blastoma: pathology and biology study of 51 cases from the international pleuropulmonary blastoma registry. Am J Surg Pathol. 2008;32:282–95.
77. MacSweeney F, Papagiannopoulos K, Goldstraw P, Sheppard MN, Corrin B, Nicholson AG. An assessment of the expanded classification of congenital cystic adenomatoid malformations and their relationship to malignant transformation. Am J Surg Pathol. 2003;27:1139–46.
78. Kukkady A, Upadhyay V, Pease PW, Chan YF. Pleuropulmonary blastoma: four cases. Pediatr Surg Int. 2000;16:595–8.
79. Parsons SK, Fishman SJ, Hoorntje LE, et al. Aggressive multimodal treatment of pleuropulmonary blastoma. Ann Thorac Surg. 2001;72:939–42.
80. Indolfi P, Bisogno G, Casale F, et al. Prognostic factors in pleuropulmonary blastoma. Pediatr Blood Cancer. 2007;48:318–23.
81. Papagiannopoulos K, Hughes S, Nicholson AG, Goldstraw P. Cystic lung lesions in the pediatric and adult population: surgical experience at the Brompton Hospital. Ann Thorac Surg. 2002;73:1594–8.
82. Dosios T, Stinios J, Nicolaides P, Spyrakos S, Androulakakis E, Constantopoulos A. Pleuropulmonary blastoma in childhood. A malignant degeneration of pulmonary cysts. Pediatr Surg Int. 2004;20:863–5.
83. Kika G. Gann. 1908:2:84.
84. Saphir O, Vass A. Carcinosarcoma. Am J Cancer. 1938;33:331–61.
85. Addis BJ, Corrin B. Pulmonary blastoma, carcinosarcoma and spindle-cell carcinoma: an immunohistochemical study of keratin intermediate filaments. J Pathol. 1985;147:291–301.
86. Humphrey PA, Scroggs MW, Roggli VL, Shelburne JD. Pulmonary carcinomas with a sarcomatoid element: an immunocytochemical and ultrastructural analysis. Hum Pathol. 1988;19:155–65.
87. Bergmann M, Ackerman LV, Kemler RL. Carcinosarcoma of the lung; review of the literature and report of two cases treated by pneumonectomy. Cancer. 1951;4:919–29.
88. Huszar M, Herczeg E, Lieberman Y, Geiger B. Distinctive immunofluorescent labeling of epithelial and mesenchymal elements of carcinosarcoma with antibodies specific for different intermediate filaments. Hum Pathol. 1984;15:532–8.
89. Thompson L, Chang B, Barsky SH. Monoclonal origins of malignant mixed tumors (carcinosarcomas). Evidence for a divergent histogenesis. Am J Surg Pathol. 1996;20:277–85.
90. Dacic S, Finkelstein SD, Sasatomi E, Swalsky PA, Yousem SA. Molecular pathogenesis of pulmonary carcinosarcoma as determined by microdissection-based allelotyping. Am J Surg Pathol. 2002;26:510–6.
91. Pardo J, Aisa G, Alava E, et al. Primary mixed squamous carcinoma and osteosarcoma (carcinosarcomas) of the lung have a CGH mapping similar to primitive squamous carcinomas and osteosarcomas. Diagn Mol Pathol. 2008;17:151–8.
92. Stackhouse EM, Harrison Jr EG, Ellis Jr FH. Primary mixed malignancies of lung: carcinosarcoma and blastoma. J Thorac Cardiovasc Surg. 1969;57:385–99.
93. Gabriel Jr JB, Ibanez I, Kondlapoodi P, Chauhan PM, Hagstrom JW. Carcinosarcoma of the lung with spindle-cell epithelial component: report of a case. J Surg Oncol. 1984;25:116–8.
94. Battifora H. Spindle cell carcinoma: ultrastructural evidence of squamous origin and collagen production by the tumor cells. Cancer. 1976;37:2275–82.
95. Nappi O, Glasner SD, Swanson PE, Wick MR. Biphasic and monophasic sarcomatoid carcinomas of the lung. A reappraisal of 'carcinosarcomas' and 'spindle-cell carcinomas'. Am J Clin Pathol. 1994;102:331–40.
96. Davis MP, Eagan RT, Weiland LH, Pairolero PC. Carcinosarcoma of the lung: Mayo Clinic experience and response to chemotherapy. Mayo Clin Proc. 1984;59:598–603.
97. Cabarcos A, Gomez Dorronsoro M, Lobo Beristain JL. Pulmonary carcinosarcoma: a case study and review of the literature. Br J Dis Chest. 1985;79:83–94.
98. Heremans A, Verbeken E, Deneffe G, Demedts M. Carcinosarcoma of the lung. Report of two cases and review of the literature. Acta Clin Belg. 1989;44:110–5.
99. Koss MN, Hochholzer L, Frommelt RA. Carcinosarcomas of the lung: a clinicopathologic study of 66 patients. Am J Surg Pathol. 1999;23:1514–26.
100. Sato S, Koike T, Yamato Y, et al. A case of rapidly growing pulmonary carcinosarcoma. Int J Clin Oncol. 2010;15:319–24.
101. Nappi O, Wick MR. Sarcomatoid neoplasms of the respiratory tract. Semin Diagn Pathol. 1993;10:137–47.
102. Moore TC. Carcinosarcoma of the lung. Surgery. 1961;50:886–93.
103. Ludwigsen E. Endobronchial carcinosarcoma. A case with osteosarcoma of pulmonary invasive part, and a review with respect to prognosis. Virchows Arch A Pathol Anat Histol. 1977;373:293–302.
104. Mayall FG, Gibbs AR. 'Pleural' and pulmonary carcinosarcomas. J Pathol. 1992;167:305–11.
105. Kim KI, Flint JD, Müller NL. Pulmonary carcinosarcoma: radiologic and pathologic findings in three patients. AJR Am J Roentgenol. 1997;169:691–4.
106. Meade P, Moad J, Fellows D, Adams CW. Carcinosarcoma of the lung with hypertrophic pulmonary osteoarthropathy. Ann Thorac Surg. 1991;51:488–90.
107. Reynolds S, Jenkins G, Akosa A, Roberts CM. Carcinosarcoma of the lung: an unusual cause of empyema. Respir Med. 1995;89:73–5.
108. Vidal Losada MJ, Bernal Monterde V, Amores Arriaga B, Ferrer Pérez AI, Serrano Solares S, Tobeña Puyal M. Lung carcinosarcoma. Clin Transl Oncol. 2010;12:303–5.
109. Zimmerman KG, Sobonya RE, Payne CM. Histochemical and ultrastructural features of an unusual pulmonary carcinosarcoma. Hum Pathol. 1981;12:1046–51.
110. Kitazawa R, Kitazawa S, Nishimura Y, Kondo T, Obayashi C. Lung carcinosarcoma with liposarcoma element: autopsy case. Pathol Int. 2006;56:449–52.
111. Tsubota YT, Kawaguchi T, Hoso T, Nishino E, Travis WD. A combined small cell and spindle cell carcinoma of the lung. Report of a unique case with immunohistochemical and ultrastructural studies. Am J Surg Pathol. 1992;16:1108–15.
112. Rainosek DE, Ro JY, Ordonez NG, Kulaga AD, Ayala AG. Sarcomatoid carcinoma of the lung. A case with atypical carcinoid and rhabdomyosarcomatous components. Am J Clin Pathol. 1994;102:360–4.

113. Koss MN, Moran CA, Stocker JT. Mixed epithelial-mesenchymal tumors. In: Saldana MJ, editor. Pathology of pulmonary disease. Philadelphia: Lippincott; 1994. p. 618–9.
114. Huwer H, Kalweit G, Straub U, Feindt P, Volkmer I, Gams E. Pulmonary carcinosarcoma: diagnostic problems and determinants of the prognosis. Eur J Cardiothorac Surg. 1996;10:403–7.
115. Haraguchi S, Fukuda Y, Sugisaki Y, Yamanaka N. Pulmonary carcinosarcoma: immunohistochemical and ultrastructural studies. Pathol Int. 1999;49:903–8.
116. Yamazaki K. Electron microscopy and immunohistochemistry studies of pulmonary carcinosarcomas expressing the transcription factor MEF-2 and showing significant cell-to-cell, cell-to-matrix, and epithelial-mesenchymal interactions. Virchows Arch. 2004; 444:542–53.
117. Davis PW, Briggs JC, Seal RM, Storring FK. Benign and malignant mixed tumours of the lung. Thorax. 1972;27:657–73.
118. Petrov DB, Vlassov VI, Kalaydjiev GT, et al. Primary pulmonary sarcomas and carcinosarcomas – postoperative results and comparative survival analysis. Eur J Cardiothorac Surg. 2003;23: 461–6.
119. Langer F, Wintzer HO, Werner M, Weber C, Brümmendorf TH, Bokemeyer C. A case of pulmonary carcinosarcoma (squamous cell carcinoma and osteosarcoma) treated with cisplatin and doxorubicin. Anticancer Res. 2006;26:3893–7.

6 Salivary Gland and Adnexal Type Tumors of the Lungs

Introduction

Salivary gland type tumors have been described in many locations of the body including the bronchopulmonary system. In the lungs, they are thought to arise from the minor salivary gland tissue of the tracheobronchial tree. Morphologically, histochemically, and immunohistochemically, these tumors share similar characteristics with their counterparts in the salivary glands; however, some differences have been observed in their histologic spectrum and biologic behavior. In addition, contrary to primary salivary gland tumors, the tumors arising in the lungs are uncommon, representing <1 % of all pulmonary neoplasms [1, 2]. Therefore, careful clinical and radiological investigations in patients presenting with a pulmonary salivary gland type tumor are essential to rule out metastasis from a salivary gland primary. The salivary gland type tumors known to originate in the lungs include mucoepidermoid carcinoma, adenoid cystic carcinoma, acinic cell carcinoma, pleomorphic adenoma, carcinoma ex pleomorphic adenoma, epithelial-myoepithelial carcinoma, and oncocytoma. Another rare adnexal type neoplasm, sebaceous carcinoma, is also included in this chapter. The most pertinent histochemical, immunohistochemical, ultrastructural, and molecular features of these tumors are summarized in Table 6.1.

Pulmonary Mucoepidermoid Carcinoma

Clinical Features

Mucoepidermoid carcinoma is the most common salivary gland type tumor occurring in the lung. It presents over a wide age range and has been described in patients aged 6–78 years with a peak in the fourth and fifth decade [3–8]. When the tumors are divided into low- and high-grade categories, high-grade tumors are more commonly seen in individuals older than 30 years [5]. Males appear to be slightly more commonly affected than females [3, 5, 6, 8]. The tumors often occur endobronchially, and symptoms are mainly due to bronchial obstruction and include cough, fever, shortness of breath, hemoptysis, and postobstructive pneumonia. On imaging, a solitary lung mass or nodule can be identified, which may be associated with postobstructive pneumonia or atelectasis [5].

Gross Features

Low-grade mucoepidermoid carcinomas are centrally located tumors that are well-circumscribed, exophytic, and polypoid lesions with a smooth surface that are attached to the bronchial wall by a small base. The tumor size ranges from 1–6 cm with an average of 2.2 cm. The cut surface often reveals a solid cystic lesion and variable mucoid material. High-grade lesions are grossly similar to the low-grade tumors but tend to show more obvious infiltration into the lung parenchyma and more commonly demonstrate solid rather than cystic growth [5].

Histological Features

Mucoepidermoid carcinomas of the lung are divided into low- and high-grade variants based primarily on cytologic criteria but generally show similar histologic features (Table 6.2). They are composed of three different cellular components: epidermoid cells, mucus-secreting glandular cells, and the so-called intermediate cells. Low-grade lesions usually display a close association with the submucosal bronchial glands and airway and are composed of solid and cystic tumor elements (Fig. 6.1). The solid areas are composed

A. Weissferdt, C.A. Moran, *Diagnostic Pathology of Pleuropulmonary Neoplasia*,
DOI 10.1007/978-1-4419-0787-5_6, © Springer Science+Business Media New York 2013

Table 6.1 Histochemical, immunohistochemical, ultrastructural, and molecular features of pulmonary salivary gland and adnexal type tumors

Tumor	Histochemical features	Immunohistochemical features	Ultrastructural features	Molecular features
Mucoepidermoid carcinoma	Mucicarmine	Similar to conventional non-small cell carcinoma	Not routinely used	t(11;19), MECT1-MAML2 fusion oncogene, EGFR mutations variable, EML4-ALK fusion oncogene
Adenoid cystic carcinoma	Not routinely used	CK, CAM5.2, vimentin, SMA, S100 variable	Not routinely used	EGFR, Kras negative
Acinic cell carcinoma	PAS, mucicarmine	CK, EMA, α-1-antichymotrypsin, amylase	Zymogen-type granules	Not investigated
Pleomorphic adenoma/ carcinoma ex pleomorphic carcinoma	Not routinely used	CK, CAM5.2, CK7 in epithelial elements; CK14, SMA, S100, GFAP, and CD56 in myoepithelial cells	Not routinely used	Not investigated
Epithelial-myoepithelial carcinoma	Not routinely used	CK, CAM 5.2, and c-kit in epithelial cells; SMA, S100, vimentin, and p63 in myoepithelial cells	Not routinely used	EGFR, Kras negative
Oncocytoma	Not routinely used	CK, vimentin, and α-1-antitrypsin	Mitochondrial hyperplasia	Not investigated
Sebaceous carcinoma	Oil Red O	CK, EMA, CEA	Not routinely used	Not investigated

CK cytokeratin, *EMA* epithelial membrane antigen, *SMA* smooth muscle actin, *CEA* carcinoembryonic antigen, *GFAP* glial fibrillary acidic protein, *PAS* periodic acid-Schiff, *EGFR* epidermal growth factor receptor, *MECT1-MAML2* mucoepidermoid carcinoma translocated 1-mastermind-like2, *EML4-ALK* echinoderm microtubule-associated protein-like 4-anaplastic lymphoma kinase, *Kras* Kirsten rat sarcoma viral oncogene homolog

Table 6.2 Diagnostic criteria of low and high-grade mucoepidermoid carcinoma of the lung

	Low-grade pulmonary mucoepidermoid carcinoma	High-grade pulmonary mucoepidermoid carcinoma
Gross features	Central location, well circumscribed, exophytic, polypoid, smooth surface, solid cystic	Central location, less well circumscribed, infiltrative, solid
Histological features	Solid and cystic elements, mix of epidermoid, intermediate, and mucus cells, bland cytologic features, <4 mitoses/10 HPF, no necrosis/hemorrhage	Predominantly solid growth, predominantly epidermoid and intermediate cells, marked cytologic atypia, nuclear hyperchromatism, increased mitotic activity (>4/10HPF), necrosis, and hemorrhage

HPF high-power fields

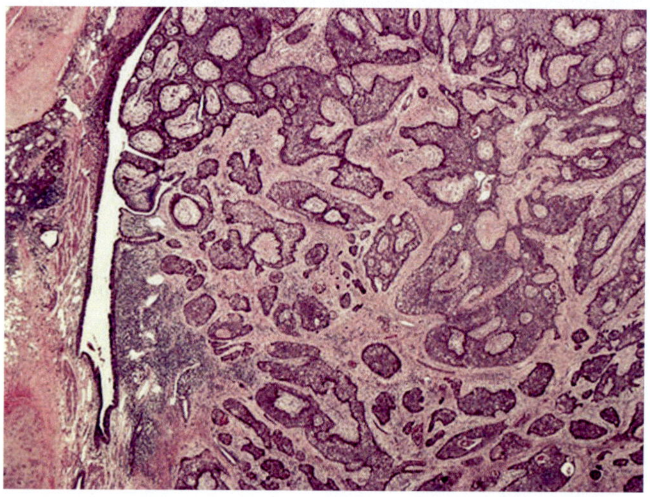

Fig. 6.1 Low power view of endobronchial mucoepidermoid carcinoma

of epidermoid cells, which are variably admixed with mucus-secreting glandular and intermediate cells (Fig. 6.2). The epidermoid cells in mucoepidermoid carcinoma contain intercellular bridges, but keratinization in any form is usually absent (Fig. 6.3). The intermediate cells show neither squamous nor glandular differentiation and are characterized by abundant amphophilic or eosinophilic cytoplasm and bland nuclear features (Figs. 6.4 and 6.5). The mucus-secreting cells are large with ample bluish cytoplasm and may occasionally show columnar, oncocytic, clear cell, or goblet cell change (Fig. 6.6). The cystic spaces can be of varying size and shape and may resemble gland-like or tubular structures (Fig. 6.7). The cysts are typically lined by the mucus-secreting cells and contain pools of either basophilic wispy mucin or hard eosinophilic mucinous material reminiscent of colloid (Figs. 6.8 and 6.9). The epidermoid component usually predominates, but at times the mucinous component may be

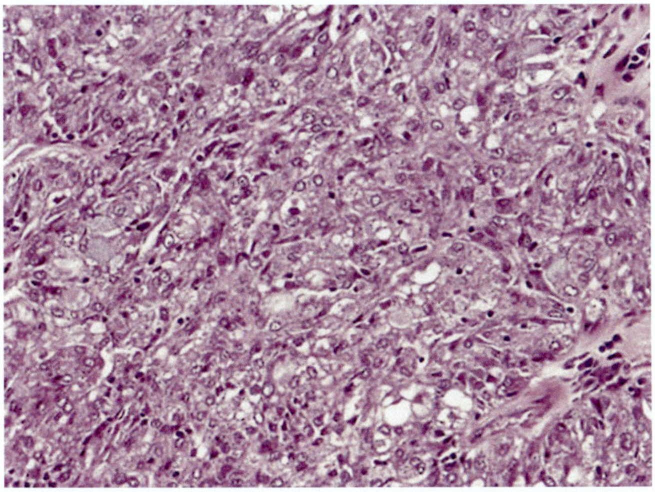

Fig. 6.2 Solid areas of bronchial mucoepidermoid carcinoma showing a mix of all cell types

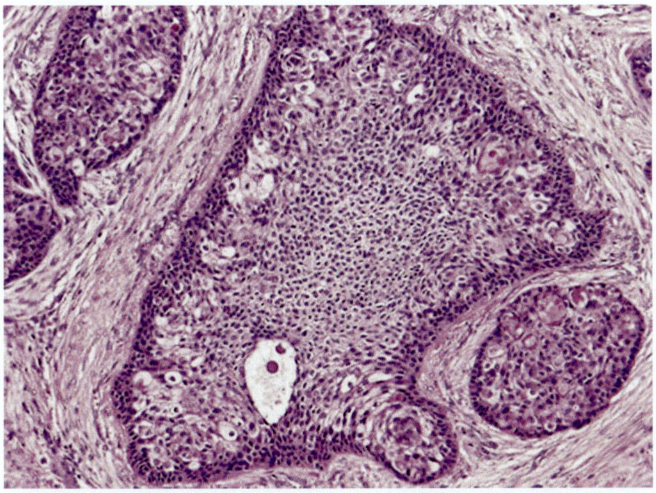

Fig. 6.3 Prominent epidermoid component in mucoepidermoid carcinoma lacking keratinization

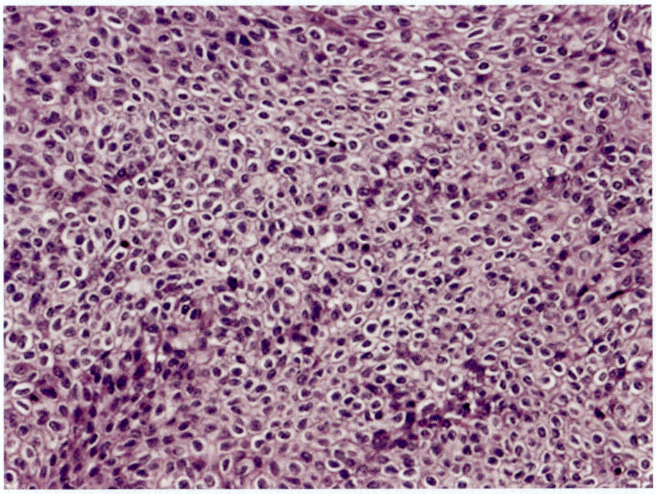

Fig. 6.4 Intermediate cells with lack of cytologic atypia or mitotic activity

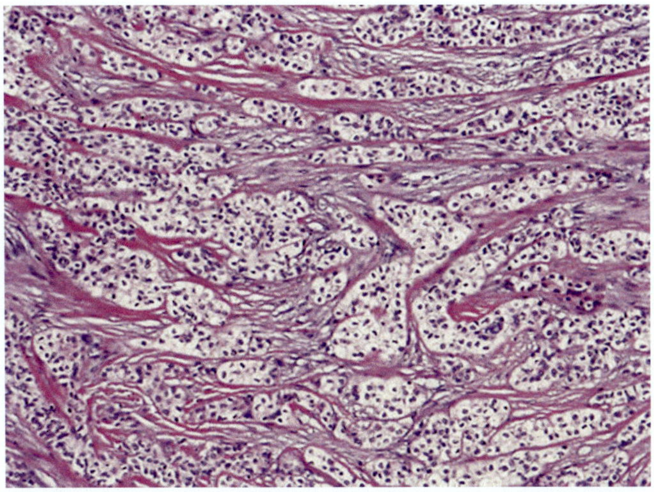

Fig. 6.5 Clear cell change in intermediate cells of mucoepidermoid carcinoma

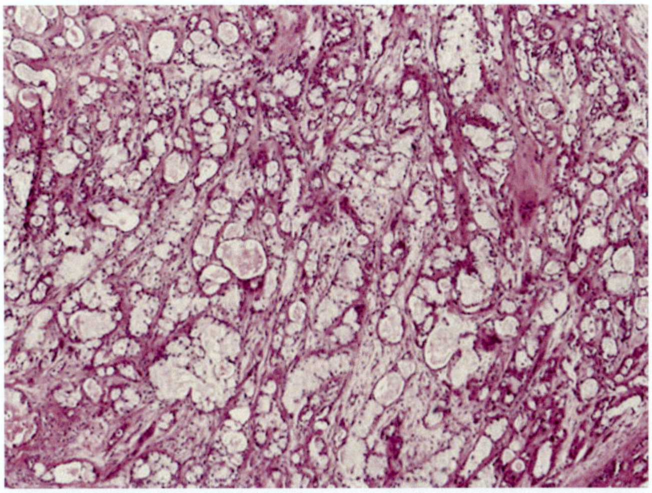

Fig. 6.6 Mucinous cells in bronchial mucoepidermoid carcinoma

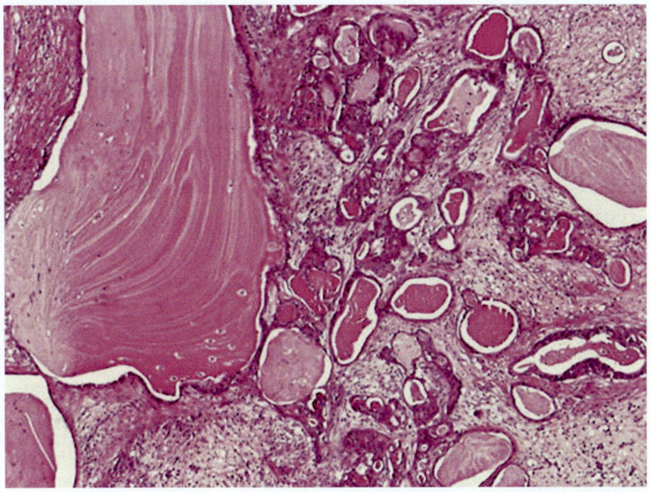

Fig. 6.7 Cysts of varying size are a typical finding in mucoepidermoid carcinoma

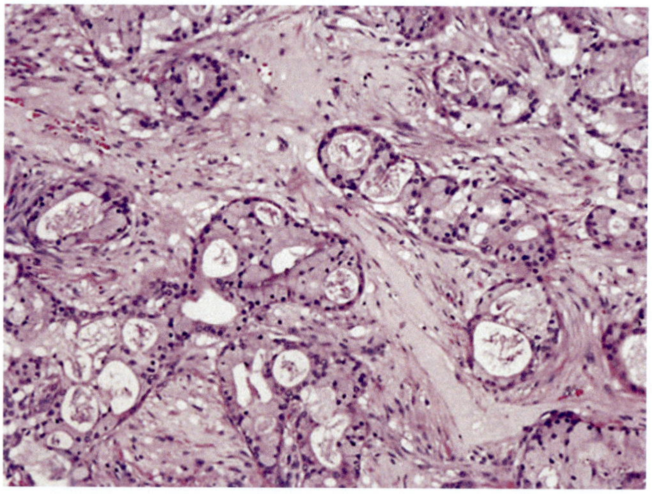

Fig. 6.8 Cystic spaces lined by mucinous cells in mucoepidermoid carcinoma

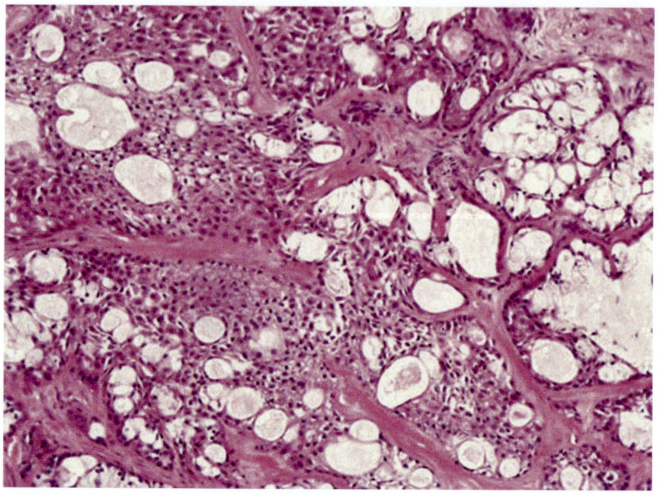

Fig. 6.10 Pulmonary mucoepidermoid carcinoma showing equal proportions of epidermoid and mucinous areas

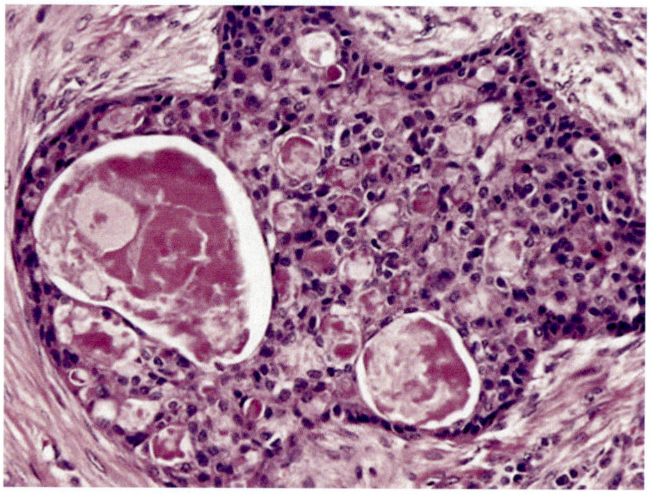

Fig. 6.9 Colloid-like material in the cystic lumina in mucoepidermoid carcinoma

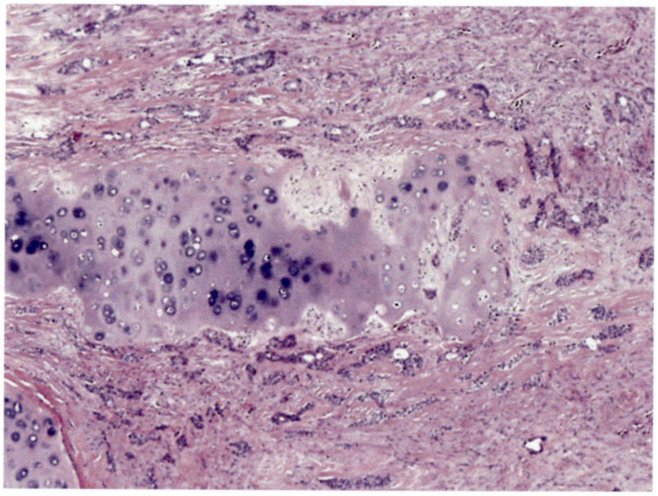

Fig. 6.11 High-grade mucoepidermoid carcinoma showing invasion of the bronchial cartilage

so prominent as to reach equal proportions (Fig. 6.10). High-grade mucoepidermoid tumors show a higher incidence of infiltration into the lung parenchyma and more often display extensive solid growth of epidermoid or intermediate cells (Fig. 6.11). On a cytologic level, they show more marked atypia, nuclear hyperchromatism, and mitotic activity (>4 per 10 high-power fields) (Fig. 6.12). In addition, areas of necrosis and hemorrhage are more often seen in these higher-grade neoplasms (Fig. 6.13). Papillary areas may also be identified, and the stroma often shows sclerotic changes, dense hyalinized "amyloid-like" material, or prominent lymphoid infiltration [9, 10] (Figs. 6.14 and 6.15). Areas of calcification are another typical finding in these tumors [5] (Fig. 6.16).

Immunohistochemical Features and Molecular Features

Immunohistochemical investigations do not play a prominent role in the diagnosis of pulmonary mucoepidermoid carcinoma as they show a similar immunohistochemical phenotype as conventional non-small cell carcinoma. Of more practical use in difficult cases would be a histochemical stain, like mucicarmine or periodic acid-Schiff (PAS), to confirm the presence of intracytoplasmic mucin in the glandular component of the tumor (Fig. 6.17). Recent cytogenetic analysis has demonstrated the presence of multiple reciprocal translocations among mucoepidermoid carcinomas of salivary gland and lung origin. These include t(11;19)

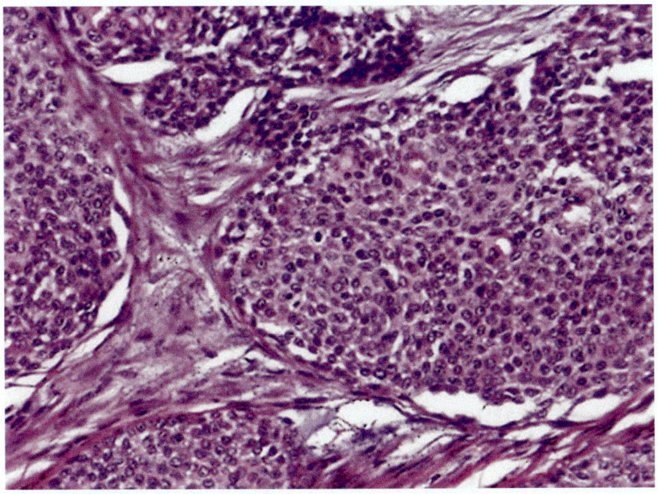

Fig. 6.12 High-grade mucoepidermoid carcinoma displaying mitotic activity

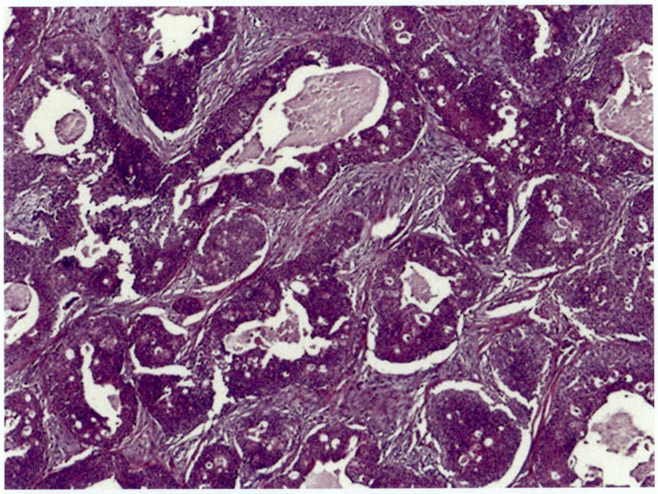

Fig. 6.13 Comedo-type necrosis is high-grade mucoepidermoid carcinoma

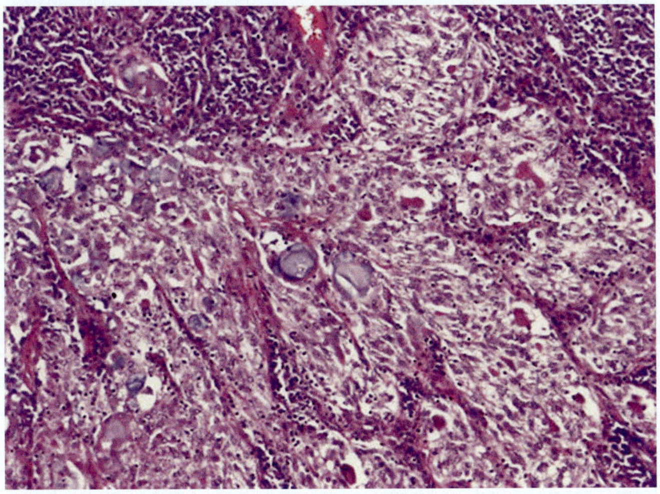

Fig. 6.14 Infiltration by lymphoid cells in high-grade mucoepidermoid carcinoma

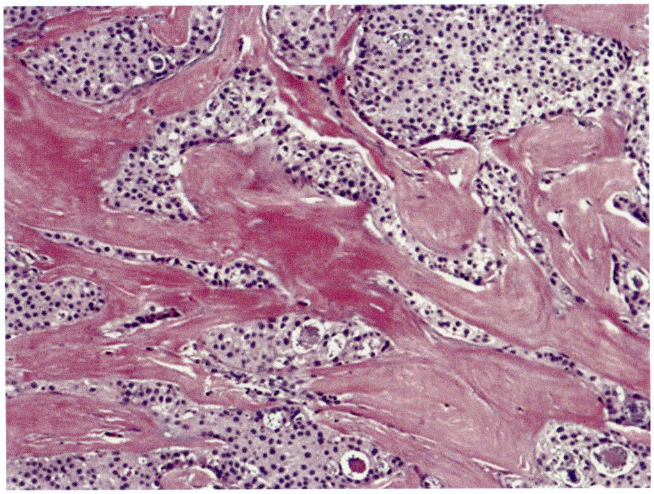

Fig. 6.15 Prominent stromal sclerosis in mucoepidermoid carcinoma

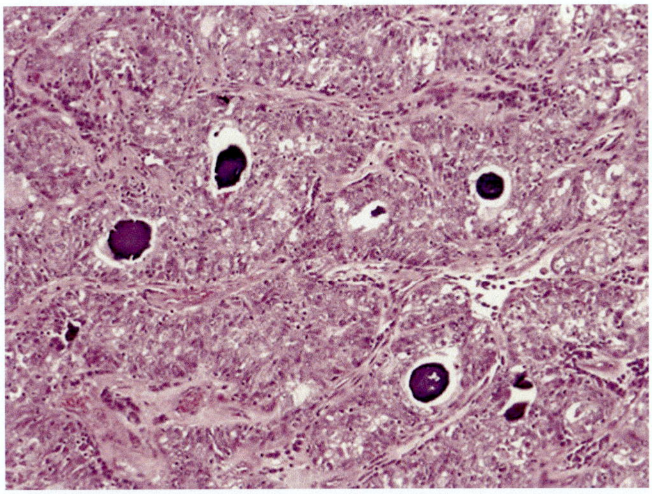

Fig. 6.16 Focal calcification is a common finding in bronchial mucoepidermoid carcinoma

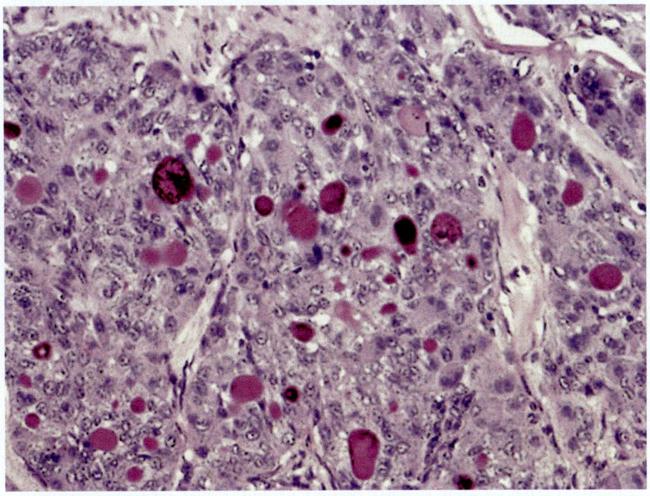

Fig. 6.17 PAS histochemical stain highlighting areas of mucinous differentiation in mucoepidermoid carcinoma

leading to a fusion product, the mucoepidermoid carcinoma translocated 1-mastermind-like2 (MECT1-MAML2) and t(1;11), resulting in cyclin D1 overexpression [11, 12]. Mutational status for epidermal growth factor receptor (EGFR) and Kras has been investigated in several small series with variable results. Whereas some authors found EGFR mutations in up to 40 % of their cases [13], other groups demonstrated an absence of EGFR and Kras mutations in these tumors [14, 15]. Echinoderm microtubule-associated protein-like 4-anaplastic lymphoma kinase (EML4-ALK) fusion oncogene was recently identified in one mucoepidermoid carcinoma of the lung in a study investigating the mutational status of 266 lung carcinomas [16].

Differential Diagnosis

Low-grade mucoepidermoid carcinoma can be confused with mucous gland adenoma. Mucous gland adenoma is a benign proliferation of the bronchial glands, which may closely resemble the low-grade variant of mucoepidermoid carcinoma especially in small biopsy specimens. The most distinguishing feature between these lesions is the confinement of mucous gland adenoma to the bronchial wall, whereas mucoepidermoid carcinoma often invades beyond the cartilage. High-grade mucoepidermoid carcinoma may be mistaken for adenosquamous carcinoma. The former is characterized by its central location, absence of an in situ component, and areas of low-grade mucoepidermoid carcinoma associated with the high-grade elements. Microcystic squamous cell carcinoma of the lung is an unusual variant of squamous cell carcinoma histologically mimicking tumors with glandular or adnexal differentiation. The presence of intermediate cells and absence of keratinization should be the most distinguishing features in favor of mucoepidermoid carcinoma in this context. Lastly, complete clinical history is an important tool to rule out metastatic disease from a salivary gland primary.

Treatment and Prognosis

The prognosis of these tumors is related to their grade and stage. Patients with low-grade mucoepidermoid carcinoma are expected to be cured following complete surgical resection, whereas high-grade tumors require lymph node sampling and dissection as well as close clinical follow-up [5, 6]. The role and efficacy of irradiation or chemotherapy is not well defined; however, recent reports indicate that tyrosine kinase inhibitors like gefitinib may be effective in pulmonary mucoepidermoid carcinoma despite an absence of sensitizing EGFR mutations [13, 14]. Low-grade mucoepidermoid carcinomas of the lung have a relatively good prognosis with reported 5-year survival rates ranging from 57.1 to 80 % [6, 8]. High-grade lesions have a worse clinical outcome reflected in a 5-year survival rate of only 31 % [6]. One of the most important prognostic factors for high-grade mucoepidermoid carcinoma appears to be lymph node involvement emphasizing the significance of tumor-nodes-metastasis (TNM) staging and adequate lymph node sampling in these tumors [5, 6].

Pulmonary Adenoid Cystic Carcinoma

Clinical Features

Adenoid cystic carcinoma is the second most frequent salivary gland type tumor of the lung. It predominantly affects adults with a reported age range from 21 to 79 years and a peak incidence in the sixth decade [4, 7, 17]. There appears to be a slight male predominance [17]. The tumors most often arise in the proximal bronchial tree [18, 19] although isolated cases (<10 %) have been described to originate in the peripheral lung [20]. Symptoms are typically related to bronchial obstruction due to the endobronchial location of the tumors and include cough, wheezing, hemoptysis, shortness of breath, and pneumonia [7, 17]. The most common abnormality on chest X-ray is a single endobronchial mass associated with obstructive pneumonia, atelectasis, or pleural effusion [4]. Peripheral solitary lung masses that are often incidental findings are less commonly seen [4].

Gross Features

The common gross presentation is that of an endobronchial, soft tan-colored, and well-circumscribed mass. The size of the lesions ranges from less than 1–4 cm. In some instances the tumors are less well defined and show infiltrative borders [17].

Histological Features

Histologically, three growth patterns have been described in keeping with those seen in adenoid cystic carcinoma of the salivary glands. The cribriform pattern is the most common and predominant one and can be seen in up to 74.4 % of cases [7, 17] (Fig. 6.18). This pattern is characterized by nests of tumor cells that have abundant sharply punched-out pseudoluminal spaces that contain mucinous or basement-membrane-like material (Figs. 6.19 and 6.20). The individual tumor cells are small with hyperchromatic round to angulated nuclei and a sparse rim of amphophilic cytoplasm (Fig. 6.21). Peripheral palisading in the tumor islands can be

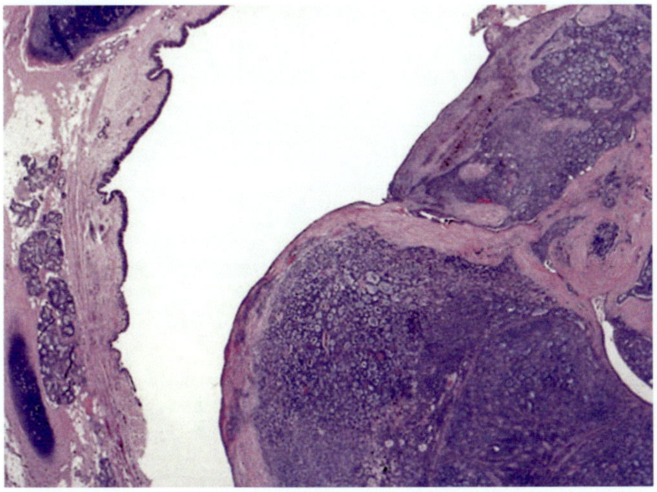

Fig. 6.18 Low-power view of bronchial adenoid cystic carcinoma with cribriform growth pattern

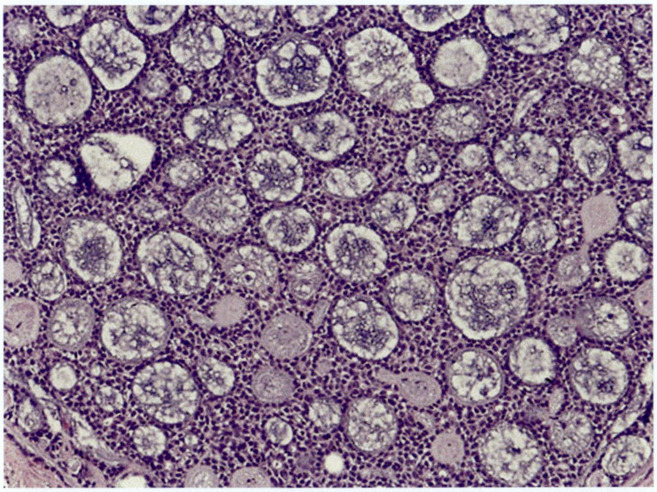

Fig. 6.19 Cribriform pattern of pulmonary adenoid cystic carcinoma showing sharply punched-out spaces separating the tumor cells

identified in some cases imparting a basaloid appearance. The second most common pattern (17.9 %) is the tubular type [7, 17]. This consists of cells forming scattered gland-like spaces with central lumina lined by cells that have identical features to those seen in the cribriform pattern (Figs. 6.22 and 6.23). Pink amorphous material is often noted in the luminal spaces. The least frequently seen type is the solid one amounting to about 7.7 % of cases [7, 17] (Fig. 6.24). Here, the cells form sheets and nests of tumor with few or no luminal spaces and more vesicular nuclei with an open chromatin pattern (Fig. 6.25). Contrary to the cribriform and tubular patterns, where mitotic activity is virtually absent, occasional mitotic figures can be identified in the solid variant [17]. Although perineural invasion is a frequent finding, necrosis, hemorrhage, and nuclear pleomorphism are not common features (Fig. 6.26).

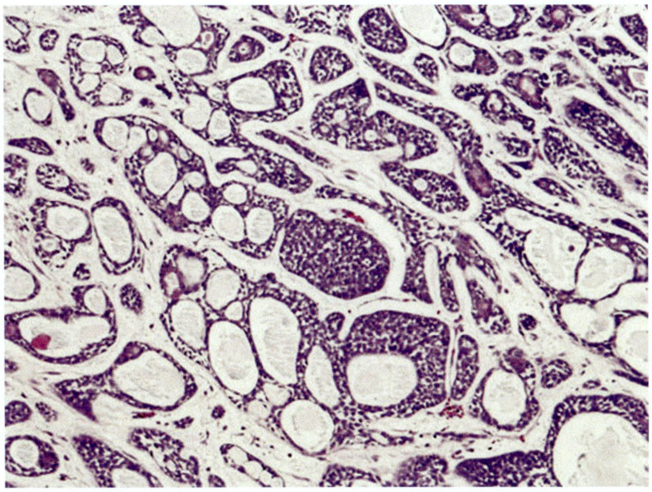

Fig. 6.20 Adenoid cystic carcinoma showing predominantly cribriform growth pattern, smaller areas of more solid growth can be appreciated focally

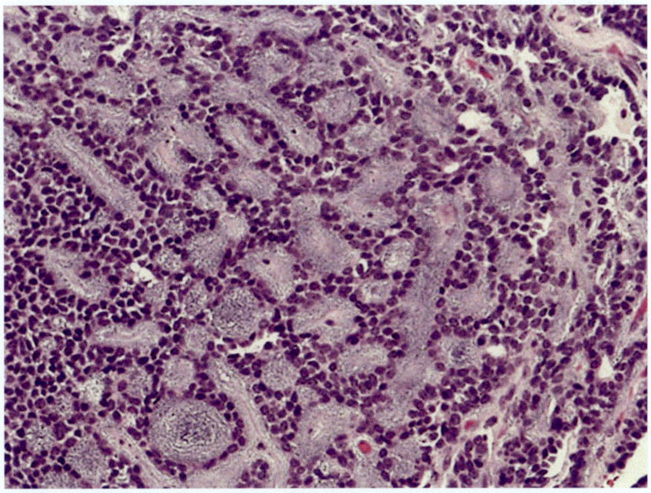

Fig. 6.21 Tumor cells are composed of small angulated cells with scant cytoplasm and bland nuclear features

Metastatic deposits in lymph nodes or other organs typically show the same histologic appearance as the main tumor.

Immunohistochemical and Molecular Features

Immunohistochemically, adenoid cystic carcinomas show evidence of epithelial and myoepithelial differentiation [2]. Therefore, the tumor cells express cytokeratin, CAM5.2, vimentin, and smooth muscle actin and show variable reactivity for S100 [17, 21, 22]. More recently, c-kit and EGFR protein expression has been demonstrated in the majority of these tumors [15, 23]. C-kit and EGFR mutations, however, have not been identified in these tumors, casting doubt on any clinical benefit from tyrosine kinase inhibitors [15, 23].

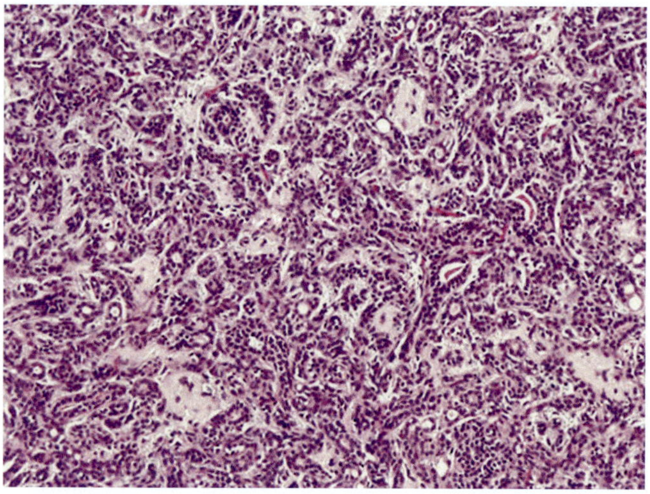

Fig. 6.22 Tubular pattern in adenoid cystic carcinoma containing numerous tubular or gland-like structures

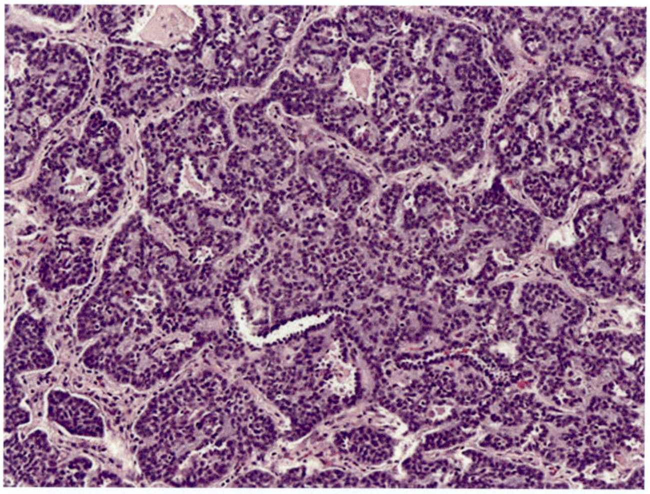

Fig. 6.23 The tumor cells in the tubular growth pattern show similar characteristics to those in the cribriform type

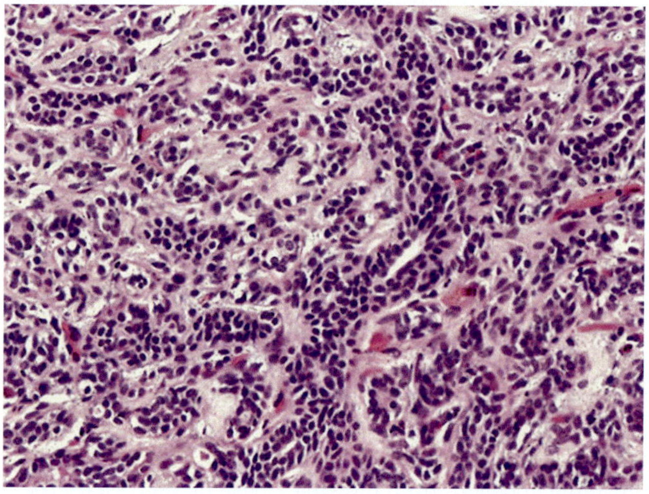

Fig. 6.24 Solid pattern in bronchial adenoid cystic carcinoma

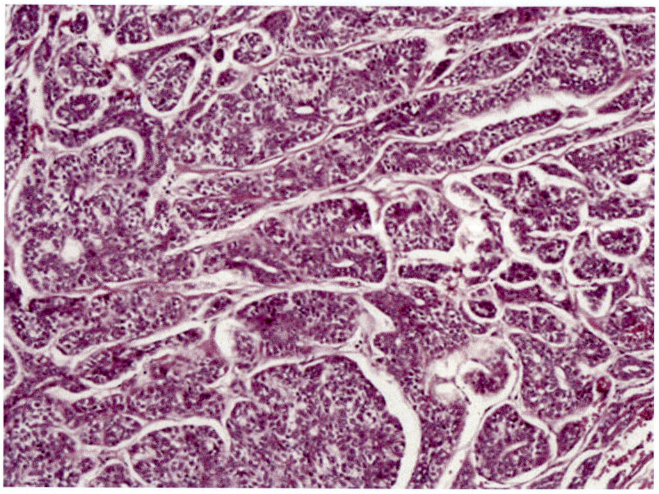

Fig. 6.25 Cytologic features in the solid variant of adenoid cystic carcinoma with slightly larger tumor cells and more vesicular nuclear chromatin pattern

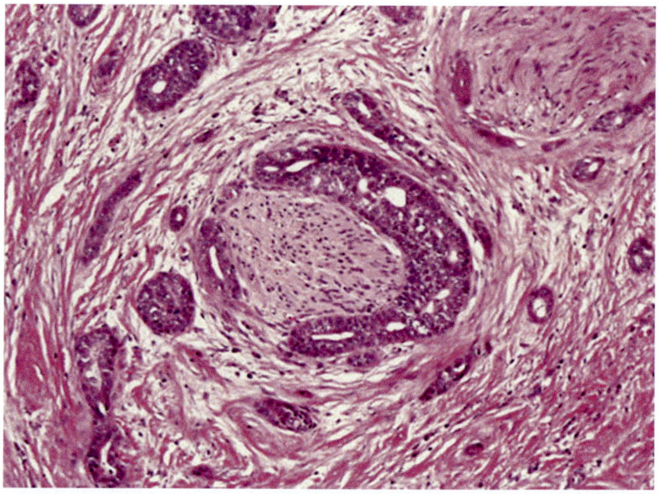

Fig. 6.26 Characteristic perineural invasion in pulmonary adenoid cystic carcinoma

Differential Diagnosis

Although the morphologic features of adenoid cystic carcinoma are often distinctive enough to allow correct diagnosis, the tumor may sometimes be mistaken for other neoplasms like conventional pulmonary adenocarcinoma and other salivary gland type tumors of the lung such as pleomorphic adenoma. Pulmonary adenocarcinoma does not contain myoepithelial cells and lacks coexpression of cytokeratin, smooth muscle actin, and vimentin. In addition, adenocarcinoma typically displays more nuclear pleomorphism, necrosis, and hemorrhage—features that are usually absent in adenoid cystic carcinoma. Pleomorphic adenoma is a rare lesion of the lung that can share similar histological and immunohistochemical characteristics with adenoid cystic carcinoma. Careful evaluation of the lesion for the more typical cribriform growth pattern of adenoid cystic carcinoma may be the only distinguishing feature. Importantly, exclusion of metastasis from a primary adenoid cystic carcinoma of the salivary gland is essential in the assessment of these tumors.

Treatment and Prognosis

Although initially thought to be a slow-growing and indolent neoplasm, adenoid cystic carcinoma of the lung has been shown to pursue a more aggressive clinical course than its counterpart in the salivary glands, and complete surgical resection is the treatment of choice [4, 17, 24]. Since these tumors are known to show a high incidence of submucosal extension and tendency to recur locally, frozen section at the time of surgery is recommended to assess the margin status [20]. In addition, postoperative radiotherapy is often administered in cases of incomplete resection or residual disease [25–27]. Lymph node involvement and metastasis are frequent phenomena in these tumors, and survival rates are 73 % at 3 years, 57 % at 5 years, and 45 % at 10 years [7]. Overall, tumor stage and complete surgical resection seem to be the most predictive determinants of outcome [4, 7, 17].

Pulmonary Acinic Cell Carcinoma

Clinical Features

Acinic cell carcinoma of the lung or "Fechner tumor" was first described by Fechner et al. in 1972 as a solitary lung tumor that was histologically, immunohistochemically, and ultrastructurally identical to acinic cell carcinoma of the salivary gland [28]. This tumor is one of the rarest salivary gland type neoplasms occurring in the lung, with less than 20 cases of primary tracheal or bronchopulmonary tumors described to date [28–41]. Adults are affected more commonly, but several cases have also been described in children (age range 4–75, average age 45 years). The male-to-female ratio is 5:4. The tumors may arise in the trachea, central bronchial system, distal airways, or pulmonary parenchyma. Presenting symptoms include hemoptysis, dyspnea, cough, or recurrent pneumonia, although patients with parenchymal lesions are often asymptomatic. On chest X-ray, the lesions are either solitary masses or present with secondary changes such as pneumonia or atelectasis. In some rare instances, combined acinic cell carcinomas and typical carcinoid tumors have been described in the lung [42–44].

Gross Features

Acinic cell carcinomas of the lung may present as endotracheal or endobronchial lesions or as parenchymal or subpleural nodules. The tumors are well-circumscribed but unencapsulated masses ranging in size from 1.2 to 4.2 cm [28, 30]. The cut surface is usually tan-white or yellow in color and of rubbery or soft consistency.

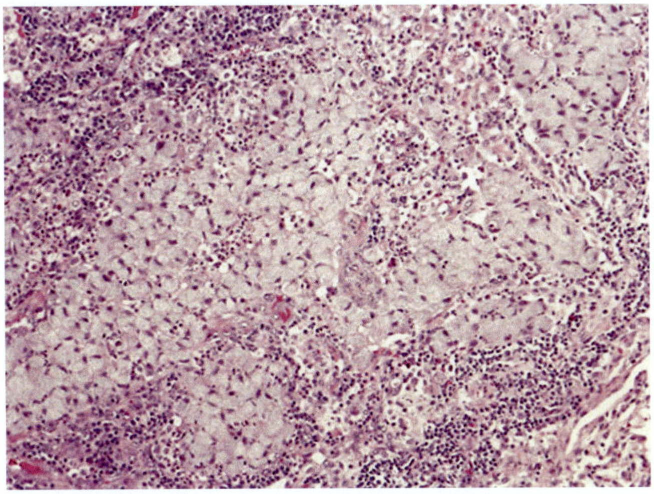

Fig. 6.27 Pulmonary acinic cell carcinoma composed of sheets of polygonal cells with prominent granular cytoplasm

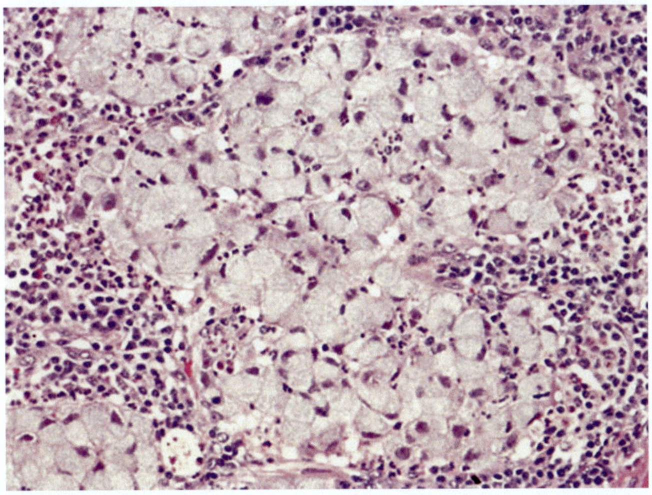

Fig. 6.28 High-power view of acinic cell carcinoma with tumor cells mimicking signet ring cell carcinoma

Histological Features

Histologically, the tumors are characterized by a solid proliferation of large, cohesive cells of polygonal shape and abundant granular cytoplasm (Fig. 6.27). The nuclei are small, round to oval shaped, and either centrally placed or diplaced toward the periphery, imparting a signet ring cell appearance (Fig. 6.28). Large vesicular nuclei with marked nuclear pleomorphism and prominent nucleoli may be identified in isolated cases (Fig. 6.29). In addition to a solid arrangement of these cells, areas showing acinar,

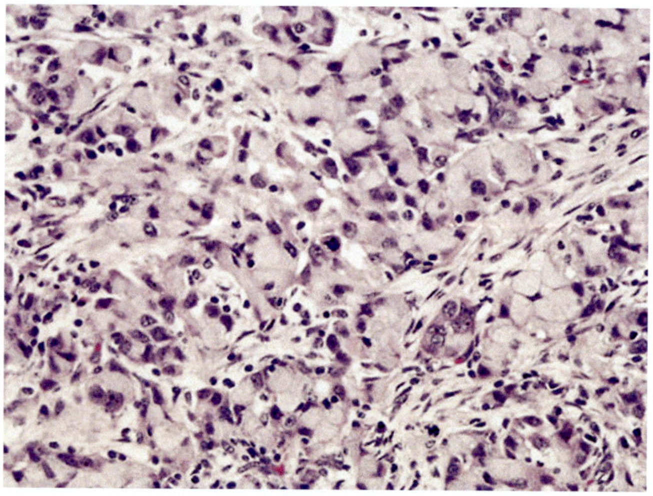

Fig. 6.29 Acinic cell carcinoma demonstrating areas of nuclear pleomorphism and rare mitotic figures

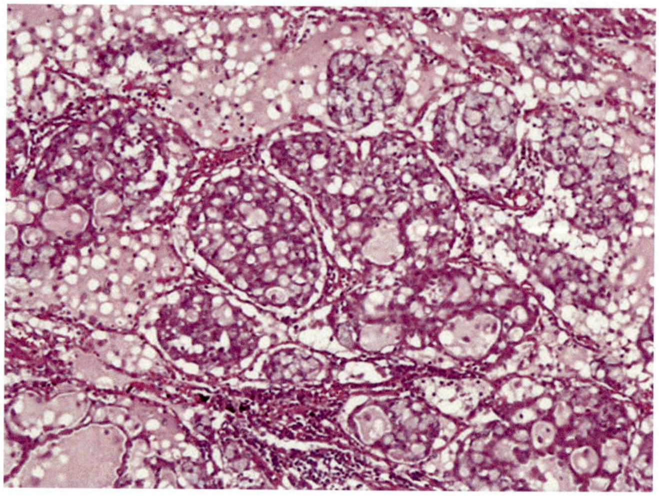

Fig. 6.31 Microcystic change in acinic cell carcinoma of the lung

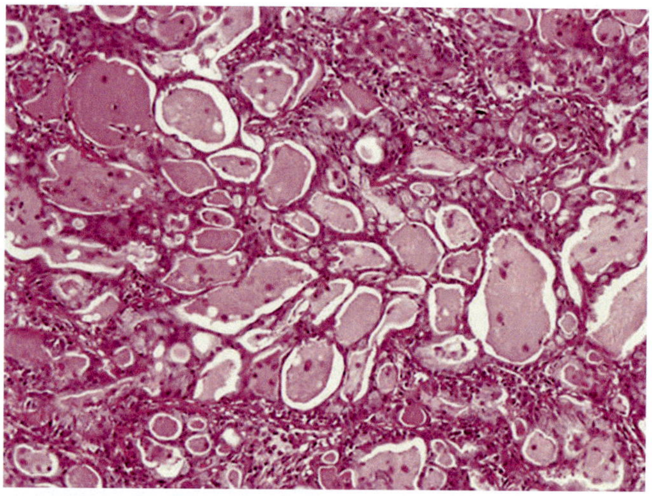

Fig. 6.30 Acinar pattern in pulmonary acinic cell carcinoma

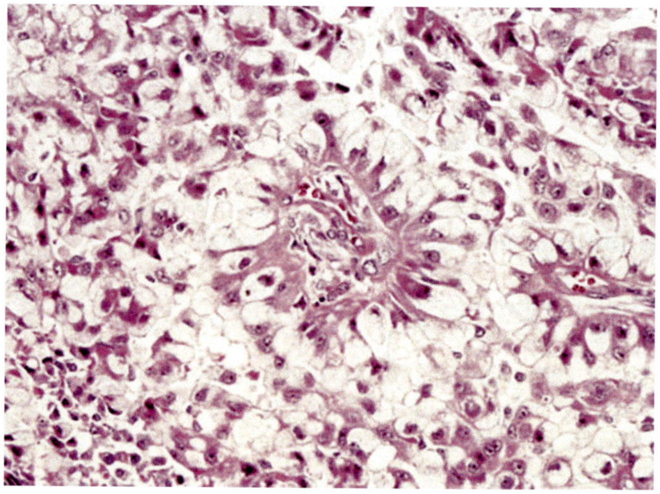

Fig. 6.32 Papillary areas can sometimes be identified in pulmonary acinic cell carcinoma

microcystic, or papillocystic growth patterns may be seen (Figs. 6.30, 6.31, and 6.32). Mitotic activity is usually low to absent and necrosis is not typically seen. The cells are often traversed by bands of connective tissue carrying a lymphoplasmacytic infiltrate or are separated by a prominent vasculature [30, 32] (Fig.6.33). Perineural invasion has been described in a single case [29].

Immunohistochemical and Ultrastructural Features

Acinic cell carcinomas of the lung show an epithelial immunohistochemical phenotype with reactivity for low molecular weight cytokeratins (CAM5.2), epithelial membrane antigen, and cytokeratin. Occasionally, the tumor may also express markers like α(alpha)-1-antichymotrypsin and

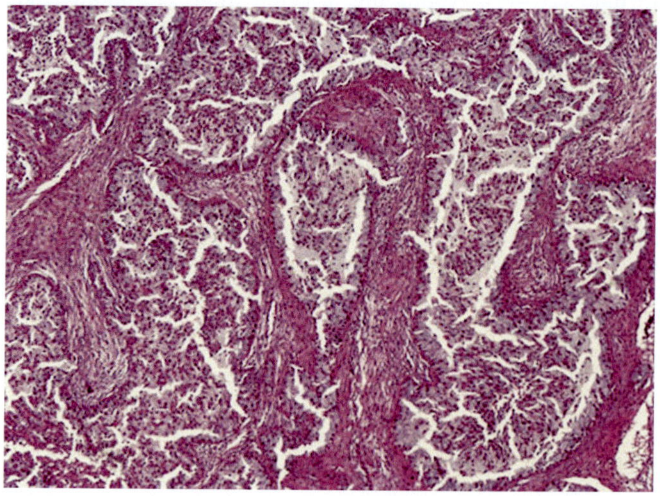

Fig. 6.33 Acinic cell carcinoma traversed by fibrous stromal bands

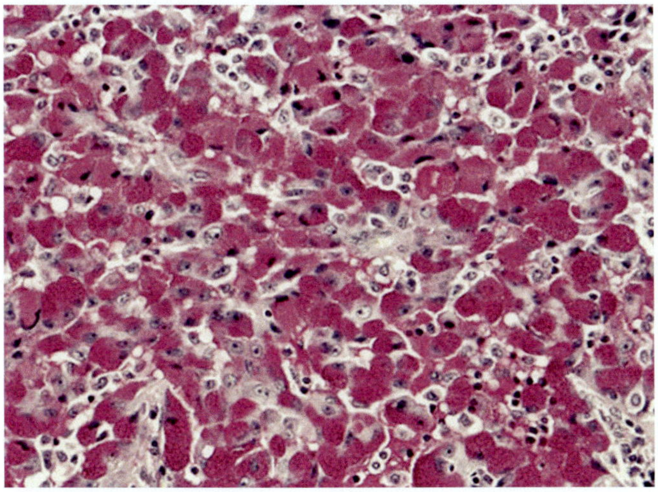

Fig. 6.34 Strong positivity with a PAS histochemical stain is usually seen in acinic cell carcinoma

amylase, while vimentin, S100, HMB45, chromogranin, and synaptophysin are usually negative. A characteristic finding is diffuse positivity of the tumor cells for PAS histochemical staining, which is resistant to diastase digestion. Mucicarmine histochemical stain is usually negative, however, focal positive staining may be seen. [28–30] (Fig. 6.34). Ultrastructurally, the tumor cells contain abundant zymogen-type cytoplasmic granules each measuring 600–800 nm in size characteristic of acinar-type secretory cells [28–30, 32].

Differential Diagnosis

Since acinic cell carcinoma of the lung is such a rare neoplasm, the tumor is often confused with other lesions in which the tumor cells show granular or clear cell change features. These include granular cell tumor, sugar tumor, oncocytic carcinoid tumor, pulmonary oncocytoma, clear cell adenocarcinoma, and metastatic renal cell carcinoma. Granular cell tumor has a granular cytoplasm with eosinophilic appearance contrary to the basophilic color of acinic cell carcinoma. In addition, granular cell tumors display immunoreactivity with S100 protein and are negative for epithelial markers and PAS histochemical staining. Sugar tumor of the lung is another rare neoplasm with bland cytologic features and clear cell appearance. Sugar tumor, although also positive for PAS, is typically positive for HMB45 and negative for epithelial immunomarkers. Ultrastructural examinations are the most important tool to differentiate acinic cell carcinoma of the lung from oncocytic carcinoid and pulmonary oncocytoma. Oncocytic carcinoid tumors contain cytoplasmic electron-dense neurosecretory granules, and oncocytomas are characterized by mitochondrial hyperplasia; these features are distinct from the zymogen-type granules typically seen in acinic cell carcinoma. Primary clear cell adenocarcinoma will display a higher degree of cytologic atypia and mitotic activity as well as an absence of distinctive granules on ultrastructural examination. Lastly, metastatic renal cell carcinoma may be mistaken for acinic cell carcinoma of the lung. Metastatic renal cell carcinoma is usually found in patients with a clinical history of a renal tumor. A PAS stain in renal cell carcinoma may also show a positive reaction although not as strong as that seen acinic cell carcinoma. Nevertheless, the morphological appearance of both tumors is distinct enough to separate them.

Treatment and Prognosis

Similar to acinic cell carcinomas of the salivary glands, their counterparts in the lungs are considered indolent neoplasms that carry a favorable prognosis and complete surgical resection is the treatment of choice. However, local recurrence and lymph node metastasis have been reported in isolated cases advocating close clinical follow-up for all patients [29, 32, 36, 45]. Due to the small number of cases of primary pulmonary acinic cell carcinoma, the role of radiation or chemotherapy is still unknown and the assessment of adverse prognostic factors is limited. The presence of mitotic activity, perineural invasion, and lymph node metastasis has been proposed as negative prognostic markers in this context [45].

Pulmonary Pleomorphic Adenoma/Carcinoma Ex Pleomorphic Adenoma

Clinical Features

While pleomorphic adenoma is the most common neoplasm in the salivary glands, it is exceedingly rare in the tracheobronchial tree. To date, only 35 of these neoplasms have been reported in the literature [46]. Even smaller is the number of pleomorphic adenomas displaying malignant features (carcinoma ex pleomorphic adenoma) in this location [47–51]. Together, these tumors affect mainly adults and rarely children with an age range from 8 to 76 years and a peak in the sixth decade [46–48, 51]. Whereas there is no clear gender predominance in pleomorphic adenoma [46], carcinoma ex pleomorphic adenoma is slightly more common in men [51]. Although most tumors are connected to the tracheobronchial system, lesions arising in the peripheral lung have also been described [48]. Symptoms depend on tumor location: Endobronchial lesions may cause shortness of breath, cough, hemoptysis, fever, and pleural effusion, while peripheral tumors are often incidental findings [48, 51]. Recently, the simultaneous occurrence of a bronchial pleomorphic adenoma with conventional non-small cell lung cancer has been reported [46].

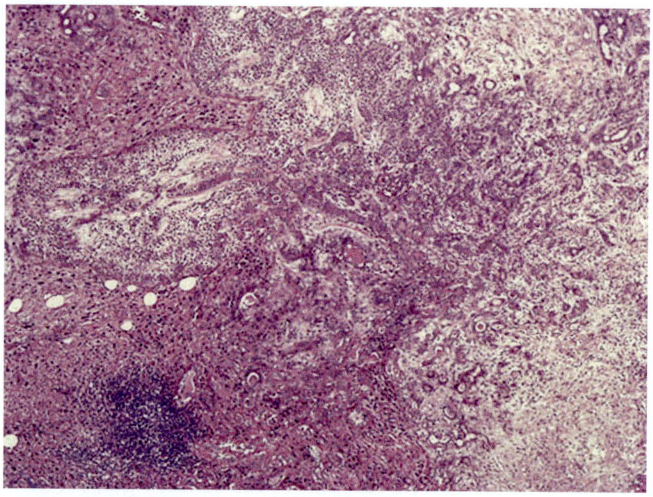

Fig. 6.35 Pulmonary pleomorphic adenoma composed of mixed epithelial, myoepithelial, and stromal components

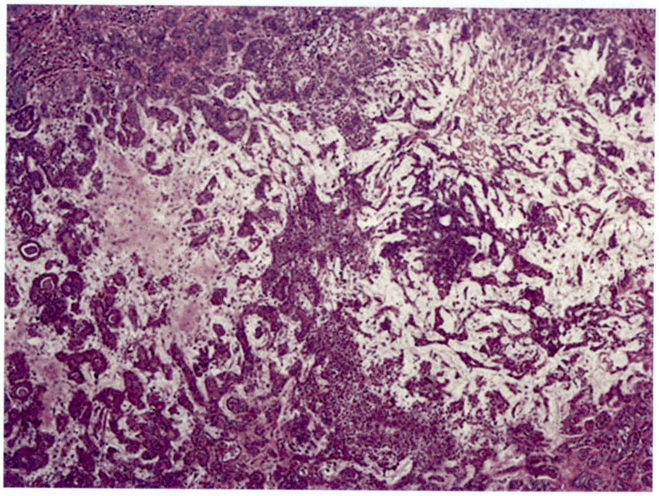

Fig. 6.36 Prominent myxoid stroma, solid myoepithelial proliferation, and scattered duct-like structures in pleomorphic adenoma of the lung

Gross Features

On gross inspection endobronchial tumors often present as polypoid masses protruding into the bronchial lumen, while peripheral lesions are usually well-circumscribed and sometimes lobulated tumors. The size can range from 2 cm to more than 15 cm. The cut surface is gray-white in color and often has a soft or rubbery or myxoid appearance. Areas of hemorrhage can be seen in the malignant lesions [48, 51].

Histological Features

Pleomorphic adenomas are biphasic tumors characterized by benign epithelial, myoepithelial, and stromal components (Figs. 6.35, 6.36, and 6.37). The histological composition of these tumors arising in the lung is similar to those seen in the salivary glands. On low power, endobronchial tumors present as well-defined polypoid masses protruding into the luminal space, while peripheral tumors are circumscribed lesions clearly separated from the surrounding lung parenchyma (Fig. 6.38). On higher magnification, the epithelial component is growing in nests, tubules, or duct-like structures (Fig. 6.39). These ducts are typically composed of two cell layers, inner cuboidal luminal cells and an outer rim of myoepithelial cells (Fig. 6.40). Some tumors may show a more solid and cellular proliferation of predominantly myoepithelial cells reminiscent of the cellular variant of pleomorphic adenoma of the salivary glands (Fig. 6.41). The myoepithelial cells may further display the whole spectrum of changes typically attributed to them including plasmacytoid, spindle cell, or clear cell change (Figs. 6.42 and 6.43). This epithelial component merges with a characteristic chondromyxoid stroma containing bland spindle or stellate cells

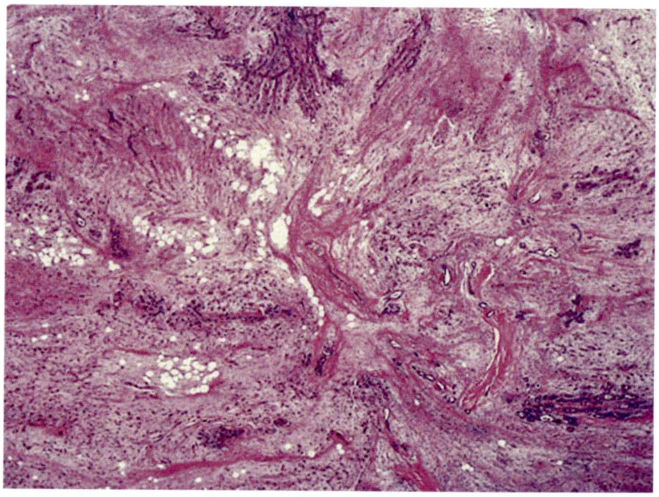

Fig. 6.37 Pulmonary pleomorphic adenoma composed of myxoid stroma, fat, and myoepithelial proliferation

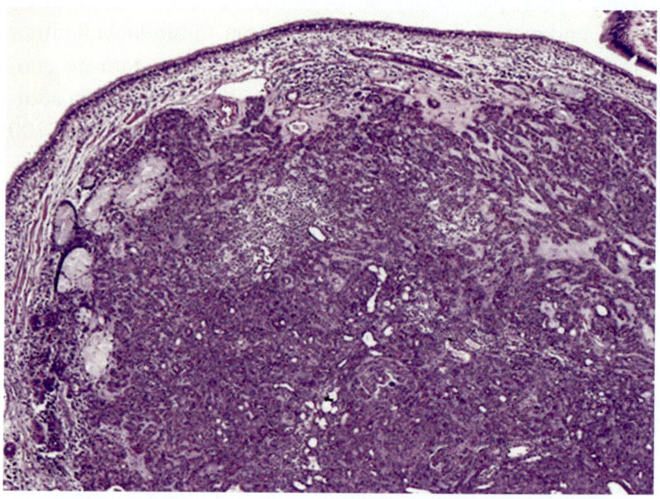

Fig. 6.38 Endobronchial growth of bronchial pleomorphic adenoma

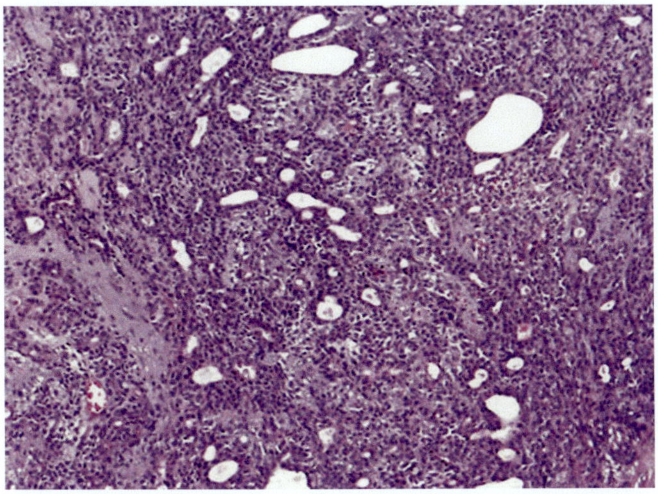

Fig. 6.39 Epithelial component of pleomorphic adenoma characterized by gland-like structures

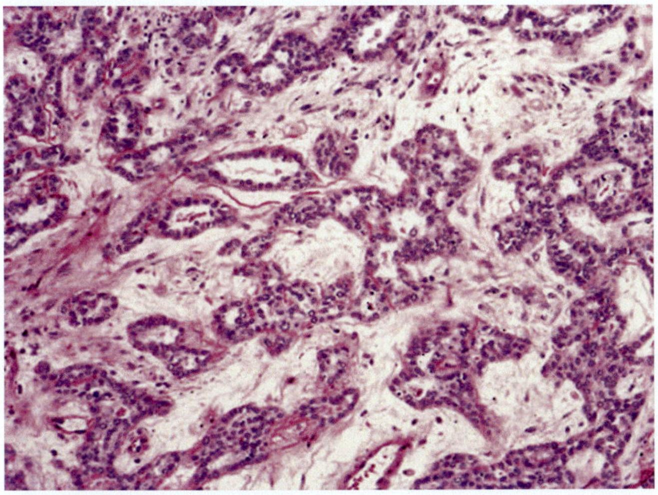

Fig. 6.40 Tubular structures in pulmonary pleomorphic adenoma composed of inner epithelial and inner myoepithelial cells

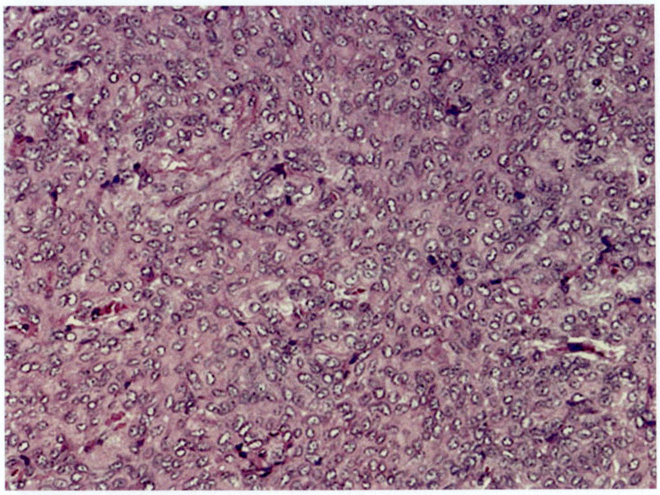

Fig. 6.41 Solid proliferation of myoepithelial cells in pulmonary pleomorphic adenoma

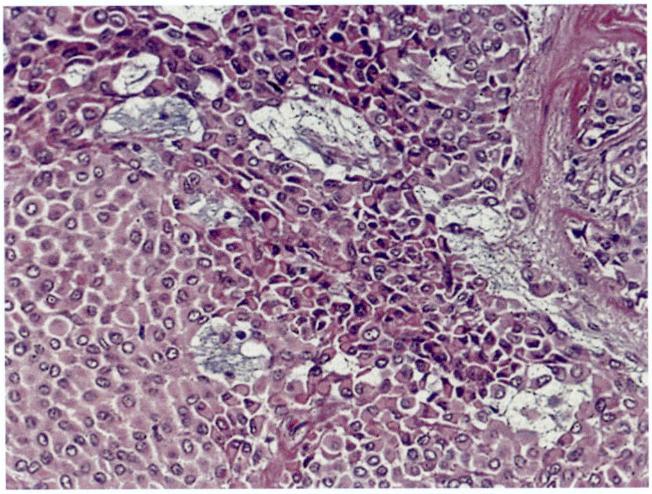

Fig. 6.42 Myoepithelial elements displaying a plasmacytoid appearance

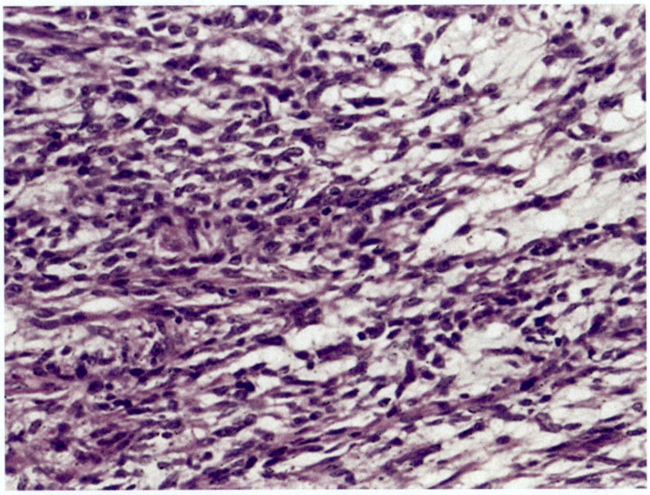

Fig. 6.43 Spindle cell formation in myoepithelial cells of pulmonary pleomorphic adenoma

and occasional inflammatory cells (Figs. 6.44 and 6.45). Cytologic atypia, mitotic activity, necrosis, or hemorrhage are usually lacking in these tumors; however, squamous metaplasia may be prominent (Fig. 6.46). Contrary to pleomorphic adenoma of salivary gland origin, well-developed cartilage is not a prominent feature in their pulmonary counterparts and ductal structures are also less conspicuous [48].

Carcinoma ex pleomorphic adenoma of the lung resembles benign pleomorphic adenoma in many aspects like cellular composition and a benign chondromyxoid stroma; however, carcinoma ex pleomorphic carcinoma shows subtle infiltrative margins and malignant features of the myoepithelial component characterized by cytologic atypia, mitotic activity, hemorrhage, necrosis, and vascular invasion (Figs. 6.47, 6.48, and 6.49). In some cases residual pleomorphic adenoma may be identified in addition to the malignant

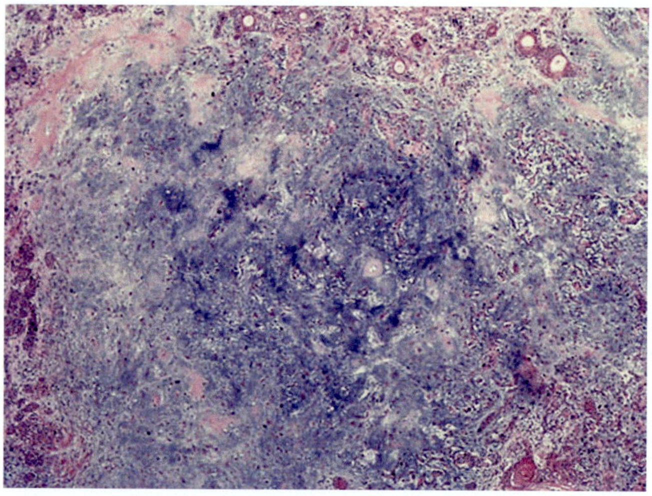

Fig. 6.44 Pleomorphic adenoma with prominent chondroid stroma

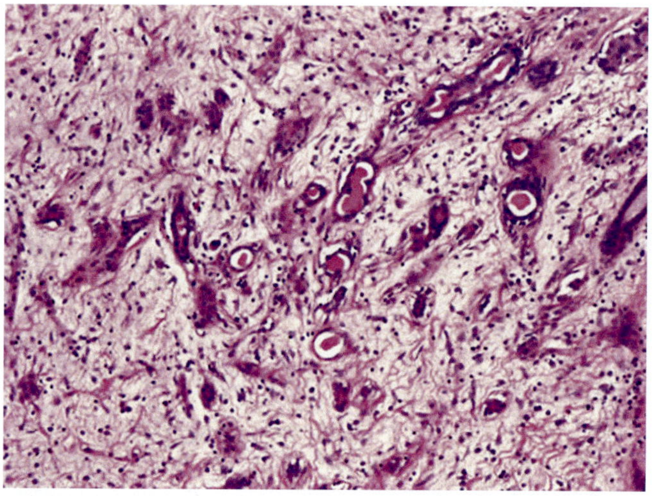

Fig. 6.45 Myxoid stromal background in pulmonary pleomorphic adenoma

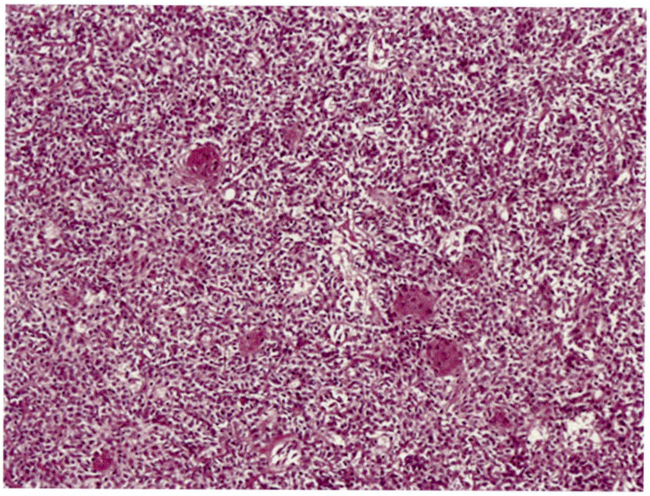

Fig. 6.46 Foci of squamous metaplasia in pleomorphic adenoma

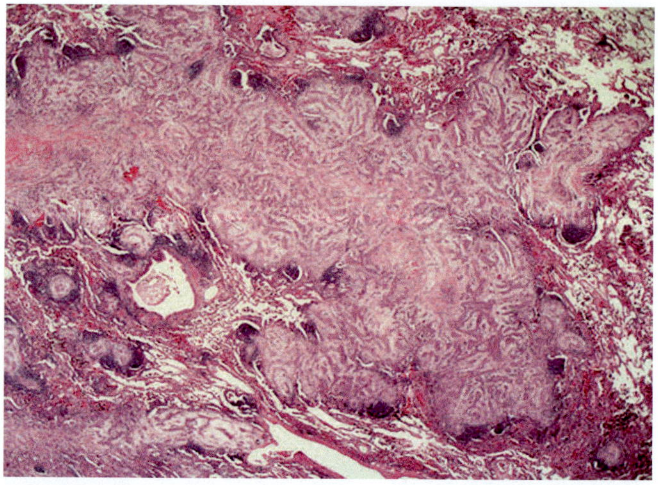

Fig. 6.47 Carcinoma ex pleomorphic adenoma showing infiltration into the surrounding lung parenchyma

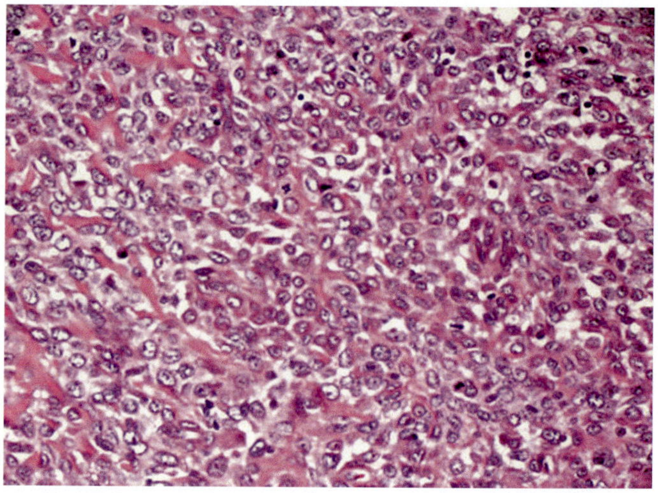

Fig. 6.48 Myoepithelial component showing increased mitotic activity in carcinoma ex pleomorphic adenoma of the lung

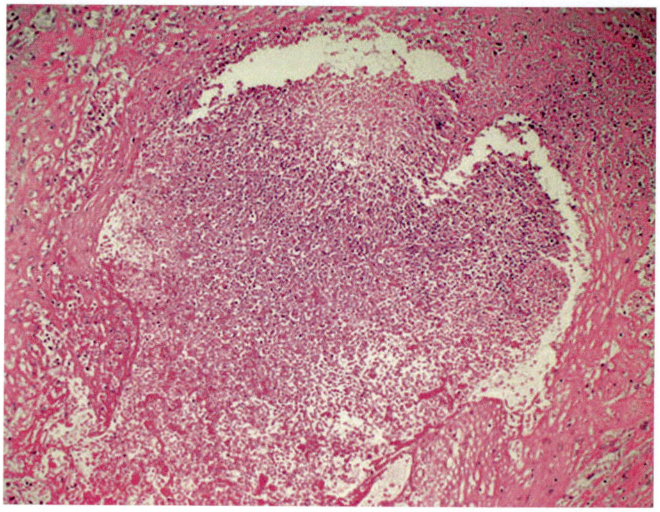

Fig. 6.49 Extensive necrosis in pulmonary carcinoma ex pleomorphic adenoma

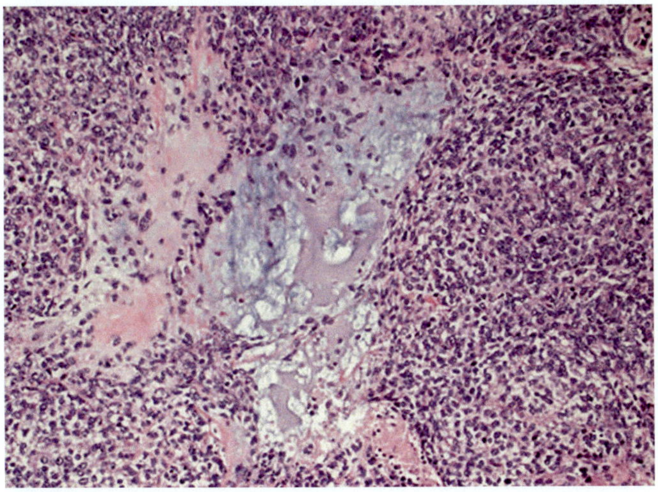

Fig. 6.50 Malignant myoepithelial proliferation in carcinoma ex pleomorphic adenoma

elements. Of note, whereas the malignant component in carcinoma ex pleomorphic adenoma is most often adenocarcinoma or salivary duct carcinoma, primary carcinoma ex pleomorphic adenoma of the lung most often shows malignant myoepithelial differentiation [47, 49–51] (Fig. 6.50).

Immunohistochemical Features

The immunohistochemical phenotype reflects the myoepithelial differentiation of pleomorphic adenoma and carcinoma ex pleomorphic adenoma. Positive markers include pancytokeratin, CAM5.2, CK7, CK14, SMA, S100, GFAP, and CD56.

Differential Diagnosis

The differential diagnosis largely depends on the type of specimen with which one is dealing. On small biopsy specimens, pleomorphic adenoma may be confused with chondroid hamartoma or other salivary gland type neoplasms, depending on which component is sampled. In chondroid hamartoma, the cartilaginous component is well developed and sharply demarcated from any glandular components contrary to pleomorphic adenoma. Adenoid cystic carcinoma is another salivary gland type tumor that may mimic pleomorphic adenoma. Here, the tumor nests are clearly separated from the connective tissue lacking the gradual transition seen in pleomorphic adenoma. In resection specimens, the biphasic pattern should be typical enough as to point to the correct diagnosis; however, tumors with a predominantly solid pattern may be mistaken for conventional non-small cell carcinoma of the lung. The latter tumors lack myoepithelial differentiation and will not show reactivity for the respective myoepithelial markers.

Two other biphasic tumors that may resemble carcinoma ex pleomorphic adenoma are carcinosarcoma and biphasic pulmonary blastoma. In carcinosarcoma, the presence of a malignant epithelial component (most often squamous cell carcinoma) and a differentiated malignant mesenchymal component (rhabdomyosarcoma, chondrosarcoma, etc.) should facilitate correct diagnosis. Biphasic pulmonary blastoma is characterized by a malignant glandular component with an embryonic-like appearance and areas of undifferentiated sarcoma separating this tumor from carcinoma ex pleomorphic adenoma.

Treatment and Prognosis

Complete surgical excision is the treatment of choice for both the benign and malignant variants of pulmonary pleomorphic adenoma. Whereas surgical intervention should be curative in the former due to the generally indolent behavior of this tumor, carcinoma ex pleomorphic adenoma displays an aggressive clinical course with early distant metastasis [48–51]. In this instance, patients may benefit from additional adjuvant treatment.

Pulmonary Epithelial-Myoepithelial Carcinoma

Clinical Features

To date, less than 30 primary pulmonary epithelial-myoepithelial carcinomas have been described [24, 52–66]. Epithelial-myoepithelial carcinoma of the lung is a low-grade malignant neoplasm composed of epithelial and myoepithelial elements. Although most cases affect the adult population (34–73 years) with a slight female predominance, a single case has been reported in a 7-year-old boy [65]. Like most other salivary gland type neoplasms, patients with pulmonary epithelial-myoepithelial carcinomas present with symptoms of bronchial obstruction (shortness of breath, cough, hemoptysis) due to the often endobronchial location of these tumors.

Gross Features

Grossly, epithelial-myoepithelial carcinomas present as polypoid endobronchial lesions with a size ranging from 0.6 to 16 cm (average 3.2 cm) [64]. The tumors are well circumscribed but unencapsulated. The cut surface is white to tan in color and of solid and firm consistency. Areas of necrosis or hemorrhage are not usually appreciated.

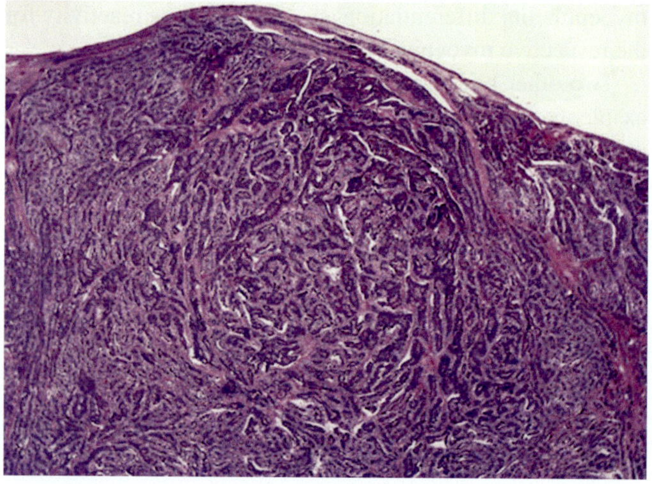

Fig. 6.51 Low-power view of endobronchial epithelial-myoepithelial carcinoma

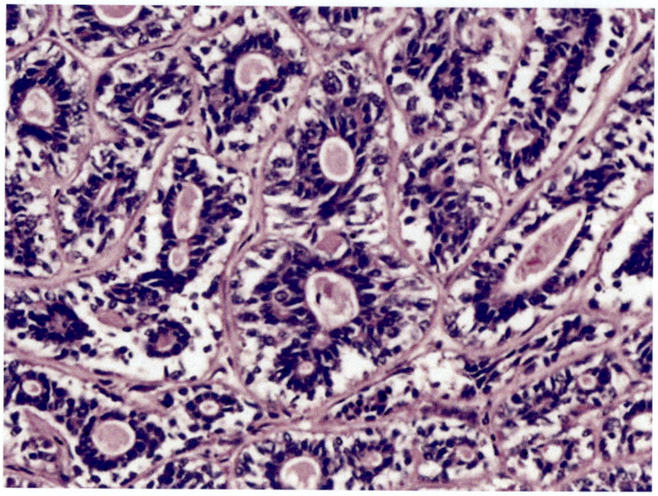

Fig. 6.53 Epithelial-myoepithelial carcinoma of the lung demonstrating the typical dual cellular proliferation with an inner epithelial and outer clear myoepithelial layer

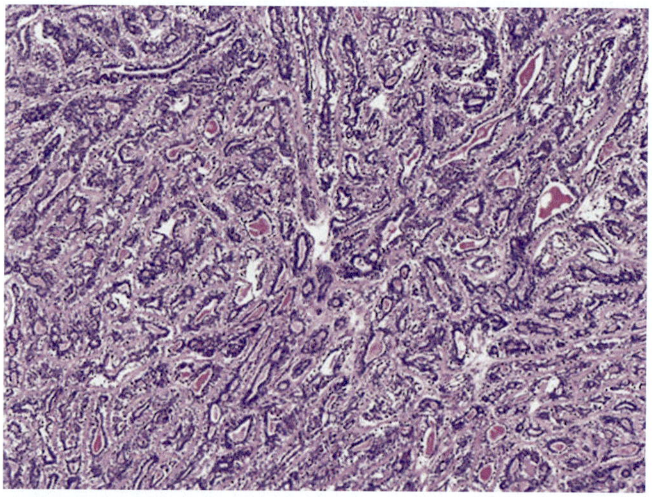

Fig. 6.52 Biphasic architecture of epithelial-myoepithelial carcinoma of the lung

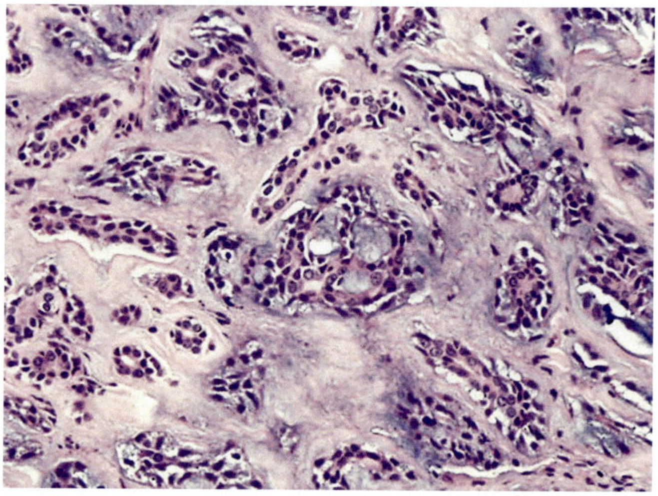

Fig. 6.54 Bland acellular stroma separating the epithelial-myoepithelial components

Histological Features

The histological hallmark of epithelial-myoepithelial carcinoma is a biphasic architecture composed of epithelial cells and myoepithelial cells set in a fibrous stroma (Fig. 6.51). Typically the tumor consists of glands, ducts, and tubular structures with a bilayered composition (Fig. 6.52); the inner luminal cells consist of cuboidal or columnar epithelial cells with pink cytoplasm and bland nuclei, whereas the outer layer is composed of round to polygonal myoepithelial cells with clear or eosinophilic cytoplasm (Fig. 6.53). In the periphery of the glands, the tumor cells often blend with a stroma composed of bland fibrous spindle cells (Fig. 6.54). Mitotic activity is only rarely seen and if present is not restricted to a particular cell type. The lumina of the gland or duct-like structures often contain a dense eosinophilic colloid-like material or basophilic granular debris (Fig. 6.55). In some tumors the cell composition may vary and the myoepithelial component may be prominent or inconspicuous (Figs. 6.56, 6.57 and 6.58). In addition, the biphasic arrangement of the glands and duct-like structures may appear lost in some areas because the outer cells merge with the surrounding tissues (Fig. 6.59). Although nuclear atypia has been described in isolated cases, this is not a common feature and necrosis, if present, is only seen very focally [54, 58, 60, 64, 65]. As in many other salivary gland type tumors, squamous metaplasia can be seen (Fig. 6.60).

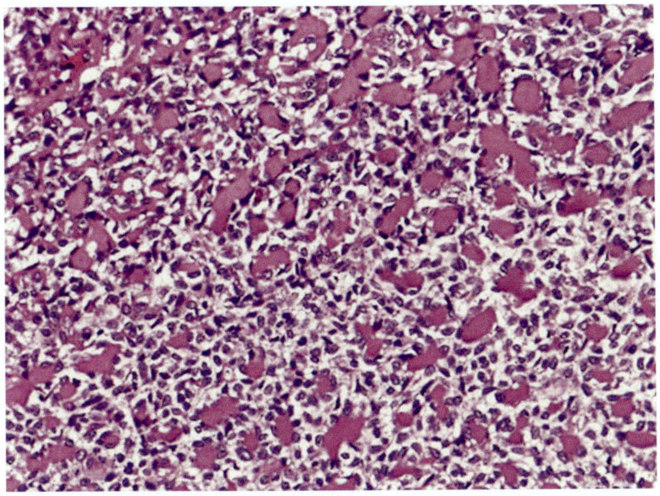

Fig. 6.55 Dense eosinophilic material in lumina of epithelial-myoepithelial carcinoma

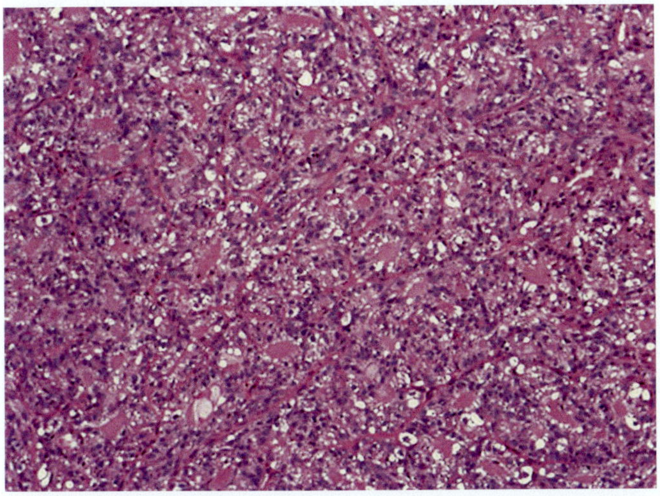

Fig. 6.56 The dual cell composition may be less conspicuous in some epithelial-myoepithelial carcinomas

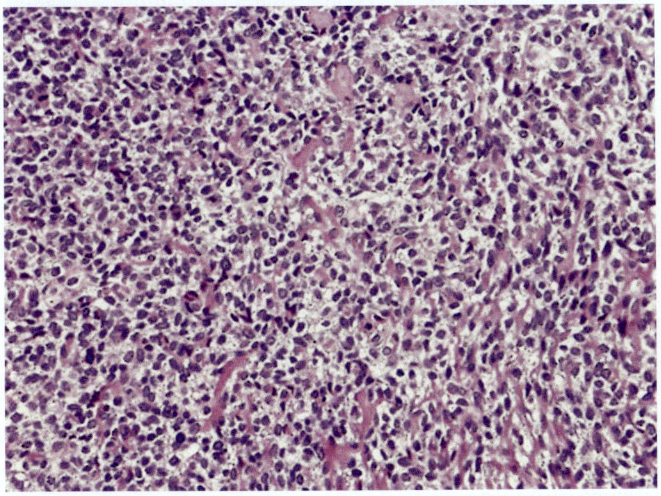

Fig. 6.57 Spindle cell change in myoepithelial component of epithelial-myoepithelial carcinoma of the lung

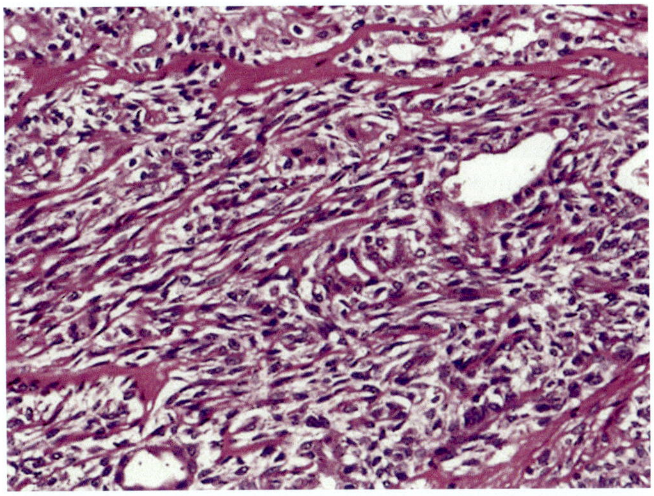

Fig. 6.58 Solid proliferation of myoepithelial cells in epithelial-myoepithelial carcinoma

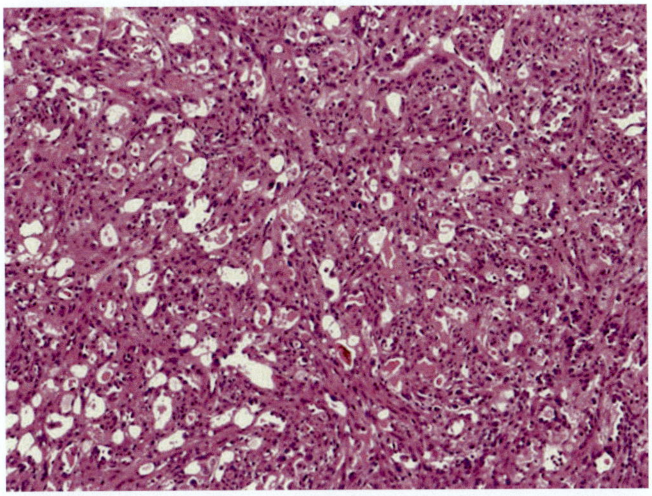

Fig. 6.59 Loss of the biphasic arrangement of epithelial-myoepithelial carcinoma may be seen in some cases

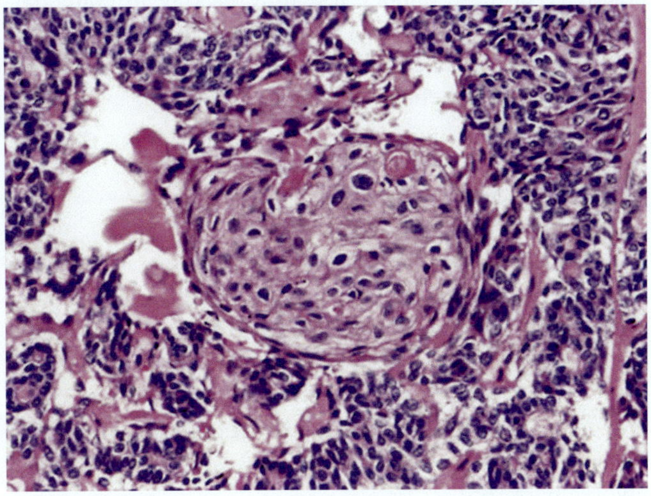

Fig. 6.60 Squamous metaplasia in epithelial-myoepithelial carcinoma

Immunohistochemical and Molecular Features

Immunohistochemical studies confirm the biphasic pattern of these tumors. The epithelial component shows strong immunoreactivity for pancytokeratin, CAM 5.2, and c-kit and is negative for smooth muscle actin, S100 protein, HMB45, GFAP, vimentin, p63, and TTF-1 [64, 66]. The outer layer of myoepithelial cells on the other hand shows strong staining with SMA, S100, vimentin, and p63 and is focally positive for pancytokeratin and GFAP, while TTF1 and c-kit are negative [64, 66]. Polymerase chain reaction (PCR) performed on a single case failed to identify any EGFR or Kras mutations [65].

Differential Diagnosis

The differential diagnosis for epithelial-myoepithelial carcinoma of the lung is quite broad. Importantly, metastatic epithelial-myoepithelial carcinoma from the salivary glands has to be ruled out clinically. Other tumors that may mimic epithelial-myoepithelial carcinoma include adenoid cystic carcinoma, pleomorphic adenoma, myoepithelial tumors, sugar tumor, and primary or metastatic clear cell carcinomas. Adenoid cystic carcinoma, although also composed of tubules and gland-like structures, often demonstrates at least focal areas of its typical cribriform pattern and shows extensive infiltrative growth and prominent perineural invasion. Pleomorphic adenoma usually shows a characteristic myxoid or chondroid stroma, which is not normally seen in pulmonary epithelial-myoepithelial carcinoma. Pure myoepithelial tumors are composed of only one cell type and lack the typical biphasic pattern of epithelial-myoepithelial carcinoma. Sugar tumors of the lung arise peripherally and are composed of a monotypic proliferation of large clear cells. Immunohistochemical stains will demonstrate HMB45 positivity in these tumors, a feature lacking in epithelial-myoepithelial carcinomas. Clear cell carcinoma of the lung and metastatic renal cell carcinoma are monophasic tumors lacking a myoepithelial component.

Treatment and Prognosis

Although epithelial-myoepithelial carcinoma of the lung is generally considered a low-grade neoplasm, cases with regional lymph node metastasis have recently been described and the long-term prognosis is therefore somewhat uncertain [64, 65]. Complete surgical excision is the current treatment of choice. Regular radiological follow-up is recommended in cases of lymph node involvement [65].

Pulmonary Oncocytoma

Clinical Features

Oncocytes are defined as cells containing abundant granular eosinophilic cytoplasm. A variety of cytoplasmic organelles can cause this eosinophilic appearance including abundant smooth endoplasmic reticulum, lysosome-like bodies, or neurosecretory granules; however, only those cells showing mitochondrial hyperplasia are considered oncocytes. Thus, ultrastructural studies are needed to confirm true oncocytic differentiation. Oncocytomas are thought to express epithelial differentiation and are presumed to arise from serous glands or duct-like epithelium [67]. Based on these criteria, less than 10 true primary oncocytomas of the lung have been described [67–72]. Pulmonary oncocytomas affect adults with an age range from 22 to 68 years and no specific sex predilection. Presenting symptoms include malaise, pneumonia, and weight loss. In at least one case, the tumor was found incidentally [67]. Although most tumors are endobronchial lesions, tumors may also occur in the lung parenchyma [69].

Gross Features

Grossly, most tumors measure around 3 cm in size and are circumscribed tumors of soft to firm consistency and yellow-tan color. One tumor described as malignant was characterized by a more infiltrative growth pattern showing multiple confluent nodules adjacent to the main bronchus [72].

Histological Features

Histologically, the tumor cells are arranged in sheets, cords, or alveolar-like clusters. Most individual tumor cells are large and of ovoid or polygonal shape containing abundant eosinophilic granular cytoplasm. Other cells have a more vacuolated cytoplasm, and smaller cells with indistinct cytoplasmic borders can also be identified. The nuclei may be small and uniform or larger with prominent nucleoli. Mitotic activity and necrosis are generally not identified. Focal calcification and a lymphoplasmacytic infiltrate can occasionally be seen.

Immunohistochemical and Ultrastructural Features

Rare immunohistochemical studies have demonstrated immunoreactivity of the oncocytes with cytokeratin, vimentin, and α(alpha)-1-antitrypsin [67]. The most characteristic feature of oncocytoma is seen by ultrastructural examination. The tumor cells will typically contain abundant mitochondria in the cytoplasm. These mitochondria are large, swollen, and distended and will show loss of mitochondrial cristae. Golgi apparatus, lysosomes, and endoplasmic reticulum profiles are inconspicuous. The presence of microvilli and junctional complexes seem to suggest epithelial differentiation, and these features are similar to those seen in serous oncocytes of the salivary glands [73].

Differential Diagnosis

A range of neoplasms with oncocytic change need to be differentiated from oncocytoma. One of the most common tumors with oncocytic differentiation in the lung is oncocytic carcinoid tumor. In fact, some of the earlier descriptions of "pulmonary oncocytoma" were later found to be oncocytic neuroendocrine tumors. In oncocytic carcinoid tumors, the eosinophilic appearance of the cytoplasm is due to a combination of mitochondrial hyperplasia and electron-dense neurosecretory granules. The presence of the latter will point toward neuroendocrine differentiation, and their presence precludes classification as oncocytoma. Other tumors with a similar light microscopic appearance are granular cell tumor and acinic cell carcinoma of the lung. Granular cell tumor will be positive for S100 by immunohistochemistry and will show an abundance of cytoplasmic lysosomes by electron microscopy. Acinic cell carcinoma of the lung is another rare salivary gland type tumor that shows characteristic PAS positivity of the cytoplasm and abundant zymogen-type granules on ultrastructural examination thereby differentiating this tumor from oncocytoma. Lastly, metastatic oncocytic tumors will have to be excluded by clinical history and supportive immunohistochemical examinations.

Treatment and Prognosis

Complete surgical excision is the treatment of choice for pulmonary oncocytomas. Although initially thought to be entirely benign tumors, a single case of "malignant" pulmonary oncocytoma has been reported showing an infiltrative growth pattern and metastasis to a peribronchial lymph node implying at least low-grade malignant potential [72].

Sebaceous Carcinoma of the Lung

Clinical Features

Sebaceous neoplasms are tumors of adnexal derivation most commonly found in the orbital area. These lesions have rarely been described in an extraorbital location [74, 75]. A single case report has recently described a primary sebaceous carcinoma arising in the bronchus [76]. The tumor occurred in a 78-year-old male who was investigated for weight loss. The patient did not have any previous history of sebaceous carcinoma.

Gross Features

The tumor was a well-circumscribed mass arising in a segmental bronchus and a tumor size of 2.2 cm. The cut surface was yellowish-white and of friable consistency.

Histological Features

Microscopy revealed a cellular tumor composed of uniform cells arranged in undulating rows. A range of cytological features were seen ranging from small basaloid cells to cells with more eosinophilic cytoplasm and finally clear vacuolated cells with distinct cytoplasmic borders. In addition, focal squamous differentiation was noted. The mitotic rate was up to four mitoses per ten high-power fields, and focal areas of necrosis were also appreciated.

Immunohistochemical Features

Immunohistochemical results revealed an epithelial phenotype showing staining for keratin, epithelial membrane antigen, and carcinoembryonic antigen. Importantly, Oil Red O showed a positive reaction, while mucicarmine and diastase PAS stains were negative, confirming sebaceous differentiation.

Differential Diagnosis

The differential diagnosis includes salivary gland type tumors showing sebaceous differentiation, squamous cell carcinoma with sebaceous differentiation, and metastatic sebaceous carcinoma. Sebaceous differentiation in salivary gland type tumors is usually focal and will be identified against a background of an otherwise typical salivary gland neoplasm. In sebaceous carcinoma, the sebaceous change is usually diffuse and other salivary gland type elements are absent. Similar criteria apply when differentiating sebaceous carcinoma from squamous cell carcinoma with sebaceous differentiation. Whereas squamous cell carcinoma with sebaceous differentiation will only show focal sebaceous change and the majority of the tumor will be composed of typical squamous cell carcinoma, sebaceous carcinoma will only show focal squamous change if any. As with all other salivary gland or adnexal type neoplasms arising in the bronchopulmonary system, metastasis from an extrapulmonary primary has to be excluded before a primary sebaceous carcinoma of the lung can be diagnosed.

Treatment and Prognosis

Complete surgical excision by lobectomy was carried out and the patient remains disease-free 3 years after presentation.

References

1. Moran CA. Primary salivary gland-type tumors of the lung. Semin Diagn Pathol. 1995;12:106–22.
2. Bennett AK, Mills SE, Wick MR. Salivary-type neoplasms of the breast and lung. Semin Diagn Pathol. 2003;20:279–304.
3. Turnbull AD, Huvos AG, Goodner JT, Foote Jr FW. Mucoepidermoid tumors of bronchial glands. Cancer. 1971;28:539–44.
4. Conlan AA, Payne WS, Woolner LB, Sanderson DR. Adenoid cystic carcinoma (cylindroma) and mucoepidermoid carcinoma of the bronchus. Factors affecting survival. J Thorac Cardiovasc Surg. 1978;76:369–77.
5. Yousem SA, Hochholzer L. Mucoepidermoid tumors of the lung. Cancer. 1987;60:1346–52.
6. Vadasz P, Egervary M. Mucoepidermoid bronchial tumors: a review of 34 operated cases. Eur J Cardiothorac Surg. 2000;17:566–9.
7. Molina JR, Aubry MC, Lewis JE, Wampfler JA, Williams BA, Midthun DE, Yang P, Cassivi SD. Primary salivary gland-type lung cancer: spectrum of clinical presentation, histopathologic and prognostic factors. Cancer. 2007;110:2253–9.
8. Chin CH, Huang CC, Lin MC, Chao TY, Liu SF. Prognostic factors of tracheobronchial mucoepidermoid carcinoma–15 years experience. Respirology. 2008;13:275–80.
9. Kim TS, Lee KS, Han J, Im JG, Seo JB, Kim JS, Kim HY, Han SW. Mucoepidermoid carcinoma of the tracheobronchial tree: radiographic and CT findings in 12 patients. Radiology. 1999;212:643–8.
10. Shilo K, Foss RD, Franks TJ, DePeralta-Venturina M. Travis WDPulmonary mucoepidermoid carcinoma with prominent tumor-associated lymphoid proliferation. Am J Surg Pathol. 2005;29:407–11.
11. Barrett W, Heaps LS, Diaz S, Sharma P, Arbuckle S, Smith A. Mucoepidermoid carcinoma of the bronchus in a 15-year-old girl with complex cytogenetic rearrangement involving 11q and overexpression of cyclin D1. Med Pediatr Oncol. 2002;39:49–51.
12. Tonon G, Gehlhaus KS, Yonescu R, Kaye FJ, Kirsch IR. Multiple reciprocal translocations in salivary gland mucoepidermoid carcinomas. Cancer Genet Cytogenet. 2004;152:15–22.
13. Han SW, Kim HP, Jeon YK, Oh DY, Lee SH, Kim DW, Im SA, Chung DH, Heo DS, Bang YJ, Kim TY. Mucoepidermoid carcinoma of lung: potential target of EGFR-directed treatment. Lung Cancer. 2008;61:30–4.
14. Rossi G, Sartori G, Cavazza A, Tamberi S. Mucoepidermoid carcinoma of the lung, response to EGFR inhibitors, EGFR and K-RAS mutations, and differential diagnosis. Lung Cancer. 2009;63:159–60.
15. Macarenco RS, Uphoff TS, Gilmer HF, Jenkins RB, Thibodeau SN, Lewis JE, Molina JR, Yang P, Aubry MC. Salivary gland-type lung carcinomas: an EGFR immunohistochemical, molecular genetic and mutational analysis study. Mod Pathol. 2008;21:1168–75.
16. Wong DW, Leung EL, So KK, Tam IY, Sihoe AD, Cheng LC, Ho KK, Au JS, Chung LP, Pik Wong M. University of Hong Kong lung cancer study group. The EML4-ALK fusion gene is involved in various histologic types of lung cancers from non-smokers with wild-type EGFR and KRAS. Cancer. 2009;115:1723–33.
17. Moran CA, Suster S, Koss MN. Primary adenoid cystic carcinoma of the lung. A clinicopathologic and immunohistochemical study of 16 cases. Cancer. 1994;73:1390–7.
18. Reid JD. Adenoid cystic carcinoma (cylindroma) of the bronchial tree. Cancer. 1952;5:685–94.
19. Payne WS, Ellis Jr FH, Woolner LB, Moersch HJ. The surgical treatment of cylindroma (adenoid cystic carcinoma) and mucoepidermoid tumors of the bronchus. J Thorac Cardiovasc Surg. 1959;38:709–26.
20. Inoue H, Iwashita A, Kanegae H, Higuchi K, Fujinaga Y, Matsumoto I. Peripheral pulmonary adenoid cystic carcinoma with substantial submucosal extension to the proximal bronchus. Thorax. 1991;46:147–8.
21. Kitada M, Ozawa K, Sato K, Hayashi S, Tokusashi Y, Miyokawa N, Sasajima T. Adenoid cystic carcinoma of the peripheral lung: a case report. World J Surg Oncol. 2010;8:74.
22. Yokouchi H, Otsuka Y, Otoguro Y, Takemoto N, Ito K, Uchida Y, Okamoto K, Nishimura M, Kimura K, Kaji H. Primary peripheral adenoid cystic carcinoma of the lung and literature comparison of features. Intern Med. 2007;46:1799–803.
23. Aubry MC, Heinrich MC, Molina J, Lewis JE, Yang P, Cassivi SD, Corless CL. Primary adenoid cystic carcinoma of the lung: absence of KIT mutations. Cancer. 2007;110:2507–10.
24. Kang DY, Yoon YS, Kim HK, Choi YS, Kim K, Shim YM, Kim J. Primary salivary gland-type lung cancer: surgical outcomes. Lung Cancer. 2011;72:250–4.
25. Kawashima O, Hirai T, Kamiyoshihara M, Ishikawa S, Morishita Y. Primary adenoid cystic carcinoma in the lung: report of two cases and therapeutic considerations. Lung Cancer. 1998;19:211–7.
26. Haresh KP, Prabhakar R, Rath GK, Sharma DN, Julka PK, Subramani V. Adenoid cystic carcinoma of the trachea treated with PET-CT based intensity modulated radiotherapy. J Thorac Oncol. 2008;3:793–5.
27. Chopra R, Mendenhall WM, Morris CG, Zlotecki RA. Olivier KR surgery and postoperative radiotherapy for adenoid cystic carcinoma of the lung. Am J Clin Oncol. 2006;29:420–1.
28. Fechner RE, Bentinck BR, Askew Jr JB. Acinic cell tumor of the lung. A histologic and ultrastructural study. Cancer. 1972;29:501–8.
29. Lee HY, Mancer K, Koong HN. Primary acinic cell carcinoma of the lung with lymph node metastasis. Arch Pathol Lab Med. 2003;127:e216–9.
30. Moran CA, Suster S, Koss MN. Acinic cell carcinoma of the lung ("Fechner tumor"). A clinicopathologic, immunohistochemical, and ultrastructural study of five cases. Am J Surg Pathol. 1992;16:1039–50.
31. Sabaratnam RM, Anunathan R, Govender D. Acinic cell carcinoma: an unusual cause of bronchial obstruction in a child. Pediatr Dev Pathol. 2004;7:521–6.
32. Ukoha OO, Quartararo P, Carter D, Kashgarian M, Ponn RB. Acinic cell carcinoma of the lung with metastasis to lymph nodes. Chest. 1999;115:591–5.
33. Watanabe K, Ono N, Hoshi T, Hanzawa M, Ishida T. Fine-needle aspiration cytology of bronchial acinic cell carcinoma: a case report. Diagn Cytopathol. 2004;30:359–61.
34. Heard BE, Dewar A, Firmin RK, Lennox SC. One very rare and one new tracheal tumour found by electron microscopy: glomus tumour and acinic cell tumour resembling carcinoid tumours by light microscopy. Thorax. 1982;37:97–103.
35. Horowitz Z, Kronenberg J. Acinic cell carcinoma of the trachea. Auris Nasus Larynx. 1994;21:193–5.

36. Martin H, Abboud A, Nawka T. Predominantly mucous-differentiated acinic cell adenocarcinoma of the trachea. Zentralbl Allg Pathol. 1989;135(8):751–6.
37. Murakami M, Ochi T, Tokunaga H, Nagata M, Kawahara H, Odagiri S, Ishikura Y, Yoshimatsu H. Acinic cell carcinoma of the trachea–a case report. Gan No Rinsho. 1984;30:1412–6.
38. Ansari MA, Marchevsky A, Strick L, Mohsenifar Z. Upper airway obstruction secondary to acinic cell carcinoma of the trachea. Use of Nd: YAG laser. Chest. 1996;110:1120–2.
39. Katz DR, Bubis JJ. Acinic cell tumor of the bronchus. Cancer. 1976;38:830–2.
40. Gharpure KJ, Deshpande RK, Vlshweshvara RN, Raghu CR, Bhargava MK. Acinic cell tumour of the bronchus (a case report). Indian J Cancer. 1985;22:152–6.
41. Yoshida K, Koyama I, Matsui T, Tsukiyama M, Mizushima M. Acinic cell tumor of the bronchial gland. Nippon Geka Gakkai Zasshi. 1989;90:1810–3.
42. Miura K, Morinaga S, Horiuchi M, Shimosato Y, Tsuchiya R. Bronchial carcinoid tumor mimicking acinic cell tumor. Acta Pathol Jpn. 1988;38:523–30.
43. Rodriguez J, Diment J, Lombardi L, Dominoni F, Tench W, Rosai J. Combined typical carcinoid and acinic cell tumor of the lung: a heretofore unreported occurrence. Hum Pathol. 2003;34: 1061–5.
44. Sano A, Takeuchi E, Hebisawa A, Nakajima Y. Combined typical carcinoid and acinic cell tumor of the lung. Interact Cardiovasc Thorac Surg. 2011;12:311–2.
45. Chuah KL, Yap WM, Tan HW, Koong HN. Recurrence of pulmonary acinic cell carcinoma. Arch Pathol Lab Med. 2006;130: 932–3.
46. Goto T, Maeshima A, Akanabe K, Hamaguchi R, Wakaki M, Oyamada Y, Kato R. Bronchial pleomorphic adenoma coexisting with lung cancer. Ann Thorac Cardiovasc Surg. 2011;17:174–7.
47. Hemmi A, Hiraoka H, Mori Y, Wataya T, Sato H, Jinnai M, Yamaguchi H, Arai Y. Malignant pleomorphic adenoma (malignant mixed tumor) of the trachea. Report of a case. Acta Pathol Jpn. 1988;38:1215–26.
48. Moran CA, Suster S, Askin FB, Koss MN. Benign and malignant salivary gland-type mixed tumors of the lung. Clinicopathologic and immunohistochemical study of eight cases. Cancer. 1994;73: 2481–90.
49. Demirağ F, Topçu S, Kurul C, Memiş L, Altinok T. Malignant pleomorphic adenoma (malignant mixed tumor) of the trachea: a case report and review of the literature. Eur Arch Otorhinolaryngol. 2003;260:96–9.
50. Ding CS, Yap WM, Teo CH, Giron D, Chuah KL. Tracheal carcinoma ex pleomorphic adenoma: a rare tumour with potential problems in diagnosis. Histopathology. 2007;51:868–71.
51. Weissferdt A, Moran CA. Pulmonary salivary gland-type tumors with features of malignant mixed tumor (carcinoma ex pleomorphic adenoma): a clinicopathological study of 5 cases. Am J Clin Pathol. 2011;136(5):793–8.
52. Nistal M, García-Viera M, Martínez-García C, Paniagua R. Epithelial-myoepithelial tumor of the bronchus. Am J Surg Pathol. 1994;18:421–5.
53. Tsuji N, Tateishi R, Ishiguro S, Terao T, Higashiyama M. Adenomyoepithelioma of the lung. Am J Surg Pathol. 1995;19: 956–62.
54. Wilson RW, Moran CA. Epithelial-myoepithelial carcinoma of the lung: immunohistochemical and ultrastructural observations and review of the literature. Hum Pathol. 1997;28:631–5.
55. Ryska A, Kerekes Z, Hovorková E, Barton P. Epithelial-myoepithelial carcinoma of the bronchus. Pathol Res Pract. 1998;194:431–5.
56. Shanks JH, Hasleton PS, Curry A, Rahman A. Bronchial epithelial-myoepithelial carcinoma. Histopathology. 1998;33:90–1.
57. Papla B, Gałazka K, Malinowski E. Epithelial-myoepithelial carcinoma of the bronchus. Pol J Pathol. 2000;51:153–7.
58. Pelosi G, Fraggetta F, Maffini F, Solli P, Cavallon A, Viale G. Pulmonary epithelial-myoepithelial tumor of unproven malignant potential: report of a case and review of the literature. Mod Pathol. 2001;14:521–6.
59. Fulford LG, Kamata Y, Okudera K, Dawson A, Corrin B, Sheppard MN, Ibrahim NB, Nicholson AG. Epithelial-myoepithelial carcinomas of the bronchus. Am J Surg Pathol. 2001;25:1508–14.
60. Doganay L, Bilgi S, Ozdil A, Yoruk Y, Altaner S, Kutlu K. Epithelial-myoepithelial carcinoma of the lung. A case report and review of the literature. Arch Pathol Lab Med. 2003;127:e177–80.
61. Ru K, Srivastava A, Tischler AS. Bronchial epithelial-myoepithelial carcinoma. Arch Pathol Lab Med. 2004;128:92–4.
62. Chang T, Husain AN, Colby T, Taxy JB, Welch WR, Cheung OY, Early A, Travis W, Krausz T. Pneumocytic adenomyoepithelioma: a distinctive lung tumor with epithelial, myoepithelial, and pneumocytic differentiation. Am J Surg Pathol. 2007;31(4):562–8.
63. Chao TY, Lin AS, Lie CH, Chung YH, Lin JW, Lin MC. Bronchial epithelial-myoepithelial carcinoma. Ann Thorac Surg. 2007;83: 689–91.
64. Nguyen CV, Suster S, Moran CA. Pulmonary epithelial-myoepithelial carcinoma: a clinicopathologic and immunohistochemical study of 5 cases. Hum Pathol. 2009;40:366–73.
65. Rosenfeld A, Schwartz D, Garzon S, Chaleff S. Epithelial-myoepithelial carcinoma of the lung: a case report and review of the literature. J Pediatr Hematol Oncol. 2009;31:206–8.
66. Okudela K, Yazawa T, Tajiri M, Omori T, Takahashi K, Woo T, Shimoyamada H, Ogawa N, Kitamura H. A case of epithelial-myoepithelial carcinoma of the bronchus - a review of reported cases and a comparison with other salivary gland-type carcinomas of the bronchus. Pathol Res Pract. 2010;206:121–9.
67. Tashiro Y, Iwata Y, Nabae T, Manabe H. Pulmonary oncocytoma: report of a case in conjunction with an immunohistochemical and ultrastructural study. Pathol Int. 1995;45:448–51.
68. Fechner RE, Bentinck BR. Ultrastructure of bronchial oncocytoma. Cancer. 1973;31:1451–7.
69. Santos-Briz A, Terrón J, Sastre R, Romero L, Valle A. Oncocytoma of the lung. Cancer. 1977;40:1330–6.
70. Fernandez MA, Nyssen J. Oncocytoma of the lung. Can J Surg. 1982;25:332–3.
71. Tesluk H, Dajee A. Pulmonary oncocytoma. J Surg Oncol. 1985;29: 173–5.
72. Nielsen AL. Malignant bronchial oncocytoma: case report and review of the literature. Hum Pathol. 1985;16:852–4.
73. Hamperl H. Benign and malignant oncocytoma. Cancer. 1962;15: 1019–27.
74. Rao NA, Hidayat AA, McLean IW, Zimmerman LE. Sebaceous carcinomas of the ocular adnexa: a clinicopathologic study of 104 cases, with five-year follow-up data. Hum Pathol. 1982;13:113–22.
75. Wick MR, Goellner JR, Wolfe 3rd JT, Su WP. Adnexal carcinomas of the skin. II. Extraocular sebaceous carcinomas. Cancer. 1985;56:1163–72.
76. Borczuk AC, Sha KK, Hisler SE, Mann JM, Hajdu SI. Sebaceous carcinoma of the lung: histologic and immunohistochemical characterization of an unusual pulmonary neoplasm: report of a case and review of the literature. Am J Surg Pathol. 2002;26:795–8.

7 Tumors Derived from Presumed Ectopic Tissues

Introduction

The occurrence of these types of neoplasms as primary intrapulmonary tumors is rather rare. It is assumed that these tumors occur in the lung under the assumption that they may originate from ectopically occurring tissues that may have remained in the lung during embryogenesis. Although an interesting and provocative theory, it is only a theory as from a practical aspect this is rather difficult to prove. On other hand, for practical purposes, it remains a viable theory to account for these tumors, which otherwise could be misconstrued as metastatic tumors to the lung. This particular issue must be considered not only for making a diagnosis of primary lung neoplasm but also to ensure that patients do not undergo unnecessary work-ups or treatments. This chapter highlights the occurrence of these tumors and emphasizes the importance of being familiar with these lesions in order to avoid misdiagnosis.

The histopathological criteria for the diagnosis of these tumors are essentially the same as for their counterparts in their more common anatomic site. However, knowing that the pulmonary system is often a site for metastasis and given the unusual occurrence of these tumors as primary lung neoplasms, it is always important to rule out a possible metastasis before rendering a diagnosis of primary pulmonary neoplasm for these tumors. Thus, careful clinicopathological correlations including radiographic imaging are important parameters in the evaluation and diagnosis of these tumors.

Although, theoretically speaking, any tumor can occur at any time and in any anatomic site, in this chapter we will address those tumors that appear to be a relatively more common occurrence in the lung parenchyma. The tumoral conditions that will be discussed are the following:

- Pulmonary meningioma
- Bronchial/pulmonary melanoma
- Pulmonary glomangioma/glomangiosarcoma
- Intrapulmonary thymoma
- Intrapulmonary teratoma

Tables 7.1 and 7.2 depict some of the most important histological, immunohistochemical, and differential diagnostic features of these tumors.

Pulmonary Meningioma

The occurrence of meningiomas outside of the central nervous systems is rare but well known. Their occurrence as primary intrapulmonary tumors, although it has been known for some time, still remains a rare occurrence. In addition, meningiomas are also well known to arise in ectopic locations such as the head and neck area in sites like the scalp, orbital fossa, maxillary antrum, and frontal sinus [1]. Another unusual phenomenon is the simultaneous occurrence of pulmonary and central nervous system (CNS) meningiomas with "benign histology"; this has been regarded by some as benign metastasizing meningioma [2]. In other patients late metastasis to the lung from a previous CNS meningioma has been reported [3]. The time period from first diagnosis of a CNS neoplasm and development of metastasis has been as long as 19 years [3]. In 1960, Hoye et al. [4] suggested possible explanations for the occurrence of extracranial meningiomas, which included four possibilities:

1. Direct extension from an intracranial tumor
2. Extracranial growth from arachnoid cell rests along cranial nerve sheaths
3. Proliferation of ectopic embryonic rests of arachnoid cells
4. Extracranial metastases from intracranial tumors

It appears that the most logical explanation for the appearance of meningiomas in the lung may be best explained by the proliferation of ectopic embryonic rests of arachnoid cells. However, as stated before, although an interesting theory, it still remains unproved.

Because of the unusual occurrence of these neoplasms as primary lung tumors, most of what has been reported in the literature is in the form of case reports. Kemnitz et al. [5] is given credit for the first description of a primary pul-

A. Weissferdt, C.A. Moran, *Diagnostic Pathology of Pleuropulmonary Neoplasia*,
DOI 10.1007/978-1-4419-0787-5_7, © Springer Science+Business Media New York 2013

Table 7.1 Commonly used immunohistochemical stains in the diagnosis of tumors derived from presumed ectopic tissues

Tumor	Keratin	EMA	Vimentin	LCA	TdT	Pax8	Actin	S100 protein	Melan A
Meningioma	neg/pos	pos	pos	neg	neg	neg	neg	neg	neg
Glomus/ glomangiosarcoma	neg	neg	pos	neg	neg	neg	pos	neg	neg
Melanoma	neg	neg	pos	neg	neg	neg	neg	pos	pos
Thymoma	pos	neg	neg/pos	pos	pos	pos	neg	neg	neg

EMA epithelial membrane antigen, *LCA* leukocyte common antibody, *TdT* terminal deoxynucleotidyl transferase, *neg* negative, *pos* positive

Table 7.2 Commonly considered neoplams in the differential diagnosis of tumors derived from presumed ectopic tissues

Tumor	Differential diagnosis
Meningioma	Carcinoma Spindle cell sarcoma Carcinoid tumor Thymoma Metastatic meningioma
Melanoma	Carcinoma Spindle cell sarcoma Neuroendocrine carcinoma Metastatic melanoma
Glomangioma/ glomangiosarcoma	Sugar tumor Oncocytic carcinoid tumor Paraganglioma Leiomyoma Leiomyosarcoma
Thymoma	Carcinoma Spindle cell carcinoid tumor Monophasic synovial sarcoma Meningioma

monary meningioma in a 59-year-old female patient. Since then, numerous case reports describing similar findings have been presented [6–16]. Drawn from the cases described in the literature, the patients encountered are adult individuals and predominantly female. In the majority of patients, their tumors were discovered incidentally during a routine physical examination. Only in a few cases, patients suffered symptoms related to their tumors. In the largest series reported of intrapulmonary meningiomas, the authors were able to describe ten such cases [17]. The authors' findings somewhat mirrored those reported in the prior literature. The patients were adult individuals between the ages of 30 and 72 years (mean: 51 years) whose tumors were discovered incidentally. Only one patient in this series of cases had symptoms (cough) related to the intrapulmonary tumor. However, interestingly, the female predominance previously reported was not apparent in this study. Although the authors [17] stated that the occurrence of intrapulmonary meningiomas remains speculative, they acknowledge the occurrence of the so-called meningothelial-like nodules in the lung as a possible and more logical origin for pulmonary meningiomas. However, in the reported ten cases, none of the cases had associated meningothelial-like nodules in addition to the pulmonary meningioma.

More recently, we have been able to study more cases of intrapulmonary meningiomas in which an association of meningothelial-like nodules and meningioma was apparent. Interestingly, such an association has been made in some other reported cases, supporting the theory of a histogenetic link between meningothelial-like nodules and meningioma [18, 19]. On the other hand, one still needs to explain the occurrence of meningothelial-like nodules, which revives the previous theory of ectopic embryonic rests. Although the great majority of intrapulmonary meningiomas reported are of the "benign" type, reports of malignant intrapulmonary meningiomas have been published [20, 21]. This raises the issue of specific criteria for the diagnosis of malignancy in intrapulmonary meningiomas. For instance, in the case described by Prayson and Farver [20], the histological features of the tumors, like nuclear pleomorphism, and increased mitotic activity (15 mitoses × 10 high-power fields) lead the authors to classify this case as malignant. However, in the case described by van der Meij [21], it appears that the authors designated their case as malignant based on the invasiveness of the tumor (the tumor invaded pleura, esophagus, intrapulmonary vessels, hilar lymph nodes, peribronchial fat, and caused destruction of bronchial cartilage) rather than on the histological features of the tumor, which showed 0–1 mitotic figures per square millimeter. It is logical that when these tumors occur in an intrapulmonary location, all of these features need to be taken into account in order to possibly predict behavior.

Macroscopic Features

In the majority of cases reported, the tumors are well circumscribed and in many cases are found in a subpleural location. The tumors are solid and whitish in color with a homogenous cut surface. Areas of necrosis and/or hemorrhage are not common, except in cases that have malignant features. The

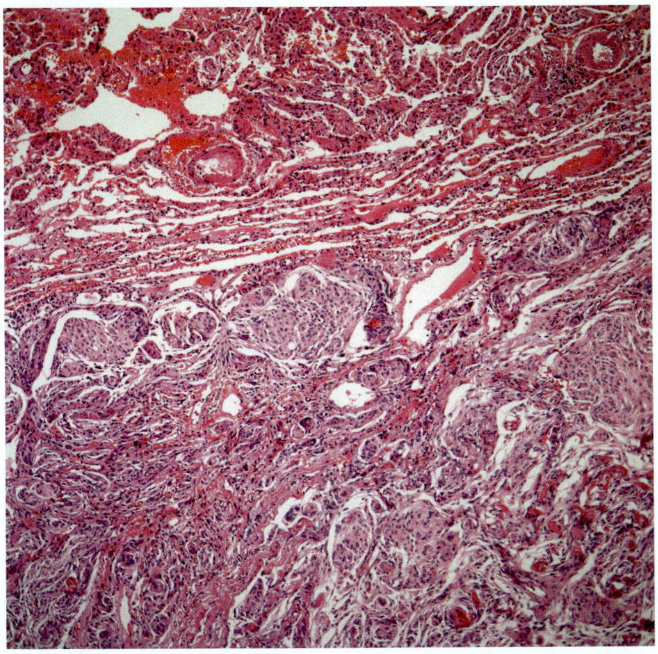

Fig. 7.1 Low power view of a primary pulmonary meningioma showing a well circumscribed but unencapsulated lesion. The tumor grows in small nests

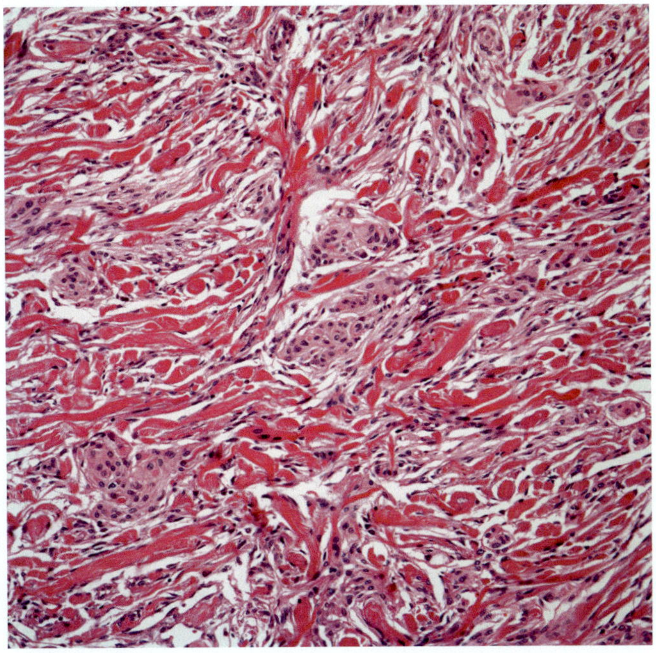

Fig. 7.2 Pulmonary meningioma showing tumor cells dissecting bundles of fibroconnective tissue

size of the tumors varies from 1 cm to more than 5 cm; however, the majority of cases are in the 3–4 cm range.

Histological Features

The histological features of intrapulmonary meningiomas recapitulate those seen in CNS tumors. Transitional meningiomas (Figs. 7.1, 7.2, 7.3, 7.4, 7.5, 7.6, and 7.7) are characterized by the presence of a well-circumscribed but not encapsulated tumor mass surrounded by normal lung parenchyma. The cellular proliferation is composed of plump, slightly spindle-shaped cells arranged in lobules or whorls interspersed by collagenized vascular structures. At high-power magnification, the plump cells have indistinct cell borders, pale eosinophilic cytoplasm, round to oval nuclei, and inconspicuous nucleoli. Psammoma bodies may be present toward the periphery of the tumor, but they may be completely absent in some cases. Areas resembling microcystic meningioma or clusters of xanthoma cells may be seen focally in some cases. Cellular atypia if present may be only focal, and mitotic activity is absent. The fibrous variant of meningioma (Figs. 7.8, 7.9, 7.10, and 7.11) is characterized by the presence of a spindle cell proliferation composed of fusiform cells with indistinct cell borders, pale eosinophilic cytoplasm, elongated nuclei, and inconspicuous nucleoli. However, the presence of more conventional areas of transitional meningiomas may be seen in the periphery of these tumors. Just like the cases of transitional meningioma, mitotic activity is absent in fibrous meningiomas. Recently, Rowsell et al. [22] described an intrapulmonary meningioma characterized by cords and fascicles of spindle cells and epithelioid cells surrounded by abundant mucoid stroma that led the authors to classify the case as chordoid meningioma.

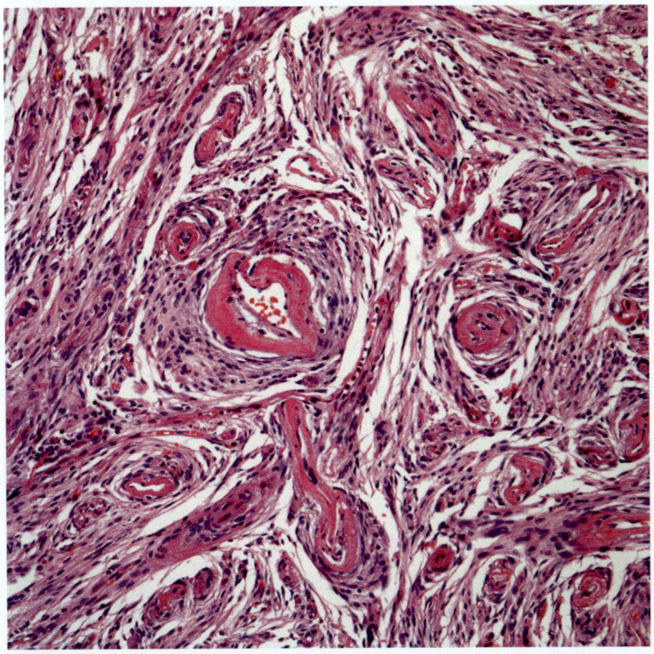

Fig. 7.3 Pulmonary meningioma showing prominent dilated vascular structures surrounded by tumor cells

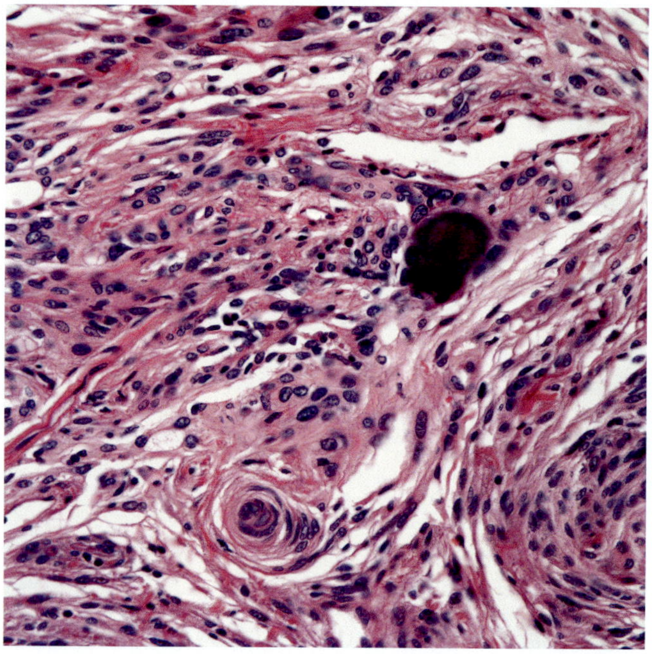

Fig. 7.4 Pulmonary meningioma showing a single psammoma body

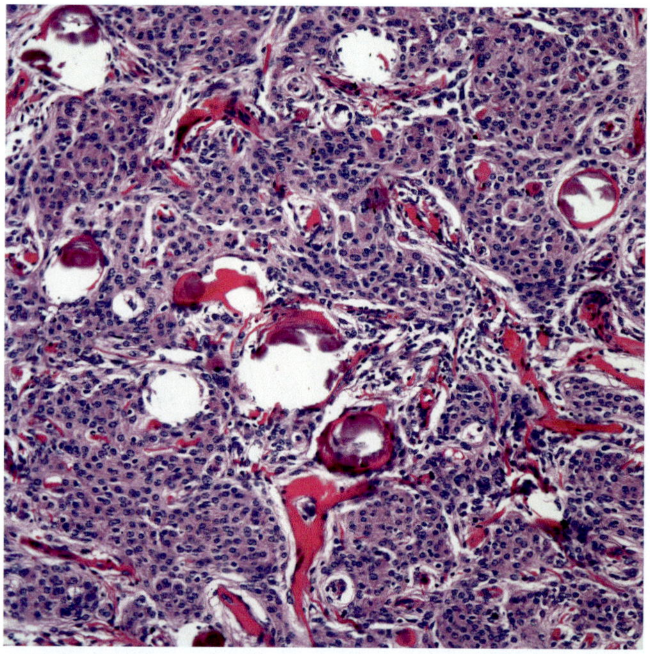

Fig. 7.5 Pulmonary meningioma showing calcifications admixed with fibroconnective tissue

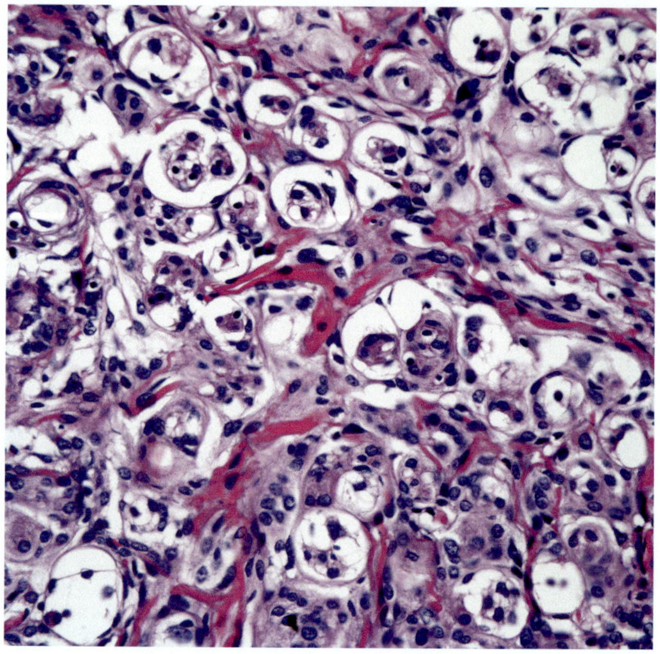

Fig. 7.6 Pulmonary meningioma showing the typical whirling and a subtle clear cell component

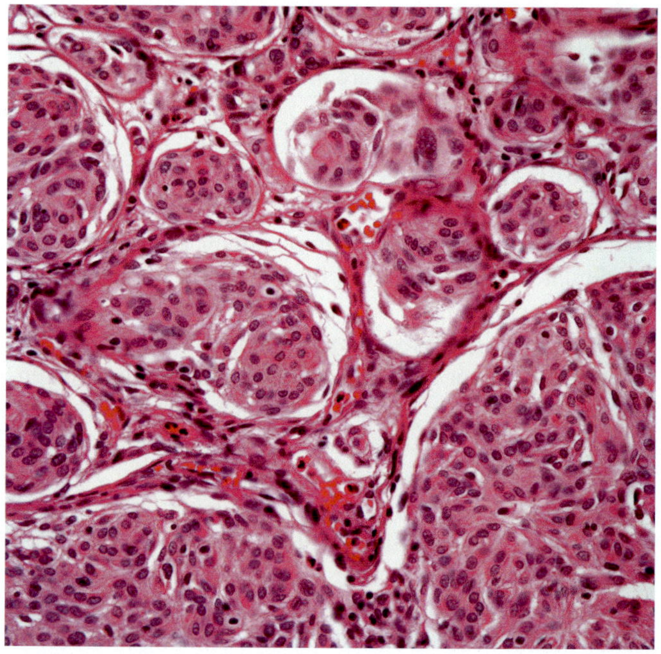

Fig. 7.7 Close magnification of a pulmonary meningioma showing a homogenous cellular proliferation without nuclear atypia or mitotic activity

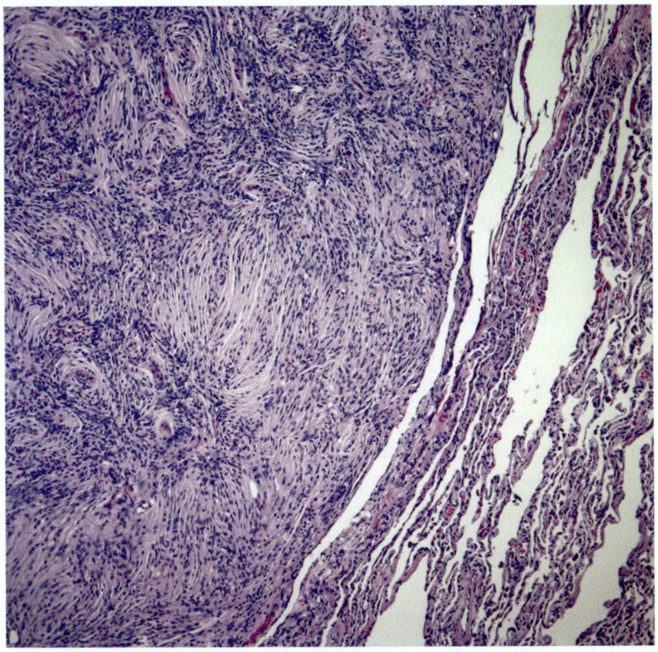

Fig. 7.8 Pulmonary fibrous meningioma characterized by a prominent spindle cell proliferation destroying normal lung parenchyma

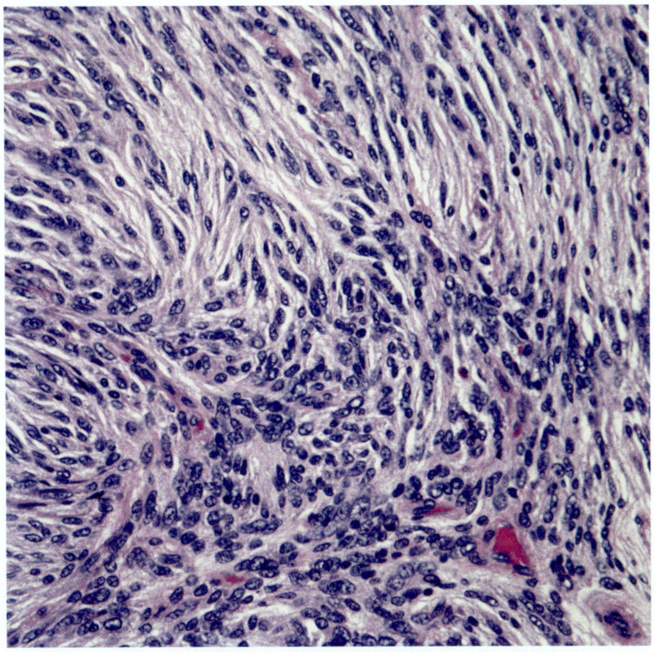

Fig. 7.10 High-power magnification of a fibrous meningioma showing a spindle cell proliferation without significant nuclear atypia

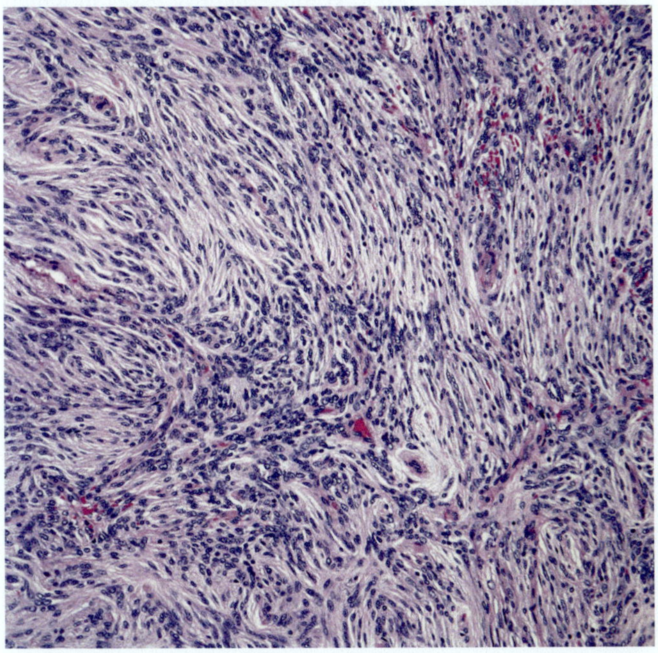

Fig. 7.9 Fibrous meningioma with a subtle schwannoma-like appearance

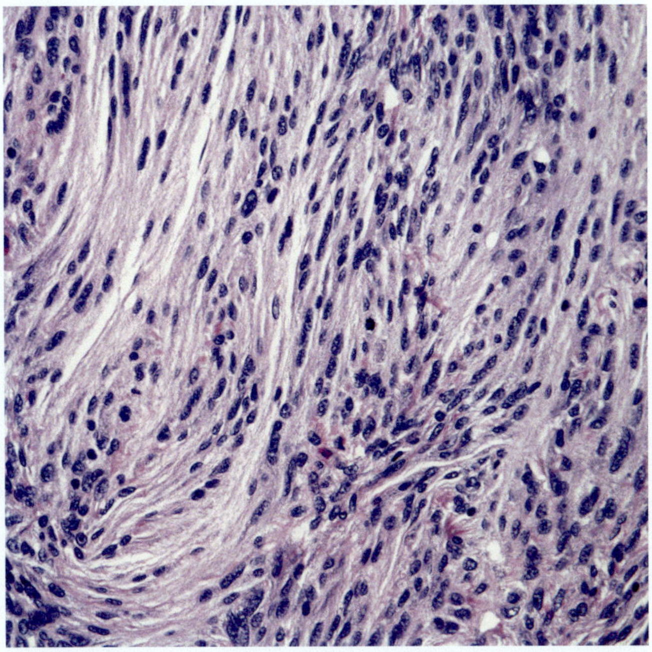

Fig. 7.11 High-power magnification of a fibrous meningioma showing a single mitotic figure

In one of the cases described as malignant meningioma, the tumor displayed more cytological atypia and increased mitotic activity [20], while in another, the tumor did not show increased mitotic activity but had a rather infiltrative growth pattern.

Immunohistochemical Features

The two most consistent immunohistochemical stains that will aid in the diagnosis of meningiomas are vimentin and epithelial membrane antigen (EMA). However, in the reported cases of intrapulmonary meningiomas, other stains that have been reported as weakly or focally positive include CD34, S100 protein, keratin, and progesterone receptors. However, in all those tumors in which some of these stains have been reported as positive, vimentin and EMA have also always been reported as positive. Therefore, it is important to carefully evaluate the histological features of the tumor and the respective immunohistochemical profile.

Differential Diagnosis

The most important differential diagnosis is to determine whether the tumor is not a metastasis from a cranial meningioma. Once that is established, then there are several other diagnostic considerations depending on the particular histology of the meningioma. Intrapulmonary spindle cell thymoma is one important differential diagnosis. Although rare, thymomas may present as an intrapulmonary tumor. In this setting, the presence of psammoma bodies and whorling of cells would be unusual features for thymoma. In addition, thymomas would show a strong positive reaction for keratin and either weak or negative staining for EMA. Inflammatory pseudotumor may also enter the differential diagnosis in cases of fibrous meningioma. However, the absence of plasma cells or a more meaningful inflammatory component would be unusual in cases of inflammatory pseudotumor. Intrapulmonary solitary fibrous tumor is one other possibility; however, solitary fibrous tumors will display more characteristic histological features and likely will display positive staining for CD34 and be negative for EMA.

Treatment and Prognosis

The treatment of choice for intrapulmonary meningioma is complete surgical resection. In the majority of cases reported, the tumor has followed an indolent behavior. However, there is not enough data to determine what the best treatment is for cases that display more aggressive clinical behavior or for those cases that are deemed malignant from the beginning.

Meningothelial-Like Nodules and Diffuse Pulmonary Meningotheliomatosis

Meningothelial-like nodules are small tumors that are commonly encountered randomly in resected lungs for other conditions (Figs. 7.12, 7.13, and 7.14). Their occurrence has been known for more than 50 years, and in the past, they were referred to as minute chemodectomas [23–30]. Although the concept of chemodectomas of the lung was essentially for lesions found incidentally in autopsy material, there are several reports in which the patients presented with "coin lesions" that were deemed to represent this particular entity. In addition, some authors considered that these "chemodectomas" were induced by pulmonary thromboemboli [31, 32], while others studying similar tumors in the head and neck considered that the occurrence of these lesions was due to prolonged and severe hypoxia [33]. However, it is important to note that in the past, these lesions were studied mainly in cases in which they did not represent the main pathology, as pulmonary resections were performed for other reasons and the nodules were encountered by chance. Although in the majority of cases reported, these small tumor nodules were reported as single nodules, there are several reports of multiple lesions. Zak and Chabes [34] reported three autopsy cases in which the authors described multiple lung lesions, which the authors referred to as "pulmonary chemodectomatosis." Unfortunately, no detailed description as to the number and distribution of these nodules was provided.

In 1975, Kuhn and Askin [35] using electron microscopy evaluated several tumors from one patient, which histologically were in keeping with the so-called minute chemodectomas of the lung. The authors concluded that these lesions had little resemblance to paragangliomas and their features were more akin to meningiomas. Churg and Warnock recorded similar findings [36] after the authors studied 26 cases with electron microscopy. The authors concluded that these so-called minute chemodectomas are not related to paragangliomas and their findings also suggested origin from meningeal arachnoid cells. Gaffey et al. [37], using electron microscopy and immunohistochemistry, studied 23 of these tumors and concluded that a more accurate term for these lesions is that of "meningothelial-like nodule." In addition, the authors found that these lesions are more common in women and in the majority of cases are found at autopsy. Also important to mention is that the authors estimated their incidence at approximately 1 in every 60 autopsies. No particular association to any specific disease was determined, and the tumor nodules varied in size from 1 to 3 mm, with pleural or parenchymal location. These clinical findings mirrored those reported in the previous literature, namely, the occurrence of these lesions in a wide spectrum of ages (range: 12–91) and with predominance in females.

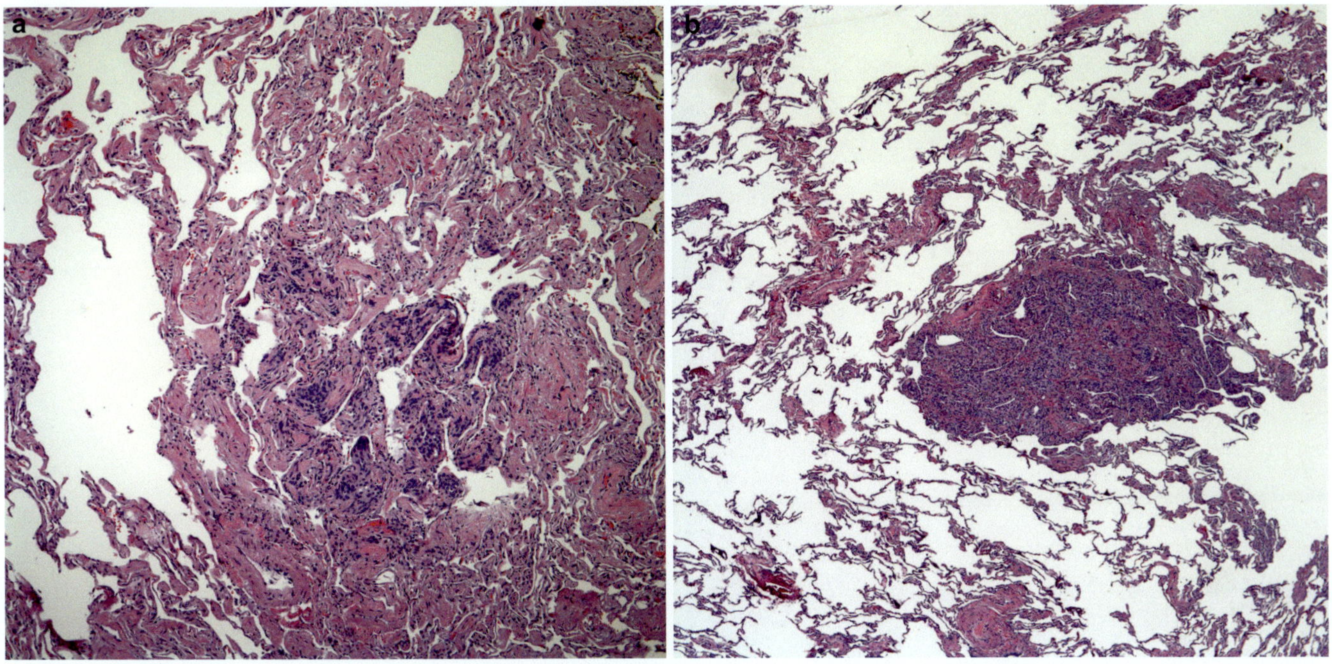

Fig. 7.12 (**a**) Pulmonary parenchyma with an incidental small tumor nodule typical of a meningothelial-like nodule of the lung. (**b**) In some cases, the nodules may be more conspicuous in the lung parenchyma

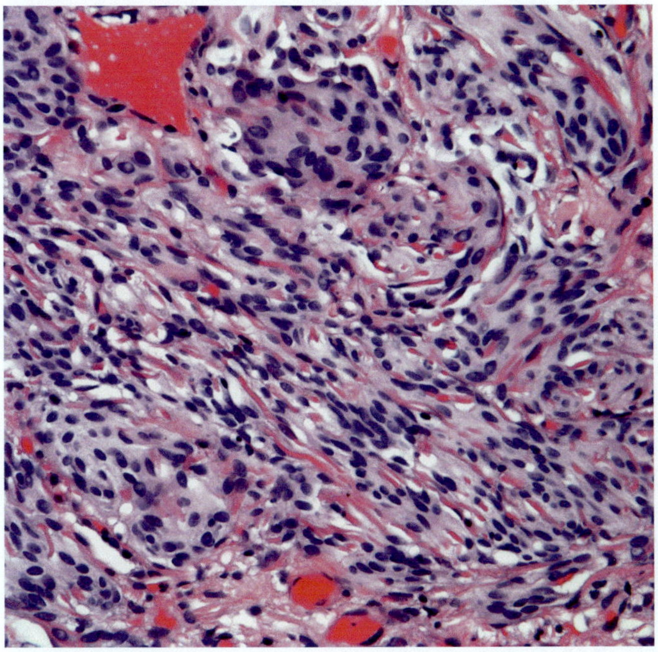

Fig. 7.13 High-power magnification of a meningothelial-like nodule showing a spindle cell growth pattern

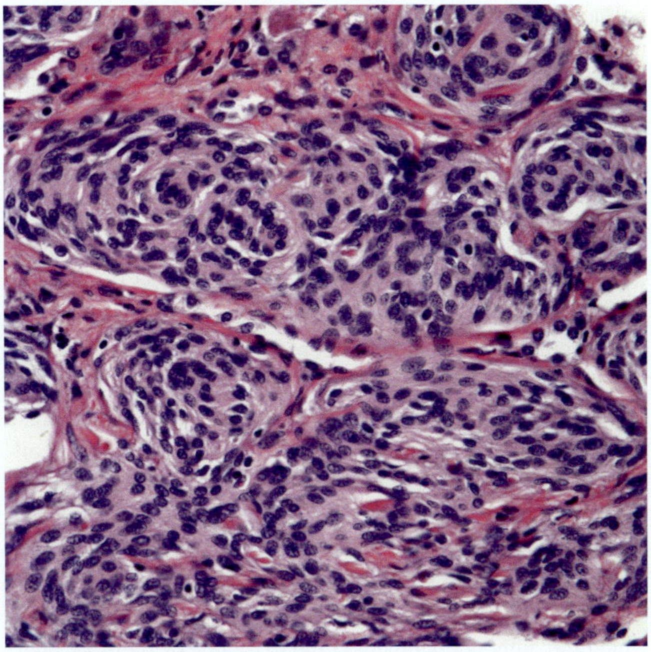

Fig. 7.14 High-power magnification of a meningothelial-like nodule with more conventional "transitional" features

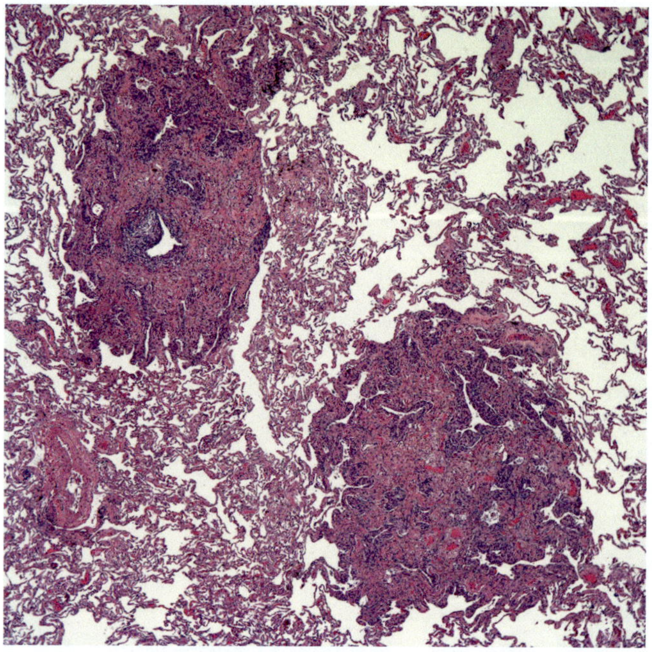

Fig. 7.15 Pulmonary meningotheliomatosis showing two distinct nodules in the lung parenchyma

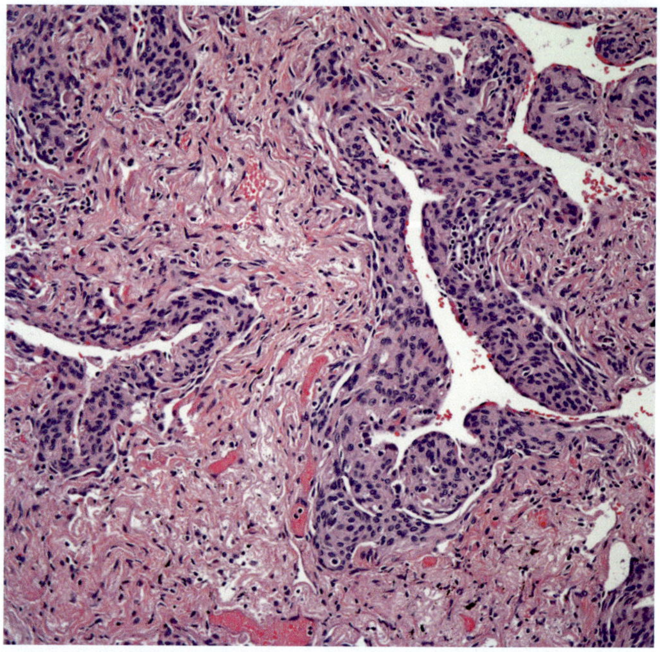

Fig. 7.16 The meningothelial nodules show the conventional "transitional" features in this particular case with moderate amounts of fibroconnective tissue

More recently, a new entity under the designation of diffuse pulmonary meningotheliomatosis was presented in the literature [38]. The authors reported five patients who presented with bilateral diffuse pulmonary involvement (Figs. 7.15, 7.16, and 7.17). Female patients predominated (4 women and 1 man) ranging in age from 54 to 75 years. Clinically, some patients presented with symptoms of dyspnea and shortness of breath, and open lung biopsies were obtained for their diagnosis. In three of the reported patients, a history of previous malignancy was noted, and these patients were being followed for possible metastatic disease. The lesions are the same as those reported as meningothelial-like nodules, except that the patients were symptomatic, had bilateral lung involvement, with clinical evidence of restrictive lung disease, and radiological evidence of diffuse reticulonodular pulmonary infiltrates. These findings are in contrast to the ones observed in meningothelial-like nodules in which the nodules are often an incidental finding and do not cause any symptoms. Nevertheless, cases of multiple pulmonary nodules of the type of meningothelial-like nodules have been reported. Ionescu et al. [39] reported a series of 35 cases in which the authors documented the existence of multiple bilateral nodules in three of their patients. Also Kukoki and Sellawi [40, 41] have documented cases in which the imaging demonstrated multiple bilateral pulmonary nodules.

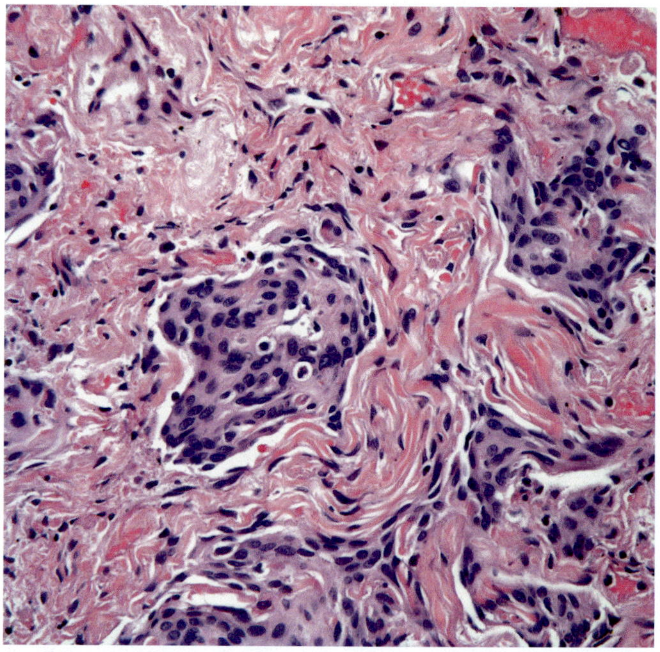

Fig. 7.17 High-power view of pulmonary meningotheliomatosis showing the classic features of a meningiomatous cellular proliferation

Histological Features

Low-power magnification of meningothelial-like nodules shows small aggregates or interstitial nodules distributed in a subpleural or parenchymal location. These nodules range in size from 1 to 3 mm in greatest diameter. High-power magnification shows that these nodules are composed of oval to spindle cells with moderate amounts of eosinophilic cytoplasm, indistinct cell borders, oval nuclei with finely dispersed chromatin, and inconspicuous nucleoli. In some areas, whorling of the tumor cells may be apparent, while in other areas, the cells may show pseudonuclear inclusions.

These tumor nodules show no evidence of mitotic activity, prominent cellular atypia, necrosis, or hemorrhage. However, many of these nodules may be close to dilated blood vessels. The adjacent lung parenchyma may show areas of hemosiderin-laden macrophages or be completely normal. These nodules may be solitary or numerous in the lung parenchyma.

In cases of meningotheliomatosis, the presence of these nodules is more obvious, and, depending on the number of sections available for study, one may be able to identify many of these nodules disseminated throughout the lung parenchyma.

Immunohistochemical and Molecular Biology Features

The immunohistochemical findings of meningothelial-like nodules and meningotheliomatosis are similar to the findings described for pulmonary meningiomas. In essence, these nodules are positive for vimentin and epithelial membrane antigen (EMA), which are the most consistent positive markers. In addition, the tumor cells are negative for keratins, muscle-specific actin, smooth muscle actin, chromogranin, synaptophysin, and CD34.

In a molecular study by Niho et al. [42], the authors concluded that meningothelial-like nodules may represent reactive proliferations after demonstrating monoclonal expansion of the X chromosome-linked human androgen receptor gene (HUMARA) in 7 of the 11 cases studied. Ionescu et al. [39], in a comparative study of intracranial meningiomas and pulmonary meningothelial-like nodules, using mutational analysis demonstrated loss of heterozygosity alterations at different chromosomal loci in both lesions, thus, concluding that both of these conditions are unrelated and that the lesions in the lung may represent a reactive process.

Differential Diagnosis

The differential diagnosis of these lesions may be divided into clinical and histological. Due to the small size of meningothelial nodules, they may easily be confused with carcinoid tumorlets. However, the histological features of carcinoid tumorlets are similar to those seen in neuroendocrine tumors, mainly an organoid, nested pattern, in which the cells react with epithelial markers like keratins, and also with neuroendocrine markers such as chromogranin and synaptophysin. One other possibility considerations would include metastatic disease mainly from a neuroendocrine tumor such as paraganglioma. However, the use of immunohistochemical studies for epithelial and neuroendocrine markers will lead to the correct interpretation. In cases in which the number of intrapulmonary lesions is large, the clinical impression may be of a metastatic process. As evidenced by some of the cases presented under meningotheliomatosis, cases in which there is a previous history of malignancy, the clinical impression may be suggestive of metastatic disease.

Treatment and Prognosis

These tumors are benign, and complete surgical resection is curative. One needs to keep in mind that approximately 65 % of the cases reported are derived from autopsy material, while 35 % stems from surgically resected material unrelated to these lesions. However, with new modalities and techniques in diagnostic imaging, it is very likely that these tumor nodules may become part of daily diagnostic surgical pathology.

Bronchial/Pulmonary Melanoma

Primary bronchial melanomas are rare, and their mere existence as a primary malignant pulmonary neoplasm is rather controversial. Not only are the criteria for diagnosis as a primary lung neoplasm difficult to apply but also is late metastasis from an extrapulmonary primary a known occurrence. The lungs are not unusual sites for metastatic disease from melanomas. Gromet et al. [43], in a study of 324 patients with malignant melanoma with a follow up period of 24 months, noted that the thorax was the initial site of relapse in 13 patients, 12 of whom were asymptomatic. The authors concluded that the thorax is a common site for relapse and that early detection of resectable metastases correlates with longer survival. Also Panagopoulos and Murray [44] evaluated 30 patients with metastatic melanoma of unknown primary and found that 5 patients (16 %) presented with lung metastases. From those reports it is evident that before a diagnosis of primary pulmonary malignant melanoma can be rendered, a detailed history mainly to assess the issue of previous skin or ocular tumors should be obtained.

Even though the existence of primary melanomas of the lung is well known, most of what is in the literature corresponds to case reports [45–71]. Some of these reports date back to the older literature in which there is not enough clinical, radiological, or histological information to properly define those tumors as of lung origin, while in others, there is a history of a skin tumor [45–48]. The first case of primary melanoma of the lung appears to be reported by Reid and Metha [49]. Although the authors reported two cases, one of the cases presented was a tracheal melanoma. One case of bronchial melanoma corresponded to a 60-year-old woman who during a bronchoscopic examination was found to have a mass in the posterior basal bronchus. The patient denied any previous history of tumor, and no other malignancy was found. The patient was treated with pneumonectomy.

The criteria set forward for the diagnosis of primary pulmonary melanoma were presented by Jensen and Egedorf [72] who stated that in order for a melanoma to be accepted as of lung origin, certain requirements had to be met. These can be summarized as follows:

1. No history of cutaneous lesion
2. No history of ocular tumor
3. Single tumor in the lung
4. Morphology of the lung tumor compatible with primary neoplasm
5. No spread of melanoma in other organs at the time of diagnosis
6. Autopsy proven

In addition to these criteria, Allen and Drash [51] reiterated previous criteria of melanomas in other sites and suggested that in order to accept melanomas as primary lung neoplasms, the following features had to be present:

1. Junctional change with "dropping off" or "nesting" of malignant cells just beneath the bronchial epithelium
2. Invasion of the bronchial epithelium in an area where the bronchial epithelium is not ulcerated
3. Obvious melanoma beneath the epithelium

Needless to say, in numerous reports, the issue of primary pulmonary melanoma has been diminished because of the possibility of a previous cutaneous melanoma that has undergone spontaneous regression. Based on all the required parameters for the diagnosis of primary bronchial/pulmonary melanoma, it is obvious that such a diagnosis is very difficult to apply in real practice, therefore, leaving such assessment to a more conventional clinicopathological approach in which a detailed clinical history is of utmost importance.

Interestingly, in one of the largest series of primary melanomas of the lung, Wilson [73] encountered that all the criteria for the diagnosis of bronchial/pulmonary melanomas are often not present or difficult to obtain in any given patient. The authors assessed the incidence of primary malignant melanoma of the lung to be 0.01 % in a period of 45 years. Even though the eight cases reported mirrored to some extent what had been reported in the literature through case reports, the authors clearly stated that not all the parameters were met in each individual case. For instance, one of the "strongest" criteria for the diagnosis of pulmonary melanoma is the finding of an in situ melanoma. However, it is well known that some metastatic melanomas to the lung will not only present as a single pulmonary mass but also will display histological features of in situ melanoma [74].

If we were to analyze in more detail the set clinical and histological criteria for the diagnosis of pulmonary melanoma, we could discover that some of the items stated in the 1967 criteria may not necessarily apply in today's more modern practice of medicine. One example would be the use of autopsy to confirm the diagnosis, which is less relevant today as it may have been 30 years ago. In today's practice, it is possible to evaluate a patient for the possibility of an occult tumor in the eye or elsewhere. Also today it is possible to evaluate the possibility of widespread metastatic disease at the time of diagnosis. Therefore we may conclude that these criteria do not apply to today's practice. Recently, de Wilt et al. [75] analyzed the subject of metastatic versus primary pulmonary melanoma in a study of 15 patients with no history of melanoma and who presented with tumors in the lung. The authors acknowledged that this group of patients may represent approximately 5 % of all patients in whom the primary melanoma site is unknown. Of the 15 patients reported, 11 patients presented with a single tumor, and further analysis produced seven cases in which the diagnosis of primary pulmonary melanoma was very likely. The authors concluded that the distinction between primary and metastatic melanoma is best accomplished by clinical behavior (pattern of spread) rather than by histopathological criteria. Similar to the series of cases presented by Wilson [73], de Wilt et al. [75] were not able to match the entire set of criteria proposed for the diagnosis of primary pulmonary melanomas and stated that although the dilemma of primary versus metastatic disease was of considerable interest, it may be irrelevant in terms of optimal management of these patients. Therefore, each case should be evaluated on an individual basis.

Clinical Features

The clinical symptoms of patients with primary melanomas of the lung are in no way specific and are similar to those seen in primary lung carcinomas. Therefore, it is very likely that patients with these unusual tumors will present with symptoms of cough, dyspnea, fever, chest pain, hemoptysis, or any other sign of bronchial obstruction. Bronchoscopic findings may suggest the possibility of melanoma if the lesion in question is pigmented; however, such a finding is not always present. The tumor does not have any predilection for a particular gender and usually is diagnosed in adult patients with a mean age of 51 years. One of the most important parameters that needs to be excluded by history or physical and radiological evaluations is the presence of past or present skin or ocular tumors.

Macroscopic Features

Ideally, the presence of a single tumor has been proposed as an important parameter, and in many ways such information will bias toward the possibility of a primary neoplasm. However, it should be kept in mind that such occurrence can take place in cases of metastatic melanoma to the lung, limiting the use of that information in the assessment of primary versus metastatic disease. The tumors appear well defined with or without obvious pigmentation. The cut surface may be tan in color with a

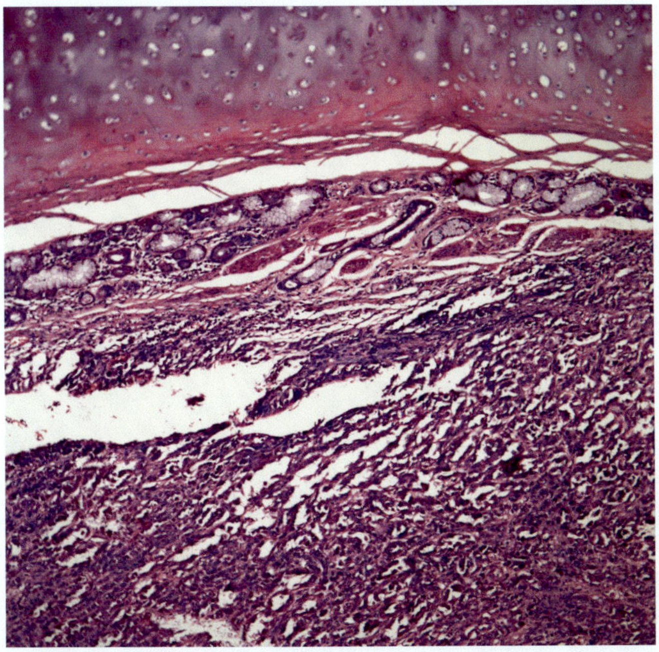

Fig. 7.18 Bronchial melanoma with an in situ component. Note the presence of uninvolved bronchial glands and bronchial cartilage

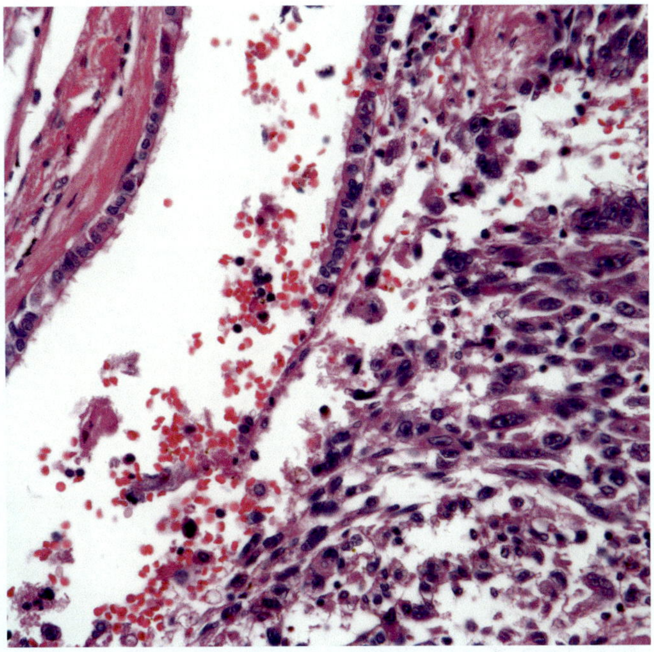

Fig. 7.19 Different view of a bronchial melanoma with an in situ component. Note the presence of ciliated bronchial epithelium being replaced by tumor

homogenous surface with or without areas of hemorrhage and/or necrosis. The tumors may vary in size from 1 cm to more than 5 cm in greatest diameter. The tumors may appear as polypoid bronchial lesions obstructing the lumen or may appear as an intraparenchymal mass.

Microscopic Features

The spectrum of histopathological features of primary melanomas of the lung is similar to that seen in melanomas of the skin (Figs. 7.18, 7.19, 7.20, 7.21, 7.22, and 7.23). The tumor may show in situ changes of the bronchial epithelium in many cases but not in all. These in situ changes may mimic in situ changes of carcinomas. Underneath the bronchial epithelium, the tumor may grow in an organoid or nested, diffuse, or spindle cell pattern. The neoplastic cellular proliferation may be composed of medium-size cells with moderate amounts of eosinophilic cytoplasm, round to oval nuclei, prominent nucleoli, and easily identifiable mitotic activity. The tumor may also display a cellular proliferation composed of rather small cells with round nuclei and inconspicuous nucleoli mimicking the growth pattern of a small cell carcinoma. In spindle cell melanomas, the tumors may be composed of fusiform cells with elongated nuclei and inconspicuous nucleoli. Pseudonuclear inclusions and mitotic activity can be easily identified. Areas of necrosis and/or hemorrhage may be seen in pulmonary melanomas regardless of the growth pattern. Melanin pigment is present in the majority of cases; however, in a few cases, its presence may only be focal.

Immunohistochemical Features

The use of immunohistochemical stains is generally helpful in the diagnosis of pulmonary melanoma. Since these tumors are very unusual as primary lung neoplasms and since melanomas may also share some immunophenotypic features with lung carcinomas, it is important to perform a panel of immunohistochemical stains that may allow for proper characterization of these tumors. It is known that melanomas react positively with S100 protein, HMB45, and Melan A; thus, these stains should be part of the panel. Important to recognize is that some spindle cell melanomas may be negative for HMB45 [76] and some may also be positive for carcinoembryonic antigen (CEA) [50], thus the importance of adding putative epithelial markers such as keratins and EMA. Recently, Sox2-positive staining in melanomas has been described.

Differential Diagnosis

The wide spectrum of histopathological patterns that melanoma may display is well known, thus making a differential diagnosis rather impractical since melanoma can mimic any primary tumor in the lung, namely, carcinomas that do not show the conventional features of squamous or adenocarcinomatous features. For instance, the histology observed in some cases of pleomorphic or sarcomatoid carcinomas of the lung can easily be applied to some cases of melanomas. Also some neuroendocrine tumors may share some histopathological

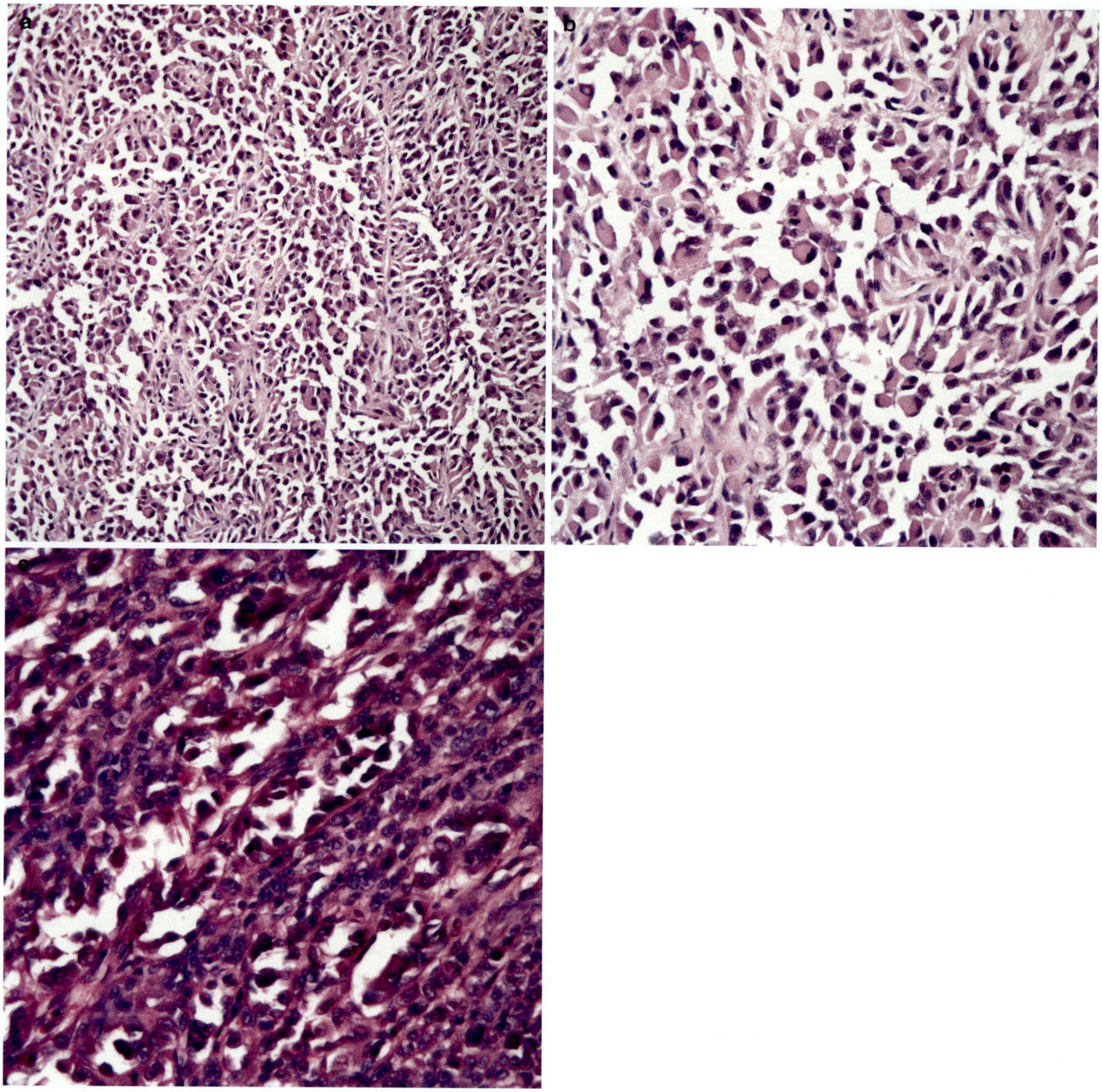

Fig. 7.20 (**a**) Low-power view of a melanoma with prominent "rhabdoid" features. (**b**) High-power view showing neoplastic cells with ample eosinophilic cytoplasm and peripherally situated nucleus. (**c**) Alveolar-like areas alternating with a more solid component

features with melanomas. Even the presence of melanin pigment can be seen in some neuroendocrine carcinomas; therefore, the recommended use of an immunohistochemical panel in cases in which the index of suspicion is high for a non-epithelial malignancy. The only issue left is whether the tumor represents primary or metastatic disease, which to some extent cannot be solved by a histopathological assessment but rather by good clinical and radiological evaluation of the patient.

Treatment and Prognosis

The treatment of choice is complete surgical resection of the tumor. The prognosis of primary melanomas of the lung may be variable. In the cases described, some patients had an aggressive behavior of the tumors, while others had a protracted clinical course. In the series of eight patients reported by Wilson and Moran [73], five patients died of disease 4–32 months after initial diagnosis, two patients were alive with

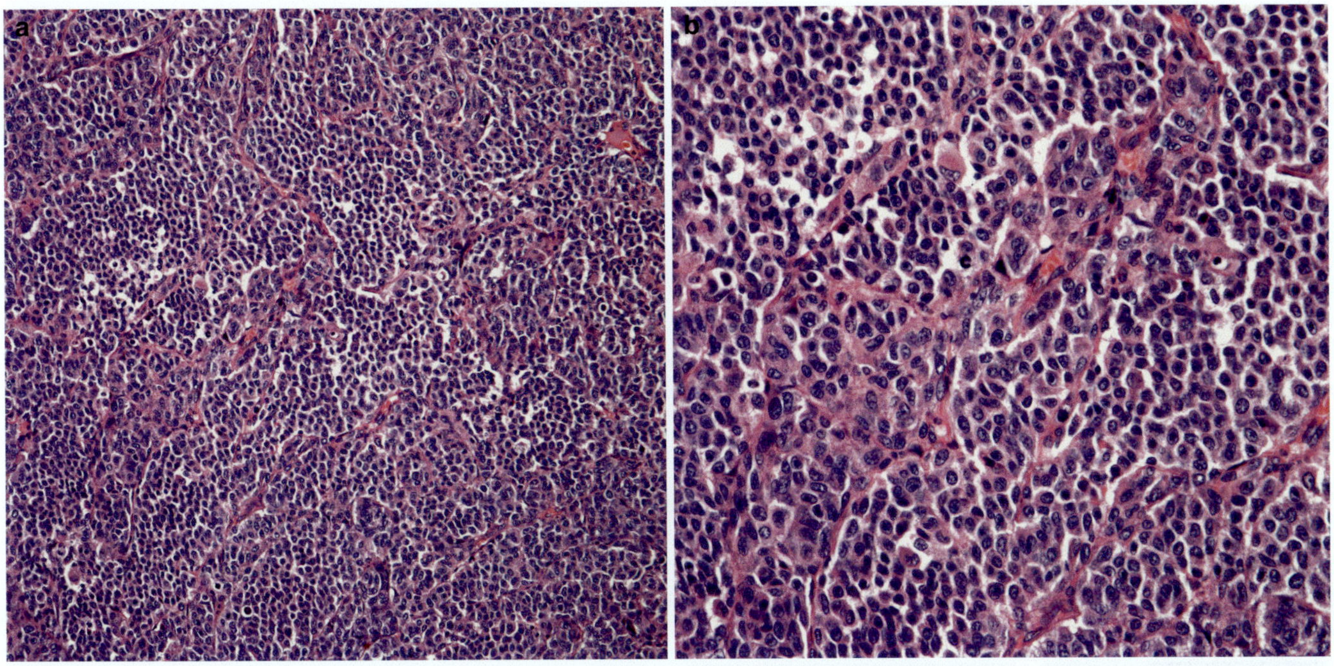

Fig. 7.21 (**a**) Low-power view of pulmonary melanoma with prominent neuroendocrine-like growth pattern. (**b**) High-power view showing a subtle nested pattern with a homogenous cellular proliferation admixed with numerous mitotic figures

metastasis 4–30 months after initial diagnosis, and one patient was alive without evidence of metastatic disease 108 months after initial diagnosis. In the cases described by de Wilt et al. [75], the 5-year survival was 42 %, which led the authors to state that resection of pulmonary disease in melanoma patients without a known primary can result in long-term survival.

Pulmonary Glomangioma/Glomangiosarcoma

Of these two tumors, glomangioma is by far the most common. Glomangiomas occur more often in the nail bed, superficial, and deep soft tissue but have also been described in a more ubiquitous distribution that includes the gastrointestinal and gynecological systems and the head and neck area [77–82]. The tumors are assumed to originate from the glomus body, which represents a specialized arteriovenous anastomosis made up of the Sucquet-Hoyer canals. Over the years, there has been considerable debate regarding whether glomangioma represents a true tumor or a hyperplasia. However, the fact that there is an entity known as glomangiosarcoma that can behave in an aggressive manner seems to favor that both of these conditions represent true neoplasms and not just a hyperplastic process.

Primary glomus tumor in the respiratory system is a very unusual neoplasm despite several reports in the lung or other respiratory structures. In the respiratory system, the trachea is the most common location, and although most of the cases described are of the benign type (glomangioma), cases of glomangiosarcoma have also been described [83–86]. Herein, we will focus only on those tumors of the lower respiratory tract, namely, those occurring in the bronchus and in the lung.

Primary pulmonary and/or bronchial glomangiomas and glomangiosarcomas are very rare, and for the most part, are tumors reported as a curiosity or in small series of cases [87–94]. Tang et al. [87] are given the credit for the first description of a glomangioma in the lung. The authors reported a 67-year-old woman who on radiographic evaluation showed the presence of a mass in the left lung. Two important aspects about this report are that the authors suggested the possibility of glomera in the lung; the other important aspect is of the possible multicentricity of glomangiomas as their patient had two distinct intrapulmonary nodules. Mackay et al. [88] also described a 19-year-old with a coin lesion in the lung. However, more detailed history disclosed that the patient also had a soft tissue tumor with similar histology as that in the lung; therefore, in this particular case, it is most likely that the lesion in the lung represented metastatic disease from an extrapulmonary origin. Alt et al. [89] reported a 34-year-old asymptomatic man with a coin lesion in the lung. The authors proposed that the term glomus tumor be reserved for those tumors composed of endothelial-lined vascular spaces surrounded by smooth muscle. Koss et al. [90] added two additional cases of intrapulmonary glomangiomas in two asymptomatic adult patients 40 and 51 years old, respectively. Gaetner et al. [91]

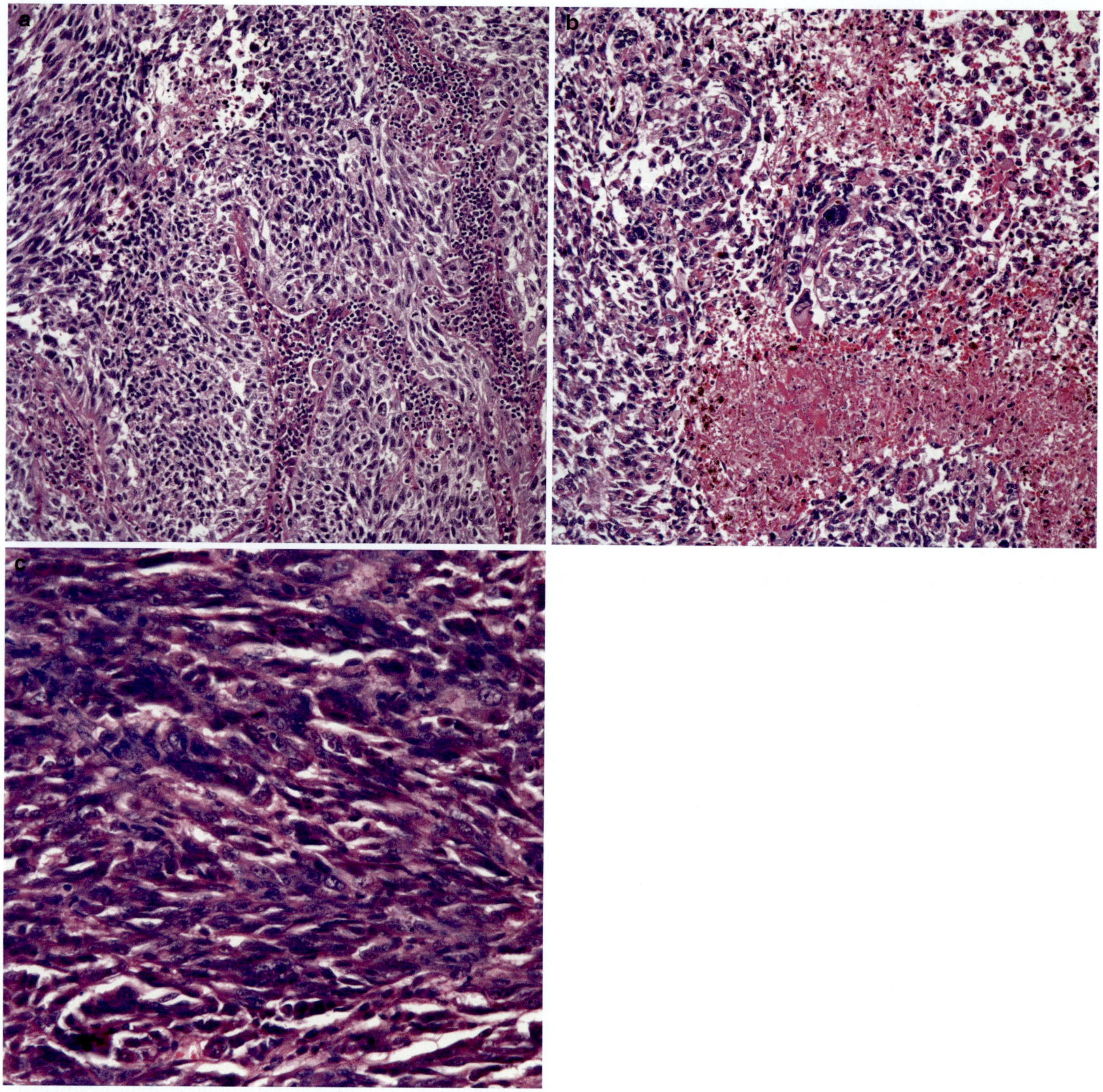

Fig. 7.22 (**a**) Spindle cell growth pattern of a pulmonary melanoma with a subtle neural-like appearance. (**b**) Spindle cell melanoma with focal multinucleated malignant giant cells and necrosis. (**c**) More solid spindle cell component with nuclear pleomorphism

was able to collect five cases; however, one of those cases originated in the mediastinum and one case was a glomangiosarcoma. The three patients with glomangiomas were adults and their intrapulmonary lesion was discovered incidentally while being followed for different reasons. On the other hand, the patient diagnosed with glomangiosarcoma appeared to have symptoms related to the tumor such as hemoptysis. More recently, three additional reports of glomangiomas have been presented [92–94] and, contrary to previous cases in which the tumor has been in the lung parenchyma, these cases have been reported within the bronchus, obstructing its lumen.

Clinical Features

There are no specific clinical features that can be correlated with glomangioma or glomangiosarcoma. In the reported

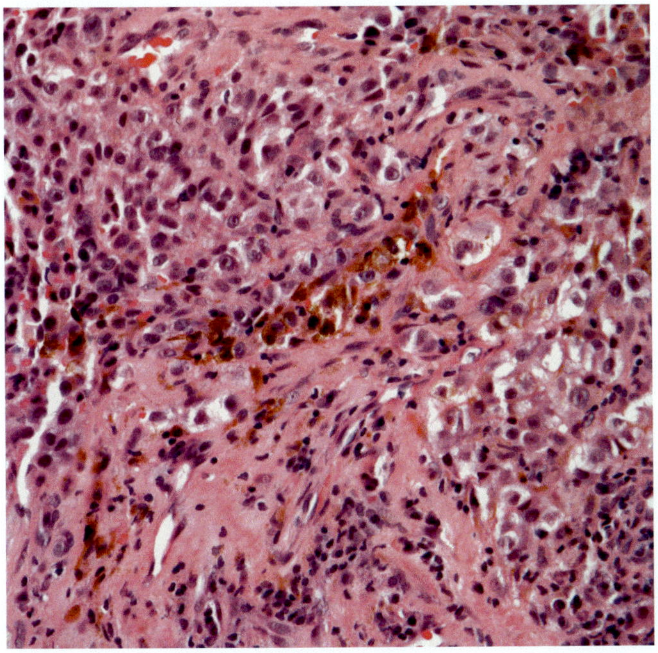

Fig. 7.23 Pulmonary melanoma with focal areas of melanin pigment deposition

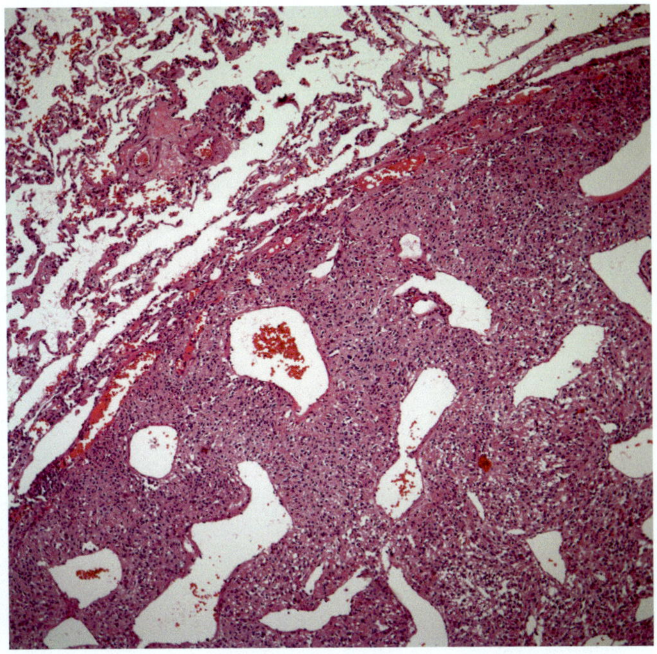

Fig. 7.24 Pulmonary glomus tumor showing a well circumscribed but unencapsulated lesion. Note the presence of numerous dilated vessels

cases, many patients have been asymptomatic and their tumors have been found either during a routine radiographic evaluation or during the course of evaluating a different problem. On the contrary, when these tumors occur in a central location, it is more likely that these patients may present with some symptomatology related to bronchial obstruction, namely, cough, chest pain, and/or hemoptysis. Since glomangiomas are very unusual tumors, the clinical impression is of that of a different, more common bronchial neoplasm. These tumors can be seen in young adult individuals or in older patients, approximately between the ages of 20 and 65 years. The tumors also appear not to discriminate based on gender or racial background as they have been described in men and women and in Caucasian, Black, or Asian individuals.

Macroscopic Features

These tumors can occur either as central or peripheral tumors. The majority of cases appear to be within the lung proper, and they have been described as well-circumscribed tumor nodules that may range in size from 1 cm to 6 cm in greatest diameter. In a few cases, the description has been of two separate nodules. The tumors are described as being of soft consistency, tan in color, with a smooth homogenous surface. In a few cases, the description has been of "encapsulated" tumor nodules with dilated spaces on cut surface. Glomangiomas characteristically do not show areas of necrosis and/or hemorrhage. Glomangiosarcomas appear to be larger tumors with areas of hemorrhage and/or necrosis.

Microscopic Features

The histopathological spectrum of glomangiomas in the soft tissue appears to be wider than that observed in the lung. Those tumors occurring in the lung appear to be more of the solid mucohyaline type (Figs. 7.24, 7.25, 7.26, 7.27, 7.28, 7.29, 7.30, 7.31, and 7.32). The low-power view is that of a well-demarcated tumor nodule surrounded by normal lung parenchyma. At low-power magnification, the tumor is characterized by the presence of a fairly homogenous cellular proliferation admixed with dilated vascular spaces. Those arising in a central location will show partial obstruction of the bronchial lumen with similar histopathological features as those present within the lung parenchyma. Higher magnification of these tumors show a homogenous cellular proliferation composed of medium-size cells, with round to oval nuclei, clear to lightly eosinophilic cytoplasm, and presence of ectatic vascular spaces. The cellular proliferation is characterized by clear cytoplasm and elicits the so-called fried egg appearance, while the vascular spaces characteristically show perivascular hyalinization. Glomangiomas characteristically do not show evidence of necrosis and/or mitotic activity.

Glomangiosarcoma will display areas reminiscent of glomangiomas (Figs. 7.33, 7.34, 7.35, 7.36, 7.37, and 7.38). However, at low-power magnification, it is possible to

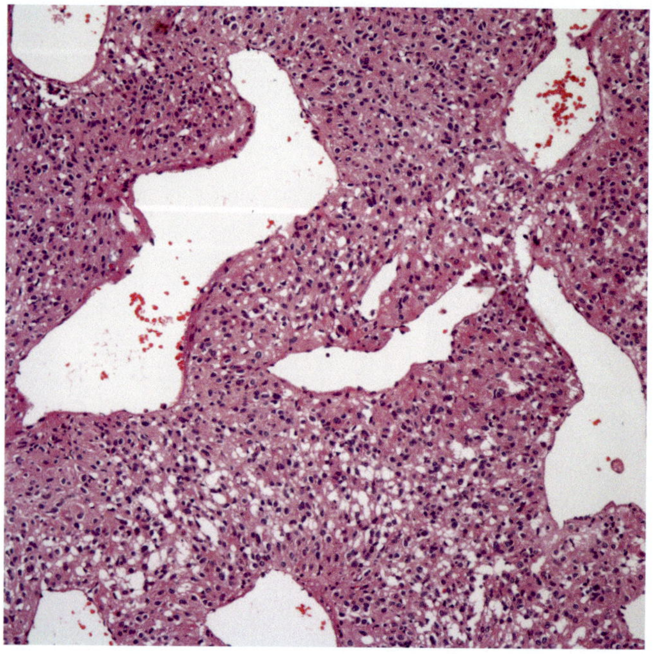

Fig. 7.25 Pulmonary glomus tumor showing a homogenous cellular proliferation admixed with prominent dilated vessels

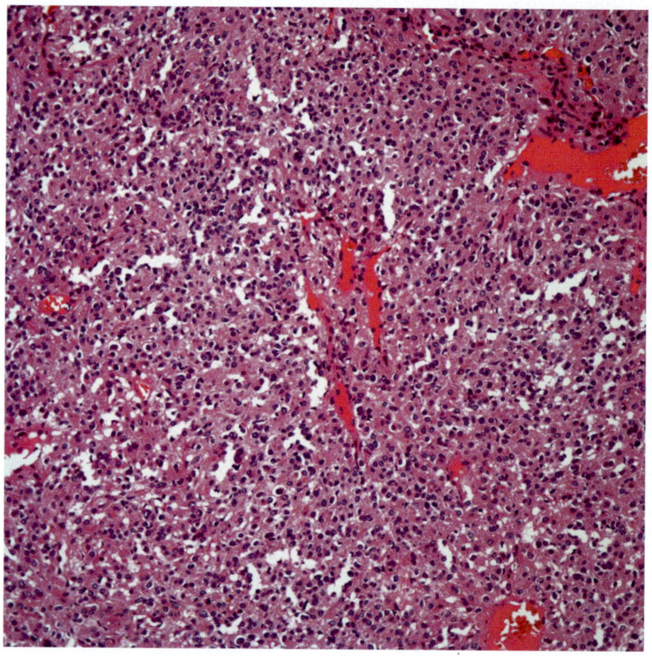

Fig. 7.26 Pulmonary glomus tumor composed of more solid areas

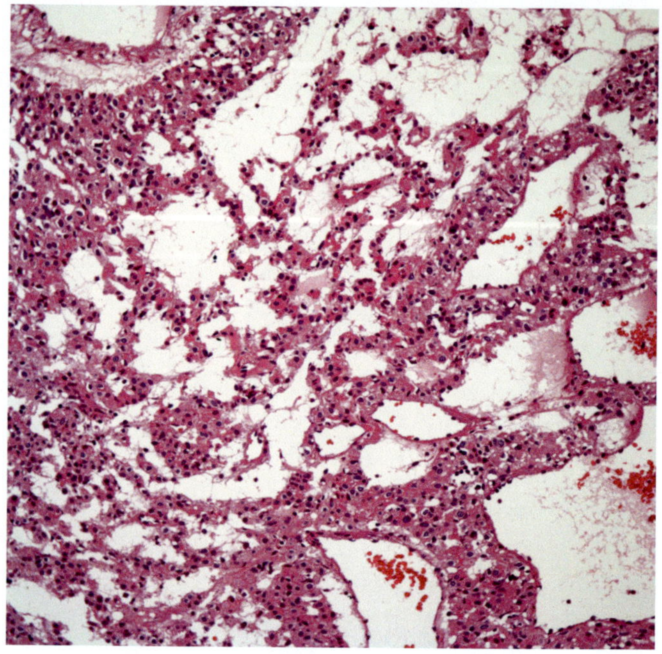

Fig. 7.27 Pulmonary glomus tumor with a more discohesive cellular proliferation and subtle hyaline changes

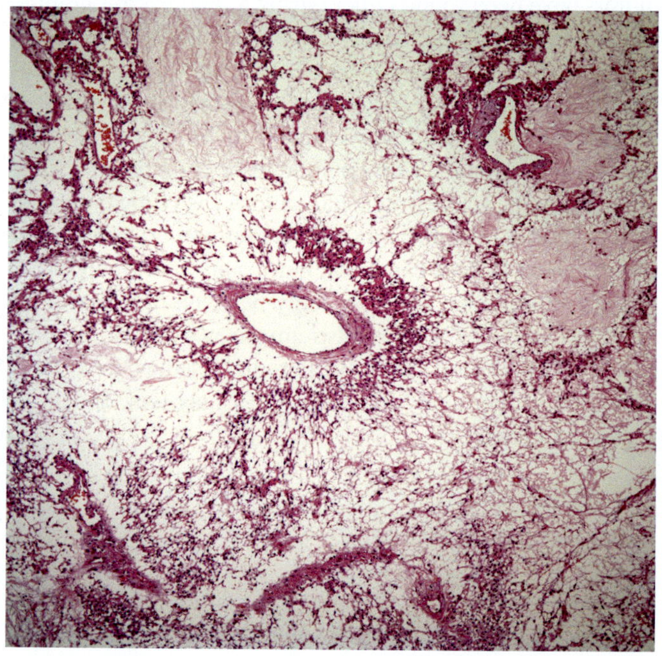

Fig. 7.28 Pulmonary glomus tumor with prominent hyaline changes and dilated vessels

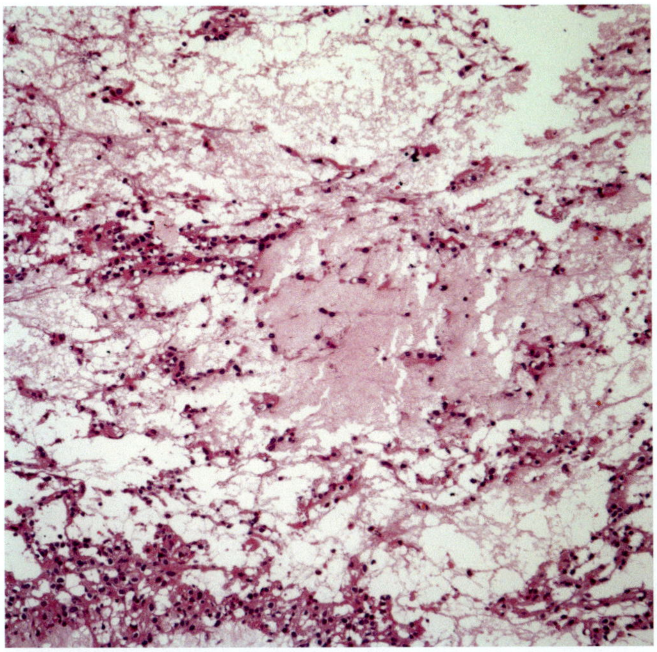

Fig. 7.29 Pulmonary glomus tumor with prominent hyaline changes and scant cellularity

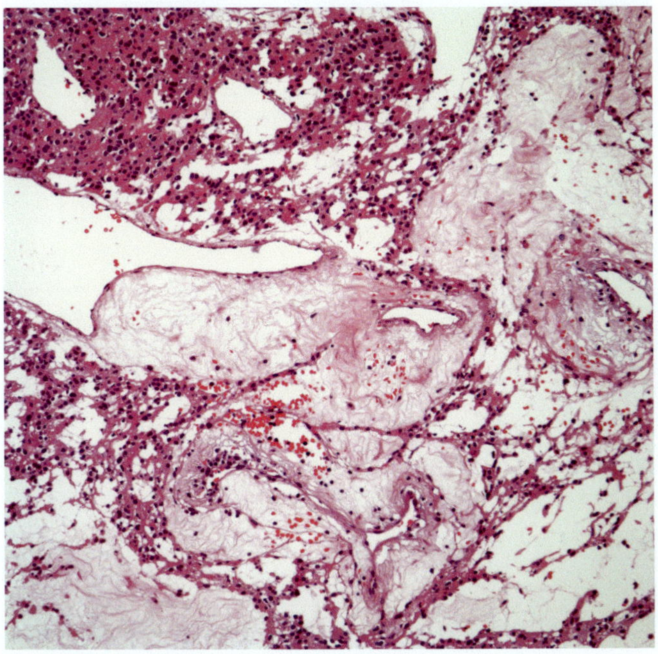

Fig. 7.30 Pulmonary glomus tumor with prominent hyaline changes in the walls of vessels

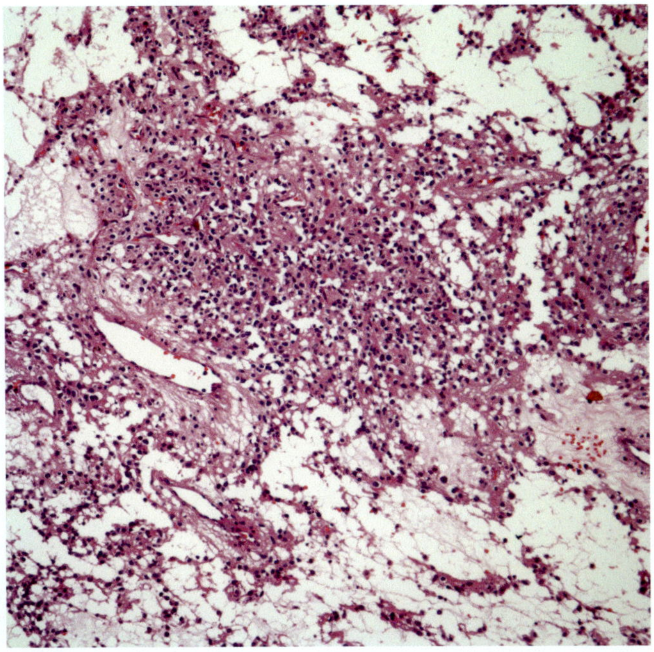

Fig. 7.31 Pulmonary glomus tumor showing a combination of hyaline changes with solid areas and clear cell changes

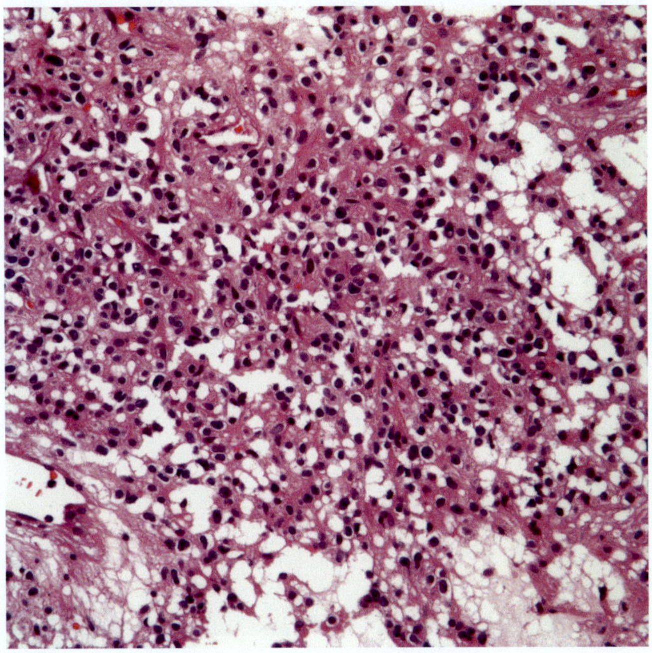

Fig. 7.32 Closer view at the cellular proliferation of a pulmonary glomus tumor showing prominent clear cell changes

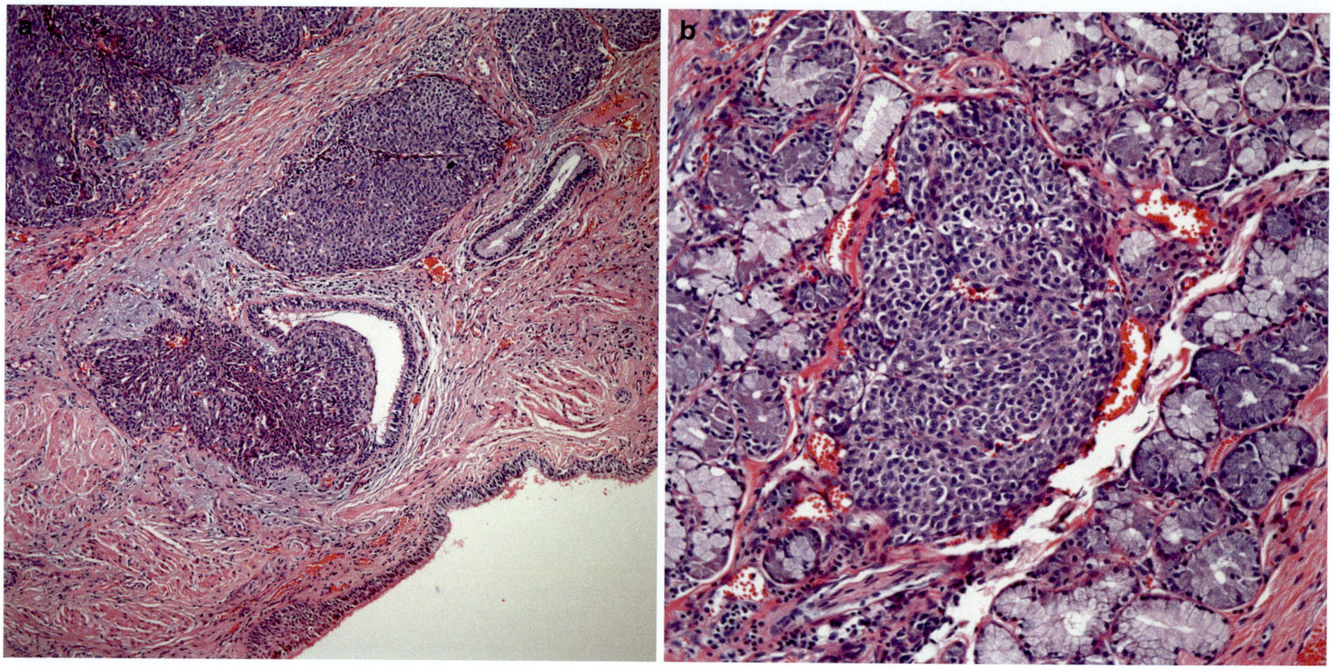

Fig. 7.33 (**a**) Low-power view of a pulmonary glomangiosarcoma. Note the ciliated respiratory epithelium. (**b**) Glomangiosarcoma invading bronchial glands

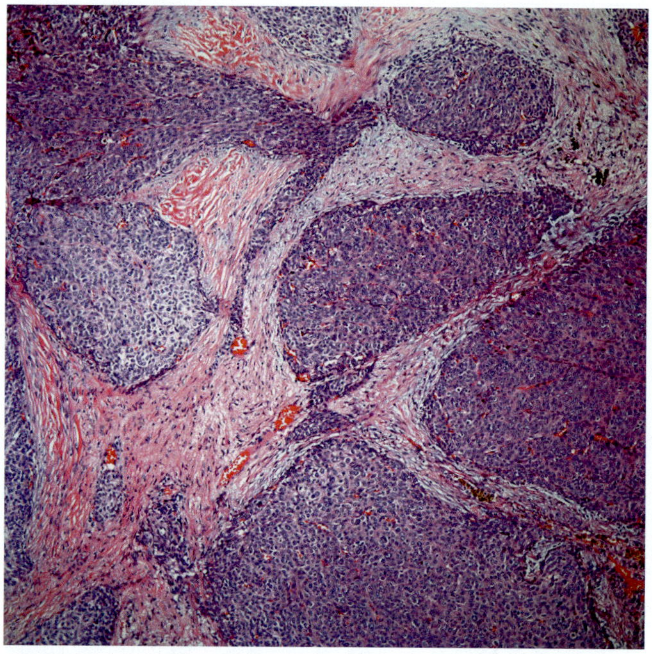

Fig. 7.34 Pulmonary glomangiosarcoma showing prominent lobulation

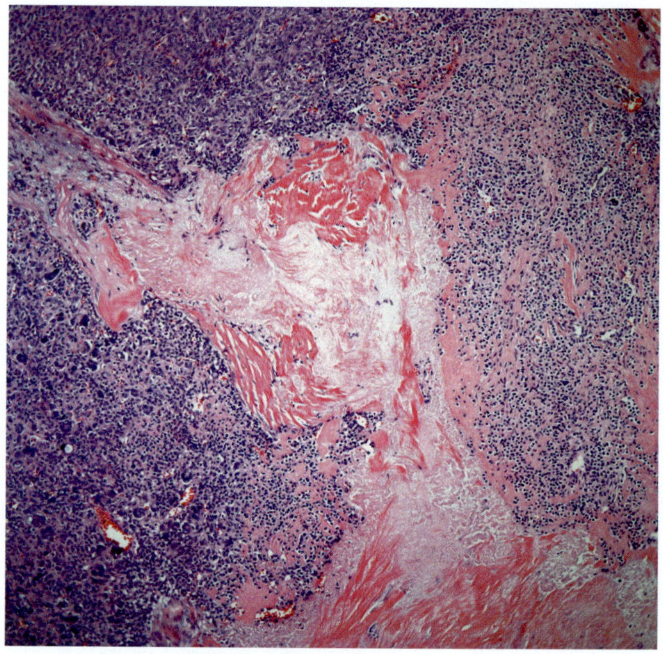

Fig. 7.35 Glomangiosarcoma with extensive hyalinization and focal areas of conventional benign glomus tumor

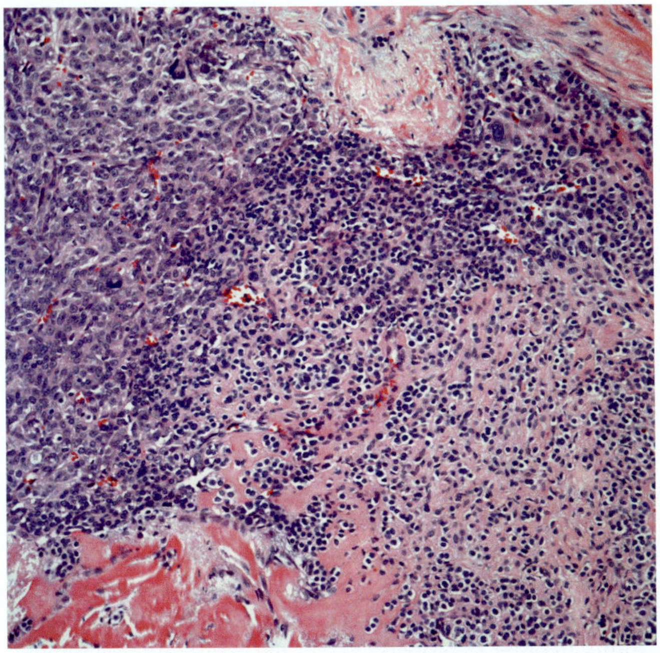

Fig. 7.36 Higher magnification of malignant areas (glomangiosarcoma) with transition to benign areas (glomangioma)

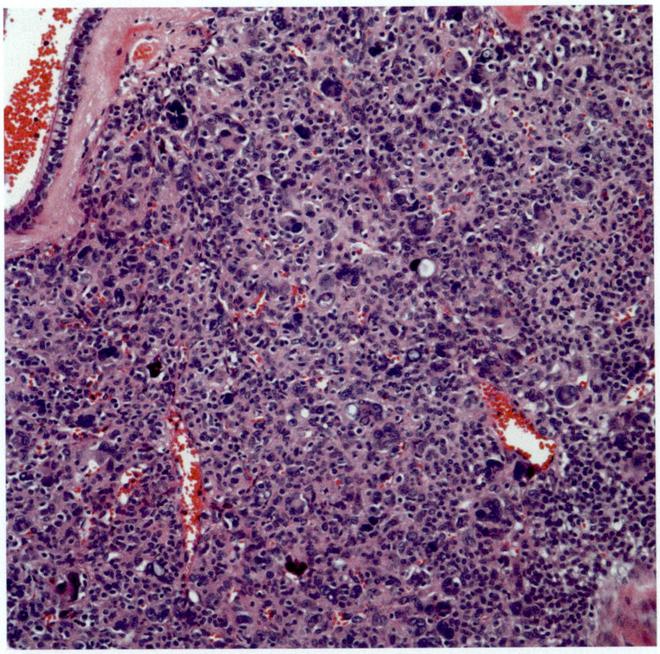

Fig. 7.37 Glomangiosarcoma with prominent nuclear atypia

observe areas of necrosis, which may not necessarily be extensive. Closer magnification of glomangiosarcomas shows areas of nuclear atypia and mitotic activity. Transitional areas from conventional glomangioma into glomangiosarcoma may be observed and are helpful in arriving at the correct interpretation.

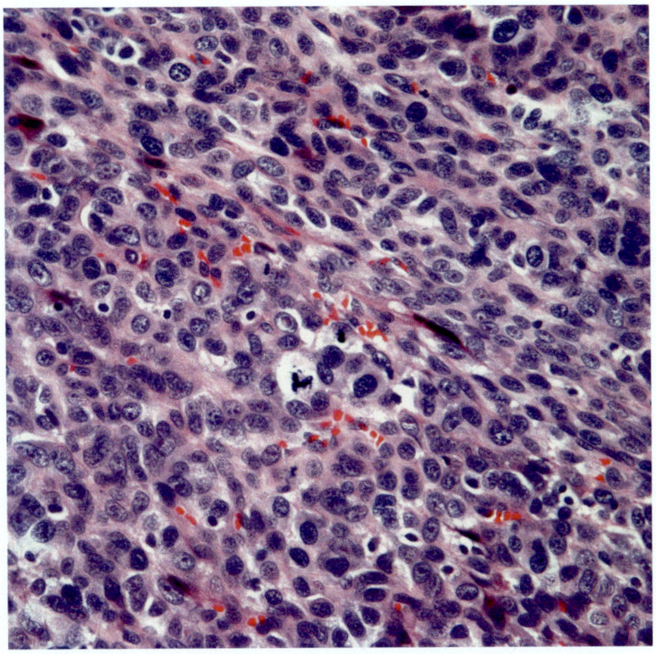

Fig. 7.38 Glomangiosarcoma showing a spindle cellular proliferation with marked nuclear atypia and mitotic activity

Immunohistochemical Features

The most consistent immunohistochemical characteristics for these tumors are positive staining for vimentin and muscle-specific actin (Fig. 7.39). However, these tumors may show positive staining for other markers including smooth muscle actin, desmin, neuron-specific enolase, and CD57. Glomangiomas and glomangiosarcomas characteristically show negative staining for keratins, EMA, myoglobin, chromogranin, S100 protein, and HMB45. Hatori et al. [95] reported a study of six cases of glomus tumors (subungual tumors) in which the authors reported positive staining in vascular endothelial cells as well as in tumor cells for CD34. However, other authors have reported negative staining for CD34 [90].

Differential Diagnosis

The differential diagnosis of glomangiomas in the lung may be challenging due to the rarity of these tumors as primary lung neoplasms. Tumors that may pose a challenge and that may share some macroscopic as well as histopathological features with glomangiomas include clear cell "sugar tumor" and well-differentiated neuroendocrine carcinoma (carcinoid tumor). Both of these tumors may show dilated vascular spaces, lack of mitotic activity and necrosis and may show a cellular proliferation composed of medium-size cells with clear or lightly eosinophilic cyto-

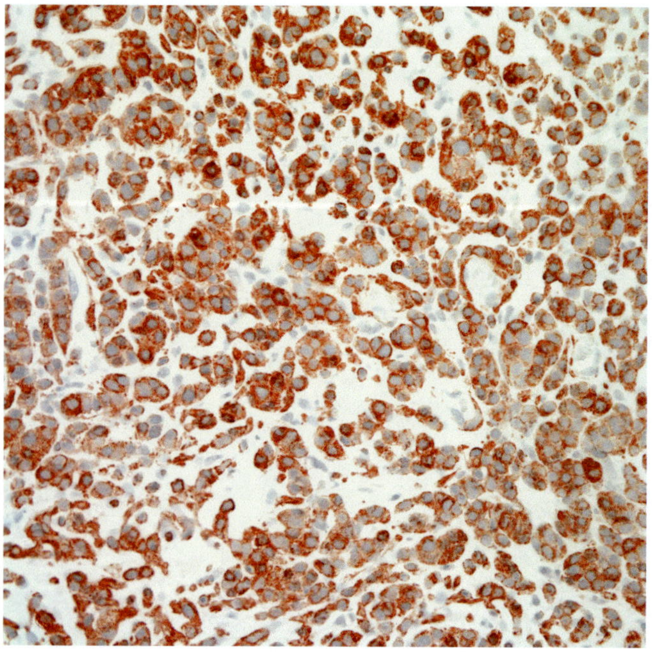

Fig. 7.39 Muscle specific actin immunohistochemical stain showing strong positive reaction in tumor cells

plasm. However, the use of immunohistochemical studies, mainly the positive staining of tumor cells for muscle-specific actin, will lead to the correct interpretation as sugar tumor or neuroendocrine carcinomas are negative for muscle markers. In addition, sugar tumors may show positive staining for CD34, S100 protein, and HMB45, while neuroendocrine carcinomas will show positive staining for keratin, EMA, and neuroendocrine markers such as chromogranin and/or synaptophysin. In cases of glomangiosarcoma, the main issue will be the identification of more conventional areas of glomangioma and positive staining for muscle-specific actin. Nevertheless, a valid differential diagnosis will be with leiomyosarcoma, which may show a similar immunophenotype. In this setting, the identification of more conventional areas of glomangioma is crucial in arriving at a more specific diagnosis.

Treatment and Prognosis

In cases of glomangioma, complete surgical resection of the tumor is curative. This procedure may be in the form of wedge resection or lobectomy, depending on the clinical and radiological evaluation. For those cases diagnosed as glomangiosarcoma, surgical resection followed by chemotherapy appears to be a reasonable approach; however, since the number of cases of this tumor in the lung is exceedingly low, there is not enough cumulative information to properly determine the exact nature of these tumors. However, it is possible that these tumors may follow an aggressive behavior with widespread metastasis.

Intrapulmonary Thymoma

Thymomas are more often found in the anterior mediastinal compartment. However, the occurrence of thymomas outside of the mediastinal structures is well known, and thymomas have been recorded to present as primary tumors in the neck, trachea, and thyroid gland [96–98]. In the thoracic area, thymomas have been described as primary tumors in the pleura [99] and in the lung [100–114]. One important issue to keep in mind before rendering the diagnosis of primary ectopic thymoma is to rule out the presence of a primary thymoma the mediastinal compartment. Thymomas can become infiltrative and spread outside of the mediastinal compartment into the pleura, lung, or outside of the thoracic cavity. Therefore, the most important issue is to rule out such possibility in order to properly assess the origin of these tumors. In addition, there are two additional aspects that need to be kept in mind in the evaluation of intrapulmonary thymomas: (1) although capsular integrity is the most important parameter to evaluate in mediastinal thymomas, such aspect is irrelevant when these tumors occur in an intrapulmonary location; (2) the histopathological subtype of thymomas is another aspect that becomes irrelevant when these tumors occur in an intrapulmonary location. However, a diagnostic challenge may arise in cases of atypical thymoma in an intrapulmonary location, as these tumors will require careful evaluation in order to separate them from non-small cell carcinomas of the lung, namely, squamous cell carcinoma. Nevertheless, it would be highly important to distinguish thymoma from thymic carcinoma, as thymic carcinoma not only is a separate clinicopathological entity but it also follows a more aggressive behavior.

Different theories have been presented to account for the occurrence of thymomas in an intrapulmonary location; however, there is not a single one that can completely explain such occurrence. Although links have been made to the embryologic development of the thymus, one may encounter that such theory may explain the occurrence of ectopic thymic tissue in the neck area but not in an intrapulmonary location. Therefore, the occurrence of these tumors in the lung cannot be fully explained and remains only in a speculative form.

Clinical Features

Clinically, intrapulmonary thymomas have been described in a wide range of individuals from teenagers to patients older than 70 years. Although there may be a slight predilection for these tumors to occur in females, the tumor has been described in men and women almost equally. Clinically, the patients may present completely asymptomatic or with a wide variety of symptoms that may include chest pain, fatigue, hemoptysis, dyspnea, dysphagia, dysarthria, nephrotic syndrome, cough, fever, chills, hyperhomocysteinemia, and more unusually myasthenia gravis.

Macroscopic Features

Intrapulmonary thymomas can be seen in two different forms: (1) as a hilar tumor and (2) as an intrapulmonary peripheral tumor. The tumor size may vary from 1 to more than 10 cm in greatest diameter. The tumors appear well-circumscribed, firm, white to tan, with or without focal areas of hemorrhage and/or necrosis. In unusual cases, the tumor may also show additional lesions in the pulmonary parenchyma.

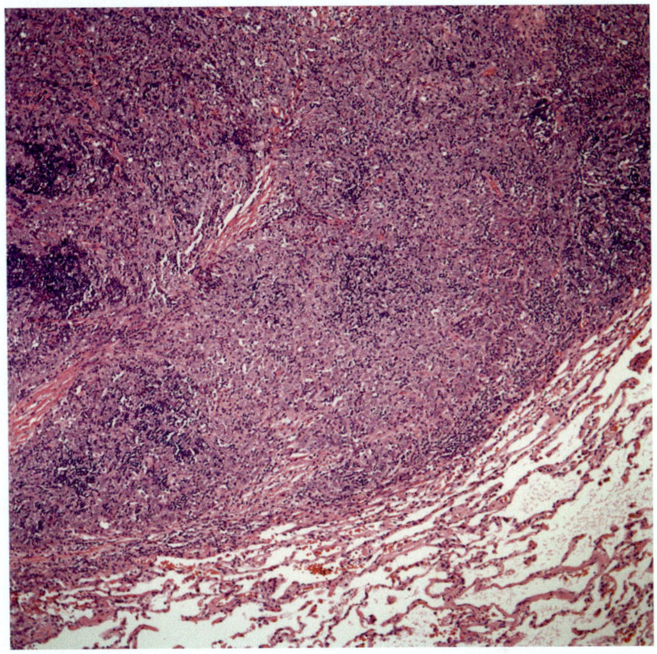

Fig. 7.40 Intrapulmonary thymoma showing a well-demarcated tumor mass. The classic biphasic cellular growth pattern is apparent

Histopathological Features

The histopathological features seen in intrapulmonary thymomas are the same as those described for mediastinal thymomas (Figs. 7.40, 7.41, 7.42, 7.43, 7.44, 7.45, 7.46, and 7.47). Essentially, the tumor may show a biphasic cellular proliferation composed of lymphocytes and epithelial cells in different proportions. In some cases, either of these components may appear as the predominant component. The tumor may show the characteristic fibrous bands separating the cellular proliferation into different islands of tumor cells of different sizes. The epithelial cellular proliferation is composed of medium-size cells with round to oval nuclei and small or inconspicuous nucleoli. Mitotic activity in the epithelial component may be seen, but it is not high, while mitotic figures may be seen in the lymphocytic component. In spindle cell thymoma, the cellular proliferation is composed of fusiform cells with indistinct cell borders, elongated nuclei, and inconspicuous nucleoli. The cells may be arranged in a subtle storiform pattern with numerous easily identifiable dilated vessels, reminiscent of a hemangiopericytic pattern of growth. Mitotic figures and nuclear atypia are absent, while the presence of lymphocytes is inconspicuous.

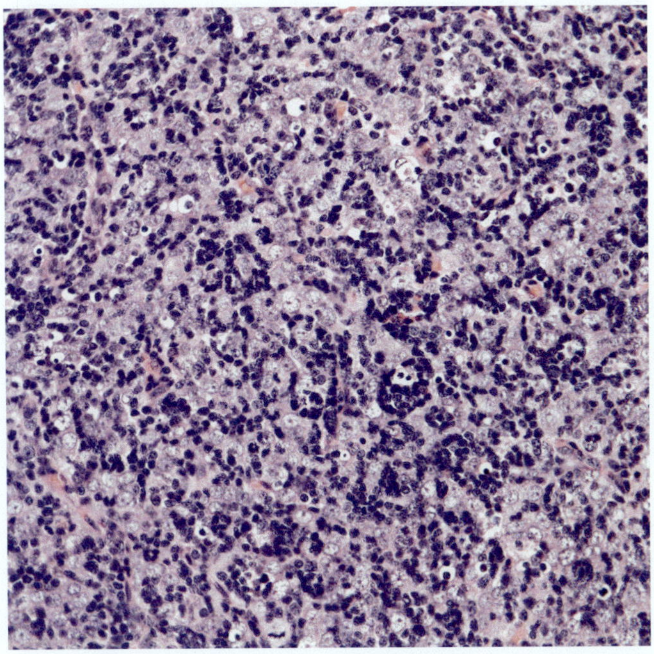

Fig. 7.41 Intrapulmonary thymoma showing a dual cell population of lymphocytes and epithelial cells

Immunohistochemical Features

The use of immunohistochemical studies may aid and help in separating intrapulmonary thymomas from other more common intrapulmonary neoplasms. Thymomas show positive staining for keratin, and, in cases in which the lymphocytic component is present, the lymphocytes may also show positive staining for leukocyte common antibody and T and B cell markers such as CD20 and TdT. Although thymomas are epithelial tumors, EMA may show only weak positive staining, and in a high number of cases, it is negative. Other markers that may show positive staining for thy-

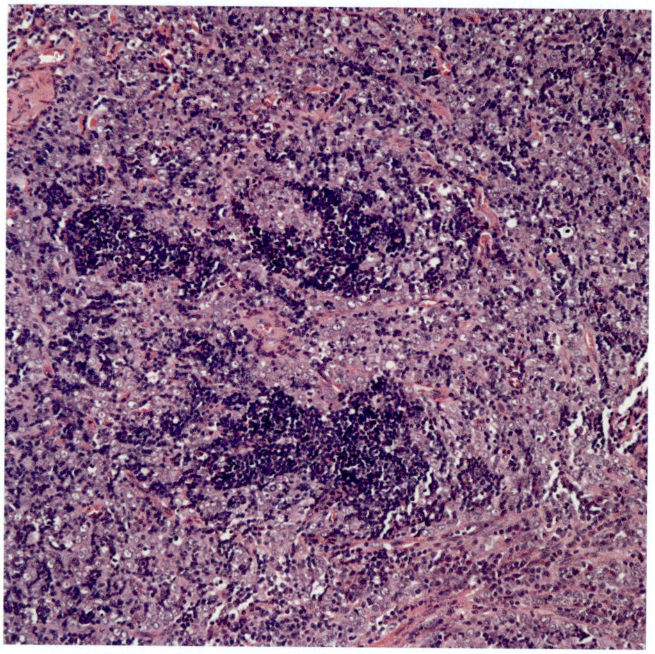

Fig. 7.42 Intrapulmonary thymoma showing clusters of lymphocytes in a predominantly epithelial neoplasm

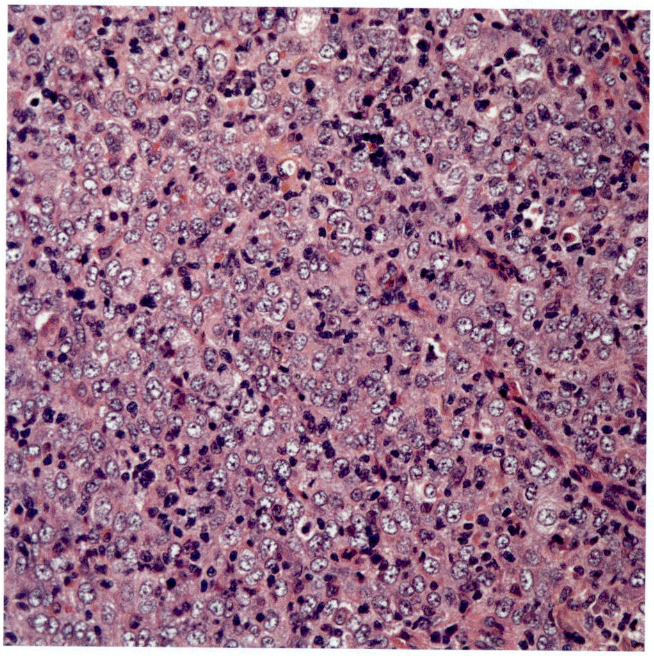

Fig. 7.43 Intrapulmonary thymoma with a predominantly epithelial component

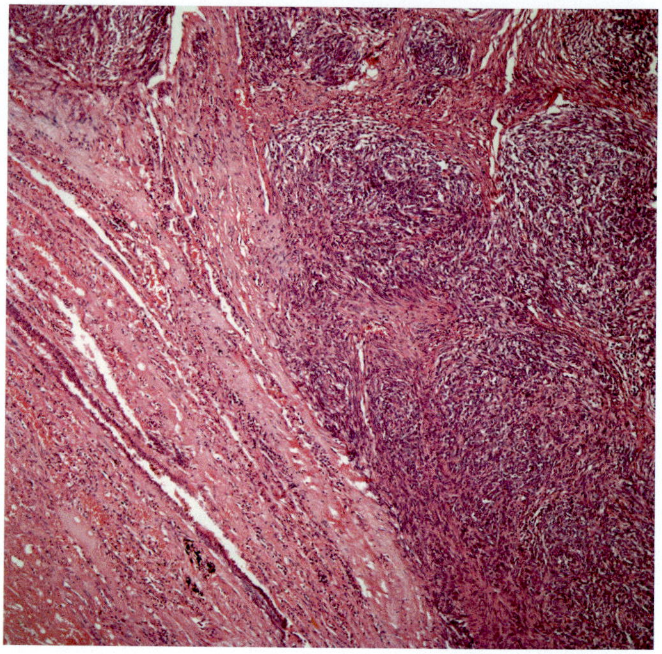

Fig. 7.44 Intrapulmonary thymoma with spindle cell growth pattern. Note the presence of lung parenchyma and bronchial epithelium

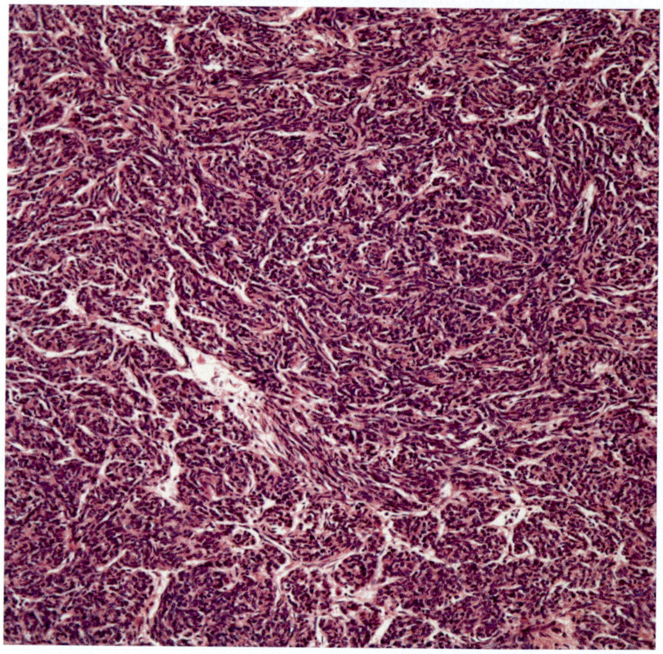

Fig. 7.45 Intrapulmonary spindle cell thymoma with subtle vascular-like growth pattern

momas include keratin 5/6, calretinin, CD5, and CD117. More recently, Pax8 has been found to show positive staining in thymomas. This latter stain may be important as intrapulmonary carcinomas are generally negative for this antibody.

Differential Diagnosis

Because of the presence of prominent lymphocytic component and proliferation of T cells, one important differential diagnosis is lymphoblastic lymphoma. In addition, the positive

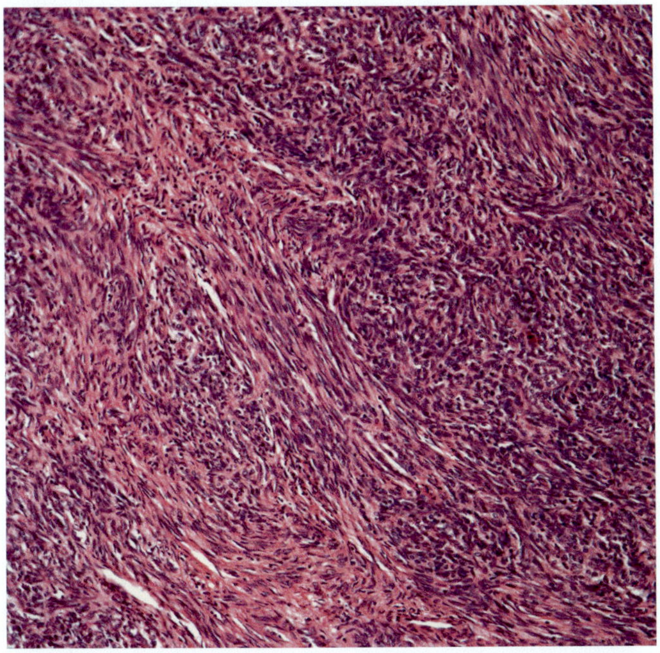

Fig. 7.46 Intrapulmonary spindle cell thymoma with areas mimicking a mesenchymal spindle cell tumor

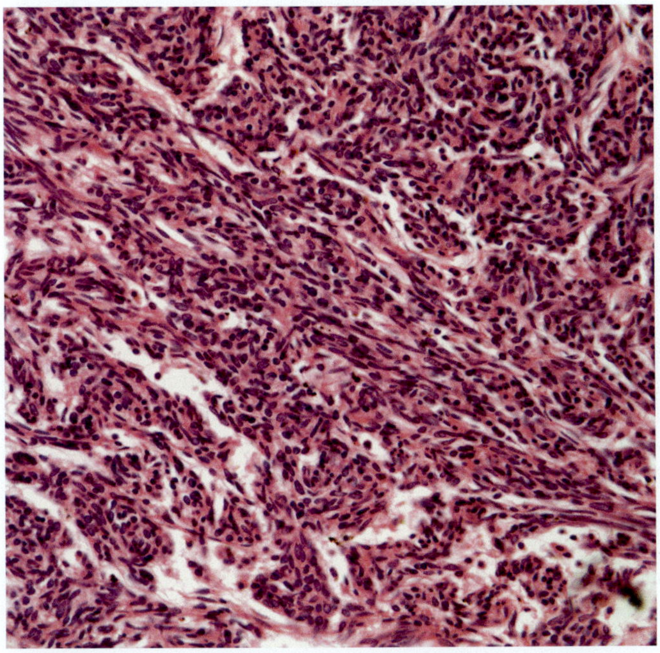

Fig. 7.47 High-power view of a spindle cell thymoma showing a cellular proliferation with lack of nuclear atypia or mitotic activity

staining using markers for T cells (TdT) may obscure the diagnosis of thymoma. In this setting, the use of epithelial markers, namely, keratin may be of great help in properly classifying the tumor as thymoma. In cases in which the predominant cell population is composed of epithelial cells, the main differential diagnosis is with a non-small cell lung carcinoma. However, the absence of marked nuclear atypia and mitotic activity coupled with the presence of lobulation and presence of perivascular spaces interspersed with the cellular proliferation are features more often seen in thymomas. When the tumors show a spindle cell growth pattern, the main differential diagnosis would be with a primary spindle cell sarcoma, namely, those sarcomas that may display a hemangiopericytic pattern. One of those sarcomas that may pose a specific problem would be synovial sarcoma, which may show positive staining for keratin and weak positive staining for EMA. However, other stains such as Bcl-2 may help in this setting. More importantly, the absence of marked nuclear atypia and mitotic activity should lead to the correct interpretation.

Treatment and Prognosis

The treatment of choice for intrapulmonary thymomas is complete surgical resection of the tumor. In most of the cases reported, the behavior of the tumor has been indolent. In the largest series published of these tumors [114], seven patients were followed for a period of time ranging from 10 months to 8 years showing that only one patient had recurrence of the tumor. However, in that particular case, the patient did not have complete surgical resection of the tumor, and the patient was treated with radiation therapy. In those patients who died, the cause of death was unrelated to the intrapulmonary thymoma. The authors concluded that intrapulmonary thymomas are slow-growing neoplasms with good prognosis when the tumor is amenable to complete surgical resection. For those patients with a non-resectable tumor, adjuvant treatment should be considered as well as for those patients with invasive tumors. Myers et al. [113] in a review of the literature on this topic concluded that complete resection appears sufficient for the treatment of intrapulmonary thymoma. The authors also found that the presence of paraneoplastic syndromes decreases survival, while histological type and tumor size do not.

Intrapulmonary Teratoma

Germ cell tumors in an intrapulmonary location are exceedingly rare. Germ cell tumors occur more often along the midline, and in the thorax, they are by far more common in the anterior mediastinum. When these tumors occur in the lungs, teratomas are the most common of this family of tumors. Nevertheless, it is important to be cautious about making a definitive diagnosis of primary intrapulmonary teratoma as germ cell tumors of either testicular or ovarian origin may metastasize to the lung. These can either show malignant components or as mature teratomatous elements [115] and distinction between a primary versus a metastatic neoplasm can be difficult. In addition, it is highly important to properly rule out the possibility of an anterior mediastinal teratoma with extension into the lung parenchyma as in some rare cases the teratomatous lesion may have intrapulmonary and mediastinal involvement [116].

In general, intrapulmonary teratomas are exceedingly rare and their occurrence has been reported in the literature only in the form of case reports [117–132]. There is not a single series of cases dealing with these tumors; thus, their exact incidence, is difficult to assess. Clinically, intrapulmonary teratomas have been described in a wide range of individuals from childhood to adulthood varying in age from a few months old to patients older than 60 years. The symptomatology reported by patients with intrapulmonary teratomas is also wide and includes symptoms that may be seen in patients with other pulmonary neoplasms such as cough, hemoptysis, chest pain, fever, dyspnea, pneumonia, weight loss, and vomiting. One of the most salient signs of intrapulmonary teratomas is the presence of trichoptysis (expectoration of hair). However, this latter sign is seen in less than 20 % of the cases. Also important to mention is that a small number of patients may not present with any symptomatology. Although it appears that the tumors are more common in female patients, the tumor has been also described in male patients in almost the same number.

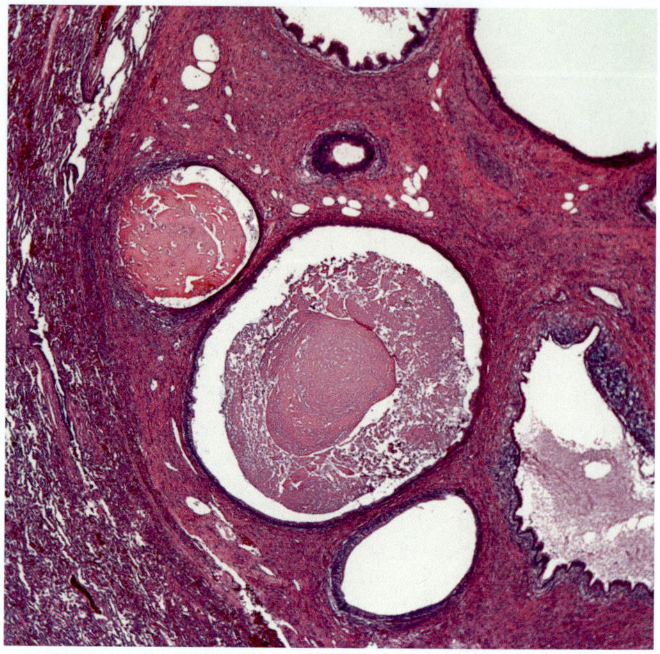

Fig. 7.48 Intrapulmonary teratoma showing prominent cystic changes and tissues from different germ cell layers

Macroscopic Features

Intrapulmonary teratomas may occur as an intraparenchymal tumor or as an endobronchial lesions [133–135]. In many cases, the diagnosis becomes evident by finding hair during a bronchoscopic examination. In addition, gross examination of the tumors can reveal the diagnosis. The tumors are cystic with focal solid areas, and in a minority of cases, the tumor may appear predominantly solid. The size of the tumors vary but they can reach up to 10 cm in greatest diameter. The cut surface of the tumor may disclose the presence of hair, cartilage, teeth, and sebaceous material.

Histopathological Features

The criteria for the diagnoses of intrapulmonary teratoma are the same as for gonadal teratomas, which is mainly the presence of tissue from the three germinal layers. Intrapulmonary teratomas just like their counterparts in the gonads may show a wide variety of tissues (Figs. 7.48, 7.49, 7.50, and 7.51). The majority of the cases reported have been of the mature type, which is resembled by the presence of appendage, squamous epithelium, mature glial tissue, cartilage, bone, pancreatic tissue, and enteric epithelium. Several cases in which thymic tissue has been present as a component of mature teratomas have also been described.

Cases of malignant teratoma have also been reported [136–140]. However, in some of these cases, the malignant component has only been reported as undifferentiated, while in other cases, the other germ cell tumors such as yolk sac tumor, or sarcomatous components in the form of malignant cartilage or undifferentiated sarcomatous component have been identified. In a case described as teratocarcinoma by Stair et al. [140], the tumor showed areas of adenocarcinoma with cartilage and also areas of a spindle cell proliferation. Such findings in an intrapulmonary neoplasm may raise the question of either a pulmonary carcinosarcoma or the so-called carcinoma ex pleomorphic adenoma.

Differential Diagnosis

The diagnosis of teratoma is rather simple and straightforward. However, in a small biopsy, the diversity of conditions that may enter the differential diagnosis is rather wide, and very likely one is not going to be able to make a definitive diagnosis. The differential diagnosis will be directly related to the sample of tissue obtained.

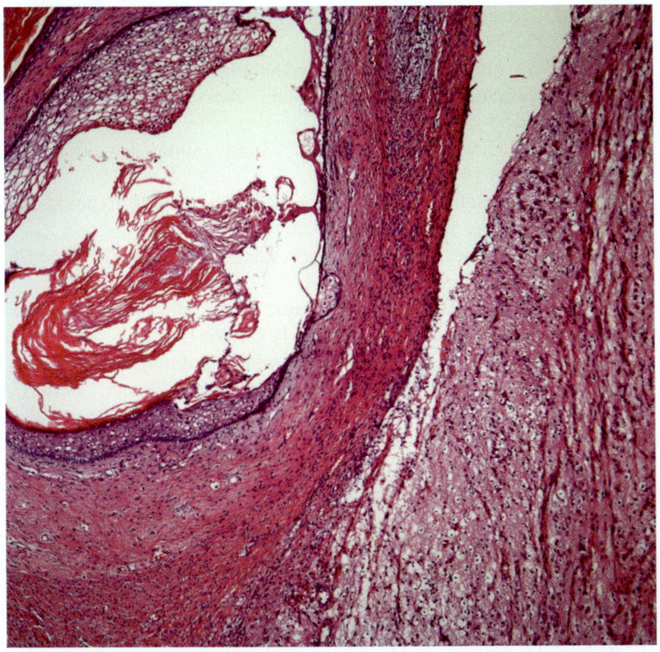

Fig. 7.49 Intrapulmonary teratoma showing a mixture of an epidermal cystic component and neural areas

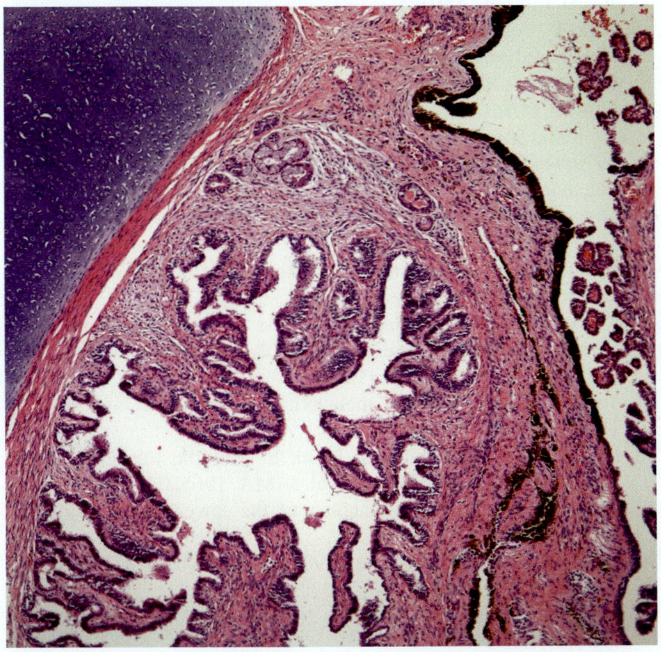

Fig. 7.50 Intrapulmonary teratoma showing cartilage, pigmented epithelium, and low columnar epithelium lining a glandular structure—all mature elements

Immunohistochemical Features

For the purpose of diagnosis, the use of immunohistochemistry is not necessary. However, the use of immunohistochemical stains may be to identify specific tissues that may

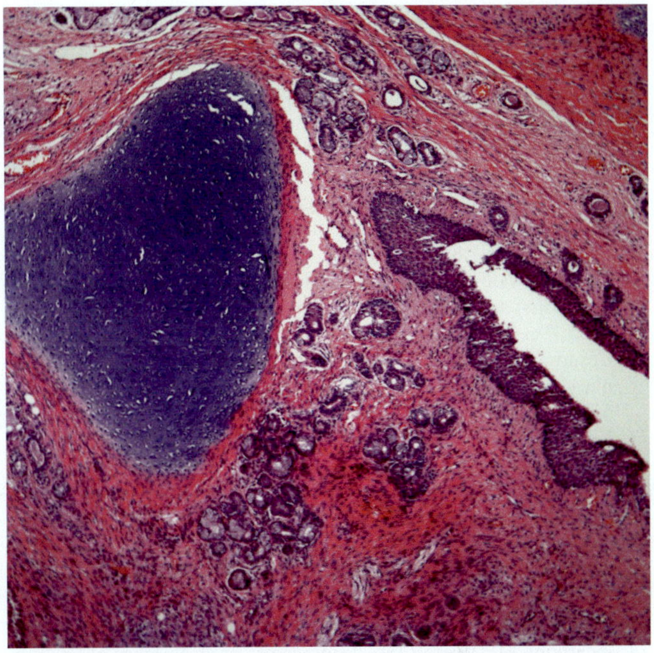

Fig. 7.51 Intrapulmonary teratoma showing a mixture of cartilage, glandular, and epidermal structures

be part of the tumor. The use of neural markers such as S100 protein, muscle markers such as desmin and actin, and vascular markers such as factor VIII, CD34, and CD31 may be of help in the identification of a particular tissue component of the tumor.

Treatment and Prognosis

Complete surgical resection via lobectomy or pneumonectomy is the treatment of choice and is curative in cases of mature teratomas. The patients may also be followed with additional therapy. The behavior of teratoma with malignant components may be aggressive mainly in cases in which the malignant elements are sarcomatous. In some of the reported cases of malignant teratoma, recurrences, metastatic disease, and fatal outcome have been documented despite aggressive therapy.

References

1. Shuangshoti A, Panyathanya R. Ectopic meningiomas. Arch Otolaryngol. 1973;98:102–5.
2. Miller DC, Ojeman RG, Proppe KH, et al. Benign metastasizing meningioma. J Neurosurg. 1985;62:763–6.
3. Kodama K, Doi O, Higashiyama M, et al. Primary and metastatic meningioma. Cancer. 1991;67:1412–7.
4. Hoye SJ, Hoar CS, Murray JE. Extracranial meningioma presenting as a tumor of the neck. Am J Surg. 1960;100:486–9.

5. Kemnitz P, Spormann H, Heinrich P. Meningioma of lung: first report with light and electron microscopic findings. Ultrastruct Pathol. 1982;3:359–65.
6. Chumas JC, Lorelle CA. Pulmonary meningioma: a light and electron microscopic study. Am J Surg Pathol. 1982;6:795–801.
7. Strimlan CV, Golembiewski RS, Celko DA, Fino GJ. Primary pulmonary meningioma. Surg Neurol. 1988;29:410–3.
8. Robinson PG. Pulmonary meningioma: report of a case with electron microscopic and immunohistochemical findings. Am J Clin Pathol. 1992;97:814–7.
9. Piquet J, Valo I, Jousset Y, Enon B. Primary pulmonary meningioma first suspected of being a lung metastasis. Ann Thorac Surg. 2005;79:1407–9.
10. Cesario A, Galetta D, Margaritora S, Granone P. Unsuspected primary pulmonary meningioma. Eur J Cardiothorac Surg. 2002;21: 553–5.
11. Kaleem Z, Fitzpatrick MM, Ritter J. Primary pulmonary meningioma: report of a case and review of the literature. Arch Pathol Lab Med. 1997;121:631–6.
12. Maiorana A, Ficarra G, Fano RA, Spagna G. Primary solitary meningioma of the lung. Patologica. 1996;88:457–62.
13. Falleni M, Roz E, Dessy E, et al. Primary intrathoracic meningioma: histological, immunohistochemical and ultrastructural study of two cases. Virchows Arch. 2001;439:196–200.
14. Incarbone M, Ceresoli GL, Tommaso L, et al. Primary pulmonary meningioma: report of a case and review of the literature. Lung Cancer. 2008;62:401–7.
15. Drlicek M, Grisold W, Lorber J, et al. Pulmonary meningioma: immunohistochemical and ultrastructural features. Am J Surg Pathol. 1991;15:455–9.
16. Flynn SD, Yousem SA. Pulmonary meningiomas: report of two cases. Hum Pathol. 1991;22:469–74.
17. Moran CA, Hochholzer L, Rush W, Koss MN. Primary intrapulmonary meningiomas: a clinicopathologic and immunohistochemical study of ten cases. Cancer. 1996;78:2328–33.
18. Spinelli M, Claren R, Colombi R, Sironi M. Primary pulmonary meningioma may arise from meningothelial-like nodules. Adv Clin Path. 2000;4:35–9.
19. Gomez-Aracil V, Mayayo E, Alvira R, et al. Fine needle aspiration cytology of primary pulmonary meningioma associated with minute meningothelial nodules: report of a case with histologic, immunohistochemical, and ultrastructural studies. Acta Ctyol. 2002;46:899–903.
20. Prayson RA, Farver CF. Primary pulmonary malignant meningioma. Am J Surg Pathol. 1999;23:722–6.
21. Van der Meij JJ, Boomars KA, van den Bosch JM, et al. Primary pulmonary malignant meningioma. Ann Thorac Surg. 2005;80:1523–5.
22. Rowsell C, Sirbovan J, Rosemblum MK, Perez-Ordonez B. Primary chordoid meningioma of lung. Virchows Arch. 2005;446:333–7.
23. Heppleston AG. A carotid-body-like tumour in the lung. J Pathol Bacteriol. 1958;75:461–4.
24. Prior JT. Minute peripheral pulmonary tumors: observations on their histogenesis. Am J Pathol. 1953;29:703–19.
25. Fawcett FJ, Husband EM. Chemodectoma of lung. J Clin Pathol. 1967;20:260–2.
26. Korn D, Bensch K, Liebow AA, Castleman B. Multiple minute tumors resembling chemodectomas. Am J Pathol. 1960;37: 641–72.
27. Goodman ML, Laforet EG. Solitary primary chemodectomas of the lung. Chest. 1972;61:48–50.
28. Lee YT, Hori JM. Chemodectoma of the lung. J Surg Oncol. 1972;4:33–6.
29. Laustela E, Mattila S, Fransilla K. Chemodectoma of the lung. Scand J Thorac Cardiovasc Surg. 1969;3:59–62.
30. Prior JT, Jones DB. Minute peripheral pulmonary tumors. J Thorac Surg. 1952;23:224–36.
31. Spain DM. Intrapulmonary chemodectomas in subjects with organizing pulmonary thromboemboli. Am Rev Respir Dis. 1967;96:1158–69.
32. Ichinose H, Hewitt RL, Drapanas T. Minute pulmonary chemodectoma. Cancer. 1971;28:692–700.
33. Saldana MJ, Salem LE, Travezan R. High altitude hypoxia and chemodectomas. Hum Pathol. 1973;4:251–63.
34. Zak FG, Chabes A. Pulmonary chemodectomatosis. JAMA. 1963;183:887–9.
35. Kuhn C, Askin FB. The fine structure of so-called minute pulmonary chemodectomas. Hum Pathol. 1975;6:681–91.
36. Churg AM, Warnock ML. So-called minute pulmonary chemodectoma: a tumor not related to paraganglioma. Cancer. 1976;37: 1759–69.
37. Gaffey MJ, Mills SE, Askin FB. Minute pulmonary meningothelial-like nodules: a clinicopathologic study of so-called minute pulmonary chemodectoma. Am J Surg Pathol. 1988;12:167–75.
38. Suster S, Moran CA. Diffuse pulmonary meningotheliomatosis. Am J Surg Pathol. 2007;31:624–31.
39. Ionescu DN, Sastomi E, Aldeeb D, et al. Pulmonary meningothelial-like nodules. A genotypic comparison with meningiomas. Am J Surg Pathol. 2004;28:207–14.
40. Kukoki M, Nakata H, Masuda T, et al. Minute pulmonary meningothelial-like nodules: high-resolution computer tomography and pathologic correlations. J Thorac Imaging. 2002;17:227–9.
41. Sellawi D, Gotway MB, Hawks DK, et al. Minute pulmonary meningothelial-like nodules: thin section CT appearance. J Comput Assist Tomogr. 2001;25:311–3.
42. Niho S, Yokose T, Nishiwaki Y, et al. Immunohistochemical and clonal analysis of minute pulmonary meningothelial-like nodules. Hum Pathol. 1999;30:425–9.
43. Gromet MA, Ominsky SH, Epstein WL, Blois MS. The thorax as the initial site for systemic relapse in malignant melanoma. Cancer. 1979;44:776–84.
44. Paganopoulos E, Murray D. Metastatic malignant melanoma of unknown primary origin: a study of 30 cases. J Surg Oncol. 1983;23:8–10.
45. Carlucci GA, Schleussner RC. Primary melanoma of the lung. J Thorac Surg. 1942;11:643–9.
46. Kunkel OF, Torrey E. Report of a case of primary melanotic sarcoma of lung presenting difficulties in differentiating from tuberculosis. NY J Med. 1916;16:198–201.
47. Todd FW. Two cases of melanotic tumors in the lung. JAMA. 1888;11:53–4.
48. Rosenberg LM, Polanco G, Blank S. Multiple tracheobronchial melanomas with ten-year survival. JAMA. 1965;192:133–5.
49. Reid JD, Mehta VT. Melanoma of the lower respiratory tract. Cancer. 1966;19:627–31.
50. Taboada CF, McMurray JD, Jordan RA, Seybold WD. Primary melanoma of the lung. Chest. 1972;62:629–31.
51. Allen SM, Drash EC. Primary melanoma of the lung. Cancer. 1968;21:154–9.
52. Mori K, Cho H, Som M. Primary "flat" melanoma of the trachea. J Pathol. 1977;121:101–5.
53. Robertson AJ, Sinclair DJM, Sutton PP, Guthrie W. Primary melanocarcinoma of the lower respiratory tract. Thorax. 1980;35:158–9.
54. Gephardt GN. Malignant melanoma of the bronchus. Hum Pathol. 1981;12:671–3.
55. Cagle P, Mace ML, Judge DM, et al. Pulmonary melanoma: primary vs metastatic. Chest. 1984;85:125–6.
56. Angel R, Prados M. Primary bronchial melanoma. J La State Med Soc. 1984;136:13–5.

57. Carstens PH, Kuhns JG, Ghazi C. Primary malignant melanoma of the lung and adrenal. Hum Pathol. 1984;15:910–4.
58. Demeter SL, Fuenning C, Miller JB. Primary malignant melanoma of the lower respiratory tract: endoscopic identification. Cleve Clin J Med. 1987;54:305–8.
59. Santos F, Entrenas LM, Sebastian F, et al. Primary bronchopulmonary malignant melanoma. Scand J Thorac Cardiovasc Surg. 1987;21:187–9.
60. Alhanem AA, Mehan J, Hassan AA. Primary malignant melanoma of the lung. J Surg Oncol. 1987;34:109–12.
61. Bertola G, Pasquotti B, Morassut S, et al. Primary lung melanoma. Italian J Surg Sci. 1989;19:187–9.
62. Bagwell SP, Flynn SD, Cox PM, Davison JA. Primary malignant melanoma of the lung. Am Rev Respir Dis. 1989;139:1543–7.
63. Jennings TA, Axiotis CA, Kress Y, Carter D. Primary malignant melanoma of the lower respiratory tract: report of a case and literature review. Am J Clin Pathol. 1990;94:649–55.
64. Pasquini E, Rastelli E, Mureto P, et al. Primary bronchial malignant melanoma: a case report. Pathologica. 1994;86:546–8.
65. Farrell DJ, Kashyap AP, Ashcroft T, Morritt GN. Primary malignant melanoma of the bronchus. Thorax. 1996;51:223–4.
66. Ost D, Joseph C, Sogoloff H, Menezes G. Primary pulmonary melanoma: case report and literature review. Mayo Clin Proc. 1999;74:62–6.
67. Dountsis A, Zisis C, Karagianni E, Dahabreh J. Primary malignant melanoma of the lung: a case report. World J Surg Oncol. 2003;1:26–9.
68. Lie CH, Chao TY, Chung YH, Lin MC. Primary pulmonary malignant melanoma presenting with haemoptysis. Melanoma Res. 2005;15:219–21.
69. Kundranda MN, Clark CT, Chaudhry AA, et al. Primary malignant melanoma of the lung: a case report and review of the literature. Clin Lung Cancer. 2006;4:279–81.
70. Reddy VS, Mykytenko J, Giltman LI, Mansour KA. Primary malignant melanoma of the lung: review of the literature and report of a case. Am Surg. 2007;73:287–9.
71. Ozdemir N, Cangir AK, Kutlay H, Yavuzer S. Primary malignant melanoma of the lung in oculocutaneous albino patient. Eur J Cardiothorac Surg. 2001;20:864–7.
72. Jensen OW, Egedorf J. Primary malignant melanoma of the lung. Scand J Respir Dis. 1967;48:127–35.
73. Wilson RW, Moran CA. Primary melanoma of the lung: a clinicopathologic and immunohistochemical study of eight cases. Am J Surg Pathol. 1997;21:1196–202.
74. Littman CD. Metastatic melanoma mimicking primary bronchial melanoma. Histopathology. 1991;18:561–3.
75. De Wilt JHW, Farmer SEJ, Scolyer RA, et al. Isolated melanoma in the lung where there is no known primary site: metastatic disease or primary lung tumour. Melanoma Res. 2005;15:531–7.
76. Wick MR, Swanson PE, Rocamora A. Recognition of malignant melanoma by monoclonal antibody HMB-45. An immunohistochemical study of 200 paraffin-embedded cutaneous tumors. J Cutan Pathol. 1988;15:201–7.
77. Gerughty JM, Thomas RW. Glomus tumor of the palate: case report and review of the literature. Br J Oral Maxillofac Surg. 1992;30:398–400.
78. Hayes MM, van der Westhuizen N, Holden GP. Aggressive glomus tumor of the nasal region: report of a case with multiple local recurrences. Arch Pathol Lab Med. 1993;117:649–52.
79. Almagro UA, Schulte WJ, Norback DH. Glomus tumor of the stomach: histologic and ultrastructural features. Am J Clin Pathol. 1981;75:415–9.
80. Haque A, Modlin IM, West AB. Multiple glomus tumors of the stomach with intravascular spread. Am J Surg Pathol. 1992;16:291–9.
81. Gould EW, Manivel JC, Albores-Saavedra J, Monteforte H. Locally infiltrative glomus tumors and glomangiosarcomas: a clinical, ultrastructural, and immunohistochemical study. Cancer. 1990;65:310–8.
82. Folpe AL, Fanburg-Smith JC, Miettienen M, Weiss SW. Atypical and malignant glomus tumors: analysis of 52 cases with proposal for the classification of glomus tumors. Am J Surg Pathol. 2001;25:1–12.
83. Watanabe M, Takagi K, Ono K, et al. Successful resection of a glomus tumor arising from the lower trachea: report of a case. Jpn J Surg. 1998;28:332–4.
84. Koshiken SK, Niemi PT, Ekfors TO, et al. Glomus tumor of the trachea. Eur Radiol. 1998;8:364–6.
85. Altinok T, Cakir E, Gulhan E, Tastepe I. Tracheal glomus tumor. J Thorac Cardiovasc Surg. 2006;132:201–2.
86. Yu DK, Cho KH, Kim YJ, Heo DS. Tracheal glomangiosarcoma with multiple skin metastases. J Dermatol. 2004;31:776–8.
87. Tang CK, Toker C, Foris N, Trump BF. Glomangioma of the lung. Am J Surg Pathol. 1978;2:103–9.
88. Mackay B, Legha SS, Pickler GM. Coin lesion of the lung in a 19-year-old male. Ultrastruct Pathol. 1981;2:289–94.
89. Alt B, Huffer WE, Belchis DA. A vascular lesion with smooth muscle differentiation presenting as a coin lesion in the lung: glomus tumor versus hemangiopericytoma. Am J Clin Pathol. 1983;80:765–71.
90. Koss MN, Hochholzer L, Moran CA. Primary pulmonary glomus tumor: a clinicopathologic and immunohistochemical study of two cases. Mod Pathol. 1998;11:253–8.
91. Gaetner EM, Steinberg DM, Huber M, et al. Pulmonary and mediastinal glomus tumors: report of five cases including a pulmonary glomangiosarcoma: a clinicopathologic study with literature review. Am J Surg Pathol. 2000;24:1105–14.
92. Kapur U, Helenowski M, Zayaad A, et al. Pulmonary glomus tumor. Ann Diagn Pathol. 2007;11:457–9.
93. Lange TH, Magee MJ, Boley TM, et al. Tracheobronchial glomus tumor. Ann Thorac Surg. 2000;70:292–5.
94. Oizumi S, Kon Y, Ishida T, et al. A rare case of bronchial glomus tumor. Respiration. 2001;68:95–8.
95. Hatori M, Aiba S, Kato M, et al. Expression of CD34 in glomus tumors. Tohoku J Exp Med. 1997;182:241–7.
96. Asa SL, Dardick I, Van Nostrand PAW, et al. Primary thyroid thymoma: a distinct clinicopathologic entity. Hum Pathol. 1988;19:1463–6.
97. Martin JME, Rundhawa G, Temple WJ. Cervical thymoma. Arch Pathol Lab Med. 1986;110:354–7.
98. Wadon A. Thymoma intratracheal. Am J Pathol. 1934;60:308–12.
99. Moran CA, Travis WD, Rosado-de-Christenson M, et al. Thymomas presenting as pleural tumors: report of eight cases. Am J Surg Pathol. 1992;16:138–44.
100. McBurney RP, Clagett OT, McDonald JR. Primary intrapulmonary neoplasm (Thymoma?) associated with myasthenia gravis: report of case. Mayo Clin Proc. 1951;26:345–53.
101. Thorburn JD, Stephens HB, Grimes OF. Benign thymoma in the hilus of the lung. J Thorac Surg. 1952;24:540–3.
102. Crane AR, Carrigan PT. Primary subpleural intrapulmonary thymoma. J Thorac Surg. 1953;25:600–5.
103. Kalish PE. Primary intrapulmonary thymoma. N Y State J Med. 1963;63:1705–8.
104. Yeoh CB, Ford JM, Lattes R, Wylie RH. Intrapulmonary thymoma. J Thorac Cardiovasc Surg. 1966;51:131–6.
105. Kung ITM, Loke SL, So SY, et al. Intrapulmonary thymoma: report of two cases. Thorax. 1985;40:471–4.
106. Green WR, Pressoir R, Gumbs RV, et al. Intrapulmonary thymoma. Arch Pathol Lab Med. 1987;111:1074–6.
107. Fukayama M, Maeda Y, Funata N, et al. Pulmonary and pleural thymoma: diagnostic application of lymphocyte markers to the thymoma of unusual site. Am J Clin Pathol. 1988;89:617–21.
108. James CL, Iyer PV, Leong ASY. Intrapulmonary thymoma. Histopathology. 1992;21:175–7.

109. Stefani A, Boulenger E, Mehaut S, et al. Primary intrapulmonary thymoma associated with congenital hyperhomocysteinemia. J Thorac Cardiovasc Surg. 2007;134:799–801.
110. Ishibashi H, Takahashi S, Hosaka T, et al. Primary intrapulmonary thymoma successfully resected with vascular reconstruction. Ann Thorac Surg. 2003;76:1735–7.
111. Srivastava A, Padilla O, Alroy J, et al. Primary intrapulmonary spindle cell thymoma with marked granulomatous reaction: report of a case with review of literature. Int J Surg Pathol. 2003;11:353–6.
112. Veynovich B, Masetti P, Kaplan PD, et al. Primary pulmonary thymoma. Ann Thorac Surg. 1997;64:1471–3.
113. Myers PO, Kritikos N, Bongiovani M, et al. Primary intrapulmonary thymoma: a systematic review. Eur J Surg Oncol. 2007;33:1137–41.
114. Moran CA, Suster S, Fishback NF, Koss MN. Primary intrapulmonary thymoma: a clinicopathologic and immunohistochemical study of eight cases. Am J Surg Pathol. 1995;19:304–12.
115. Moran CA, Travis WD, Carter D, Koss MN. Metastatic mature teratoma in lung following testicular embryonal carcinoma and teratocarcinoma. Arch Pathol Lab Med. 1993;117:641–4.
116. Smith CJ. A teratoma of the lung containing teeth. Ann R Coll Surg Engl. 1967;41:413–5.
117. Trivedi SA, Mehta KN, Nanavaty JM. Teratoma of the lung: report of a case. Br J Dis Chest. 1966;60:156–9.
118. Day DW, Taylor SA. An intrapulmonary teratoma associated with thymic tissue. Thorax. 1975;30:582–7.
119. Holt S, Deverall PB, Boddy JE. A teratoma of the lung containing thymic tissue. J Pathol. 1978;126:85–9.
120. Saruk M, Stern H, Tronic BS, et al. Intrapulmonary benign cystic teratoma. Conn Med. 1980;44:687–90.
121. Prauer HW, Mack D, Babic R. Intrapulmonary teratoma 10 years after removal of a mediastinal teratoma in a young man. Thorax. 1983;38:632–4.
122. Berghout A, Mallens WMC, Velde J, Haak HL. Teratoma of the lung in a hemophilic patient. Acta Haematol. 1983;70:330–4.
123. Iwasaki T, Iuchi K, Matsumura A, et al. Intrapulmonary mature teratoma. Jpn J Thorac Cardiovasc Surg. 2000;48:468–72.
124. Groeger AM, Baldi A, Caputi M, et al. Intrapulmonary teratoma associated with thymic tissue. Anticancer Res. 2000;20:3919–22.
125. Asano S, Hoshikawa Y, Yamane Y, et al. An intrapulmonary teratoma associated with bronchiectasia containing various kinds of primordium: a case report and review of the literature. Virchows Arch. 2000;436:384–8.
126. Eren MN, Balci AE, Eren S. Benign intrapulmonary teratoma: report of a case. J Thorac Cardiovasc Surg. 2003;126:855–7.
127. Zenker D, Aleksic I. Intrapulmonary cystic benign teratoma: a case report and review of the literature. Ann Thorac Cardiovasc Surg. 2004;10:290–2.
128. Khan JA, Aslam F, Fatimi SH, Ahmed R. Cough, fever, and a cavitary lung lesion – an intrapulmonary teratoma. J Postgrad Med. 2005;51:330–1.
129. Alper F, Kaynar H, Kantarci M, et al. Trichoptysis caused by intrapulmonary teratoma: computed tomography and magnetic resonance imaging findings. Australas Radiol. 2005;49:53–6.
130. Faria RA, Bizon JA, Juior RS, et al. Intrapulmonary teratoma. J Bras Pneumol. 2007;33:612–5.
131. Agarwal R, Srinivas R, Saxena AK. Trichoptysis due to an intrapulmonary teratoma. Respir Care. 2007;52:1779–81.
132. Rana SS, Swami N, Mehta S, et al. Intrapulmonary teratoma: an exceptional disease. Ann Thorac Surg. 2007;83:1194–6.
133. Bateson EM, Hayes JA, Woo-Ming M. Endobronchial teratoma associated with bronchiectasis and bronchiolectasis. Thorax. 1968;23:69–75.
134. Jamieson MPG, McGowan AR. Endobronchial teratoma. Thorax. 1982;37:157–9.
135. Cai C, Zeng Y, Chen H, et al. Fibrobronchoscopic evidence of endobronchial hairs in intrapulmonary teratoma with hemoptysis but without trichoptysis. Am J Med Sci. 2008;336:441–4.
136. Pound AW, Willis RA. A malignant teratoma of the lung in an infant. J Pathol. 1969;98:111–4.
137. Kakkar N, Vasishta RK, Banerjee AK, et al. Primary pulmonary malignant teratoma with yolk sac element associated with hematologic neoplasia. Respiration. 1996;63:52–4.
138. Gautam HP. Intrapulmonary malignant teratoma. Am Rev Respir Dis. 1969;100:863–5.
139. Maasilta PK, Ulla-Stina E, Salminen E, Taskinen EI. Malignant teratoma of the lung. Acta Oncol. 1999;38:1113–5.
140. Stair JM, Stevenson R, Schaefer RF, et al. Primary teratocarcinoma of the lung. J Surg Oncol. 1986;33:262–7.

8 Vascular Tumors of the Lungs

Introduction

Contrary to their counterparts in other organ systems, primary vascular neoplasms of the lung are rare. Because of the rarity of these lesions, the clinical and radiological features are often mistaken for other, more common lesions. Both benign and malignant vascular tumors have been described. Before a diagnosis of a primary malignant vascular neoplasm can be rendered, metastasis from extrapulmonary sites will have to be excluded through thorough clinical and radiological investigations. Primary vascular tumors of the lungs include hemangioma, lymphangioma, angiolymphoid hyperplasia with eosinophilia, and capillary hemangiomatosis among the benign lesions and epithelioid hemangioendothelioma, angiosarcoma, and Kaposi's sarcoma among the malignant ones (Table 8.1).

Hemangioma

Clinical Features

Hemangiomas are frequently seen in the soft tissue, skin, and liver and can occasionally occur in the subglottic region or in the mediastinum [1, 2]. In the lung, however, these tumors are rare. To date, only 24 cases of pulmonary hemangioma have been described in the English and Japanese literature [3, 4]. Hemangiomas have been described in patients of all ages with no specific sex predilection and can present as solitary or multiple lesions [3–9]. Patients are either asymptomatic or present with respiratory symptoms such as hemoptysis, pneumonia, or cyanosis [10–12]. Hemangiomas may arise anywhere in the lower respiratory tract from the lung parenchyma to the airways and the bronchial tree [13–16]. Although only few hemangiomas of the lung have been reported, a case with partial trisomy D has been described. In addition, it has been stated that pulmonary hemangiomas may be complicated by conditions such as Kasabach-Merritt syndrome [17, 18].

Gross Features

Macroscopically, hemangiomas present as well-demarcated or ill-defined hemorrhagic nodules, cysts, or cavernous spaces filled with hemorrhagic porous or thrombotic material [9–11, 19, 20]. The tumors may measure between 1 and 3 cm in size. Tumors with a bronchial component often display a polypoid growth pattern with protrusion into the bronchial lumen.

Histological Features

Histologically, pulmonary hemangiomas are identical to those seen elsewhere in the body. They are encapsulated and lobulated masses composed of numerous cavernous or capillary vessels lined by bland endothelial cells [9, 10, 19, 20] (Fig. 8.1). Cytologic atypia and mitotic activity are usually absent, although rare mitotic figures may be present in isolated cases (Figs. 8.2 and 8.3). As is true for all other vascular tumors, the adjacent pulmonary parenchyma may show intra-alveolar hemorrhage and abundant hemosiderin-laden macrophages (Fig. 8.4).

Immunohistochemical and Molecular Features

The endothelial cells of hemangioma show immunoreactivity for factor VIII related antigen, CD31, and CD34 [10, 12]. Due to the rarity of pulmonary hemangiomas, molecular investigations are lacking; however, studies performed on hemangiomas of the skin and soft tissue showed VEGF and TEM8 signaling pathway mutations [21, 22].

A. Weissferdt, C.A. Moran, *Diagnostic Pathology of Pleuropulmonary Neoplasia*,
DOI 10.1007/978-1-4419-0787-5_8, © Springer Science+Business Media New York 2013

Table 8.1 Clinical, histological, and immunohistochemical features of vascular lung tumors

Tumor	Age and sex	Clinical presentation	Histology	Immunohistochemical phenotype	Clinical associations
Hemangioma	All ages, M=F	Hemoptysis, pneumonia, cyanosis, or asymptomatic	Proliferation of cavernous or capillary vessels lined by bland endothelial cells	Factor VIII, CD31, CD34	Trisomy D, Kasabach-Merritt-syndrome
Lymphangioma	Mostly pediatric population, M=F	Respiratory distress, pneumothorax, or asymptomatic	Proliferation of capillary, cavernous, or cystic lymphatic vessels lined by bland endothelial cells	Factor-VIII-related antigen, CD31, D2-40, VEGFR3, and LYVE1	Maffucci's and Klippel-Trenaunay-Weber syndromes
Angiolymphoid hyperplasia with eosinophilia	Adults, M=F	Cough, dyspnea	Proliferation of small vessels with prominent eosinophilic infiltrate and lymphoid hyperplasia	CD31 in vessels, CD20 and CD45 in lymphoid cells	Asthma
Capillary hemangiomatosis	Young adults, M=F	Pulmonary hypertension with dyspnea, cough, hemoptysis, fatigue, and weight loss or asymptomatic	Proliferation of capillary-sized blood vessels distributed along the interstitium and alveolar septa	CD31 and CD34	Hypertrophic cardiomyopathy, systemic lupus erythematosus, and Takayasu aortoarteritis
Epithelioid hemangioendothelioma	Young adults, F>M	Dyspnea, cough, pleuritic chest pain, or asymptomatic	Nodular proliferation of endothelial cells with bland cytologic features set in myxoid stroma	Factor VIII, CD31, CD34; CK may be positive in up to 50 % of cases	–
Angiosarcoma	Adults, mean age 54 years	Dyspnea, chest pain, hemoptysis, cough, pulmonary hemorrhage, or hemothorax	Proliferation of endothelial cells with cytologic atypia and mitotic activity	Factor VIII, CD31, CD34; CK may be positive in the epithelioid type	Maffucci's and Klippel-Trenaunay-Weber syndromes
Kaposi's sarcoma	Adults, M>F	Dyspnea, cough, hemoptysis, fatigue, fever, or respiratory failure	Spindle cells, inflammatory cells, and red blood cells forming infiltrative nodular masses	CD34, CD31, D2-40, VEGFR3, and HHV8	HIV/AIDS, immunocompromised state, HHV8

M male, *F* female, *VEGFR3* vascular endothelial growth factor receptor 3, *LYVE1* vessel endothelial receptor 1, *CK* cytokeratin, *HIV* human immunodeficiency virus, *AIDS* acquired immunodeficiency syndrome, *HHV8* human herpes virus 8

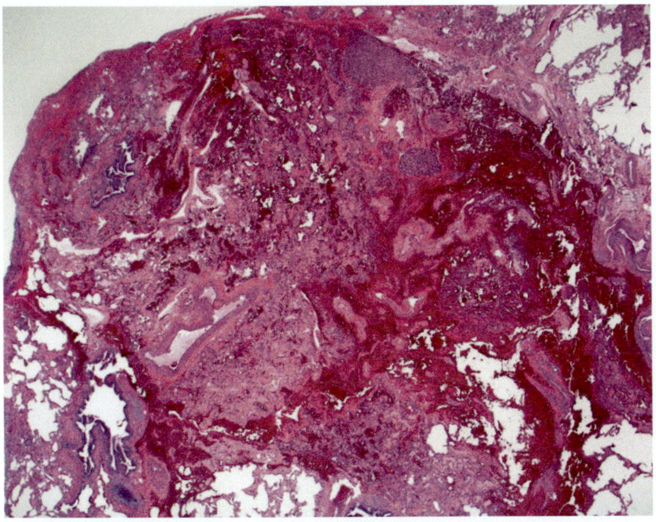

Fig. 8.1 Low power view of pulmonary hemangioma with cavernous pattern

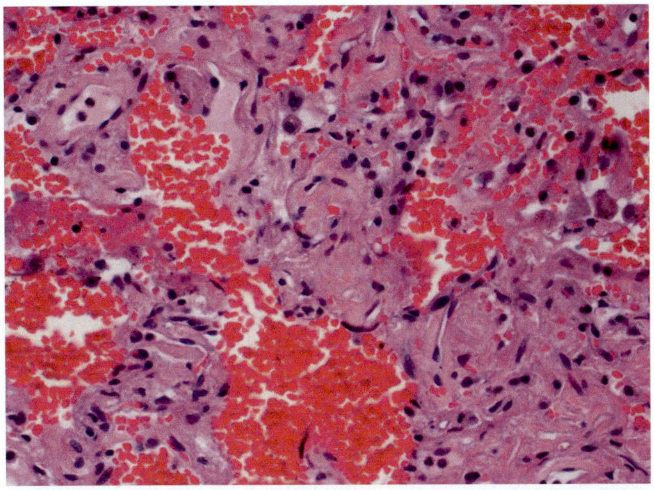

Fig. 8.3 High power view of pulmonary hemangioma demonstrating no cytologic atypia

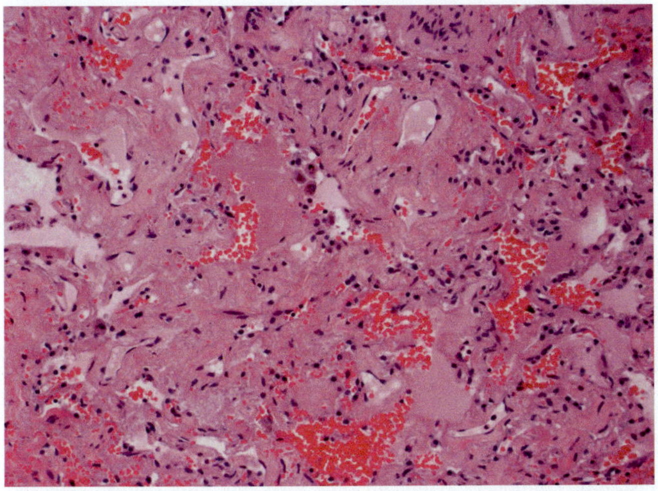

Fig. 8.2 Pulmonary hemangioma composed of cavernous blood vessels

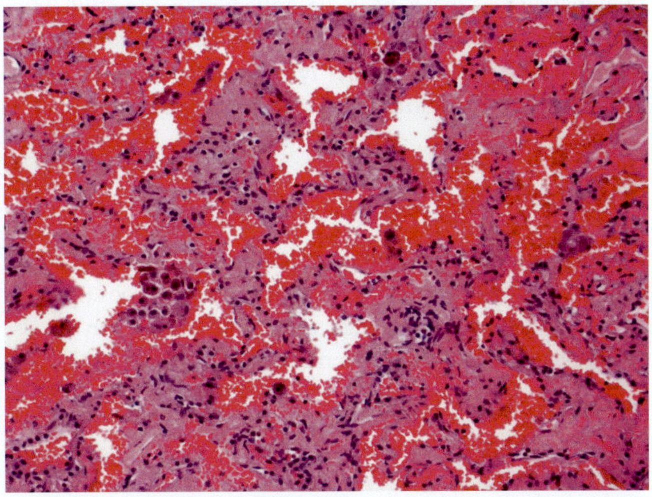

Fig. 8.4 Pulmonary hemangioma showing intra-alveolar hemorrhage and hemosiderin-laden macrophages

Differential Diagnosis

Pulmonary hemangioma should be distinguished from lymphangioma, pulmonary capillary hemangiomatosis, and sclerosing hemangioma. Lymphangioma may resemble hemangioma closely; the absence of red blood cells in the vascular lumina and presence of smooth muscle in the vessel walls are supportive of the former. Pulmonary capillary hemangiomatosis is a distinct entity presenting as a multifocal angiomatous proliferation associated with pulmonary hypertension and poor long-term survival. The angiomatoid pattern of sclerosing hemangioma may mimic the cavernous type of hemangioma; however, the cavernous spaces in this tumor are separated by a cellular proliferation of cells displaying an epithelial immunohistochemical phenotype.

Treatment and Prognosis

Localized hemangiomas are best treated with surgical excision, whereas interferon-α(alpha)-2a or coil embolization may be considered for multifocal lesions [11]. In asymptomatic cases, radiologic follow-up may be sufficient [3, 9]. Whereas localized pulmonary hemangiomas tend to have a favorable outcome, multifocal lesions may cause significant loss of lung function, resulting in poorer clinical course [11].

Lymphangioma

Clinical Features

Lymphangiomas can occur at any age but present most often in the pediatric population. The median age at presentation is 36.6 years. Males and females are equally affected [23–25]. Most patients are asymptomatic unless compression of vital structures occurs. In the latter case, patients may present with respiratory distress or rarely pneumothorax [26, 27]. Radiologically, lymphangiomas may be mistaken for benign cystic lung disease on computed tomography (CT) [25, 26, 28]. Predominant involvement of the right lung has been reported [25]. Several etiologies have been proposed for the development of these tumors including developmental abnormalities, cystic change in response to infection, surgery, and radiation treatment or embryologic remnants of lymphatic tissue that failed to connect to efferent lymph channels [29, 30]. Lymphangiomas have been described in association with Maffucci's and Klippel-Trenaunay-Weber syndromes, and further investigations for other lymphangiomatous lesions or anomalies may be warranted in this context [29, 31, 32].

Gross Features

Lymphangiomas grossly often present as multiloculated cystic masses containing gelatinous or sanguinous secretions [25, 33]. These tumors can reach a large size (up to 10 cm). Cavernous, capillary, or cystic growth patterns may be observed [29].

Histological Features

The histological features are very similar to hemangiomas, and capillary, cavernous, or cystic growth patterns can be seen [29] (Figs. 8.5 and 8.6). The lesions are composed of dilated lymphatic channels lined by flat endothelial cells (Figs. 8.7 and 8.8). Serous material may be present in the cystic lumina [25, 30, 34–36]. In addition, foci of hyperplastic smooth muscle and admixed lymphoid tissue are often identified in the interstitial spaces [28, 37] (Fig. 8.9).

Immunohistochemical and Molecular Features

Lymphangiomas are positive for factor VIII related antigen, CD31, D2-40, vascular endothelial growth factor receptor 3 (VEGFR3), and vessel endothelial receptor 1 (LYVE1) [25, 38]. Lymphangiomas do not show reactivity for cytokeratin (CK), epithelial membrane antigen (EMA), or CD34 [25, 33, 37]. Molecular investigations performed on lymphangiomas of the skin and soft tissue showed VEGFR3 mutations in these tumors [39].

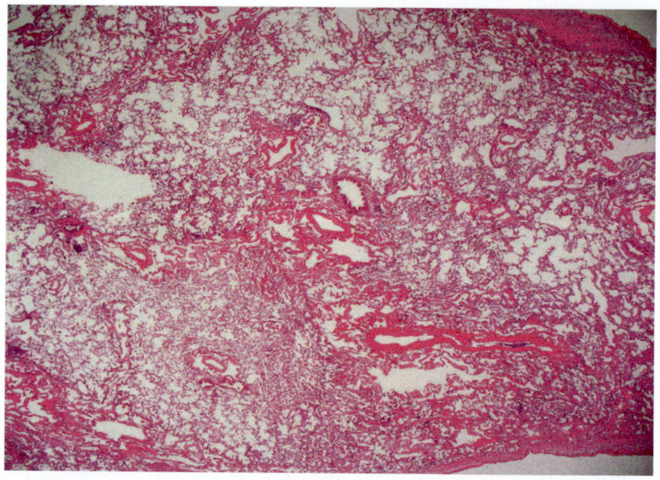

Fig. 8.5 Subtle histological features of pulmonary lymphangioma

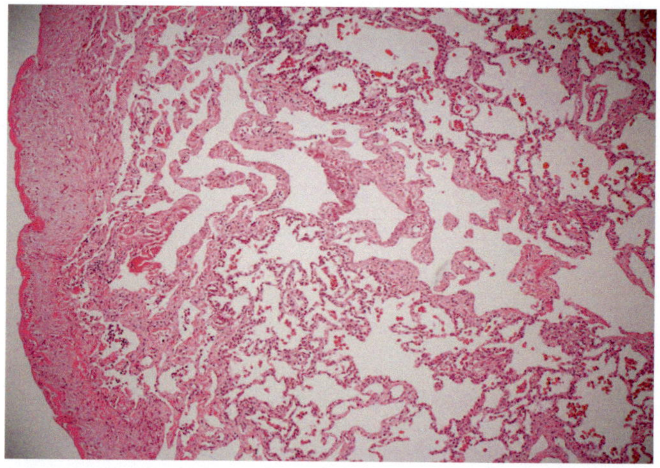

Fig. 8.6 Pulmonary lymphangioma involving lung parenchyma and pleural surface

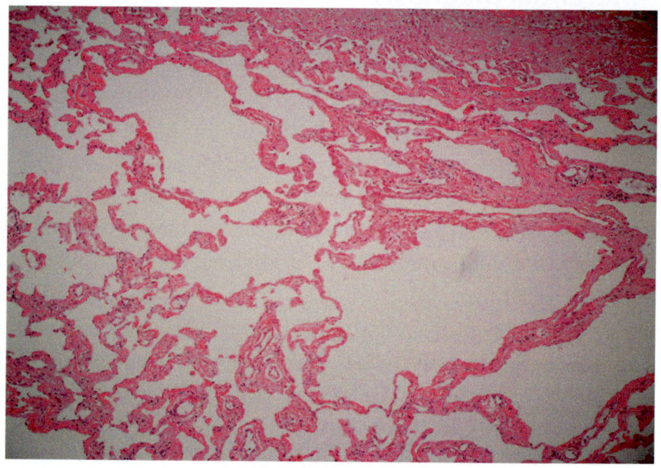

Fig. 8.7 Dilated lymphatic channels replacing the normal lung parenchyma

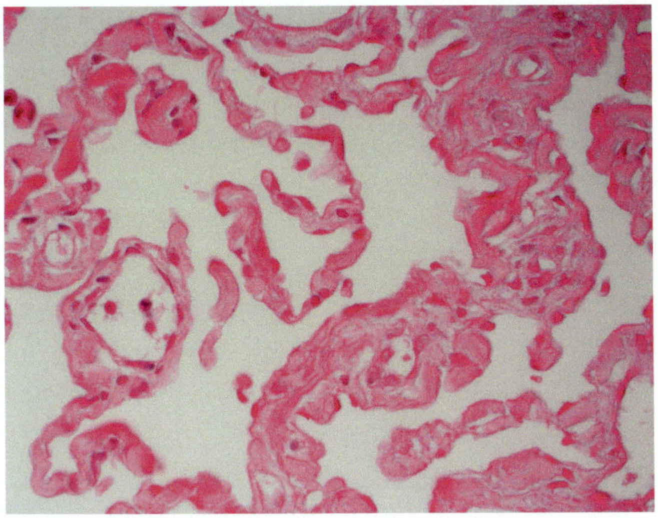

Fig. 8.8 High power view of pulmonary lymphangioma lined by bland endothelial cells

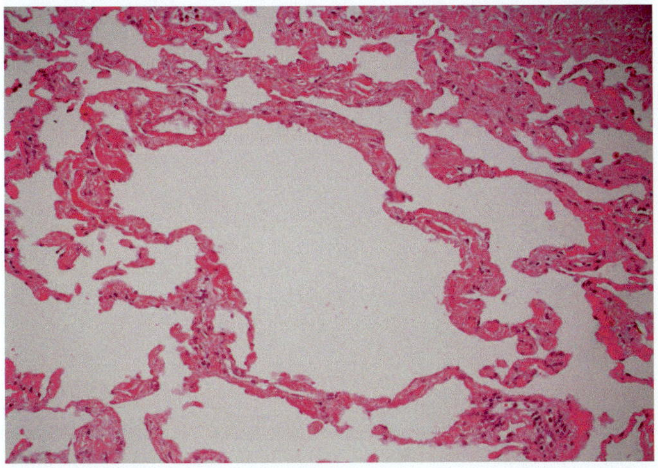

Fig. 8.9 Pulmonary lymphangioma with focal smooth muscle proliferation involving vessel walls

Differential Diagnosis

The differential diagnosis for lymphangiomas includes hemangioma, alveolar adenoma, and lymphangioleiomyomatosis. Hemangiomas are characterized by blood-filled cystic space lined by bland endothelium. Smooth muscle is normally not seen in the vessel walls of this tumor. Alveolar adenoma is composed of large cystic spaces containing clear acellular secretions. The cystic spaces are lined by pneumocytes with a hobnailing pattern and are separated by fibrous septa containing inflammatory cells. Alveolar adenomas are positive for CK and EMA by immunohistochemistry contrary to the endothelial phenotype of lymphangioma [40, 41]. Lastly, lymphangioleiomyomatosis is a condition that primarily occurs in women of reproductive age. It typically presents as a cystic lung process that is not limited to the lymphatic routes but rather involves the alveoli and contains a relatively large proportion of smooth muscle. Immunohistochemically, the spindle cells in lymphangioleiomyomatosis express immunoreactivity for estrogen and progesterone receptors and HMB45, further distinguishing this lesion from lymphangioma [42–44].

Treatment and Prognosis

As spontaneous regression has not been described and the tumors have a tendency to recur if incompletely excised, the therapy of choice for lymphangioma consists of surgical resection or sclerotherapy [29, 45, 46]. If complete excision of lymphangioma is achieved, surgery alone should be curative with no reported recurrences to date [25].

Angiolymphoid Hyperplasia with Eosinophilia (Epithelioid Hemangioma)

Angiolymphoid hyperplasia with eosinophilia or "epithelioid hemangioma" is an entity that was first described by Wells and Whimster in 1969 as an inflammatory angiomatous lesion affecting the subcutaneous tissues of the head and neck area of young to middle-aged adults [47]. Angiolymphoid hyperplasia with eosinophilia has since been reported in other sites such as the lymph nodes, bone, heart, salivary glands, and orbit [48–51]. There has been contention in the literature in the past as to whether angiolymphoid hyperplasia with eosinophilia and Kimura's disease represent the same disease entity; however, recent evidence seems to suggest that these two lesions represent different clinicopathological entities [52–54]. To date, only two of these lesions have been described in the lung [55].

Clinical Features

The two cases described have occurred in a 60-year-old man and a 27-year-old woman. Cough and dyspnea were the presenting symptoms in the first case, and the second patient had a long history of asthma. Radiologically, right upper lobe lesions were identified in both cases [55].

Gross Features

Both lesions were situated in the lung parenchyma and were described as well-circumscribed but unencapsulated tumors with a soft gray and partly cystic cut surface. The lesions measured 2 and 3 cm, respectively. Hemorrhage and necrosis were not identified [55].

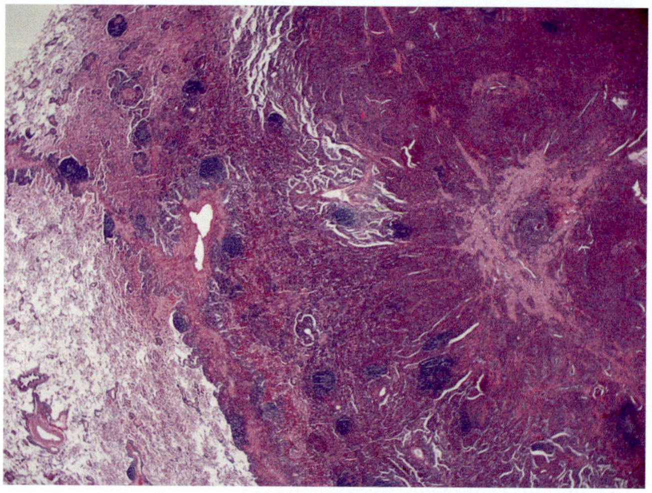

Fig. 8.10 Low power view of angiolymphoid hyperplasia with eosinophilia arising in the lung

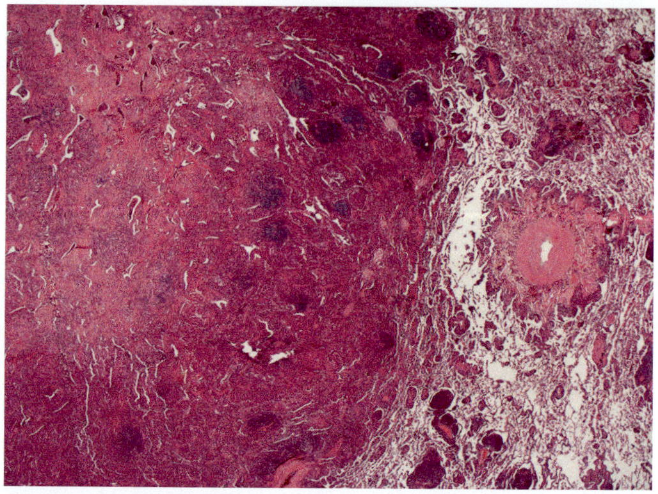

Fig. 8.11 Circumscribed nature of pulmonary angiolymphoid hyperplasia with eosinophilia

Histological Features

Histologically, the lesions are similar to the ones seen in the skin. They are well-delineated and non-encapsulated tumors composed of a proliferation of small caliber vessels lined by plump epithelioid endothelial cells (Figs. 8.10, 8.11, and 8.12). These endothelial cells possess eosinophilic cytoplasm, prominent nucleolus, and occasional cytoplasmic vacuoles (Fig. 8.13). The vascular proliferation is accompanied by a prominent inflammatory infiltrate composed predominantly of eosinophils (Fig. 8.14). Lymphoid aggregates often accompany the vascular proliferation [55] (Fig. 8.15). Involvement of larger vessels can occasionally be identified (Fig. 8.16).

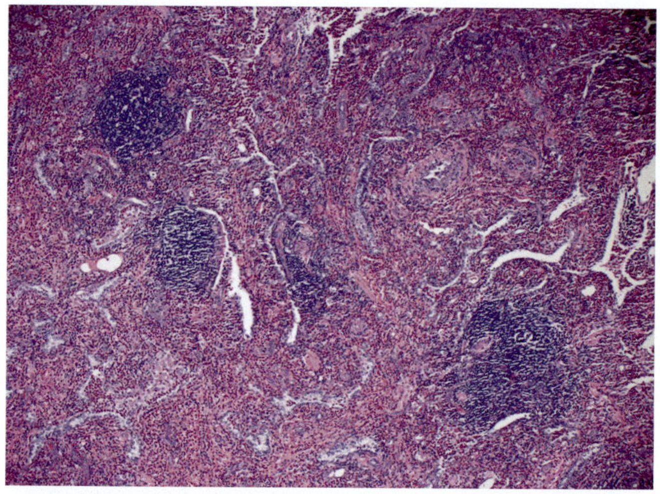

Fig. 8.12 Proliferation of small caliber vessels in pulmonary angiolymphoid hyperplasia with eosinophilia

Immunohistochemical and Molecular Features

The vascular proliferation is reactive for endothelial markers like CD31, whereas the lymphocytic component shows positive staining for CD20 and CD45 [55]. More recently, it has been shown that some cases of angiolymphoid hyperplasia with eosinophilia of the skin harbor a clonal T-cell population and may therefore represent a T-cell lymphoproliferative disorder of benign or low-grade malignant nature [56].

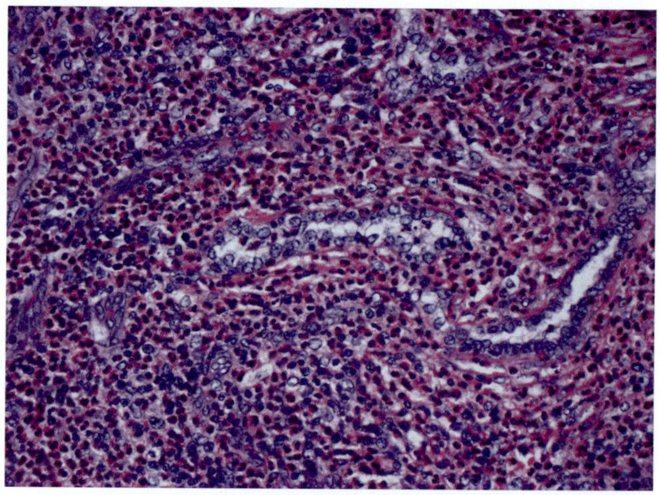

Fig. 8.13 High power view of plump endothelial cells lining the vessel walls in angiolymphoid hyperplasia with eosinophilia of the lung

Differential Diagnosis

Angiolymphoid hyperplasia with eosinophilia must be distinguished from other benign or malignant vascular tumors of the lungs. Hemangioma is a benign lesion that is rarely found in the lung. This tumor is composed of a proliferation of capillary or cavernous blood vessels lined by bland endothelial cells. Lymphoid follicles or a prominent eosinophilic cell infiltrate are not seen in this tumor. More important

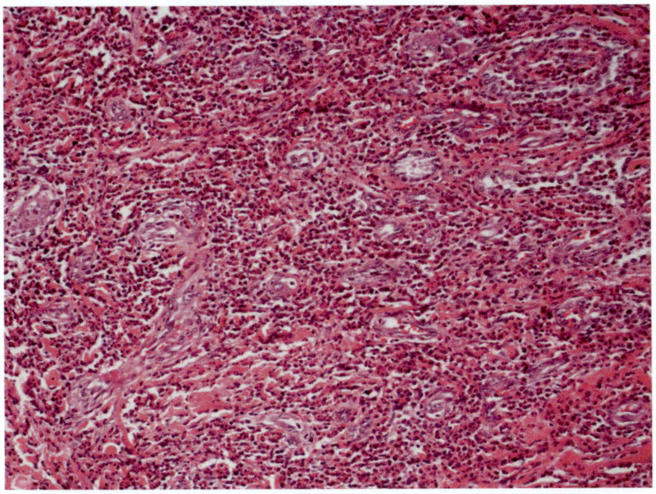

Fig. 8.14 Prominent eosinophilic infiltrate in pulmonary angiolymphoid hyperplasia with eosinophilia

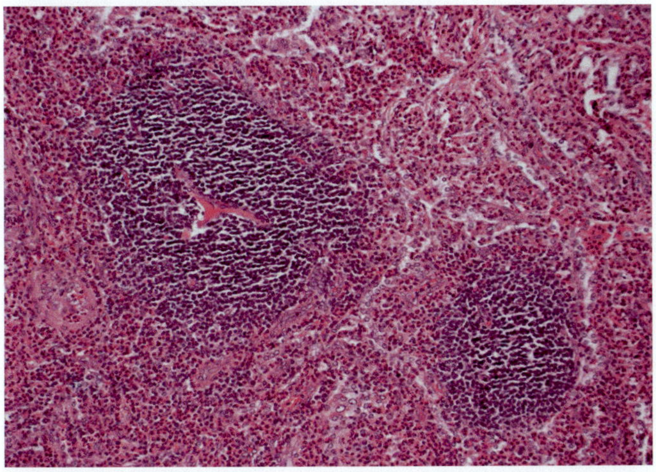

Fig. 8.15 Lymphoid follicles in pulmonary angiolymphoid hyperplasia with eosinophilia

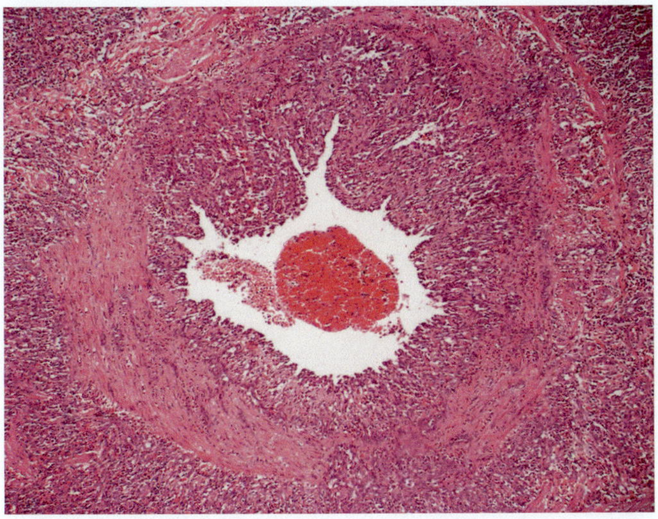

Fig. 8.16 Large vessel involvement in pulmonary angiolymphoid hyperplasia with eosinophilia

is the distinction from angiosarcoma. Primary angiosarcomas of the lung as well as metastatic angiosarcomas are often multifocal lesions that show malignant cytologic features and are not typically accompanied by the lymphoid and eosinophilic infiltrate seen in angiolymphoid hyperplasia with eosinophilia. Other conditions to include in the differential diagnosis comprise lymphoproliferative disorders. These include benign lesions like nodular lymphoid hyperplasia or lymphocytic interstitial pneumonia. Both affect the lung in a diffuse manner and are characterized by a prominent lymphoid infiltrate, whereas eosinophils are not a prominent feature. Among the malignant lymphoid lesions are the low-grade mucosa-associated lymphoid tissue (MALT) lymphoma and Hodgkin's disease. These tumors lack the vascular component seen in angiolymphoid hyperplasia with eosinophilia and would show a more prominent atypical lymphoid proliferation including the typical Reed-Sternberg cells in Hodgkin's disease.

Treatment and Prognosis

Similar to the lesions in the skin, complete surgical excision appears to be the treatment of choice for these tumors and should be curative. The behavior for these lesions is generally benign; however, tumor recurrence has been observed.

Capillary Hemangiomatosis

Capillary hemangiomatosis was first described by Wagenvoort et al. in 1978, and since then fewer than 50 cases have been described in the literature [57]. It is a disorder characterized by a proliferation of thin capillary-sized blood vessels in the lung parenchyma often leading to pulmonary hypertension. Many cases are initially mistaken for pulmonary veno-occlusive disease or primary pulmonary hypertension, and the diagnosis is often only established at autopsy. More recently, cases have been described in patients that did not have signs and symptoms of pulmonary hypertension and where the lesion was merely an incidental finding [58, 59].

Clinical Features

Capillary hemangiomatosis can affect patients of all age groups (birth to 71 years) but is most often seen in young adults [57, 58, 60]. There is no specific gender predilection. In its diffuse form, capillary hemangiomatosis manifests as pulmonary hypertension with an indolent onset but eventual progression to cor pulmonale. Dyspnea, cough, hemoptysis, fatigue, and weight loss are often the presenting symptoms in these cases [61–65]. In focal capillary hemangiomatosis, the patients may be entirely asymptomatic and the lesion is often an incidental finding [58, 59, 66]. Radiologically, capillary hemangiomatosis is characterized by bilateral ill-defined micronodular densities with equal distribution of lower and upper lobes and radiological findings associated with pulmonary hypertension such as right ventricular hypertrophy or enlarged proximal pulmonary arteries [61, 67]. Although most cases appear to be sporadic, familial cases have also been described [65]. In addition, associations with hypertrophic cardiomyopathy, systemic lupus erythematosus and Takayasu aortoarteritis have been described [68–70].

Gross Features

Grossly, capillary hemangiomatosis presents as multiple small hemorrhagic nodules or firm patchy areas with prominent pulmonary vessels [65, 67–68, 71–73]. While microscopic lesions ranged from 0.6 to 1.8 cm in size, grossly visible lesions can measure up to 3 cm [58].

Histological Features

Microscopically, the characteristic finding is a proliferation of capillary-sized blood vessels distributed along the interstitium and alveolar septa preserving the overall lung architecture (Figs. 8.17 and 8.18). This process may be diffused and involve both lungs or be solitary and restricted to a single lung. The capillaries are arranged forming at least a double row on both sides of the alveolar walls (Fig. 8.19). The abnormal capillaries may occasionally protrude into the alveolar spaces or invade the walls of small veins resulting in compression and obstruction of these structures and resulting in pulmonary hypertension (Figs. 8.20 and 8.21). The capillary proliferation may also involve the bronchial tree.

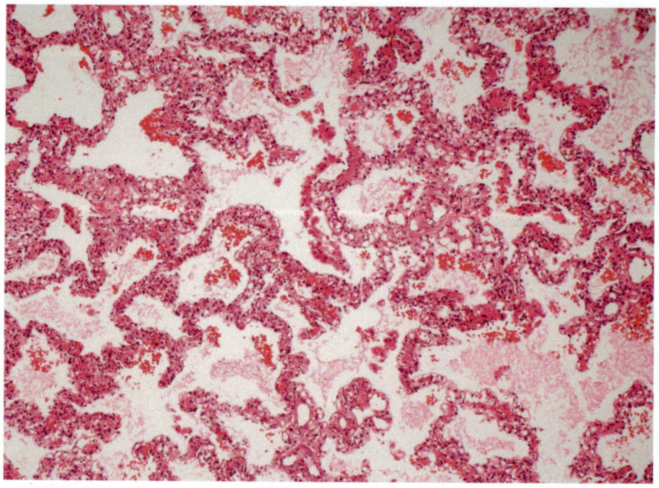

Fig. 8.18 At higher magnification, a capillary proliferation affecting the alveolar walls can be appreciated

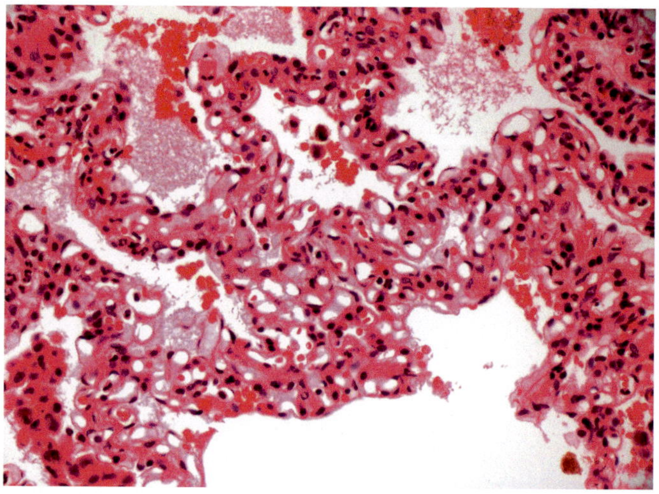

Fig. 8.19 High power view of capillary hemangiomatosis showing the multiple layers of capillary blood vessels within alveolar septa

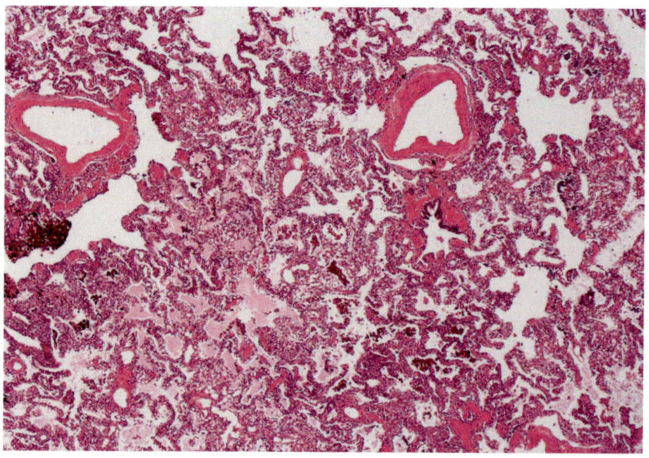

Fig. 8.17 Low power view of pulmonary capillary hemangiomatosis with relative preservation of the normal architecture

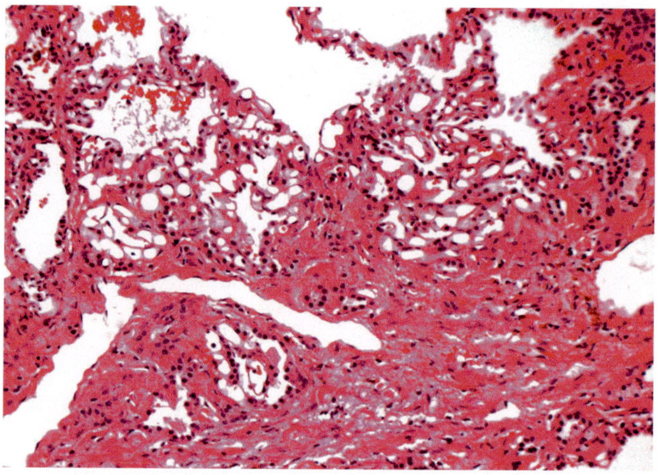

Fig. 8.20 Capillary proliferation affecting the peribronchial areas in capillary hemangiomatosis

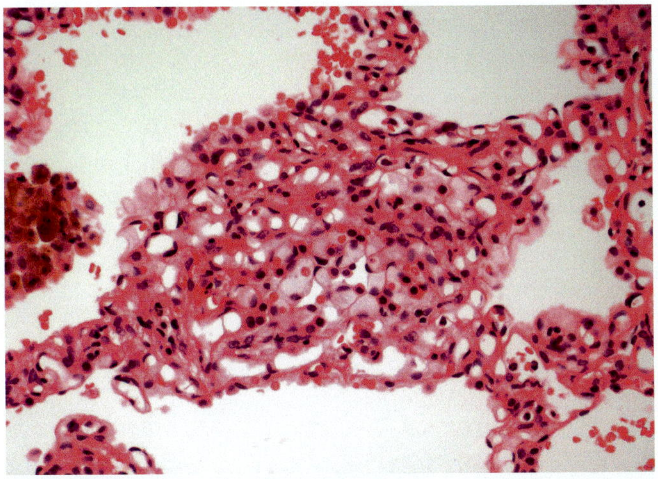

Fig. 8.21 Nodular proliferation of capillary blood vessels protruding into alveolar spaces in capillary hemangiomatosis

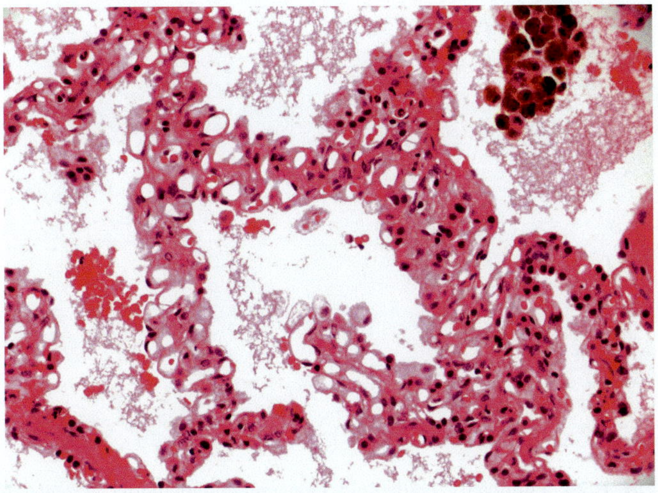

Fig. 8.22 Pulmonary capillary hemangiomatosis showing an absence of cytologic atypia or mitotic activity

The cytologic features are generally bland with no evidence of atypia or mitotic activity; only rare cases can display mild endothelial atypia and pleomorphism [57, 63, 73, 74] (Fig. 8.22). Collections of red blood cells and hemosiderin-laden macrophages are often seen filling the alveolar spaces in the periphery of the process [58, 63, 70, 71].

Immunohistochemical and Molecular Features

The proliferating capillaries are positive for CD31 and CD34 and negative for D2-40 [65]. On a molecular level, capillary hemangiomatosis is characterized by overexpression of platelet-derived growth factor (PDGF)-B and PDGF-β(beta) genes [75].

Differential Diagnosis

The most important differential diagnosis for capillary hemangiomatosis is pulmonary veno-occlusive disease, a process it can be confused with both clinically and histologically. Contrary to capillary hemangiomatosis, pulmonary veno-occlusive disease originates from small pulmonary venules and veins and is characterized by fibrous obliteration of the vascular lumina with secondary dilatation of pulmonary capillaries and small vessels. A proliferation of vessels as such is not identified, and only a single layer of dilated capillaries is observed in the alveolar walls. Furthermore, invasion of capillaries into vascular walls is not seen in pulmonary veno-occlusive disease [58, 64]. Pulmonary angiopathy is another entity that enters the differential diagnosis. This process involves predominantly the small arteries with sparing of the veins. The localized form of capillary hemangiomatosis can mimic conventional capillary hemangioma. The latter lesion is a nodular proliferation of vessels that is not restricted to the alveolar septa or vascular structures.

Treatment and Prognosis

Surgical resection of affected lung tissue is the treatment of choice and may result in pneumonectomy or lung transplantation [58, 73, 77]. In addition, interferon-α(alpha)-2a has been successfully used in the treatment of capillary hemangiomatosis due to its antiangiogenic properties [78–79]. Furthermore, supportive therapy consisting of angiotensin-converting enzyme (ACE) inhibitors, diuretics, oxygen, and warfarin may be indicated in cases associated with pulmonary hypertension [80]. When associated with the clinical signs and symptoms of pulmonary hypertension, capillary hemangiomatosis usually has a slowly progressive and unrelenting clinical course eventually leading to death. The focal type, however, is normally identified incidentally at autopsy or during lung resection for other causes and does not seem to have an influence on life expectancy [58, 66].

Epithelioid Hemangioendothelioma

Epithelioid hemangioendothelioma was first described as "intravascular bronchioloalveolar tumor" (IVBAT) by Dail and Liebow in 1975, suggesting that this tumor was of epithelial origin [81]. Using ultrastructural techniques, several groups subsequently demonstrated that the lesion was in fact a vascular tumor [82–83]. After Weiss and Enzinger used the term "epithelioid hemangioendothelioma" to describe a similar tumor in the soft tissue in 1982, it soon became clear that these lesions were essentially identical and the term "epithelioid hemangioendothelioma" has since been used to describe these tumors regardless of their location [84–86]. To date, more than 80 cases have been described in the lung [87].

Clinical Features

Epithelioid hemangioendothelioma primarily occurs in younger individuals with 50 % of patients being younger than 40 years of age at diagnosis (median age 36 years). Females account for approximately 80 % of cases [88–90]. Patients are often asymptomatic or present with dyspnea, cough, or pleuritic chest pain. Rare cases are symptomatic with alveolar hemorrhage and pleural effusions [91–95]. Radiologically, epithelioid hemangioendothelioma is characterized by multiple small nodular lesions in both lungs mimicking granulomatous or metastatic disease processes. In rare cases, ground glass opacities are identified on CT suggestive of interstitial lung disease. Epithelioid hemangioendothelioma is always a multifocal process and composed of multiple discrete nodules that individually measure less than 2 cm in diameter [96]. A single case report describes the presence of pulmonary epithelioid hemangioendothelioma in association with hypertrophic pulmonary osteoarthropathy, and approximately 5 % of cases can be seen with concurrent bronchioloalveolar carcinoma raising the possibility of an association between these lesions [89, 91, 97].

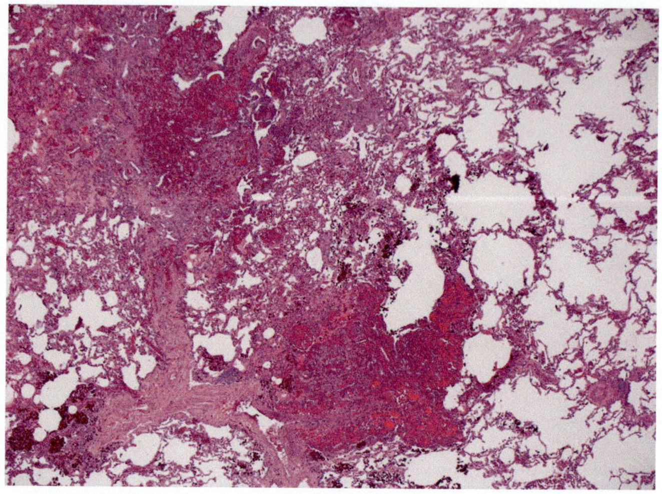

Fig. 8.23 Low power view showing the multifocal nature of pulmonary epithelioid hemangioendothelioma

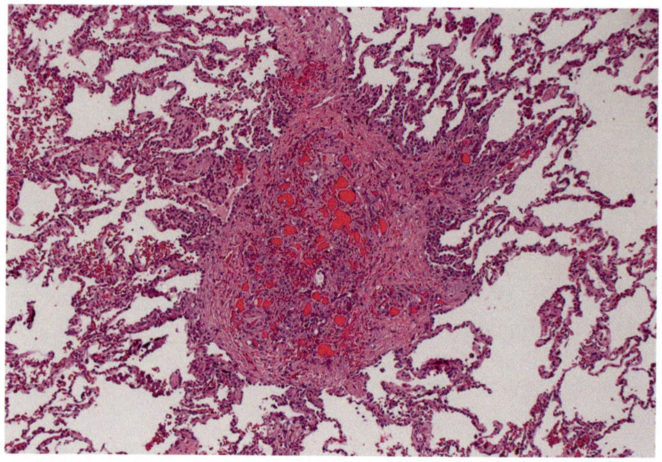

Fig. 8.24 Pulmonary epithelioid hemangioendothelioma associated with pulmonary vessels

Gross Features

Macroscopically, epithelioid hemangioendothelioma presents as multiple nodules that on their own can measure up to 2 cm in diameter. The nodules have a gray-white cut surface and a mucoid, chondroid, or calcified appearance. Pleural involvement may occasionally be seen.

Histological Features

Histologically, epithelioid hemangioendothelioma is often closely associated with vascular structures and is characterized by the presence of multiple nodules (Figs. 8.23, 8.24, and 8.25). These tumor nodules often display an intra-alveolar growth pattern, hence the original term of "IVBAT" (Fig. 8.26). The individual nodules often have hypocellular centers surrounded by rims of more cellular tissue (Fig. 8.27). The cellular areas are composed of short strands or solid nests of rounded or spindled endothelial cells (Fig. 8.28). They have central round to ovoid nuclei and characteristic intracytoplasmic lumina or vacuoles that may contain erythrocytes (Fig. 8.29). The cells are set in a prominent myxochondroid or hyaline stroma (Fig. 8.30). Overall, the cytologic features are bland with minimal nuclear pleomorphism and virtually

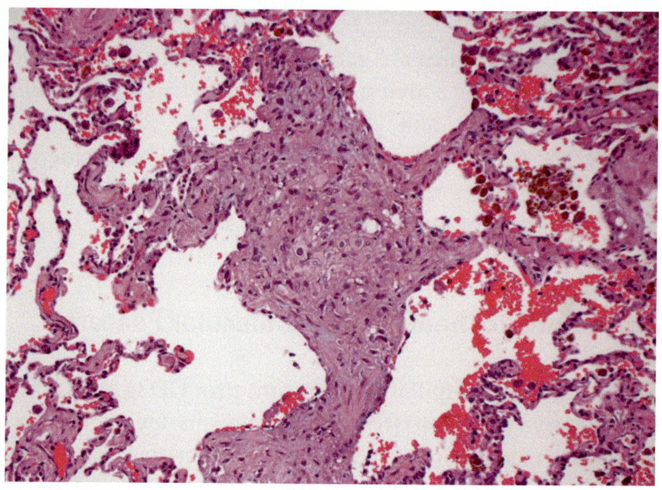

Fig. 8.25 Nodular nature of pulmonary epithelioid hemangioendothelioma

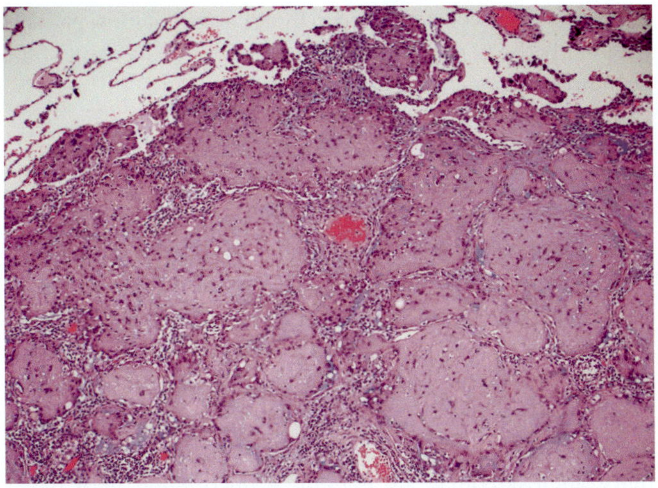

Fig. 8.26 Prominent intra-alveolar growth pattern in pulmonary epithelioid hemangioendothelioma

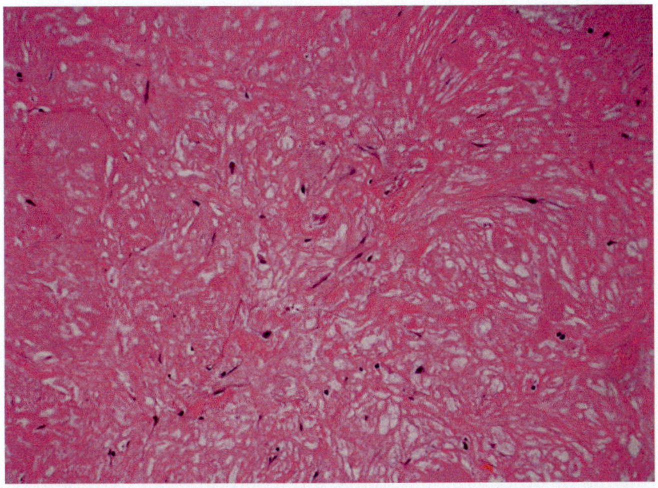

Fig. 8.27 Hypocellular centers in pulmonary epithelioid hemangioendothelioma

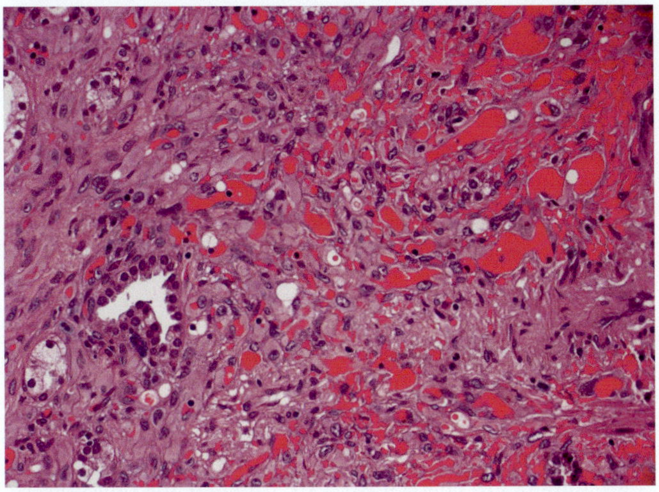

Fig. 8.28 Solid proliferation of epithelioid cells in pulmonary epithelioid hemangioendothelioma

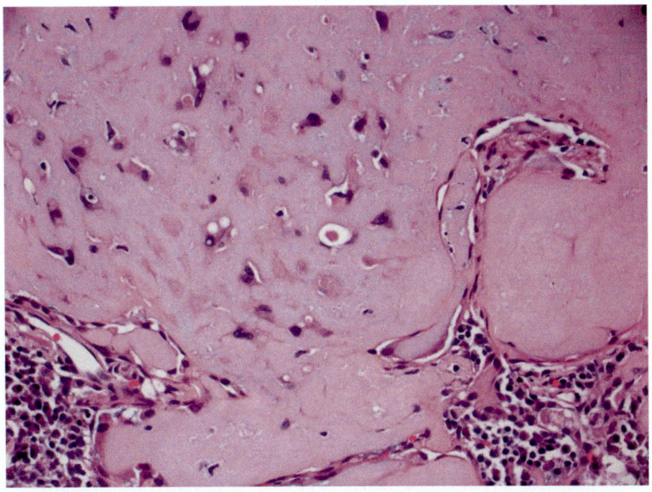

Fig. 8.29 Tumor cells of pulmonary epithelioid hemangioendothelioma showing cytoplasmic vacuoles containing red blood cells

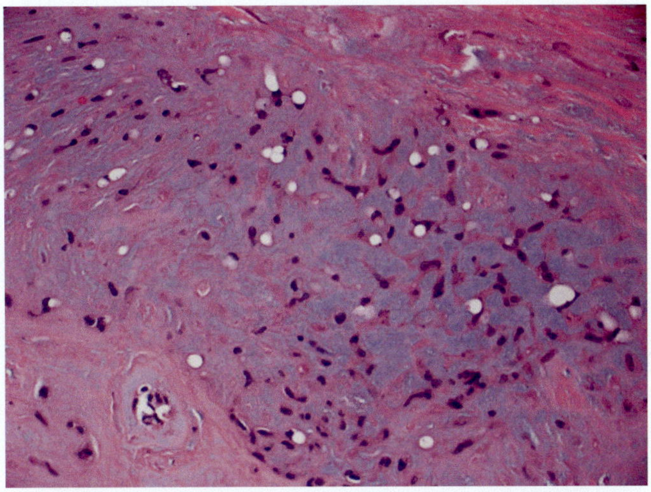

Fig. 8.30 Tumor cells set in a prominent myxochondroid stroma in pulmonary epithelioid hemangioendothelioma

no mitotic activity [96, 98]. In the soft tissue, up to one-fourth of cases may display a degree of cytologic atypia, mitotic activity, spindling of cells, or necrosis [98]. These features have not been described in primary lung lesions.

Immunohistochemical and Molecular Features

Immunohistochemically, epithelioid hemangioendothelioma shows the typical phenotype of endothelial cells demonstrated by reactivity for factor VIII related antigen (up to 99 % of cases), CD31 (up to 86 %), and CD34 (up to 94 %) [85, 99–100]. However, it should be noted that up to 50 % of cases may show positivity for cytokeratins so that this marker may not be helpful in distinguishing hemangioendothelioma from certain types of carcinoma [101]. At the molecular level, isolated case reports have described (1;3)(p36.3;q25) or (7;22) translocations in epithelioid hemangioendothelioma of the soft tissue [102–103], but larger series have yet to be investigated.

Differential Diagnosis

The differential diagnosis for epithelioid hemangioendothelioma includes adenocarcinoma, sarcomas with a chondroid or epithelioid appearance, sclerosing hemangioma, and metastatic cardiac myxoma [91, 98]. Adenocarcinomas usually have a glandular growth pattern and show a greater degree of nuclear pleomorphism and increased mitotic activity. Sarcomas may demonstrate prominent intra-alveolar growth, but unequivocal areas of sarcomatous differentiation as well as cellular pleomorphism and mitotic activity are normally identifiable. Sclerosing hemangioma is a peculiar tumor presenting as an isolated lung mass; it is composed of bland-looking cells set in a sclerotic background. In contrast to epithelioid hemangioendothelioma, however, this lesion is more cellular, displays a greater variety of growth patterns, and often contains large telangiectatic vessels. In addition, sclerosing hemangioma is a misnomer as the tumor is not vascular, thus, the tumor fails to stain with the typical endothelial immunomarkers as described for epithelioid hemangioendothelioma. Finally, metastatic cardiac myxomas, although typically positive for factor VIII related antigen, have a more myxomatous background and an irregular cellular arrangement. These tumors are normally contained within vascular structures and do not display an intra-alveolar growth pattern. Most of the tumors considered in the differential diagnosis carry a worse prognosis and require different treatment modalities, making accurate diagnosis highly important for patient management.

Treatment and Prognosis

If the disease burden is limited, surgical excision is the treatment of choice for epithelioid hemangioendothelioma. Lung transplantation may be considered in cases of aggressive tumor growth [87]. Unfortunately, both chemotherapy and radiation have not proven to be effective in the treatment of this tumor, although antiangiogenic therapy with bevacizumab has been successful in one case [86, 91, 104–105]. In general terms, epithelioid hemangioendothelioma is considered a low-grade malignant tumor associated with a protracted clinical course and non-aggressive behavior but metastatic potential [85–86]. Life expectancy spans 1–20 years with a 5-year survival rate of 60 % [87, 106–107]. Factors of poor prognosis include extensive intrapulmonary and pleural spread, weight loss, anemia, pulmonary symptoms, and hemorrhagic pleural effusions [86–87, 91]. Partial regression has been described in three cases, but most patients eventually die of respiratory failure due to replacement of the pulmonary parenchyma by tumor [90].

Angiosarcoma

Angiosarcomas represent less than 1 % of all sarcomas and develop most often in the skin, soft tissue, or liver. Associations have been described with prior radiation treatment, environmental carcinogens, foreign body material, or lymphedema [108–115]. The lungs are more often the site of metastasis from extrapulmonary tumors, most frequently from the heart and the pulmonary artery trunk [116–119]. In the lung, primary angiosarcomas are extremely uncommon with fewer than 20 cases reported in the English literature to date.

Clinical Features

Pulmonary angiosarcomas affect adults with an age range from 22 to 79 years (mean 54.0 years) and a male-to-female ratio of 3:1. Presenting symptoms include dyspnea, chest pain, hemoptysis, cough, pulmonary hemorrhage, or hemothorax [120–123]. Radiologically, bilateral interstitial or parenchymal infiltrates, pleural effusions, or solid masses are identified that may mimic inflammatory processes or metastatic carcinoma [120, 122, 124–126]. The tumors arise in the parenchyma, the pulmonary artery trunk, or the bronchus [120, 124, 127]. Although often presenting as a diffuse process, single mass lesions may also be seen [121, 124, 126]. While pulmonary angiosarcomas may rarely be seen in association with concurrent malignant neoplasms of other organ systems, angiosarcomas of extrapulmonary sites have been described in association with Maffucci's and Klippel-Trenaunay-Weber syndromes [128–130].

Gross Features

In angiosarcoma, the lungs appear diffusely hemorrhagic and studded with multiple dark-red nodules [121, 124]. The tumors have a predilection for the interlobular septa and bronchovascular bundles and tend to grow along the lymphatic or venous routes.

Histological Features

Primary angiosarcomas of the lung have similar histological growth patterns to those seen in other sites (Fig. 8.31). Low-grade tumors are characterized by irregular interanastomosing vascular channels dissecting the lung parenchyma (Fig. 8.32). In contrast to benign vascular neoplasms, these

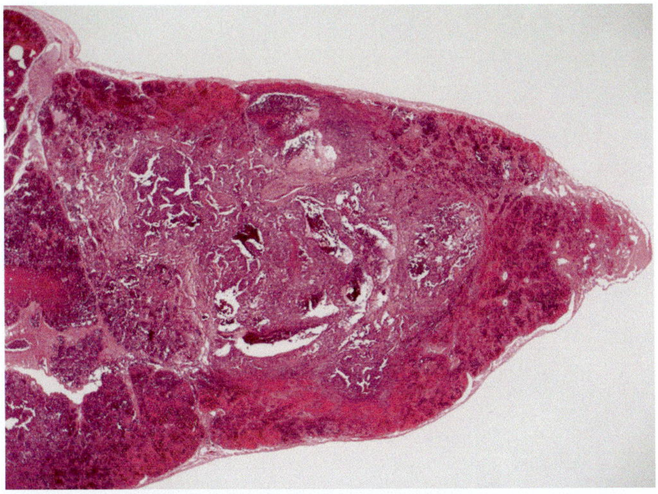

Fig. 8.31 Pulmonary angiosarcoma arising in the lung periphery

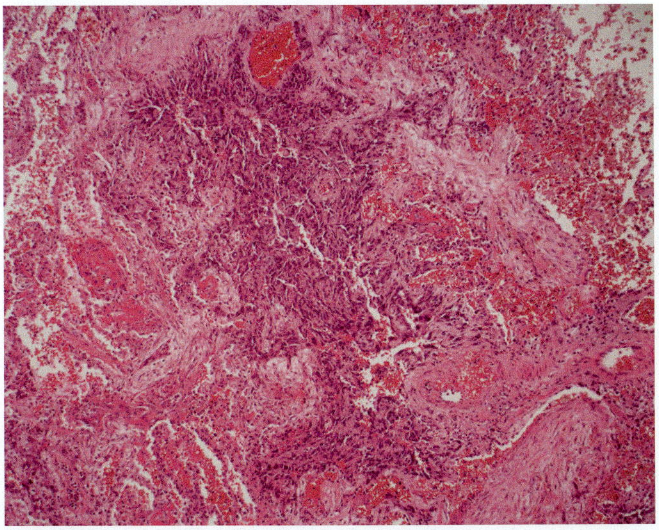

Fig. 8.32 Low-grade angiosarcoma of lung characterized by small slit-like vessels replacing the lung parenchyma

channels are lined by more atypical endothelial cells that display crowding or hobnailing along the vessel walls (Figs. 8.33 and 8.34). In some areas, the crowding is so pronounced as to form papillary projections similar to those seen in papillary endothelial hyperplasia (Fig. 8.35). Further patterns of growth include the formation of capillary, cavernous, or slit-like vascular spaces. In high-grade tumors, the vascular nature of the neoplasms may be difficult to identify. These tumors are commonly composed of solid sheets of epithelioid or spindled tumor cells (Fig. 8.36). Cytologically, these cells show obvious malignant features. In the epithelioid variant, the tumor cells are large and pleomorphic with vesicular and hyperchromatic nuclei and abundant pale cytoplasm (Figs. 8.37 and 8.38), while the conventional spindle cell type is characterized by fusiform and hyperchromatic nuclei, inconspicuous

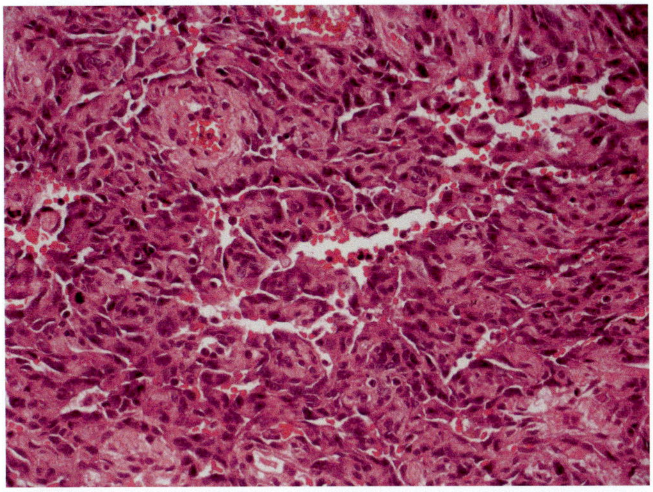

Fig. 8.33 Low-grade pulmonary angiosarcoma showing crowding of atypical endothelial cells

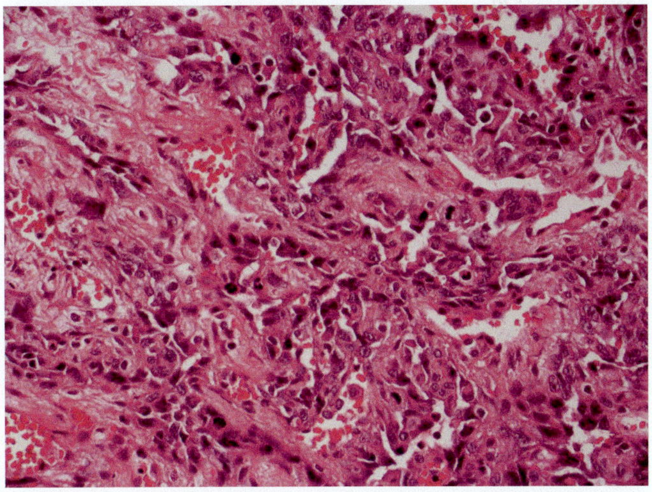

Fig. 8.34 Low-grade pulmonary angiosarcoma demonstrating mild cytologic atypia and increased mitotic activity

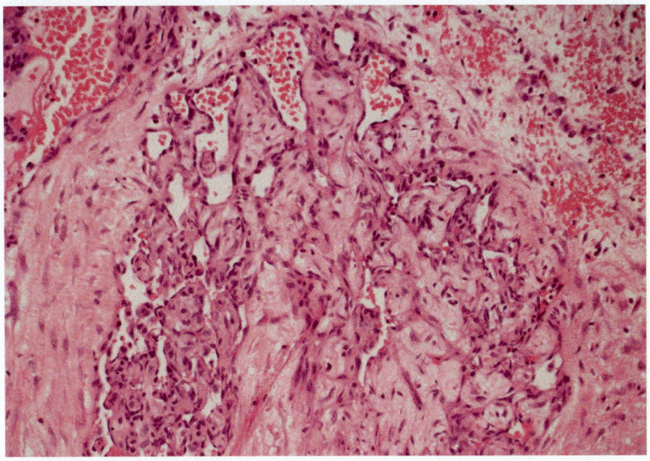

Fig. 8.35 Low-grade angiosarcoma of lung resembling papillary endothelial hyperplasia

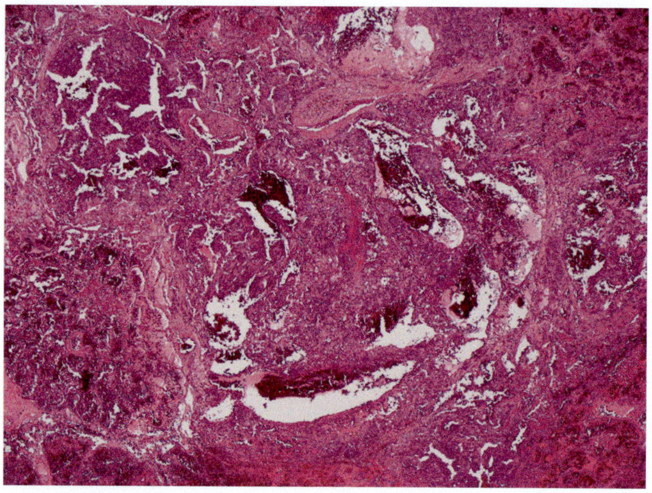

Fig. 8.36 Low power view of high-grade angiosarcoma with more solid growth pattern

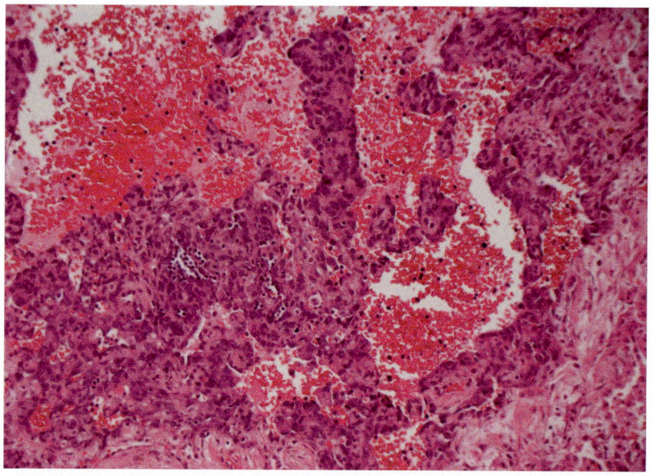

Fig. 8.37 High-grade angiosarcoma composed of a proliferation of epithelioid tumor cells

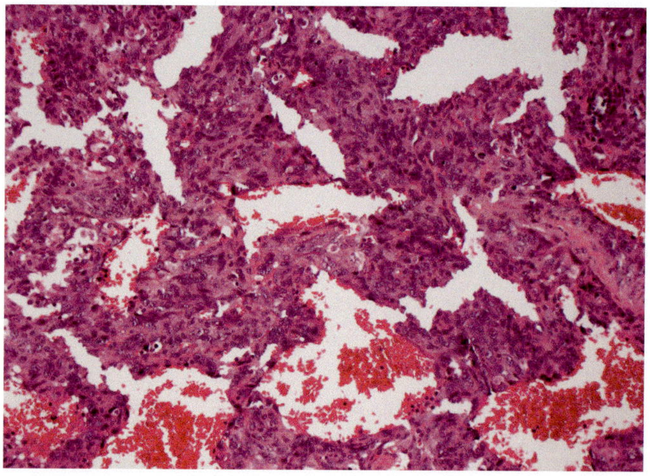

Fig. 8.38 Prominent cytologic atypia and mitotic activity in high-grade pulmonary angiosarcoma

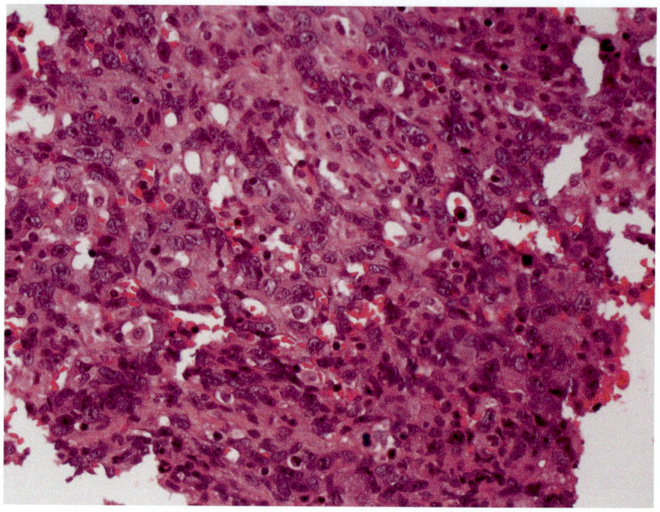

Fig. 8.39 Rudimentary lumen formation in high-grade pulmonary angiosarcoma

nucleoli, and moderate amounts of eosinophilic cytoplasm. Mitoses are generally easily found. Intracytoplasmic vacuoles containing red blood cells or rudimentary lumen formation may occasionally be seen facilitating distinction from other neoplasms (Fig. 8.39). The parenchyma surrounding the tumors is often intensely hemorrhagic and may contain abundant hemosiderin-laden macrophages [120, 123, 127, 131]. Prominent concentric rings of tumor around intact blood vessels were described in one case [120].

Immunohistochemical and Molecular Features

Angiosarcomas are positive for the endothelial markers factor VIII related antigen, CD34, and CD31 [122–137]; immunoreactivity for cytokeratin has been identified in a subset of the epithelioid angiosarcomas [138–139]. Studies investigating the molecular events in hepatic and cardiac angiosarcomas suggest that K-ras-2, p53, ras oncogene, or PTEN gene mutations play a role in the development of these tumors [140–143]. In addition, cases with chromosomal structural rearrangement and polysomy of chromosome 8 or increased expression of VEGFR and mdm-2-protooncogene have been reported [144–145]. In angiosarcomas of the soft tissues, abnormal chromosome numbers have been identified characterized by gains of chromosomes 5, 8, and 20 and losses of chromosomes 7 and 22 and Y-chromosome [146–147].

Differential Diagnosis

The main differential diagnoses include organizing thromboemboli and the plexiform lesions of pulmonary hypertension. These processes have a tendency to form intravascular papillae and anastomosing vascular channels and may be mistaken for a malignant tumor. The lack of cytologic atypia, mitoses, and confinement of the lesions to the vascular lumina should help to distinguish these reactive processes from angiosarcoma. Among the neoplastic lesions, lymphangitis carcinomatosa, pseudoangiomatous carcinomas, and especially other vascular neoplasms such as Kaposi's sarcoma and epithelioid hemangioendothelioma need to be excluded. Lymphangitis carcinomatosa is normally associated with a known primary tumor, lacks a vasoformative component, and reacts with epithelial immunohistochemical markers. Pseudoangiomatous carcinomas likewise should show positivity for epithelial markers and do not react with vascular immunohistochemical stains. Kaposi's sarcoma is a tumor characterized by a proliferation of spindle cells showing prominent extravasation of red blood cells but no blood vessel formation as such. Epithelioid hemangioendothelioma shows a different growth pattern or distribution with a largely intra-alveolar growth pattern, a conspicuous myxoid background, and a bland cytological morphology.

Treatment and Prognosis

Current treatment for angiosarcoma consists of systemic chemotherapy with various combinations of doxorubicin, vincristine, cyclophosphamide, dacarbazine, and methotrexate, and radiotherapy [120, 148]. One case report has shown treatment with interleukin-2 to be successful [126]. The prognosis is generally poor with survival dates ranging from <1 to 15 months (median 5.1 months) [129, 126, 127, 148].

Kaposi's Sarcoma

Before 1981, Kaposi's sarcoma was mainly known as an indolent neoplasm affecting the skin of the lower extremities of elderly men of Mediterranean or Ashkenazi Jewish origin [149]. Sporadic disseminated Kaposi's sarcoma was rare and pulmonary involvement even rarer [150–151]. Kaposi's sarcoma, however, was soon recognized to be the most common neoplasm in patients with acquired immune deficiency syndrome (AIDS) and in this setting often presenting with nodal and visceral involvement and a more aggressive behavior [152–153]. As many as 47–90 % of AIDS patients were found to have Kaposi's sarcoma involving the lungs at autopsy, but only isolated case reports describe the presence of Kaposi's sarcoma as a primary pulmonary tumor [154–166].

Clinical Features

The main presenting symptoms in patients with pulmonary Kaposi's sarcoma include dyspnea, cough, hemoptysis, fatigue, fever, or respiratory failure [150, 163, 167]. Radiologically, Kaposi's sarcoma is characterized by diffuse reticulonodular pulmonary infiltrates, solitary lung nodules, or pleural effusions [154–155, 164, 168–169]. Central symmetrical bronchial wall thickening particularly in association with septal lines is a common finding; unusual features include the presence of larger peripherally located nodules, the predominance of which should prompt investigations into a different etiology [152]. The disease may be widespread with involvement of the tracheobronchial tree, lung parenchyma, mediastinal lymph nodes, and pleura [170–171]. Although most cases of Kaposi's sarcoma of the lung present in association with AIDS, cases may also develop after organ transplantation, in association with other immunocompromised states and less commonly in healthy individuals [160, 166]. Kaposi's sarcoma in AIDS and in transplant patients is closely associated with human herpes virus 8 (HHV8) infection, and the detection of HHV8-DNA is thought to be highly specific and sensitive for a diagnosis of this tumor, adding an important diagnostic tool in this setting [172–173].

Gross Features

Macroscopically, the lung parenchyma in Kaposi's sarcoma is infiltrated by discrete dark-red hemorrhagic nodules with associated intra-alveolar hemorrhage. Endobronchial lesions may present as multiple dark-red raised lesions on bronchoscopy [154, 174–176]. Individual tumor nodules can measure from a few millimeters to 3 cm in size and may involve the pleural surfaces.

Histological Features

The histological hallmark of Kaposi's sarcoma is its lymphatic distribution with growth along the septa and infiltration of small airways, pulmonary arteries, and veins (Fig. 8.40). The tumor is composed of spindle cells, inflammatory cells, and red blood cells forming infiltrative nodular masses of varying size (Figs. 8.41 and 8.42). The histological spectrum ranges from hypocellular areas in the periphery of the nodules to cellular areas composed of spindled tumor cells, nonspecific plump mesenchymal cells, lymphocytes, and plasma cells centrally. The spindle cells have elongated nuclei, only mild nuclear atypia, dense chromatin, and indistinct nucleoli (Fig. 8.43). Cytoplasmic hyaline globules are often conspicuous. The spindle cells are arranged either without a specific pattern or as intersecting fascicles. Cleft-like spaces may be identified containing extravasated red blood cells and hemosiderin (Fig. 8.44). Mitoses are often present but not plentiful, and necrosis is only occasionally detected [96, 115, 177].

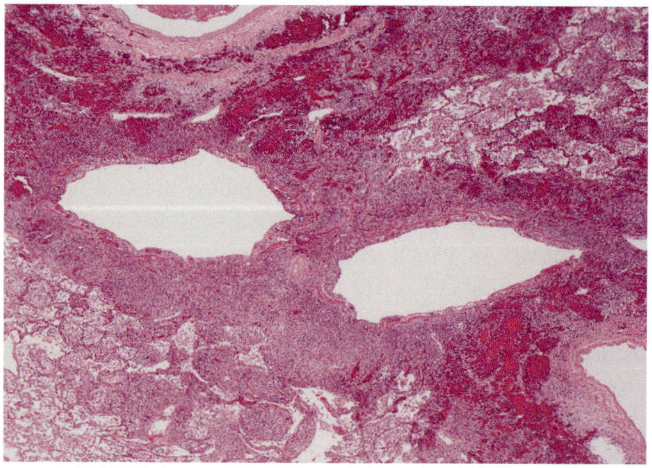

Fig. 8.40 Low power view of pulmonary Kaposi's sarcoma growing along the pulmonary vasculature

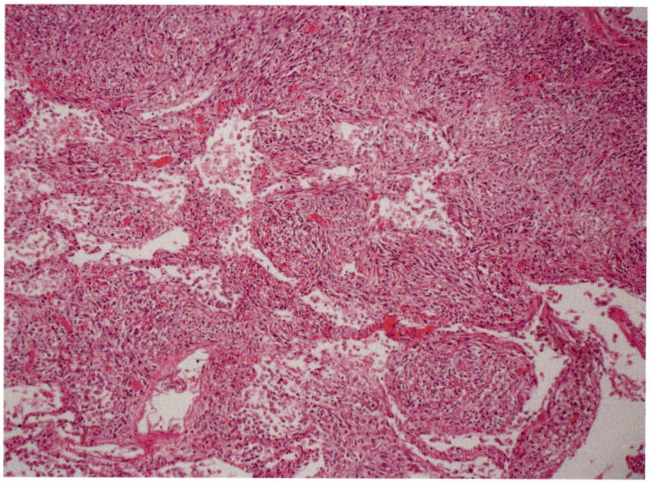

Fig. 8.41 Formation of nodular masses by pulmonary Kaposi's sarcoma

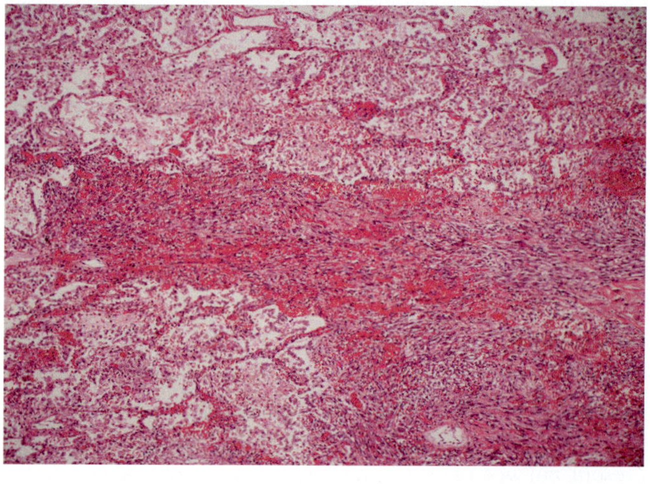

Fig. 8.42 Pulmonary Kaposi's sarcoma involving the lung parenchyma

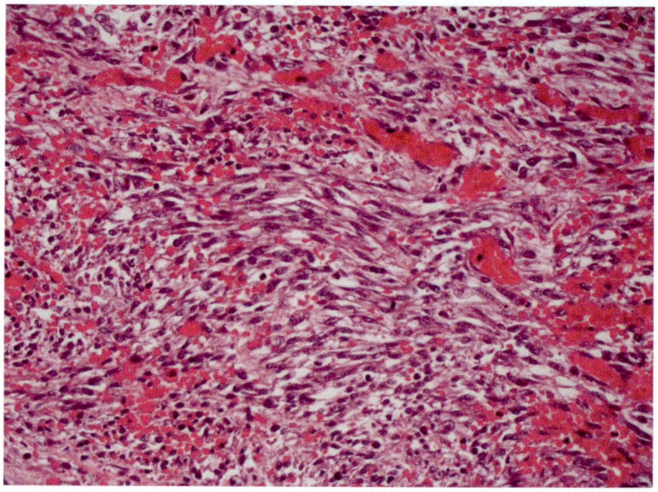

Fig. 8.43 High power view of pulmonary Kaposi's sarcoma composed of spindle cells intermixed with numerous inflammatory cells

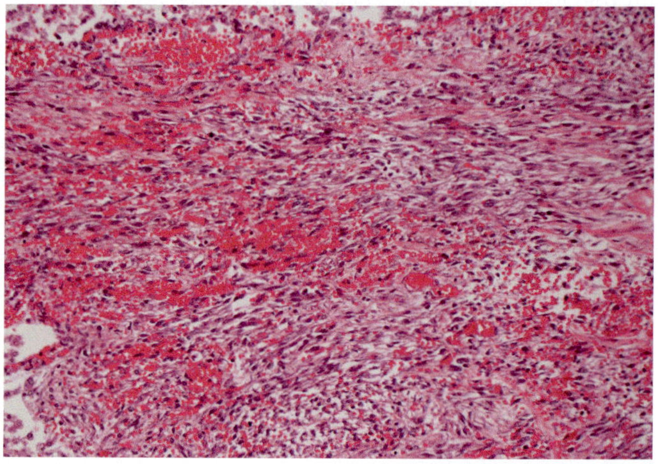

Fig. 8.44 Characteristic red blood cell extravasation in pulmonary Kaposi's sarcoma

Immunohistochemical and Molecular Features

Immunohistochemical characteristics of Kaposi's sarcoma include reactivity of tumor cells for CD34, CD31, D2-40, VEGFR-3, and HHV8 [39, 178–184]. Molecular characteristics include deletion and translocation of chromosome 3, int-2 oncogene expression, and overexpression of Bcl-2 [185–187].

Differential Diagnosis

The differential diagnosis for Kaposi's sarcoma of the lung includes entities like angiosarcoma, spindle cell carcinoma, melanoma, and inflammatory lesions like organizing pneumonia. Angiosarcoma forms definitive vascular structures and lacks the spindle cell component and red blood cell extravasation seen in Kaposi's sarcoma. The lack of red blood cells, prominent inflammatory cells, hyaline globules, and immunoreactivity with endothelial markers makes a diagnosis of other spindle cell lesions such as carcinoma or melanoma unlikely. Organizing pneumonia, although containing variable amounts of inflammatory or spindle cells, does not have the growth pattern of Kaposi's sarcoma and does not react with endothelial immunomarkers.

Treatment and Prognosis

Due to its multifocal growth pattern, surgical treatment is of limited use in Kaposi's sarcoma and cytotoxic chemotherapy with doxorubicin, bleomycin, vincristine, taxol, or liposomal doxorubicin is considered the treatment of choice [155, 188–189]. In addition, highly active antiretroviral treatment (HAART) is thought to be an important component in the prevention and treatment of Kaposi's sarcoma in patients with AIDS [190]. Furthermore, targeted antiviral treatment with zidovudine and immune response modifiers are thought to be effective but are still at an experimental stage [191–192]. Radiotherapy plays only a minor role in the palliation of symptoms and has not shown to be beneficial with curative intent. Untreated pulmonary Kaposi's sarcoma has a poor prognosis with a median survival of only 2–6 months [154–155, 193]; treatment with chemotherapy may increase median survival to up to 10 months [188]. The most important factor, however, for the prognosis of patients with pulmonary Kaposi's sarcoma appears to be their serologic human immunodeficiency virus (HIV) status, as patients with AIDS are likely to have an accelerated clinical course of their disease [96].

References

1. Shikhani AH, Jones MM, Marsh BR, et al. Infantile subglottic hemangiomas. An update. Ann Otol Rhinol Laryngol. 1986; 95:336–47.
2. Moran CA, Suster S. Mediastinal hemangiomas: a study of 18 cases with emphasis on the spectrum of morphological features. Hum Pathol. 1995;26:416–21.
3. Maeda R, Isowa N, Sumitomo S, et al. Pulmonary cavernous hemangioma. Gen Thorac Cardiovasc Surg. 2007;55:177–9.
4. Capizzani TR, Patel H, Hines MH, Mott RT, Petty JK. A unique case of a giant congenital pulmonary hemangioma in a newborn. J Pediatr Surg. 2008;43:574–8.
5. Harding JR, Williams J, Seal RM. Pedunculated capillary haemangioma of the bronchus. Br J Dis Chest. 1978;72:336–42.
6. Mori A, Obata K, Tada T, et al. A case of multiple cavernous hemangiomas of the lung. Gan No Rinsho. 1985;31:1433–8.
7. Wu JM, Lin CS, Wang JN, et al. Pulmonary cavernous hemangiomatosis treated with interferon alfa-2a. Pediatr Cardiol. 1996;17:332–4.
8. Kase M, Sakamoto K, Yamagata T, et al. A case of pulmonary cavernous hemangioma: immunohistological examination revealed its endothelial cell origin. Kyobu Geka. 2000;53:1055–7.
9. Fine SW, Whitney KD. Multiple cavernous hemangiomas of the lung: a case report and review of the literature. Arch Pathol Lab Med. 2004;128:1439–41.
10. Galliani CA, Beatty JF, Grosfeld JL. Cavernous hemangioma of the lung in an infant. Pediatr Pathol. 1992;12:105–11.
11. Abrahams NA, Colby TV, Pearl RH, et al. Pulmonary hemangiomas of infancy and childhood: report of two cases and review of the literature. Pediatr Dev Pathol. 2002;5:283–92.
12. Sirmali M, Demirağ F, Aydin E, et al. A pulmonary cavernous hemangioma causing massive hemoptysis. Ann Thorac Surg. 2003;76:1275–6.
13. Paul KP, Börner C, Müller KM, et al. Capillary hemangioma of the right main bronchus treated by sleeve resection in infancy. Am Rev Respir Dis. 1991;143:876–9.
14. Cohen MC, Kaschula RO. Primary pulmonary tumors in childhood: a review of 31 years' experience and the literature. Pediatr Pulmonol. 1992;14:222–32.
15. Kayser K, Zink S, Link B, et al. Endobronchial juvenile hemangioma – a case report of a neonate including immunohistochemical monitoring and nuclear, cellular, and vascular morphometry. Virchows Arch. 2001;438:192–7.
16. Rose AS, Mathur PN. Endobronchial capillary hemangioma: case report and review of the literature. Respiration. 2008;76:221–4.
17. Quijano G, Drut R. Multiple congenital infantile hemangiomas of the lung in partial trisomy D. J Clin Pathol. 2007;60:943–5.
18. Kobayashi A, Ohno S, Bando M, et al. Cavernous hemangiomas of lungs and liver in an asymptomatic girl. Respiration. 2003;70: 647–50.
19. Bowyer JJ, Sheppard M. Capillary haemangioma presenting as a lung pseudocyst. Arch Dis Child. 1990;65:1162–4.
20. Fugo K, Matsuno Y, Okamoto K, et al. Solitary capillary hemangioma of the lung: report of 2 resected cases detected by high-resolution CT. Am J Surg Pathol. 2006;30:750–3.
21. Walter JW, North PE, Waner M, Mizeracki A, et al. Somatic mutation of vascular endothelial growth factor receptors in juvenile hemangioma. Genes Chromosomes Cancer. 2002;33:295–303.
22. Jinnin M, Medici D, Park L, et al. Suppressed NFAT-dependent VEGFR1 expression and constitutive VEGFR2 signaling in infantile hemangioma. Nat Med. 2008;14:1236–46.
23. Bill Jr AH, Sumner DS. A unified concept of lymphangioma and cystic hygroma. Surg Gynecol Obstet. 1965;120:79–86.
24. Kransdorf MJ. Benign soft tissue tumors in a large referral population: distribution of specific diagnoses by age, sex, and location. AJR Am J Roentgenol. 1994;164:395–402.
25. Limmer S, Krokowski M, Kujath P. Pulmonary lymphangioma. Ann Thorac Surg. 2008;85:336–9.
26. Kim WS, Lee KS, Kim I, et al. Cystic intrapulmonary lymphangioma: HRCT findings. Pediatr Radiol. 1995;25:206–7.
27. Drut R, Mosca HH. Intrapulmonary cystic lymphangioma. Pediatr Pulmonol. 1996;22:204–6.
28. Takahara T, Morisaki Y, Torigoe T, et al. Intrapulmonary cystic lymphangioma: report of a case. Surg Today. 1998;28:1310–2.
29. Faul JL, Berry GJ, Colby TV, et al. Thoracic lymphangiomas, lymphangiectasis, lymphangiomatosis, and lymphatic dysplasia syndrome. Am J Respir Crit Care Med. 2000;161:1037–46.
30. Hernanz-Schulman M. Cysts and cystlike lesions of the lung. Radiol Clin North Am. 1993;31:631–49.
31. Suringa DW, Ackerman AB. Cutaneous lymphangiomas with dyschondroplasia (Maffucci's syndrome). A unique variant of an unusual syndrome. Arch Dermatol. 1970;101:472–4.
32. Weber PF. Angioma formation in connection with hypertrophy of the limbs and hemihypertrophy. Br J Dermatol. 1907;19:231.
33. Nagayasu T, Hayashi T, Ashizawa K, et al. A case of solitary pulmonary lymphangioma. J Clin Pathol. 2003;56:396–8.
34. Wada A, Tateishi R, Terazawa T, et al. Case report: lymphangioma of the lung. Arch Pathol. 1974;98:211–3.

35. Milovic I, Oluic D. Lymphangioma of the lung associated with respiratory distress in a neonate. Pediatr Radiol. 1992;22:156.
36. Hilliard RI, McKendry JB, Phillips MJ. Congenital abnormalities of the lymphatic system: a new clinical classification. Pediatrics. 1990;86:988–94.
37. Hamada K, Ishii Y, Nakaya M, et al. Solitary lymphangioma of the lung. Histopathology. 1995;27:482–3.
38. Folpe AL, Veikkola T, Valtola R, et al. Vascular endothelial growth factor receptor-3 (VEGFR-3): a marker of vascular tumors with presumed lymphatic differentiation, including Kaposi's sarcoma, kaposiform and Dabska-type hemangioendotheliomas, and a subset of angiosarcomas. Mod Pathol. 2000;13:180–5.
39. Irrthum A, Karkkainen MJ, Devriendt K, et al. Congenital hereditary lymphedema caused by a mutation that inactivates VEGFR3 tyrosine kinase. Am J Hum Genet. 2000;67:295–301.
40. Yousem SA, Hochholzer L. Alveolar adenoma. Hum Pathol. 1986;17:1066–71.
41. Burke LM, Rush WI, Khoor A, Mackay B, Oliveira P, Whitsett JA, Singh G, Turnicky R, Fleming MV, Koss MN, Travis WD. Alveolar adenoma: a histochemical, immunohistochemical, and ultrastructural analysis of 17 cases. Hum Pathol. 1999;30:158–67.
42. Berger U, Khaghani A, Pomerance A, et al. Pulmonary lymphangioleiomyomatosis and steroid receptors. An immunocytochemical study. Am J Clin Pathol. 1990;93:609–14.
43. Ohori NP, Yousem SA, Sonmez-Alpan E, et al. Estrogen and progesterone receptors in lymphangioleiomyomatosis, epithelioid hemangioendothelioma, and sclerosing hemangioma of the lung. Am J Clin Pathol. 1991;96:529–35.
44. Bonetti F, Pea M, Martignoni G, et al. Cellular heterogeneity in lymphangiomyomatosis of the lung. Hum Pathol. 1991;22:727–8.
45. Molitch HI, Unger EC, Witte CL, et al. Percutaneous sclerotherapy of lymphangiomas. Radiology. 1995;194:343–7.
46. Wilson C, Askin FB, Heitmiller RF. Solitary pulmonary lymphangioma. Ann Thorac Surg. 2001;71:1337–8.
47. Wells GC, Whimster IW. Subcutaneous angiolymphoid hyperplasia with eosinophilia. Br J Dermatol. 1969;81:1–14.
48. Suster S. Nodal angiolymphoid hyperplasia with eosinophilia. Am J Clin Pathol. 1987;88:236–9.
49. Hidayat AA, Cameron JD, Font RL, Zimmerman LE. Angiolymphoid hyperplasia with eosinophilia (Kimura's disease) of the orbit and ocular adnexa. Am J Ophthalmol. 1983;96:176–89.
50. Kuo TT, Hsueh S, Su IJ, Gonzalez-Crussi F, Chen JS. Histiocytoid hemangioma of the heart with peripheral eosinophilia. Cancer. 1985;55:2854–61.
51. Nielsen GP, Srivastava A, Kattapuram S, Deshpande V, O'Connell JX, Mangham CD, Rosenberg AE. Epithelioid hemangioma of bone revisited: a study of 50 cases. Am J Surg Pathol. 2009;33: 270–7.
52. Urabe A, Tsuneyoshi M, Enjoji M. Epithelioid hemangioma versus Kimura's disease. A comparative clinicopathologic study. Am J Surg Pathol. 1987;11:758–66.
53. Ahn HJ, Lee KG. A clinicopathological study of Kimura's disease and epithelioid hemangioma. Yonsei Med J. 1990;31:205–11.
54. Weiss SW, Ishak KG, Dail DH, Sweet DE, Enzinger FM. Epithelioid hemangioendothelioma and related lesions. Semin Diagn Pathol. 1986;3:259–87.
55. Moran CA, Suster S. Angiolymphoid hyperplasia with eosinophilia (epithelioid hemangioma) of the lung: a clinicopathologic and immunohistochemical study of two cases. Am J Clin Pathol. 2005; 123:762–5.
56. Kempf W, Haeffner AC, Zepter K, Sander CA, Flaig MJ, Mueller B, Panizzon RG, Hardmeier T, Adams V, Burg G. Angiolymphoid hyperplasia with eosinophilia: evidence for a T-cell lymphoproliferative origin. Hum Pathol. 2002;33:1023–9.
57. Wagenvoort CA, Beetstra A, Spijker J. Capillary haemangiomatosis of the lungs. Histopathology. 1978;2:401–6.
58. Havlik DM, Massie LW, Williams WL, Crooks LA. Pulmonary capillary hemangiomatosis-like foci. An autopsy study of 8 cases. Am J Clin Pathol. 2000;113:655–62.
59. Umezu H, Naito M, Yagisawa K, Hattori A, Aizawa Y. An autopsy case of pulmonary capillary hemangiomatosis without evidence of pulmonary hypertension. Virchows Arch. 2001;439: 586–92.
60. Oviedo A, Abramson LP, Worthington R, Dainauskas JR, Crawford SE. Congenital pulmonary capillary hemangiomatosis: report of two cases and review of the literature. Pediatr Pulmonol. 2003;36: 253–6.
61. Lawler LP, Askin FB. Pulmonary capillary hemangiomatosis: multidetector row CT findings and clinico-pathologic correlation. J Thorac Imaging. 2005;20:613.
62. Silva CJ, Massie J, Mandelstam SA. Pulmonary capillary haemangiomatosis in a premature infant. Pediatr Radiol. 2005;35: 635–40.
63. Whittaker JS, Pickering CA, Heath D, Smith P. Pulmonary capillary haemangiomatosis. Diagn Histopathol. 1983;6:77–84.
64. Tron V, Magee F, Wright JL, Colby T, Churg A. Pulmonary capillary hemangiomatosis. Hum Pathol. 1986;17:1144–50.
65. Langleben D, Heneghan JM, Batten AP, Wang NS, Fitch N, Schlesinger RD, Guerraty A, Rouleau JL. Familial pulmonary capillary hemangiomatosis resulting in primary pulmonary hypertension. Ann Intern Med. 1988;109:106–9.
66. Moritani S, Ichihara S, Seki Y, Kataoka M, Yokoi T. Pulmonary capillary hemangiomatosis incidentally detected in a lobectomy specimen for a metastatic colon cancer. Pathol Int. 2006;56: 350–7.
67. Lippert JL, White CS, Cameron EW, Sun CC, Liang X, Rubin LJ. Pulmonary capillary hemangiomatosis: radiographic appearance. J Thorac Imaging. 1998;13:49–51.
68. Fernández-Alonso J, Zulueta T, Reyes-Ramirez JR, Castillo-Palma MJ, Sanchez-Román J. Pulmonary capillary hemangiomatosis as cause of pulmonary hypertension in a young woman with systemic lupus erythematosus. J Rheumatol. 1999;26:231–3.
69. Kakkar N, Vasishta RK, Banerjee AK, Singh S, Kumar L. Pulmonary capillary haemangiomatosis as a cause of pulmonary hypertension in Takayasu's aortoarteritis. Respiration. 1997;64:381–3.
70. Jing X, Yokoi T, Nakamura Y, Nakamura M, Shan L, Tomimoto S, Hano T, Kakudo K. Pulmonary capillary hemangiomatosis: a unique feature of congestive vasculopathy associated with hypertrophic cardiomyopathy. Arch Pathol Lab Med. 1998;122(1): 94–6.
71. al-Fawaz IM, al Mobaireek KF, al-Suhaibani M, Ashour M. Pulmonary capillary hemangiomatosis: a case report and review of the literature. Pediatr Pulmonol. 1995;19:243–8.
72. Ishii H, Iwabuchi K, Kameya T, Koshino H. Pulmonary capillary haemangiomatosis. Histopathology. 1996;29:275–8.
73. Faber CN, Yousem SA, Dauber JH, Griffith BP, Hardesty RL, Paradis IL. Pulmonary capillary hemangiomatosis. A report of three cases and a review of the literature. Am Rev Respir Dis. 1989;140:808–13.
74. Masur Y, Remberger K, Hoefer M. Pulmonary capillary hemangiomatosis as a rare cause of pulmonary hypertension. Pathol Res Pract. 1996;192:290–5.
75. Domingo C, Encabo B, Roig J, López D, Morera J. Pulmonary capillary hemangiomatosis: report of a case and review of the literature. Respiration. 1992;59:178–80.
76. Assaad AM, Kawut SM, Arcasoy SM, Rosenzweig EB, Wilt JS, Sonett JR, Borczuk AC. Platelet-derived growth factor is increased in pulmonary capillary hemangiomatosis. Chest. 2007;131: 850–5.
77. Wagenaar SS, Mulder JJ, Wagenvoort CA, van den Bosch JM. Pulmonary capillary haemangiomatosis diagnosed during life. Histopathology. 1989;14:212–4.

78. White CW, Sondheimer HM, Crouch EC, Wilson H, Fan LL. Treatment of pulmonary hemangiomatosis with recombinant interferon alfa-2a. N Engl J Med. 1989;320:1197–200.
79. White CW. Treatment of hemangiomatosis with recombinant interferon alfa. Semin Hematol. 1990;27:15–22.
80. Almagro P, Julià J, Sanjaume M, González G, Casalots J, Heredia JL, Martínez J, Garau J. Pulmonary capillary hemangiomatosis associated with primary pulmonary hypertension: report of 2 new cases and review of 35 cases from the literature. Medicine (Baltimore). 2002;81:417–24.
81. Dail DH, Liebow AA. Intravascular bronchioloalveolar tumor. Am J Pathol. 1975;78:6a(abstr).
82. Corrin B, Manners B, Millard M, et al. Histogenesis of the so-called "intravascular bronchioloalveolar tumour". J Pathol. 1979;128:163–7.
83. Weldon-Linne CM, Victor TA, Christ ML, et al. Angiogenic nature of the "intravascular bronchioloalveolar tumor" of the lung: an electron microscopic study. Arch Pathol Lab Med. 1981;105:174–9.
84. Weiss SW, Enzinger FM. Epithelioid hemangioendothelioma: a vascular tumor often mistaken for a carcinoma. Cancer. 1982;50:970–81.
85. Bhagavan BS, Dorfman HD, Murthy MS, et al. Intravascular bronchiolo-alveolar tumor (IVBAT): a low-grade sclerosing epithelioid angiosarcoma of lung. Am J Surg Pathol. 1982;6:41–52.
86. Weiss SW, Ishak KG, Dail DH, et al. Epithelioid hemangioendothelioma and related lesions. Semin Diagn Pathol. 1986;3:259–87.
87. Bagan P, Hassan M, Le Pimpec Barthes F, et al. Prognostic factors and surgical indications of pulmonary epithelioid hemangioendothelioma: a review of the literature. Ann Thorac Surg. 2006;82:2010–3.
88. Rock MJ, Kaufman RA, Lobe TE, et al. Epithelioid hemangioendothelioma of the lung (intravascular bronchioloalveolar tumor) in a young girl. Pediatr Pulmonol. 1991;11:181–6.
89. Kitaichi M, Nagai S, Nishimura K, et al. Pulmonary epithelioid haemangioendothelioma in 21 patients, including three with partial spontaneous regression. Eur Respir J. 1998;12:89–96.
90. Einsfelder B, Kuhnen C. Epithelioid hemangioendothelioma of the lung (IVBAT) – clinicopathological and immunohistochemical analysis of 11 cases. Pathologe. 2006;27:106–15.
91. Dail DH, Liebow AA, Gmelich JT, et al. Intravascular, bronchiolar, and alveolar tumor of the lung (IVBAT). An analysis of twenty cases of a peculiar sclerosing endothelial tumor. Cancer. 1983;51:452–64.
92. Miettinen M, Collan Y, Halttunen P, et al. Intravascular bronchioloalveolar tumor. Cancer. 1987;60:2471–5.
93. Bevelaqua FA, Valensi Q, Hulnick D. Epithelioid hemangioendothelioma. A rare tumor with variable prognosis presenting as a pleural effusion. Chest. 1988;93:665–6.
94. Carter EJ, Bradburne RM, Jhung JW, et al. Alveolar hemorrhage with epithelioid hemangioendothelioma. A previously unreported manifestation of a rare tumor. Am Rev Respir Dis. 1990;142:700–1.
95. Struhar D, Sorkin P, Greif J, et al. Alveolar haemorrhage with pleural effusion as a manifestation of epithelioid haemangioendothelioma. Eur Respir J. 1992;5:592–3.
96. Wick MR, Leslie KO, Cerilli LA, Mills SE. Sarcomas and sarcomatoid neoplasms of the lungs and pleural surfaces. In: Leslie KO, Wick MR, editors. Practical pulmonary pathology. A diagnostic approach. Philadelphia: Churchill Livingstone/Elsevier; 2005. p. 465–517.
97. Ledson MJ, Convery R, Carty A, et al. Epithelioid haemangioendothelioma. Thorax. 1999;54:560–1.
98. Enzinger FM, Weiss SW. Hemangioendothelioma: vascular tumors of intermediate malignancy. In: Weiss SW, Goldblum JR, editors. Soft tissue tumors. St. Louis: Mosby/Elsevier; 2008. p. 681–702.
99. Bollinger BK, Laskin WB, Knight CB. Epithelioid hemangioendothelioma with multiple site involvement. Literature review and observations. Cancer. 1994;73:610–5.
100. Makhlouf HR, Ishak KG, Goodman ZD. Epithelioid hemangioendothelioma of the liver: a clinicopathologic study of 137 cases. Cancer. 1999;85:562–82.
101. Miettinen M, Fetsch JF. Distribution of keratins in normal endothelial cells and a spectrum of vascular tumors: implications in tumor diagnosis. Hum Pathol. 2000;31:1062–7.
102. Boudousquie AC, Lawce HJ, Sherman R, et al. Complex translocation [7;22] identified in an epithelioid hemangioendothelioma. Cancer Genet Cytogenet. 1996;92:116–21.
103. Mendlick MR, Nelson M, Pickering D, et al. Translocation t(1;3)(p36.3;q25) is a nonrandom aberration in epithelioid hemangioendothelioma. Am J Surg Pathol. 2001;25:684–7.
104. Emery RW, Fox AL, Raab DE. Intravascular bronchioloalveolar tumour. Thorax. 1982;37:472–3.
105. Belmont L, Zemoura L, Couderc LJ. Pulmonary epithelioid haemangioendothelioma and bevacizumab. J Thorac Oncol. 2008;3:557–8.
106. Cronin P, Arenberg D. Pulmonary epithelioid hemangioendothelioma: an unusual case and a review of the literature. Chest. 2004;125:789–93.
107. Schattenberg T, Pfannschmidt J, Herpel E, et al. Bilateral surgical resection in pulmonary epitheloid hemangioendothelioma. Thorac Cardiovasc Surg. 2007;55:199–200.
108. Chen KT, Hoffman KD, Hendricks EJ. Angiosarcoma following therapeutic irradiation. Cancer. 1979;44:2044–8.
109. Maddox JC, Evans HL. Angiosarcoma of skin and soft tissue: a study of forty-four cases. Cancer. 1981;48:1907–21.
110. Thomas LB, Popper H. Pathology of angiosarcoma of the liver among vinyl chloride-polyvinyl chloride workers. Ann N Y Acad Sci. 1975;246:268–77.
111. Thomas LB, Popper H, Berk PD, et al. Vinyl-chloride-induced liver disease. From idiopathic portal hypertension (Banti's syndrome) to angiosarcomas. N Engl J Med. 1975;292:17–22.
112. Milby TH. Preventive medicine and public health-epitomes of progress: vinyl chloride-related cancer. West J Med. 1979;130:247–8.
113. Baxter PJ. The British hepatic angiosarcoma register. Environ Health Perspect. 1981;41:115–6.
114. Jennings TA, Peterson L, Axiotis CA, et al. Angiosarcoma associated with foreign body material. A report of three cases. Cancer. 1988;62:2436–44.
115. Enzinger FM, Weiss SW. Malignant vascular tumors. In: Weiss SW, Goldblum JR, editors. Soft tissue tumors. St. Louis: Mosby/Elsevier; 2008. p. 703–20.
116. Glancy DL, Morales Jr JB, Roberts WC. Angiosarcoma of the heart. Am J Cardiol. 1968;21:413–9.
117. Edwards RL, Chalk SM, McEvoy JD, et al. Pulmonary haemorrhage in disseminated cardiac haemangiosarcoma. Br J Dis Chest. 1977;71:127–31.
118. Ali MY, Lee GS. Sarcoma of the pulmonary artery. Cancer. 1964;17:1220–4.
119. Wackers FJ, van der Schoot JB, Hampe JF. Sarcoma of the pulmonary trunk associated with hemorrhagic tendency. A case report and review of the literature. Cancer. 1969;23:339–51.
120. Yousem SA. Angiosarcoma presenting in the lung. Arch Pathol Lab Med. 1986;110:112–5.
121. Segal SL, Lenchner GS, Cichelli AV, et al. Angiosarcoma presenting as diffuse alveolar hemorrhage. Chest. 1988;94:214–6.
122. Pandit SA, Fiedler PN, Westcott JL. Primary angiosarcoma of the lung. Ann Diagn Pathol. 2005;9:302–4.
123. Campione A, Forte G, Luzzi L, et al. Pulmonary angiosarcoma presenting as spontaneous recurrent hemothorax. Asian Cardiovasc Thorac Ann. 2009;17:84–5.

124. Spragg RG, Wolf PL, Haghighi P, et al. Angiosarcoma of the lung with fatal pulmonary hemorrhage. Am J Med. 1983;74:1072–6.
125. Primack SL, Hartman TE, Lee KS, et al. Pulmonary nodules and the CT halo sign. Radiology. 1994;190:513–5.
126. Kojima K, Okamoto I, Ushijima S, et al. Successful treatment of primary pulmonary angiosarcoma. Chest. 2003;124:2397–400.
127. Palvio DH, Paulsen SM, Henneberg EW. Primary angiosarcoma of the lung presenting as intractable hemoptysis. Thorac Cardiovasc Surg. 1987;35:105–7.
128. Ott RA, Eugene J, Kollin J, et al. Primary pulmonary angiosarcoma associated with multiple synchronous neoplasms. J Surg Oncol. 1987;35:269–76.
129. Davidson TI, Kissin MW, Bradish CF, et al. Angiosarcoma arising in a patient with Maffucci syndrome. Eur J Surg Oncol. 1985;11: 381–4.
130. Ploegmakers MJ, Pruszczynski M, De Rooy J, et al. Angiosarcoma with malignant peripheral nerve sheath tumour developing in a patient with Klippel-Trénaunay-Weber syndrome. Sarcoma. 2005;9:137–40.
131. Sheppard MN, Hansell DM, Du Bois RM, et al. Primary epithelioid angiosarcoma of the lung presenting as pulmonary hemorrhage. Hum Pathol. 1997;28:383–5.
132. Mukai K, Rosai J, Burgdorf WH. Localization of factor VIII-related antigen in vascular endothelial cells using an immunoperoxidase method. Am J Surg Pathol. 1980;4:273–6.
133. Burgdorf WH, Mukai K, Rosai J. Immunohistochemical identification of factor VIII-related antigen in endothelial cells of cutaneous lesions of alleged vascular nature. Am J Clin Pathol. 1981;75:167–71.
134. Sehested M, Hou-Jensen K. Factor VII related antigen as an endothelial cell marker in benign and malignant diseases. Virchows Arch A Pathol Anat Histol. 1981;391:217–25.
135. Guarda LA, Ordonez NG, Smith Jr JL, et al. Immunoperoxidase localization of factor VIII in angiosarcomas. Arch Pathol Lab Med. 1982;106:515–6.
136. DeYoung BR, Swanson PE, Argenyi ZB, et al. CD31 immunoreactivity in mesenchymal neoplasms of the skin and subcutis: report of 145 cases and review of putative immunohistologic markers of endothelial differentiation. J Cutan Pathol. 1995;22: 215–22.
137. Orchard GE, Zelger B, Jones EW, et al. An immunocytochemical assessment of 19 cases of cutaneous angiosarcoma. Histopathology. 1996;28:235–40.
138. Fletcher CD, Beham A, Bekir S, et al. Epithelioid angiosarcoma of deep soft tissue: a distinctive tumor readily mistaken for an epithelial neoplasm. Am J Surg Pathol. 1991;15:915–24.
139. Meis-Kindblom JM, Kindblom LG. Angiosarcoma of soft tissue: a study of 80 cases. Am J Surg Pathol. 1998;22:683–97.
140. Przygodzki RM, Finkelstein SD, Keohavong P, et al. Sporadic and thorotrast-induced angiosarcomas of the liver manifest frequent and multiple point mutations in K-ras-2. Lab Invest. 1997;76:153–9.
141. Marion MJ, Froment O, Trépo C. Activation of Ki-ras gene by point mutation in human liver angiosarcoma associated with vinyl chloride exposure. Mol Carcinog. 1991;4:450–4.
142. De Vivo I, Marion MJ, Smith SJ, et al. Mutant c-Ki-ras p21 protein in chemical carcinogenesis in humans exposed to vinyl chloride. Cancer Causes Control. 1994;5:273–8.
143. Tate G, Suzuki T, Mitsuya T. Mutation of the PTEN gene in a human hepatic angiosarcoma. Cancer Genet Cytogenet. 2007;178:160–2.
144. Zu Y, Perle MA, Yan Z, et al. Chromosomal abnormalities and p53 gene mutation in a cardiac angiosarcoma. Appl Immunohistochem Mol Morphol. 2001;9:24–8.
145. Zietz C, Rössle M, Haas C, et al. MDM-2 oncoprotein overexpression, p53 gene mutation, and VEGF up-regulation in angiosarcomas. Am J Pathol. 1998;153:1425–33.
146. Mandahl N, Jin YS, Heim S, et al. Trisomy 5 and loss of the Y chromosome as the sole cytogenetic anomalies in a cavernous hemangioma/angiosarcoma. Genes Chromosomes Cancer. 1990;1: 315–6.
147. Schuborg C, Mertens F, Rydholm A. Cytogenetic analysis of four angiosarcomas from deep and superficial soft tissue. Cancer Genet Cytogenet. 1998;100:52–6.
148. Patel AM, Ryu JH. Angiosarcoma in the lung. Chest. 1993;103: 1531–5.
149. Cox FH, Helwig EB. Kaposi's sarcoma. Cancer. 1959;12:289–98.
150. Dantzig PI, Richardson D, Rayhanzadeh S, et al. Thoracic involvement of non-African Kaposi's sarcoma. Chest. 1974;66:522–5.
151. Epstein DM, Gefter WB, Conard K, et al. Lung disease in homosexual men. Radiology. 1982;143:7–10.
152. Gruden JF, Huang L, Webb WR, et al. AIDS-related Kaposi sarcoma of the lung: radiographic findings and staging system with bronchoscopic correlation. Radiology. 1995;195:545–52.
153. Mitsuyasu RT, Groopman JE. Biology and therapy of Kaposi's sarcoma. Semin Oncol. 1984;11:53–9.
154. Meduri GU, Stover DE, Lee M, et al. Pulmonary Kaposi's sarcoma in the acquired immune deficiency syndrome. Clinical, radiographic, and pathologic manifestations. Am J Med. 1986;81: 11–8.
155. Ognibene FP, Steis RG, Macher AM, et al. Kaposi's sarcoma causing pulmonary infiltrates and respiratory failure in the acquired immunodeficiency syndrome. Ann Intern Med. 1985;102: 471–5.
156. Wallis JM, Hannah J. Pulmonary disease found at autopsy in patients with the acquired immunodefiencency syndrome (AIDS). Am Rev Respir Dis. 1985;131:A222.
157. Nesbitt S, Mark PF, Zimmerman HF. Dissemintated visceral idiopathic hemorrhagic sarcoma (Kaposi's disease): report of case with necropsy findings. Ann Intern Med. 1945;22:601–5.
158. Loring WE, Wolman SR. Idiopathic multiple hemorrhagic sarcoma of lung (Kaposi's sarcoma). N Y State J Med. 1965;65:668–76.
159. Mesmin F, Gomes H, Behar C, et al. Lymphoblastic leukaemia and Kaposi's sarcoma. Pediatr Radiol. 1979;8:185–7.
160. Misra DP, Sunderrajan EV, Hurst DJ, et al. Kaposi's sarcoma of the lung: radiography and pathology. Thorax. 1982;37:155–6.
161. Friedman-Kien AE, Laubenstein LJ, Rubinstein P, et al. Disseminated Kaposi's sarcoma in homosexual men. Ann Intern Med. 1982;96:693–700.
162. Kornfeld H, Axelrod JL. Pulmonary presentation of Kaposi's sarcoma in a homosexual patient. Am Rev Respir Dis. 1983;127:248–9.
163. Bach MC, Bagwell SP, Fanning JP. Primary pulmonary Kaposi's sarcoma in the acquired immunodeficiency syndrome: a cause of persistent pyrexia. Am J Med. 1988;85:274–5.
164. Roux FJ, Bancal C, Dombret MC, et al. Pulmonary Kaposi's sarcoma revealed by a solitary nodule in a patient with acquired immunodeficiency syndrome. Am J Respir Crit Care Med. 1994;149:1041–3.
165. Huang L, Schnapp LM, Gruden JF, et al. Presentation of AIDS-related pulmonary Kaposi's sarcoma diagnosed by bronchoscopy. Am J Respir Crit Care Med. 1996;153:1385–90.
166. Martinez S, McAdams HP, Youens KE. Kaposi sarcoma after bilateral lung transplantation. J Thorac Imaging. 2008;23:50–3.
167. Sadaghdar H, Eden E. Pulmonary Kaposi's sarcoma presenting as fulminant respiratory failure. Chest. 1991;100:858–60.
168. Stover DE, White DA, Romano PA, et al. Spectrum of pulmonary diseases associated with the acquired immune deficiency syndrome. Am J Med. 1985;78:429–37.
169. Davis SD, Henschke CI, Chamides BK, et al. Intrathoracic Kaposi sarcoma in AIDS patients: radiographic-pathologic correlation. Radiology. 1987;163:495–500.
170. Stats D. The visceral manifestations of Kaposi's sarcoma. J Mt Sinai Hosp N Y. 1946;12:971–83.

171. Zibrak JD, Silvestri RC, Costello P, et al. Bronchoscopic and radiologic features of Kaposi's sarcoma involving the respiratory system. Chest. 1986;90:476–9.
172. Chang Y, Cesarman E, Pessin MS, et al. Identification of herpesvirus-like DNA sequences in AIDS-associated Kaposi's sarcoma. Science. 1994;266:1865–9.
173. Tamm M, Reichenberger F, McGandy CE, et al. Diagnosis of pulmonary Kaposi's sarcoma by detection of human herpes virus 8 in bronchoalveolar lavage. Am J Respir Crit Care Med. 1998;157: 458–63.
174. Pitchenik AE, Fischl MA, Saldana MJ. Kaposi's sarcoma of the tracheobronchial tree. Clinical, bronchoscopic, and pathologic features. Chest. 1985;87:122–4.
175. Garay SM, Belenko M, Fazzini E, et al. Pulmonary manifestations of Kaposi's sarcoma. Chest. 1987;91:39–43.
176. Hanson PJ, Harcourt-Webster JN, Gazzard BG, et al. Fibreoptic bronchoscopy in diagnosis of bronchopulmonary Kaposi's sarcoma. Thorax. 1987;42:269–71.
177. Purdy LJ, Colby TV, Yousem SA, et al. Pulmonary Kaposi's sarcoma. Premortem histologic diagnosis. Am J Surg Pathol. 1986;10: 301–11.
178. Nadji M, Morales AR, Ziegles-Weissman J, et al. Kaposi's sarcoma: immunohistologic evidence for an endothelial origin. Arch Pathol Lab Med. 1981;105:274–5.
179. Weninger W, Partanen TA, Breiteneder-Geleff S, et al. Expression of vascular endothelial growth factor receptor-3 and podoplanin suggests a lymphatic endothelial cell origin of Kaposi's sarcoma tumor cells. Lab Invest. 1999;79:243–51.
180. Kahn HJ, Bailey D, Marks A. Monoclonal antibody D2-40, a new marker of lymphatic endothelium, reacts with Kaposi's sarcoma and a subset of angiosarcomas. Mod Pathol. 2002;15:434–40.
181. Patel RM, Goldblum JR, Hsi ED. Immunohistochemical detection of human herpes virus-8 latent nuclear antigen-1 is useful in the diagnosis of Kaposi sarcoma. Mod Pathol. 2004;17:456–60.
182. Cheuk W, Wong KOY, Wong CSC, et al. Immunostaining for human herpesvirus 8 latent nuclear antigen-1 helps distinguish Kaposi sarcoma from its mimickers. Am J Clin Pathol. 2004;121:335–42.
183. Hammock L, Reisenauer A, Wang W, et al. Latency-associated nuclear antigen expression and human herpesvirus-8 polymerase chain reaction in the evaluation of Kaposi sarcoma and other vascular tumors in HIV-positive patients. Mod Pathol. 2005;18: 463–8.
184. Fukunaga M. Expression of D2-40 in lymphatic endothelium of normal tissues and in vascular tumours. Histopathology. 2005;46:396–402.
185. Popescu NC, Zimonjic DB, Leventon-Kriss S, et al. Deletion and translocation involving chromosome 3 (p14) in two tumorigenic Kaposi's sarcoma cell lines. J Natl Cancer Inst. 1996;88:450–5.
186. Huang YQ, Li JJ, Moscatelli D, et al. Expression of int-2 oncogene in Kaposi's sarcoma lesions. J Clin Invest. 1993;91:1191–7.
187. Simonart T, Degraef C, Noel JC, et al. Overexpression of Bcl-2 in Kaposi's sarcoma-derived cells. J Invest Dermatol. 1998;111: 349–53.
188. Gill PS, Akil B, Colletti P, et al. Pulmonary Kaposi's sarcoma: clinical findings and results of therapy. Am J Med. 1989;87:57–61.
189. Stewart S, Jablonowski H, Goebel FD, et al. Randomized comparative trial of pegylated liposomal doxorubicin versus bleomycin and vincristine in the treatment of AIDS-related Kaposi's sarcoma. International Pegylated Liposomal Doxorubicin Study Group. J Clin Oncol. 1998;16:683–91.
190. International Collaboration on HIV and Cancer. Highly active antiretroviral therapy and incidence of cancer in human immunodeficiency virus-infected adults. J Natl Cancer Inst. 2000;92: 1823–30.
191. Wick MR. Kaposi's sarcoma unrelated to the acquired immunodeficiency syndrome. Curr Opin Oncol. 1991;3:377–82.
192. Cadranel J, Naccache J, Wislez M, et al. Pulmonary malignancies in the immunocompromised patient. Respiration. 1999;66:289–309.
193. Kaplan LD, Hopewell PC, Jaffe H, et al. Kaposi's sarcoma involving the lung in patients with the acquired immunodeficiency syndrome. J Acquir Immune Defic Syndr. 1988;1:23–30.

9 Mesenchymal Tumors of the Lungs

Introduction

Primary mesenchymal tumors of the lung are uncommon tumors that often resemble their counterparts in the soft tissue. Both benign and malignant tumors of mesenchymal origin may arise from the bronchopulmonary system. These may be of single lineage differentiation and show fibroblastic, muscle, cartilage and bone, adipose, myxoid, neurogenic, or neuroectodermal features or be composed of heterogenous cell types like hamartomas or malignant triton tumor. The incidence for these tumors is very low and based on the current literature it appears that primary pulmonary sarcomas account for less than 1 % of all primary lung tumors.

Tumors of Fibroblastic Origin

Primary lung tumors of fibroblastic origin encompass a group of heterogenous neoplasms that range from benign to malignant neoplasms. Included among this group of tumors are lesions, the histogenetic origins of which are still somewhat uncertain, like solitary fibrous tumor or synovial sarcoma.

Pulmonary Adenofibroma

Pulmonary adenofibromas are tumorous lesions histologically resembling the adenofibroma of the female genital tract. Only two well-documented cases have been described in the literature [1], although several other cases using a different terminology ("fibroadenoma" or "pulmonary hamartoma") histologically also appeared to represent this lesion [2, 3]. Pulmonary adenofibromas are tumors composed of a combination of glandular and spindle cell stromal elements. Since the lesions comprise two elements native to the lung, a hamartomatous origin was proposed in terms of histogenesis [1].

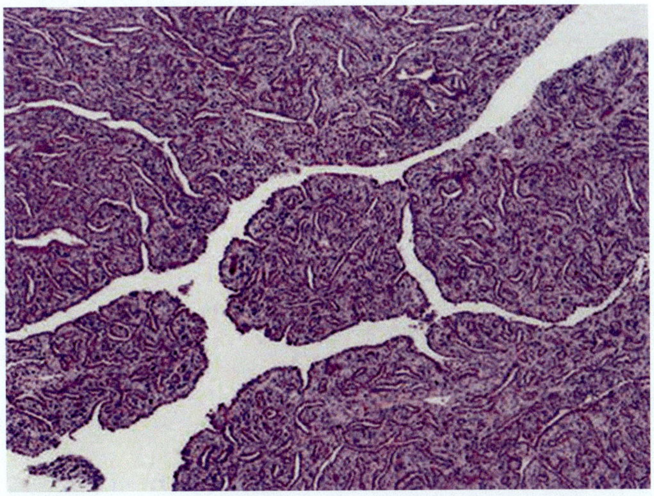

Fig. 9.1 Low-power view of pulmonary adenofibroma composed of glandular and spindle cell elements

Clinical Features

Pulmonary adenofibromas occur in an adult population and are usually incidental findings on routine chest X-ray as so-called coin lesions.

Gross Features

Grossly, adenofibromas are well-circumscribed lesions in the lung parenchyma measuring 1–2 cm in maximum dimension. The lesions are firm, rubbery intraparenchymal masses that display a homogenous tan-pink cut surface.

Histological Features

Histological examination shows complex branching spaces lined by a single layer of cuboidal to columnar epithelium (Figs. 9.1 and 9.2). These spaces are surrounded by a dense sclerotic stroma protruding into the epithelium-lined spaces as

A. Weissferdt, C.A. Moran, *Diagnostic Pathology of Pleuropulmonary Neoplasia*,
DOI 10.1007/978-1-4419-0787-5_9,

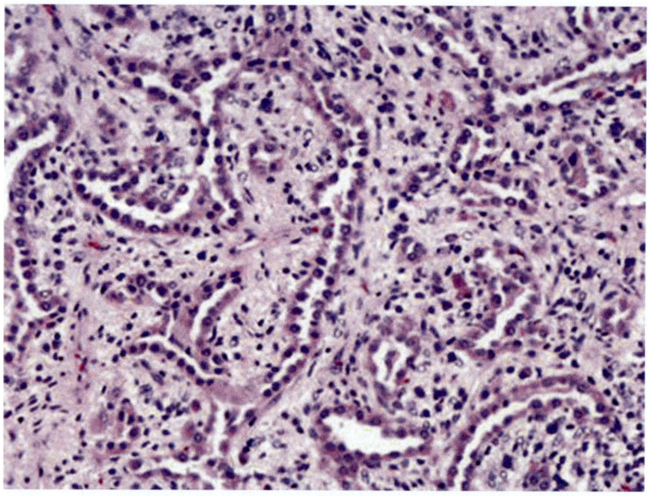

Fig. 9.2 The glands of pulmonary adenofibroma are lined by bland cuboidal- to columnar-shaped epithelial cells and are surrounded by scanty stromal spindle cells

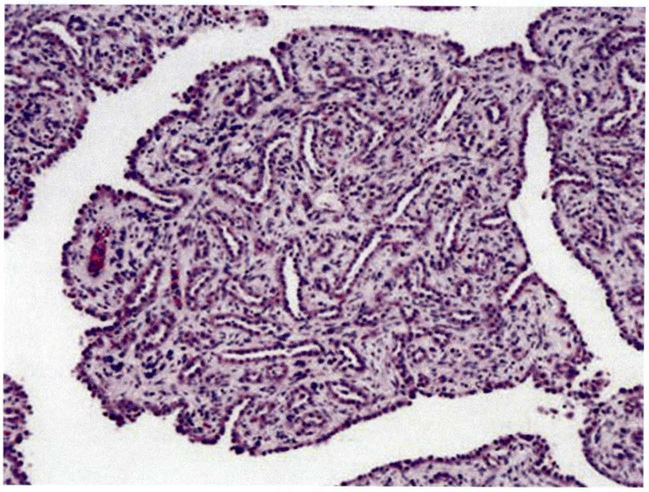

Fig. 9.3 Typical club-shaped papillary projections in pulmonary adenofibroma

club-shaped papillary projections (Fig. 9.3). The stroma is composed of a hypocellular proliferation of bland spindle-shaped cells. The spindle cells have elongated nuclei with tapered ends and no discernible cytoplasm. Mitotic activity or cytologic atypia is not seen in any component. On occasion, isolated gland-like structures or myxoid change can be identified. Overall, the histological features are reminiscent of the adenofibromas typically seen in the female genital tract.

Immunohistochemical Features

The lining epithelial cells in adenofibroma stain are positive for epithelial markers (keratin, EMA), while the spindled stromal cells are reactive with vimentin. The spindle cells are negative for SMA, desmin, S-100, and CD34.

Differential Diagnosis

Another tumor that is characterized by a bland spindle cell proliferation is intrapulmonary solitary fibrous tumor. This lesion may frequently entrap benign respiratory epithelium in the tumor periphery, hence mimicking the biphasic composition of pulmonary adenofibroma. However, adenofibroma shows a diffuse distribution of the epithelial-lined spaces that are not restricted to a certain area within the lesion. This and the fact that the spindle cells of solitary fibrous tumor display immunoreactivity for CD34 should help guide toward the correct diagnosis. In addition, metastatic sarcomas may enter the differential diagnosis. Histologically, these can be quite bland but should at least focally display some degree of cytologic atypia or mitotic activity. Furthermore, the clinical history should aid in arriving at the correct diagnosis.

Treatment and Prognosis

Surgical excision is the treatment of choice for pulmonary adenofibroma. The few cases described have been entirely benign; therefore, complete resection should be curative.

Intrapulmonary Solitary Fibrous Tumor

Solitary fibrous tumor was first described by Klemperer in 1931, describing a neoplasm arising from the pleura [4]. Since then, solitary fibrous tumors have been identified in numerous extrapleural sites including the meninges, orbit, peritoneum, liver, skin, and soft tissues, to name but a few [5]. Solitary fibrous tumors originating from the lung parenchyma with no obvious connection to the pleural surface are exceedingly rare with less than 15 cases reported in the English literature so far [6–13]. While the pleural tumors are thought to arise from the subpleural mesenchyma [4, 14, 15], two theories have been proposed as to the origin of intrapulmonary solitary fibrous tumors [6, 7]. First, the subpleural mesenchyme is in direct continuity with the connective tissue of the interlobular septa of the lung and the intrapulmonary tumors may arise from this septal mesenchyme. Second, fibroblastic elements in pulmonary parenchyma may give rise to the tumors. Regardless of their site of origin, intrapulmonary solitary fibrous tumors display very similar histological and immunohistochemical characteristics to their pleural counterparts. Another interesting observation is that, similarly to their counterparts in the soft tissue, cases of lung tumors previously diagnosed as "hemangiopericytoma" [16] probably belong to the same spectrum of tumors as solitary fibrous tumors, most likely representing a cellular variant of these lesions.

Clinical Features

Intrapulmonary solitary fibrous tumors affect mainly adults (age range 20–82 years) but have also been described in two children (7- and 8-year-old boys). Males appear to be slightly more commonly affected than females. Most tumors are incidental findings ("coin lesions") on chest X-ray during workup for non-related health issues; however, some patients presented with symptoms including cough, hemoptysis, chest pain, and arthralgia [11, 13].

Gross Features

The tumors range in size from 1.0 to 15.0 cm, with a mean size of 5.0 cm. They are well-defined, white, firm, elastic masses that on cut section have a bulging whorled appearance. Focal areas of hemorrhage may be identified, but necrosis is usually absent.

Histological Features

Microscopic examination reveals a hypo- or hypercellular proliferation of spindle cells arranged in various patterns (Figs. 9.4 and 9.5). In some areas, the cells are arranged in short interdigitating fascicles (Fig. 9.6), whereas in others they are arranged haphazardly, the so-called patternless pattern (Figs. 9.7 and 9.8). The individual-spindled tumor cells are bland with medium-sized and elongated nuclei with inconspicuous nucleoli (Fig. 9.9). The cellularity can vary from area to area and show closely apposed cells (Fig. 9.10) or separation of cells by coarse, wavy collagen bundles (Fig. 9.11). In hypocellular areas the collagen may appear hyalinized and have a whorled or cartwheel configuration. Other areas may have a more loose or myxoid stroma (Fig. 9.12). The vessels may consist of narrow cleft-like spaces or gaping vascular channels similar to those seen in hemangiopericytoma (Fig. 9.13). A feature unique to intrapulmonary solitary fibrous tumors is the presence of entrapped alveolar or bronchial epithelium in the periphery of the lesion. The presence of different growth patterns in solitary fibrous tumor is a good indicator as to the correct diagnosis. Malignant features as described for extrapulmonary solitary fibrous tumors—including high cellularity (Fig. 9.14), nuclear pleomorphism, necrosis, and increased mitotic activity (Fig. 9.15)—have not been described in the published cases of intrapulmonary solitary fibrous tumors. However, a large series of these cases has recently been collected from different medical centers expanding the morphological spectrum of these tumors (Publication In Press).

Immunohistochemical and Molecular Features

The immunohistochemical characteristics mirror those described for pleural solitary fibrous tumors. The spindle stains will be positive for CD34, bcl-2, and vimentin and negative for cytokeratin, S-100 protein, desmin, EMA, and TTF-1. In one of the reported cases, cytogenetic studies were performed to exclude a pulmonary hamartoma and found that high mobility group AT-hook-1 and −2 (HMGA-1 and −2) translocations, which are commonly found in pulmonary hamartoma, are absent in intrapulmonary solitary fibrous tumor [10].

Differential Diagnosis

Due to the multiple histological patterns that solitary fibrous tumor may show, the differential diagnosis can be quite extensive. Perhaps some of the most important consider-

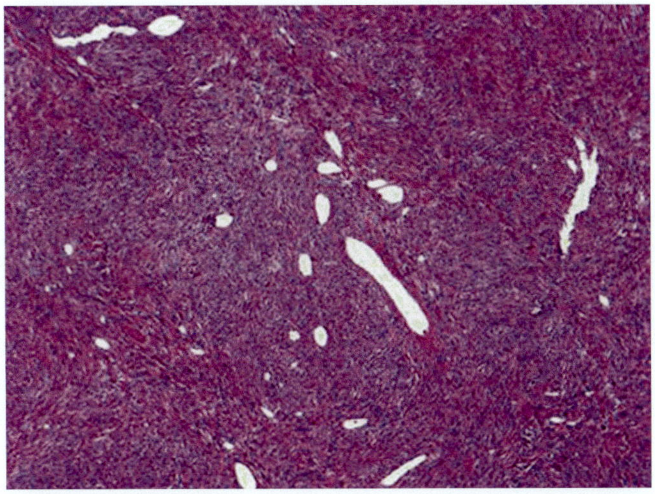

Fig. 9.4 Low magnification of hypercellular proliferation of intrapulmonary solitary fibrous tumor

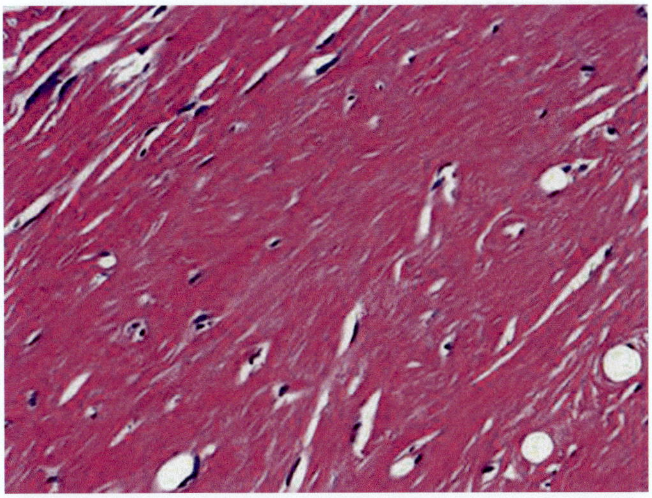

Fig. 9.5 Hypocellular sclerotic areas are typical findings in intrapulmonary solitary fibrous tumor

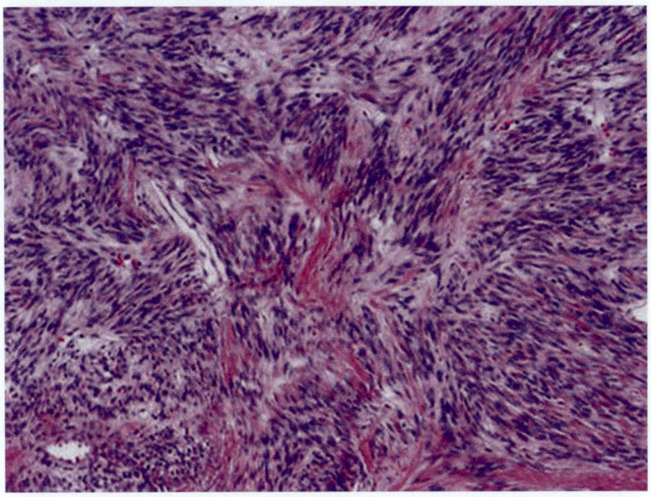

Fig. 9.6 Spindle cells in intrapulmonary solitary fibrous tumor arranged in short intersecting fascicles

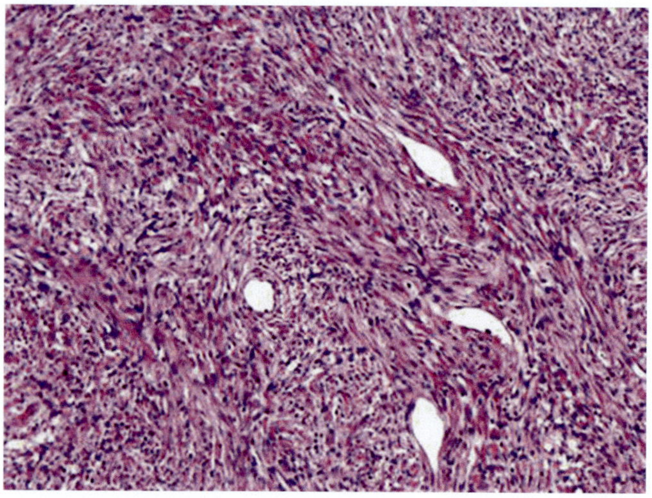

Fig. 9.7 Spindle cells in intrapulmonary solitary fibrous tumor arranged in a disorderly short storiform (so-called patternless) pattern

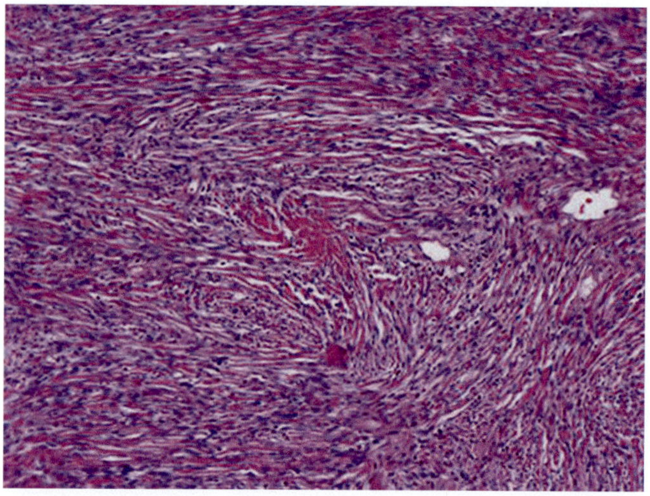

Fig. 9.8 Intrapulmonary solitary fibrous tumor composed of haphazardly arranged spindle cells

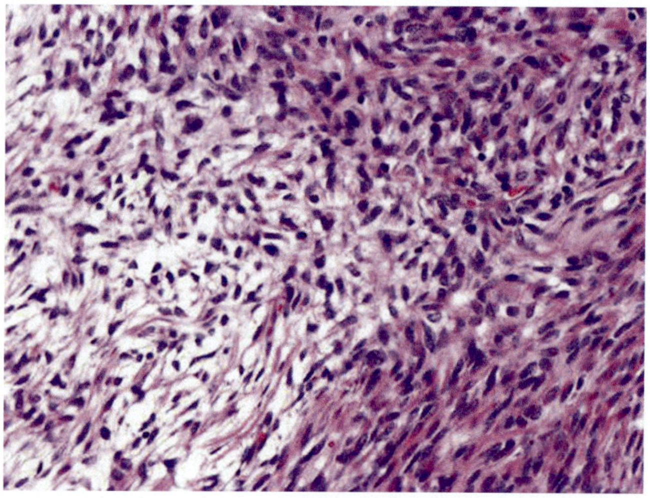

Fig. 9.9 Bland spindle cells in intrapulmonary solitary fibrous tumor showing no cytologic atypia or mitotic activity

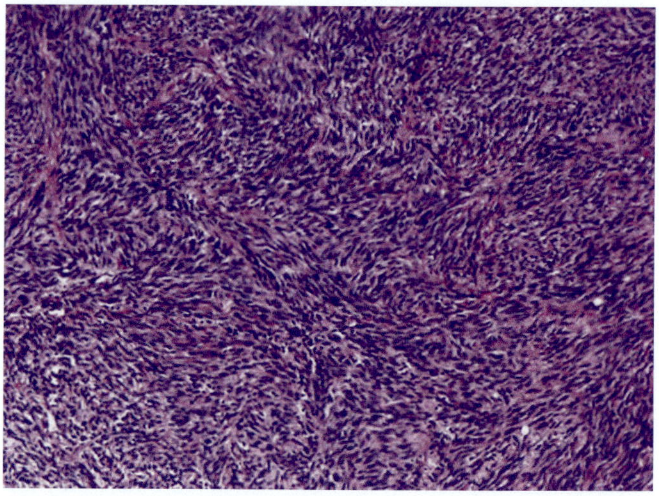

Fig. 9.10 Dense spindle cell proliferation in hypercellular area of intrapulmonary solitary fibrous tumor

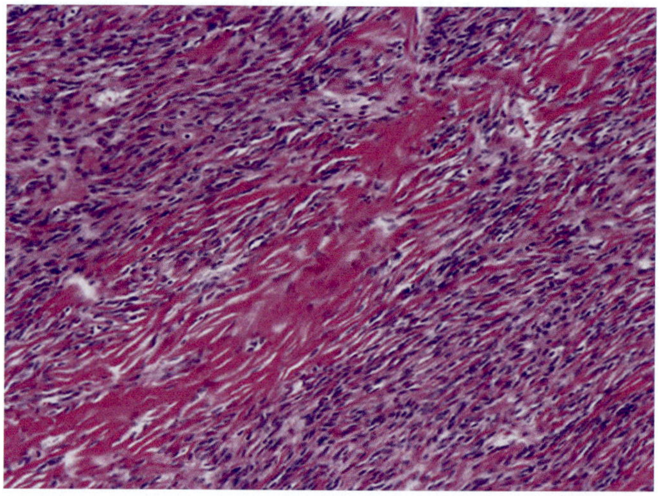

Fig. 9.11 Rope-like collagen separating the spindle cells of intrapulmonary solitary fibrous tumor

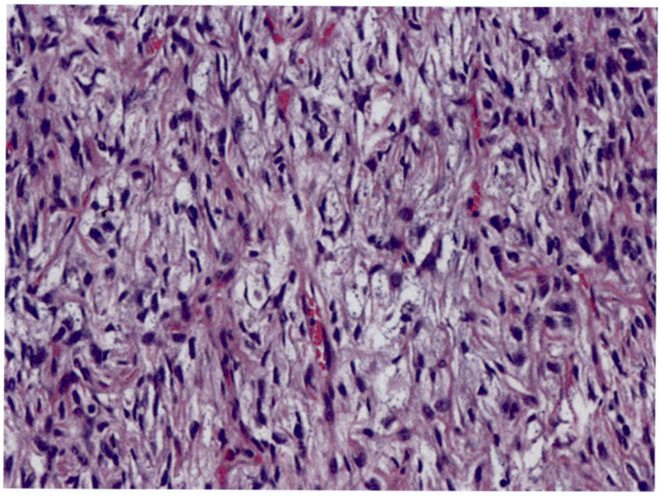

Fig. 9.12 Myxoid stroma in hypocellular area of intrapulmonary solitary fibrous tumor

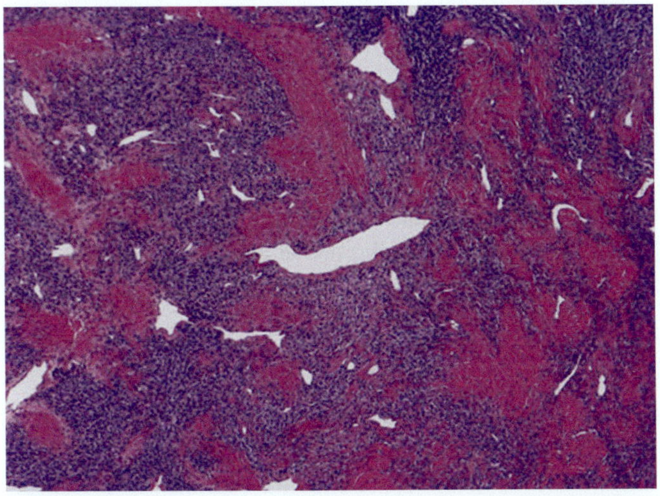

Fig. 9.13 Intrapulmonary solitary fibrous tumor with characteristic hemangiopericytoma-like pattern

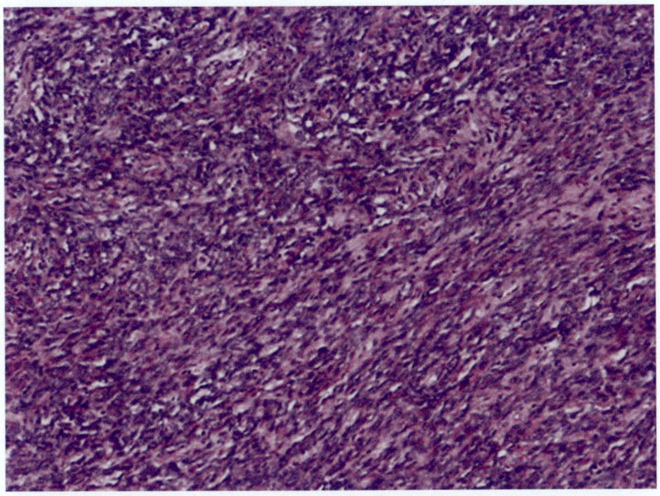

Fig. 9.14 High cellularity and increased cytologic atypia in a malignant intrapulmonary solitary fibrous tumor

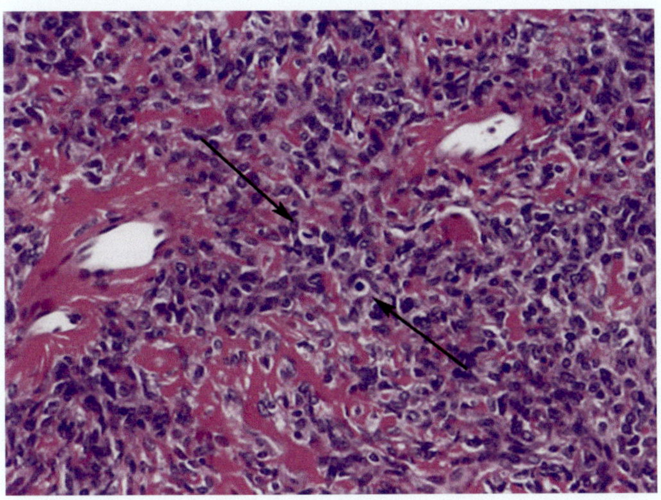

Fig. 9.15 Increased mitotic activity (*arrows*) in the malignant variant of intrapulmonary solitary fibrous tumor

ations would include monophasic synovial sarcoma and fibrosarcoma. Both of these tumors will show a prominent "herringbone" histological pattern, which can closely mimic some areas of solitary fibrous tumor. This issue may be even more compounded by the fact that monophasic synovial sarcoma may show positive staining for Bcl-2 just like solitary fibrous tumor does. However, monophasic synovial sarcoma may also show in addition focal positive staining for EMA and keratin. In cases in which such distinction may be difficult on morphological grounds, the use of molecular techniques, especially the demonstration of the typical SYT-SSX translocation will ultimately confirm the diagnosis of monophasic synovial sarcoma.

Treatment and Prognosis

Complete surgical resection has been the treatment of choice in the described cases of intrapulmonary solitary fibrous tumor. Although follow-up has been rather limited in most cases, the tumors appear to behave in a benign fashion with no reported recurrences or metastasis to date.

Pulmonary Fibrosarcoma

Fibrosarcomas are very rare primary lung tumors accounting for only 12 % of all primary lung sarcomas [17]. However, it is very likely that most of the cases reported in the past as fibrosarcomas may represent what is today known as monophasic synovial sarcoma. The diagnosis of these tumors is largely one of exclusion requiring differentiation from other spindle cell neoplasms often using immunohistochemical techniques [18]. Primary pulmonary fibrosarcoma is a tumor affecting all age groups. In children and adolescents, these tumors, especially when in an endobronchial location, appear to be low-grade malignancies with a favorable prognosis; these lesions have been referred to as the bronchopulmonary counterpart of the congenital–infantile fibrosarcoma of the soft tissues [19]. In adults, the tumor prognosis is more varied, depending on location, size, and mitotic activity [20].

Clinical Features

Pulmonary fibrosarcomas are neoplasms affecting the whole age range, from neonates to older adults with no specific gender predilection [19, 20]. Patients present complaining of cough, chest pain, or hemoptysis, especially those with endobronchial lesions. Peripherally located tumors are often asymptomatic and discovered incidentally during workup for unrelated conditions. On imaging, the tumors present as sharply defined and sometimes lobulated homogenous densities [20].

Gross Features

Endobronchial tumors are normally restricted to the bronchial wall with minimal involvement of the lung parenchyma.

These tumors are usually small in size ranging from 1 to 2.5 cm in greatest dimension. Peripheral lesions may exceed 20 cm in size. Regardless of location, the tumors are well circumscribed but not encapsulated and may have lobulated or nodular outlines. The cut surface is white to yellowish in color and firm to rubbery in consistency. Areas of hemorrhage or necrosis may be identified.

Histological Features

Pulmonary fibrosarcomas are highly cellular tumors composed of sheets and interlacing fascicles of spindle cells often arranged in a herringbone pattern. The individual tumor cells are oval or fusiform in shape and contain vesicular nuclei, granular chromatin, and inconspicuous nucleoli. The cytoplasm is scant and ill-defined with short cytoplasmic processes. Areas containing cells with a less spindled and more epithelioid appearance growing in patternless sheets may be identified in some tumors. The stromal component is usually minimal but may show hyalinization or calcification in some cases. The mitotic activity can range from 0 to 12 mitoses per 10 high-power fields (hpf) and is usually less in endobronchial tumors compared to parenchymal lesions. Foci of hemorrhage or necrosis may be identified occasionally.

Immunohistochemical Features

There is no specific immunohistochemical marker for pulmonary fibrosarcoma, and therefore, several immunohistochemical stains may have to be applied to rule out other spindle cell neoplasms of similar morphology. The cells of pulmonary fibrosarcoma show strong and diffuse cytoplasmic staining for vimentin. Markers that are typically negative in fibrosarcoma include cytokeratin, EMA, SMA, desmin, and S-100 protein, thereby excluding epithelial, muscle, or neural neoplasms [19, 21].

Differential Diagnosis

Pulmonary fibrosarcoma is often a diagnosis of exclusion after ruling out other spindle cell neoplasms that may arise in the lungs. These include leiomyosarcoma, monophasic synovial sarcoma, sarcomatoid carcinoma, and malignant peripheral nerve sheath tumor. The use of immunohistochemical stains in this context should lead to the correct diagnosis. Pulmonary fibrosarcomas will only stain for vimentin and be negative for muscle-related, epithelial, or neural markers. In cases where monophasic synovial sarcoma enters the differential diagnosis, immunocytochemical studies using cytokeratin, EMA, and bcl-2 may be used to identify this tumor; in equivocal cases, molecular studies to identify the typical translocation specific to synovial sarcoma may be applied.

Treatment and Prognosis

Complete surgical resection is the main treatment modality for pulmonary fibrosarcoma. The efficacy of adjuvant chemotherapy or irradiation is still questionable [19, 22]. The prognosis for these tumors has been associated with tumor size, mitotic count, and location (endobronchial tumors demonstrating better survival) [20]. Generally, pulmonary fibrosarcomas of childhood are associated with a better prognosis (5-year overall survival 84 %) than those affecting adults, and this is especially true for those pediatric tumors arising in an endobronchial location [19].

Pulmonary Synovial Sarcoma

Synovial sarcoma accounts for up to 10 % of soft tissue sarcomas with the most common sites of origin being the thigh, knee, ankle, foot, and upper extremity. Primary synovial sarcoma of the lung was first described in 1995 in a series of 25 cases from the Armed Forces Institute of Pathology (AFIP) [23]. The advent of modern immunohistochemical and cytogenetic techniques has increased the recognition of synovial sarcoma as a distinct subtype of sarcoma in the lung, and this tumor has since also been described in various other thoracic locations including the chest wall, pleura, and mediastinum [24–28]. Although pulmonary synovial sarcomas resemble their soft tissue counterparts in many ways, the tumors in the lung seem to affect a slightly older patient population and appear to have a more aggressive clinical course than those tumors arising in the soft tissues.

Clinical Features

Pulmonary synovial sarcoma presents primarily in young or middle-aged patients with a peak in the fourth and fifth decade of life and an age range from 12 to 77 years [23, 29]. The tumors affect men and women equally with no specific sex predilection. Clinically, patients most often present with cough, chest pain, shortness of breath, or hemoptysis, and in a subset of cases, the tumors are incidental findings. Less frequent forms of presentation are pneumothorax [30], fever, or weight loss [31]. One reported case is associated with a history of radiation therapy to the chest [32]. On computed tomography (CT) scanning, the tumors are typically well-defined heterogenous masses with no calcifications and no associated lymphadenopathy [33].

Gross Features

On gross examination, the tumors are well circumscribed but unencapsulated tumors of white or gray color and soft to rubbery or fleshy consistency. The tumors may measure less than 1 cm or more than 20 cm in maximum dimension with a mean size of 4–5 cm. Most primary pulmonary synovial sarcomas are solitary lesions in the lung parenchyma, although rarely, central tumors with an endobronchial polypoid appearance may be identified [34, 35]. Hemorrhage, necrosis, and cystic change can be seen in the majority of cases.

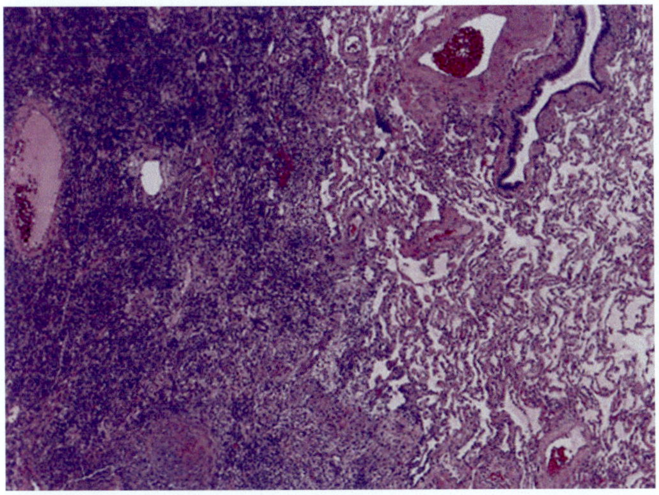

Fig. 9.16 Demarcation of monophasic synovial sarcoma from surrounding lung parenchyma

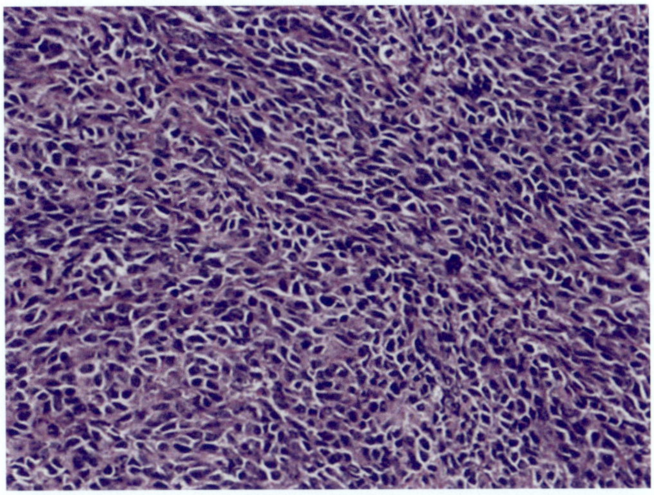

Fig. 9.17 Highly cellular proliferation of spindle cells in pulmonary monophasic synovial sarcoma

Histological Features

Generally, synovial sarcomas can be subtyped into the monophasic and biphasic variant. In the lungs, however, the vast majority of synovial sarcomas are monophasic neoplasms with only isolated cases of the biphasic variant reported [36]. On low magnification, the tumors impress as circumscribed tumors with pushing borders (Fig. 9.16). Higher power reveals a highly cellular proliferation of spindle cells composed of relatively uniform plump spindle cells with scanty cytoplasm and elongated oval nuclei. Cell borders are typically indistinct. The cells are often arranged in interlacing fascicles with densely packed tumor cells and little intervening stroma (Figs. 9.17, 9.18, and 9.19). Myxoid degeneration, cystic change, osteoid/cartilaginous metaplasia, Verocay-like bodies, rosette-like structures, rhabdoid cytoplasmic inclusions, and papillary, tigroid, or adenomatoid areas have all been described (Figs. 9.20, 9.21, 9.22, 9.23, and 9.24) [23, 27, 37, 38]. The mitotic activity varies and may range from less than 2 to more than 20 mitoses per 10 high-power fields (Fig. 9.25) [23]. Necrosis, hemorrhage, and a prominent hemangiopericytoma-like vasculature are common findings (Figs. 9.26 and 9.27). Infiltration by mast cells is another typical finding in these tumors (Fig. 9.28). Some cases may demonstrate areas of cells with a more round cell epithelioid appearance with a greater degree of nuclear pleomorphism and high mitotic rate qualifying for classification of poorly differentiated synovial sarcoma [27].

Immunohistochemical and Molecular Features

Pulmonary synovial sarcomas display an identical immunohistochemical phenotype to their soft tissue counterparts. The most characteristic finding is the positivity of tumor cells for epithelial markers including cytokeratin, EMA, and Cam5.2. Other markers typically expressed by these tumors include bcl-2, CD99, and vimentin, while SMA, desmin, and CD34 are negative. Staining for S-100 protein may show variable results. Synovial sarcomas are characterized cytogenetically by a specific chromosomal translocation t(X;18) and the consequent fusion genes SYT-SSX1 or SYT-SSX2 present in about 90 % of cases [39], and the same is true for primary pulmonary synovial sarcomas [24, 25, 27, 31].

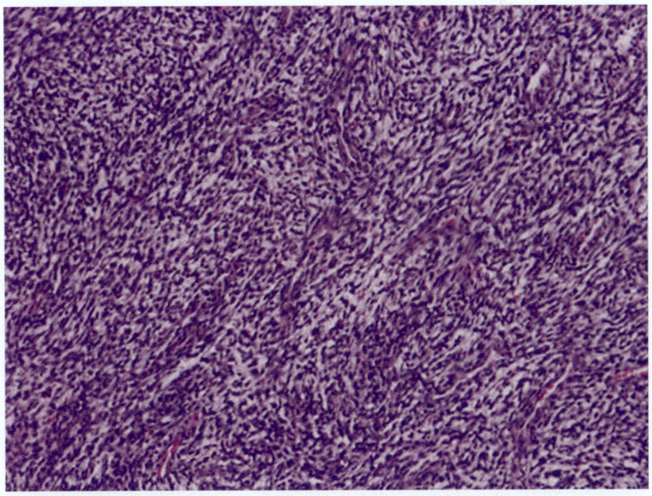

Fig. 9.18 Monophasic synovial sarcoma composed of a uniform spindle cell proliferation

Differential Diagnosis

The differential diagnosis for pulmonary synovial sarcoma is broad and includes primary and metastatic spindle cell tumors. The most important distinction is whether the tumor is primary or a metastatic deposit from a soft tissue primary as the latter tumors have a tendency to spread to the lungs. In this instance, solitary tumors and a negative clinical history as to a soft tissue neoplasm speak in favor

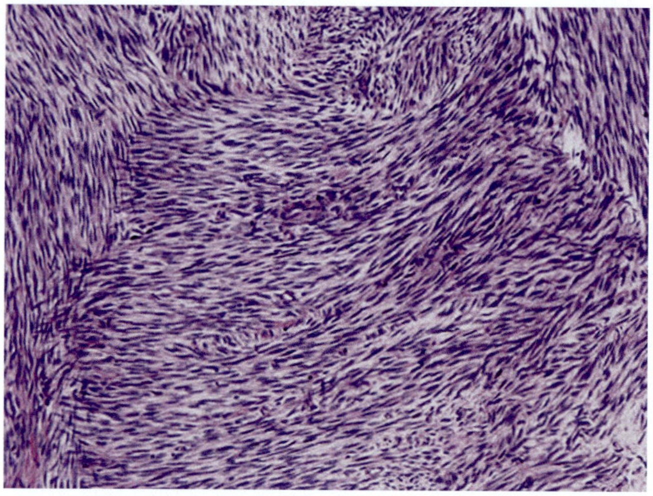

Fig. 9.19 Interlacing fascicles of tumor cells in monophasic synovial sarcoma of the lung

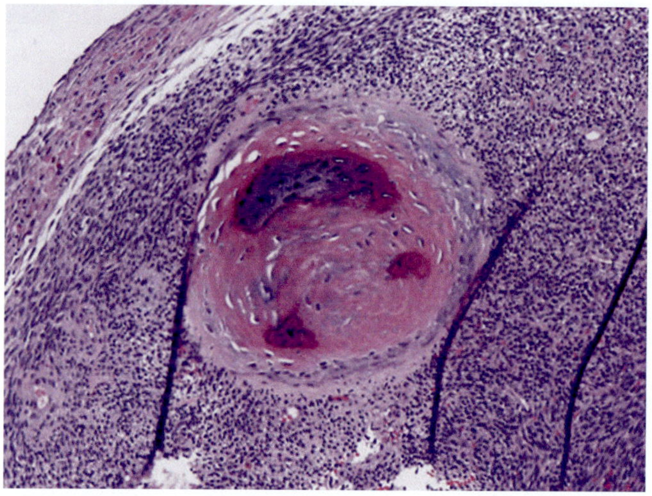

Fig. 9.20 Osseous metaplasia in monophasic synovial sarcoma of the lung

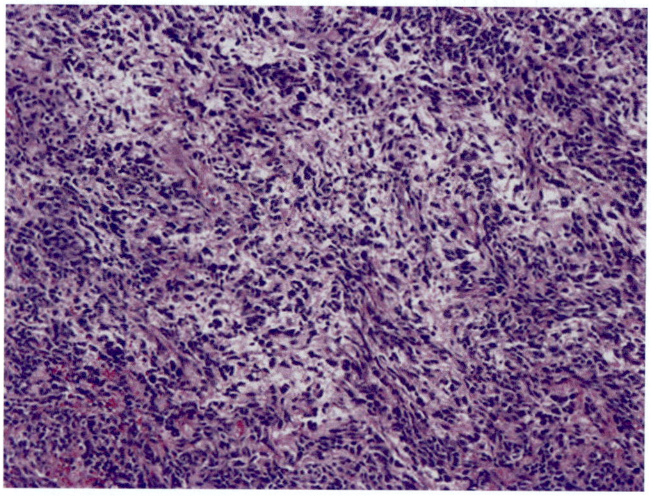

Fig. 9.21 Pulmonary monophasic synovial sarcoma with myxoid stromal changes

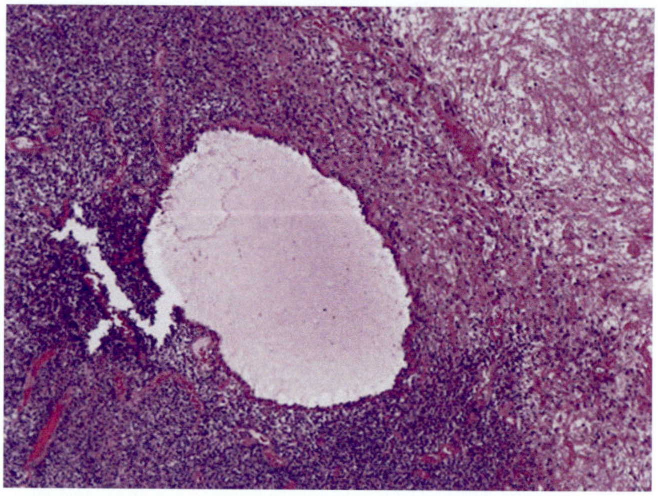

Fig. 9.22 Cystic change in monophasic synovial sarcoma of the lung

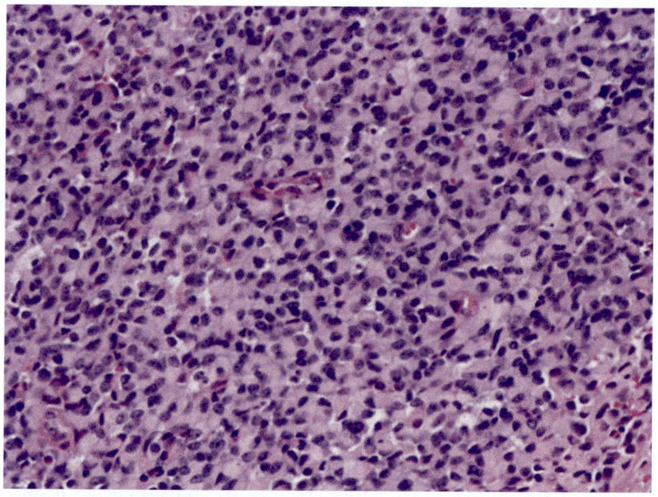

Fig. 9.23 Prominent rhabdoid cytoplasmic inclusions in monophasic synovial sarcoma of the lung

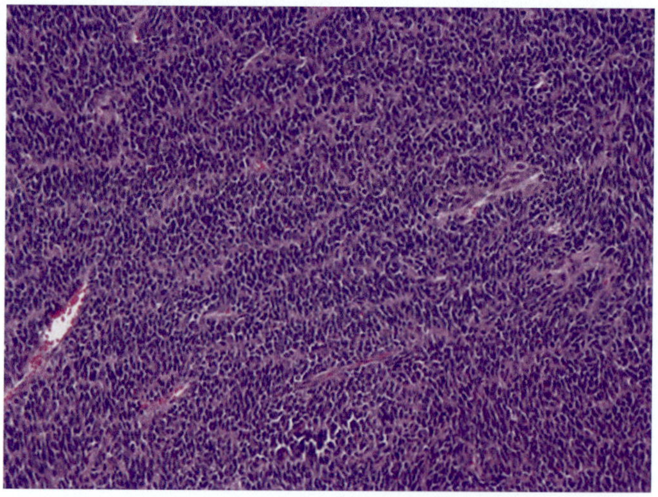

Fig. 9.24 So-called tigroid pattern in pulmonary monophasic synovial sarcoma

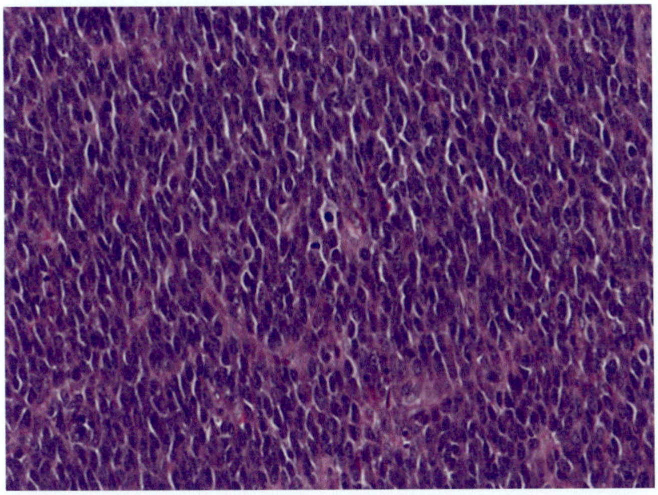

Fig. 9.25 Mitotic activity in monophasic synovial sarcoma of the lung

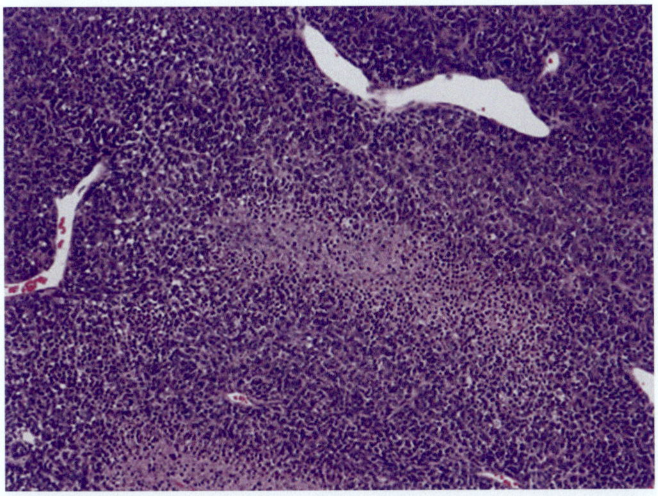

Fig. 9.26 Areas of necrosis are not an uncommon finding in pulmonary synovial sarcoma

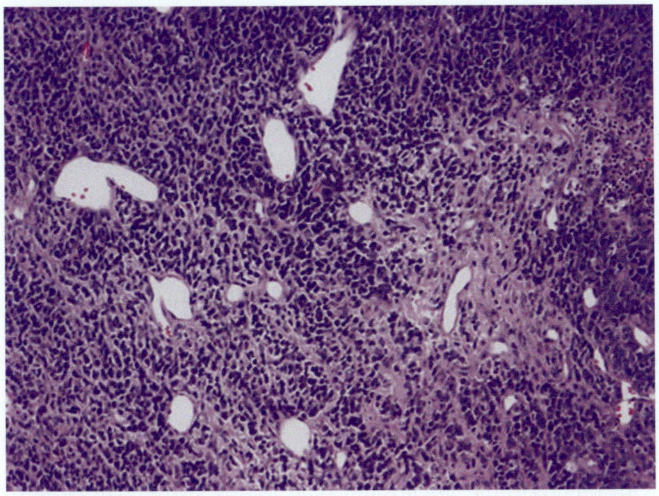

Fig. 9.27 Hemangiopericytoma-like vasculature in monophasic synovial sarcoma of the lung

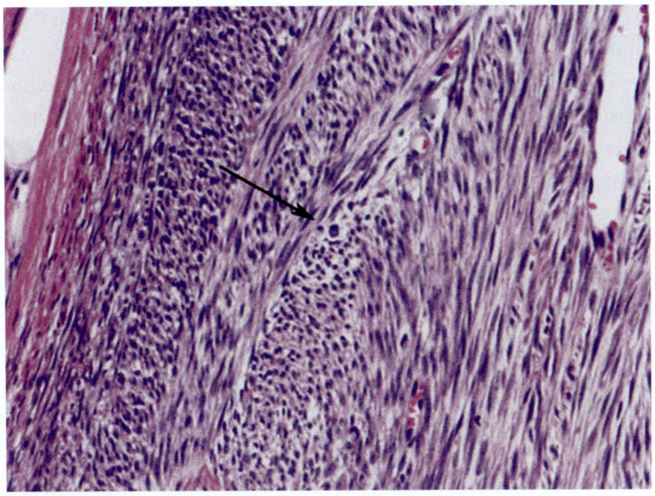

Fig. 9.28 Scattered mast cells (*arrow*) are typical for pulmonary monophasic synovial sarcoma

of a primary lung tumor. The tumors should also be differentiated from the more common spindle cell tumors of the lung like leiomyosarcoma, fibrosarcoma, hemangiopericytoma, solitary fibrous tumor, and spindle cell carcinoma. Application of immunohistochemical stains is of value in this setting. Leiomyosarcomas will show diffuse positivity for muscle markers including SMA and desmin, stains that will be negative in synovial sarcomas. Fibrosarcomas will not display epithelial differentiation contrary to synovial sarcoma. Cellular areas in hemangiopericytoma and solitary fibrous tumor may closely resemble synovial sarcoma histologically; however, these tumors express CD34 and typically do not show a positive reaction with epithelial markers. Lastly, sarcomatoid carcinoma shows spindle cell morphology. Immunohistochemically, both sarcomatoid carcinoma and synovial sarcoma are reactive with epithelial markers. Sarcomatoid carcinoma, however, typically affects an older age group, shows prominent cytologic atypia, and often shows transition with squamous or adenocarcinoma, thereby allowing differentiation from synovial sarcoma. Importantly, cytogenetic studies for the typical t(X;18) translocation specific for synovial sarcoma can be performed in any equivocal cases.

Treatment and Prognosis

Multimodality treatment including complete surgical resection, chemotherapy, and radiation therapy is the treatment of choice for pulmonary synovial sarcoma [40, 41] with the main determinant for prognosis being the completeness of surgical resection. Pulmonary synovial sarcomas appear to run a more aggressive clinical course than those tumors arising in the soft tissue, a feature attributed to the large size and difficulty to achieve complete resection of the pulmonary lesions [24]. The recurrence rate is generally high (up to 75 %), and 39.4 % of cases are known to produce distant metastasis [24, 25]. The 5-year survival rate ranges from

31.6 % to around 50 % [25, 27]. Some authors have suggested that the type of fusion gene is important in terms of prognosis, reporting that SYT-SSX1 lesions behave more aggressively than SYT-SSX2 tumors in synovial sarcomas of the soft tissues [42–44]. This difference could not be demonstrated in a study of 40 primary intrathoracic synovial sarcomas [25].

Pulmonary Malignant Fibrous Histiocytoma

Malignant fibrous histiocytoma is one of the most common soft tissue sarcomas of adulthood but is exceedingly uncommon as a primary lung tumor. Among all primary lung cancers, the incidence for malignant fibrous histiocytoma is only 0.04 % [45]. Fewer than 100 cases have been reported on review of the English and Japanese literature [46] since the first three cases were published almost simultaneously in 1979 [47, 48]. Histologically, these tumors are characterized by an admixture of malignant fibroblasts, myofibroblasts, and histiocytes, which are probably derived from primitive multipotent mesenchymal cells [49].

Clinical Features

Malignant fibrous histiocytoma appears to affect men and women equally, with a peak in the sixth decade of life and an age range from 12 to 80 years [50, 51]. Single case reports have also described this tumor in the pediatric population [52–54]. The main presenting symptoms include cough, shortness of breath, chest pain, hemoptysis, or weight loss, although patients may also be entirely asymptomatic and their tumors are incidental findings on a routine chest X-ray. Radiographically, primary malignant fibrous histiocytoma tends to be large solitary non-cavitating lesions situated mostly in the lung periphery [50].

Macroscopic Features

The tumors are large and can measure from 1 cm to more than 14 cm in size [51]. The majority of tumors appear to arise in the lung periphery, but smaller numbers of cases can also be identified in an endobronchial location [51]. There is a slight preponderance for the tumors to occur in the middle and lower lobes [50]. Grossly, the tumors are well circumscribed, but unencapsulated masses on cut section have a tan fleshy or rubbery appearance. Areas of hemorrhage or necrosis can be identified.

Histological Features

Malignant fibrous histiocytoma of the lung have similar histological features to their soft tissue counterparts and can be classified into the corresponding subtypes [51]. The majority of cases arising in the lung are of the storiform-pleomorphic type, which is characterized by cytologically malignant slender spindle cells arranged in short intersecting fascicles or swirls around blood vessels resulting in a cartwheel or storiform pattern (Figs. 9.29 and 9.30). Admixed with these are larger, more pleomorphic spindle cells with irregular vesicular nuclei and prominent nucleoli as well as tumor giant cells showing multinucleation (Figs. 9.31 and 9.32). In some areas, a more fascicular arrangement of slim spindle cells arranged in parallel bands can be seen. The neoplastic cells are separated by a variable amount of fibrous stroma, which may contain a scattered mononuclear inflammatory infiltrate. In some cases, a prominent myxoid matrix can predominate containing stellate pleomorphic cells with deeply eosinophilic cytoplasm or signet-ring cell appearance (myxoid variant) (Figs. 9.33 and 9.34). The inflammatory variant is composed of sheets of histiocytic and xanthomatous cells with pleomorphic nuclei and pale foamy cytoplasm (Reed-Sternberg-like cells) and a prominent inflammatory cell

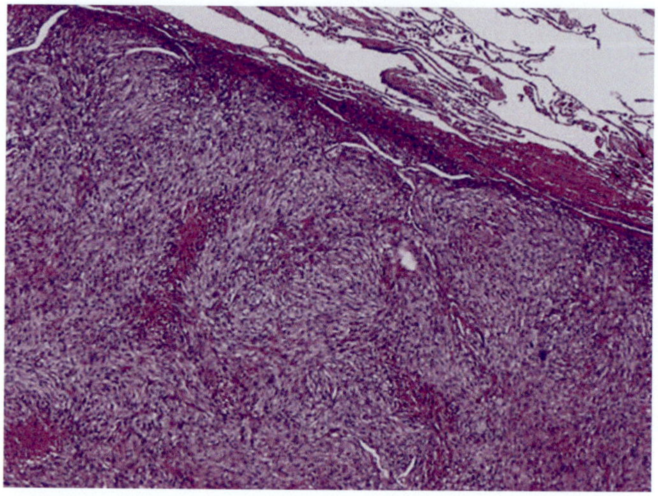

Fig. 9.29 Malignant fibrous histiocytoma arising from the lung parenchyma

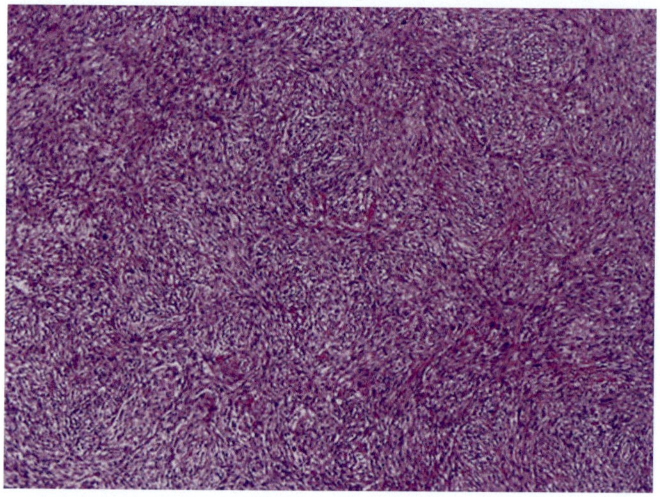

Fig. 9.30 Storiform pattern of pulmonary malignant fibrous histiocytoma

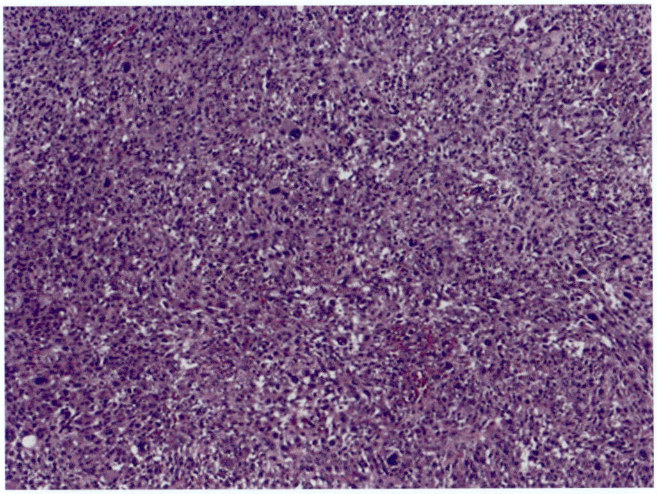

Fig. 9.31 Malignant fibrous histiocytoma of lung showing an admixture of malignant spindle cells and pleomorphic giant cells

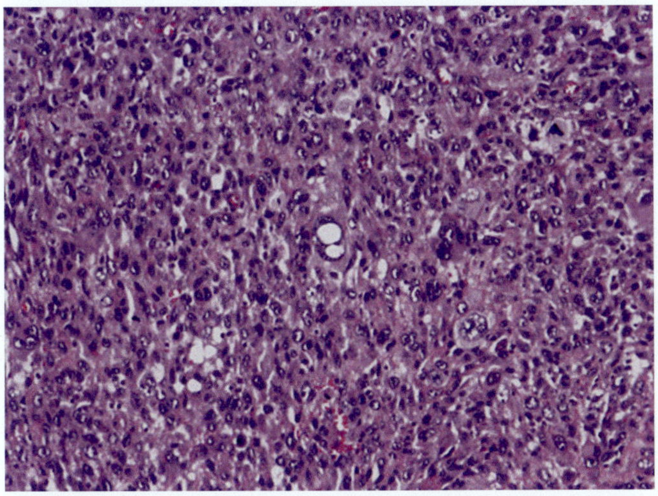

Fig. 9.32 Multinucleated tumor giant cells in malignant fibrous histiocytoma of the lung

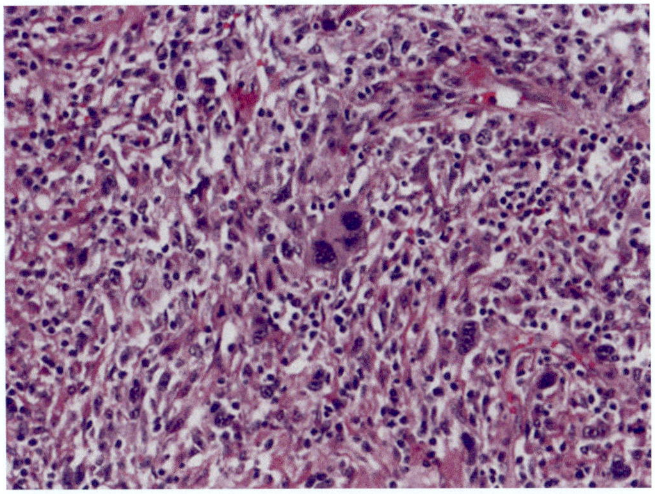

Fig. 9.33 High-power view of malignant fibrous histiocytoma showing numerous pleomorphic tumor cells

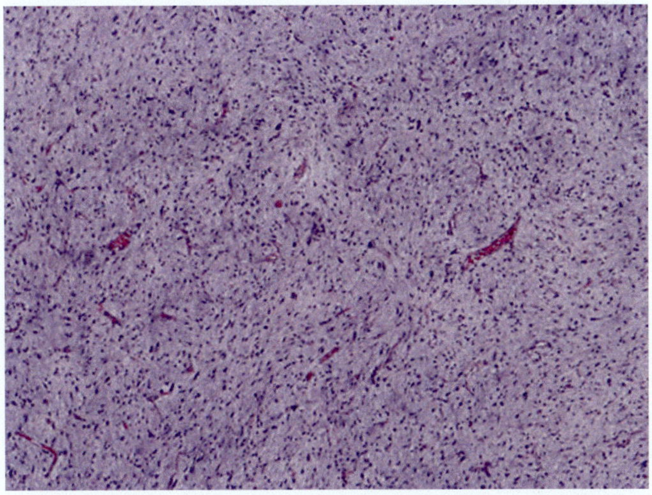

Fig. 9.34 Myxoid variant of malignant fibrous histiocytoma of the lung showing a prominent myxoid stromal background

infiltrate composed of large numbers of neutrophils, eosinophils, and lymphyocytes. Very rarely, the giant cell variant of malignant fibrous histiocytoma may be diagnosed in the lung. This type is characterized by a large number of osteoclast-like giant cells among a diffuse proliferation of malignant histiocyte-like cells (Fig. 9.35) [45]. Areas of coagulative tumor necrosis and hemorrhage are frequently seen in these tumors, and the mitotic activity is high and may exceed >20 mitoses per hpf (Figs. 9.36, 9.37, 9.38, and 9.39). Vascular invasion is another very common finding being present in up to 50 % of cases (Fig. 9.40) [51].

Immunohistochemical Features

No specific immunohistochemical marker exists to diagnose malignant fibrous histiocytoma, but histiocytic stains like CD68, factor XIII, α(alpha)-1-antitrypsin, and α(alpha)-1-antichymotrypsin as well as vimentin are generally positive in the tumor cells. Markers to detect more specific differentiation like cytokeratins, smooth muscle actin, desmin, myoglobin, and S-100 protein are generally negative.

Differential Diagnosis

The differential diagnosis for pulmonary malignant fibrous histiocytoma includes a range of other spindle cell proliferations. First and foremost, metastatic disease from a soft tissue primary has to be excluded based on clinical history and radiological investigations as malignant fibrous histiocytoma of the soft tissue has a high propensity to metastasize to the lungs. Other primary spindle cell lesions of the lung that have similar morphologic features include benign fibrohistiocytic proliferations as well as inflammatory

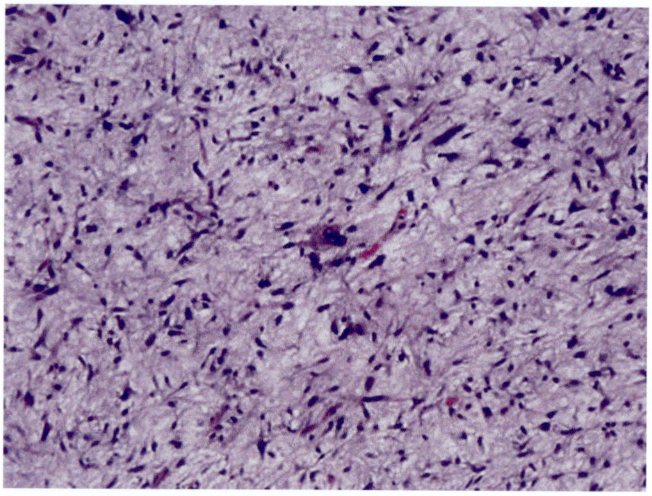

Fig. 9.35 Myxoid malignant fibrous histiocytoma of the lung containing pleomorphic stellate-shaped tumor cells

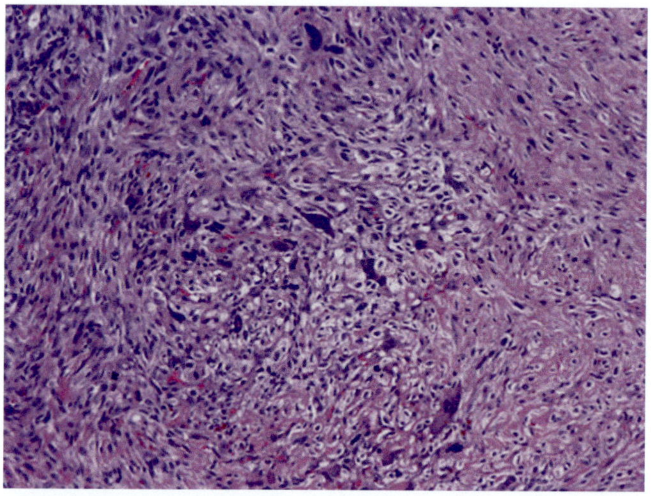

Fig. 9.36 Scattered osteoclast-like giant cells in the giant cell type of malignant fibrous histiocytoma of the lung

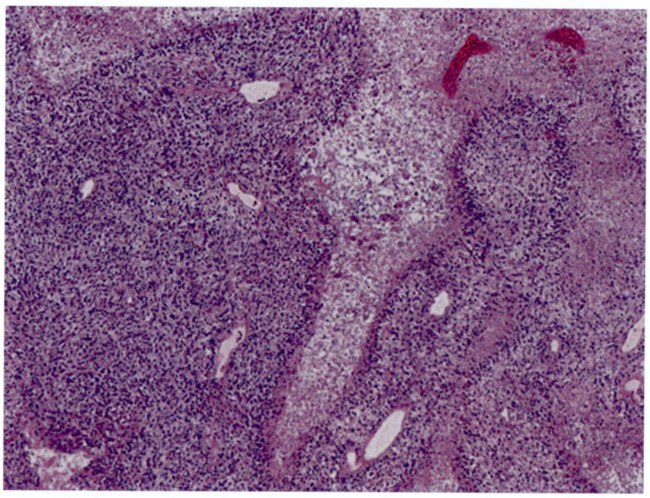

Fig. 9.37 Coagulative necrosis in malignant fibrous histiocytoma of the lung

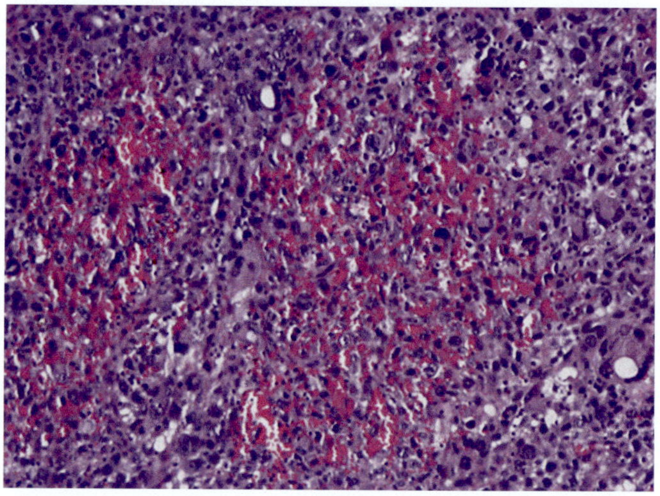

Fig. 9.38 Areas of hemorrhage may be identified in pulmonary malignant fibrous histiocytoma

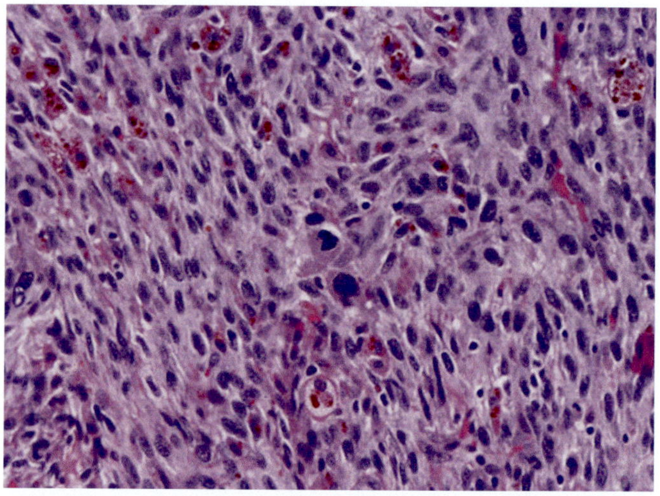

Fig. 9.39 High-power view of malignant fibrous histiocytoma of the lung showing increased mitotic activity

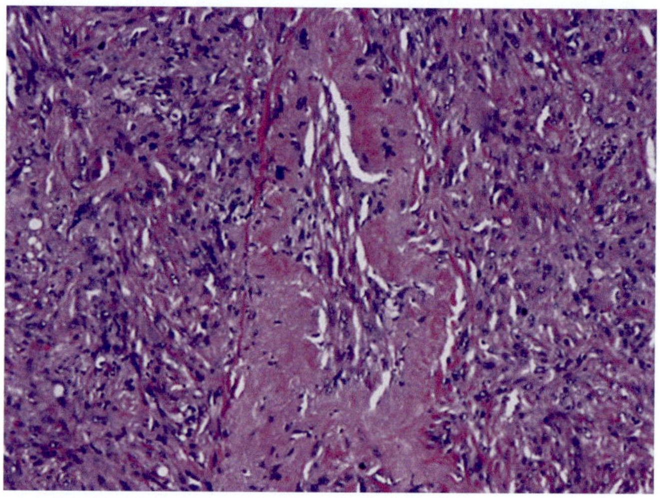

Fig. 9.40 Malignant fibrous histiocytoma of the lung with vascular invasion

pseudotumor or pleomorphic carcinoma. The presence of nuclear pleomorphism and increased mitotic activity will favor malignant fibrous histiocytoma from other fibrohistiocytic lesions. Pleomorphic carcinoma is a malignant epithelial tumor composed of a mix of spindle cells and giant cells. The use of immunohistochemical markers to detect epithelial differentiation in these tumors as well as residual areas of conventional non-small cell carcinoma should allow correct diagnosis.

Treatment and Prognosis

Complete surgical resection with lymph node dissection is the treatment of choice for these tumors [46]. Although no consistent data are available on the effectiveness of chemotherapy or irradiation in patients with malignant fibrous histiocytoma, adjuvant treatment may be considered for some patients [55]. The prognosis is generally poor, with a 5-year survival rate of 43 % in resected patients [46] and frequent metastasis to lymph nodes and distant sites [46, 50].

Tumors of Muscle Origin

Primary pulmonary tumors with muscle differentiation can be either of smooth muscle differentiation (leiomyoma and leiomyosarcoma) or skeletal muscle differentiation (rhabdomyosarcoma). Interestingly and contrary to their soft tissue counterparts, leiomyosarcomas by far outnumber benign smooth muscle tumors when arising in the lung.

Pulmonary Leiomyoma

Leiomyoma is a benign tumor of smooth muscle origin. These tumors are thought to represent less than 2 % of the benign tumors involving the lower respiratory tract [56]. Approximately 70 cases have been described in the literature; however, a number of these cases were described in patients who had a prior history of primary uterine or soft tissue smooth muscle neoplasm, raising the suspicion that these cases represented metastatic disease to the lungs rather than being primary lung neoplasms (so-called benign metastasizing leiomyoma) [56, 57]. The true incidence of primary pulmonary leiomyoma is thus likely to be lower. Primary leiomyomas may arise anywhere in the lower respiratory tract. Tumors involving the trachea or bronchus often grow in an endobronchial fashion, whereas parenchymal lesions are often solitary lesions in the lung periphery [56]. The tumors are thought to arise from the smooth muscle of the bronchi or bronchioles in the central lesions or from vessel walls in the periphery of the lung in parenchymal tumors [58]. The trachea is the least common site for these tumors in the respiratory tract, with the majority of cases arising in the lung parenchyma and about a third of tumors presenting as endobronchial lesions.

Clinical Features

Leiomyomas are tumors predominantly affecting middle-aged patients with a mean age around 35 years; however, pediatric as well as older patients may also be affected. Patients with tracheal lesions are normally slightly older (mean age 40.6 years) [56, 59–62]. Leiomyomas of the lung and bronchi are more frequently reported to occur in females, while tracheal lesions are more commonly seen in men [59, 61]. The higher incidence in females for the pulmonary lesions should be approached with care though, as many of these tumors likely represent metastatic disease from the uterus. Whereas tracheal and endobronchial lesions often cause obstructive symptoms (dyspnea, cough, chest pain, fever, pneumonia, and atelectasis), peripheral lesions are often incidental findings [59, 63]. On imaging, leiomyomas do not show any specific features and cannot be distinguished completely from other benign or malignant tumors [56].

Gross Features

Tumor size usually ranges from 2 to 4 cm but may rarely exceed 10 cm in maximum dimension. Tracheal and endobronchial lesions are usually polypoid, protruding into the tracheal or bronchial lumen. Often these tumors are connected to the tracheal/bronchial wall by a broad base. Intraparenchymal tumors are generally well circumscribed but not encapsulated. On sectioning, the tumor is characterized by white-yellow firm cut surface that shows a homogenous or whorled pattern. Prominent cystic change has been described in isolated cases [64].

Histological Features

Histologically, leiomyomas of the lower respiratory tract are identical to those arising in the soft tissue. The tumors are composed of bundles of spindle cells arranged in fascicles intersecting at wide angles (Figs. 9.41 and 9.42). The nuclei are pale and elongated, show blunt-ended tips, and contain a moderate amount of eosinophilic cytoplasm. Nucleoli are not a prominent feature (Fig. 9.43). Entrapped respiratory epithelium may mimic gland-like spaces or clefts (Fig. 9.44). Features of malignancy like cytologic atypia, mitotic activity, or areas of hemorrhage and necrosis are usually missing.

Immunohistochemical Features

Leiomymomas of the bronchopulmonary system show reactivity for markers specific for muscle differentiation. These include primarily smooth muscle actin, muscle specific actin, desmin, calponin, and caldesmon, while keratin is usually negative but may be focally positive in isolated cases.

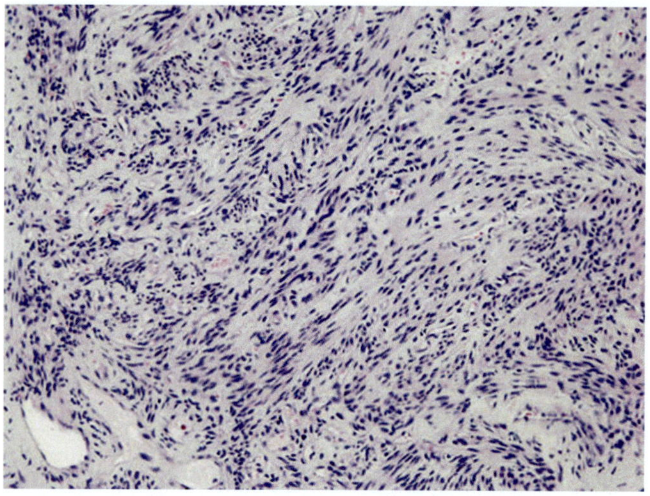

Fig. 9.41 Fascicular arrangement of spindle cells in pulmonary leiomyoma

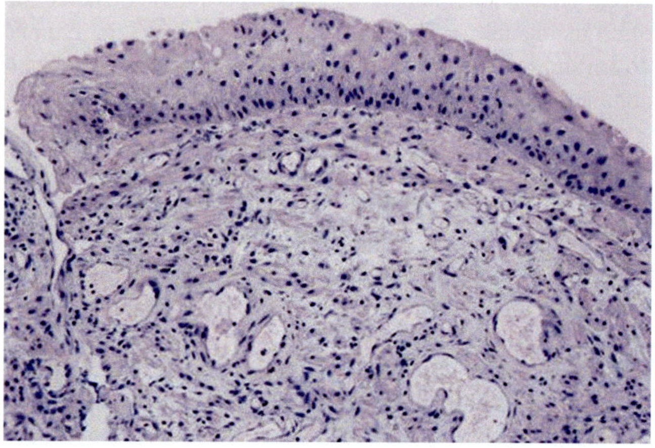

Fig. 9.42 Spindle cells of pulmonary leiomyoma growing underneath the bronchial epithelium

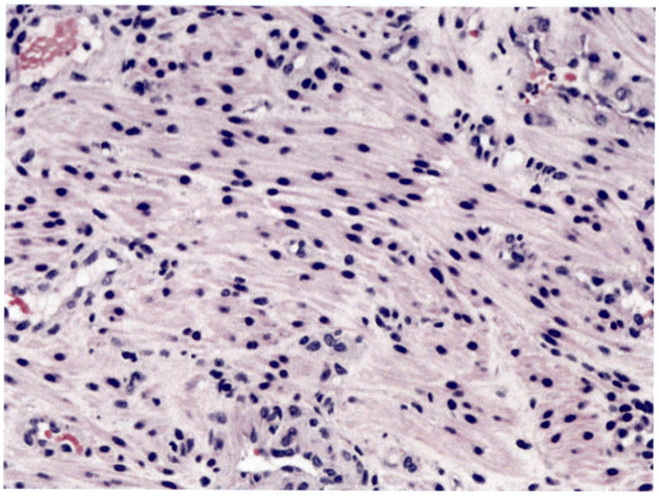

Fig. 9.43 Bland cytologic features of pulmonary leiomyoma characterized by spindle cells with blunt-ended nuclei and eosinophilic cytoplasm

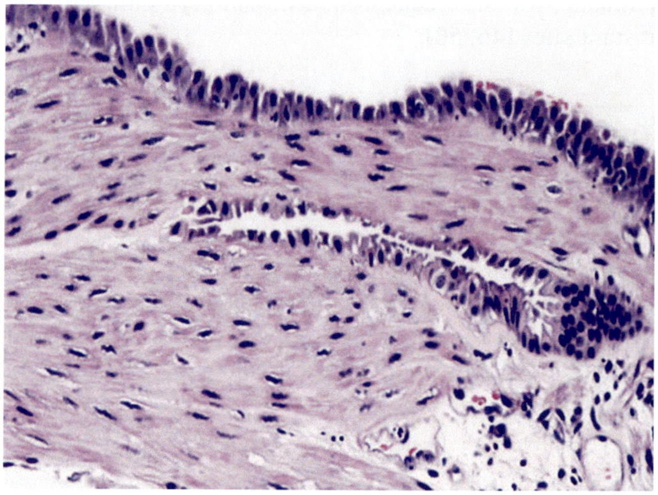

Fig. 9.44 Entrapped respiratory epithelium in pulmonary leiomyoma

Differential Diagnosis

Primary pulmonary leiomyomas must be distinguished from their malignant counterpart leiomyosarcoma. The biggest challenge represent low grade leiomyosarcomas in which nuclear atypia and mitotic activity is not high. In these cases a search for mitotic figures is highly important. In addition, peripheral nerve sheath tumors such as schwannomas may mimic a smooth muscle neoplasm. However, primary schwannomas of the lung parenchyma are exceedingly rare and the cases reported appear to show the classical histology similar to those occurring in more common locations. In addition, peripheral nerve sheath tumors such as schwannomas may mimic a smooth muscle neoplasm. The aid of immunohistochemical markers in this context, S-100 protein versus muscle markers, should allow differentiation. Another important diagnostic consideration is the exclusion of metastatic disease from the so-called benign metastasizing leiomyoma of the uterus. The presence of multiple nodules in a female patient coupled with a history of uterine leiomyomas should lead to the correct diagnosis.

Treatment and Prognosis

Bronchoscopic intervention can be considered in tumors that present as endotracheal or endobronchial lesions. In cases of wide-based tumors or larger lesions, however, surgical excision (lobectomy or pneumonectomy) should be performed in order to prevent incomplete resection or tumor recurrence. Parenchymal tumors usually require segmentectomy or lobectomy for complete surgical resection [65]. The prognosis for pulmonary leiomyoma is favorable if surgical excisions result in complete resection.

Pulmonary Leiomyosarcoma

Malignant smooth muscle tumors of the lung are more common than their benign counterparts; however, generally speaking they are still rare tumors. Approximately 100 cases have been described in adults and 15 cases in children under

16 years of age [66, 67]. Leiomyosarcomas may arise from the pulmonary vasculature, the bronchial tree, or the pulmonary parenchyma [20, 68–78]. As with most sarcomas, metastatic disease from an extrapulmonary primary will have to be excluded by clinical and radiological investigations as the tumors show the same histological features like the ones originating in the soft tissue.

Clinical Features

Pulmonary leiomyosarcoma is a tumor primarily affecting adult patients with an average age around 50 years [79]. The tumors may rarely affect children and even newborns [67, 78, 80, 81]. The tumors may arise as endobronchial, parenchymal, or subpleural lesions [79]. Cough, chest pain, dyspnea, hemoptysis, fatigue, or weight loss have been described as presenting symptoms, although peripheral lesions may often be incidental findings [79, 82]. More rarely, pulmonary leiomyosarcoma may present as a pancoast tumor [83], cause hemorrhagic pleural effusion and digital clubbing [84], produce paraneoplastic symptoms [85], or be associated with Epstein-Barr virus infection [86].

Gross Features

Macroscopically, the tumor size ranges from less than 2 cm to more than 20 cm [79, 87]. The size often correlates with the degree of histological differentiation with low- or intermediate-grade tumors being smaller (mean 3.2 cm) than high-grade tumors (up to 10 cm) [79]. Irrespective of tumor location, the lesions are well-circumscribed, gray-white, firm rubbery masses, which may show areas of hemorrhage or necrosis. Rare tumors have been described, showing central cavitation [88], arising within an emphysematous bulla [89] or arteriovenous fistula [75], or having a pedunculated appearance [73, 90].

Histological Features

Pulmonary leiomyosarcomas are proliferations of spindle cells that grow in characteristic broad fascicles that intersect at right angles (Fig. 9.45). Leiomyosarcomas can be divided into low-, intermediate-, and high-grade tumors. Low-grade tumors are characterized by a well-developed fascicular pattern of growth composed of interlacing fascicles of tumor cells. The individual cells have a lightly eosinophilic cytoplasm and show the typical blunt-ended "cigar-shaped" nuclei with little cytologic atypia (Fig. 9.46). The mitotic activity does not exceed 3 mitoses per 10 high-power fields. Prominent cellular pleomorphism, hemorrhage, or necrosis is not usually identified [79]. Intermediate-grade tumors have a preserved fascicular growth pattern, a slightly higher cellularity than low-grade tumors, and an increased mitotic activity (4–8 mitoses per 10 high-power fields). Cytologic atypia is more pronounced than in low-grade leiomyosarcoma but not pronounced (Fig. 9.47). Neither hemorrhage nor necrosis is usually seen. High-grade leiomyosarcomas show a predominantly solid spindle cell proliferation with more scanty areas showing the typical fascicular arrangement. The cellularity is high and focally as storiform pattern may be observed. There is marked cytologic atypia with large hyperchromatic nuclei and frequent mitotic figures (8–12 mitoses per 10 high-power fields) (Figs. 9.48 and 9.49). Besides the hemangiopericytic growth pattern, the stroma may show degenerative changes such as myxoid change or hyalinization, while hemorrhage or necrosis is present in most cases (Figs. 9.50 and 9.51) [79].

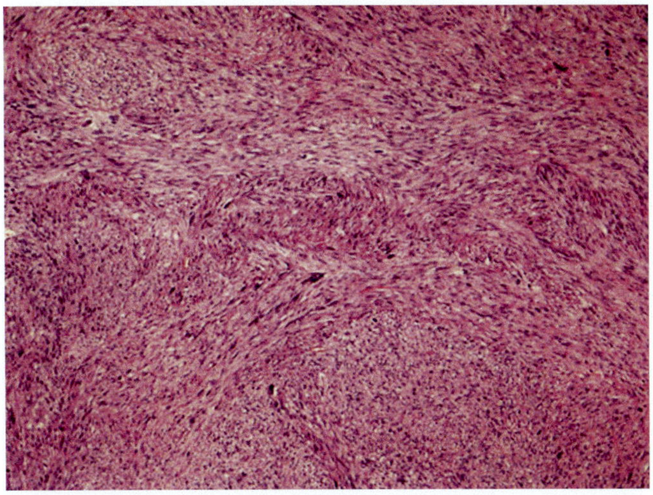

Fig. 9.45 High-power view of pulmonary leiomyosarcoma consisting of a malignant spindle cell proliferation

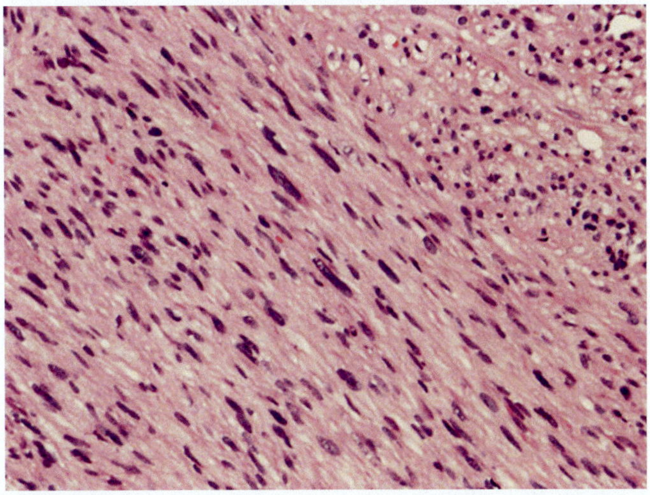

Fig. 9.46 Low-grade pulmonary leiomyosarcoma showing little cytologic atypia

Immunohistochemical and Molecular Features

Immunohistochemical markers for muscle differentiation are positive in most cases of pulmonary leiomyosarcoma. These include smooth muscle actin and desmin. While high grade

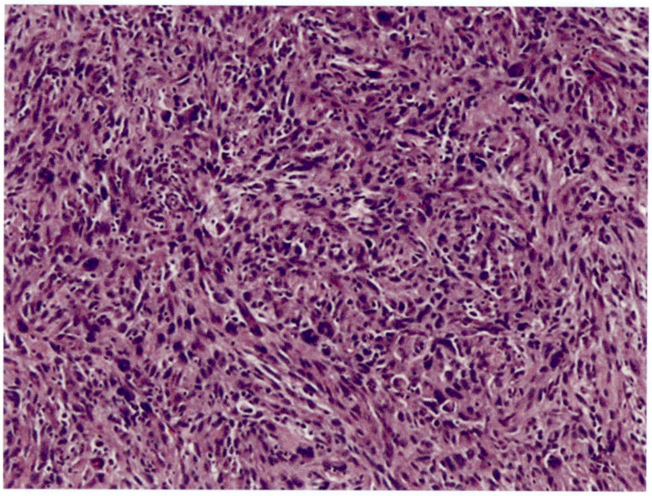

Fig. 9.47 Intermediate-grade leiomyosarcoma showing more cellular atypia

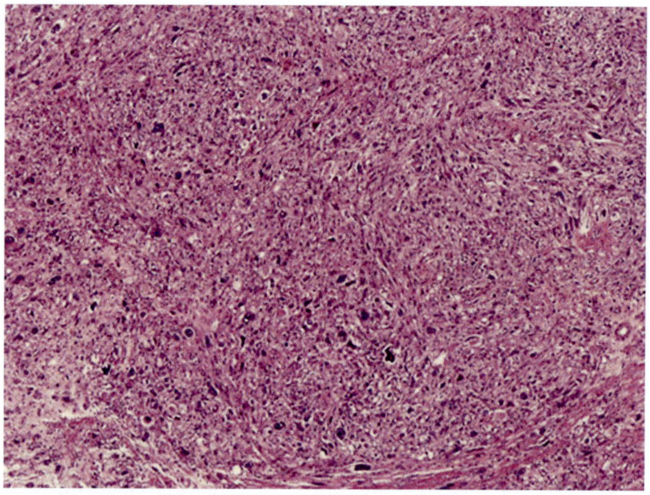

Fig. 9.48 High cellularity and obvious cytologic atypia in high-grade leiomyosarcoma of the lung

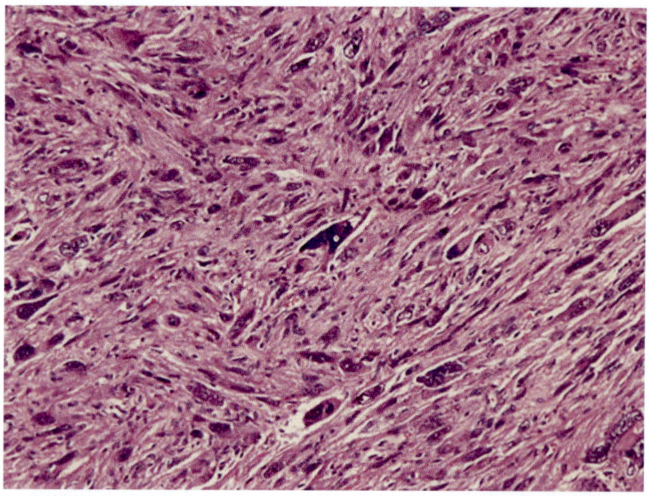

Fig. 9.49 Pleomorphic tumor cells in high-grade pulmonary leiomyosarcoma

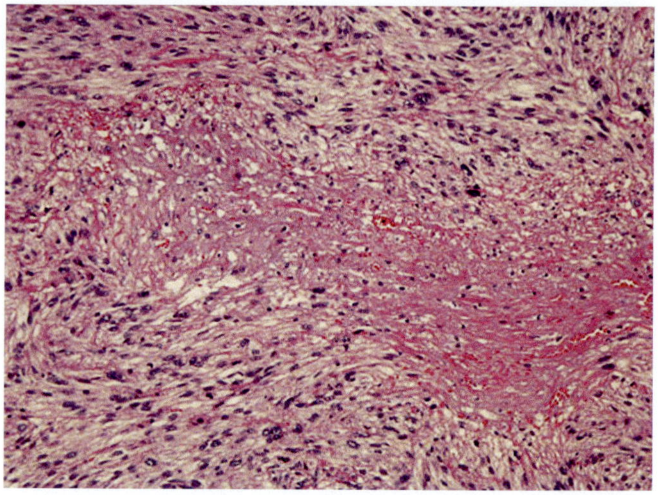

Fig. 9.50 Necrosis is often seen in high-grade leiomyosarcoma of the lung

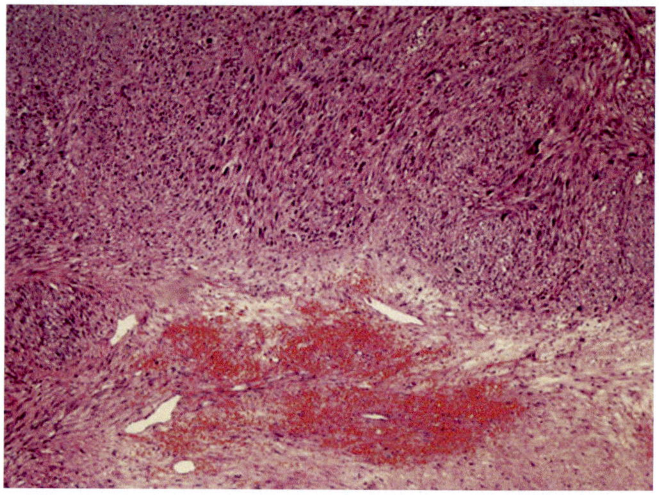

Fig. 9.51 Pulmonary leiomyosarcoma with areas of hemorrhage

tumors may only show focal positive staining for these muscle markers. It has been demonstrated that keratin can also be focally positive in these tumors. Generally, the staining pattern for muscle markers is stronger in the better differentiated tumors. S-100 protein is generally negative [79]. Cytogenetic abnormalities have been described for single case of pulmonary leiomyosarcoma in an 8-year-old boy [91]. The karyotype of the tumor demonstrated complex structural abnormalities involving chromosomes 1, 5, 6, and 7, gains of chromosomes 2 and 11, and losses of chromosomes 9, 19, 20, and 22.

Differential Diagnosis

Pulmonary leiomyosarcoma must be distinguished from leiomyoma, and from other malignant spindle cell neoplasms. Pulmonary leiomyoma may have an identical clinical presentation but lacks the cytologic atypia, mitotic activity, and areas of hemorrhage or necrosis that leiomyosarcoma usually displays. Other spindle cell neoplasms of the lung primarily include sarcomatoid carcinoma, monophasic synovial sarcoma, and malignant peripheral nerve sheath tumor. In this scenario, immunohistochemical studies may aid in arriving at the correct diagnosis. Sarcomatoid carcinoma and monophasic synovial sarcoma will stain with keratin and will lack positive smooth muscle markers. Malignant peripheral nerve sheath tumor will show S-100 protein expression and be negative for smooth muscle markers contrary to leiomyosarcoma. Lastly, in every case of pulmonary leiomyosarcoma, metastasis from an extrapulmonary leiomyosarcoma, mainly from the uterus or soft tissue, has to be excluded through a complete clinical and radiological workup.

Treatment and Prognosis

There is insufficient evidence that chemotherapy or radiation is beneficial for patients with pulmonary leiomyosarcomas either as the primary treatment or in an adjuvant setting [92], and hence, complete surgical resection remains the only curative form of treatment. It has been shown that the clinical outcome depends on histological grade and to a certain degree on the size of the tumors. Generally, lesions of smaller size (<4 cm) and low or intermediate grade tend to have a better prognosis than tumors of larger size or high-grade histology [79]. The 5-year overall survival rate is approximately 43 % [93].

Pulmonary Rhabdomyosarcoma

To date less than 50 primary pulmonary rhabdomyosarcomas have been described in the English literature. Of these, around 15 cases were diagnosed in adults and 31 in the pediatric population. In adults rhabdomyosarcomatous elements may be components of other tumors, for instance rhabdomyosarcomatous elements in carcinosarcoma or pulmonary blastoma, requiring extensive sampling and careful histological evaluation to arrive at the correct diagnosis. Likewise, all cases of pediatric primary pulmonary rhabdomyosarcoma should be examined with care as many of the cases reported, especially when associated with cystic features, have now been reclassified as pleuropulmonary blastomas, casting some doubt on the reported incidence of these tumors [94].

The absence of skeletal muscle in the bronchopulmonary system has raised speculation about the origin of these tumors. Some authors believe that primitive mesenchymal cells in the bronchial walls and interstitium undergo myoblastic differentiation [95, 96], while other hypotheses conclude that tumor cells are the result of metaplastic transformation of pluripotent non-myoblastic mesenchymal cells [97]. An alternative view is provided by other groups that believe in the misplacement of striated muscle or embryonic rests into the pulmonary system during fetal development [98–100].

Clinical Features

In the adult population, primary pulmonary rhabdomyosarcoma affects predominantly male patients with a median age of 57 years [101]. The tumors can present as endobronchial or intraparenchymal masses, and symptoms are often related to the location of the neoplasm within the lung. For tumors arising in the bronchial tree, cough and dyspnea are the most frequent complaints, while tumors in the lung periphery most often cause chest pain. Rarely, pulmonary rhabdomyosarcomas may be seen in association with other conditions such as other lung tumors [96] or neurofibromatosis type 1 [102].

Gross Features

The tumors are large and may exceed 10 cm in maximum dimension. They are well circumscribed and may show cystic changes [96]. The cut surface is tan-gray and of soft to firm or rubbery consistency. Areas of hemorrhage or necrosis are frequently seen [103].

Histological Features

Primary pulmonary rhabdomyosarcoma occurs as the pleomorphic variant in adults. On low magnification, the tumors are characterized by a proliferation of loosely arranged, discohesive spindle cells alternating with more cellular areas arranged in a fascicular or storiform patterns (Figs. 9.52 and 9.53). Foci of necrosis and hemorrhage are frequently found (Fig. 9.54). On higher power, the neoplastic spindle cells are large to medium sized, contain irregular hyperchromatic nuclei and prominent nucleoli, and have a densely eosinophilic cytoplasm that in some cases may display prominent cross striations (Figs. 9.55 and 9.56). Typical rhabdomyoblasts are a frequent finding (Figs. 9.57 and 9.58) and atypical mitoses are abundant (Fig. 9.59). In some cases, the stroma can show edematous or myxoid changes (Fig. 9.60) [101, 103].

Immunohistochemical and Molecular Features

Immunoperoxidase studies typically show strong staining of the neoplastic cells with desmin, myoglobin, myogenin, and myo-D1 [101, 103, 104]. Although keratin, EMA, and S-100 protein are negative in most cases, keratin can sometimes be focally positive in these tumors, emphasizing the need for an expanded immunopanel in the diagnosis of pleomorphic spindle cell lesions in the lung. Trisomy 8 has been reported for rhabdomyosarcomas of soft tissue origin [105] and has also been demonstrated in primary pulmonary rhabdomyosarcoma [104].

Differential Diagnosis

Due to the low incidence of primary pulmonary rhabdomyosarcoma, it is important to consider other primary pulmonary

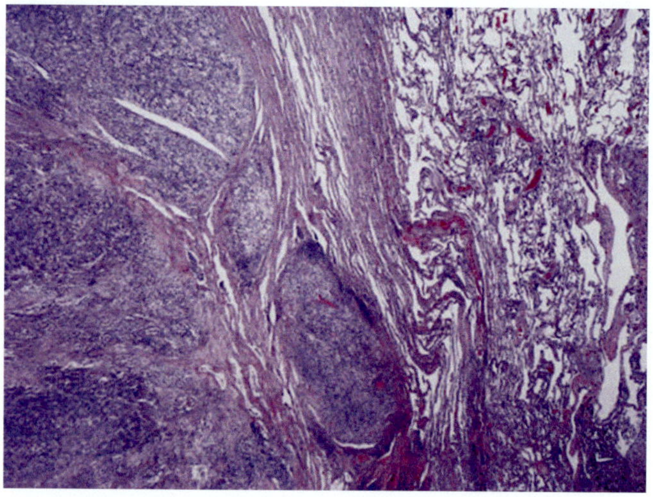

Fig. 9.52 Low-power view of pulmonary rhabdomyosarcoma composed of a loosely arranged spindle cell proliferation

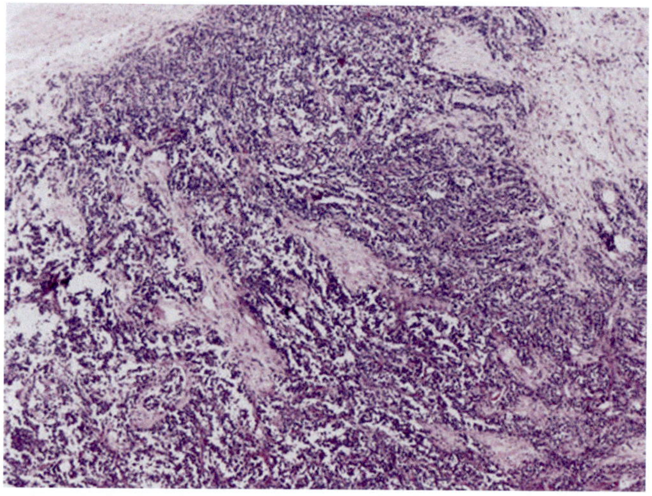

Fig. 9.53 Pulmonary rhabdomyosarcoma composed of discohesive tumor cells

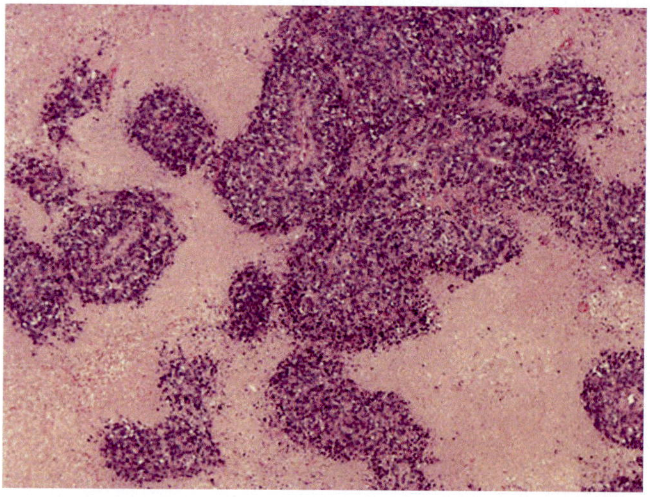

Fig. 9.54 Extensive areas of necrosis may be identified in rhabdomyosarcoma of the lung

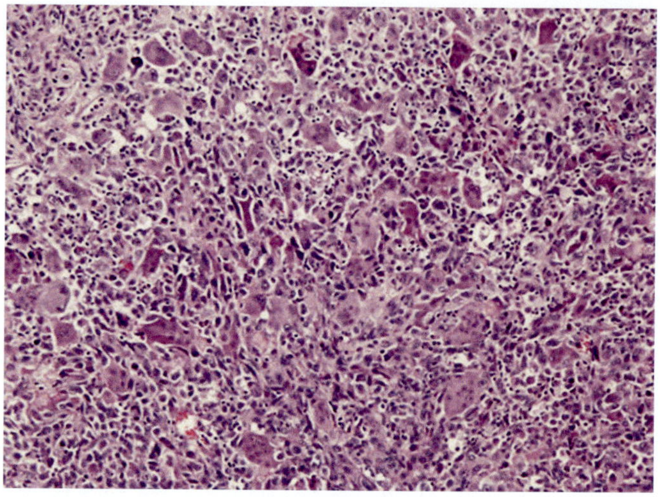

Fig. 9.55 Pulmonary rhabdomyosarcoma composed of large pleomorphic tumor cells

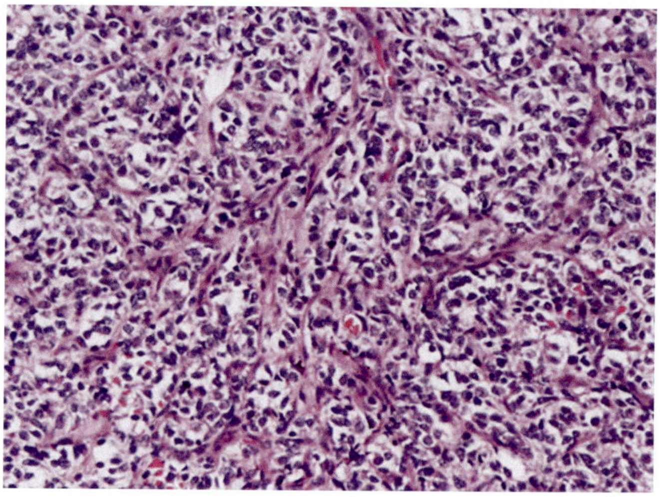

Fig. 9.56 Intermediate-sized ovoid to spindled tumor cells in pulmonary rhabdomyosarcoma

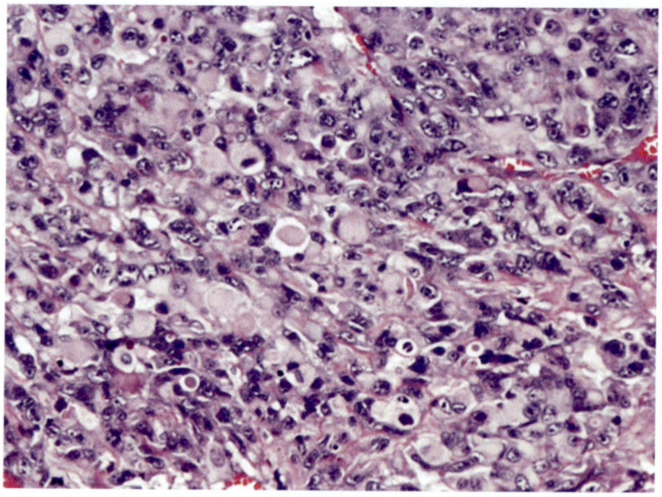

Fig. 9.57 At higher magnification, numerous rhabdomyoblasts are readily apparent

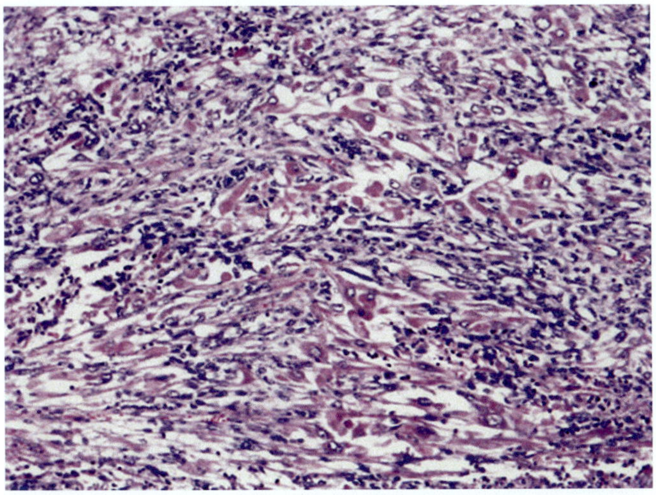

Fig. 9.58 Mixture of spindle cells and rhabdomyoblasts in pulmonary rhabdomyosarcoma

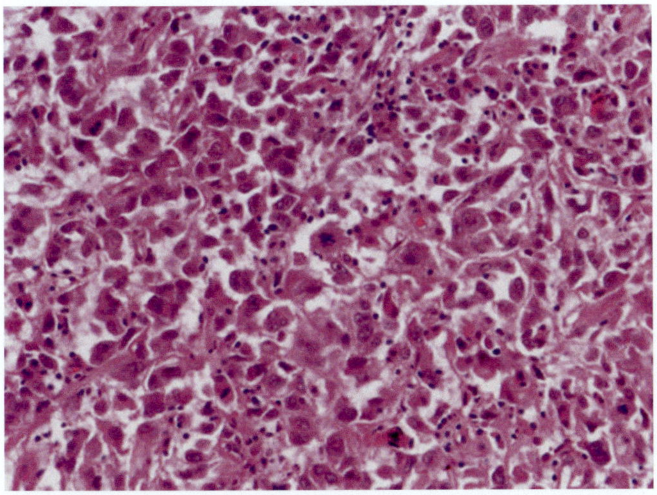

Fig. 9.59 High mitotic activity is often found in pulmonary rhabdomyosarcoma

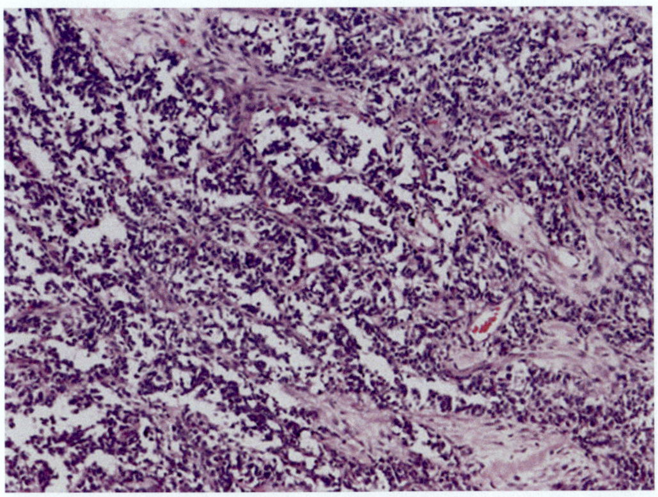

Fig. 9.60 Myxoid stromal changes may be focally identified in rhabdomyosarcoma of the lung

tumors that may resemble rhabdomyosarcoma or to exclude metastatic disease from a soft tissue or bone primary. While exclusion of metastatic rhabdomyosarcoma requires careful clinical and radiological correlation, other primary lung tumors to consider include carcinosarcoma, pulmonary blastoma, and pleomorphic carcinoma. Carcinosarcoma and pulmonary blastoma can show areas containing rhabdomyoblastic elements along with the typical malignant epithelial elements characterizing these tumors. Extensive tumor sampling should lead to the correct diagnosis in these cases. Pleomorphic carcinoma of the lung is a neoplasm composed of malignant epithelial spindle cells intermixed with tumor giant cells, thereby mimicking a sarcomatous tumor. The use of immunohistochemical studies using epithelial in combination with muscle markers should help in classifying the tumors accordingly.

Treatment and Prognosis

Complete surgical resection is the treatment of choice for primary pulmonary rhabdomyosarcoma. Chemotherapy or radiation may be used in an adjuvant setting. More than half of the adult patients reported have died with widespread metastasis and most of them within 24 months [101, 103]. However, rare long-term survivors (up to 12 years) have also been reported [96].

Tumors of Cartilage or Bone Origin

Malignant cartilage or bone is most often identified as an element in malignant biphasic lung tumors; however, primary lung tumors composed entirely of cartilaginous or osseous components represent only a very small subset of lung neoplasms.

Pulmonary Chondroma

The terms "pulmonary chondroma" and "pulmonary chondroid hamartoma" are often used interchangeably; however, it has been demonstrated that these lesions differ morphologically [106]. Pulmonary chondromas may occur as sporadic neoplasms or as part of Carney's triad, clinical association of gastrointestinal stromal tumors, pulmonary chondromas, and extra-adrenal paragangliomas [107]. Sporadic tumors tend to affect a different clinical group than tumors associated with Carney's triad as they are more commonly detected in middle-aged men, while patients with Carney's triad are usually young women. In addition, sporadic tumors are generally single endobronchial lesions, whereas tumors of the triad are often multiple lesions that arise in the lung periphery. Overall, the clinical features of sporadic pulmonary chondromas are therefore very similar to those identified in patients with pulmonary hamartomas [106].

Clinical Features

As mentioned previously, the clinical features differ for sporadic pulmonary chondromas and those associated with Carney's triad [106]. Sporadic chondromas are tumors arising in middle-aged patients with a male-to-female ratio of 2:1 and an age range from 12 to 93 years (average age 53 years). These tumors are single lesions and normally arising in an endobronchial location or being related to the bronchus. The minority of these tumors are found in the lung periphery. Patients with Carney's triad, on the other hand, are predominantly young women (male-to-female ratio 1:9) with a mean age of 24.8 years (range 12–44 years). In addition, triad-associated chondromas are often multiple and only rarely found in an endobronchial location but are rather seen in the lung periphery. Radiologically, the tumors impress as well-circumscribed round or lobulated tumors with popcorn-like calcification irrespective of sporadic or syndromic origin [106].

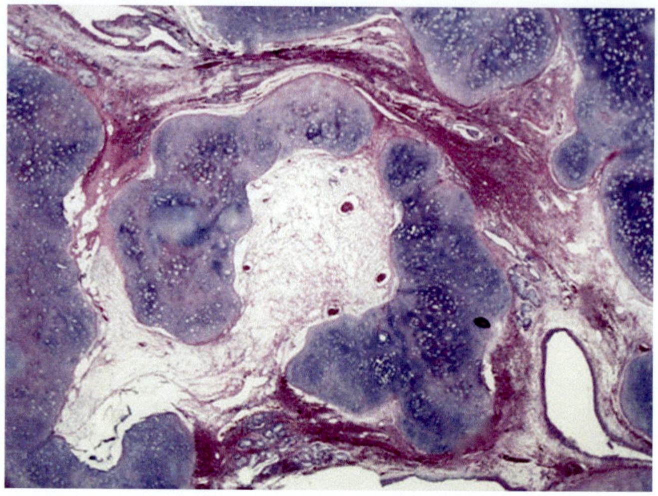

Fig. 9.61 Low magnification of pulmonary chondroma

Gross Features

The macroscopic features show well-circumscribed tumors with bosselated or lobulated outlines and a gritty or cartilaginous appearance [106]. The cut surface is gray-white or gray-blue in color and has a firm or gelatinous consistency. Cystic change, hemorrhage, or necrosis is rarely identified [106].

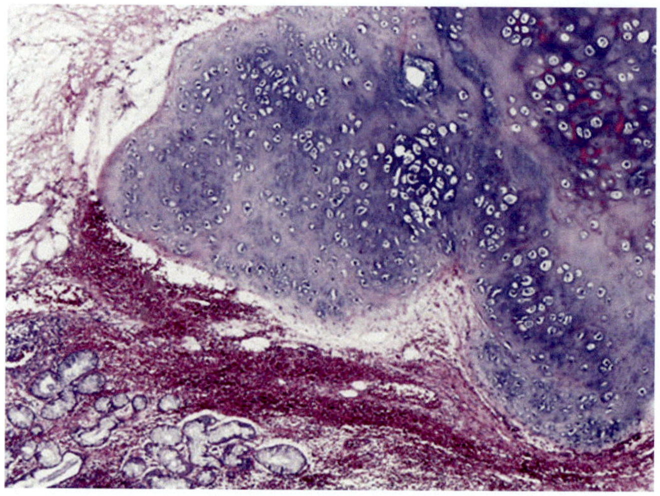

Fig. 9.62 Pulmonary chondroma composed of mature hyaline cartilage

Histological Features

Pulmonary chondromas are well circumscribed and separated from the surrounding tissues by a fibrous pseudocapsule [106]. The characteristic feature of pulmonary chondromas is that they are almost exclusively composed of cartilage, either of hyaline or myxoid type (Figs. 9.61 and 9.62). This cartilage typically shows areas of calcification or ossification. Cytologic atypia or mitotic activity is absent (Fig. 9.63). Most importantly and contrary to pulmonary hamartomas, pulmonary chondromas lack the entrapped respiratory epithelium, fatty, fibrous, or smooth muscle components typically identified in the former tumors.

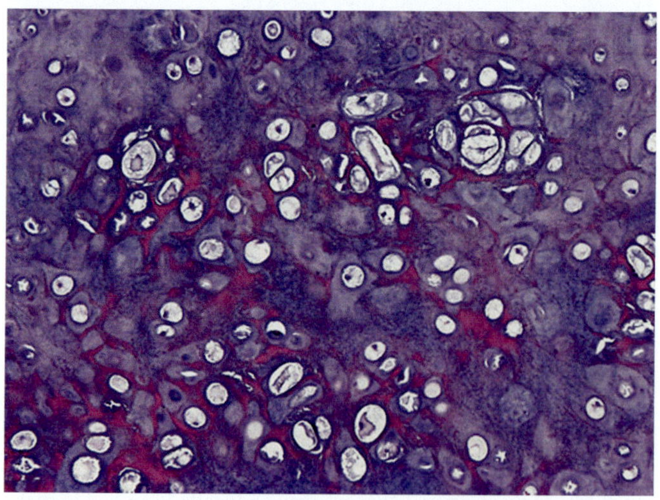

Fig. 9.63 Pulmonary chondroma lacking cytologic atypia

Differential Diagnosis

The most important differential diagnosis for pulmonary chondroma is its malignant counterpart pulmonary chondrosarcoma. Chondrosarcoma, either as a pulmonary primary or metastatic disease will show malignant properties of the cartilage characterized by prominent chondrocyte atypia but not necessarily mitotic activity. Close clinical correlation, especially in cases of multifocal pulmonary lesions, will help exclude metastatic chondrosarcoma from a bone primary. As mentioned earlier, the term pulmonary chondroma is often used interchangeably with pulmonary hamartoma. Hamartomas, however, are lesions composed of several different elements (cartilage, fat, fibrous or smooth muscle tissue, and entrapped respiratory epithelium), whereas pulmonary chondromas are composed of cartilage only.

Treatment and Prognosis

Surgical resection in the form of tumor enucleation, wedge biopsy, segmentectomy, lobectomy, or pneumonectomy is the treatment of choice for pulmonary chondromas. Although in some patients additional chondromas will develop, the lesions are considered entirely benign as metastatic disease and tumor-related deaths have not occurred [106]. Importantly, if these tumors are detected in a young female, thorough investigations to rule out Carney's triad are advised, as the other lesions associated with this syndrome carry a significant risk of morbidity and mortality.

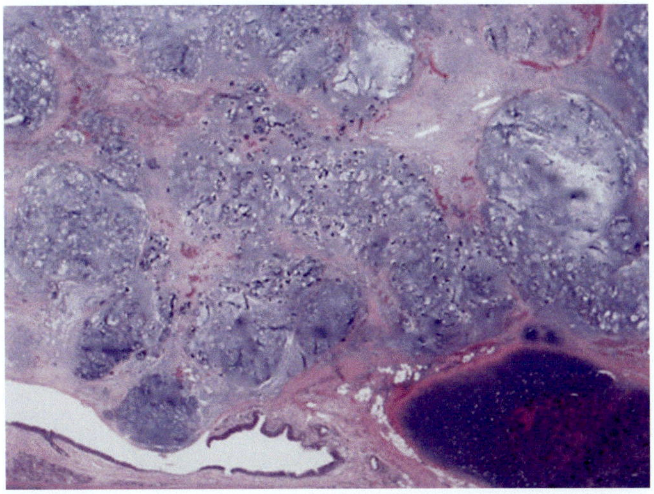

Fig. 9.64 Low-power view of conventional pulmonary chondrosarcoma of the lung characterized by a lobulated proliferation of hyaline cartilage

Pulmonary Chondrosarcoma

Pulmonary chondrosarcoma is an uncommon primary lung tumor. These tumors may arise from the tracheobronchial system or originate from the bronchial cartilage in the lung parenchyma [97, 108–124]. Since the lungs are a common site for metastatic disease, careful clinical assessment is required before a diagnosis of primary pulmonary chondrosarcoma can be rendered. Furthermore, chondrosarcomas of the lung may arise "de novo" (also called "primary" pulmonary chondrosarcoma) or from a preexisting benign chondroid neoplasm such a chondroma or hamartoma ("secondary" pulmonary chondrosarcoma) [125, 126].

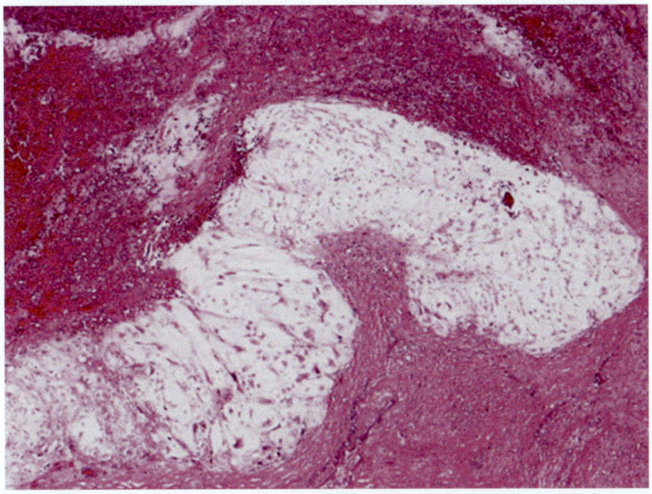

Fig. 9.65 Pulmonary chondrosarcoma with myxoid change of the cartilage

Clinical Features

Pulmonary chondrosarcomas affect the adult age group, predominantly patients in the sixth decade (age range 23–74 years) [110]. No specific gender predilection has been observed. Symptoms depend on the site of involvement, and for tracheobronchial (central) lesions include signs of bronchial obstruction characterized by cough, dyspnea, and chest pain. Parenchymal (peripheral) tumors, on the other hand, are often incidental findings or present late with symptoms of dyspnea and chest pain [97, 108, 114].

Gross Features

The tumors may vary in size and range from 1 cm to more than 10 cm in maximum dimension. The tumors are usually sharply defined and lobulated or irregular in shape. Depending on tumor subtype, the cut surface is white in color with a firm consistency (conventional hyaline type), tan colored, and soft to mucoid (myxoid type), or yellow-brown with patchy glossy white areas (dedifferentiated type) [110, 119, 121]. Areas of hemorrhage or necrosis are rarely identified.

Histological Features

The morphology of pulmonary chondrosarcomas shows similar features to those seen in the skeleton. The most common form of pulmonary chondrosarcoma is the conventional hyaline type, which is characterized by lobules of hyaline cartilage containing chondrocytes with plump nuclei, binucleated forms, and coarse nuclear chromatin (Figs. 9.64, 9.65, and 9.66). Some of the lacunae may contain two or more cells (Figs. 9.67 and 9.68). These hyaline areas may be associated with more myxoid areas. Hemorrhage, necrosis, and mitotic activity are not common in this variant [110]. Other subtypes that have been identified in primary chondrosarcomas of the lung include myxoid, mesenchymal, and dedifferentiated types [110, 119, 121–123, 127]. These show lobulated masses of cords or strands of round cells embedded in a basophilic matrix (myxoid type), combined hypercellular zones of anaplastic small cells alternating with islands of cartilage (mesenchymal type) (Figs. 9.69, 9.70, and 9.71), and areas of highly atypical cartilaginous tumor intermingled

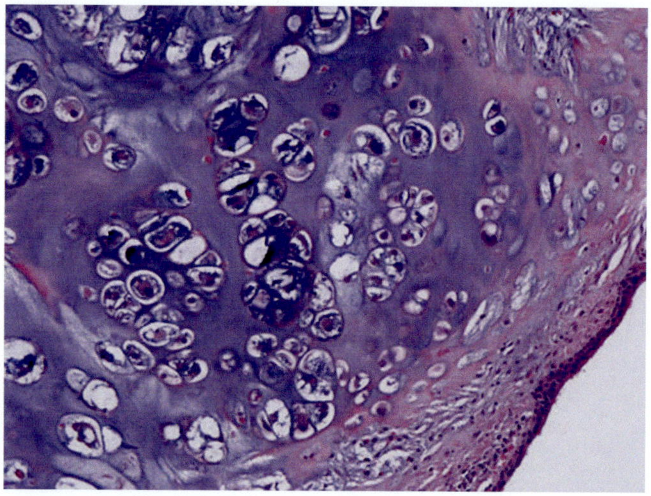

Fig. 9.66 Malignant cartilage in pulmonary chondrosarcoma showing chondrocyte atypia

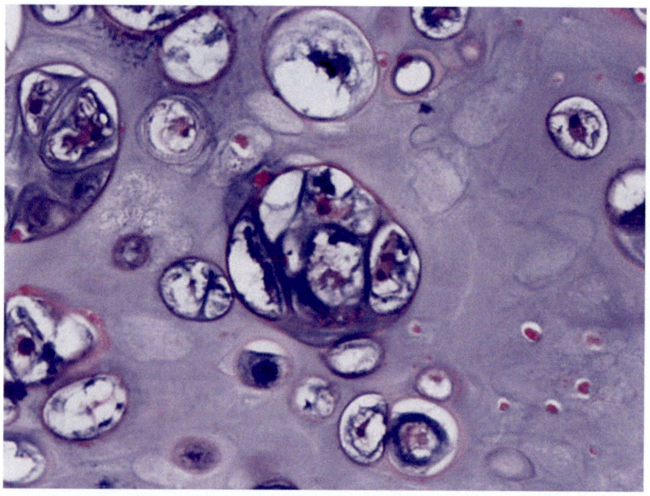

Fig. 9.67 High-power view of pulmonary chondrosarcoma with hypercellularity in chondrocyte lacunae

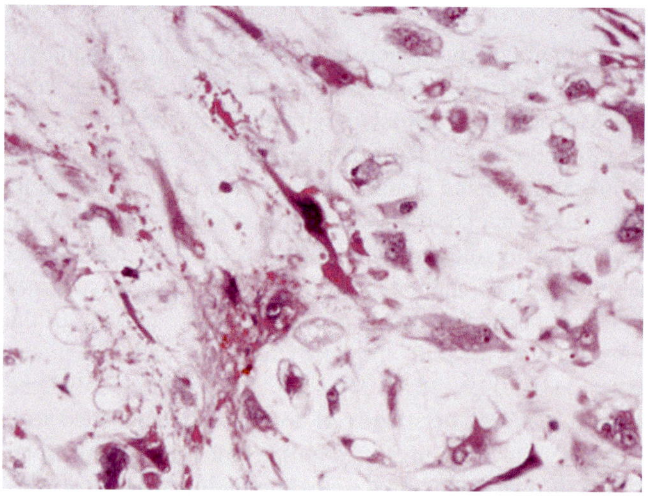

Fig. 9.68 Prominent chondrocyte atypia in pulmonary chondrosarcoma

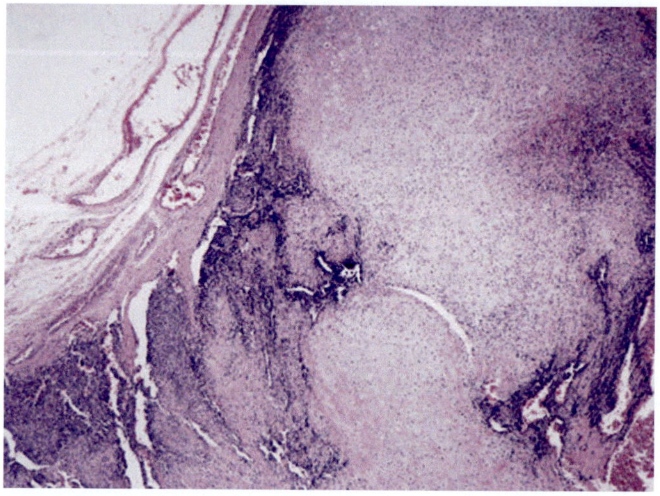

Fig. 9.69 Low-power view of mesenchymal variant of pulmonary chondrosarcoma composed of mesenchymal and cartilaginous areas

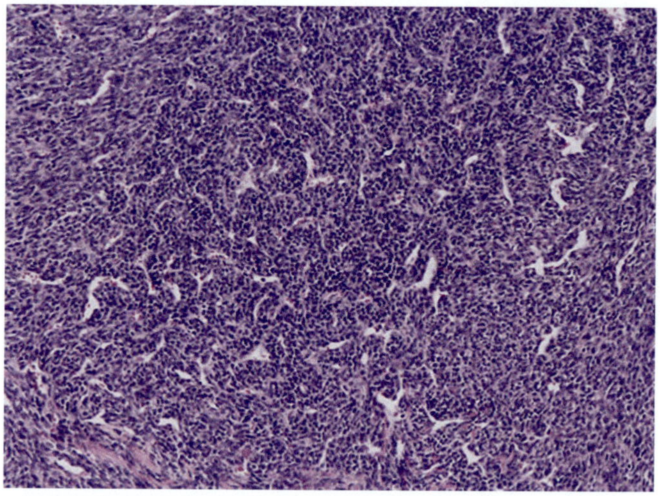

Fig. 9.70 Anaplastic small cell component in mesenchymal pulmonary chondrosarcoma

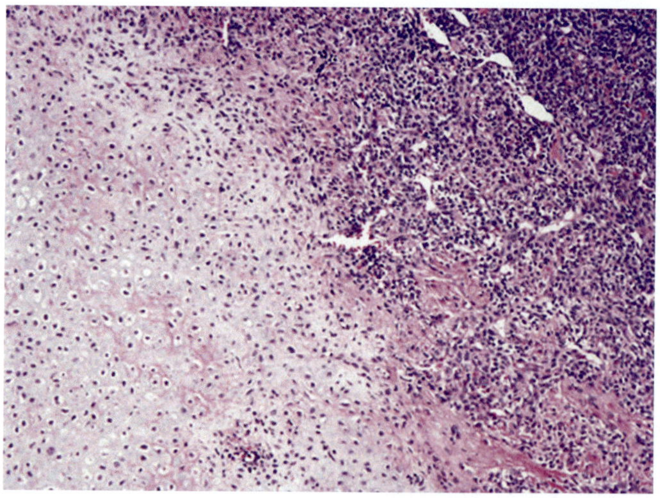

Fig. 9.71 Alternating small cells and islands of cartilage in mesenchymal pulmonary chondrosarcoma

with a malignant spindle cell component (dedifferentiated type) [110, 119, 121]. Foci of necrosis and increased mitotic activity may be observed in these latter types.

Immunohistochemical Features

Although a diagnosis of pulmonary chondrosarcoma is often a histological one, immunohistochemical techniques may aid in equivocal cases or in cases where other mesenchymal components are present (mesenchymal or dedifferentiated subtypes). The chondrocytes of the conventional hyaline type will show positive staining with S-100 protein and vimentin and will generally be negative for markers associated with epithelial and muscle differentiation [109, 110, 116]. Mesenchymal chondrosarcomas have been shown to express Sox-9 reactivity in both the small round cell and cartilaginous areas [128]. Dedifferentiated chondrosarcomas may show various sarcomatous differentiations and will show an immunohistochemical staining pattern according to the dedifferentiated sarcoma component present in the individual tumors.

Differential Diagnosis

Exclusion of metastatic chondrosarcoma to the lung is the most important differential diagnosis for primary pulmonary chondrosarcoma and should be taken care of by complete physical history and radiological investigations. Another important aspect is the separation from the benign counterpart, pulmonary chondroma. Pulmonary chondromas may be multiple and associated with Carney's triad and are usually composed of benign cartilage with areas of ossification. Chondrosarcomas, on the other hand, are usually solitary sporadic tumors that only rarely show areas of osseous differentiation. Chondroid hamartomas may also enter the differential diagnosis. These are tumors composed of several benign tissue types including cartilage, entrapped respiratory epithelium, and fat and fibrous tissue, features that are not typically seen in chondrosarcoma. Myxoid chondrosarcomas may be confused with other neoplasms showing a myxoid stroma such as epithelioid hemangioendothelioma. Immunohistochemical staining with vascular markers such as CD31 and CD34 in the tumor cells will help in making a diagnosis in favor of the latter. An important issue in the assessment of pulmonary chondrosarcoma is sufficient histological sampling of the tumors in order to exclude an epithelial component as part of the slightly more common carcinosarcomas.

Treatment and Prognosis

Complete surgical resection is the primary treatment for pulmonary chondrosarcoma. Adjuvant chemotherapy or irradiation has been used in isolated cases; however, due to the rarity of these tumors, the effectiveness of such therapy is still uncertain. The prognosis of pulmonary chondrosarcoma appears to vary depending on site of origin (tracheobronchial versus peripheral tumors) [97, 108, 114]. Central lesions are usually localized at the time of diagnosis and detected early, whereas peripheral lesions tend to be asymptomatic with the risk of more rapid growth and distant metastasis [109, 114, 120]. Furthermore, nonconventional chondrosarcomas of the lung are more likely to show aggressive behavior [110].

Pulmonary Osteosarcoma

Extraskeletal osteosarcomas represent 1–2 % of soft tissue sarcomas and approximately 4 % of all osteosarcomas [129]. Primary osteosarcomas arising in the lung are among the rarest human cancers with less than 25 reported cases in the literature [130–143]. There is still some debate about the pathogenesis of these tumors with the most popular hypothesis postulating an origin from pluripotent pulmonary mesenchymal cells [133]. Importantly, pulmonary osteosarcomas affect an older age group than their osseous equivalent.

Clinical Features

Primary pulmonary osteosarcoma usually occurs in older adults with an age range from 33 to 83 years and an average age in the seventh decade. Men and women are equally affected. The main presenting symptoms are chest pain, cough, and hemoptysis [144]. Many of the tumors are centrally located, but peripheral lesions have also been described. Interestingly, there is a striking predominance of involvement of the left lung and especially the upper lobe. On CT scanning, the tumors can be suspected by the presence of a heterogenous mass with dense calcification [142]. In addition, increased uptake can be demonstrated in the tumor mass by technetium-99 m methylene diphosphonate bone scintigraphy [142].

Gross Features

The tumors are firm and solid masses of large size (range 4–30 cm, average 10 cm). They are well defined but not encapsulated. On cut surface, the tumors may show bony or cartilaginous change. Cystic areas as well as areas of hemorrhage and necrosis may be identified.

Histological Features

The tumors are similar to the ones diagnosed in the bone (Figs. 9.72, 9.73, and 9.74). They are predominantly composed of a malignant pleomorphic spindle cell proliferation. These spindle cells have hyperchromatic nuclei and scant cytoplasm and are admixed with an osteoid or bony matrix as well as scattered osteoclast-like giant cells (Figs. 9.75, 9.76, 9.77, and 9.78). Cytologic atypia and mitotic activity are usually readily identified (Fig. 9.79). Some tumors may exhibit areas resembling fibrosarcoma or malignant cartilage, in a similar pattern to those tumors arising in the bone (Fig. 9.80).

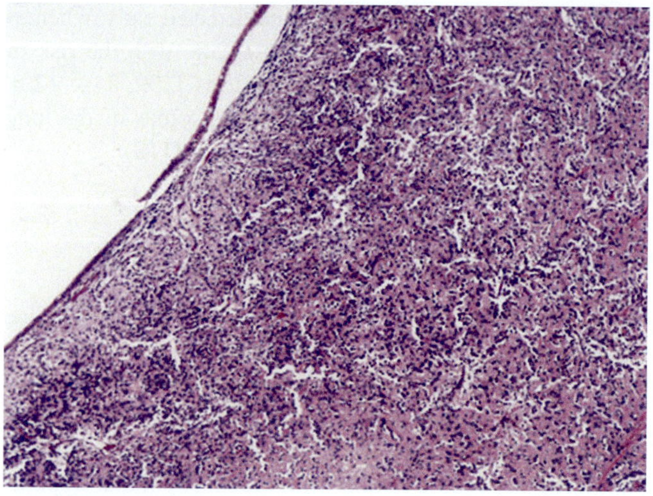

Fig. 9.72 Low-power view of pulmonary osteosarcoma undermining the bronchial epithelium

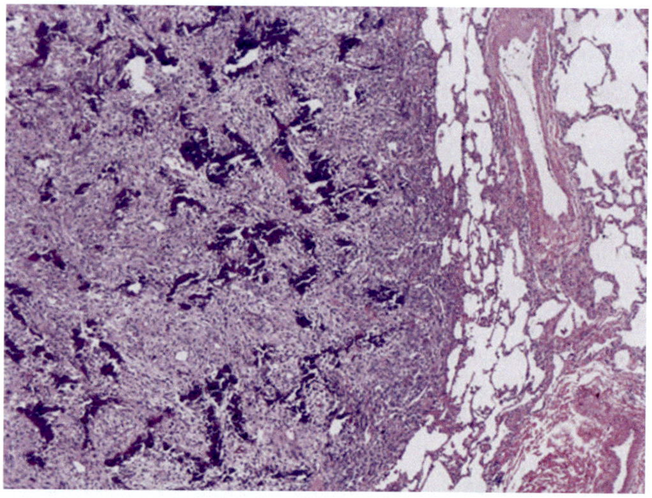

Fig. 9.73 Pulmonary osteosarcoma sharply circumscribed from the surrounding pulmonary parenchyma

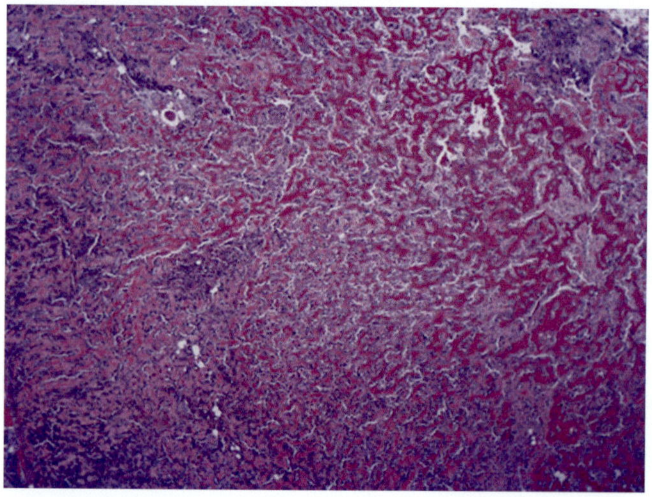

Fig. 9.74 Pulmonary osteosarcoma characterized by a bony matrix and pleomorphic spindle cell proliferation.

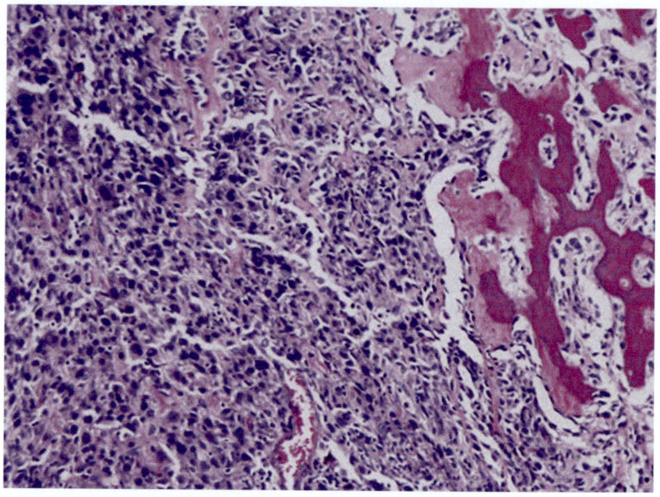

Fig. 9.75 Malignant spindle cell proliferation in close apposition with malignant bone in pulmonary osteosarcoma

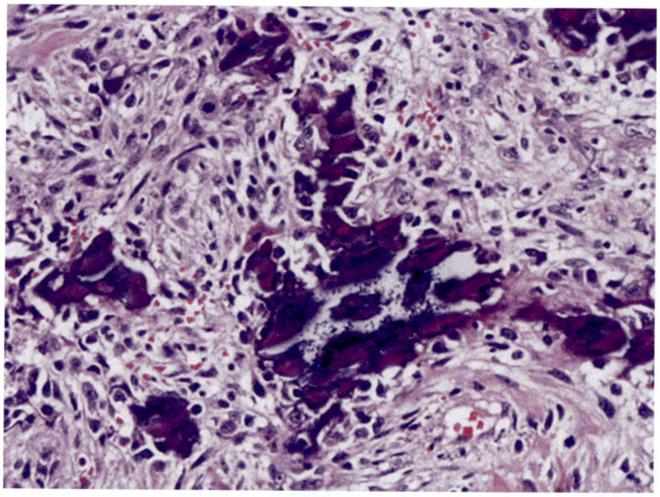

Fig. 9.76 High-power view of malignant osteoid lacking osteoblastic rimming in pulmonary osteosarcoma

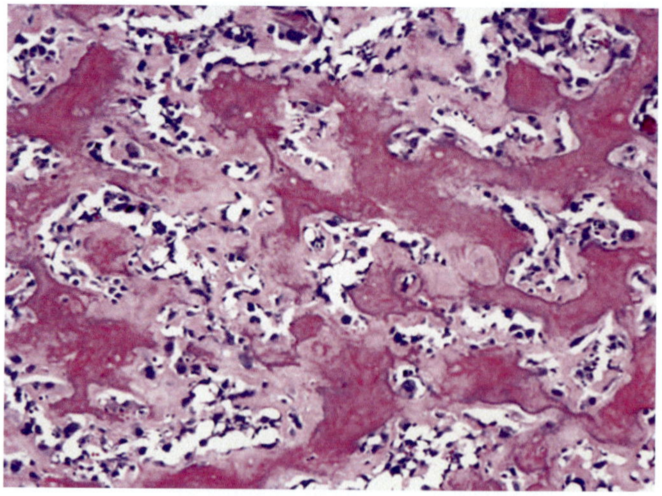

Fig. 9.77 Prominent osteoid formation in pulmonary osteosarcoma

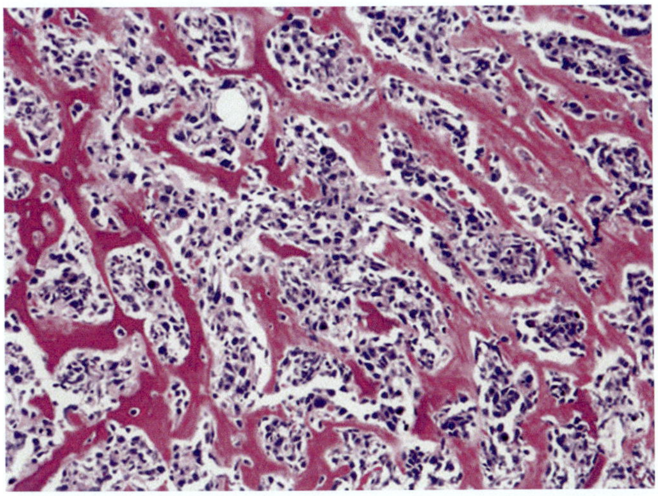

Fig. 9.78 Pulmonary osteosarcoma showing malignant spindle cells intermixed with osteoid

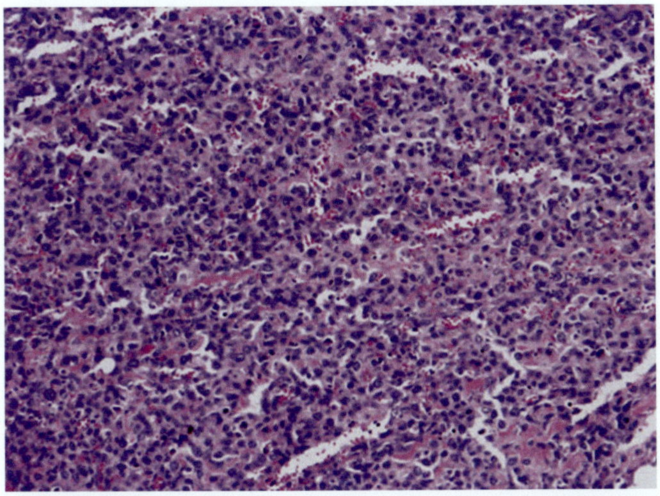

Fig. 9.79 High mitotic activity and cytologic atypia in pulmonary osteosarcoma

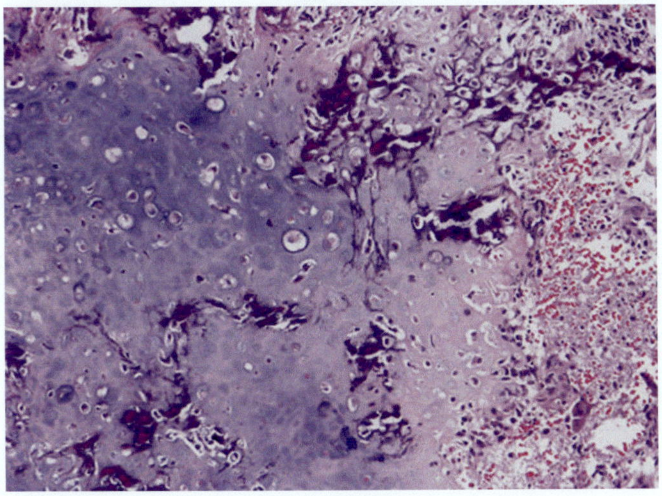

Fig. 9.80 Malignant cartilage in pulmonary osteosarcoma

Immunohistochemical and Molecular Features

The spindle cells in pulmonary osteosarcoma are positive for vimentin and osteonectin and negative for a range of other markers including epithelial markers, desmin, myoglobin, CD34, S-100, SMA, TTF-1, and osteopontin [143, 144]. A single case of primary pulmonary osteosarcoma has been investigated for molecular abnormalities using immunohistochemical and cytogenetic techniques [139]. By immunohistochemistry, strong expression of bcl-2 and cyclin D1 was observed, while comparative genomic hybridization of this case demonstrated a higher degree of genetic gains or losses than in cases of other extraskeletal osteosarcomas [139].

Differential Diagnosis

As with other lung sarcomas, metastatic disease from a bone or extraskeletal primary has to be excluded by complete clinical history and imaging techniques. In addition, an important differential diagnosis for pulmonary osteosarcoma is carcinosarcoma. Pulmonary carcinosarcoma is a biphasic neoplasm composed of epithelial and mesenchymal elements. Since the mesenchymal element often takes the form of osteosarcoma, extensive sampling and examination of the tissue is required to detect even small foci of a malignant epithelial component and to exclude carcinosarcoma. Bone formation may also be seen in some other primary lung neoplasms including carcinomas and other types of sarcoma. However, the bone in these cases will be metaplastic in nature rather than malignant osteoid.

Treatment and Prognosis

Complete surgical resection is the main treatment for patients with primary osteosarcoma of the lung. Chemotherapy and radiation have been reported to be useful in some cases of extraosseous osteosarcoma [145], but the effects of adjuvant therapy have not been proven for the pulmonary variant due to the rarity of these tumors [143]. Pulmonary osteosarcomas are highly aggressive tumors that show a high propensity to recur and metastasize, and most patients die within a year of diagnosis [142]. The longest surviving patient has been reported to be alive 42 months after resection, albeit with widespread metastasis [140].

Tumors of Adipocytic Origin

Tumors showing adipocytic differentiation are very common lesions in the soft tissue; however, in the lung these tumors are rare. Pulmonary lipomas are the most common tumors of this group, while primary pulmonary angiomyolipomas or liposarcomas have only been sporadically reported.

Pulmonary Lipoma

Although lipomas are the most common tumors of the soft tissues, their presentation as a primary lung tumor is infrequent and their incidence is estimated to range from 0.1 to 0.5 % of all lung tumors [146, 147]. The vast majority of pulmonary lipomas are endobronchial lesions and are thought to arise from the submucosal adipose tissue [146]; intraparenchymal lipomas are extremely uncommon with approximately ten reported cases in the world literature. These tumors may originate from the fatty tissue in the wall of peripheral bronchi or arise from subpleural adipose tissue [148, 149]. Interestingly, only 31 % of pulmonary lipomas are diagnosed correctly on bronchial biopsy, thereby often delaying definitive diagnosis until after surgical resection [150].

Clinical Features

Pulmonary lipomas preferentially arise in middle-aged adults with a mean age of 60 years. There is a strong male predominance. The majority of patients present with symptoms of bronchial obstruction (productive cough, hemoptysis, dyspnea, fever, obstructive pneumonia) while others are asymptomatic and the tumors are incidental findings on chest radiographs [150]. On CT scanning, the tumors are well-defined homogenous lesions of fat density and endoscopically present as pedunculated, sessile, or dumbbell-shaped masses with a soft yellowish appearance [149].

Gross Features

Pulmonary lipomas are well-circumscribed tumors with a homogeneous yellow, soft cut surface. Endobronchial lesions often have a polypoid configuration, while parenchymal tumors are surrounded by lung parenchyma. The average tumor size is around 2 cm, but some may grow larger than 7 cm [150, 151].

Histological Features

The tumors are well-circumscribed lesions and most show the classical morphology of lipomas as described in more common locations: lobules of mature adipocytes traversed by thin fibrovascular septa (Figs. 9.81, 9.82, and 9.83). In an endobronchial location, the lesions are often covered by a rim of overlying normal respiratory epithelium. The lesions lack cytologic atypia, mitotic activity, hemorrhage, or necrosis. Rarely, some neoplasms may contain a prominent but bland spindle cell proliferation or floret-like giant cells reminiscent of the changes seen in the so-called spindle cell and pleomorphic variants of lipoma of the soft tissue [151, 152].

Differential Diagnosis

The differential diagnosis for pulmonary lipoma primarily includes chondroid hamartoma. The latter is characterized by a proliferation of various tissue types including cartilage, fat, smooth muscle, and fibrous tissue. In some of these cases the fatty component may predominate, requiring close examination to identify the other elements in order to arrive at the correct diagnosis. In those rare cases, in which a spindle cell

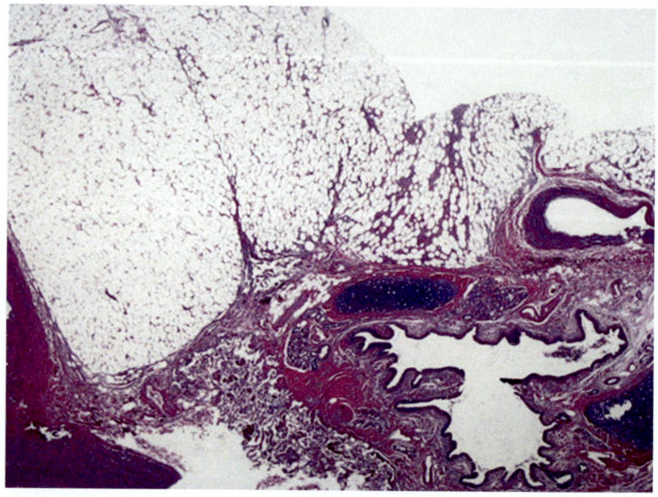

Fig. 9.81 Low-power view of pulmonary lipoma composed of mature adipose tissue

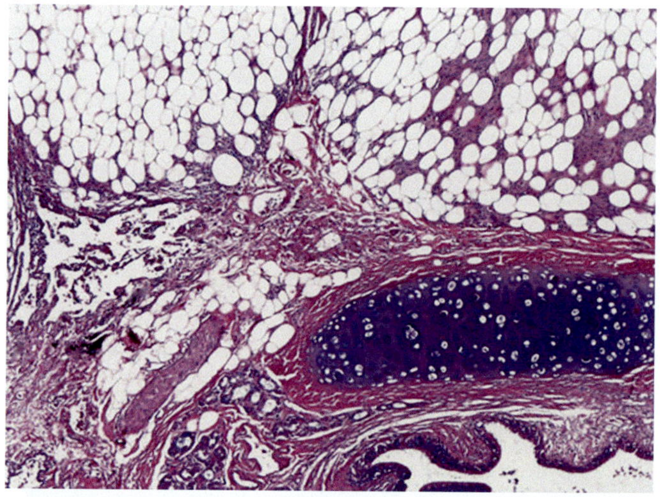

Fig. 9.82 Pulmonary lipoma in close association to bronchial system

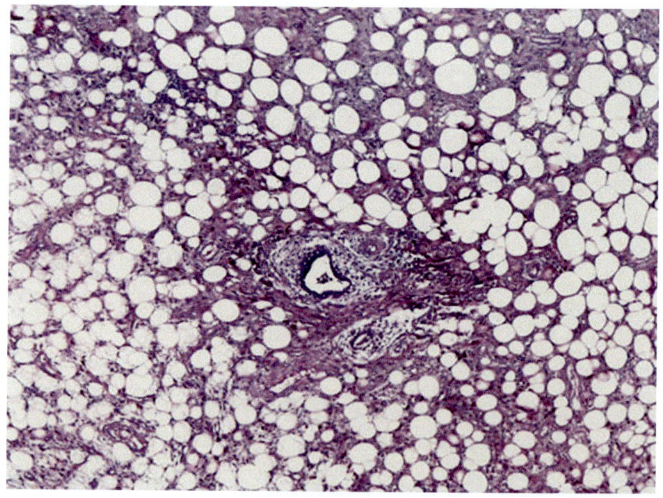

Fig. 9.83 Lipoma of the lung with sparing of the bronchial structures

component is present, malignant spindle cell tumors (sarcoma or sarcomatoid carcinoma) may enter the differential diagnosis. The lack of cytologic atypia, mitotic activity and the presence of areas of more conventional lipoma will usually lead to the correct diagnosis.

Treatment and Prognosis

Since pulmonary lipomas are considered entirely benign lesions that do not harbor any risk for malignant transformation [151, 153], a conservative surgical approach in the form of bronchoscopic resection is the treatment of choice [150]. In cases of peripheral tumors or contraindications for bronchoscopic treatment, more extensive surgical intervention may be necessary [150].

Pulmonary Angiomyolipoma

Angiomyolipoma is a rare tumor that most often occurs in the kidney and in 50 % of cases is associated with tuberous sclerosis [154]. Extrarenal angiomyolipomas are uncommon tumors and have been described in various organ systems including the lung. The number of cases of pulmonary angiomyolipomas, however, is small with less than ten reported cases in the English literature [155–160]. Contrary to renal angiomyolipomas, extrarenal tumors are well demarcated, easily resectable, and not necessarily associated with the tuberous sclerosis complex [155, 156]. Pulmonary angiomyolipomas may present as solitary or multifocal lesions and may be seen in association with other extrarenal angiomyolipomas [158, 159].

Clinical Features

Pulmonary angiomyolipomas have been described in patients ranging in age from 36 to 68 years with slight female predilection. Chest pain, fatigue, or back pain is the most common presenting symptoms; in patients with tuberous sclerosis, the tumors may be detected during workup of other lesions associated with this complex. On CT the lesions present as small, well-demarcated low-density non-enhancing nodules.

Gross Features

On gross examination pulmonary angiomyolipomas present as a well demarcated but unencapsulated nodules of tan-yellow color and rubbery consistency. The lesions may be solitary or multifocal.

Histological Features

The tumors are composed of mature fat cells admixed with numerous thick-walled blood vessels and bundles of smooth muscle cells (Figs. 9.84 and 9.85) [155, 156]. The smooth muscle cells often show accentuation around blood vessels and possess an oval shape with clear cytoplasm and irregular nuclei (Figs. 9.86 and 9.87). The vessels vary in size and may show walls of uneven thickness. An elastic lamina is usually not identified in the vessel wall. Mitotic figures and necrosis are generally absent.

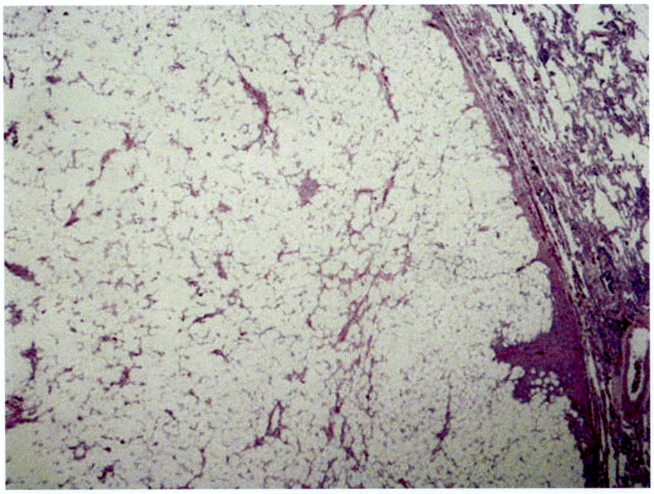

Fig. 9.84 Low-power view of angiomyolipoma of lung

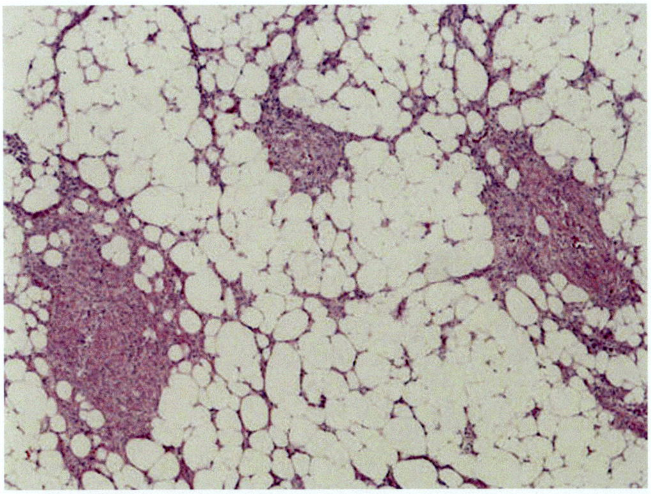

Fig. 9.85 Pulmonary angiomyolipoma of lung composed of mature fat, thick-walled blood vessels, and smooth muscle proliferation

Immunohistochemical and Molecular Features

Although histologically identical to renal angiomyolipomas, pulmonary angiomyolipomas may differ slightly in their immunohistochemical profile [155]. The smooth muscle cells of renal angiomyolipomas often show reactivity for HMB45, whereas the pulmonary tumors may [158–160] or may not express this marker [155–157]. The smooth muscle bands may further stain positive with muscle markers like SMA, desmin, and caldesmon [155–158]. Pancytokeratin and S-100 protein are usually negative [155–160]. In renal angiomyolipomas associated with the tuberous sclerosis complex, allelic loss of tuberous sclerosis complex (TSC) 1

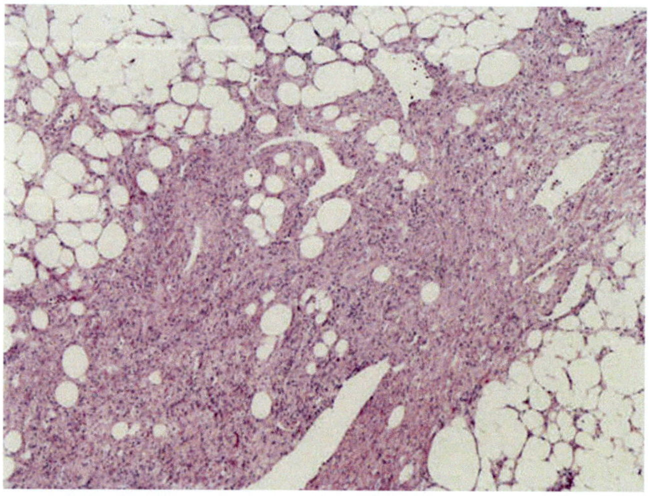

Fig. 9.86 Prominent smooth muscle component in pulmonary angiomyolipoma

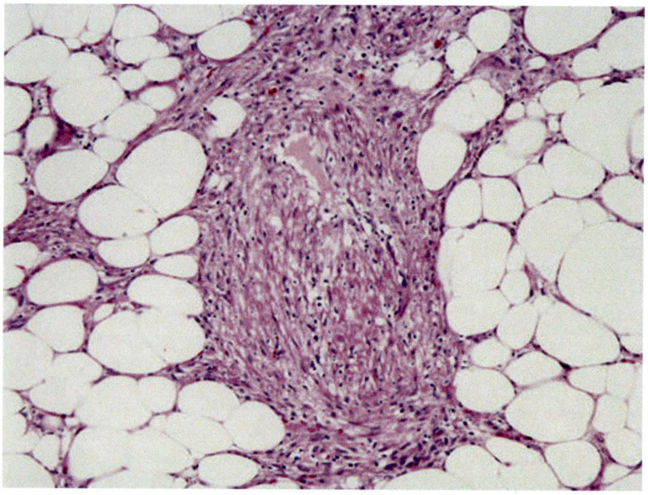

Fig. 9.87 Higher power view of pulmonary angiomyolipoma with prominent smooth muscle cells surrounding blood vessels

or 2 has been described [161]; however, this association has so far not been identified in pulmonary angiomyolipoma [159].

Differential Diagnosis

Angiomyolipomas of the lung have to be differentiated from other fat-containing lesions occurring in the pulmonary system. Among these, lipomas are rare neoplasms involving the lung. Lipomas, however, are composed entirely of mature adipocytes and lack the vascular and smooth muscle components that characterize angiomyolipoma. Pulmonary hamartoma is another lesion that is composed of various tissue elements including cartilage, fat, entrapped respiratory epithelium, smooth muscle, and fibrous tissue. Contrary to angiomyolipoma, these tumors, in addition to their typical cartilaginous elements, are devoid of a prominent vascular component.

Treatment and Prognosis

In contrast to renal angiomyolipomas, pulmonary angiomyolipomas are noninvasive lesions that are easily resected and run a benign clinical course [155, 156]. Despite this, some authors have argued that since some renal and hepatic angiomyolipomas have shown malignant behavior, pulmonary angiomyolipomas should be viewed as tumors with uncertain malignant potential, at least until more follow-up becomes available in a larger number of cases [159].

Pulmonary Liposarcoma

Pulmonary liposarcomas have only been reported in a handful of case reports, and some of them are either not well documented or may have arisen from the pulmonary artery or mediastinum [162–166]. Indeed, in the thorax liposarcomas are more commonly found originating in the mediastinum or from the chest wall. Due to the scarcity of this tumor in the lung, reliable data especially about treatment and prognosis are still lacking.

Clinical Features

Primary pulmonary liposarcomas have been described in patients with an age range from 18 to 49 years with no specific gender predilection. The most common presenting symptoms are cough, dyspnea, and chest pain. CT scanning shows well-defined lobulated masses of low density [163].

Gross Features

Liposarcomas of the lung are usually well-defined lesions that may either arise in an endobronchial location or in the peripheral lung. When associated with a bronchus, the tumors may have a polypoid configuration. Generally, the tumors have a homogenous soft and yellow cut surface. The tumor size can range from 1.5 cm to very large tumors involving the whole hemithorax.

Histological Features

Liposarcomas of the lung show very similar morphological features to their soft tissue counterparts. In addition to the classical well-differentiated variant of liposarcoma, myxoid (Figs. 9.88, 9.89, and 9.90) and pleomorphic subtypes have also been described in the lung [162–165].

Differential Diagnosis

The most important issue when encountering a liposarcoma in the lung is exclusion of metastatic disease from an extrapulmonary primary. In cases of well-differentiated liposarcoma, pulmonary lipoma may be included in the differential

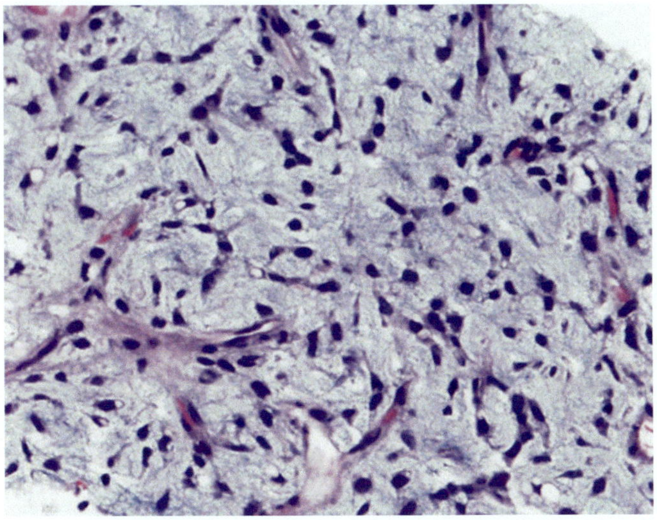

Fig. 9.88 Myxoid variant of pulmonary liposarcoma of lung

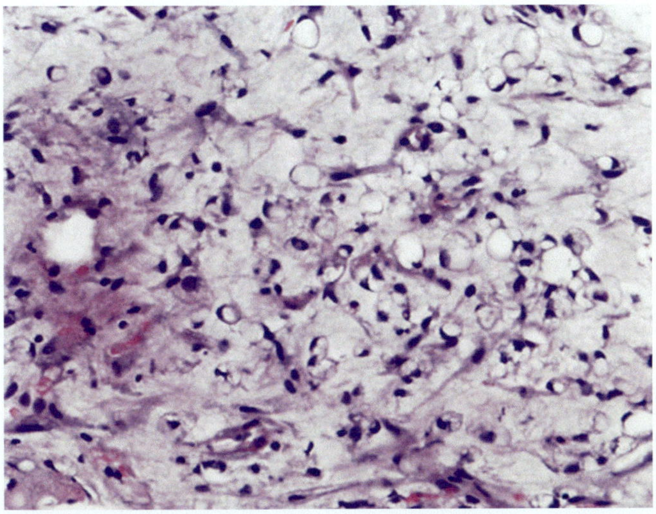

Fig. 9.89 Scattered lipoblasts embedded in a myxoid matrix in pulmonary liposarcoma of the lung

diagnosis. The latter will usually not show any lipoblasts, atypical stromal cells, and variation in cell size and shape—features that are commonly seen in liposarcomas.

Treatment and Prognosis

In the few cases described in the literature, the primary treatment of choice for pulmonary liposarcoma is complete surgical resection. Adjuvant chemoradiaton has been applied in isolated cases, with varying success [162, 165]. Liposarcomas of the lungs are considered aggressive neoplasms, which appear to have high intraoperative mortality [163, 166] and low survival rates (6–8 months) [162, 165]. Only a single patient was alive and free of disease 1 year after the operation [164].

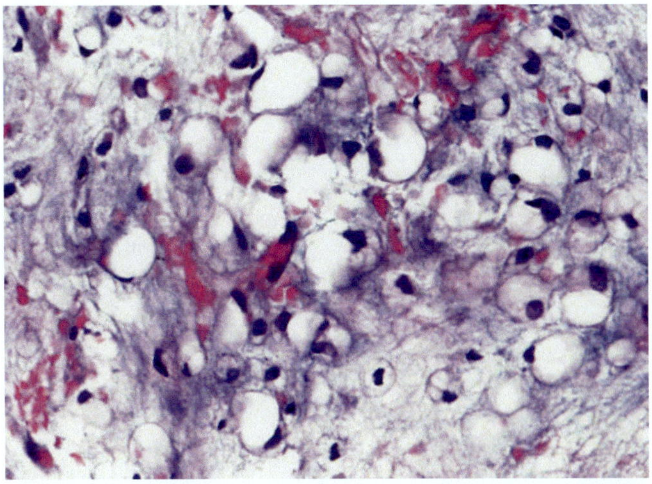

Fig. 9.90 High-power view of myxoid liposarcoma of lung showing adipocytes embedded in a prominent myxoid matrix

Tumors with Myxoid Features

Myxoid tumors of the lung encompass a group of very rare benign and malignant neoplasms that have only sporadically been reported. Among these, myxomas, angiomyxoma, aggressive angiomyxoma, and malignant myxoid endobronchial tumors have been described [167–173]. The latter have not been characterized fully and may actually represent examples of malignant salivary-gland-type tumors such as carcinoma ex-pleomorphic adenoma [173].

Myxoma, Angiomyxoma, Aggressive Angiomyxoma, and Malignant Myxoid Endobronchial Tumor

Clinical Features

Primary myxoid tumors of the lungs arise in the adult age group (27–70 years) with a slight female predominance. Presenting symptoms include cough, chest pain, and dyspnea. Some patients are asymptomatic and their tumors are found during a routine radiographic evaluation. Radiologically the tumors present as well-defined homogenous nodules, either in an endobronchial location or in the lung periphery.

Gross Features

Macroscopically, the benign and malignant myxoid tumors show similar features. The tumors are characterized by fairly well-circumscribed masses with a soft to rubbery consistency and glistening or gelatinous cut surface. Cystic degeneration may be focally observed. Areas of hemorrhage and necrosis should raise the suspicion for a more aggressive clinical course. The tumor size can range from 1.3 cm to more than 6 cm.

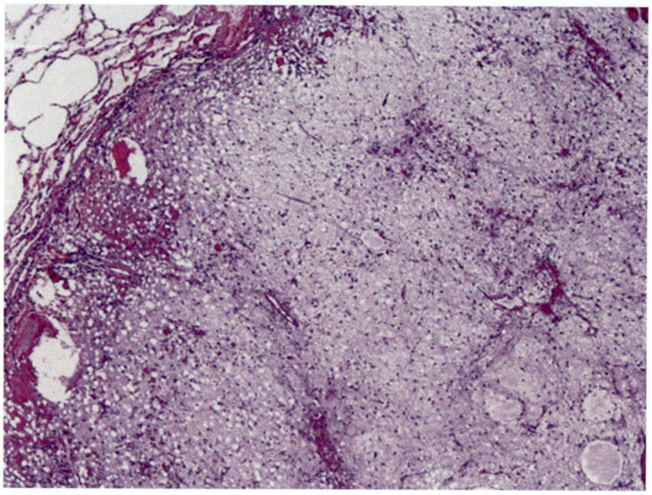

Fig. 9.91 Low-power view of pulmonary myxoma demonstrating the circumscribed nature of the lesion

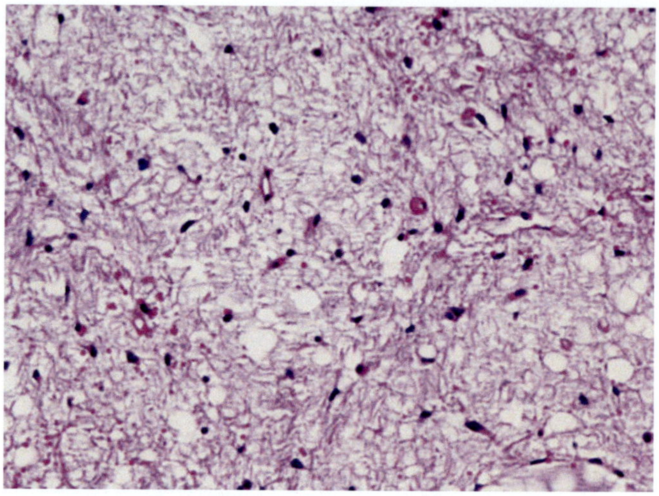

Fig. 9.93 High-power view of pulmonary myxoma showing lack of cytologic atypia or mitotic activity

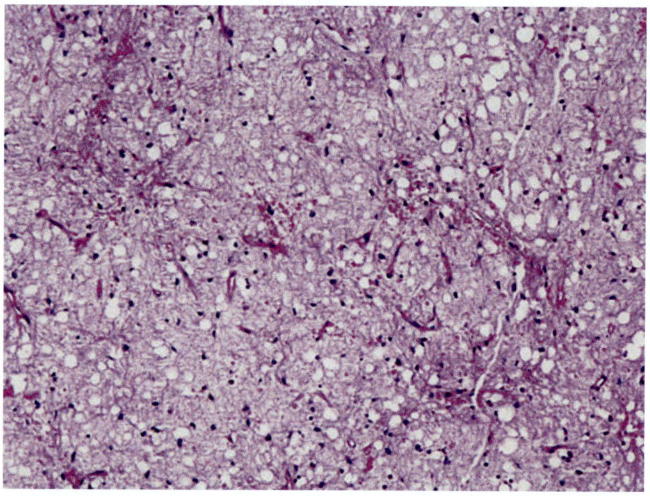

Fig. 9.92 Bland stellate-shaped cells are embedded in a hypovascular myxoid matrix in pulmonary myxoma

Histological Features

Pulmonary myxomas are well circumscribed but unencapsulated tumors composed of bland spindle or stellate cells embedded in a myxoid stroma (Figs. 9.91 and 9.92) [167, 170]. The lesions are distinctly hypocellular and lack a prominent vascular component (Fig. 9.93). Necrosis, hemorrhage, or mitotic activity is not identified in these lesions.

Pulmonary angiomyxomas show ill-defined borders to the surrounding lung parenchyma. In these tumors, the neoplastic stellate-shaped cells are dispersed in a prominent myxoid stroma. Contrary to pulmonary myxomas, an arborescent network of thin-walled small vessels and capillaries is characteristic [171].

Aggressive angiomyxoma of the lung is composed of scattered oval to spindle-shaped cells and variably sized thin- and thick-walled blood vessels embedded in a prominent myxoid stroma. The cellularity is generally low to moderate but may be increased around blood vessels. The vessels often show striking hyalinization in addition to medial hypertrophy. Mitotic figures and necrosis are generally not identified [172].

The so-called malignant myxoid endobronchial tumors are described as ill-defined nodules composed of myxoid stroma containing interweaving cords of small uniform round cells with scanty eosinophilic cytoplasm. The nodules are traversed by thin fibrous septa imparting a lobulated architecture. Occasional mitoses are typically seen. Overall, the histological features are reminiscent to those of extraskeletal myxoid chondrosarcoma or malignant salivary-gland-type tumors [173].

Immunohistochemical Features

The spindle cells of pulmonary myxoid neoplasms express vimentin but are negative for a range of other immunohistochemical markers like cytokeratin, S-100 protein, desmin, SMA, bcl-2, neurofilament, HMB45, and CD34 [170, 172, 173].

Differential Diagnosis

Myxoid changes can be seen in other primary lung neoplasm, for example, solitary fibrous tumor or pulmonary hamartoma. Immunohistochemical stains using CD34 and bcl-2 will be helpful in excluding solitary fibrous tumor, which will show positive reactivity for these markers contrary to myxoid neoplasms. The cartilage in pulmonary hamartoma can show prominent myxoid changes mimicking a true myxoid neoplasm. However, hamartomas will show additional tissue elements (fat, respiratory epithelium, fibrous tissue, smooth muscle), whereas myxoid neoplasms are composed of one tissue type only.

Treatment and Prognosis

The treatment of choice for primary myxoid neoplasms of the lung is complete surgical resection. For pulmonary myxomas surgical resection should be curative [170], while aggressive angiomyxomas have a tendency for local recurrence [171]. Based on individual circumstances, malignant myxoid tumors of the lung may require adjuvant treatment in addition to surgical resection.

Pulmonary Hyalinizing Spindle Cell Tumor with Giant Rosettes

Hyalinizing spindle cell tumor with giant rosettes is a rare tumor occurring mainly in the deep soft tissues of the extremities and is considered a variant of low-grade fibromyxoid sarcoma [174, 175]. Very occasionally this tumor can be identified in other sites; however, a lung origin has only been proposed for two cases [176, 177]. It has to be noted, though, that in the first reported case, the tumor was described as multiple bilateral nodules raising the possibility of metastatic disease despite a negative clinical history [176]. In the second case report, the tumor was a solitary lung lesion with associated small pleural metastasis [177].

Clinical Features

The two reported cases of pulmonary hyalinizing spindle cell tumor with giant rosettes involved two female patients aged 20 and 50 years. In one patient, the tumor was an incidental finding, whereas the other presented with chest pain. CT scanning shows a lobulated mass with focal calcification [177].

Gross Features

The tumors are described as well-circumscribed multinodular and firm masses surrounded by a thin pseudocapsule. The largest single tumor mass measured 7.5 cm in size [177]. The cut surface demonstrates a white to tan whorled appearance with focal myxoid change, cystic degeneration, and extensive calcification.

Histological Features

On histological examination, the tumors are composed of a proliferation of bland spindle cells arranged in various patterns that may show hyaline or myxoid areas (Fig. 9.94). The cellularity may vary in different areas of the same tumor. Hypocellular areas may be composed of hyalinized stroma, whereas in more cellular areas, the spindle cells may be arranged in crisscrossing fascicles (Fig. 9.95). The most characteristic finding is the presence of large collagen rosettes consisting of a central collagen core surrounded by a rim of spindle cells (Fig. 9.96). The tumor periphery may show hemangiopericytoma-like vessels and scattered giant cells. Mild cytologic atypia may be seen, but mitotic activity is

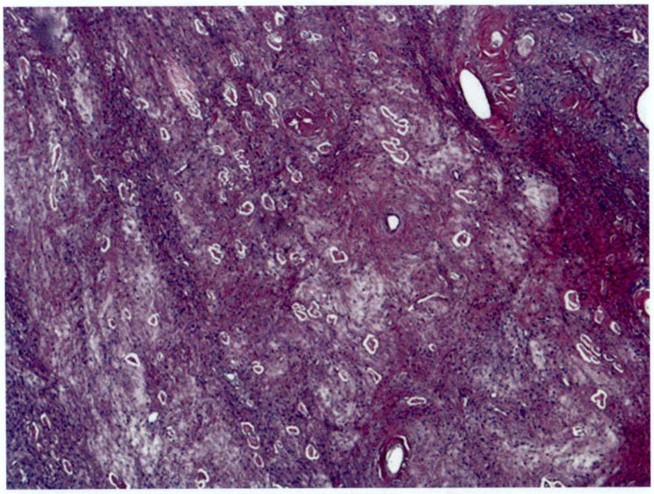

Fig. 9.94 Low-power view of hyalinizing spindle cell tumor with giant rosettes composed of a bland spindle cell proliferation demonstrating hyaline and myxoid areas

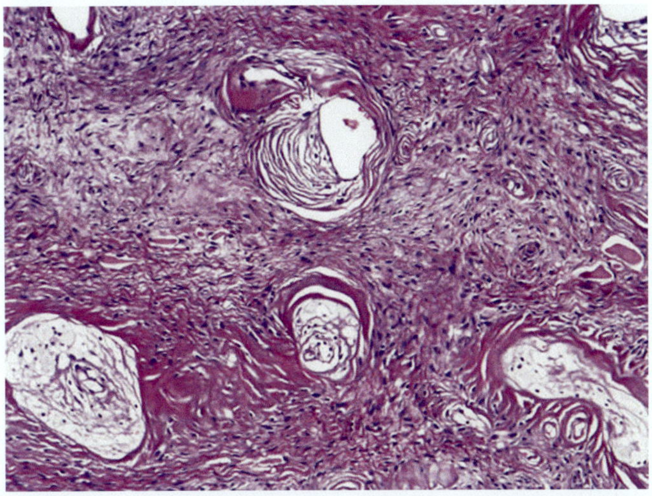

Fig. 9.95 Hyalinizing spindle cell tumor with giant rosettes showing stromal and vascular hyalinization

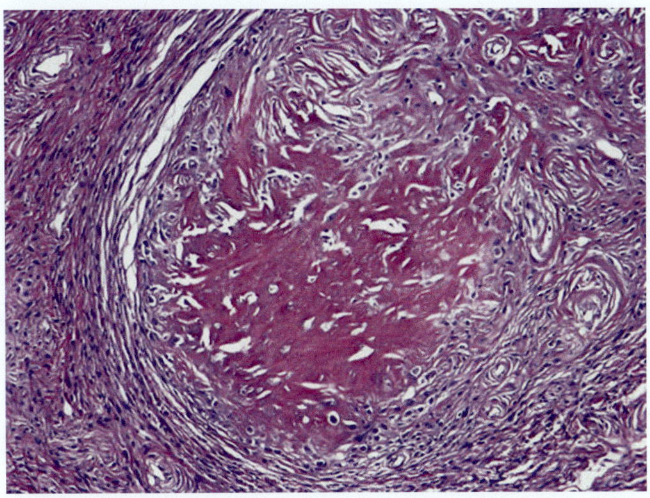

Fig. 9.96 Characteristic large collagen rosette in hyalinizing spindle cell tumor with giant rosettes

usually absent. Osseous metaplasia, foci of necrosis, and cystic degeneration are focally identified [176, 177].

Immunohistochemical and Molecular Features

The neoplastic cells of hyalinizing spindle cell tumor with giant rosettes stain positive for vimentin. S-100 protein may be focally positive in the rosette-like structures. Pancytokeratin, SMA, desmin, CD34, EMA, NSE, and calretinin are generally negative. One of the cases was examined cytogenetically and demonstrated the FUS-CREB3L2 fusion gene product resulting from a reciprocal translocation t (7;16), the same characteristic fusion transcript that has been described for their soft tissue counterparts [177–179].

Differential Diagnosis

First and foremost, metastatic soft tissue hyalinizing spindle cell tumor with giant rosettes has to be excluded by complete clinical and radiological examination. Furthermore, pulmonary solitary fibrous tumor may enter the differential diagnosis. Immunohistochemical studies may be of use in this setting demonstrating expression of CD34 and bcl-2 in solitary fibrous tumors but not in hyalinizing spindle cell tumor with giant rosettes.

Treatment and Prognosis

Although initially believed to be benign, hyalinizing spindle cell tumor with giant rosettes has been shown to be a low-grade sarcoma that may produce metastasis over time [175, 180, 181] and, indeed, in one of the reported cases of the lung metastasis to the pleura, was present at the time of diagnosis [177]. Complete surgical excision is therefore the treatment of choice, and long-term follow-up is advised.

Tumors of Neurogenic Origin

Primary lung tumors of neurogenic origin may be sporadic neoplasms or genetic lesions associated with neurofibromatosis. Whether benign or malignant, these tumors are very uncommon with an estimated incidence of 0.2–0.5 % of all pulmonary neoplasms [182, 183].

Pulmonary Neurofibroma

Thoracic neurofibromas are most commonly seen in the posterior mediastinum and only rarely present as primary pulmonary tumors. Although most of these are sporadic tumors, the possibility of these tumors arising in association with neurofibromatosis should be kept in mind.

Clinical Features

Pulmonary neurofibromas are predominantly tumors of the adult age group (18–67 years) but can rarely be seen in children as well [184]. The tumors present with symptoms such as cough, expectoration, and dyspnea, owing to their often endobronchial location. Radiologically, they are described as circumscribed lung masses that may be associated with a major bronchus. Generally, the tumors are solitary neoplasms; however, a case of multiple pulmonary tumors has also been reported [185].

Gross Features

Grossly, the tumors are well-defined masses that may range in size from less than 3 cm to more than 9 cm [186, 187]. When located endobronchially, the lesions appear as smooth polypoid intraluminal masses [188]. Parenchymal lesions are often encapsulated. On cut surface, the tumors are white to gray colored and of firm consistency.

Histological Features

The typical histological findings include a well-circumscribed spindle cell proliferation embedded in a fibrocollagenous stroma (Fig. 9.97). The neoplastic cells have elongated to pear-shaped nuclei and scant eosinophilic cytoplasm (Fig. 9.98). Mitotic activity or cytologic atypia is absent. In some areas, the stroma can show prominent myxoid or fibrotic changes (Fig. 9.99). Hemorrhage and necrosis are not usually identified.

Immunohistochemical Features

The neoplastic cells in pulmonary neurofibromas show positive staining for S-100 and neurofilament protein [188].

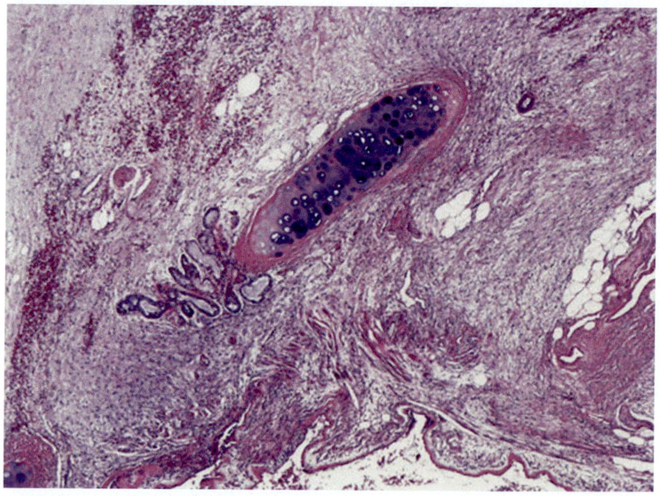

Fig. 9.97 Low magnification of neurofibroma of the lung

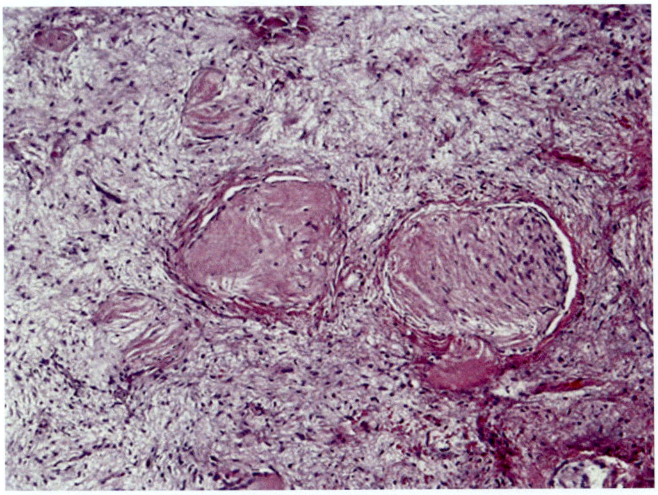

Fig. 9.98 Bland spindle cell proliferation surrounding nerve trunks in pulmonary neurofibroma

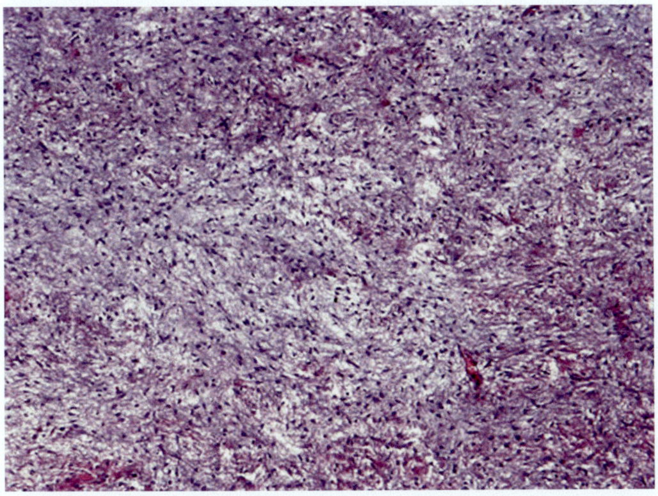

Fig. 9.99 Myxoid change in pulmonary neurofibroma

Differential Diagnosis

Other spindle cell lesions with similar morphology enter the differential diagnosis for pulmonary neurofibroma. Tumors like pulmonary leiomyoma or intrapulmonary solitary fibrous tumor are composed of a bland spindle cell proliferation similar to the features of neurofibroma. Immunohistochemical studies may aid in the differential diagnosis of these lesions; leiomyomas typically show strong and diffuse positivity of smooth muscle markers like SMA and desmin, and solitary fibrous tumor is generally positive for CD34 and bcl-2. These markers will not be expressed by neurofibroma, which will show staining for S-100 and neurofilament protein only.

Treatment and Prognosis

The treatment of pulmonary neurofibroma consists of complete surgical resection. In endobronchial tumors this may be achieved by transbronchial snaring and laser abrasion [188]. Complete surgical resection is regarded as curative in these patients.

Pulmonary Schwannoma

Schwannomas are benign tumors of peripheral nerve sheath origin. In the thoracic cavity, these tumors are commonly found in the posterior mediastinum and the chest wall [189]. Primary intrapulmonary schwannomas, originating from nerve fibers associated with the bronchopulmonary system, however, are uncommon tumors, accounting for 0.2–0.5 % of all pulmonary neoplasms [182, 183].

Clinical Features

Pulmonary schwannomas can arise in any age group and have been described in patients ranging from 5 to 83 years of age [189]. Females are slightly more commonly affected than males. The presenting symptoms largely depend on tumor location and for endobronchial tumors consist of cough, shortness of breath, obstructive pneumonia, or hemoptysis, whereas peripheral tumors are often asymptomatic [189]. Radiographically, the tumors present as rounded or lobulated masses with well-defined margins [189, 190]. Although most pulmonary schwannomas are sporadic lesions, some tumors may be associated with neurofibromatosis [191, 192].

Gross Features

The tumors are well encapsulated and of firm consistency. The cut surface is homogenous and may show cystic areas; hemorrhage, necrosis, and calcification are not usually identified [190]. The tumor size averages 4 cm with a range from 1.5 to 10 cm [189]. Intrapulmonary schwannomas most often arise in the peripheral lung, but endobronchial lesions are also more frequently described.

Histological Features

Pulmonary schwannomas are sharply circumscribed and surrounded by a thin capsule (Fig. 9.100). The characteristic morphologic feature is the presence of two growth patterns: Antoni A and Antoni B areas (Fig. 9.101). Antoni A areas are composed of compactly arranged spindle cells with elongated nuclei arranged in parallel rows creating a palisaded pattern with the formation of Verocay bodies (Figs. 9.102, 9.103, and 9.104). Antoni B areas are less cellular and show elongated spindle cells arranged in an irregular fashion and embedded in an edematous stroma (Figs. 9.105 and 9.106).

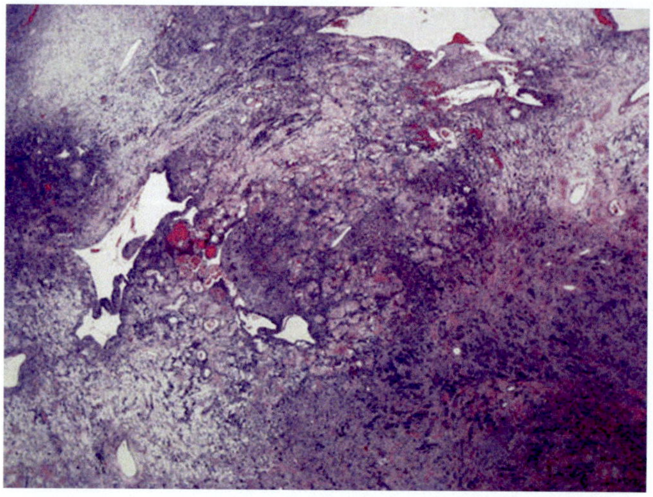

Fig. 9.100 Low-power view of pulmonary schwannoma

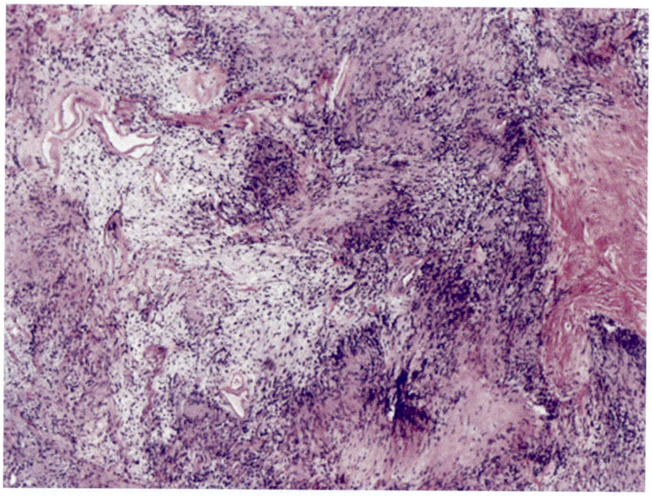

Fig. 9.101 Typical hypo- and hypercellular areas in pulmonary schwannoma

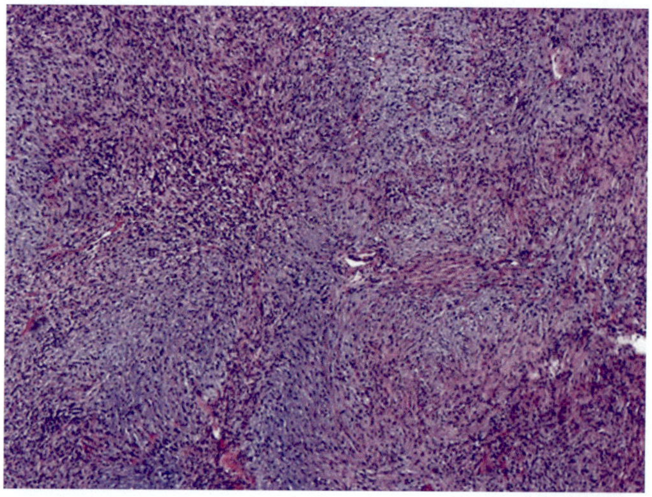

Fig. 9.102 Antoni A area in schwannoma characterized by a hypercellular spindle cell proliferation

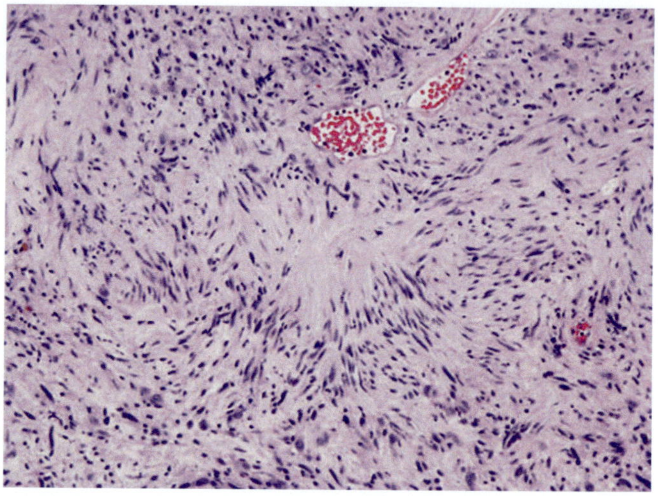

Fig. 9.103 Subtle palisading in pulmonary schwannoma

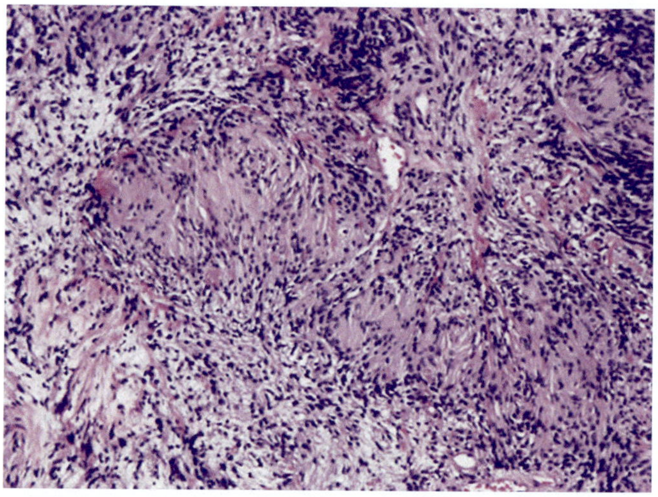

Fig. 9.104 Verocay body formation can be seen in pulmonary schwannoma

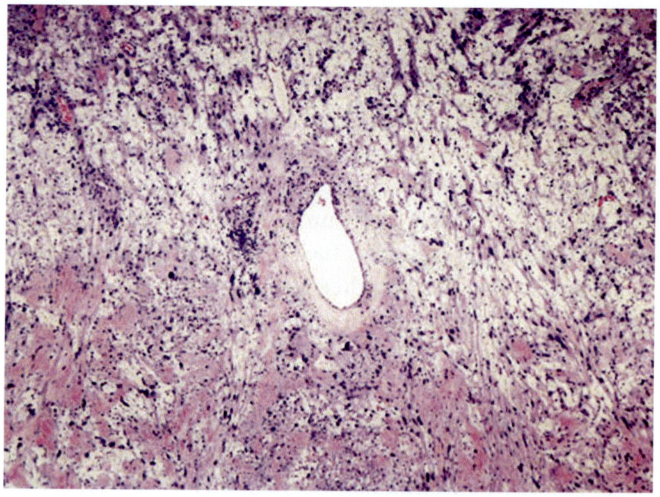

Fig. 9.105 Myxoid stroma in Antoni B areas of pulmonary schwannoma

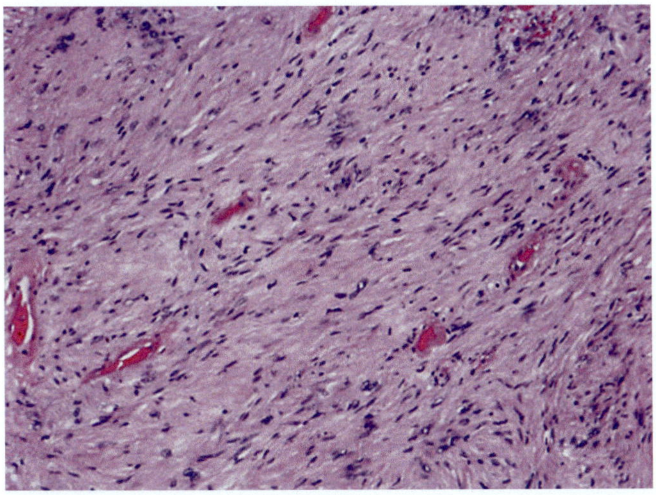

Fig. 9.106 Antoni B areas in pulmonary schwannoma composed of a hypocellular spindle cell proliferation

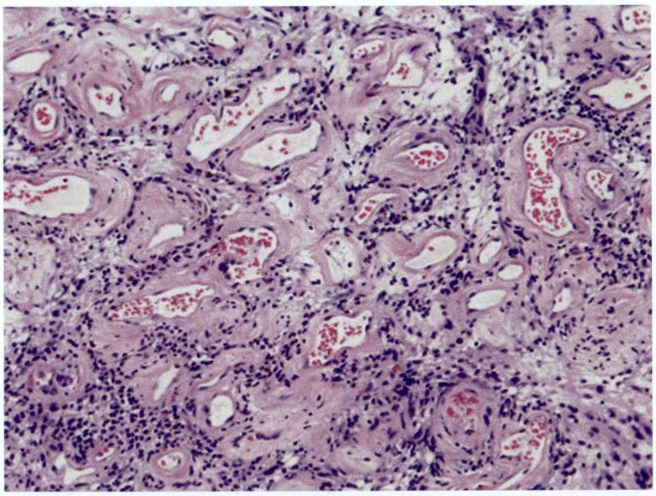

Fig. 9.107 Prominent hyalinized blood vessels are a characteristic finding in pulmonary schwannoma

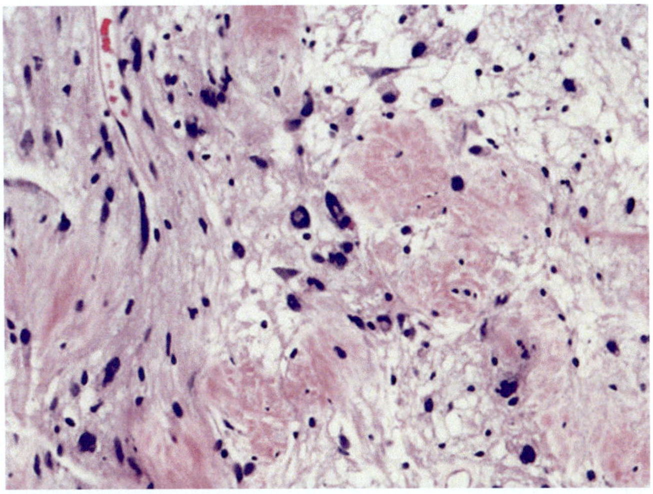

Fig. 9.108 Ancient type of pulmonary schwannoma characterized by atypical hyperchromatic spindle cells

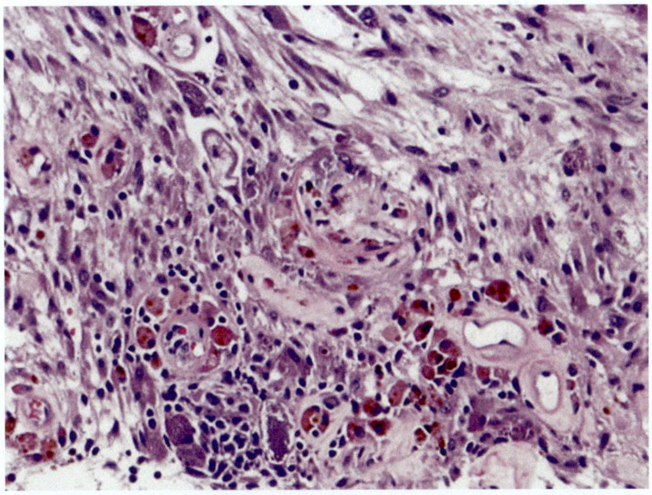

Fig. 9.109 Melanotic pigment can be identified in melanotic schwannomas

Microcyst formation and prominent hyalinized blood vessels are another typical finding in these areas (Fig. 9.107). Hemorrhage, necrosis, and mitotic activity are not typical findings in these tumors. Variants of schwannoma like the ancient type (Fig. 9.108), psammomatous melanotic type (Fig. 9.109), or cellular type have also been described in a primary pulmonary location [183, 193–195].

Immunohistochemical and Molecular Features

Pulmonary schwannomas demonstrate strong and diffuse nuclear and cytoplasmic positivity for S-100 protein and are negative for cytokeratin, desmin, HHF35, c-kit, and CEA [183, 189–193]. Flow cytometry performed on two cases showed diploid DNA profiles [183].

Differential Diagnosis

Pulmonary schwannomas may resemble other spindle cell tumors arising in the bronchopulmonary system. Among these, neurofibroma, leiomyoma, and spindle cell neuroendocrine carcinoma (carcinoid tumor) enter the differential diagnosis. Neurofibroma is another type of benign neurogenic tumor that infrequently affects the lung. Neurofibromas lack the typical Antoni A and B areas seen in schwannoma and only show focal immunohistochemical reactivity with S-100 protein in contrast to the diffuse staining characteristic for schwannoma. Leiomyomas can easily be differentiated using immunohistochemical studies; these tumors will express muscle markers including SMA and desmin and will lack reactivity with S-100 protein. Lastly, spindle cell neuroendocrine carcinoma can mimic pulmonary schwannoma. The use of immunohistochemical markers to detect neuroendocrine differentiation in the former can aid in the differential diagnosis.

Treatment and Prognosis

Surgical resection is the treatment of choice for pulmonary schwannomas as these are entirely benign tumors with an excellent prognosis.

Pulmonary Ependymoma

Extra-axial ependymomas are rare tumors that have been reported predominantly in the gynecologic tract, the pelvic area, and the mediastinum. To date, only two primary ependymomas of the lung have been described [196, 197], one of which arose near the site of a previously treated small cell lung carcinoma [196]. Despite various hypotheses including origin from heterotopic glial tissue, monodermal differentiation of a pulmonary teratoma, or a metaplastic event related to therapy, the histogenesis for these tumors in the lung is still uncertain [196].

Clinical Features

In the cases described, the patients affected have been females aged 48 and 64 years. In one patient the tumor was detected at routine surveillance for small cell carcinoma of the lung diagnosed and treated by chemo- and radiotherapy 2½ years earlier [196]. The other patient presented with dyspnea on exertion [197]. Radiographically, the tumors were solitary lung lesions with no evidence of hilar adenopathy.

Gross Features

The tumors have been described as circumscribed but unencapsulated masses which measured 2 and 17.5 cm in maximum dimension. The cut surface appears lobulated or multinodular and pale gray in color. Areas of hemorrhage, necrosis, and cystic degeneration can be appreciated.

Histological Features

The tumors are composed of plump and pleomorphic spindle cells with round to oval nuclei, prominent nucleoli, and abundant eosinophilic cytoplasm containing fine fibrils [196]. The tumors can show solid or pseudopapillary patterns or can be arranged in ill-defined fascicles with nuclear palisading. Perivascular pseudorosettes, increased mitotic activity, and foci of calcification are a common finding. Cystic changes and areas of necrosis may also be identified [196, 197].

Immunohistochemical Features

Positive immunohistochemical markers for pulmonary ependymoma include glial fibrillary acidic protein (GFAP), CK7, estrogen and progesterone receptors, high molecular weight cytokeratin, CAM5.2, CK18, EMA, S-100 protein, and vimentin. Staining is usually negative for neuroendocrine markers and CK20 [196, 197].

Differential Diagnosis

Pulmonary ependymomas may be mistaken for other spindle cell neoplasms of the lung. Sarcomatoid carcinoma may enter the differential diagnosis but can be excluded by the presence of nuclear palisading and pseudorosettes, features that are uncommon in carcinomas. In addition, the use of immunohistochemical stains, in this context especially keratins, GFAP, S-100 protein, and vimentin, may facilitate the correct diagnosis. Schwannomas are neoplasms that may also show nuclear palisading, but pseudorosettes are not a typical finding. In addition, schwannomas will be negative for GFAP and keratins.

Treatment and Prognosis

Although surgical resection has been performed in the cases reported, little is known about the use of adjuvant therapy and the prognosis of these tumors. Of the cases reported, one patient died 6 months post diagnosis while no follow-up was obtained in the other patient (196, 197).

Pulmonary Ganglioneuroma and Ganglioneuroblastoma

Ganglioneuromas and ganglioneuroblastomas of the lung are extremely uncommon tumors attributed to arise from the sympathetic component of the posterior pulmonary plexus [198]. Only a handful of cases of pulmonary ganglioneuroma [199–201] and three cases of pulmonary ganglioneuroblastoma [198, 202] have been reported in the literature. Of the latter, one case occurred in a patient suffering from multiple endocrine neoplasia (MEN) syndrome type 1 [202].

Clinical Features

Ganglioneuromas of the lung can affect both adults and children [199–201], whereas pulmonary ganglioneuroblastomas have been exclusively described in adults [198, 202]. Depending on exact tumor location, both lesions can produce symptoms of bronchial obstruction or be entirely asymptomatic.

Gross Features

Gross examination shows well-circumscribed tumors that can range from <1 cm to up to 5 cm. The tumors are pale-pink to gray-white with a firm consistency. On cut surface, the tumors appear fleshy and may be homogenous or show focal areas of hemorrhage or cystic change in cases of ganglioneuroblastomas.

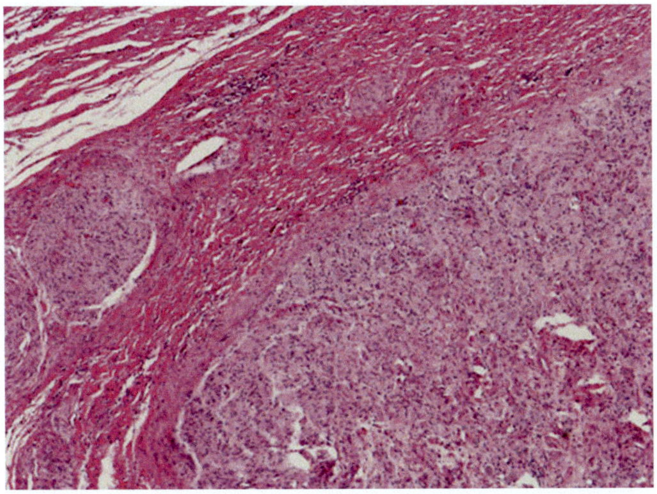

Fig. 9.110 Low-power view of pulmonary ganglioneuroma

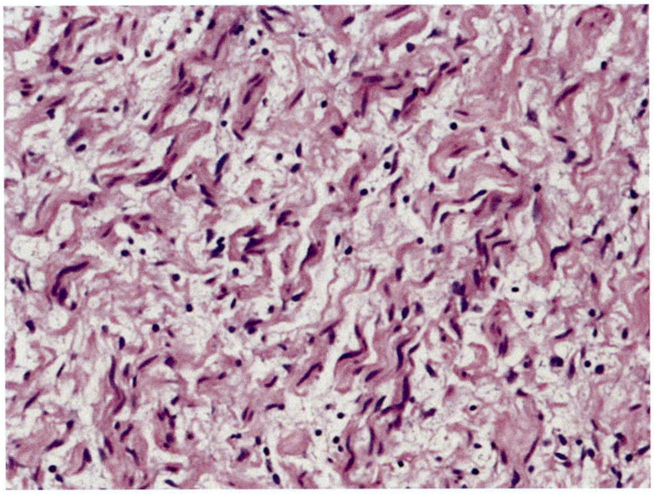

Fig. 9.112 Spindle cells embedded in a fibrocollagenous stroma in pulmonary ganglioneuroma

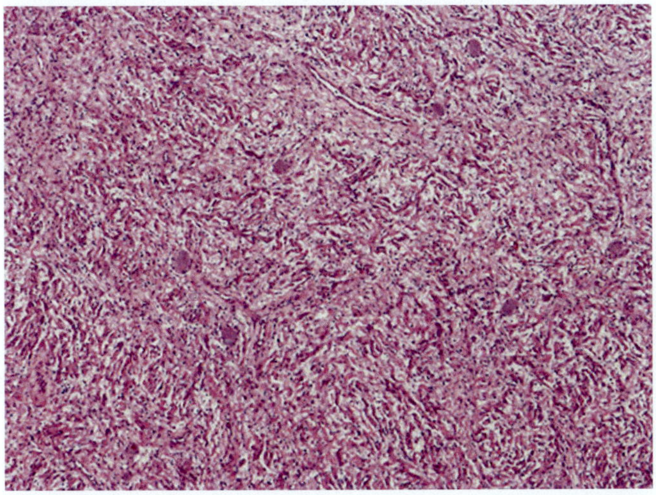

Fig. 9.111 Bland spindle cell proliferation in pulmonary ganglioneuroma

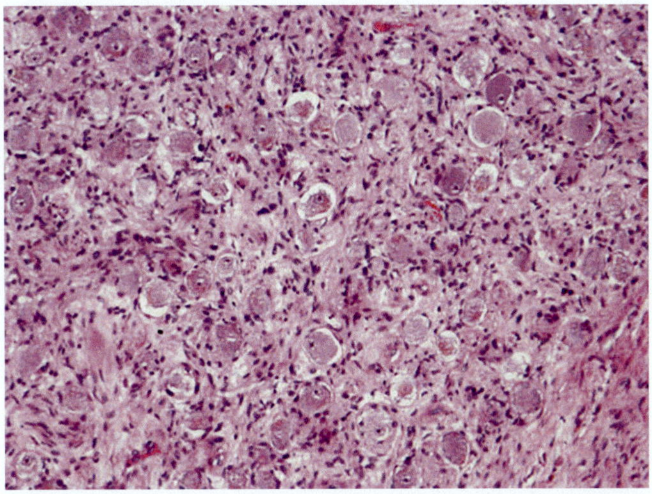

Fig. 9.113 Numerous ganglion cells are interspersed in pulmonary ganglioneuroma

Histological Features

Pulmonary ganglioneuromas are characterized by a similar spindle cell proliferation to that seen in neurofibroma (Figs. 9.110, 9.111, and 9.112). In addition, numerous ganglion cells with abundant pink cytoplasm and prominent eosinophilic nucleoli are interspersed with the spindle cell proliferation (Figs. 9.113 and 9.114). All cells have a mature appearance, and mitotic activity is absent.

Pulmonary ganglioneuroblastomas show a population of small undifferentiated cells with hyperchromatic nuclei, occasional punctuate nucleoli, and scanty cytoplasm embedded in a fibrillary neuropil matrix (Figs. 9.115, 9.116, and 9.117). Mitotic activity and nuclear atypia are usually present and occasionally Homer–Wright-type rosettes can be identified (Fig. 9.118) [202]. Areas of necrosis, cystic degeneration, and vascular invasion are also common findings [198]. Diffusely admixed with this component are prominent mature-appearing ganglion cells, hence the term "ganglioneuroblastoma" (Fig. 9.119). In some cases the presence of ganglion cells is not very conspicuous a fact that can further be challenging as these scattered ganglion cells can have an immature appearance.

Immunohistochemical Features

Immunohistochemical staining for S-100 and neurofilament protein as well as neuron-specific enolase usually show at least focal reactivity in the tumor cells; staining for cytokeratin, glial fibrillary acidic protein, and chromogranin is not observed [202]. In some cases in which the presence of ganglion cells is inconspicuous the use of NeuN may help detect these cells.

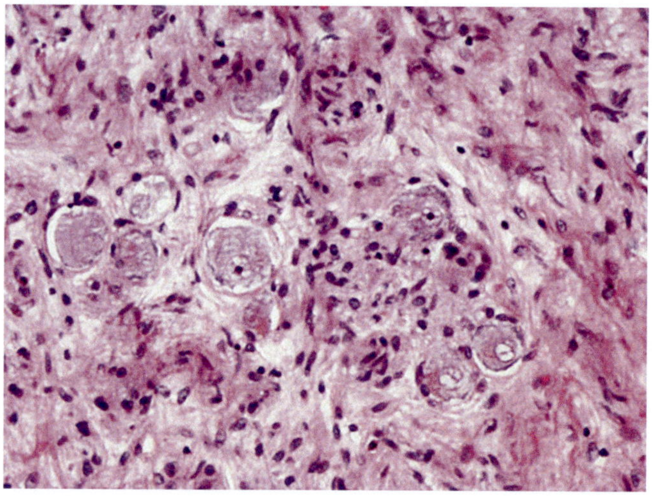

Fig. 9.114 High-power view of ganglion cells in pulmonary ganglioneuroma

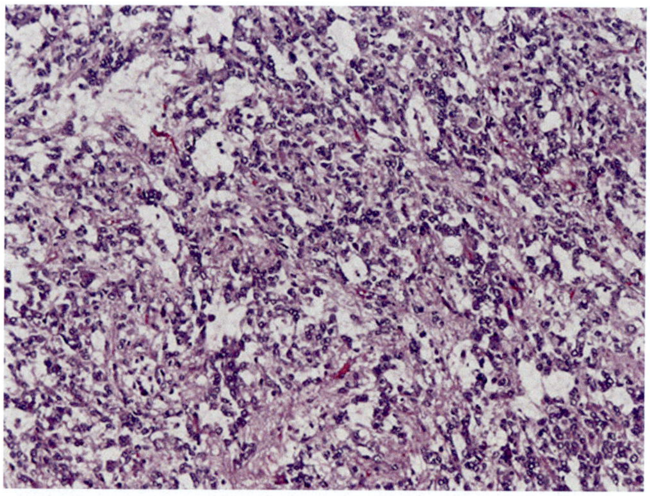

Fig. 9.115 Low-power view of pulmonary ganglioneuroblastoma showing prominent neuroblastomatous differentiation

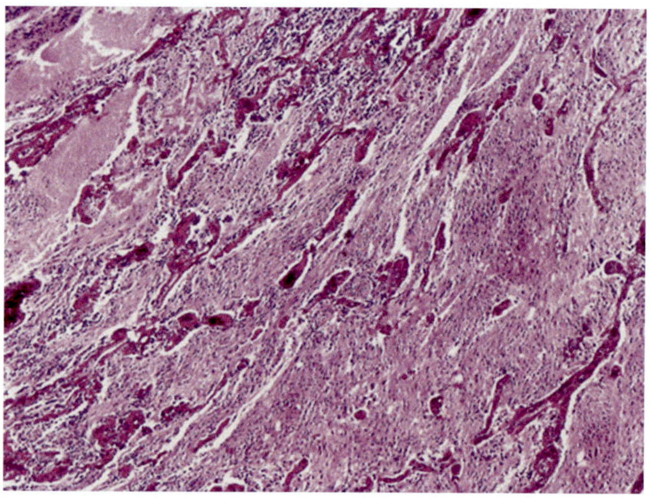

Fig. 9.116 Pulmonary ganglioneuroblastoma composed of small cells embedded in a neuropil matrix

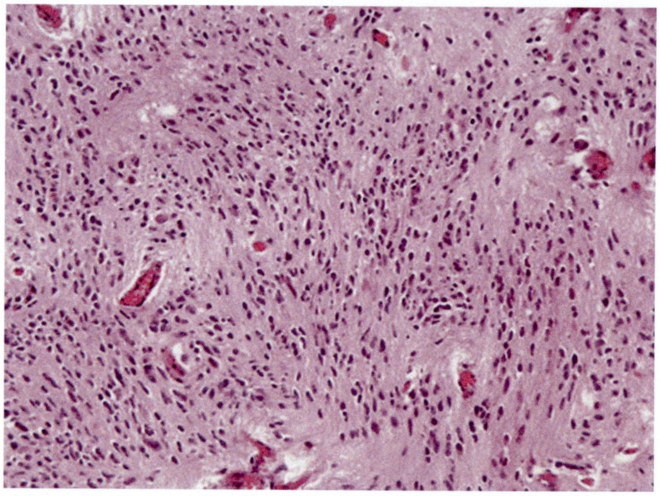

Fig. 9.117 Prominent fibrillary neuropil in pulmonary ganglioneuroblastoma

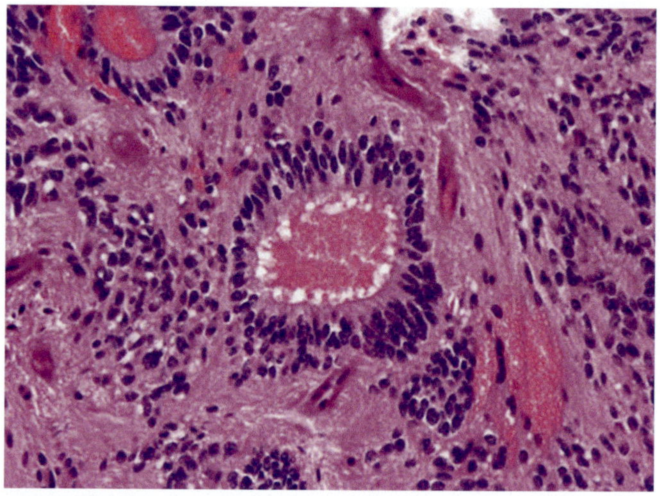

Fig. 9.118 Homer–Wright-type rosettes in pulmonary ganglioneuroblastoma

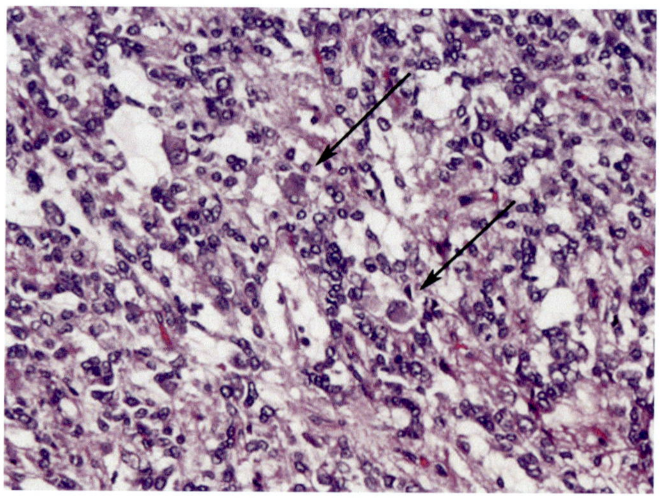

Fig. 9.119 Ganglion cells (*arrows*) interspersed with neuroblastoma cells in pulmonary ganglioneuroblastoma

Differential Diagnosis

The differential diagnosis for ganglioneuroma is similar to that for neurofibroma. The identification of ganglion cells and the use of immunohistochemical stains should aid in arriving at the correct diagnosis. Pulmonary ganglioneuroblastoma must be differentiated from other small round cell tumors of the lung. However, small cell carcinoma represents the most important tumor to exclude. In this setting the presence of ganglioneuromatous differentiation coupled with immunohistochemical staining for S-100 and neurofilament protein should favor a diagnosis of ganglioneuroblastoma.

Treatment and Prognosis

The treatment for both tumors consists of complete surgical resection. Pulmonary ganglioneuromas are benign tumors with an excellent prognosis, whereas ganglioneuroblastomas of the lung are malignant neoplasms with the potential to metastasize. The effectiveness of adjuvant treatment in these patients as well as the exact biologic behavior is difficult to assess given the low number of reported cases.

Pulmonary Malignant Peripheral Nerve Sheath Tumor

These tumors are also known as malignant schwannoma, neurogenic sarcoma, or neurofibrosarcoma. They account for approximately 10 % of soft tissue sarcomas and are often associated with neurofibromatosis [203, 204]. Malignant peripheral nerve sheath tumors originating in the lung are exceedingly rare; less than 25 cases have been described in the English literature [41, 92, 182, 183, 205–217].

Clinical Features

Primary malignant peripheral nerve sheath tumors of the lung are more common in adults with an age range from 19 to 74 years and slight male predilection. A single case has been reported, affecting a 2-year-old child without neurofibromatosis [214]. The majority of pulmonary malignant peripheral nerve sheath tumors are symptomatic and patients present with cough, chest pain, dyspnea, hemoptysis, weight loss, fever, and anorexia. More commonly the tumors arise in a peripheral location; only a few cases have been described involving the tracheobronchial system [215, 216]. CT scan of the chest often reveals a solid homogenous mass lesion that fails to show any more specific features. Very rarely, malignant peripheral nerve sheath tumor of the lung is associated with neurofibromatosis [183].

Gross Features

Malignant peripheral nerve sheath tumors of the lung can vary greatly in size and be as small as <1 cm or measure more than 20 cm in maximum dimension. The tumors are well-circumscribed masses with a white, firm, whorled cut surface. Areas of hemorrhage and necrosis may be identified.

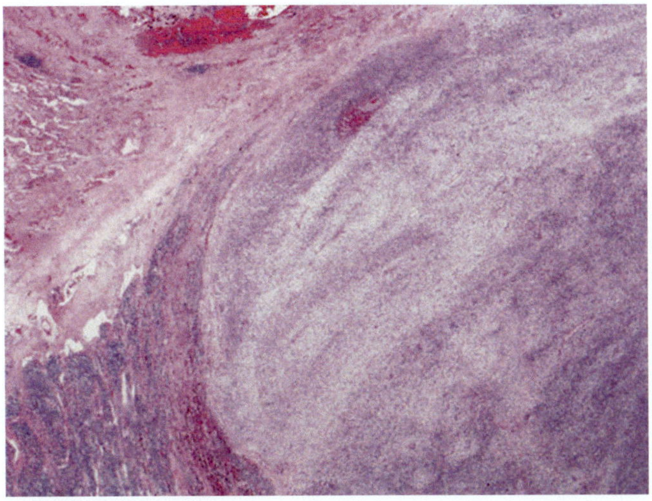

Fig. 9.120 Well-demarcated pulmonary malignant peripheral nerve sheath tumor

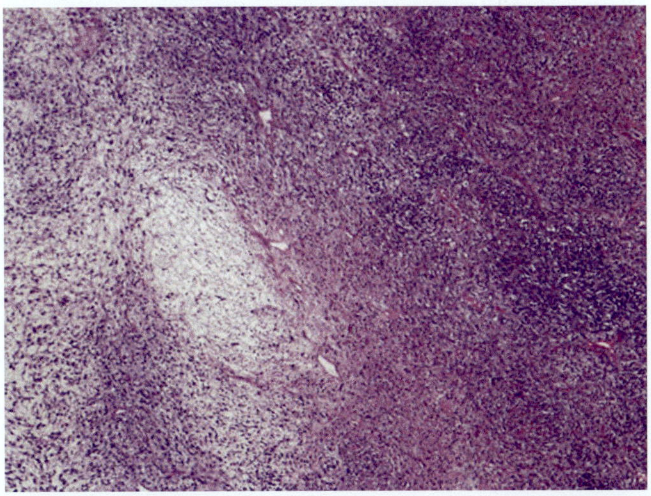

Fig. 9.121 Hypo- and hypercellular areas in pulmonary malignant peripheral nerve sheath tumor

Histological Features

Pulmonary malignant peripheral nerve sheath tumors are composed of loose fascicles of round epithelioid cells and spindle cells arranged in fascicular patterns (Fig. 9.120). The individual tumor cells show moderately or marked cytologic atypia, hyperchromatic nuclei, and occasional conspicuous nucleoli. The neoplastic cells have fine and elongated eosinophilic cytoplasm (Figs. 9.121, 9.122, 9.123, and 9.124). Multinucleated tumor giant cells are a common finding in these tumors (Fig. 9.125). The mitotic activity can be high with more than 25 mitoses per 10 hpf (Fig. 9.126).

Immunohistochemical and Molecular Features

Contrary to their benign counterparts, malignant peripheral nerve sheath tumors only show focal staining with S-100 protein but diffuse and strong positivity for vimentin [183].

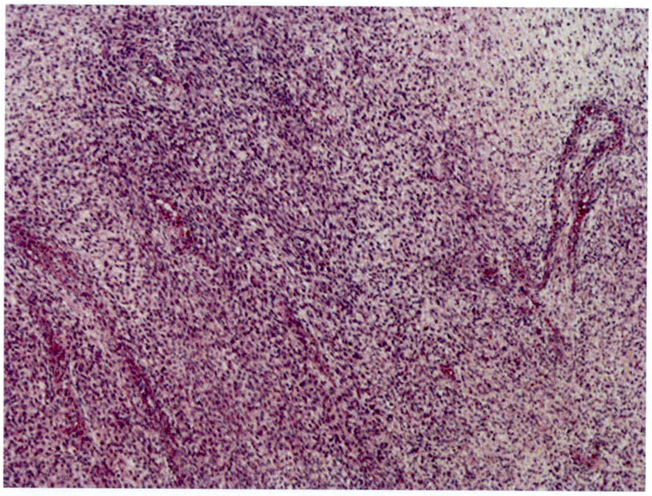

Fig. 9.122 Pulmonary malignant peripheral nerve sheath tumor characterized by a malignant spindle cell proliferation

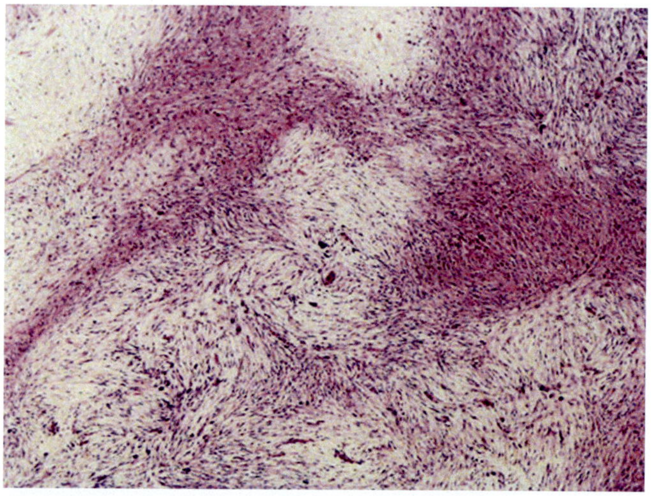

Fig. 9.123 Less cellular areas in pulmonary malignant peripheral nerve sheath tumor

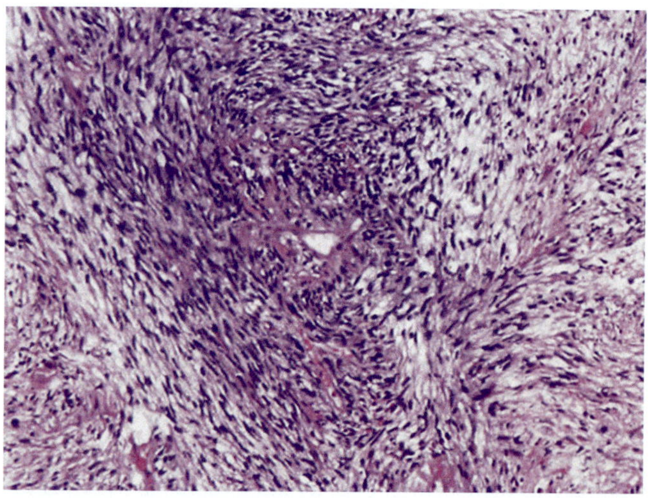

Fig. 9.124 Pulmonary malignant peripheral nerve sheath tumor showing perivascular tumor cell condensation

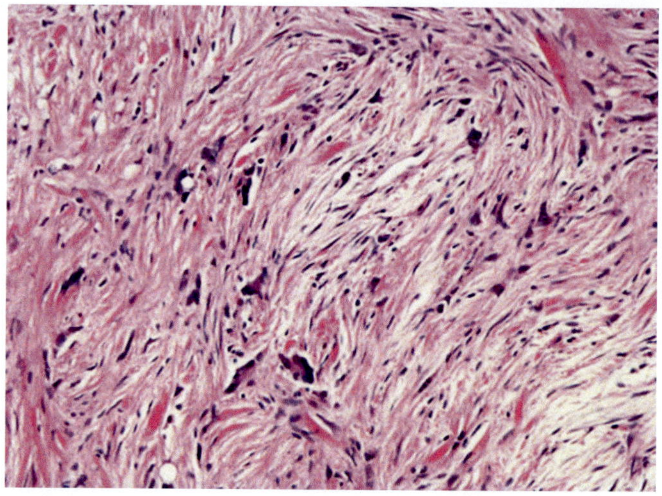

Fig. 9.125 Tumor giant cells in pulmonary malignant peripheral nerve sheath tumor

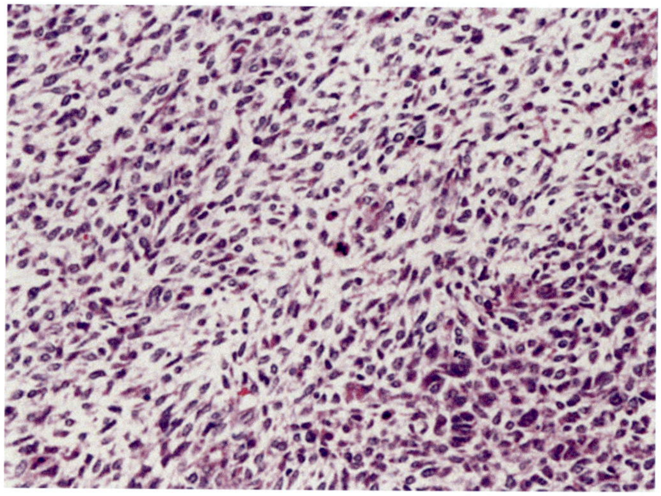

Fig. 9.126 Mitotic activity can be high in pulmonary malignant peripheral nerve sheath tumors

Cytokeratin, CEA, SMA, desmin, CD34, TTF-1, HMB45, and EMA are usually negative [183, 214, 215]. Similar to pulmonary schwannoma, flow cytometry performed on two cases failed to show any aneuploid DNA profiles [183].

Differential Diagnosis

Several other malignant spindle cell neoplasms enter the differential diagnosis for malignant peripheral nerve sheath tumors of the lung. Monophasic synovial sarcoma may closely resemble a malignant peripheral nerve sheath tumor based on their spindle cell morphology. The cells of synovial sarcoma, however, show a distinctly uniform population of spindle cells that lack morphologic variability or the presence of tumor giant cells. Cytogenetic studies may help in equivocal cases showing the typical translocation t(X;18) in synovial sarcoma but not malignant peripheral nerve sheath tumor. Another tumor that may closely mimic malignant peripheral nerve sheath tumor of the lung is malignant fibrous histiocytoma. Immunopositivity for S-100 protein in the former may be the only distinguishing feature between these tumors. Lastly, malignant melanoma can present as a spindle cell lesion. Melanoma, however, will show diffuse and strong expression of S-100 protein in addition to positivity for other melanocytic markers like HMB45 or melan A. The latter have not been shown to be positive in malignant peripheral nerve sheath tumors.

Treatment and Prognosis

Complete surgical excision is the treatment of choice for pulmonary malignant peripheral nerve sheath tumors. This can be followed by chemo and radiation therapy on an individual basis. Although isolated long-term survival has been noted [92], the prognosis for these tumors is generally poor, with most patients dying of tumor recurrence or metastatic disease within 2 years [213].

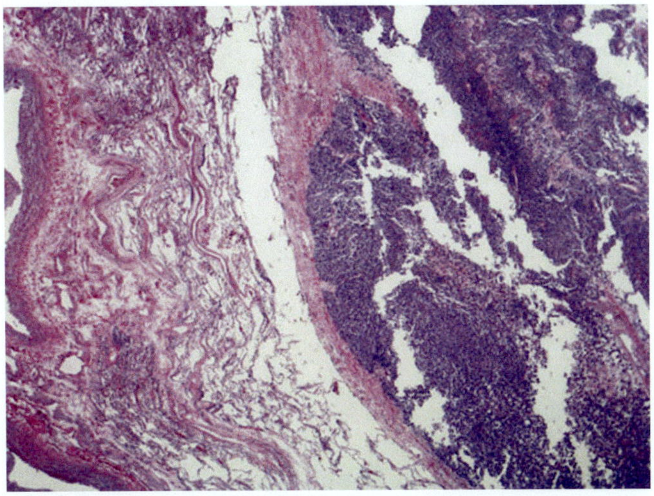

Fig. 9.127 Low-power view of pulmonary peripheral neuroectodermal tumor showing a proliferation of small cells sharply demarcated from the surrounding lung parenchyma

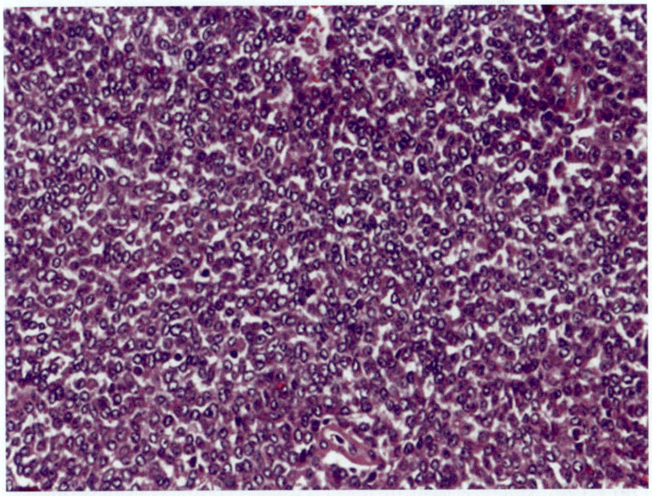

Fig. 9.128 Higher magnification of peripheral neuroectodermal tumor of the lung composed of sheets of discohesive and monotonous small cells

Tumors of Neuroectodermal Origin

Tumors composed of small neuroectodermal cells constitute a family of related malignant neoplasms including Ewing's sarcoma of bone, extraskeletal Ewing's sarcoma, and peripheral primitive neuroectodermal tumor (PNET). PNET, as these tumors are commonly referred to in an extraosseous location, have also been described in the thoracopulmonary region and are here also known under the designation "Askin tumor" [218]. Similar tumors arising in the lung parenchyma are rarities, with less than 20 cases described in the English literature.

Pulmonary Primitive Neuroectodermal Tumor (PNET)

Clinical Features

Pulmonary PNET are tumors primarily affecting a younger age group with a mean age in the fourth decade and an age range from 8 to 64 years [219–221]. Males are slightly more commonly affected than females. Presenting symptoms include dry cough, fever, hemoptysis, or back pain, although several patients were asymptomatic at presentation [219, 221–223]. Radiographically, the tumors are described as as well-circumscribed masses in the lung parenchyma, hilar area, or in an endobronchial location [219, 221, 223–225].

Gross Features

The tumors are generally large and may range in size from 3.6 to 9.0 cm [222, 223]. They are described as well-demarcated tumors with a lobulated configuration, yellow-gray cut surface, and varying amounts of necrosis [222].

Histological Features

The tumors are composed of diffuse sheets or lobules of fairly homogenous small round or ovoid tumor cells separated by thin fibrovascular septa (Fig. 9.127). Individual tumor cells are discohesive and closely packed with hyperchromatic nuclei, indistinct cytoplasm, and inconspicuous nucleoli (Fig. 9.128). Homer–Wright-like rosettes are occasionally seen (Fig. 9.129). The mitotic activity is usually high (Fig. 9.130), and areas of necrosis are commonly seen (Fig. 9.131). In some cases, perivascular accentuation can be identified (Fig. 9.132). Areas of calcification (Fig. 9.133), edematous stromal change (Fig. 9.134), and cystic degeneration (Fig. 9.135) are not uncommon. Interestingly, chondroid differentiation has been described in a single case [223].

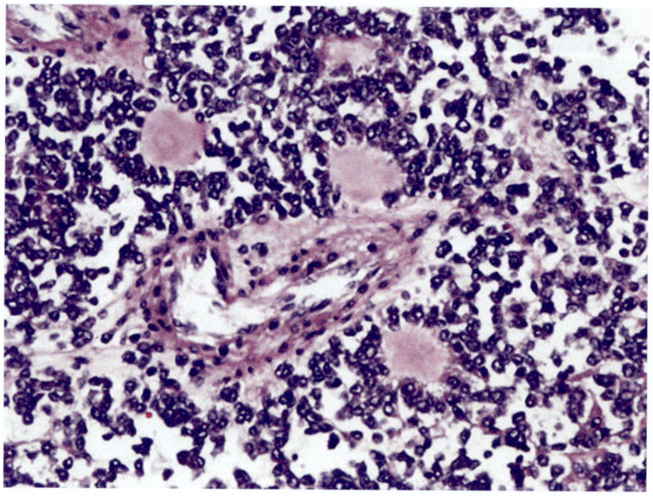

Fig. 9.129 In some cases of pulmonary peripheral neuroectodermal tumor, Homer–Wright-like rosettes may be identified

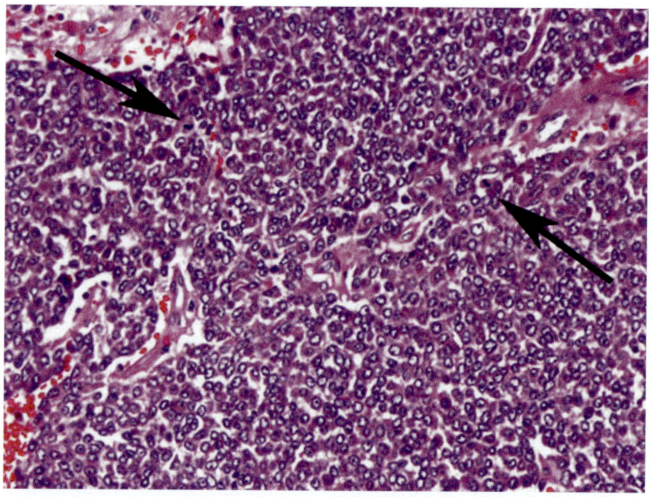

Fig. 9.130 Mitotic activity (*arrows*) is usually conspicuous in peripheral neuroectodermal tumor of the lung

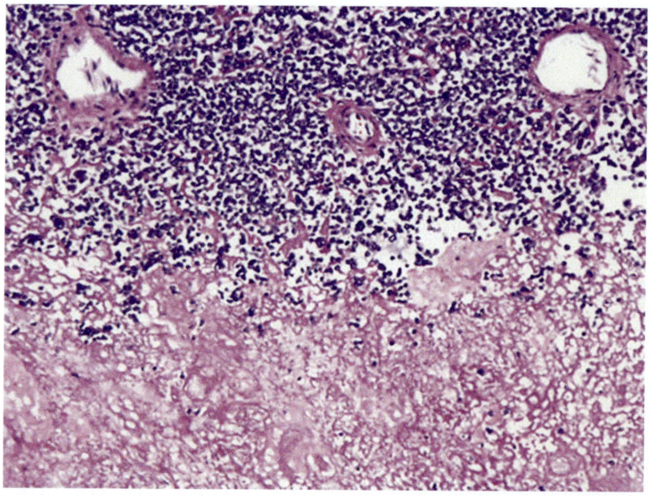

Fig. 9.131 Areas of necrosis are another common finding in pulmonary peripheral neuroectodermal tumor

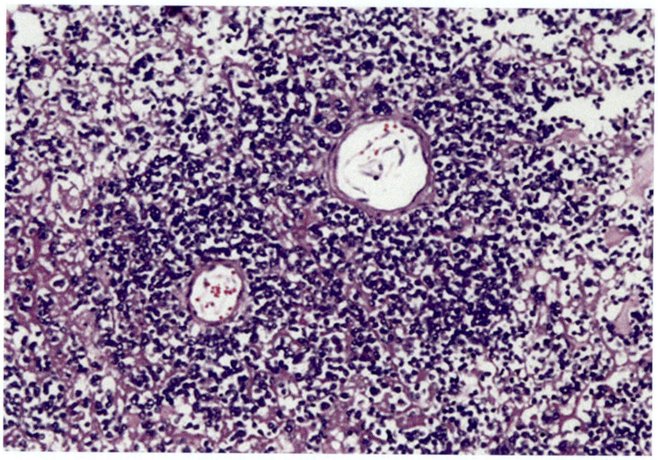

Fig. 9.132 The tumor cells sometimes show prominent arrangement around blood vessels in peripheral neuroectodermal tumor of the lung

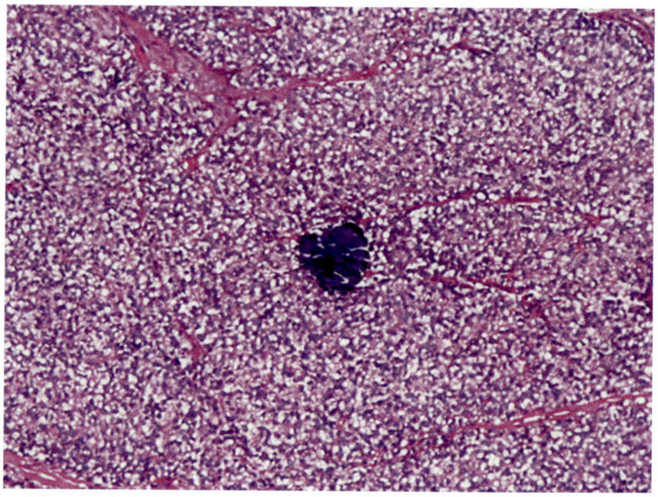

Fig. 9.133 Foci of calcification may be identified in some cases of pulmonary peripheral neuroectodermal tumor

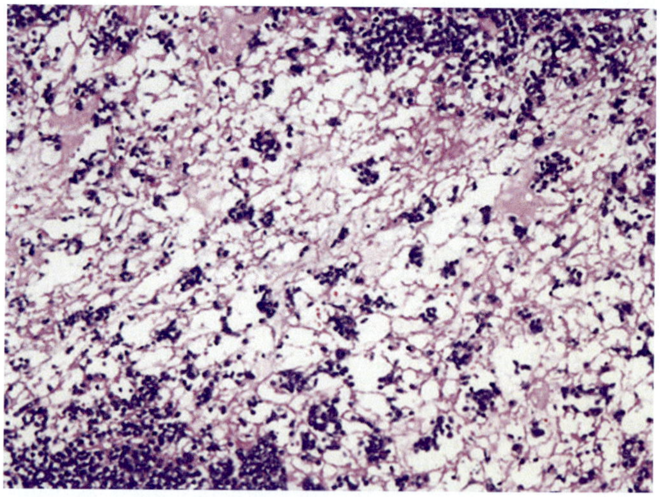

Fig. 9.134 Stromal edema in peripheral neuroectodermal tumor of the lung

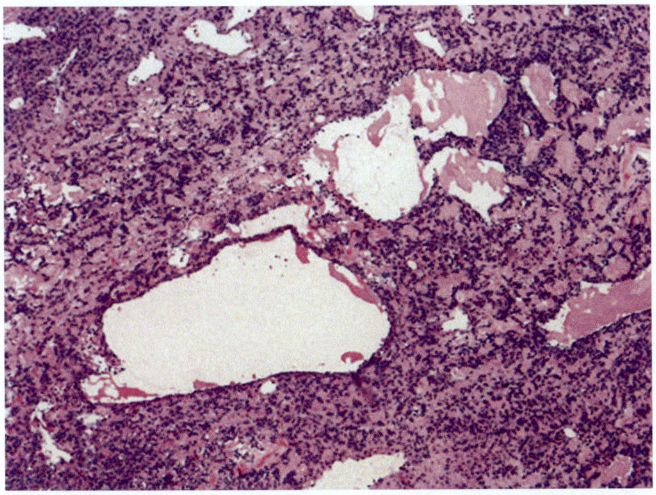

Fig. 9.135 Formation of cystic spaces in pulmonary peripheral neuroectodermal tumor

Immunohistochemical and Molecular Features

Pulmonary PNET share the same immunohistochemical and molecular characteristics as their extrapulmonary counterparts. The tumor cells are positive for CD99 and neuron specific enolase and negative for cytokeratin, chromogranin, leukocyte common antigen, smooth muscle actin, desmin, and epithelial membrane antigen [219, 221, 223, 225]. Synaptophysin, S-100 protein, and neurofilament can show varying results. Since the tumor cells often contain glycogen, a PAS histological stain may be used to confirm the diagnosis.

On a molecular level, chromosomal translocations t(11;22)(q24;q12) or t(21;22)(q22;q12) resulting in EWS-FLI1 or EWS-ERG fusion genes are a consistent finding in PNET and Ewing's sarcoma, confirming a close relationship between these tumors [226–229].

Differential Diagnosis

The differential diagnosis for PNET mainly includes other blue, round, small cell neoplasms. In the lung, small cell carcinoma is an important entity to include in the differential diagnosis. Both tumors may show similar histological features and immunohistochemical studies may be required to arrive at the correct diagnosis. In this setting, an absence of cytokeratin positivity and lack of convincing reactivity for neuroendocrine markers (especially chromogranin) would support a diagnosis of PNET. Other diagnostic considerations include rhabdomyosarcoma, neuroblastoma, or lymphoma. In cases of rhabdomyosarcoma, the presence of typical rhabdomyoblasts and immunohistochemical expression of muscle specific markers may lead to the correct interpretation. Neuroblastomas may show histological and immunohistochemical overlap with PNET; however, the latter will show CD99 positivity along with the typical cytogenetic translocation, allowing distinction from the former. Lymphoma is distinguished from PNET by its morphologic features along with positive staining of the tumor cells for LCA and B or T cell markers.

Treatment and Prognosis

PNET is an aggressive malignancy that requires multimodal therapy consisting of surgery, chemotherapy, and/or radiotherapy. In a recent study by Demir et al. [230], neoadjuvant chemotherapy led to greater complete resection rate and disease-free survival in patients with thoracic PNET. However, for patients with primary pulmonary PNET, the prognosis is still poor with a mean 2-year event-free survival rate of only 25 % [230].

Tumors of Mixed Origin

Some primary tumors of the lung are composed of a mix of two or more cell types. Pulmonary hamartoma is an example of such lesions with benign behavior, whereas triton tumor is a malignant tumor composed of neural and skeletal muscle elements. Pulmonary artery sarcoma is a rare and unusual tumor arising from pluripotent cells in the vessel wall that can show any single and even dual sarcomatous differentiation [231].

Pulmonary Hamartoma

Pulmonary hamartomas are mesenchymal lesions composed of several tissue elements. There has been debate in the past whether these lesions represent true hamartomatous lesions or rather benign neoplasms. Evidence to support one or the other opinion has been presented in various publications [232–238]. More recently, a cytogenetic analysis of seven pulmonary hamartomas demonstrated an abnormal karyotype with recombinations between chromosomal bands 6p21 and 14q24 supporting the view that these tumors are genuine neoplasms rather than developmental anomalies [239]. The incidence of pulmonary hamartoma in the general population is approximately 0.25 % [240] and it accounts for 3 % of all benign lung tumors [241]. Pulmonary hamartomas are generally composed of varying amounts of cartilage, entrapped benign respiratory epithelium, adipose tissue, smooth muscle, and fibrous tissue. Based on this, these tumors can be differentiated from two related lesions—pulmonary chondroma and pulmonary lipoma—which are composed of a single tissue type only.

Clinical Features

Pulmonary hamartomas seem to affect men slightly more than women. The age range spans 14–74 years with a peak age in the sixth decade [233]. The tumors most often occur in the periphery of the lung (92 %) and are often asymptomatic, while only 8 % arise from the bronchial tree [233]. The latter tumors may produce pulmonary symptoms (cough, hemoptysis, dyspnea, fever) due to bronchial obstruction. Solitary tumors showing partial calcification ("popcorn calcification") are a typical finding of these tumors using imaging techniques. Rarely, multiple pulmonary hamartomas may be identified in the same patient [242], may show a diffuse growth pattern along the bronchial tree [243], or the tumors may present with unusual symptoms like pneumothorax [244]. Pulmonary hamartomas have also been described in association with other tumors, especially bronchial carcinomas [233, 245, 246]. More recently, cases of carcinoid tumor, atypical lipomatous tumor, and myoepithelial tumors have been described, arising within otherwise typical hamartomas [244, 247, 248].

Gross Features

The gross features of pulmonary hamartoma are those of well-circumscribed unencapsulated lesions that usually range from 1 to 10 cm in size. Giant pulmonary hamartomas measuring more than 12 cm are sometimes seen [249]. On sectioning, the tumors appear lobulated, firm, and white and have a cartilaginous or myxoid appearance. Hemorrhage and necrosis are generally absent, but cystic change can be seen in isolated cases [250]. An unusual case arising in an extralobar location connected to the lung by a slender stalk has been described [251].

Histological Features

Pulmonary hamartomas are typically composed of a mixture of tissue types, and most often chondroid differentiation predominates (Figs. 9.136, 9.137, and 9.138). The cartilage normally grows in a lobulated pattern and may be of the myxoid type or more mature-appearing cartilage with typical chondrocytes. Intermixed with the chondroid tissue are areas of adipose tissue and entrapped benign respiratory epithelium (Figs. 9.139, 9.140, and 9.141). Smooth muscle, fibrous tissue, or endobronchial glands (in central lesions) may be present in some cases; in those lesions, in which the smooth muscle predominates, a diagnosis of leiomyomatous hamartoma may be rendered (Figs. 9.142, 9.143, and 9.144). In endobronchial tumors, the chondroid component is not usually associated with the bronchial cartilage. A mix of inflammatory cells including lymphocytes, plasma cells, and mast cells can occasionally be seen in the periphery of the tumors. Cytologic atypia, mitotic activity, hemorrhage, or necrosis are usually absent, although mild nuclear atypia of chondrocytes can be seen in large lesions.

Molecular Features

Cytogenetic studies performed in several small series of pulmonary hamartomas have demonstrated clonal chromosome aberrations and shown that recombination of chromosomes 6p21, 12q14-15, and 14q24 are common. The authors concluded from this that pulmonary hamartomas are in fact genuine neoplasms and not hamartomatous in nature [239, 252–254].

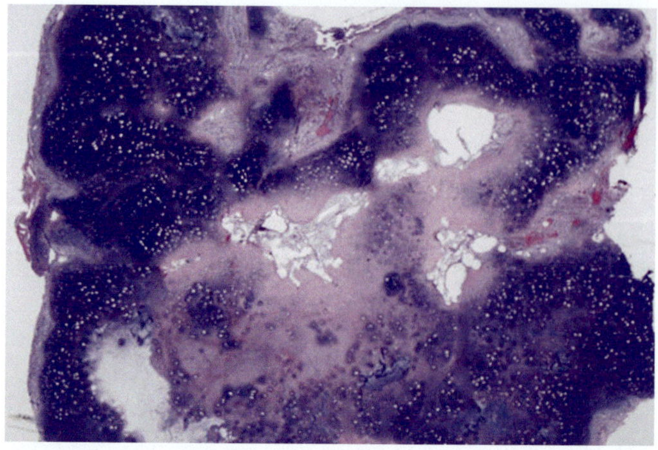

Fig. 9.136 Lobulated appearance of pulmonary chondroid hamartoma

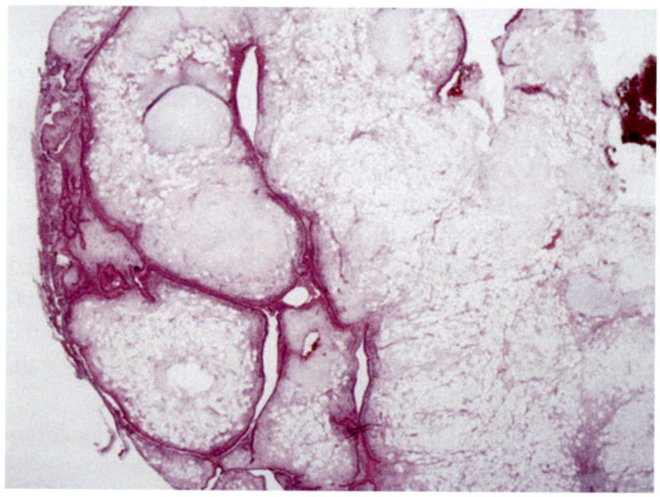

Fig. 9.137 Chondroid and adipose elements in pulmonary chondroid hamartoma

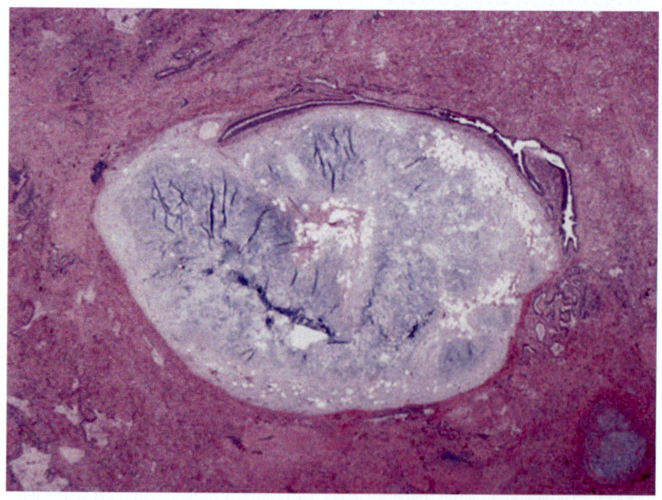

Fig. 9.138 Low-power view of small pulmonary chondroid hamartoma composed of cartilage, fat, and entrapped respiratory epithelium

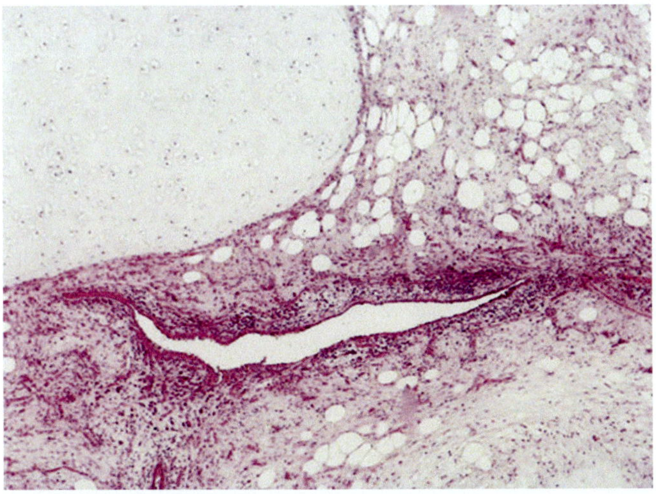

Fig. 9.139 Intermediate-power view showing typical epithelial invaginations of pulmonary chondroid hamartoma

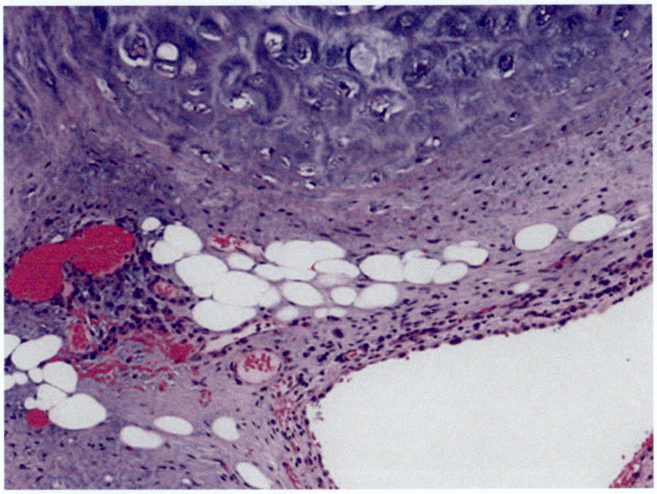

Fig. 9.140 Adipose tissue juxtaposed with cartilage in pulmonary chondroid hamartoma

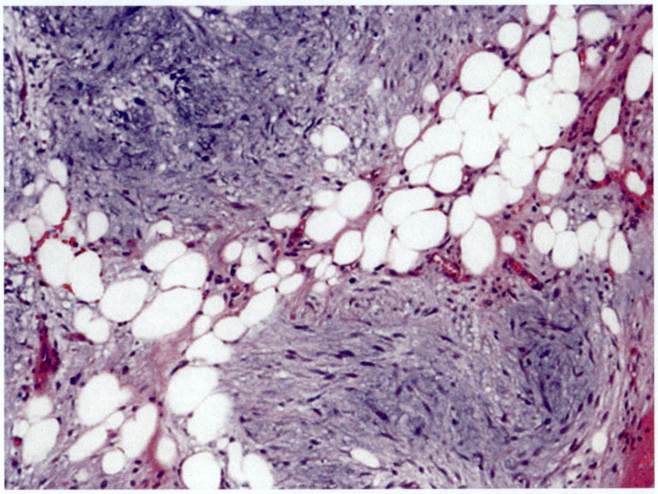

Fig. 9.141 Myxoid-type cartilage in pulmonary chondroid hamartoma

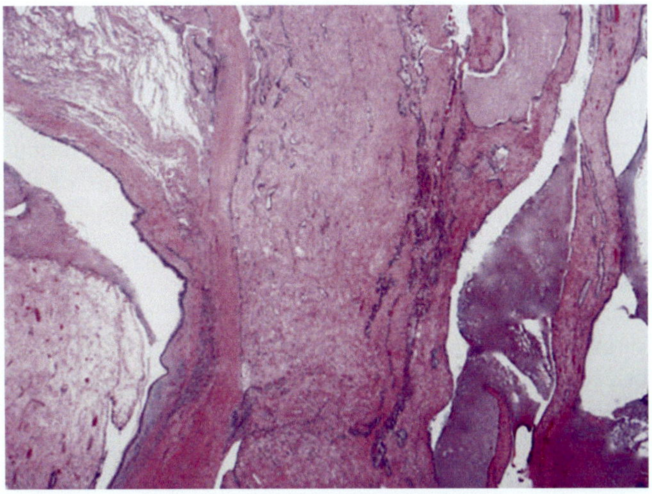

Fig. 9.142 Low-power view of pulmonary leiomyomatous hamartoma

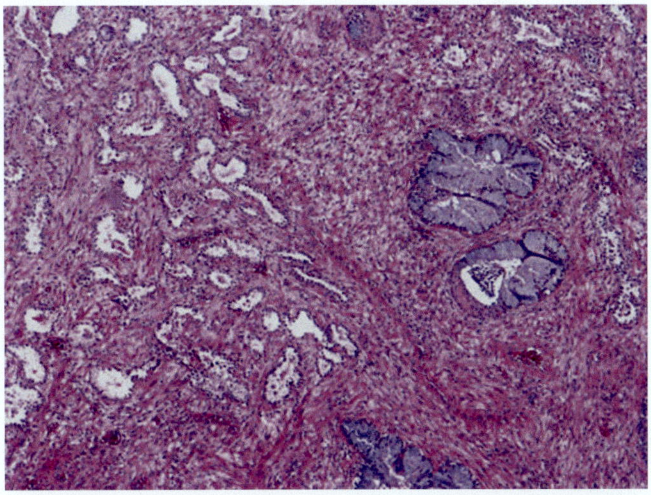

Fig. 9.143 Smooth muscle proliferation with entrapped respiratory and bronchial epithelium in leiomyomatous hamartoma of the lung

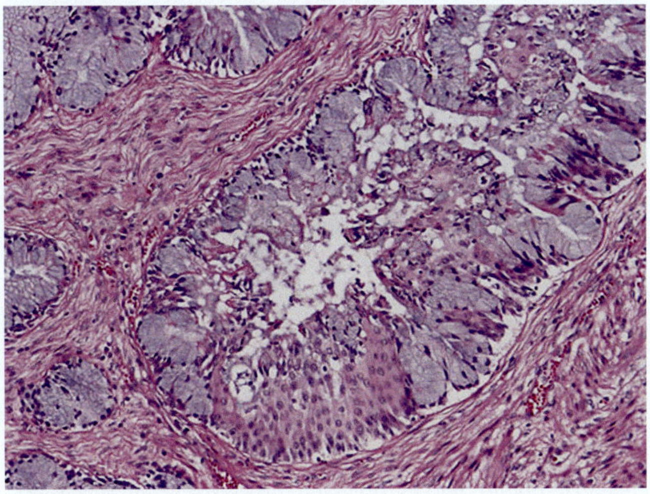

Fig. 9.144 High-power view showing a proliferation of smooth muscle surrounding bronchial epithelium

Differential Diagnosis

Pulmonary hamartomas do not usually pose a diagnostic problem. In case of endobronchial lesions, however, bronchial chondromas or bronchial lipomas may enter the differential diagnosis. Chondromas and lipomas are lesions composed of one tissue type only and lack the mix of elements typically seen in hamartomas.

Treatment and Prognosis

Pulmonary hamartomas are benign lesions, and complete surgical excision is curative. Parenchyma-saving enucleation or excision in the form of enucleation, wedge resection, or segmentectomy has been recommended as the treatment of choice [255].

Malignant Triton Tumor

Malignant triton tumors are defined as malignant neurogenic tumors with rhabdomyoblastic differentiation. These are rare tumors of the soft tissues that have occasionally been described in sites other than the soft tissues, but only three cases of primary malignant triton tumor of the lung have been reported [256, 257]. In the soft tissues, there appears to be an association with neurofibromatosis; however, in the lung cases, this association has not been observed [256].

Clinical Features

Malignant triton tumors of the lung have been described in two men, 28 and 53 years of age, as well as in a 3-year-old child [256, 257]. The patients presented with shortness of breath and demonstrated large intrapulmonary masses on chest radiographs.

Gross Features

The tumors were large (8–13 cm) and variably delineated masses with a soft and gelatinous cut surface and areas of hemorrhage and necrosis.

Histological Features

The histological features of malignant triton tumor of the lung are those of a spindle cell proliferation forming fascicles and a subtle storiform pattern embedded in a myxoid stroma. Faint nuclear palisading was observed in some areas as well as areas of perivascular hyalinization (Figs. 9.145 and 9.146). Nuclear atypia and mitotic activity varied from case to case, with the pediatric case demonstrating large bizarre tumor cells with prominent nuclear pleomorphism. Extensive areas of hemorrhage and necrosis were present in all cases. Intermixed with the spindle cell proliferation were foci containing larger cells with eosinophilic cytoplasm, eccentric nuclei, and cytoplasmic cross-striations representing rhabdomyoblastic differentiation (Fig. 9.147).

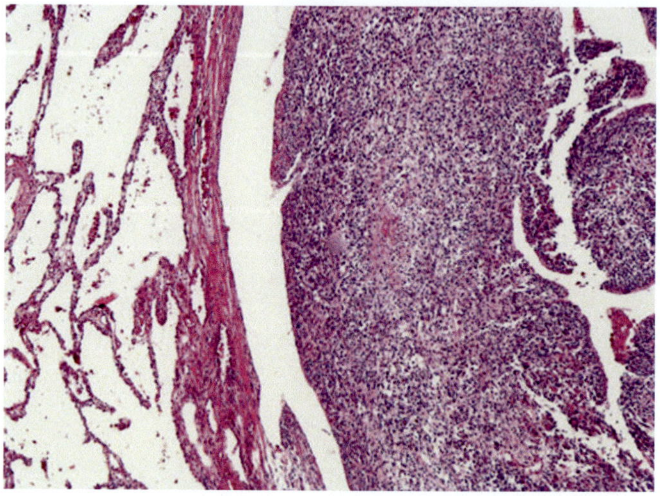

Fig. 9.145 Low-power view of malignant triton tumor of the lung

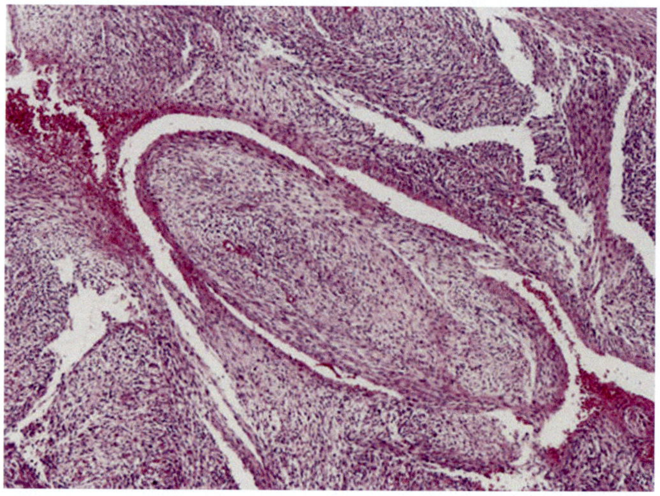

Fig. 9.146 Malignant triton tumor of the lung composed of a malignant spindle cell proliferation embedded in a myxoid stroma

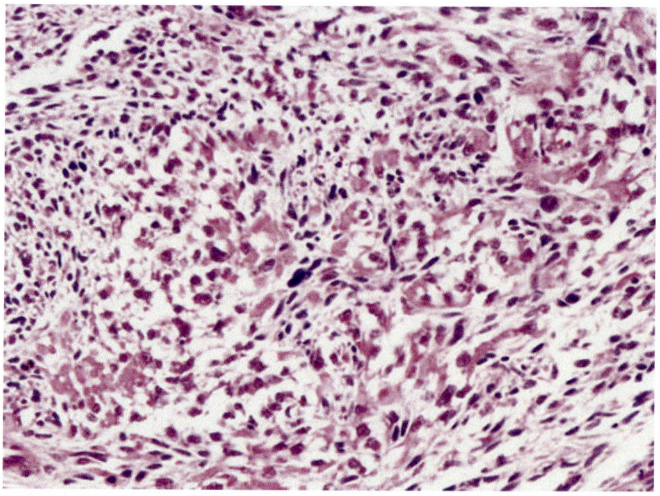

Fig. 9.147 The spindle cell proliferation of malignant triton tumor of the lung contains interspersed rhabdomyoblasts

Immunohistochemical Features

Immunohistochemically, S-100 protein is focally expressed in the neural component of the tumors, while desmin and myoglobin highlighted the rhabdomyoblasts [256]. Vimentin was positive for both components, but cytokeratin, GFAP, and neurofilament protein were negative.

Differential Diagnosis

The differential diagnosis for these lesions comprises a range of other spindle cell tumors primary or metastatic to the lung. In children, the most important differential diagnosis is pleuropulmonary blastoma, a tumor composed of undifferentiated blastemal elements and rhabdomyomatous differentiation. These tumors, however, will lack any Schwannian features typically present in malignant triton tumor. In adults, pure malignant peripheral nerve sheath tumors will lack the rhabdomyomatous elements seen in triton tumor. Other tumors that may show similar histological features include leiomyosarcoma and intrapulmonary fibrous tumor. Immunohistochemical studies detecting desmin and SMA positivity in leiomyosarcoma and CD34 and bcl-2 in solitary fibrous tumor should facilitate correct interpretation. Importantly, metastasis from a soft tissue primarily needs to be excluded by careful clinical and radiological evaluation of the patients.

Treatment and Prognosis

Complete surgical excision was performed in all cases of pulmonary malignant triton tumor. One patient died 3 months after surgical resection due to widespread intrathoracic spread [256], while one patient was alive and free of disease 1 year after diagnosis [257]. The third patient was lost to follow-up.

Pulmonary Artery Sarcoma

Pulmonary artery sarcomas are rare malignancies that most often originate in the pulmonary trunk, the pulmonary arteries (or less commonly pulmonary veins), the pulmonary valve, or the right ventricular outflow tract [258–260]. The cell of origin is believed to be a pluripotent cell in the intimal or medial layers of the vessel wall, hence the early name of "intimal sarcoma" [259, 261]. Clinically, pulmonary artery sarcoma is commonly mistaken for pulmonary embolism or primary pulmonary hypertension, and the diagnosis is delayed until thoracotomy or autopsy is performed [262, 263].

Clinical Features

Pulmonary artery sarcomas affect adults with an age range from 21 to 69 years and a peak in the fifth and sixth decades [264, 265]. Whereas in some series males appear to be predominantly affected [265], other authors report female predilection [70, 266]. Cough, chest pain, dyspnea, cyanosis, hemoptysis, and right-sided heart failure are the most common presenting symptoms. Radiographically, intravascular masses causing filling defects are seen often mimicking pulmonary embolism. Cardiomegaly and right ventricular hypertrophy are often identified on an echocardiogram [266].

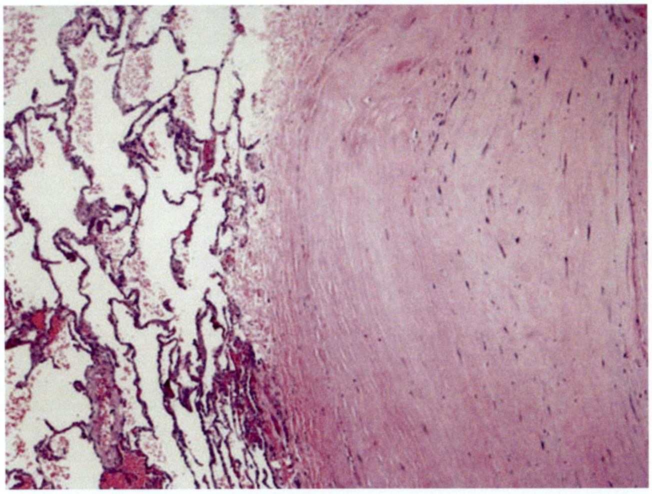

Fig. 9.148 Atypical spindle cells in the vessel wall of a pulmonary artery sarcoma

Gross Features

The tumor is seen attached to the pulmonary artery and may show extension along the vessel branches into the right heart or lung parenchyma. The tumors are white, gray, or yellow and irregular masses that, depending on the histological subtype, may contain bony, chondroid, or hemorrhagic elements.

Histological Features

Histological examination will reveal the sarcomatous nature of the tumor. Generally, any type of sarcoma may arise in the pulmonary vasculature with the most common types being leiomyosarcoma and high-grade "undifferentiated" sarcomas (Figs. 9.148 and 9.149) [70]. Less frequently, angiosarcomatous, osteosarcomatous, chondrosarcomatous, rhabdomyosarcomatous, or low-grade myofibroblastic differentiation is seen [231, 265, 267–270]. The histological features of these tumors will be identical to those described in the lung or soft tissue; however, it is essential to identify the subtype and pulmonary artery origin of these tumors because of treatment and prognostic implications.

Immunohistochemical Features

Immunohistochemical studies may be used in order to allow more definitive classification, and the use of smooth or skeletal muscle as well as vascular markers may be helpful for correct subtyping of the lesions.

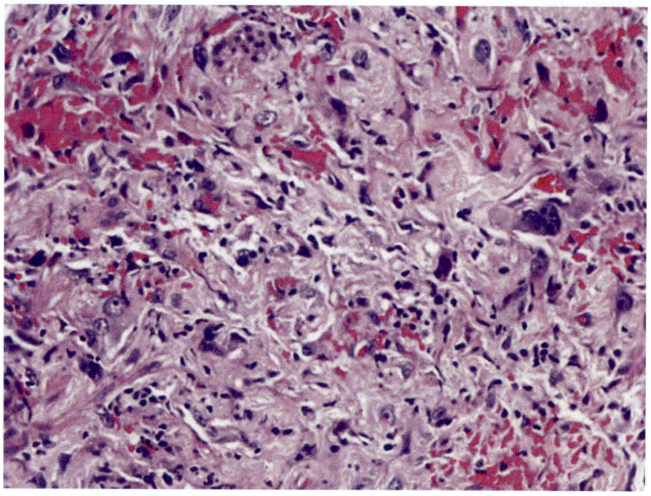

Fig. 9.149 High-grade undifferentiated tumor cells in pulmonary artery sarcoma

Treatment and Prognosis

The treatment for pulmonary artery sarcoma consists of complete surgical resection. Although the role of additional treatment is still uncertain, neoadjuvant or adjuvant chemotherapy and radiation are increasingly being used to treat these patients with potential benefit for symptom relief and survival [271]. Despite this, the prognosis for these tumors is poor with a reported median survival times of 1.5 months without surgery and 10 months with surgery and adjuvant chemotherapy [263] and an overall 1 year survival of 20 % [266]. The tumors are characterized by frequent recurrences, intrathoracic and distant metastasis, and tumor embolism [258]. Although historically, pulmonary artery sarcomas has been considered a single disease entity, more recently it could be demonstrated that survival to a certain degree also depends on tumor subtype, with better prognosis for patients with leiomyosarcoma, intermediate prognosis for high-grade undifferentiated sarcomas, and worse survival in patients with rhabdomyosarcoma [265].

References

1. Suster S, Moran CA. Pulmonary adenofibroma: report of two cases of an unusual type of hamartomatous lesion of the lung. Histopathology. 1993;23:547–51.
2. Scarff RW, Gowar FJS. Fibroadenoma of the lung. J Pathol Bacteriol. 1944;56:257–9.
3. Butler C, Kleinerman J. Pulmonary hamartoma. Arch Pathol. 1969;88:584–92.
4. Klemperer P, Rabin CP. Primary neoplasms of the pleura. Arch Pathol. 1931;11:385–412.
5. Morimitsu Y, Nakajima M, Hisaoka M, Hashimoto H. Extrapleural solitary fibrous tumor: clinicopathologic study of 17 cases and molecular analysis of the p53 pathway. APMIS. 2000;108: 617–25.
6. Yousem SA, Flynn SD. Intrapulmonary localized fibrous tumor. Intraparenchymal so-called localized fibrous mesothelioma. Am J Clin Pathol. 1988;89:365–9.
7. Aufiero TX, McGary SA, Campbell DB, Phillips PP. Intrapulmonary benign fibrous tumor of the pleura. J Thorac Cardiovasc Surg. 1995;110:549–51.
8. Caruso RA, LaSpada F, Gaeta M, Minutoli I, Inferrera C. Report of an intrapulmonary solitary fibrous tumor: fine-needle aspiration cytologic findings, clinicopathological, and immunohistochemical features. Diagn Cytopathol. 1996;14:64–7.
9. Kanamori Y, Hashizume K, Sugiyama M, Motoi T, Fukayama M, Ida K, Igarashi T. Intrapulmonary solitary fibrous tumor in an eight-year-old male. Pediatr Pulmonol. 2005;40:261–4.
10. Sagawa M, Ueda Y, Matsubara F, Sakuma H, Yoshimitsu Y, Aikawa H, Usuda K, Minato H, Sakuma T. Intrapulmonary solitary fibrous tumor diagnosed by immunohistochemical and genetic approaches: report of a case. Surg Today. 2007;37:423–5.
11. Sakurai H, Tanaka W, Kaji M, Yamazaki K, Suemasu K. Intrapulmonary localized fibrous tumor of the lung: a very unusual presentation. Ann Thorac Surg. 2008;86:1360–2.
12. Geramizadeh B, Banani A, Moradi A, Hosseini SM, Foroutan H. Intrapulmonary solitary fibrous tumor with bronchial involvement: a rare case report in a child. J Pediatr Surg. 2010;45:249–51.
13. Míguez González J, Varona Porres D, Andreu Soriano J, Montero Fernández MA. Intrapulmonary solitary fibrous tumor associated with hemoptysis: a case report. Radiologia. 2012;54(2):182–6. Epub 2011 Feb 5.
14. Hernandez FJ, Fernandez BB. Localized fibrous tumors of pleura: a light and electron microscopic study. Cancer. 1974;34:1667–74.
15. Said JW, Nash G, Banks-Schlegel S, Sassoon AF, Shintaku IP. Localized fibrous mesothelioma: an immunohistochemical and electron microscopic study. Hum Pathol. 1984;15:440–3.
16. Yousem SA, Hochholzer L. Primary pulmonary hemangiopericytoma. Cancer. 1987;59:549–55.
17. Gebauer C. The postoperative prognosis of primary pulmonary sarcomas. A review with a comparison between the histological forms and the other primary endothoracal sarcomas based on 474 cases. Scand J Thorac Cardiovasc Surg. 1982;16:91–7.
18. Suster S. Primary sarcomas of the lung. Semin Diagn Pathol. 1995;12:140–57.
19. Pettinato G, Manivel JC, Saldana MJ, Peyser J, Dehner LP. Primary bronchopulmonary fibrosarcoma of childhood and adolescence: reassessment of a low-grade malignancy. Clinicopathologic study of five cases and review of the literature. Hum Pathol. 1989;20: 463–71.
20. Guccion JG, Rosen SH. Bronchopulmonary leiomyosarcoma and fibrosarcoma. A study of 32 cases and review of the literature. Cancer. 1972;30:836–47.
21. Logrono R, Filipowicz EA, Eyzaguirre EJ, Sawh RN. Diagnosis of primary fibrosarcoma of the lung by fine-needle aspiration and core biopsy. Arch Pathol Lab Med. 1999;123:731–5.
22. Goldthorn JF, Duncan MH, Kosloske AM, Ball WS. Cavitating primary pulmonary fibrosarcoma in a child. J Thorac Cardiovasc Surg. 1986;91:932–4.
23. Zeren H, Moran CA, Suster S, Fishback NF, Koss MN. Primary pulmonary sarcomas with features of monophasic synovial sarcoma: a clinicopathological, immunohistochemical, and ultrastructural study of 25 cases. Hum Pathol. 1995;26:474–80.
24. Essary LR, Vargas SO, Fletcher CD. Primary pleuropulmonary synovial sarcoma: reappraisal of a recently described anatomic subset. Cancer. 2002;94:459–69.
25. Bégueret H, Galateau-Salle F, Guillou L, Chetaille B, Brambilla E, Vignaud JM, Terrier P, Groussard O, Coindre JM. Primary intrathoracic synovial sarcoma: a clinicopathologic study of 40 t(X;18)-positive cases from the French Sarcoma Group and the Mesopath Group. Am J Surg Pathol. 2005;29:339–46.

26. Frazier AA, Franks TJ, Pugatch RD, Galvin JR. From the archives of the AFIP: pleuropulmonary synovial sarcoma. Radiographics. 2006;26:923–40.
27. Hartel PH, Fanburg-Smith JC, Frazier AA, Galvin JR, Lichy JH, Shilo K, Franks TJ. Primary pulmonary and mediastinal synovial sarcoma: a clinicopathologic study of 60 cases and comparison with five prior series. Mod Pathol. 2007;20:760–9.
28. Suster S, Moran CA. Primary synovial sarcomas of the mediastinum: a clinicopathologic, immunohistochemical, and ultrastructural study of 15 cases. Am J Surg Pathol. 2005;29:569–78.
29. Kaplan MA, Goodman MD, Satish J, Bhagavan BS, Travis WD. Primary pulmonary sarcoma with morphologic features of monophasic synovial sarcoma and chromosome translocation t(X; 18). Am J Clin Pathol. 1996;105:195–9.
30. Cummings NM, Desai S, Thway K, Stewart S, Hill DA, Priest JR, Nicholson AG, Rintoul RC. Cystic primary pulmonary synovial sarcoma presenting as recurrent pneumothorax: report of 4 cases. Am J Surg Pathol. 2010;34:1176–9.
31. Okamoto S, Hisaoka M, Daa T, Hatakeyama K, Iwamasa T, Hashimoto H. Primary pulmonary synovial sarcoma: a clinicopathologic, immunohistochemical, and molecular study of 11 cases. Hum Pathol. 2004;35:850–6.
32. Deraedt K, Debiec-Rychter M, Sciot R. Radiation-associated synovial sarcoma of the lung following radiotherapy for pulmonary metastasis of Wilms' tumour. Histopathology. 2006;48:473–5.
33. Duran-Mendicuti A, Costello P, Vargas SO. Primary synovial sarcoma of the chest: radiographic and clinicopathologic correlation. J Thorac Imaging. 2003;18:87–93.
34. Niwa H, Masuda S, Kobayashi C, Oda Y. Pulmonary synovial sarcoma with polypoid endobronchial growth: a case report, immunohistochemical and cytogenetic study. Pathol Int. 2004;54:611–5.
35. Watanabe R, Kamiyoshihara M, Kaira K, Motegi A, Takise A. Spontaneous expectoration of primary pulmonary synovial sarcoma. J Thorac Oncol. 2006;1:1025–6.
36. Yoon GS, Park SY, Kang GH, Kim OJ. Primary pulmonary sarcoma with morphologic features of biphasic synovial sarcoma: a case report. J Korean Med Sci. 1998;13:71–6.
37. Hisaoka M, Hashimoto H, Iwamasa T, Ishikawa K, Aoki T. Primary synovial sarcoma of the lung: report of two cases confirmed by molecular detection of SYT-SSX fusion gene transcripts. Histopathology. 1999;34:205–10.
38. Noguera R, Navarro S, Cremades A, Roselló-Sastre E, Pellín A, Peydró-Olaya A, Llombart-Bosch A. Translocation (X;18) in a biphasic synovial sarcoma with morphologic features of neural differentiation. Diagn Mol Pathol. 1998;7:16–23.
39. van de Rijn M, Barr FG, Collins MH, Xiong QB, Fisher C. Absence of SYT-SSX fusion products in soft tissue tumors other than synovial sarcoma. Am J Clin Pathol. 1999;112:43–9.
40. Dennison S, Weppler E, Giacoppe G. Primary pulmonary synovial sarcoma: a case report and review of current diagnostic and therapeutic standards. Oncologist. 2004;9:339–42.
41. Etienne-Mastroianni B, Falchero L, Chalabreysse L, Loire R, Ranchère D, Souquet PJ, Cordier JF. Primary sarcomas of the lung: a clinicopathologic study of 12 cases. Lung Cancer. 2002;38: 283–9.
42. Inagaki H, Nagasaka T, Otsuka T, Sugiura E, Nakashima N, Eimoto T. Association of SYT-SSX fusion types with proliferative activity and prognosis in synovial sarcoma. Mod Pathol. 2000;13:482–8.
43. Kawai A, Woodruff J, Healey JH, Brennan MF, Antonescu CR, Ladanyi M. SYT-SSX gene fusion as a determinant of morphology and prognosis in synovial sarcoma. N Engl J Med. 1998;338: 153–60.
44. Nilsson G, Skytting B, Xie Y, Brodin B, Perfekt R, Mandahl N, Lundeberg J, Uhlén M, Larsson O. The SYT-SSX1 variant of synovial sarcoma is associated with a high rate of tumor cell proliferation and poor clinical outcome. Cancer Res. 1999;59:3180–4.
45. Kimizuka G, Okuzawa K, Yarita T. Primary giant cell malignant fibrous histocytoma of the lung: a case report. Pathol Int. 1999;49:342–6.
46. Maeda J, Ohta M, Inoue M, Okumura M, Minami M, Shiono H, Matsuda H. Surgical intervention for malignant fibrous histiocytoma of the lung: report of a case. Surg Today. 2007;37:316–9.
47. Kern WH, Hughes RK, Meyer BW, Harley DP. Malignant fibrous histiocytoma of the lung. Cancer. 1979;44:1793–801.
48. Bedrossian CW, Verani R, Unger KM, Salman J. Pulmonary malignant fibrous histiocytoma. Light and electron microscopic studies of one case. Chest. 1979;75:186–9.
49. Fu YS, Gabbiani G, Kaye GI, Lattes R. Malignant soft tissue tumors of probable histiocytic origin (malignant fibrous histiocytomas): general considerations and electron microscopic and tissue culture studies. Cancer. 1975;35:176–98.
50. Halyard MY, Camoriano JK, Culligan JA, Weiland LH, Allen MS, Pluth JR, Pairolero PC. Malignant fibrous histiocytoma of the lung. Report of four cases and review of the literature. Cancer. 1996;78:2492–7.
51. Yousem SA, Hochholzer L. Malignant fibrous histiocytoma of the lung. Cancer. 1987;60:2532–41.
52. Nistal M, Jimenez-Heffernan JA, Hardisson D, Viguer JM, Bueno J, Garcia-Miguel P. Malignant fibrous histiocytoma of the lung in a child. An unusual neoplasm that can mimick inflammatory pseudotumour. Eur J Pediatr. 1997;156:107–9.
53. Epstein NE, Sundrani S, Rosenthal AD. Cerebral metastasis from malignant pulmonary fibrous histiocytoma. A case report. Pediatr Neurosci. 1987;13:138–41.
54. Ismailer I, Khan A, Leonidas JC, Wind E, Herman P. Computed tomography of primary malignant fibrohistiocytoma of the lung. Comput Radiol. 1987;11:37–40.
55. Rzyman W, Jaskiewicz K, Murawski M, Sternau A, Marjanski T, Karmolinski A, Dziadziuszko R. Primary malignant fibrous histiocytoma of the lung. Thorac Cardiovasc Surg. 2007;55:186–9.
56. White SH, Ibrahim NB, Forrester-Wood CP, Jeyasingham K. Leiomyomas of the lower respiratory tract. Thorax. 1985;40:306–11.
57. Vera-Román JM, Sobonya RE, Gomez-Garcia JL, Sanz-Bondia JR, Paris-Romeu F. Leiomyoma of the lung. Literature review and case report. Cancer. 1983;52:936–41.
58. Shahian DM, McEnany MT. Complete endobronchial excision of leiomyoma of the bronchus. J Thorac Cardiovasc Surg. 1979;77: 87–91.
59. Orlowski TM, Stasiak K, Kolodziej J. Leiomyoma of the lung. J Thorac Cardiovasc Surg. 1978;76:257–61.
60. Sanders JS, Carnes VM. Leiomyoma of the trachea. Report of a case, with a note on the diagnosis of partial tracheal obstruction. N Engl J Med. 1961;264:277–9.
61. Foroughie E. Leiomyoma of the trachea. Dis Chest. 1962;42: 230–2.
62. Kitamura S, Maeda M, Kawashima Y, Masaoka A, Manabe H. Leiomyoma of the intrathoracic trachea. Report of a case successfully treated by primary end-to-end anastomosis following circumferential resection of the trachea. J Thorac Cardiovasc Surg. 1969;57: 126–33.
63. Taylor TL, Miller DR. Leiomyoma of the bronchus. J Thorac Cardiovasc Surg. 1969;57:284–8.
64. Gotti G, Haid MM, Paladini P, Di Bisceglie M, Volterrani L, Sforza V. Pedunculated pulmonary leiomyoma with large cyst formation. Ann Thorac Surg. 1993;56:1178–80.
65. Park JS, Lee M, Kim HK, Choi YS, Kim K, Kim J, Kim H, Shim YM. Primary leiomyoma of the trachea, bronchus, and pulmonary parenchyma – a single-institutional experience. Eur J Cardiothorac Surg. 2012;41(1):41–5.
66. Fitoz S, Atasoy C, Kizilkaya E, Başekim C, Karsli F. Radiologic findings in primary pulmonary leiomyosarcoma. J Thorac Imaging. 2000;15:151–2.

67. Takeda F, Yamagiwa I, Ohizumi H, Shiono S. Leiomyosarcoma of the main bronchus in a girl: a long-time survivor with multiple lung metastases. Pediatr Pulmonol. 2004;37:368–74.
68. Yellin A, Rosenman Y, Lieberman Y. Review of smooth muscle tumours of the lower respiratory tract. Br J Dis Chest. 1984;78:337–51.
69. Baker PB, Goodwin RA. Pulmonary artery sarcomas. A review and report of a case. Arch Pathol Lab Med. 1985;109:35–9.
70. Nerlich A, Permanetter W, Ludwig B, Remberger K. Primary leiomyosarcoma of the truncus pulmonalis. Report of a case with typical features and unusual metastases. Pathol Res Pract. 1990;186:296–9.
71. Thijs LG, Kroon TA, van Leeuwen TM. Leiomyosarcoma of the pulmonary trunk associated with pericardial effusion. Thorax. 1974;29:490–4.
72. Capewell S, Webb JN, Crompton GK. Primary leiomyosarcoma of the lung presenting with a persistent pneumothorax. Thorax. 1986;41:649–50.
73. Gil-Zuricalday C, Lor F, Gil-Turner C. Primary pedunculated leiomyosarcoma of the lung. Thorax. 1982;37:153–4.
74. Ramanathan T. Primary leiomyosarcoma of the lung. Thorax. 1974;29:482–9.
75. Wang NS, Seemayer TA, Ahmed MN, Morin J. Pulmonary leiomyosarcoma associated with an arteriovenous fistula. Arch Pathol. 1974;98:100–5.
76. Schanher Jr PW. Primary pulmonary leiomyosarcoma: case report and review of literature. Ann Surg. 1975;181:20–1.
77. Wick MR, Scheithauer BW, Piehler JM, Pairolero PC. Primary pulmonary leiomyosarcomas. A light and electron microscopic study. Arch Pathol Lab Med. 1982;106:510–4.
78. Jimenez JF, Uthman EO, Townsend JW, Gloster ES, Seibert JJ. Primary bronchopulmonary leiomyosarcoma in childhood. Arch Pathol Lab Med. 1986;110:348–51.
79. Moran CA, Suster S, Abbondanzo SL, Koss MN. Primary leiomyosarcomas of the lung: a clinicopathologic and immunohistochemical study of 18 cases. Mod Pathol. 1997;10:121–8.
80. Ownby D, Lyon G, Spock A. Primary leiomyosarcoma of the lung in childhood. Am J Dis Child. 1976;130:1132–3.
81. Lai DS, Lue KH, Su JM, Chang H. Primary bronchopulmonary leiomyosarcoma of the left main bronchus in a child presenting with wheezing and atelectasis of the left lung. Pediatr Pulmonol. 2002;33:318–21.
82. McNamara JJ, Paulson DL, Kingsley WB, Salinas-Izaquirre SF, Urschel Jr HC. Primary leiomyosarcoma of the lung. J Thorac Cardiovasc Surg. 1969;57:636–41.
83. Shoji F, Yoshino I, Takeshita M, Sumiyoshi S, Sueishi K, Maehara Y. Pulmonary leiomyosarcoma presenting as a pancoast tumor. Pathol Res Pract. 2007;203:745–8.
84. Passamonte PM, Luger AM. Primary pulmonary leiomyosarcoma with digital clubbing and pleural effusion. Case report Mo Med. 1984;81:667–8.
85. Kawai K, Fukamizu A, Kawakami Y, Matsumura M, Mitsui K, Murakami K, Yamashita K. A case of renin producing leiomyosarcoma originating in the lung. Endocrinol Jpn. 1991;38:603–9.
86. Suzuki K, Urushihara N, Fukumoto K, Watanabe K, Wada N, Takaba E. A case of Epstein-Barr virus-associated pulmonary leiomyosarcoma arising five yr after a pediatric renal transplant. Pediatr Transplant. 2011;15(7):E145–8. Epub 2010 Apr 26.
87. Randall WS, Blades B. Primary bronchiogenic leiomyosarcoma. Arch Pathol (Chic). 1946;42:543–8.
88. Lillo-Gil R, Albrechtsson U, Jakobsson B. Pulmonary leiomyosarcoma appearing as a cyst. Report of one case and review of the literature. Thorac Cardiovasc Surg. 1985;33:250–2.
89. Stark P, Frood L. Primary leiomyosarcoma of the lung originating in an emphysematous bulla. Rofo. 1989;151:738–9.
90. Patel SR, Jindrak KF, Anandarao N. Primary pedunculated leiomyosarcoma of the lung. N Y State J Med. 1991;91:30–1.
91. Schneider BF, Lovell MA, Golden WL. Cytogenetic abnormalities in primary bronchopulmonary leiomyosarcoma of childhood. Cancer Genet Cytogenet. 1998;105:145–51.
92. Janssen JP, Mulder JJ, Wagenaar SS, Elbers HR, van den Bosch JM. Primary sarcoma of the lung: a clinical study with long-term follow-up. Ann Thorac Surg. 1994;58:1151–5.
93. Morgan PG, Ball J. Pulmonary leiomyosarcomas. Br J Dis Chest. 1980;74:245–52.
94. Schiavetti A, Indolfi P, Hill DA, Priest JR. Primary pulmonary rhabdomyosarcoma in childhood: clinico-biologic features in two cases with review of the literature–erratum. Pediatr Blood Cancer. 2009;52:146.
95. Willis RA. Pathology of tumours. 3rd ed. London: Butterworth; 1960. p. 760–1.
96. Conquest HF, Thornton JL, Massie JR, Coxe 3rd JW. Primary pulmonary rhabdomyosarcoma; report of three cases and literature review. Ann Surg. 1965;161:688–92.
97. Daniels AC, Conner GH, Straus FH. Primary chondrosarcoma of the tracheobronchial tree. Report of a unique case and brief review. Arch Pathol. 1967;84:615–24.
98. McDonald Jr S, Heather JC. Neoplastic invasion of the pulmonary veins and left auricle. J Pathol Bacteriol. 1939;48:533–43.
99. Drennan JM, McCormack RJ. Primary rhabdomyosarcoma of the lung. J Pathol Bacteriol. 1960;79:147–9.
100. Aterman K, Patel S. Striated muscle in the lung. Am J Anat. 1970;128:341–58.
101. Comin CE, Santucci M, Novelli L, Dini S. Primary pulmonary rhabdomyosarcoma: report of a case in an adult and review of the literature. Ultrastruct Pathol. 2001;25:269–73.
102. Choi JS, Choi JS, Kim EJ. Primary pulmonary rhabdomyosarcoma in an adult with neurofibromatosis-1. Ann Thorac Surg. 2009;88:1356–8.
103. Przygodzki RM, Moran CA, Suster S, Koss MN. Primary pulmonary rhabdomyosarcomas: a clinicopathologic and immunohistochemical study of three cases. Mod Pathol. 1995;8:658–61.
104. Chang HL, Rosenberg AE, Friedmann AM, Ryan DP, Masiakos PT. Primary pulmonary rhabdomyosarcoma in a 5-month-old boy: a case report. J Pediatr Hematol Oncol. 2008;30:461–3.
105. Afify A, Mark HF. Trisomy 8 in embryonal rhabdomyosarcoma detected by fluorescence in situ hybridization. Cancer Genet Cytogenet. 1999;108:127–32.
106. Rodriguez FJ, Aubry MC, Tazelaar HD, Slezak J, Carney JA. Pulmonary chondroma: a tumor associated with Carney triad and different from pulmonary hamartoma. Am J Surg Pathol. 2007;31:1844–53.
107. Carney JA, Sheps SG, Go VL, Gordon H. The triad of gastric leiomyosarcoma, functioning extra-adrenal paraganglioma and pulmonary chondroma. N Engl J Med. 1977;296:1517–8.
108. Rees GM. Primary chondrosarcoma of lung. Thorax. 1970;25:366–71.
109. Hayashi T, Tsuda N, Iseki M, Kishikawa M, Shinozaki T, Hasumoto M. Primary chondrosarcoma of the lung. A clinicopathologic study. Cancer. 1993;72:69–74.
110. Kalhor N, Suster S, Moran CA. Primary pulmonary chondrosarcomas: a clinicopathologic study of 4 cases. Hum Pathol. 2011;42(11):1629–34. Epub 2011 Apr 14.
111. Morgan AD, Salama FD. Primary chondrosarcoma of the lung. Case report and review of the literature. J Thorac Cardiovasc Surg. 1972;64:460–6.
112. Sun CC, Kroll M, Miller JE. Primary chondrosarcoma of the lung. Cancer. 1982;50:1864–6.
113. Yellin A, Schwartz L, Hersho E, Lieberman Y. Chondrosarcoma of the bronchus. Chest. 1983;84:224–6.

114. Morgenroth A, Pfeuffer HP, Viereck HJ, Heine WD. Primary chondrosarcoma of the left inferior lobar bronchus. Respiration. 1989;56:241–4.
115. Jazy FK, Cormier WJ, Panke TW, Shehata WM, Amongero FJ. Primary chondrosarcoma of the lung. A report of two cases. Clin Oncol. 1984;10:273–9.
116. Watanabe A, Ito M, Nomura F, Saka H, Sakai S, Shimokata K. Primary chondrosarcoma of the lung – a case report with immunohistochemical study. Jpn J Med. 1990;29:616–9.
117. Parker LA, Molina PL, Bignault AG, Fidler ME. Primary pulmonary chondrosarcoma mimicking bronchogenic cyst on CT and MRI. Clin Imaging. 1996;20:181–3.
118. Alkotob LM, Miller R, Mehta AC. Primary endobronchial chondrosarcoma. J Bronchol. 2001;8:110–1.
119. Huang HY, Hsieh MJ, Chen WJ, Ko SF, Yang BY, Huang SC. Primary mesenchymal chondrosarcoma of the lung. Ann Thorac Surg. 2002;73:1960–2.
120. Shah ND, Diwanji SR. Primary chondrosarcoma of the lung with cutaneous and skeletal metastases. Singapore Med J. 2007;48: e196–9.
121. Steurer S, Huber M, Lintner F. Dedifferentiated chondrosarcoma of the lung: case report and review of the literature. Clin Lung Cancer. 2007;8:439–42.
122. Cao DB, Hua SC, Liu W, Feng CS. Primary giant pulmonary chondrosarcoma. Eur J Cardiothorac Surg. 2011;40:528.
123. Koh TW. Invasion of lung mesenchymal chondrosarcoma into the left atrium via the pulmonary vein detected on transoesophageal echocardiography. Eur J Echocardiogr. 2011;12:556.
124. Azimullah PC, Teengs JP, Boerma EJ. Chondrosarcoma of the lobar bronchus with prolonged postoperative survival. Eur Respir J. 1994;7:1537–8.
125. Simon MA, Ballon HC. An unusual hamartoma (so-called chondroma of the lung). J Thorac Surg. 1947;16:379–91.
126. Fasske E. On a hamartochondrosarcoma of the lung. Zentralbl Allg Pathol. 1965;107:514–9.
127. Kurotaki H, Tateoka H, Takeuchi M, Yagihashi S, Kamata Y, Nagai K. Primary mesenchymal chondrosarcoma of the lung. A case report with immunohistochemical and ultrastructural studies. Acta Pathol Jpn. 1992;42:364–7.
128. Wehrli BM, Huang W, De Crombrugghe B, Ayala AG, Czerniak B. Sox9, a master regulator of chondrogenesis, distinguishes mesenchymal chondrosarcoma from other small blue round cell tumors. Hum Pathol. 2003;34:263–9.
129. Bane BL, Evans HL, Ro JY, Carrasco CH, Grignon DJ, Benjamin RS, Ayala AG. Extraskeletal osteosarcoma. A clinicopathologic review of 26 cases. Cancer. 1990;65:2762–70.
130. Greenspan EB. Primary osteoid chondrosarcoma of the lung: report of a case. Am J Cancer. 1933;18:603–9.
131. Yamashita T, Kiyota T, Ukishima G, Hayama T, Yabuki E. Autopsy case of chondro-osteoid sarcoma originating in the lung. Showa Igakkai Zasshi. 1964;23:472–3.
132. Nosanchuk JS, Weatherbee L. Primary osteogenic sarcoma in lung. Report of a case. J Thorac Cardiovasc Surg. 1969;58:242–7.
133. Reingold IM, Amromin GD. Extraosseous osteosarcoma of the lung. Cancer. 1971;28:491–8.
134. Bagarić I, Belicza M. Extraskeletal osteogenic sarcoma of the lungs. Lijec Vjesn. 1982;104:467–70.
135. Saito H, Sakai S, Kobayashi T, Ishioroshi Y, Uno Y. Primary osteosarcoma of the lung – a case report. Nihon Kyobu Shikkan Gakkai Zasshi. 1983;21:153–6.
136. Colby TV, Bilbao JE, Battifora H, Unni KK. Primary osteosarcoma of the lung. A reappraisal following immunohistologic study. Arch Pathol Lab Med. 1989;113:1147–50.
137. Loose JH, el-Naggar AK, Ro JY, Huang WL, McMurtrey MJ, Ayala AG. Primary osteosarcoma of the lung. Report of two cases and review of the literature. J Thorac Cardiovasc Surg. 1990; 100:867–73.
138. Bhalla M, Thompson BG, Harley RA, McLoud TC. Primary extraosseous pulmonary osteogenic sarcoma: CT findings. J Comput Assist Tomogr. 1992;16:974–6.
139. Chapman AD, Pritchard SC, Yap WW, Rooney PH, Cockburn JS, Hutcheon AW, Nicolson MC, Kerr KM, McLeod HL. Primary pulmonary osteosarcoma: case report and molecular analysis. Cancer. 2001;91:779–84.
140. Sievert LJ, Elwing TJ, Evans ML. Primary pulmonary osteogenic sarcoma. Skeletal Radiol. 2000;29:283–5.
141. Magishi K, Yoshida H, Izumi Y, Ishikawa N, Kubota H. Primary osteosarcoma of the lung: report of a case. Surg Today. 2004;34: 150–2.
142. Kadowaki T, Hamada H, Yokoyama A, Katayama H, Abe M, Nishimura K, Tomiyama N, Kito K, Miyazaki T, Higaki J. Two cases of primary pulmonary osteosarcoma. Intern Med. 2005;44:632–7.
143. Yamazaki K, Okabayashi K, Hamatake D, Maekawa S, Yoshida Y, Yoshino I, Maehara Y. Primary osteosarcoma of the lung: a case report. Ann Thorac Cardiovasc Surg. 2006;12:126–8.
144. Shenjere P, Travis WD, Franks TJ, Doran HM, Hasleton PS. Primary pulmonary osteosarcoma: a report of 4 cases and a review of the literature. Int J Surg Pathol. 2011;19:225–9.
145. Sordillo PP, Hajdu SI, Magill GB, Golbey RB. Extraosseous osteogenic sarcoma. A review of 48 patients. Cancer. 1983;51: 727–34.
146. Schraufnagel DE, Morin JE, Wang NS. Endobronchial lipoma. Chest. 1979;75:97–9.
147. Jensen MS, Petersen AH. Bronchial lipoma. Scand J Thorac Cardiovasc Surg. 1970;4:131–4.
148. Allan JS. Rare solitary benign tumors of the lung. Semin Thorac Cardiovasc Surg. 2003;15:315–22.
149. Kim NR, Kim HJ, Kim JK, Han J. Intrapulmonary lipomas: report of four cases. Histopathology. 2003;42:305–6.
150. Muraoka M, Oka T, Akamine S, Nagayasu T, Iseki M, Suyama N, Ayabe H. Endobronchial lipoma: review of 64 cases reported in Japan. Chest. 2003;123:293–6.
151. Moran CA, Suster S, Koss MN. Endobronchial lipomas: a clinicopathologic study of four cases. Mod Pathol. 1994;7:212–4.
152. Matsuba K, Saito T, Ando K, Shirakusa T. Atypical lipoma of the lung. Thorax. 1991;46:685.
153. Pollefliet C, Peters K, Janssens A, Luijks A, Van Bouwel E, Van Marck E, Germonpre P. Endobronchial lipomas: rare benign lung tumors, two case reports. J Thorac Oncol. 2009;4:658–60.
154. Farrow GM, Harrison Jr EG, Utz DC, Jones DR. Renal angiomyolipoma. A clinicopathologic study of 32 cases. Cancer. 1968;22: 564–70.
155. Guinee Jr DG, Thornberry DS, Azumi N, Przygodzki RM, Koss MN, Travis WD. Unique pulmonary presentation of an angiomyolipoma. Analysis of clinical, radiographic, and histopathologic features. Am J Surg Pathol. 1995;19:476–80.
156. Ito M, Sugamura Y, Ikari H, Sekine I. Angiomyolipoma of the lung. Arch Pathol Lab Med. 1998;122:1023–5.
157. Wu K, Tazelaar HD. Pulmonary angiomyolipoma and multifocal micronodular pneumocyte hyperplasia associated with tuberous sclerosis. Hum Pathol. 1999;30:1266–8.
158. Garcia TR, Mestre de Juan MJ. Angiomyolipoma of the liver and lung: a case explained by the presence of perivascular epithelioid cells. Pathol Res Pract. 2002;198:363–7.
159. Saito M, Tsukamoto T, Takahashi T, Sai K, Fujii H, Nagashima K. Multifocal angiomyolipoma affecting the liver and lung without tuberous sclerosis. J Clin Pathol. 2004;57:221–4.
160. Marcheix B, Brouchet L, Lamarche Y, Renaud C, Gomez-Brouchet A, Hollington L, Chabbert V, Berjaud J, Dahan M. Pulmonary angiomyolipoma. Ann Thorac Surg. 2006;82:1504–6.

161. Henske EP, Neumann HP, Scheithauer BW, Herbst EW, Short MP, Kwiatkowski DJ. Loss of heterozygosity in the tuberous sclerosis (TSC2) region of chromosome band 16p13 occurs in sporadic as well as TSC-associated renal angiomyolipomas. Genes Chromosomes Cancer. 1995;13:295–8.
162. Krygier G, Amado A, Salisbury S, Fernandez I, Maedo N, Vazquez T. Primary lung liposarcoma. Lung Cancer. 1997;17:271–5.
163. Said M, Migaw H, Hafsa C, Braham R, Golli M, Moussa A, Zakhama A, Elkamel A, Gannouni A. Imaging features of primary pulmonary liposarcoma. Australas Radiol. 2003;47:313–7.
164. Uchikov A, Poriazova E, Zaprianov Z, Markova D. Low-grade pulmonary myxoid liposarcoma. Interact Cardiovasc Thorac Surg. 2005;4:402–3.
165. Sawamura K, Hashimoto T, Nanjo S, Nakamura K, Iioka S, Mori T, Furuse K, Shakudo Y. Primary liposarcoma of the lung: report of a case. J Surg Oncol. 1982;19:243–6.
166. Ruiz-Palomo F, Calleja JL, Fogue L. Primary liposarcoma of the lung in a young woman. Thorax. 1990;45:298–9.
167. Matsuoka H, Takata Y, Maeda S. Primary pulmonary myxoma. Ann Thorac Surg. 2005;79:329–30.
168. Littlefield JB, Drash EC. Myxoma of the lung. J Thorac Surg. 1959;37:745–9.
169. Abcarian H, Lee HT, Barker WL. Primary endobronchial myxoma. Ann Thorac Surg. 1973;15:287–90.
170. Kalhor N, Marom EM, Moran CA. Primary myxoma of the lung. Ann Diagn Pathol. 2010;14:178–81.
171. Wang NS, Morin J. Recurrent endobronchial soft tissue tumors. Chest. 1984;85:787–91.
172. Choi YD, Kim JH, Nam JH, Choi C, Na KJ, Song SY. Aggressive angiomyxoma of the lung. J Clin Pathol. 2008;61:962–4.
173. Nicholson AG, Baandrup U, Florio R, Sheppard MN, Fisher C. Malignant myxoid endobronchial tumour: a report of two cases with a unique histological pattern. Histopathology. 1999;35: 313–8.
174. Lane KL, Shannon RJ, Weiss SW. Hyalinizing spindle cell tumor with giant rosettes: a distinctive tumor closely resembling low-grade fibromyxoid sarcoma. Am J Surg Pathol. 1997;21:1481–8.
175. Folpe AL, Lane KL, Paull G, Weiss SW. Low-grade fibromyxoid sarcoma and hyalinizing spindle cell tumor with giant rosettes: a clinicopathologic study of 73 cases supporting their identity and assessing the impact of high-grade areas. Am J Surg Pathol. 2000;24:1353–60.
176. Magro G, Fraggetta F, Manusia M, Mingrino A. Hyalinizing spindle cell tumor with giant rosettes: a previously undescribed lesion of the lung. Am J Surg Pathol. 1998;22:1431–3.
177. Kim L, Yoon YH, Choi SJ, Han JY, Park IS, Kim JM, Chu YC, Kim YJ. Hyalinizing spindle cell tumor with giant rosettes arising in the lung: report of a case with FUS-CREB3L2 fusion transcripts. Pathol Int. 2007;57:153–7.
178. Reid R, de Silva MV, Paterson L, Ryan E, Fisher C. Low-grade fibromyxoid sarcoma and hyalinizing spindle cell tumor with giant rosettes share a common t(7;16)(q34;p11) translocation. Am J Surg Pathol. 2003;27:1229–36.
179. Matsuyama A, Hisaoka M, Shimajiri S, Hayashi T, Imamura T, Ishida T, Fukunaga M, Fukuhara T, Minato H, Nakajima T, Yonezawa S, Kuroda M, Yamasaki F, Toyoshima S, Hashimoto H. Molecular detection of FUS-CREB3L2 fusion transcripts in low-grade fibromyxoid sarcoma using formalin-fixed, paraffin-embedded tissue specimens. Am J Surg Pathol. 2006;30:1077–84.
180. Woodruff JM, Antonescu CR, Erlandson RA, Boland PJ. Low-grade fibrosarcoma with palisaded granulomalike bodies (giant rosettes): report of a case that metastasized. Am J Surg Pathol. 1999;23:1423–8.
181. Farinha P, Oliveira P, Soares J. Metastasizing hyalinizing spindle cell tumour with giant rosettes: report of a case with long survival. Histopathology. 2000;36:92–3.
182. Roviaro G, Montorsi M, Varoli F, Binda R, Cecchetto A. Primary pulmonary tumours of neurogenic origin. Thorax. 1983;38: 942–5.
183. McCluggage WG, Bharucha H. Primary pulmonary tumours of nerve sheath origin. Histopathology. 1995;26:247–54.
184. Doesel H. Intrabronchial psammous neurofibroma. Thoraxchirurgie. 1961;8:657–60.
185. Zisis C, Dountsis A, Dahabreh J. Multiple bilateral recurrent neurofibromas of the lungs. Eur J Cardiothorac Surg. 2003;24: 826.
186. Mahapatro RC, Bhavthankar AG, Kolhatkar MK. Neurofibroma of lung. J Indian Med Assoc. 1976;67:182–4.
187. Batori M, Lazzaro M, Lonardo MT, Lupi M, Annessi M, Loffredo L, Mugnaini L, Sportelli G. A rare case of pulmonary neurofibroma: clinical and diagnostic evaluation and surgical treatment. Eur Rev Med Pharmacol Sci. 1999;3:155–7.
188. Suzuki H, Sekine Y, Motohashi S, Chiyo M, Suzuki M, Haga Y, Hiroshima K, Ohwada H, Iizasa T, Saitoh Y, Baba M, Fujisawa T. Endobronchial neurogenic tumors treated by transbronchial electrical snaring and Nd-YAG laser abrasion: report of three cases. Surg Today. 2005;35:243–6.
189. Ohtsuka T, Nomori H, Naruke T, Orikasa H, Yamazaki K, Suemasu K. Intrapulmonary schwannoma. Jpn J Thorac Cardiovasc Surg. 2005;53:154–6.
190. Bosch X, Ramírez J, Font J, Bombí JA, Ferrer J, Vendrell J, Ingelmo M. Primary intrapulmonary benign schwannoma. A case with ultrastructural and immunohistochemical confirmation. Eur Respir J. 1990;3:234–7.
191. Unger PD, Geller GA, Anderson PJ. Pulmonary lesions in a patient with neurofibromatosis. Arch Pathol Lab Med. 1984;108: 654–7.
192. Chen SR, Chen MH, Ho DM, Lin FC, Chang SC. Massive hemoptysis caused by endobronchial schwannoma in a patient with neurofibromatosis 2. Am J Med Sci. 2003;325:299–302.
193. Domen H, Iwashiro N, Kimura N, Jinushi E, Komuro K, Ohara M, Ishizaka M. Intrapulmonary cellular schwannoma. Ann Thorac Surg. 2010;90:1352–5.
194. Simansky DA, Aviel-Ronen S, Reder I, Paley M, Refaely Y, Yellin A. Psammomatous melanotic schwannoma: presentation of a rare primary lung tumor. Ann Thorac Surg. 2000;70:671–2.
195. Díaz Beveridge R, Richart Aznar P, Núñez Lozano C, Chirivella Casanova M, Corbellas Aparicio M, Montalar Salcedo J. Orbital and myocardial metastases of a primary pulmonary melanotic schwannoma. Clin Transl Oncol. 2010;12:509–11.
196. Crotty TB, Hooker RP, Swensen SJ, Scheithauer BW, Myers JL. Primary malignant ependymoma of the lung. Mayo Clin Proc. 1992;67:373–8.
197. Idowu MO, Rosenblum MK, Wei XJ, Edgar MA, Soslow RA. Ependymomas of the central nervous system and adult extra-axial ependymomas are morphologically and immunohistochemically distinct – a comparative study with assessment of ovarian carcinomas for expression of glial fibrillary acidic protein. Am J Surg Pathol. 2008;32:710–8.
198. Cooney TP. Primary pulmonary ganglioneuroblastoma in an adult: maturation, involution and the immune response. Histopathology. 1981;5:451–63.
199. Markaki S, Edwards C. Intrapulmonary ganglioneuroma. A case report. Arch Anat Cytol Pathol. 1987;35:183–4.
200. Blankoff B. Primary and metastatic nervous tumors of the respiratory system. Apropos of 2 cases of ganglioneuroma in children. Acta Tuberc Pneumol Belg. 1965;56:363–92.
201. Opdedeck W, Demedtj M. Endobronchial ganglioneuroma. Lille Med. 1962;7:71.
202. Hochholzer L, Moran CA, Koss MN. Primary pulmonary ganglioneuroblastoma: a clinicopathologic and immunohistochemical study of two cases. Ann Diagn Pathol. 1998;2:154–8.

203. deCou JM, Rao BN, Parham DM, Lobe TE, Bowman L, Pappo AS, Fontanesi J. Malignant peripheral nerve sheath tumors: the St. Jude Children's Research Hospital experience. Ann Surg Oncol. 1995;2:524–9.
204. Komori M, Yabuuchi H, Kuroiwa T, Nagatoshi Y, Ichinose Y, Hachitanda Y. Thoracic malignant peripheral nerve sheath tumour mimicking a pleural tumour: a rare pedunculated appearance. Pediatr Radiol. 2003;33:578–81.
205. Bartley TD, Arean VM. Intrapulmonary neurogenic tumors. J Thorac Cardiovasc Surg. 1965;50:114–23.
206. Kitamura H, Kitamura H. Primary epithelioid malignant schwannoma of the lung. Pathol Int. 1994;44:317–24.
207. Diveley W, Daniel Jr RA. Primary solitary neurogenic tumors of the lung. J Thorac Surg. 1951;21:194–201.
208. Petriat A, Cornet L, Leger H, Castaing R, Tessier R. Primary intrapulmonary neurinoma. Presse Med. 1953;61:1526–8.
209. Neilson DB. Primary intrapulmonary neurogenic sarcoma. J Pathol Bacteriol. 1958;76:419–30.
210. Wiebe T, Schirpke C, Nicolai D, Preisler J, Wetzer K. A rare intrapulmonary tumor – malignant schwannoma. Prax Klin Pneumol. 1988;42:63–5.
211. Petrov D, Dakov Y, Strumeliev S, Wlassov W, Michowa Z. Malignant schwannoma of the lung. Z Erkr Atmungsorgane. 1990;175:32–7.
212. Kogel H, Mohr W. Malignant schwannoma of the lung. Zentralbl Chir. 1991;116:57–60.
213. Togashi K, Hirahara H, Sugawara M, Oguma F. Primary malignant schwannoma of the lung. Jpn J Thorac Cardiovasc Surg. 2003;51:692–5.
214. Muwakkit SA, Rodriguez-Galindo C, El Samra AI, Khoury R, Akel SR, Mroueh S, Razzouk B, Abboud MR. Primary malignant peripheral nerve sheath tumor of the lung in a young child without neurofibromatosis type 1. Pediatr Blood Cancer. 2006;47:636–8.
215. Tashiro T, Kawakita C, Takai C, Yoshida T, Sakiyama S, Kondo K, Sano N. Primary pulmonary malignant peripheral nerve sheath tumor: a case report. Acta Cytol. 2007;51:820–4.
216. Uchiyama M, Shimoyama Y, Usami N, Ito S, Yasuda A, Kawaguchi K, Yokoi K. Primary pulmonary malignant schwannoma with extension to the tracheal carina. J Thorac Cardiovasc Surg. 2007;133:265–7.
217. Keel SB, Bacha E, Mark EJ, Nielsen GP, Rosenberg AE. Primary pulmonary sarcoma: a clinicopathologic study of 26 cases. Mod Pathol. 1999;12:1124–31.
218. Askin FB, Rosai J, Sibley RK, Dehner LP, McAlister WH. Malignant small cell tumor of the thoracopulmonary region in childhood: a distinctive clinicopathologic entity of uncertain histogenesis. Cancer. 1979;43:2438–51.
219. Kahn AG, Avagnina A, Nazar J, Elsner B. Primitive neuroectodermal tumor of the lung. Arch Pathol Lab Med. 2001;125:397–9.
220. Hammar S, Bockus D, Remington F, Cooper L. The unusual spectrum of neuroendocrine lung neoplasms. Ultrastruct Pathol. 1989;13:515–60.
221. Takahashi D, Nagayama J, Nagatoshi Y, Inagaki J, Nishiyama K, Yokoyama R, Moriyasu Y, Okada K, Okamura J. Primary Ewing's sarcoma family tumors of the lung a case report and review of the literature. Jpn J Clin Oncol. 2007;37:874–7.
222. Mikami Y, Nakajima M, Hashimoto H, Irei I, Matsushima T, Kawabata S, Manabe T. Primary pulmonary primitive neuroectodermal tumor (PNET). A case report. Pathol Res Pract. 2001;197:113–9.
223. Tsuji S, Hisaoka M, Morimitsu Y, Hashimoto H, Jimi A, Watanabe J, Eguchi H, Kaneko Y. Peripheral primitive neuroectodermal tumour of the lung: report of two cases. Histopathology. 1998;33:369–74.
224. Baumgartner FJ, Omari BO, French SW. Primitive neuroectodermal tumor of the pulmonary hilum in an adult. Ann Thorac Surg. 2001;72:285–7.
225. Imamura F, Funakoshi T, Nakamura S, Mano M, Kodama K, Horai T. Primary primitive neuroectodermal tumor of the lung: report of two cases. Lung Cancer. 2000;27:55–60.
226. Batsakis JG, Mackay B, el-Naggar AK. Ewing's sarcoma and peripheral primitive neuroectodermal tumor: an interim report. Ann Otol Rhinol Laryngol. 1996;105:838–43.
227. Bown NP, Reid MM, Malcolm AJ, Davison EV, Craft AW, Pearson AD. Cytogenetic abnormalities of small round cell tumours. Med Pediatr Oncol. 1994;23:124–9.
228. Whang-Peng J, Triche TJ, Knutsen T, Miser J, Kao-Shan S, Tsai S, Israel MA. Cytogenetic characterization of selected small round cell tumors of childhood. Cancer Genet Cytogenet. 1986;21:185–208.
229. Lawlor ER, Mathers JA, Bainbridge T, Horsman DE, Kawai A, Healey JH, Huvos AG, Bridge JA, Ladanyi M, Sorensen PH. Peripheral primitive neuroectodermal tumors in adults: documentation by molecular analysis. J Clin Oncol. 1998;16:1150–7.
230. Demir A, Gunluoglu MZ, Dagoglu N, Turna A, Dizdar Y, Kaynak K, Dilege S, Mandel NM, Yilmazbayhan D, Dincer SI, Gurses A. Surgical treatment and prognosis of primitive neuroectodermal tumors of the thorax. J Thorac Oncol. 2009;4:185–92.
231. Huo L, Lai S, Gladish G, Czerniak BA, Moran CA. Pulmonary artery angiosarcoma: a clinicopathologic and radiological correlation. Ann Diagn Pathol. 2005;9:209–14.
232. Tomashefski Jr JF. Benign endobronchial mesenchymal tumors: their relationship to parenchymal pulmonary hamartomas. Am J Surg Pathol. 1982;6:531–40.
233. van den Bosch JM, Wagenaar SS, Corrin B, Elbers JR, Knaepen PJ, Westermann CJ. Mesenchymoma of the lung (so-called hamartoma): a review of 154 parenchymal and endobronchial cases. Thorax. 1987;42:790–3.
234. Bateson EM. So-called hamartoma of the lung – a true neoplasm of fibrous connective tissue of the bronchi. Cancer. 1973;31:1458–67.
235. Steele JD. The solitary pulmonary nodule. Report of a cooperative study of resected asymptomatic solitary pulmonary nodules in males. J Thorac Cardiovasc Surg. 1963;46:21–39.
236. Ray 3rd JF, Lawton BR, Magnin GE, Dovenbarger WV, Smullen WA, Reyes CN, Myers WO, Wenzel FJ, Sautter RD. The coin lesion story: update 1976. Twenty years' experience with thoracotomy for 179 suspected malignant coin lesions. Chest. 1976;70:332–6.
237. Anderson MN. Multicentric hamartomas of the lung – report of a case with two additional lesions nine years after primary resection. Ann Thorac Surg. 1968;6:469–72.
238. Minasian H. Uncommon pulmonary hamartomas. Thorax. 1977;32:360–4.
239. Johansson M, Dietrich C, Mandahl N, Hambraeus G, Johansson L, Clausen PP, Mitelman F, Heim S. Recombinations of chromosomal bands 6p21 and 14q24 characterise pulmonary hamartomas. Br J Cancer. 1993;67:1236–41.
240. McDonald JR, Harrington SW, Clagett OT. Hamartoma (often called chondroma) of the lung. J Thorac Surg. 1945;14:128–43.
241. Schwartz M. A biomathematical approach to clinical tumor growth. Cancer. 1961;14:1272–94.
242. Bini A, Grazia M, Petrella F, Chittolini M. Multiple chondromatous hamartomas of the lung. Interact Cardiovasc Thorac Surg. 2002;1:78–80.
243. Minami Y, Iijima T, Yamamoto T, Morishita Y, Terashima H, Onizuka M, Noguchi M. Diffuse pulmonary hamartoma: a case report. Pathol Res Pract. 2005;200:813–6.
244. Rossi G, Cavazza A, Valli R, Torricelli P, Richeldi L, Rivasi F, Brambilla E. Atypical lipomatous tumour (lipoma-like well-differentiated liposarcoma) arising in a pulmonary hamartoma and clinically presenting with pneumothorax. Lung Cancer. 2003;39:103–6.

245. Fudge TL, Ochsner JL, Mills NL. Clinical spectrum of pulmonary hamartomas. Ann Thorac Surg. 1980;30:36–9.
246. Karasik A, Modan M, Jacob CO, Lieberman Y. Increased risk of lung cancer in patients with chondromatous hamartoma. J Thorac Cardiovasc Surg. 1980;80:217–20.
247. Cavazza A, Paci M, Rossi G. Pulmonary hamartoma associated with typical carcinoid/tumorlet. Virchows Arch. 2006;449:392–3.
248. Pelosi G, Rodriguez J, Viale G, Rosai J. Salivary gland-type tumors with myoepithelial differentiation arising in pulmonary hamartoma: report of 2 cases of a hitherto unrecognized association. Am J Surg Pathol. 2006;30:375–87.
249. Saxena P, Downie S, Amanuel B, Newman M, Konstantinov IE. Giant pulmonary hamartoma: an interesting clinico-pathologic entity. Heart Lung Circ. 2010;19:573.
250. Miura K, Hori T, Yoshizawa K, Hamaguchi N, Morita J. Cystic pulmonary hamartoma. Ann Thorac Surg. 1990;49:828–9.
251. O'Connor-Harris L, Nasrallah D, Heitmiller 3rd R. Extralobar pulmonary hamartoma. J Am Coll Surg. 2006;202:378–9.
252. Fletcher JA, Pinkus GS, Weidner N, Morton CC. Lineage-restricted clonality in biphasic solid tumors. Am J Pathol. 1991;138:1199–207.
253. Johansson M, Heim S, Mandahl N, Johansson L, Hambraeus G, Mitelman F. t(3;6;14)(p21;p21;q24) as the sole clonal chromosome abnormality in a hamartoma of the lung. Cancer Genet Cytogenet. 1992;60:219–20.
254. Kazmierczak B, Meyer-Bolte K, Tran KH, Wöckel W, Breightman I, Rosigkeit J, Bartnitzke S, Bullerdiek J. A high frequency of tumors with rearrangements of genes of the HMGI(Y) family in a series of 191 pulmonary chondroid hamartomas. Genes Chromosomes Cancer. 1999;26:125–33.
255. Salminen US. Pulmonary hamartoma. A clinical study of 77 cases in a 21-year period and review of literature. Eur J Cardiothorac Surg. 1990;4:15–8.
256. Moran CA, Suster S, Koss MN. Primary malignant 'triton' tumour of the lung. Histopathology. 1997;30:140–4.
257. Suzuki T, Suzuki S, Kamio Y, Hori G, Tomita S, Suzuki H, Mitsuya T, Tate G, Sagawa F. A case of malignant Triton tumor of the lung. Thorac Cardiovasc Surg. 1996;44:319–20.
258. Cox JE, Chiles C, Aquino SL, Savage P, Oaks T. Pulmonary artery sarcomas: a review of clinical and radiologic features. J Comput Assist Tomogr. 1997;21:750–5.
259. Burke AP, Virmani R. Sarcomas of the great vessels. A clinicopathologic study. Cancer. 1993;71:1761–73.
260. Okuno T, Matsuda K, Ueyama K, Oota N, Terada Y, Hohjoh Y, Sakurai T, Nakayama T, Kitaichi M, Yamabe H. Leiomyosarcoma of the pulmonary vein. Pathol Int. 2000;50:839–46.
261. Altman NH, Shelley WM. Primary intimal sarcoma of the pulmonary artery. Johns Hopkins Med J. 1973;133:214–22.
262. Lyerly HK, Reves JG, Sabiston Jr DC. Management of primary sarcomas of the pulmonary artery and reperfusion intrabronchial hemorrhage. Surg Gynecol Obstet. 1986;163:291–301.
263. Krüger I, Borowski A, Horst M, de Vivie ER, Theissen P, Gross-Fengels W. Symptoms, diagnosis, and therapy of primary sarcomas of the pulmonary artery. Thorac Cardiovasc Surg. 1990;38: 91–5.
264. Wright EC, Wellons HA, Martin RP. Primary pulmonary artery sarcoma diagnosed noninvasively by two-dimensional echocardiography. Circulation. 1983;67:459–62.
265. Huo L, Moran CA, Fuller GN, Gladish G, Suster S. Pulmonary artery sarcoma: a clinicopathologic and immunohistochemical study of 12 cases. Am J Clin Pathol. 2006;125:419–24.
266. Berney CR, Roche B, Kurt AM, Spiliopoulos A, Mégevand R. Leiomyosarcoma of the pulmonary hilar vessels. Thorac Cardiovasc Surg. 1992;40:48–51.
267. Goldblum JR, Rice TW. Epithelioid angiosarcoma of the pulmonary artery. Hum Pathol. 1995;26:1275–7.
268. Tavora F, Miettinen M, Fanburg-Smith J, Franks TJ, Burke A. Pulmonary artery sarcoma: a histologic and follow-up study with emphasis on a subset of low-grade myofibroblastic sarcomas with a good long-term follow-up. Am J Surg Pathol. 2008;32:1751–61.
269. Kimura I, Kiuchi H, Sakamoto Y, Yamamoto K, Dohi Y, Takahama M. Primary osteogenic sarcoma of pulmonary artery. Jpn J Med. 1990;29:32–7.
270. Casullo J, Lisbona A, Palayew MJ. General case of the day. Primary sarcoma of the pulmonary artery (chondrosarcoma). Radiographics. 1992;12:401–4.
271. Faul JL, Wahl T, Ihnken K, Berry GJ, Doyle RL, Whyte RI. Superior vena cava syndrome caused by pulmonary artery sarcoma. J Thorac Cardiovasc Surg. 1999;118:749–50.

10 Lung Tumors of Uncertain Histogenesis

Introduction

The cell of origin of several rare lung tumors is still a matter of debate. Although some progress has been made in the last few decades in identifying the possible histogenesis of these tumors, their exact origins remain uncertain. Clear cell sugar tumor of lung, granular cell tumor, inflammatory pseudotumor, and sclerosing hemangioma are a group of tumors that fall into this category. A summary of the most pertinent features of these tumors is provided in Table 10.1.

Clear Cell Sugar Tumor of Lung

Clear cell sugar tumor of the lung is a rare neoplasm with less than 50 cases described in the literature to date. This tumor was first described by Liebow and Castleman in 1963 [1], reporting a benign clear cell tumor of the lung. The subsequent finding of abundant cytoplasmic glycogen in this tumor later led to its name "sugar cell tumor" [2]. The cell of origin of these tumors has long been a matter of debate. Initially believed to be of myoid origin [2], later proposals suggested neuroendocrine, epithelial, melanocytic, and pericytic differentiation [3–6]. More recently, it was noted that clear cell sugar tumors of the lung share morphologic and immunohistochemical features with a group of tumors known as perivascular epithelioid cell tumors (PEComas), which include angiomyolipoma, lymphangioleiomyomatosis, and clear cell myomelanocytic tumor of ligamentum teres/falciform ligament and that have been linked with the tuberous sclerosis complex [7, 8]. Hence, the "perivascular epithelioid cell" may be the regarded as the precursor cell of these tumors.

Clinical Features

Clear cell sugar tumors usually present in middle-aged adults (40–60 years) with no specific sex predilection; however, isolated cases have been described in children and adolescents [9, 10]. Since most of these tumors occur in the peripheral portions of the lung, patients are usually asymptomatic and the tumors are usually found incidentally. In rare cases, however, patients may present with hemoptysis, fever, anemia, and abnormal inflammatory blood serum markers [11, 12]. On imaging, a typical solitary "coin lesion" is identified on chest X-ray or computed tomography (CT) often mimicking a malignant lung tumor.

Gross Features

Clear cell sugar tumors are well circumscribed but unencapsulated neoplasms usually measuring less than 3 cm, but larger tumors (up to 12 cm) have also been described [11, 13]. The lesions are located in the lung parenchyma and are unrelated to the bronchial system. The cut surface is homogenous and of white or tan color. Necrosis, hemorrhage, or calcification is uncommon and has only rarely been described in cases that metastasized [14–16]. Cystic change has also been described in isolated cases [13].

A. Weissferdt, C.A. Moran, *Diagnostic Pathology of Pleuropulmonary Neoplasia*,
DOI 10.1007/978-1-4419-0787-5_10, © Springer Science+Business Media New York 2013

Table 10.1 Histological, immunohistochemical, ultrastructural, and molecular features of lung tumors of uncertain histogenesis

Tumor	Presumed cell of origin	Histology	Immunohistochemical features	Ultrastructural features	Molecular features
Clear cell sugar cell tumor	Perivascular epithelioid cell	Proliferation of clear cells with bland cytologic features	HMB45, S100 protein, CD1a, CD34	Abundant membrane-bound glycogen vesicles, pericytic differentiation and the presence of premelanosomes	Not investigated
Granular cell tumor	Schwann cell	Sheet-like proliferation of cells with abundant eosinophilic granular cytoplasm	S100 protein, CD68, NSE, vimentin	Abundant membrane-bound cytoplasmic granules consistent with lysosomes	Not investigated
Sclerosing hemangioma	Type II pneumocyte	Tumor composed of surface (cuboidal) and stromal (round) cells; solid, hemorrhagic, papillary, and sclerotic patterns	TTF-1, EMA; surface cells also positive for CK, CEA, surfactant protein alpha	Not routinely investigated	Loss of heterozygosity at 5q and 10q; microsatellite alterations of p16 and RB genes; t(8;18) and trisomy 14
Inflammatory pseudotumor	Myofibroblast	Fibrohistiocytic variant: myofibroblastic spindle cells admixed with an inflammatory cell infiltrate; plasma cell variant: proliferation of plasma cells admixed with smaller numbers of myofibroblastic spindle cells	ALK-1, SMA, vimentin; kappa and lambda light chains, IgG4 in plasma cells	Not routinely investigated	ALK-1 translocations

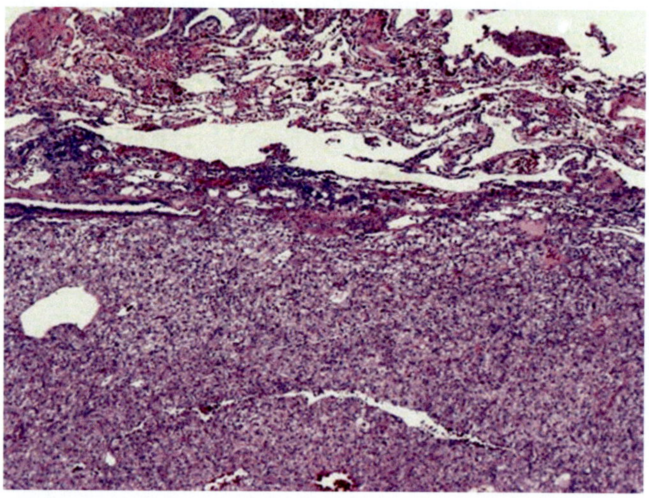

Fig. 10.1 Low-power view of sugar cell tumor of the lung demonstrating the circumscribed nature of the lesion

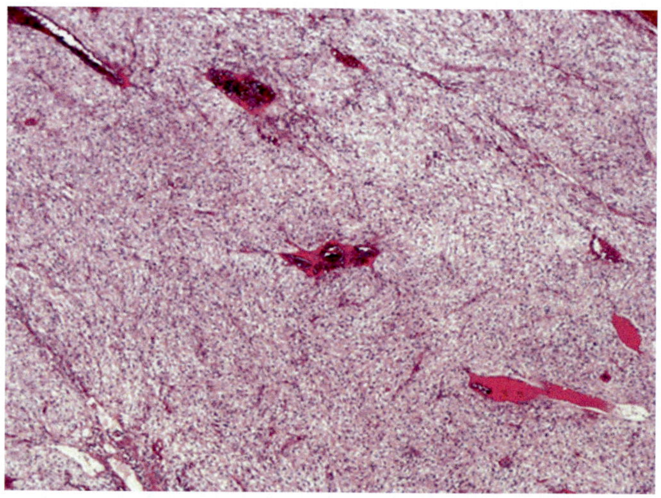

Fig. 10.2 Sugar cell tumor of the lung composed of sheets of clear cells with little stromal component

Histological Features

Clear cell sugar tumors are characterized by a sheet-like proliferation of large clear cells with little intervening stroma (Figs. 10.1 and 10.2). The cells are polygonal in shape, have distinct cell borders, and possess uniform oval-shaped nuclei and inconspicuous nucleoli (Figs. 10.3, 10.4, and 10.5). The most characteristic features are the cytoplasmic clearing of the cells and prominent sinusoidal or hemangiopericytoma-like blood vessels, which may show hyaline changes (Figs. 10.6, 10.7, and 10.8). Typically, the tumor cells are immediately juxtaposed to the vessel wall with no visible intervening stroma (Fig. 10.9). In addition, areas of spindle-shaped cells (Fig. 10.10), Touton-type or other giant cells (Fig. 10.11), calcification (Fig. 10.12), "spider cells" (large cells with granules radiating from the nucleus in a linear arrangement) (Fig. 10.13), and "neuroid cells" (round or polygonal cells with homogenous acidophilic cytoplasm resembling neural cells) (Fig. 10.14) can be observed. Mitotic activity, cellular pleomorphism,

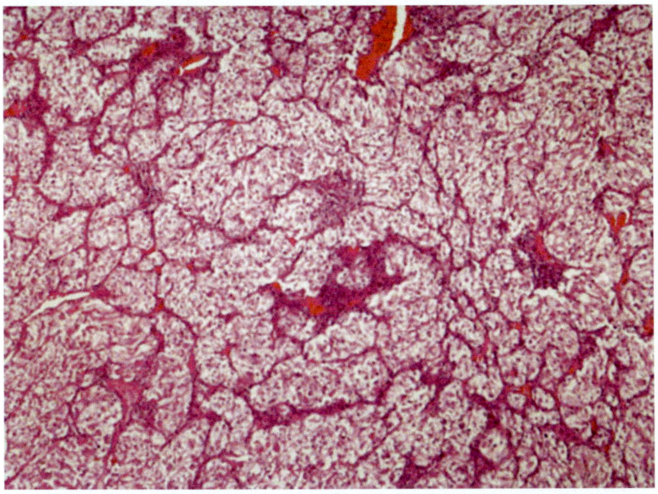

Fig. 10.3 More nested pattern composed of larger clear cells in sugar cell tumor of the lung

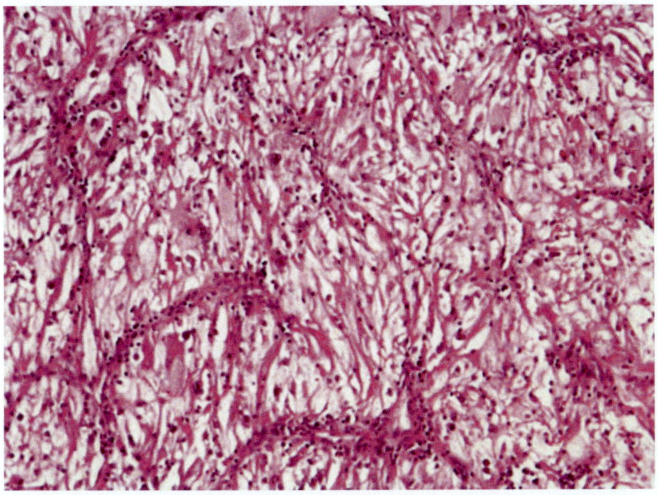

Fig. 10.4 Sugar cell tumor of lung composed of large cells with clear to eosinophilic cytoplasm

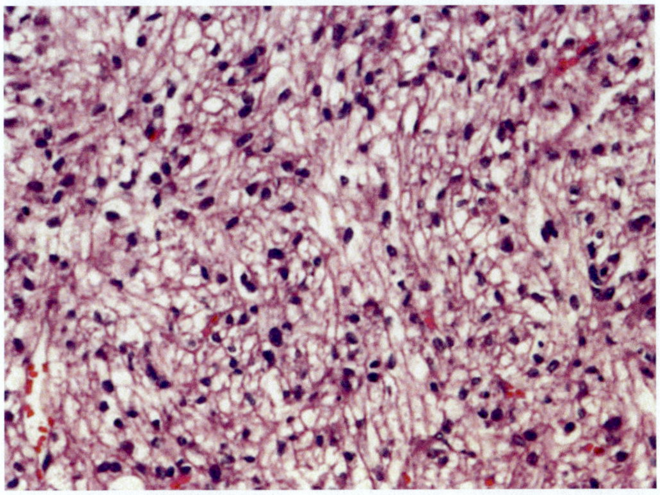

Fig. 10.5 Classic appearance of sugar cell tumor composed of monomorphic clear cells

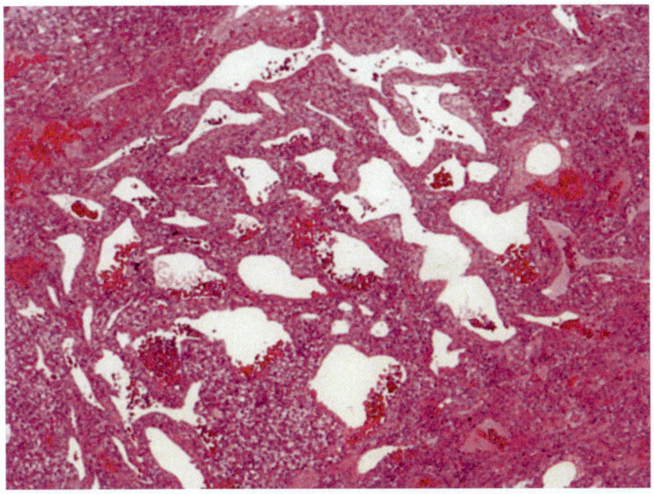

Fig. 10.6 Prominent dilated sinusoidal-like blood vessels in sugar cell tumor of the lung

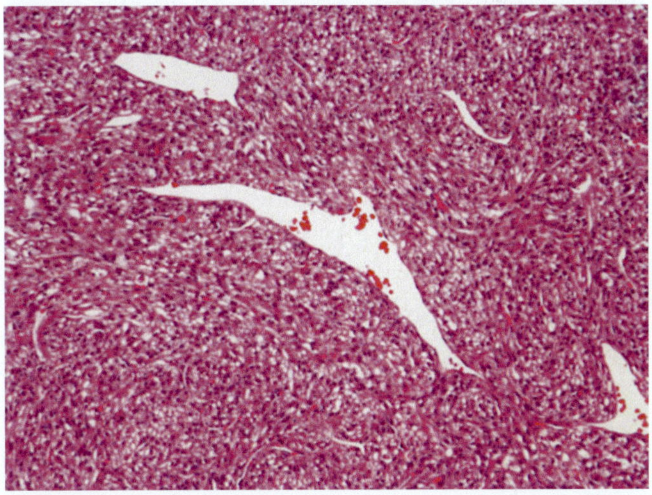

Fig.10.7 Hemangiopericytoma-like vessels are a typical finding in sugar cell tumor

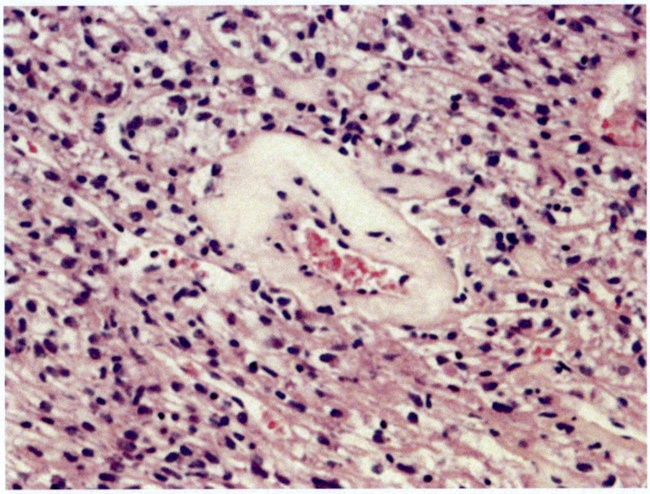

Fig. 10.8 Hyaline changes of the vessel walls are not uncommon in sugar cell tumor

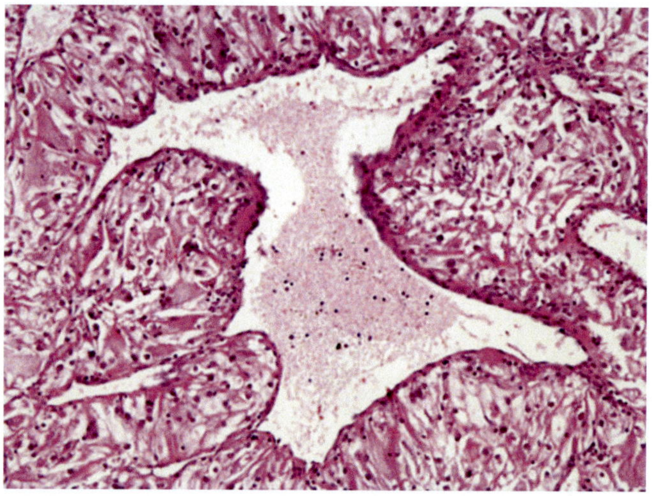

Fig. 10.9 Tumor cells of sugar cell tumor located immediately adjacent to the vessel walls

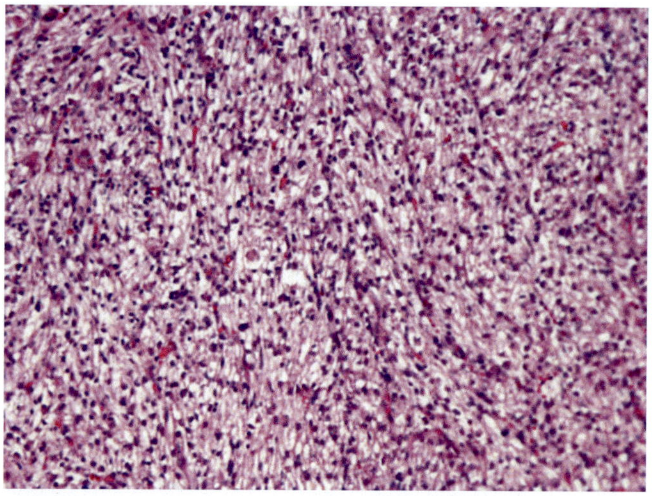

Fig. 10.10 Sugar cell tumor of lung showing slight spindling of the tumor cells

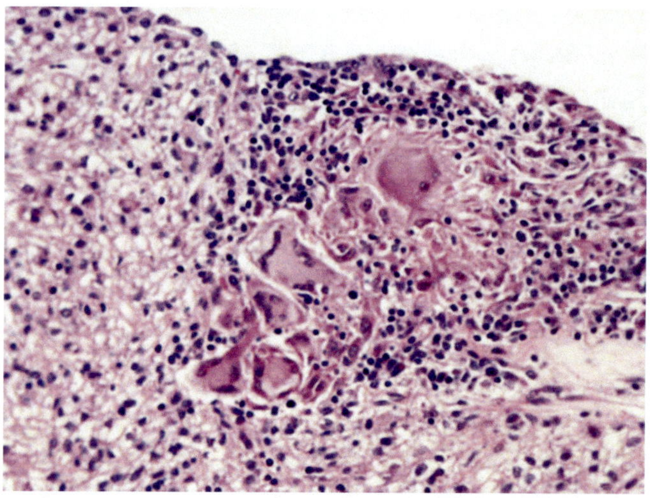

Fig. 10.11 Cluster of multinucleate giant cells forming an ill-defined granuloma in sugar cell tumor of the lung

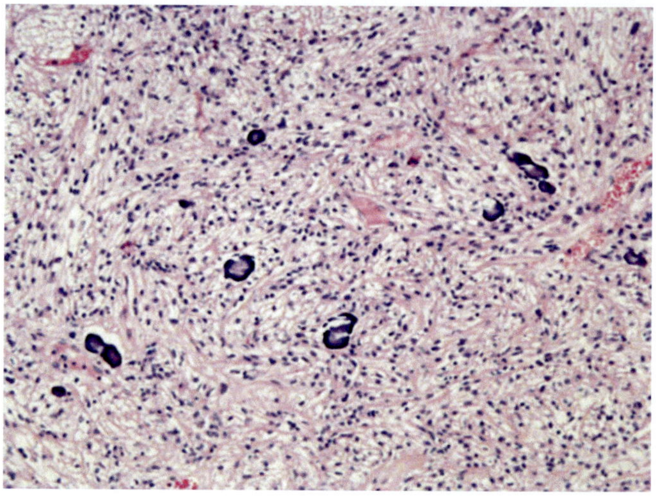

Fig. 10.12 Foci of calcification are not unusual in sugar cell tumor of lung

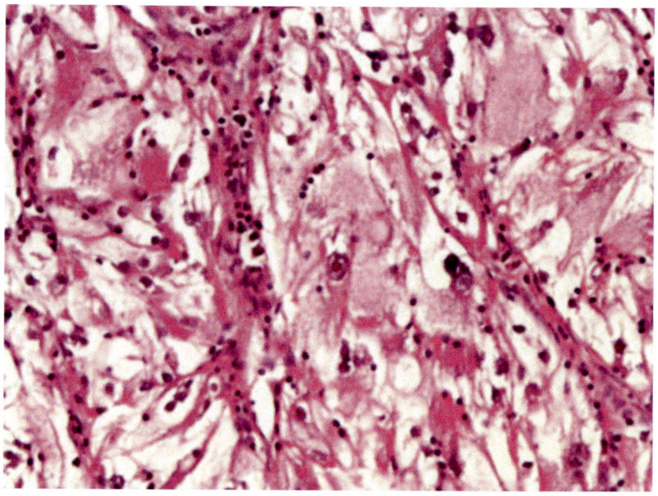

Fig. 10.13 So-called spider cells in sugar cell tumor of the lung

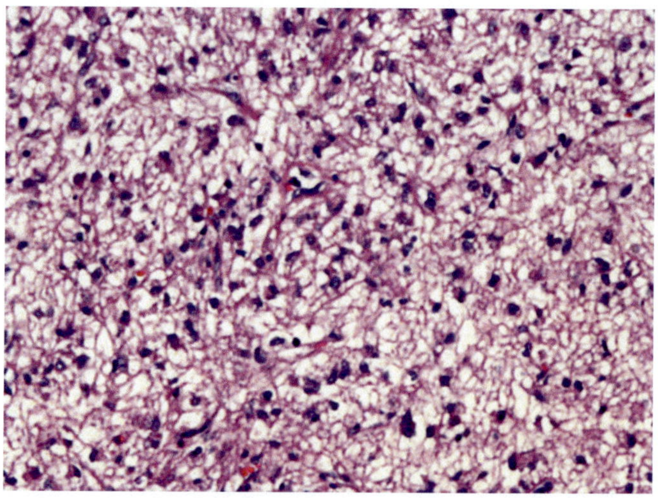

Fig. 10.14 Scattered "neuroid cells" can be identified in some sugar cell tumors

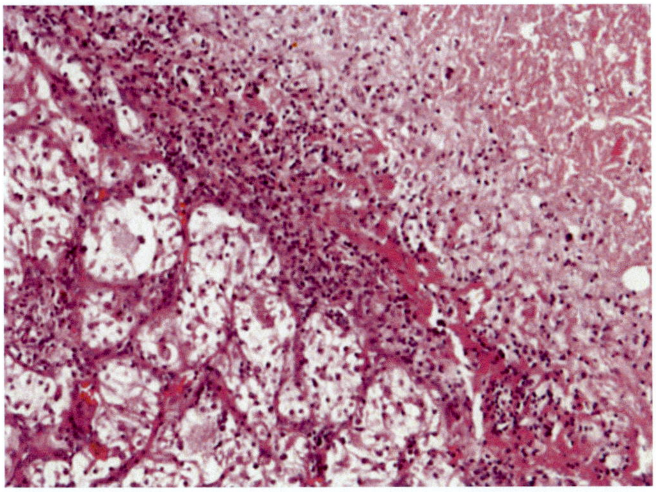

Fig. 10.15 Areas of necrosis are an unusual finding in sugar cell tumor

necrosis, and hemorrhage are usually absent but have been described in tumors that metastasized. These were therefore assumed to represent a malignant variant of clear cell sugar tumor (Fig. 10.15) [14–16].

Immunohistochemical Features and Ultrastructural Features

Clear cell sugar tumor has a characteristic immunohistochemical staining pattern. The tumors are immunoreactive for HMB45, S100 protein, CD1a, CD34, and are typically negative for epithelial markers including cytokeratin (CK), epithelial membrane antigen (EMA), and chromogranin [5, 6, 17–20]. Due to their high glycogen content, these tumors will also show positive staining for a periodic acid Schiff (PAS) histochemical stain. On an ultrastructural level, the tumors are characterized by abundant membrane-bound glycogen vesicles, pericytic differentiation, and the presence of premelanosomes [4–6, 21].

Differential Diagnosis

Clear cell sugar tumor of the lung must be distinguished from other primary or secondary lung tumors with clear cell change. Primary lung tumors with clear cell change include clear cell carcinoma and clear cell carcinoid tumor. With the aid of immunohistochemical stains, the distinction should be straightforward, as both these latter tumors will show positive staining for cytokeratins, a finding that has not been described in clear cell sugar tumor of the lung. Metastatic renal cell carcinoma is another tumor that may mimic sugar tumor of the lung, owing to its clear cell morphology and prominent vasculature. These tumors will not show the immunoreactivity for HMB45 characteristically observed for sugar tumors. In addition, the presence or absence of a tumor mass in the kidneys should facilitate correct diagnosis.

Treatment and Prognosis

Sugar tumors of the lung are generally believed to be benign neoplasms and complete excision is usually curative. However, there have been isolated case reports of sugar tumors that have metastasized or showed unequivocal malignant cytologic features [14–16], raising concern that some of these tumor may harbor malignant potential.

Granular Cell Tumor

Granular cell tumors are neoplasms that can be found in a wide anatomic distribution. Most commonly, these tumors can be found in the skin, tongue, and breast [22]. The first description of granular cell tumor is attributed to Abrikossoff [23] who described the first of these tumors in 1926. He believed granular cell tumor to be of myoid origin, hence the term "myoblastoma" in the original description. Later, other studies have proposed histiocytic, fibroblastic, or Schwannian differentiation [24–26]. Although derivation from Schwann cells seems to be supported by most authors to date, some histologic, immunohistochemical, and ultrastructural differences to the more common Schwann cell neoplasms exist, casting some doubt on this line of differentiation [27]. Based on this, granular cell tumor is currently considered a separate clinicopathologic entity. Since the first description of granular cell tumor of the lung by Kramer in 1939 [28], approximately 100 cases have been described in this location, constituting 6–10 % of all granular cell tumors [29–31]. Although most lesions run a benign clinical course, rare malignant granular cell tumors of the lung have been described [32, 33]. Of note, up to 25 % of tumors may be multifocal or may coexist with granular cell tumors outside the lung [22]. A number of granular cell tumors may also be associated with concurrent intra- or extrapulmonary malignancies including bronchogenic mucoepidermoid carcinoma, squamous cell carcinoma, adenocarcinoma, small cell carcinoma, and testicular germ cell tumors [32, 34–36]. One case report highlights the occurrence of a familial case of granular cell tumor [37].

Clinical Features

Granular cell tumors of the lungs predominantly occur in adults with equal male and female distribution and a median age of 45 years [22]. Patients of African-American descent appear to be slightly more commonly affected [22, 38]. Occasional cases have also been described in children [39, 40]. Very often these tumors are incidental findings. If symptomatic, the main presenting symptoms include obstructive symptoms (pneumonia, atelectasis) or hemoptysis [22]. Other, less specific symptoms include hypertension and neurologic symptoms [41]. The vast majority of tumors are endobronchial, while the less common parenchymal tumors often present as coin lesions on imaging.

Gross Features

Tumors range in size from less than 1 to more than 5 cm. Endobronchial lesions often have a polypoid appearance and are attached to the bronchial wall in a pedunculated or sessile manner. Although most tumors appear circumscribed, cases with infiltrative margins can also be observed. The cut surface can show white, yellow, or pink discoloration and is of firm consistency. Areas of hemorrhage and necrosis are not identified in benign granular cell tumors but may be seen in the malignant variant.

Histological Features

Most granular cell tumors contain a polypoid endobronchial component (Fig. 10.16). Although most tumors are well delineated, tumors may also show infiltrative margins (Figs. 10.17 and 10.18). Squamous metaplasia can commonly be identified in endobronchial lesions, but the pseudoepitheliomatous hyperplasia, associated with granular cell tumors of other sites, is not usually identified [22, 42]. The tumors tend to grow in sheet-like or nested patterns, and the tumor cells are round to oval shaped and possess abundant eosinophilic granular cytoplasm (Figs. 10.19 and 10.20). The nuclei tend to be small to medium sized with bland nuclear chromatin and are often displaced to the periphery of the cells (Figs. 10.21, 10.22, and 10.23). Spindling of the tumor cells may be observed in up to 40 % of cases, and a dense stroma may be present in a small subset of cases (Fig. 10.24). Connective tissue is, however, generally scarce. Involvement of regional lymph nodes by direct extension of benign granular cell tumor is not an uncommon occurrence, and perineural invasion can occasionally be identified (Fig. 10.25). Cyst formation or metaplastic bone deposits are additional features described in these tumors (Fig. 10.26). Mitotic activity, cytologic atypia, necrosis, and hemorrhage are absent in benign granular cell tumors but have been described in the rare malignant cases [32, 33].

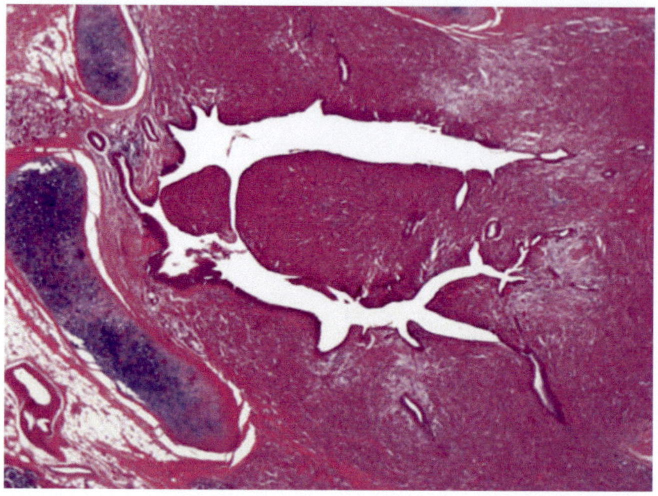

Fig. 10.16 Granular cell tumor of the lung protruding into the bronchial lumen

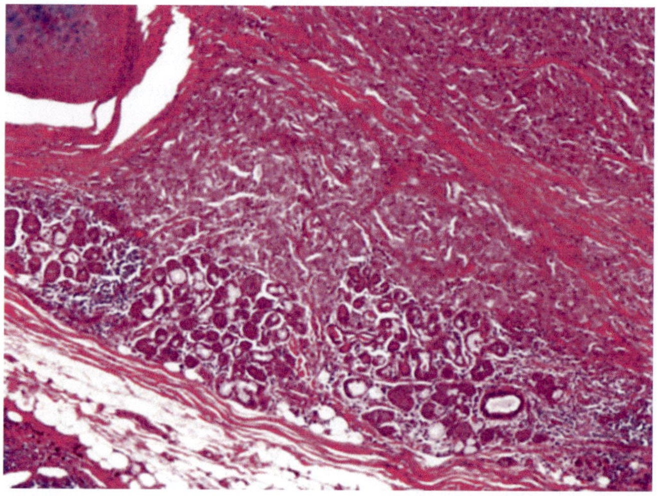

Fig.10.17 Low-power view of granular cell tumor showing an infiltrative growth pattern

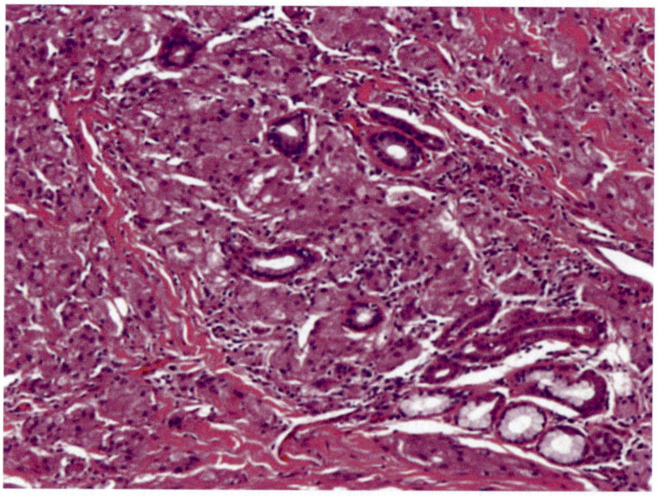

Fig. 10.18 Intermediate power view showing tumor cells of granular cell tumor infiltrating around bronchial glands

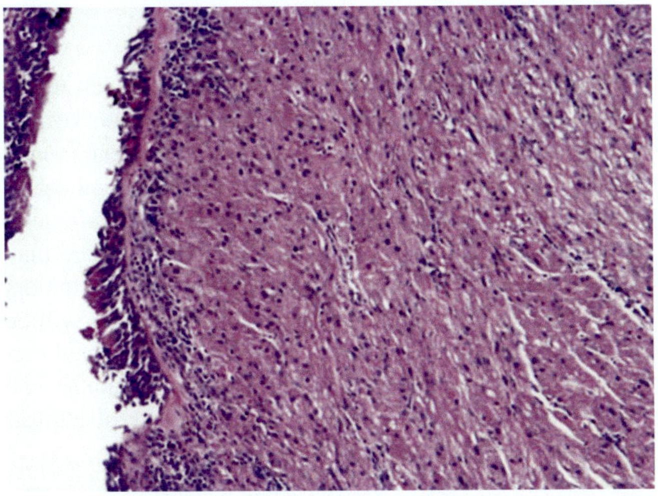

Fig. 10.19 Sheet-like proliferation of granular cells undermining the bronchial epithelium

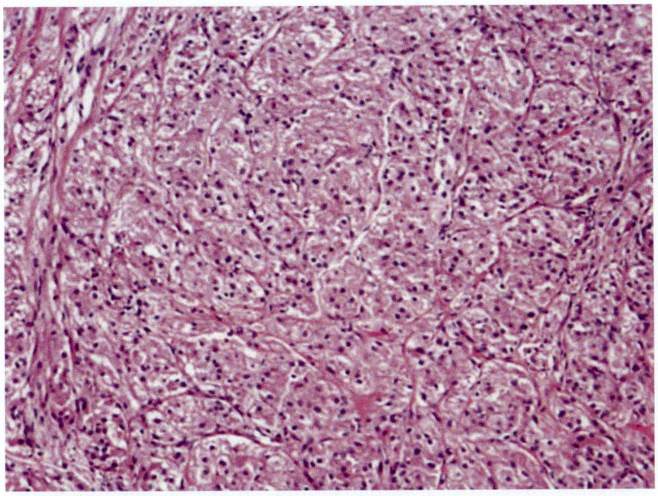

Fig. 10.20 Granular cell tumor showing the characteristic eosinophilic properties of the lesion

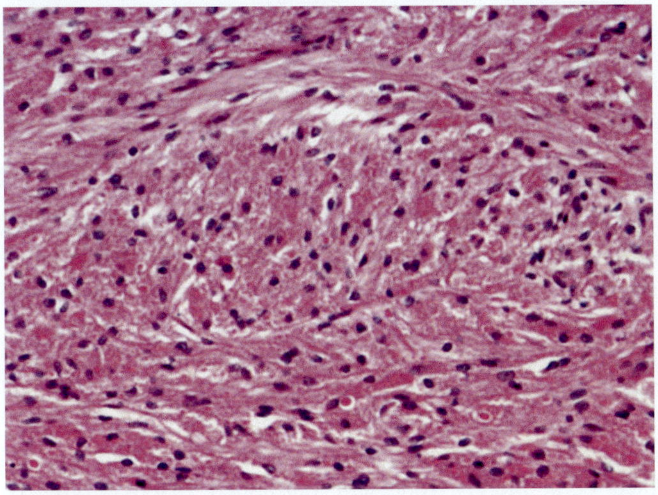

Fig.10.21 Monomorphic tumor cells with finely granular cytoplasm in granular cell tumor of the lung

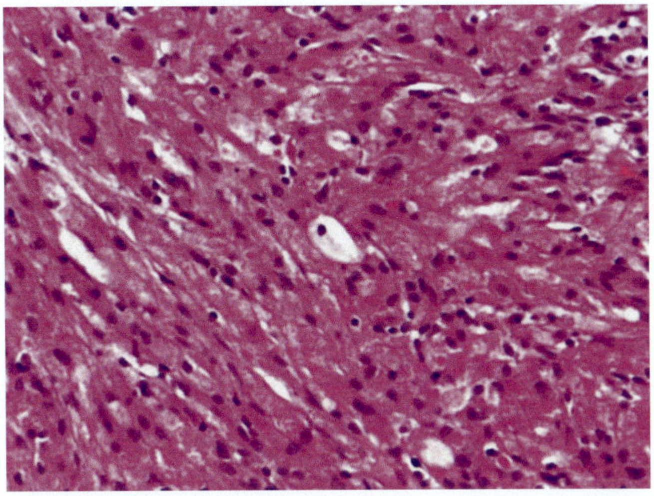

Fig. 10.22 Nuclei in granular cells are typically small round to oval and displaced to the periphery of the cell

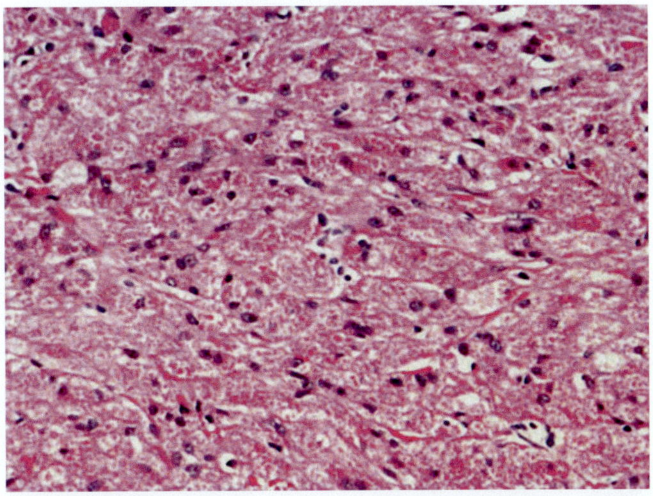

Fig. 10.23 Granular cell tumor of lung demonstrating a coarsely granular cytoplasm

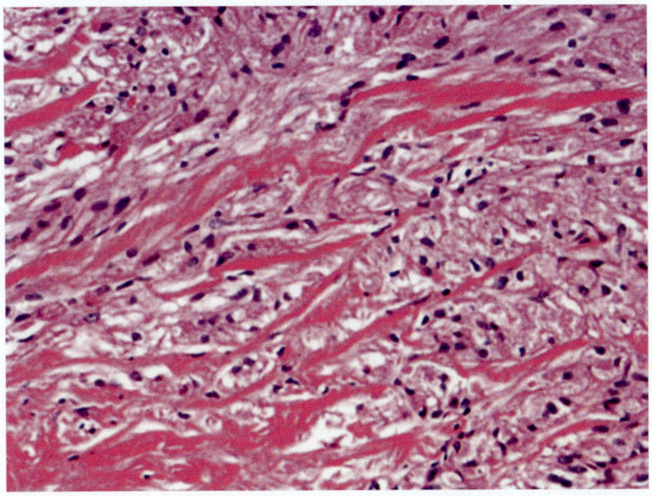

Fig. 10.24 Focal spindling of tumor cells in granular cell tumor of lung

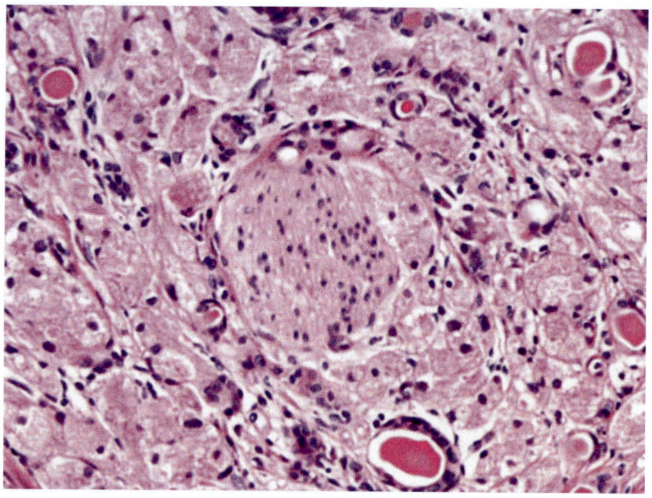

Fig. 10.25 Perineural invasion in granular cell tumor can occasionally be seen

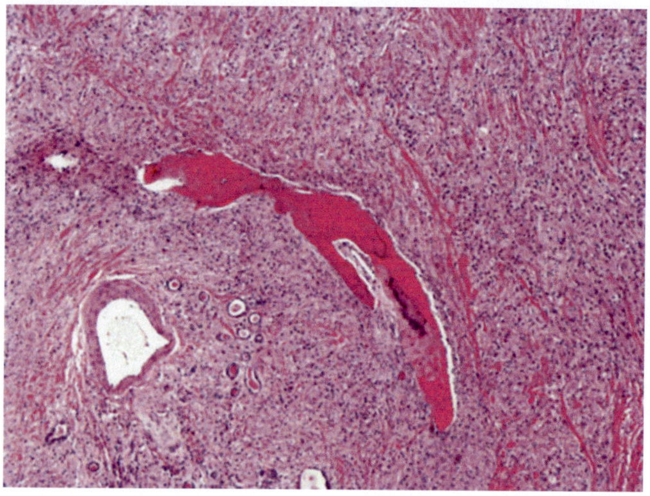

Fig. 10.26 Metaplastic bone can sometimes be identified in granular cell tumor of the lung

Immunohistochemical and Ultrastructural Features

Strong cytoplasmic reactivity of the granular cells is seen with a PAS histochemical stain. Immunohistochemical investigations show consistent reactivity for S100 protein, as well as positive reactions for neuron specific enolase, CD68, and vimentin [22, 34, 42, 43]. Negative markers include cytokeratin, EMA, smooth muscle actin, desmin, HMB45, glial fibrillary acidic protein (GFAP), thyroid transcription factor-1 (TTF-1), and chromogranin [34, 42, 44]. Ultrastructurally, the characteristic feature of granular cell tumor is abundant membrane-bound cytoplasmic granules consistent with lysosomes [34].

Differential Diagnosis

The histologic differential diagnosis of granular cell tumor includes reactive lesions like malakoplakia or tumors such as oncocytic carcinoid tumor, granular cell renal cell carcinoma, and metastatic malignant granular cell tumor to the lung. If distinction based on histologic features alone is not sufficient, the use of histochemical or immunohistochemical stains may help in making the correct diagnosis. Granular cell tumors will be strongly PAS and S100 positive; these stains will be negative in malakoplakia, carcinoid tumor, or renal cell carcinoma. Exclusion of metastatic malignant granular cell tumor from an extrathoracic site requires careful clinical assessment in order to identify the primary site.

Treatment and Prognosis

Surgical excision is the treatment of choice for pulmonary granular cell tumors including conservative approaches like bronchoscopic extirpation, laser therapy, or sleeve resection. Lobectomy can be performed for larger lesions or parenchymal tumors [22, 45]. Pulmonary granular cell tumors tend to behave in a benign fashion with slow growth and low rates of recurrence [22]. If completely resected, the patient should be cured. A more aggressive clinical course can be expected for the rare malignant variant; however, uniform treatment strategies for these lesions are still lacking [33].

Sclerosing Hemangioma (Pneumocytoma)

The term "sclerosing hemangioma" was first used describing a series of seven cases of a slow-growing lung tumor strongly resembling the so-called sclerosing hemangioma (dermatofibroma) of the skin [46]. Because of their histological appearance displaying prominent hemangiomatous structures, an endothelial origin was proposed [46]. Initially, ultrastructural investigations seemed to support this theory [47]; subsequent studies, however, suggested other origins including mesothelial [48] or mesenchymal differentiation [49]. Using ultrastructural and immunohistochemical techniques, the majority of investigators, however, have demonstrated type II pneumocyte differentiation in these tumors leading to the alternate designation "pneumocytoma" for these lesions [50–57]. Some contention still exists regarding the two cell types that form these tumors (the so-called surface cells and stromal cells). While some authors believe that both cellular elements are neoplastic in nature and share a common origin [58–60], others believe that the surface cells merely represent entrapped reactive type II pneumocytes [57, 61]. Furthermore, recent molecular studies argue for a true neoplastic process [59, 60] ending speculation that sclerosing hemangiomas represent a hamartomatous lesion [62].

Clinical Features

Sclerosing hemangiomas are more common in female patients with a male-to-female ratio of 1:5. Although these tumors may affect patients with a wide age range (10–83 years), the majority are in the fourth and fifth decade at presentation [56, 63, 64]. Approximately 80 % of patients are asymptomatic, and the tumors are found incidentally [56]. The rest of the patients often present with symptoms like hemoptysis, cough, or chest pain [56]. Radiologically, the tumors are described as peripheral, solitary, well-defined, and homogenous nodules. More rarely, sclerosing hemangiomas may present as multifocal tumors [56, 59, 63, 65–68] or may be associated with other tumors [56] or familial adenomatous polyposis [69, 70].

Gross Features

Sclerosing hemangiomas are well-circumscribed tumors of yellow to tan color located in the periphery of the lung. More rarely, tumors may be in an endobronchial or pleural location [56, 71, 72]. The tumors range in size from 0.3 to 8 cm [56, 73]. There appears to be slight predilection for the lower lobes of the lung. The cut surface is solid with some cystic change and normally displays varying degrees of hemorrhage [74].

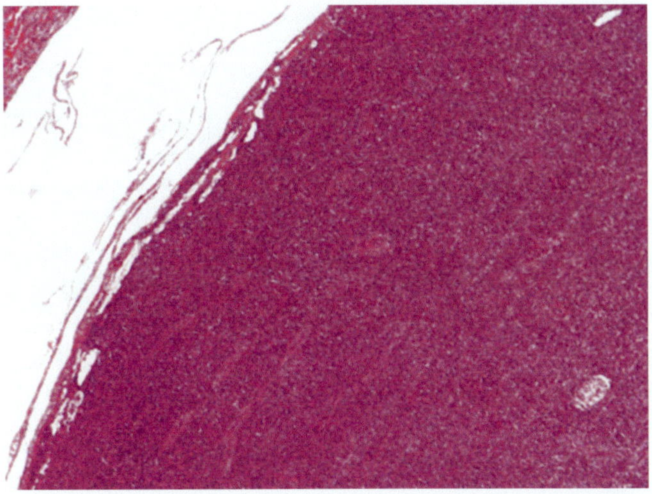

Fig. 10.27 Sclerosing hemangioma of the lung showing sharp circumscription of the lesion

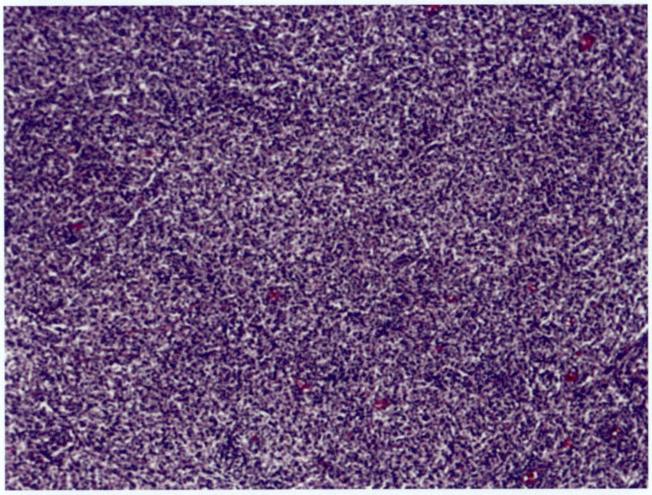

Fig. 10.28 Solid proliferation of stromal or round cells in sclerosing hemangioma of lung

Histological Features

Sclerosing hemangiomas typically display four different major histopathologic patterns or an admixture thereof [46, 56, 64]. These include solid, hemorrhagic, papillary, and sclerosing patterns. The tumors are generally composed of two cell types, surface (cuboidal) cells and stromal (round) cells. In the solid pattern, the stromal cell component is characterized by sheets of round to polygonal cells with small round nuclei, inconspicuous nucleoli, and moderate amounts of eosinophilic cytoplasm (Figs. 10.27, 10.28, 10.29, and 10.30). The cytologic features are bland lacking cytologic atypia, and the mitotic index is low (up to 1 mitosis per 10 high-power fields). Surface cells may be present lining the sheets of stromal cells peripherally. These surface cells have uniform and cuboidal shape and mirror the morphology of bronchiolar epithelium or activated type II pneumocytes (Figs. 10.31 and 10.32). The hemorrhagic pattern is composed of angiomatous spaces showing varying degrees of dilatation that are filled with blood (Figs. 10.33, 10.34, 10.35, 10.36, and 10.37). Papillae and tubular structures containing stromal cells in the stalk and surface cells lining the papillary projections are characteristic for the papillary type (Figs. 10.38, 10.39, 10.40, 10.41, and 10.42). Furthermore, the stalks may contain a myxoid or sclerotic stroma, and the interpapillary spaces may be filled with histiocytes, desquamated type II pneumocytes, or blood. Lastly, the sclerotic variant shows areas of dense hyalinization especially around vascular structures (Figs. 10.43, 10.44, and 10.45). In addition to the features described, the tumors may

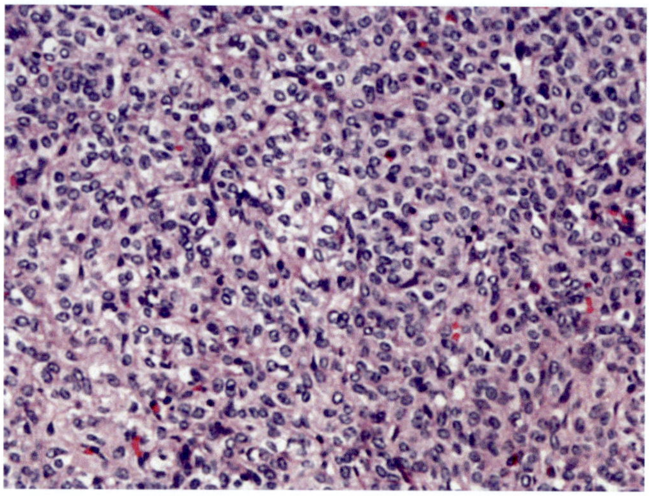

Fig. 10.29 Stromal (round) cells of sclerosing hemangioma are usually small to medium sized and lack cytologic atypia

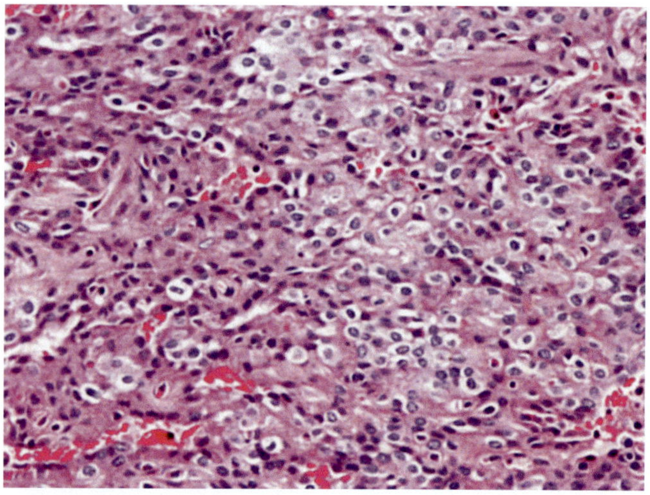

Fig. 10.30 Bland cytologic features and absence of mitotic activity in stromal (round) cells of sclerosing hemangioma

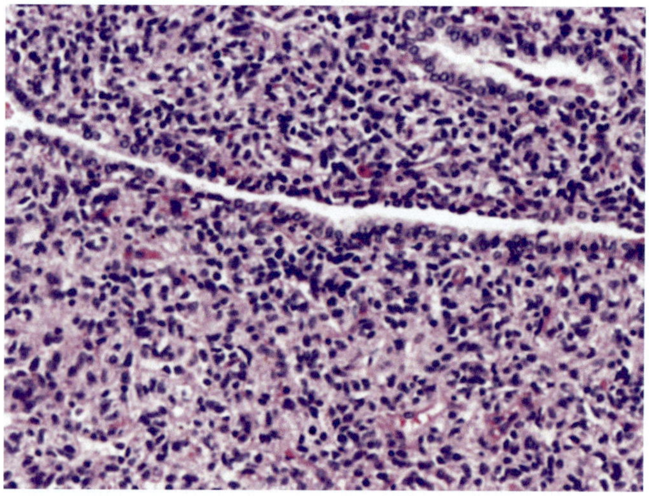

Fig. 10.31 Surface or cuboidal cells can be seen lining the proliferation of stromal (round) cells in the tumor periphery

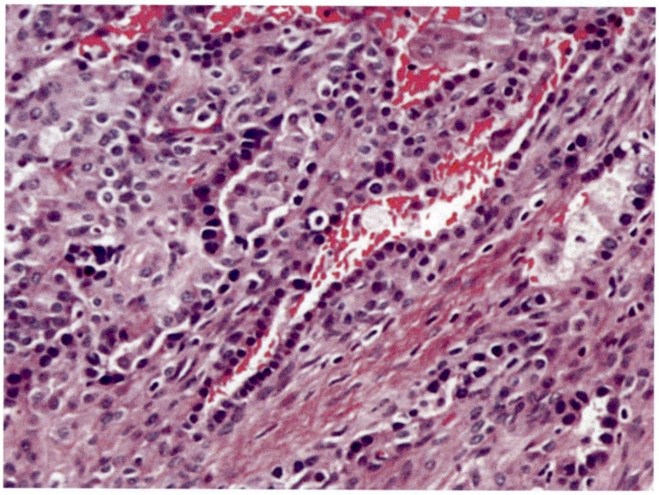

Fig. 10.32 Surface cells in sclerosing hemangioma resembling activated type II pneumocytes

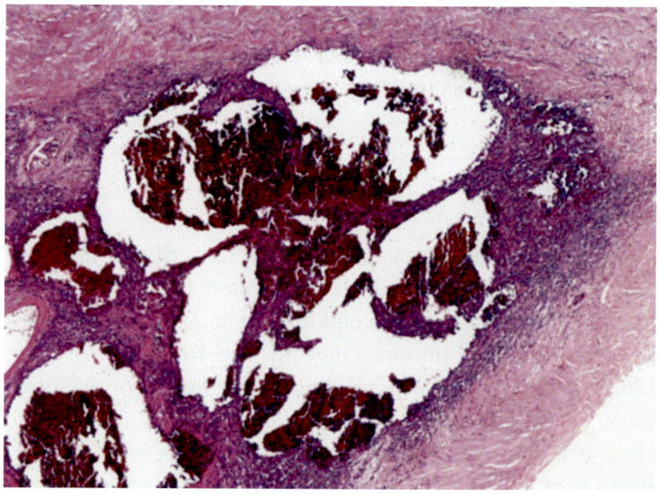

Fig. 10.33 Low-power view of the vascular or hemorrhagic pattern of sclerosing hemangioma mimicking a vascular neoplasm

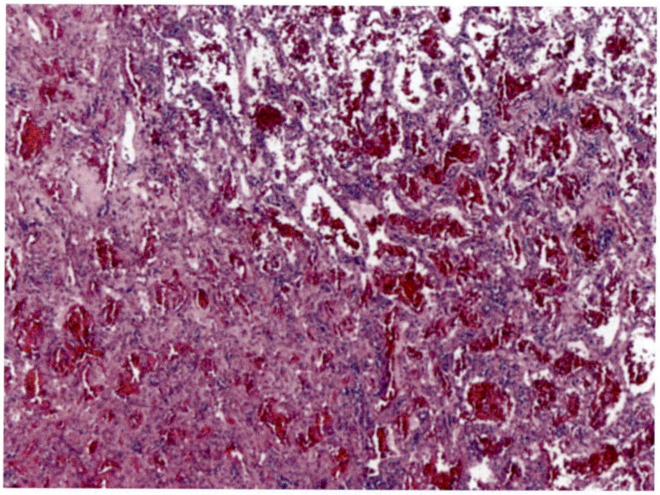

Fig. 10.34 Multiple angiomatous spaces constitute the hemorrhagic pattern of sclerosing hemangioma of lung

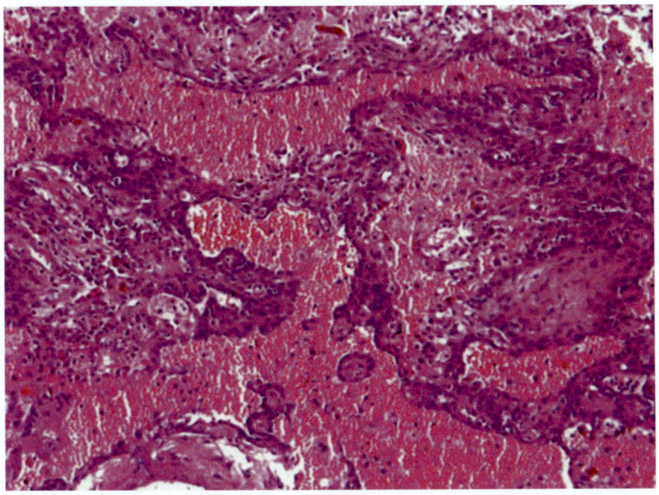

Fig. 10.35 Large dilated vascular spaces filled with blood in the hemorrhagic pattern of sclerosing hemangioma of lung

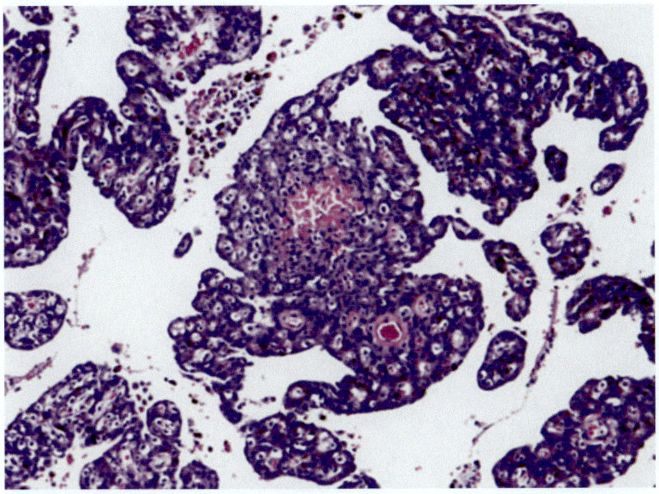

Fig. 10.36 Vascular spaces may be devoid of blood but hemosiderin deposition is seen among the tumor cells in the hemorrhagic pattern of sclerosing hemangioma of lung

show varying proportions of foamy macrophages (Figs. 10.46 and 10.47), giant cells (Fig. 10.48), cholesterol clefts (Fig. 10.49), granulomatous inflammation, adipose or sebaceous-like differentiation (Fig. 10.50), calcifications, cystic structures, or lamellar bodies [71, 75]. Small areas of necrosis as well as very occasional mitotic figures may also be identified (Fig. 10.51) [71].

Immunohistochemical and Molecular Features

The results of several immunohistochemical studies on sclerosing hemangiomas have shown that surface and stromal cells show reactivity for TTF-1 and EMA in almost all cases [53, 55, 61, 71]. While the surface cells also demonstrate positive staining for pancytokeratin, CEA, and

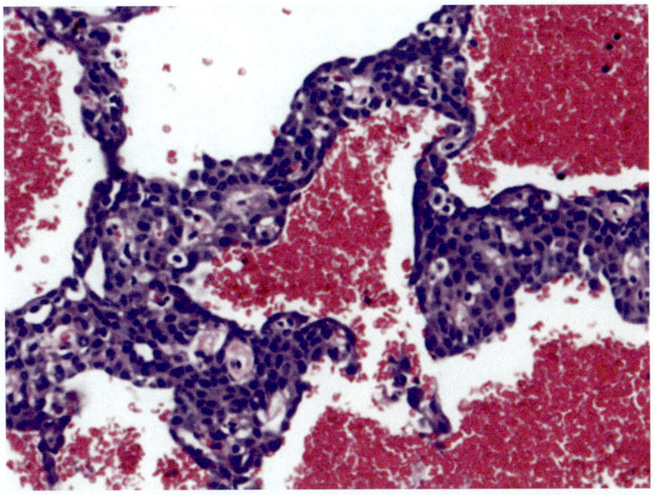

Fig. 10.37 Characteristic stromal proliferation of cells in sclerosing hemangioma of the lung

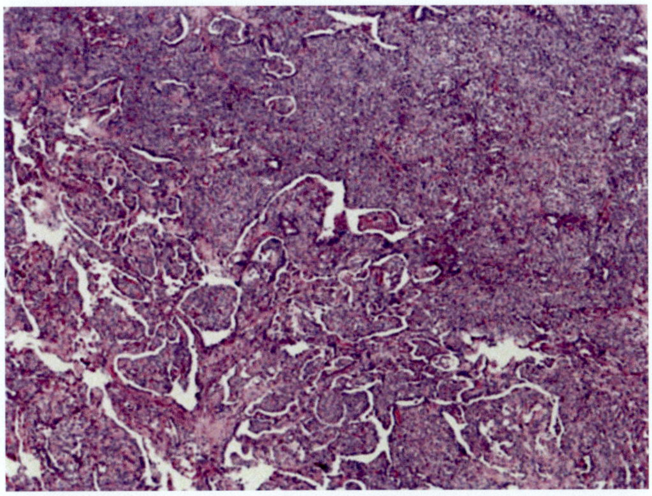

Fig. 10.38 Low-power view of the papillary pattern of sclerosing hemangioma of lung

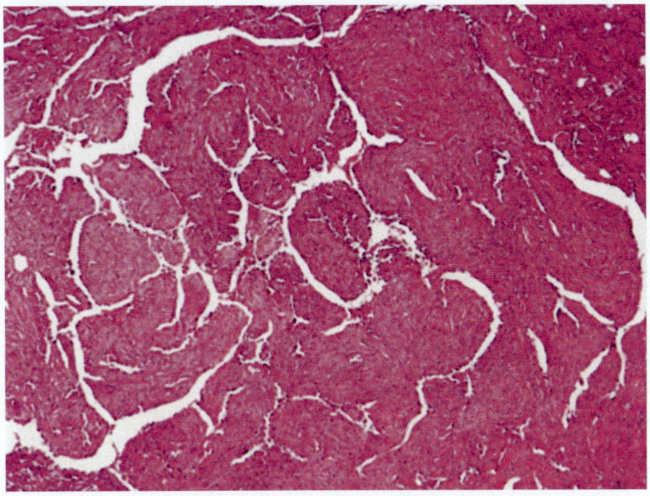

Fig. 10.39 Large broad-based papillary structures forming the papillary pattern of sclerosing hemangioma

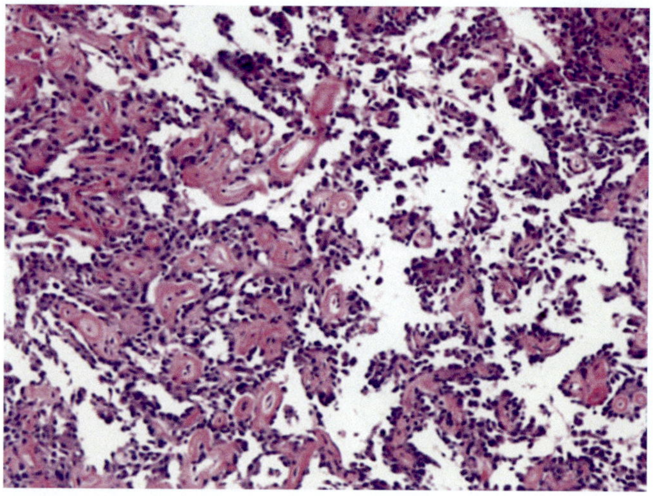

Fig. 10.40 Papillary variant of sclerosing hemangioma showing more delicate papillary structures

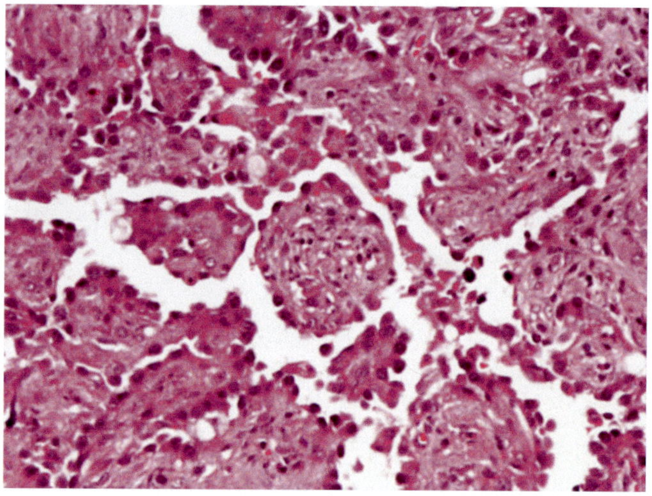

Fig. 10.41 Papillary structures in sclerosing hemangioma lined by surface (cuboidal) cells with a hobnailing appearance

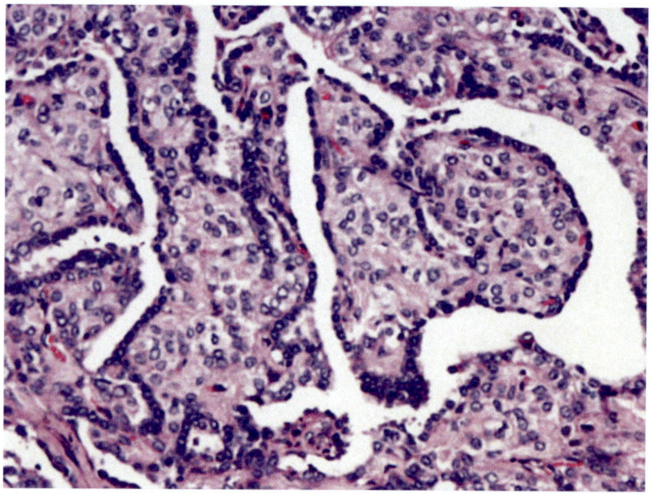

Fig. 10.42 Characteristic stromal (round) cells seen in the stalks of the papillary structures of sclerosing hemangioma

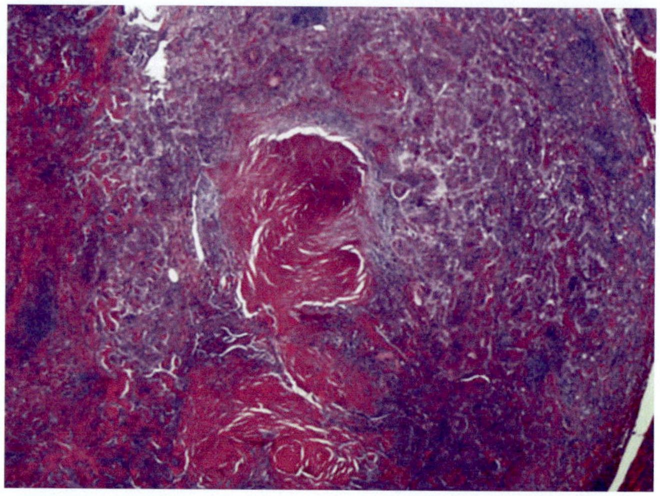

Fig. 10.43 Large areas of dense sclerosis characterize the sclerosing pattern of sclerosing hemangioma of lung

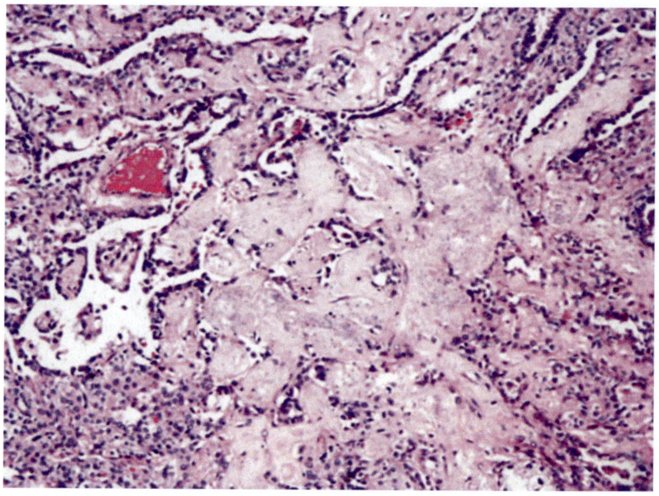

Fig. 10.44 Sclerotic mixing with papillary areas in sclerosing hemangioma of lung

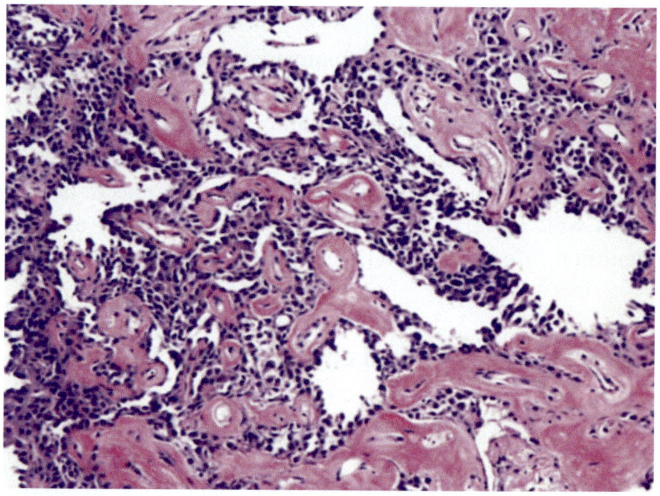

Fig. 10.45 Prominent hyalinization around vascular structures is a typical finding in sclerosing hemangioma

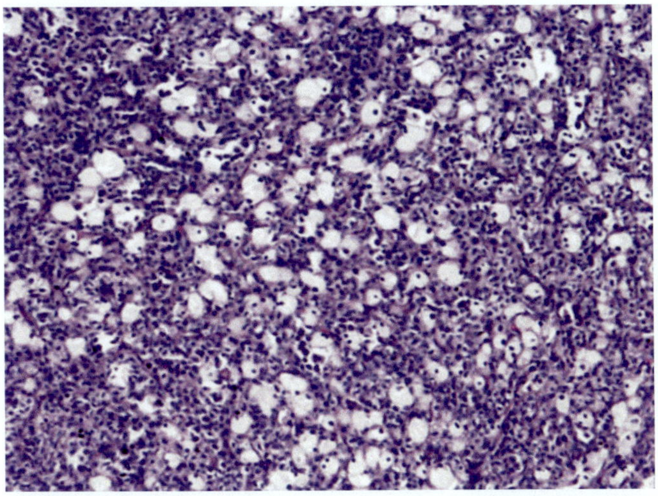

Fig. 10.46 Scattered foamy macrophages in sclerosing hemangioma of the lung imparting a starry sky appearance

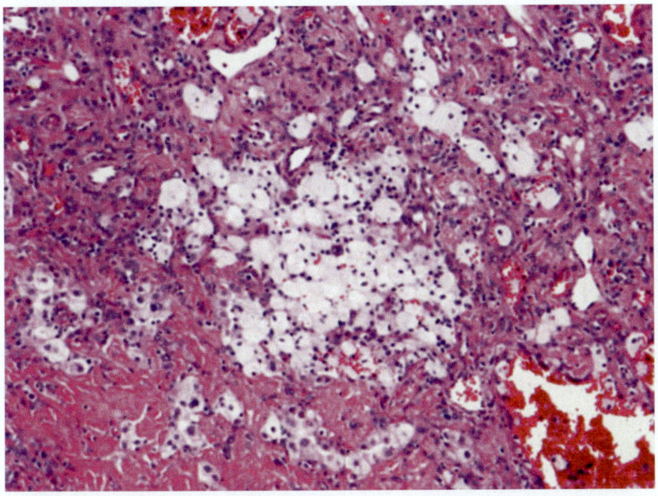

Fig. 10.47 Collections of foamy macrophages are a typical finding in sclerosing hemangioma of lung

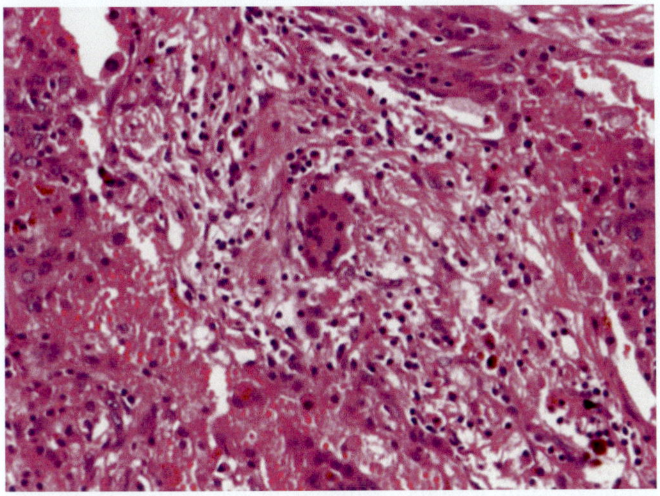

Fig. 10.48 Scattered giant cells may be identified in sclerosing hemangioma of lung

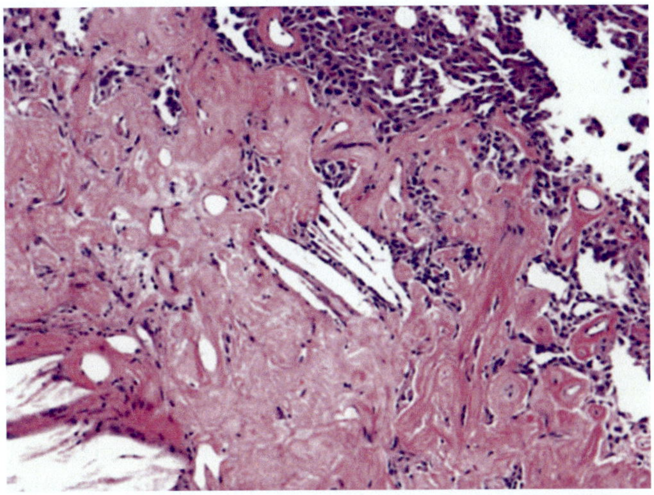

Fig. 10.49 Cholesterol clefts are frequently found in sclerosing hemangioma of lung

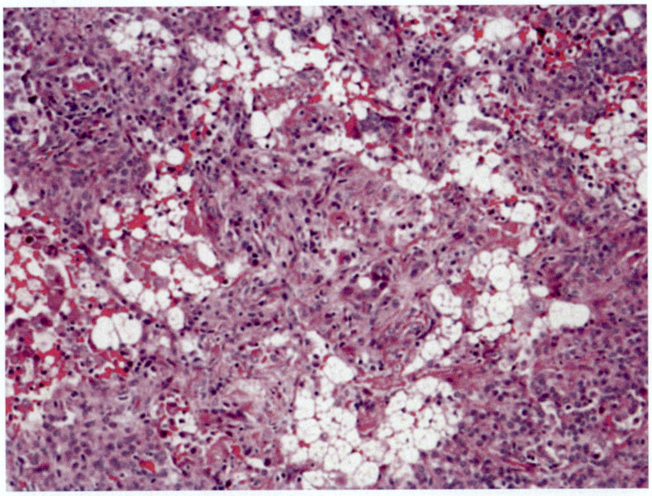

Fig. 10.50 Adipose tissue or sebaceous-like cells can occasionally be seen in sclerosing hemangioma

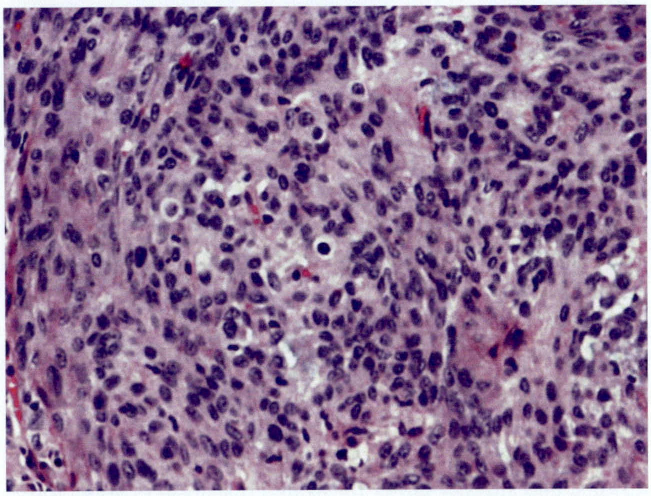

Fig. 10.51 Scattered mitotic figures in sclerosing hemangioma of lung

surfactant protein alpha, these markers are not expressed by the stromal cells [55, 61, 71]. The stromal cells may, however, react focally with cytokeratin 7 (CK7) and CAM5.2. These results have prompted some authors to believe that the cells are derived from primitive respiratory type epithelium with the surface cells being more differentiated than the stromal cells [57].

On a molecular level, sclerosing hemangioma demonstrates loss of heterozygosity at 5q and 10q, markers adjacent to APC and PTEN suppressor genes [76] as well as microsatellite alterations of p16 and RB genes [60]. These changes are similar to those seen in early lung adenocarcinoma tumorigenesis, suggesting a possible link between the two tumors. However, epidermal growth factor receptor (EGFR), Kras, and Her2 mutations could not be shown in sclerosing hemangioma, suggesting different molecular pathways [60]. The finding of monoclonality in both cellular components [59] and the fact that the microsatellite alterations were present in surface and stromal cells confirm the common origin of these cells and the neoplastic nature of the tumor [60]. Recently, cytogenetic studies identified a novel translocation t(8;18) and trisomy 14 in a single case of pulmonary sclerosing hemangioma [77].

Differential Diagnosis

The differential diagnosis depends on the predominant growth pattern of the individual tumors. Identification of more than one growth pattern may be very helpful in making the correct diagnosis. However, if the solid or papillary patterns are dominant, adenocarcinoma may enter the differential diagnosis. Adenocarcinoma will show cytologic atypia and increased mitotic activity in addition to diffuse immunoreactivity for pancytokeratin. Prominence of the hemorrhagic or angiomatous pattern may be mistaken for a low-grade vascular neoplasm. In this case, the absence of endothelial immunomarkers should point to the correct diagnosis. The rather monotonous proliferation of cells in sclerosing hemangioma may further be confused for a low-grade neuroendocrine neoplasm. The latter will often show organoid or trabecular growth patterns and will display immunoreactivity for neuroendocrine markers, features that will usually be absent in sclerosing hemangioma.

Treatment and Prognosis

Sclerosing hemangiomas are generally considered benign lesions, and surgery either by wedge resection or lobectomy is the treatment of choice and should be curative. Although multifocal disease, lymph node metastasis, and recurrent tumors have been described [55, 58, 63, 65, 71, 73, 78–80], these features do not appear to affect the prognosis, and mortality has not yet been attributed to these tumors.

Inflammatory Pseudotumor

Inflammatory pseudotumor of the lung was first described as "plasma cell granuloma" by Childress and Adie in 1950 [81] followed by the first larger series of these lesions by Bahadori and Liebow [82] describing 40 cases. Since then this tumor has been reported under a variety of different names ("inflammatory myofibroblastic tumor," "fibroxanthoma," "histiocytoma") based on its histological variability [83–85]. The lesions tend to form a spectrum of morphological patterns but are generally characterized by a proliferation of fibroblasts and myofibroblasts, plasma cells, lymphocytes, and histiocytes in varying numbers. At one end of the spectrum is the so-called fibrohistiocytic variant in which fibroblasts, myofibroblasts, and histiocytes predominate. At the other end is a type almost completely composed of plasma cells, the so-called plasma cell variant. More fundamental than nomenclature, however, is the question of the pathogenesis of these lesions. Initially, inflammatory pseudotumor was thought to be a reactive postinflammatory, infectious, or immunologic process [82, 85–88], a fact later supported by the finding that the plasma cells are polyclonal in nature by kappa and lambda immunostaining [89]. However, more recently cytogenetic studies have demonstrated a clonal origin of these lesions [90, 91]. Since cases with recurrence and metastasis have been described, a true neoplastic origin is favored for these lesions [92, 93].

Clinical Features

Inflammatory pseudotumor occurs in patients with a wide age range (less than 1 to more than 77 years) and a peak incidence in the third decade. The majority of patients are younger than 40 years of age [85]. In children, the incidence of inflammatory pseudotumor is high, representing 20 % of all pediatric primary lung tumors [94]. Generally, no significant difference in sex incidence is noted, although some reports mention slight male predominance [95]. The vast majority of patients (75 %) are asymptomatic at presentation, although some patients present with hemoptysis or abnormal laboratory tests like elevated serum immunoglobulin or ESR [85, 89, 96]. Most lesions are solitary "coin lesions" situated in the periphery of the lungs; extrapulmonary involvement of the bronchus, mediastinum, pleura, or hilum can be seen in isolated cases [85, 95, 97, 98].

Gross Features

The lesions are circumscribed but unencapsulated masses ranging in size from 1 to more than 10 cm. The lesions have a firm gray-white cut surface with a whorled appearance. Central cavitation or cystic change is infrequently identified [85, 99]. Areas of calcification may be present in up to 25 % of cases [85].

Histological Features

Two distinct histological subtypes of inflammatory pseudotumor have been described: the fibrohistiocytic variant and the plasma cell type. The fibrohistiocytic variant is characterized by a spindle cell proliferation growing in a storiform or fascicular pattern (Figs. 10.52, 10.53, and 10.54). These spindle cells are admixed with an inflammatory cell infiltrate composed of plasma cells and lymphocytes (Figs. 10.55 and 10.56). The inflammatory cells may be present in variable numbers, ranging from a sparse to prominent infiltrate. The spindle cells have elongated nuclei with blunted ends, inconspicuous nucleoli, and moderate amounts of eosinophilic cytoplasm (Fig. 10.57). Mitotic activity is usually inconspicuous and if present will not show atypical forms (Fig. 10.58). Another common feature is the presence of foamy macrophages or Touton-type giant cells in the periphery of the lesions (Figs. 10.59 and 10.60). Some cases may show a more loose arrangement of the spindle cells, a myxoid background and red blood cell extravasation reminiscent of the pattern seen in nodular fasciitis (Fig. 10.61).

As the name implies, the plasma cell variant is characterized by a nodular proliferation of plasma cells (Figs. 10.62, 10.63, and 10.64). Smaller numbers of fibrohistiocytic spindle cells may be intermixed with the inflammatory cells. The plasma cells may contain prominent Russell bodies (Fig. 10.65), and areas of sparsely cellular collagen or hyalinized stroma may be seen in this variant (Fig. 10.66). Mitotic activity is not usually identified in this subtype.

Both variants may show infiltration of adjacent anatomic structures as well as lymphoid follicles (Fig. 10.67), cholesterol clefts (Fig. 10.68), and areas of sclerosis, calcification (Fig. 10.69), or ossification (Fig. 10.70).

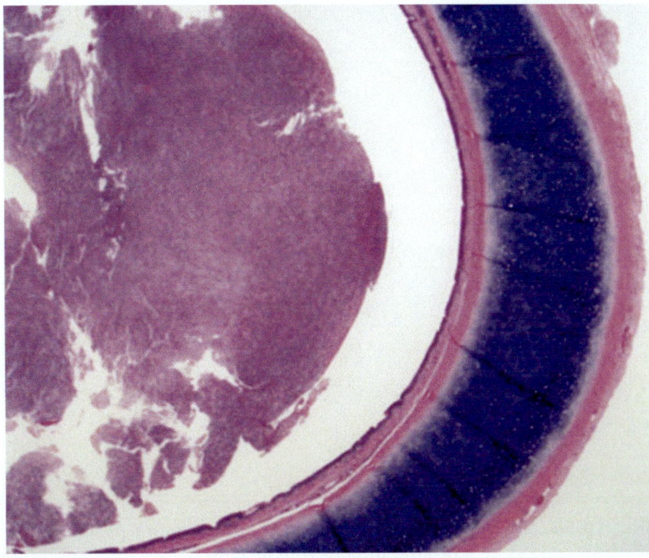

Fig. 10.52 Endobronchial component of inflammatory pseudotumor

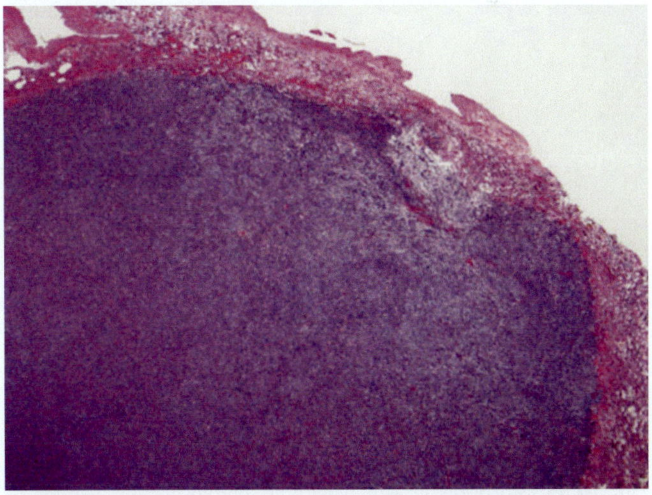

Fig. 10.53 Low-power view of fibrohistiocytic variant of inflammatory pseudotumor

Immunohistochemical and Molecular Features

In the fibrohistiocytic variant, the spindle cells show immunoreactivity for smooth muscle actin and vimentin and are negative for pancytokeratin, EMA, and S100 protein [85, 100]. More recently, anaplastic lymphoma kinase 1 (ALK-1) has been reported to be expressed immunohistochemically by up to 40 % of cases [101–106]. Corresponding to this, a range of ALK-1-associated translocations have been identified in these tumors [102, 103, 107–112]. Some authors have implicated human herpes virus 8 (HHV8) to be associated with these tumors, but this hypothesis has been refuted by others [104, 105, 113].

In the plasma cell variant, the plasma cells show a polyclonal pattern with kappa and lambda light chain stains. More recently, IgG4 positive plasma cells were found to be abundant in pulmonary inflammatory pseudotumor, raising the possibility of a link with IgG4 disease [114].

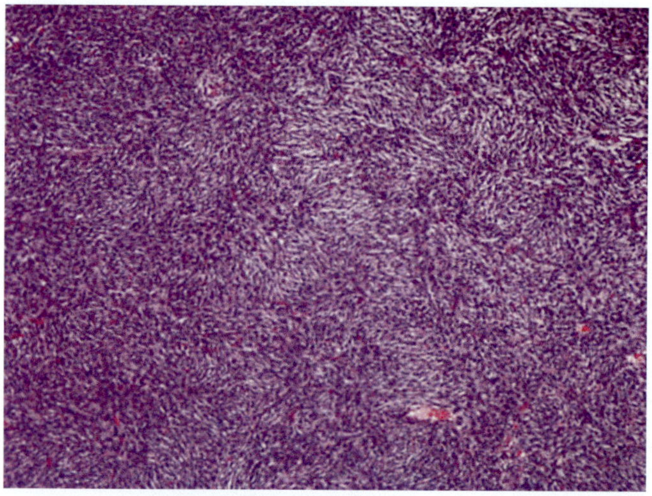

Fig. 10.54 The fibrohistiocytic variant of inflammatory pseudotumor is characterized by a proliferation of spindle cells

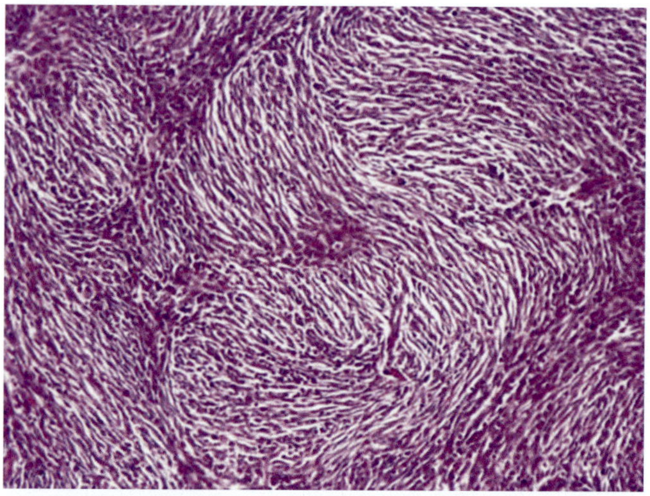

Fig. 10.55 Storiform growth pattern in fibrohistiocytic variant of inflammatory pseudotumor

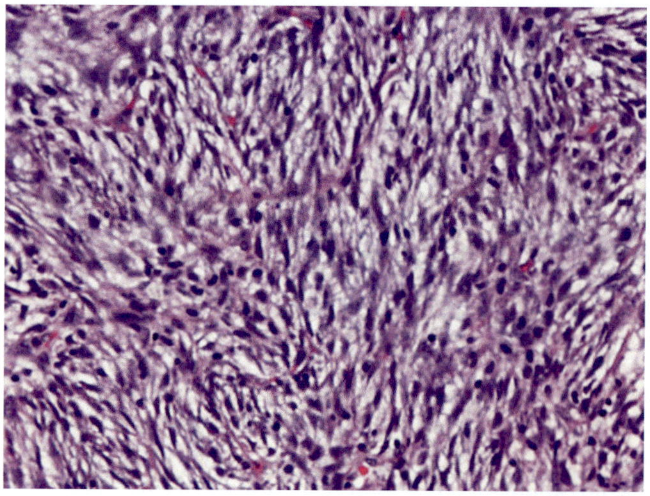

Fig. 10.56 Bland spindle cells mixed with scattered inflammatory cells are typical for the fibrohistiocytic variant of inflammatory pseudotumor

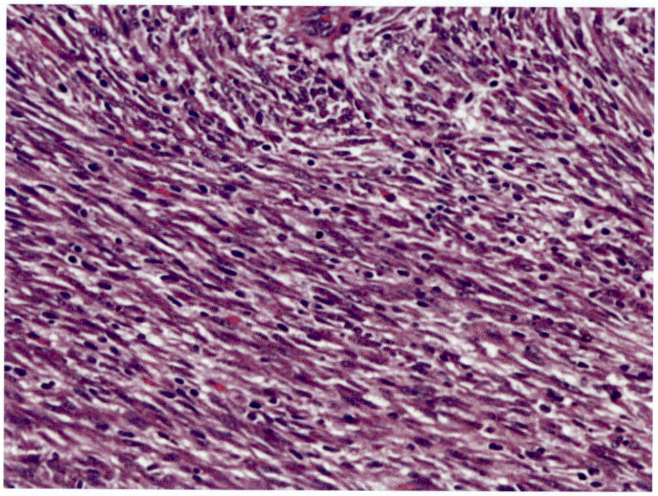

Fig. 10.57 Spindle cells with blunt elongated nuclei and eosinophilic cytoplasm in the fibrohistiocytic variant of inflammatory pseudotumor

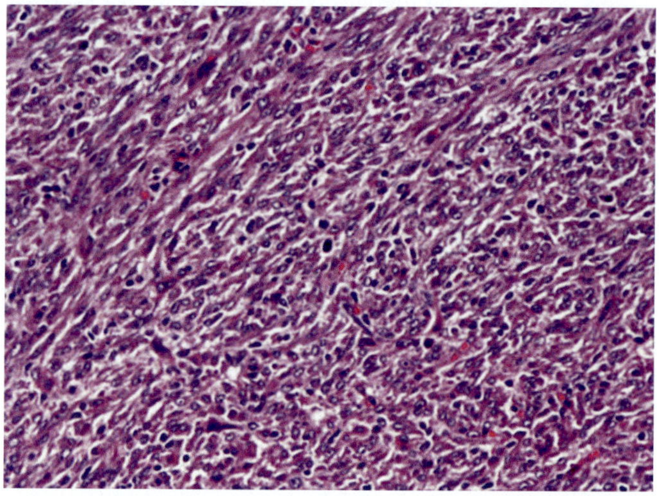

Fig. 10.58 Occasional mitotic figures can be seen in inflammatory pseudotumor of the lung

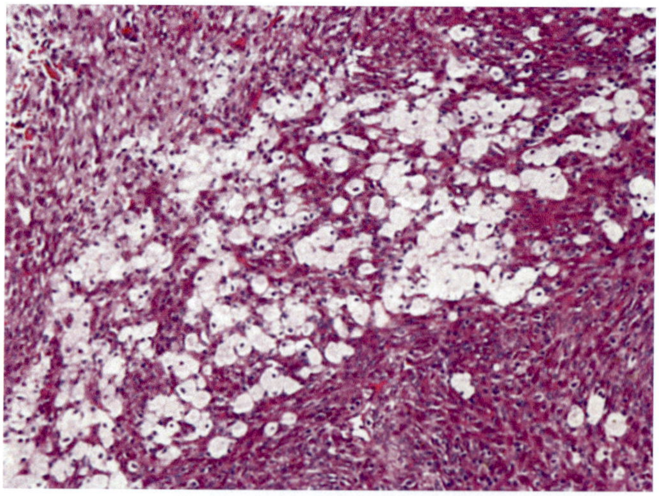

Fig. 10.59 Foamy macrophages are a typical finding in inflammatory pseudotumor of the lung

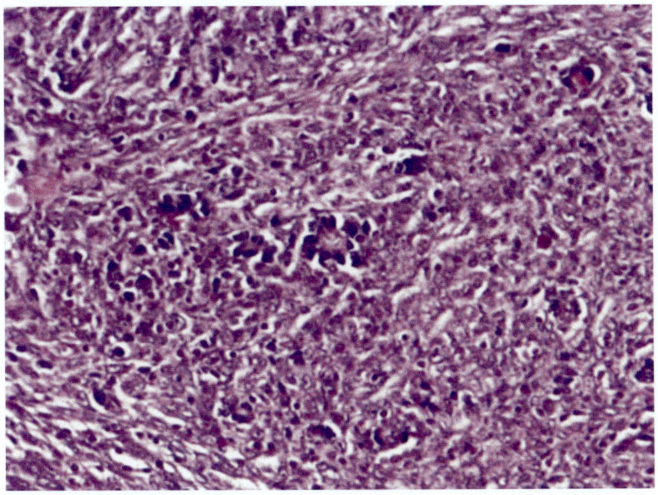

Fig. 10.60 Inflammatory pseudotumor of the lung containing scattered Touton-type giant cells

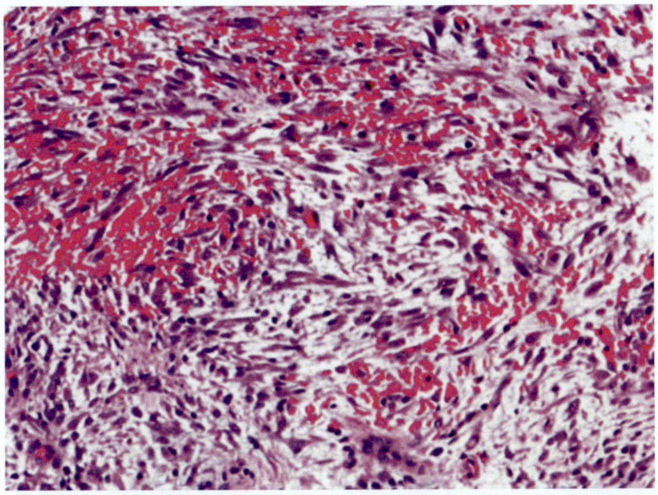

Fig. 10.61 Nodular fasciitis-like pattern in inflammatory pseudotumor of the lung characterized by loose spindle cells, myxoid stroma, and extravasated red blood cells

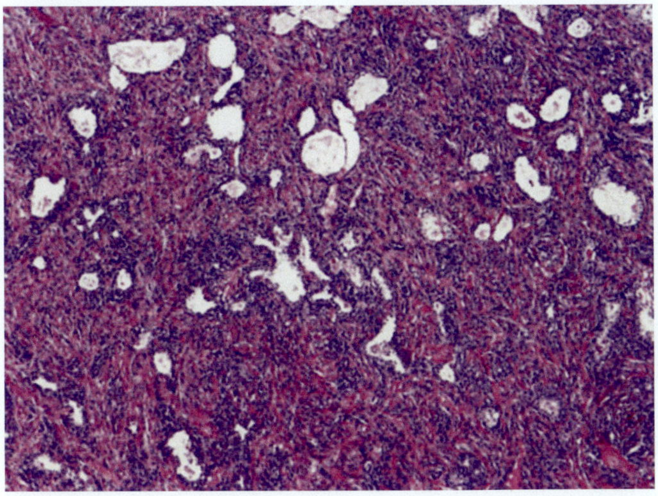

Fig. 10.62 Low-power view of the plasma cell variant of inflammatory pseudotumor

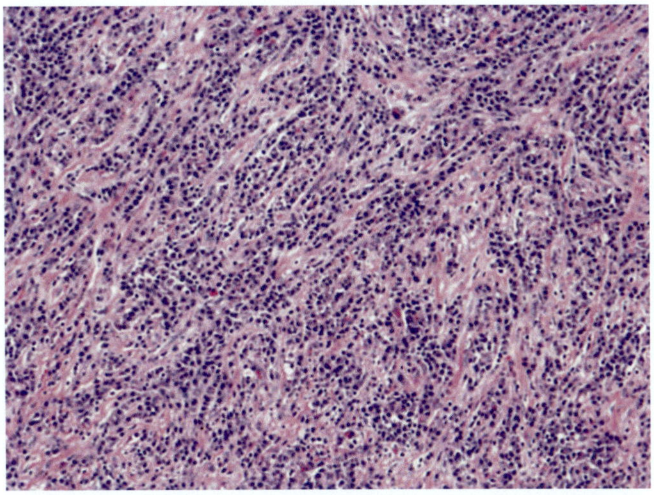

Fig. 10.63 Intermediate power view of plasma cell variant of inflammatory pseudotumor showing a sheet-like proliferation of plasma cells

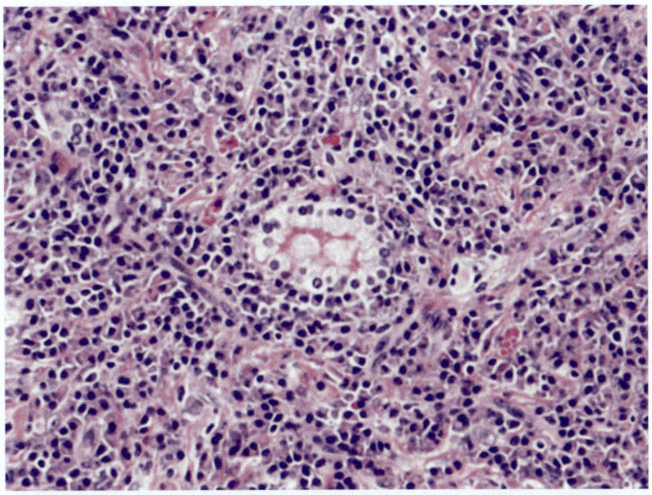

Fig. 10.64 Plasma cells infiltrating between normal bronchial structures in inflammatory pseudotumor

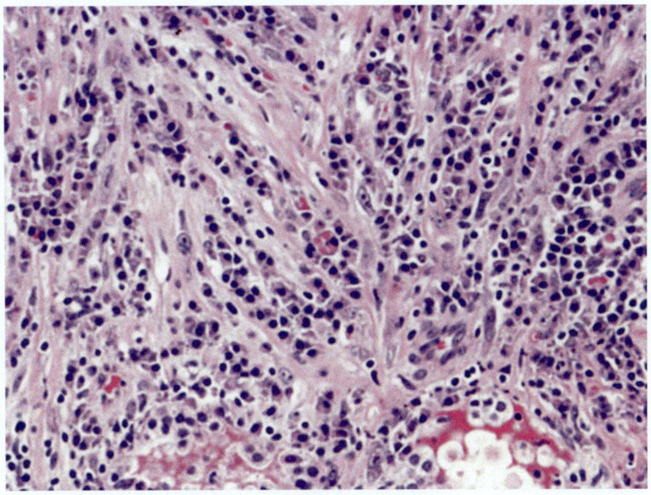

Fig. 10.65 Russell bodies can be identified in some areas of the plasma cell variant of pulmonary inflammatory pseudotumor

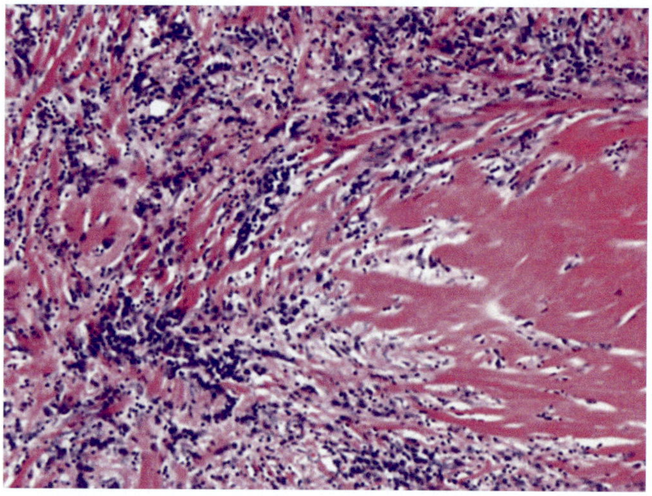

Fig. 10.66 Stromal hyalinization in the plasma cell variant of inflammatory pseudotumor

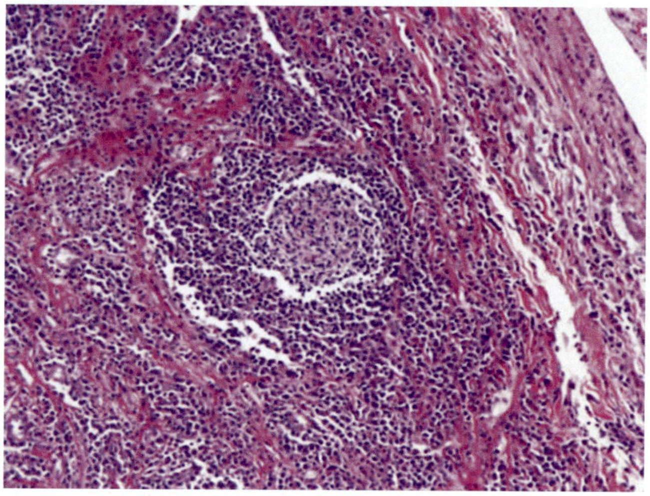

Fig. 10.67 Lymphoid follicles with germinal centers are a common finding in inflammatory pseudotumors of the lung

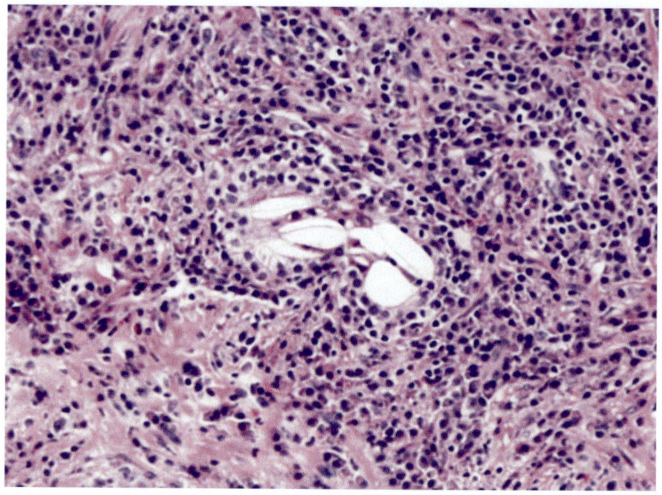

Fig. 10.68 Cholesterol cleft formation in inflammatory pseudotumor of the lung

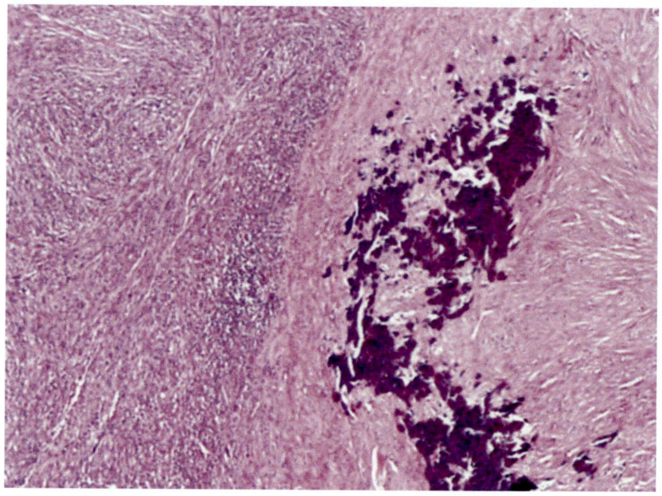

Fig. 10.69 Areas of calcification can occasionally be identified in inflammatory pseudotumor

Differential Diagnosis

The differential diagnosis for inflammatory pseudotumor largely depends on the histological subtype. In cases of the fibrohistiocytic variant, other spindle cell neoplasms enter the differential diagnosis. Among these, sarcomatoid carcinoma or pleomorphic sarcoma, are entities that must be ruled out. Both of these tumors will demonstrate more severe cytologic atypia and an increased mitotic count including atypical mitotic figures. In cases of spindle cell carcinoma, immunohistochemical stains for cytokeratin may be used to facilitate the diagnosis [100].

The plasma cell variant may be confused with an inflammatory reaction or infectious process or a malignant proliferation of plasma cells (plasmacytoma). In an infectious process, the use of histochemical stains or microbiological investigations may lead to the correct diagnosis. In plasmacytoma, the plasma cells would usually show light chain restriction confirming the presence of a clonal cell population.

Treatment and Prognosis

Complete surgical resection is the treatment of choice for pulmonary inflammatory pseudotumors. Although wedge resection is usually sufficient for peripherally located lesions, some lesions require a more extensive surgical approach (lobectomy or pneumonectomy) depending on location and degree of invasiveness. Incompletely resected cases have a tendency to recur, and in those instances, re-resection is advised. Metastasis from a pulmonary inflammatory

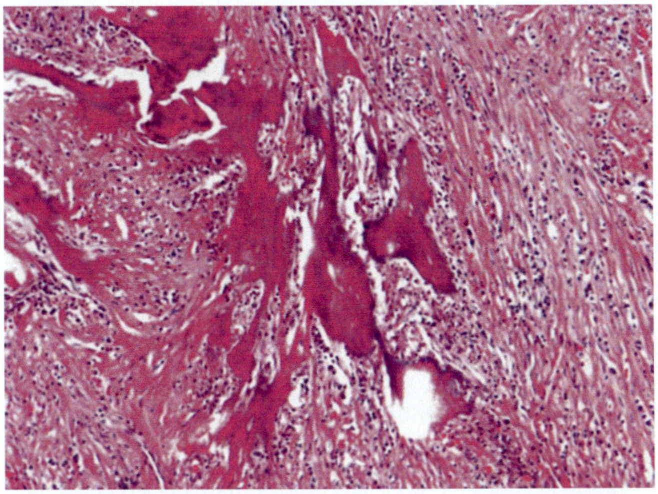

Fig. 10.70 Inflammatory pseudotumor of the lung showing metaplastic bone formation

pseudotumor is a rare event, and metastatic sites are usually the opposite lung and the brain [90, 93, 115, 116]. Interestingly, the lesions that metastasize tend to be ALK-1 negative by immunohistochemistry [93]. Overall 5-year survival is reported to be around 91 % [117].

References

1. Liebow AA, Castelman B. Benign "clear cell tumors" of the lung. Am J Pathol. 1963;43:13a–4 (abstract).
2. Liebow AA, Castleman B. Benign clear cell ("sugar") tumors of the lung. Yale J Biol Med. 1971;43:213–22.
3. Becker NH, Soifer I. Benign clear cell tumor ("sugar tumor") of the lung. Cancer. 1971;27:712–9.
4. Andrion A, Mazzucco G, Gugliotta P, Monga G. Benign clear cell (sugar) tumor of the lung. A light microscopic, histochemical, and ultrastructural study with a review of the literature. Cancer. 1985; 56:2657–63.
5. Gaffey MJ, Mills SE, Zarbo RJ, Weiss LM, Gown AM. Clear cell tumor of the lung. Immunohistochemical and ultrastructural evidence of melanogenesis. Am J Surg Pathol. 1991;15:644–53.
6. Lantuejoul S, Isaac S, Pinel N, Negoescu A, Guibert B, Brambilla E. Clear cell tumor of the lung: an immunohistochemical and ultrastructural study supporting a pericytic differentiation. Mod Pathol. 1997;10:1001–8.
7. Bonetti F, Pea M, Martignoni G, Zamboni G. PEC and sugar. Am J Surg Pathol. 1992;16:307–8.
8. Flieder DB, Travis WD. Clear cell "sugar" tumor of the lung: association with lymphangioleiomyomatosis and multifocal micronodular pneumocyte hyperplasia in a patient with tuberous sclerosis. Am J Surg Pathol. 1997;21:1242–7.
9. Fukuda T, Machinami R, Joshita T, Nagashima K. Benign clear cell tumor of the lung in an 8-year-old girl. Arch Pathol Lab Med. 1986; 110:664–6.
10. Vijayabhaskar R, Mehta SS, Deodhar KK, Pramesh CS, Mistry RC. PEComa of the lung. J Cancer Res Ther. 2010;6:109–11.
11. Santana AN, Nunes FS, Ho N, Takagaki TY. A rare cause of hemoptysis: benign sugar (clear) cell tumor of the lung. Eur J Cardiothorac Surg. 2004;25:652–4.
12. Gora-Gebka M, Liberek A, Bako W, Szumera M, Korzon M, Jaskiewicz K. The "sugar" clear cell tumor of the lung-clinical presentation and diagnostic difficulties of an unusual lung tumor in youth. J Pediatr Surg. 2006;41:e27–9.
13. Kavunkal AM, Pandiyan MS, Philip MA, Parimelazhagan KN, Manipadam MT, Cherian VK. Large clear cell tumor of the lung mimicking malignant behavior. Ann Thorac Surg. 2007;83:310–2.
14. Sale GE, Kulander BG. 'Benign' clear-cell tumor (sugar tumor) of the lung with hepatic metastases ten years after resection of pulmonary primary tumor. Arch Pathol Lab Med. 1988;112:1177–8.
15. Parfitt JR, Keith JL, Megyesi JF, Ang LC. Metastatic PEComa to the brain. Acta Neuropathol. 2006;112:349–51.
16. Ye T, Chen H, Hu H, Wang J, Shen L. Malignant clear cell sugar tumor of the lung: patient case report. J Clin Oncol. 2010;28:e626–8.
17. Gaffey MJ, Mills SE, Askin FB, Ross GW, Sale GE, Kulander BG, Visscher DW, Yousem SA, Colby TV. Clear cell tumor of the lung. A clinicopathologic, immunohistochemical, and ultrastructural study of eight cases. Am J Surg Pathol. 1990;14:248–59.
18. Gal AA, Koss MN, Hochholzer L, Chejfec G. An immunohistochemical study of benign clear cell ('sugar') tumor of the lung. Arch Pathol Lab Med. 1991;115:1034–8.
19. Adachi Y, Horie Y, Kitamura Y, Nakamura H, Taniguchi Y, Miwa K, Fujioka S, Nishimura M, Hayashi K. CD1a expression in PEComas. Pathol Int. 2008;58:169–73.
20. Adachi Y, Kitamura Y, Nakamura H, Taniguchi Y, Miwa K, Horie Y, Hayashi K. Benign clear (sugar) cell tumor of the lung with CD1a expression. Pathol Int. 2006;56:453–6.
21. Sale GF, Kulander BG. Benign clear cell tumor of lung with necrosis. Cancer. 1976;37:2355–8.
22. Deavers M, Guinee D, Koss MN, Travis WD. Granular cell tumors of the lung. Clinicopathologic study of 20 cases. Am J Surg Pathol. 1995;19:627–35.
23. Abrikossoff AI. Über Myome, ausgehend von der quergestreiften willkürlichen Muskulatur. Virchows Arch f Path Anat. 1926; 260:215–33.
24. Azzopardi JG. Histogenesis of the granular-cell myoblastoma. J Pathol Bacteriol. 1956;71:85–94.
25. Pearse AG. The histogenesis of granular-cell myoblastoma (? granular-cell perineural fibroblastoma). J Pathol Bacteriol. 1950;62: 351–62.
26. Fisher ER, Wechsler H. Granular cell myoblastoma--a misnomer. Electron microscopic and histochemical evidence concerning its Schwann cell derivation and nature (granular cell schwannoma). Cancer. 1962;15:936–54.
27. Ordóñez NG. Granular cell tumor: a review and update. Adv Anat Pathol. 1999;6:186–203.
28. Kramer R. Myoblastoma of the bronchus. Ann Otol Rhinol Laryngol. 1939;48:1083–6.
29. Wilson RW, Kirejczyk W. Pathological and radiological correlation of endobronchial neoplasms: part I, benign tumors. Ann Diagn Pathol. 1997;1:31–46.
30. De Clercq D, Van der Straeten M, Roels H. Granular cell myoblastoma of the bronchus. Eur J Respir Dis. 1983;64:72–6.
31. Ostermiller WE, Comer TP, Barker WL. Endobronchial granular cell myoblastoma. A report of three cases and review of the literature. Ann Thorac Surg. 1970;9:143–8.
32. Lauro S, Trasatti L, Bria E, Gelibter A, Larosa G, Vecchione A. Malignant bronchial Abrikossoff's tumor and small cell lung cancer: a case report and review. Anticancer Res. 2001;21:563–5.
33. Jiang M, Anderson T, Nwogu C, Tan D. Pulmonary malignant granular cell tumor. World J Surg Oncol. 2003;1:22.
34. Al-Ghamdi AM, Flint JD, Muller NL, Stewart KC. Hilar pulmonary granular cell tumor: a case report and review of the literature. Ann Diagn Pathol. 2000;4:245–51.
35. Cutlan RT, Eltorky M. Pulmonary granular cell tumor coexisting with bronchogenic carcinoma. Ann Diagn Pathol. 2001;5:74–9.

36. Gabriel Jr JB, Thomas L, Mendoza CB, Chauhan PM. Granular cell tumor of the bronchus coexisting with a bronchogenic adenocarcinoma: a case report. J Surg Oncol. 1983;24:103–6.
37. Khansur T, Balducci L, Tavassoli M. Identification of desmosomes in the granular cell tumor. Implications in histologic diagnosis and histogenesis. Am J Surg Pathol. 1985;9:898–904.
38. Robinson JM, Knoll R, Henry DA. Intrathoracic granular cell myoblastoma. South Med J. 1988;81:1453–7.
39. Vaos G, Zavras N, Priftis K, Pierrakos P. Bronchial granular cell tumor in a child: impact of diagnostic delay on the type of surgical resection. J Pediatr Surg. 2006;41:1326–8.
40. Oparah SS, Subramanian VA. Granular cell myoblastoma of the bronchus: report of 2 cases and review of the literature. Ann Thorac Surg. 1976;22:199–202.
41. Schulster PL, Khan FA, Azueta V. Asymptomatic pulmonary granular cell tumor presenting as a coin lesion. Chest. 1975;68:256–8.
42. Thomas de Montpréville V, Dulmet EM. Granular cell tumours of the lower respiratory tract. Histopathology. 1995;27:257–62.
43. Mazur MT, Shultz JJ, Myers JL. Granular cell tumor. Immunohistochemical analysis of 21 benign tumors and one malignant tumor. Arch Pathol Lab Med. 1990;114:692–6.
44. Fang HY, Wu CY, Huang HJ, Lin YM. Granular cell tumor of the lung. Lung. 2010;188:355–7.
45. Daniel TM, Smith RH, Faunce HF, Sylvest VM. Transbronchoscopic versus surgical resection of tracheobronchial granular cell myoblastomas. Suggested approach based on follow-up of all treated cases. J Thorac Cardiovasc Surg. 1980;80:898–903.
46. Liebow AA, Hubbell DS. Sclerosing hemangioma (histiocytoma, xanthoma) of the lung. Cancer. 1956;9:53–75.
47. Haas JE, Yunis EJ. Totten RS ultrastructure of a sclerosing hemangioma of the lung. Cancer. 1972;30:512–8.
48. Katzenstein AL, Weise DL, Fulling K, Battifora H. So-called sclerosing hemangioma of the lung. Evidence for mesothelial origin. Am J Surg Pathol. 1983;7:3–14.
49. Huszar M, Suster S, Herczeg E, Geiger B. Sclerosing hemangioma of the lung. Immunohistochemical demonstration of mesenchymal origin using antibodies to tissue-specific intermediate filaments. Cancer. 1986;58:2422–7.
50. Hill GS, Eggleston JC. Electron microscopic study of so-called "pulmonary sclerosing hemangioma". Report of a case suggesting epithelial origin. Cancer. 1972;30:1092–106.
51. Kennedy A. "Sclerosing haemangioma" of the lung: an alternative view of its development. J Clin Pathol. 1973;26:792–9.
52. Nagata N, Dairaku M, Ishida T, Sueishi K, Tanaka K. Sclerosing hemangioma of the lung. Immunohistochemical characterization of its origin as related to surfactant apoprotein. Cancer. 1985;55:116–23.
53. Yousem SA, Wick MR, Singh G, Katyal SL, Manivel JC, Mills SE, Legier J. So-called sclerosing hemangiomas of lung. An immunohistochemical study supporting a respiratory epithelial origin. Am J Surg Pathol. 1988;12:582–90.
54. Satoh Y, Tsuchiya E, Weng SY, Kitagawa T, Matsubara T, Nakagawa K, Kinoshita I, Sugano H. Pulmonary sclerosing hemangioma of the lung. A type II pneumocytoma by immunohistochemical and immunoelectron microscopic studies. Cancer. 1989;64:1310–7.
55. Chan AC, Chan JK. Pulmonary sclerosing hemangioma consistently expresses thyroid transcription factor-1 (TTF-1): a new clue to its histogenesis. Am J Surg Pathol. 2000;24:1531–6.
56. Devouassoux-Shisheboran M, Hayashi T, Linnoila RI, Koss MN, Travis WD. A clinicopathologic study of 100 cases of pulmonary sclerosing hemangioma with immunohistochemical studies: TTF-1 is expressed in both round and surface cells, suggesting an origin from primitive respiratory epithelium. Am J Surg Pathol. 2000;24:906–16.
57. Yamazaki K. Type-II pneumocyte differentiation in pulmonary sclerosing hemangioma: ultrastructural differentiation and immunohistochemical distribution of lineage-specific transcription factors (TTF-1, HNF-3 alpha, and HNF-3 beta) and surfactant proteins. Virchows Arch. 2004;445:45–53.
58. Tanaka I, Inoue M, Matsui Y, Oritsu S, Akiyama O, Takemura T, Fujiwara M, Kodama T, Shimosato Y. A case of pneumocytoma (so-called sclerosing hemangioma) with lymph node metastasis. Jpn J Clin Oncol. 1986;16:77–86.
59. Niho S, Suzuki K, Yokose T, Kodama T, Nishiwaki Y, Esumi H. Monoclonality of both pale cells and cuboidal cells of sclerosing hemangioma of the lung. Am J Pathol. 1998;152:1065–9.
60. Sartori G, Bettelli S, Schirosi L, Bigiani N, Maiorana A, Cavazza A. Rossi GMicrosatellite and EGFR, HER2 and K-RAS analyses in sclerosing hemangioma of the lung. Am J Surg Pathol. 2007;31:1512–20.
61. Wang E, Lin D, Wang Y, Wu G, Yuan X. Immunohistochemical and ultrastructural markers suggest different origins for cuboidal and polygonal cells in pulmonary sclerosing hemangioma. Hum Pathol. 2004;35:503–8.
62. Spencer H, Nambu S. Sclerosing haemangiomas of the lung. Histopathology. 1986;10:477–87.
63. Miyagawa-Hayashino A, Tazelaar HD, Langel DJ, Colby TV. Pulmonary sclerosing hemangioma with lymph node metastases: report of 4 cases. Arch Pathol Lab Med. 2003;127:321–5.
64. Katzenstein AL, Gmelich JT, Carrington CB. Sclerosing hemangioma of the lung: a clinicopathologic study of 51 cases. Am J Surg Pathol. 1980;4:343–56.
65. Maeda R, Isowa N, Miura H, Tokuyasu H, Kawasaki Y, Yamamoto K. Bilateral multiple sclerosing hemangiomas of the lung. Gen Thorac Cardiovasc Surg. 2009;57:667–70.
66. Lee ST, Lee YC, Hsu CY, Lin CC. Bilateral multiple sclerosing hemangiomas of the lung. Chest. 1992;101:572–3.
67. Hanaoka J, Ohuchi M, Inoue S, Sawai S, Tezuka N, Fujino S. Bilateral multiple pulmonary sclerosing hemangioma. Jpn J Thorac Cardiovasc Surg. 2005;53:157–61.
68. Soumil VJ, Navin B, Sangeeta D, Na J, Sharma S, Deshpande R. Multiple sclerosing hemangiomas of the lung. Asian Cardiovasc Thorac Ann. 2004;12:357–9.
69. de Koning DB, Drenth JP, Oyen WJ, Wagenaar M, Aliredjo RP, Nagengast FM. Pulmonary sclerosing hemangioma detected by fluorodeoxyglucose positron emission tomography in familial adenomatous polyposis: report of a case. Dis Colon Rectum. 2007;50:1987–91.
70. Hosaka N, Sasaki T, Adachi K, Sato T, Tanaka T, Miura Y, Sawai T, Toki J, Hisha H, Okamura A, Takasu K, Ikehara S. Pulmonary sclerosing hemangioma associated with familial adenomatous polyposis. Hum Pathol. 2004;35:764–8.
71. Devouassoux-Shisheboran M, de la Fouchardière A, Thivolet-Béjui F, Sourisseau-Millan ML, Guerin JC, Travis WD. Endobronchial variant of sclerosing hemangioma of the lung: histological and cytological features on endobronchial material. Mod Pathol. 2004;17:252–7.
72. Wani Y, Notohara K, Tsukayama C, Okumura N. Sclerosing hemangioma with florid endobronchial and endobronchiolar growth. Virchows Arch. 2007;450:221–3.
73. Kim KH, Sul HJ, Kang DY. Sclerosing hemangioma with lymph node metastasis. Yonsei Med J. 2003;44:150–4.
74. Khoury JD, Shephard MN, Moran CA. Cystic sclerosing haemangioma of the lung. Histopathology. 2003;43:239–43.
75. Moran CA, Zeren H, Koss MN. Sclerosing hemangioma of the lung. Granulomatous variant. Arch Pathol Lab Med. 1994;118:1028–30.
76. Dacic S, Sasatomi E, Swalsky PA, Kim DW, Finkelstein SD, Yousem SA. Loss of heterozygosity patterns of sclerosing hemangioma of the lung and bronchioloalveolar carcinoma indicate a similar molecular pathogenesis. Arch Pathol Lab Med. 2004;128:880–4.
77. Pareja MJ, Vargas MT, Sánchez A, Ibáñez J, González-Cámpora R. Cytogenetic study of a pulmonary sclerosing hemangioma. Cancer Genet Cytogenet. 2009;195:80–4.
78. Yano M, Yamakawa Y, Kiriyama M, Hara M, Murase T. Sclerosing hemangioma with metastases to multiple nodal stations. Ann Thorac Surg. 2002;73:981–3.
79. Komatsu T, Fukuse T, Wada H, Sakurai T. Pulmonary sclerosing hemangioma with pulmonary metastasis. Thorac Cardiovasc Surg. 2006;54:348–9.

80. Wei S, Tian J, Song X, Chen Y. Recurrence of pulmonary sclerosing hemangioma. Thorac Cardiovasc Surg. 2008;56:120–2.
81. Childress WG, Adie GC. Plasma cell tumors of the mediastinum and lung; report of 2 cases. J Thorac Surg. 1950;19:794–9.
82. Bahadori M, Liebow AA. Plasma cell granulomas of the lung. Cancer. 1973;31:191–208.
83. Bates T, Hull OH. Histiocytoma of the bronchus; report of case in a six-year old child. AMA J Dis Child. 1958;95:53–6.
84. Dubilier LD, Bryant LR, Danielson GK. Histiocytoma (fibrous xanthoma) of the lung. Am J Surg. 1968;115:420–6.
85. Pettinato G, Manivel JC, De Rosa N, Dehner LP. Inflammatory myofibroblastic tumor (plasma cell granuloma). Clinicopathologic study of 20 cases with immunohistochemical and ultrastructural observations. Am J Clin Pathol. 1990;94:538–46.
86. Tchertkoff V, Lee BY, Wagner BM. Plasma cell granuloma of lung; case report and review of literature. Dis Chest. 1963;44:440–3.
87. Alvarez-Fernandez E, Escalona-Zapata J. Pulmonary plasma cell granuloma – an electron microscopic and tissue culture study. Histopathology. 1983;7:279–86.
88. Berardi RS, Lee SS, Chen HP, Stines GJ. Inflammatory pseudotumors of the lung. Surg Gynecol Obstet. 1983;156:89–96.
89. Monzon CM, Gilchrist GS, Burgert Jr EO, O'Connell EJ, Telander RL, Hoffman AD, Li CY. Plasma cell granuloma of the lung in children. Pediatrics. 1982;70:268–74.
90. Biselli R, Ferlini C, Fattorossi A, Boldrini R, Bosman C. Inflammatory myofibroblastic tumor (inflammatory pseudotumor): DNA flow cytometric analysis of nine pediatric cases. Cancer. 1996;77:778–84.
91. Su LD, Atayde-Perez A, Sheldon S, Fletcher JA, Weiss SW. Inflammatory myofibroblastic tumor: cytogenetic evidence supporting clonal origin. Mod Pathol. 1998;11:364–8.
92. Janik JS, Janik JP, Lovell MA, Hendrickson RJ, Bensard DD, Greffe BS. Recurrent inflammatory pseudotumors in children. J Pediatr Surg. 2003;38:1491–5.
93. Coffin CM, Hornick JL, Fletcher CD. Inflammatory myofibroblastic tumor: comparison of clinicopathologic, histologic, and immunohistochemical features including ALK expression in atypical and aggressive cases. Am J Surg Pathol. 2007;31:509–20.
94. Hartman GE, Shochat SJ. Primary pulmonary neoplasms of childhood: a review. Ann Thorac Surg. 1983;36:108–19.
95. Agrons GA, Rosado-de-Christenson ML, Kirejczyk WM, Conran RM, Stocker JT. Pulmonary inflammatory pseudotumor: radiologic features. Radiology. 1998;206:511–8.
96. Alexiou C, Obuszko Z, Beggs D, Morgan WE. Inflammatory pseudotumors of the lung. Ann Thorac Surg. 1998;66:948–50.
97. Ishida T, Oka T, Nishino T, Tateishi M, Mitsudomi T, Sugimachi K. Inflammatory pseudotumor of the lung in adults: radiographic and clinicopathological analysis. Ann Thorac Surg. 1989;48:90–5.
98. Kim TS, Han J, Kim GY, Lee KS, Kim H, Kim J. Pulmonary inflammatory pseudotumor (inflammatory myofibroblastic tumor): CT features with pathologic correlation. J Comput Assist Tomogr. 2005;29:633–9.
99. Vujanić GM, Dojĉinov D. Inflammatory pseudotumor of the lung in children. Pediatr Hematol Oncol. 1991;8:121–9.
100. Wick MR, Ritter JH, Nappi O. Inflammatory sarcomatoid carcinoma of the lung: report of three cases and clinicopathologic comparison with inflammatory pseudotumors in adult patients. Hum Pathol. 1995;26:1014–21.
101. Coffin CM, Patel A, Perkins S, Elenitoba-Johnson KS, Perlman E, Griffin CA. ALK1 and p80 expression and chromosomal rearrangements involving 2p23 in inflammatory myofibroblastic tumor. Mod Pathol. 2001;14:569–76.
102. Debelenko LV, Arthur DC, Pack SD, Helman LJ, Schrump DS, Tsokos M. Identification of CARS-ALK fusion in primary and metastatic lesions of an inflammatory myofibroblastic tumor. Lab Invest. 2003;83:1255–65.
103. Kinoshita Y, Tajiri T, Ieiri S, Nagata K, Taguchi T, Suita S, Yamazaki K, Yoshino I, Maehara Y, Kohashi K, Yamamoto H, Oda Y, Tsuneyoshi M. A case of an inflammatory myofibroblastic tumor in the lung which expressed TPM3-ALK gene fusion. Pediatr Surg Int. 2007;23:595–9.
104. Gómez-Román JJ, Sánchez-Velasco P, Ocejo-Vinyals G, Hernández-Nieto E, Leyva-Cobián F, Val-Bernal JF. Human herpesvirus-8 genes are expressed in pulmonary inflammatory myofibroblastic tumor (inflammatory pseudotumor). Am J Surg Pathol. 2001;25:624–9.
105. Farris 3rd AB, Kradin RL. Follicular localization of dendritic cells in a xanthomatous inflammatory tumor of lung associated with human herpes virus-8 infection. Virchows Arch. 2006;449:726–9.
106. Yamamoto H, Yamaguchi H, Aishima S, Oda Y, Kohashi K, Oshiro Y, Tsuneyoshi M. Inflammatory myofibroblastic tumor versus IgG4-related sclerosing disease and inflammatory pseudotumor: a comparative clinicopathologic study. Am J Surg Pathol. 2009;33:1330–40.
107. Takeuchi K, Soda M, Togashi Y, Sugawara E, Hatano S, Asaka R, Okumura S, Nakagawa K, Mano H, Ishikawa Y. Pulmonary inflammatory myofibroblastic tumor expressing a novel fusion, PPFIBP1-ALK: reappraisal of anti-ALK immunohistochemistry as a tool for novel ALK fusion identification. Clin Cancer Res. 2011;17:3341–8.
108. Cools J, Wlodarska I, Somers R, Mentens N, Pedeutour F, Maes B, De Wolf-Peeters C, Pauwels P, Hagemeijer A, Marynen P. Identification of novel fusion partners of ALK, the anaplastic lymphoma kinase, in anaplastic large-cell lymphoma and inflammatory myofibroblastic tumor. Genes Chromosomes Cancer. 2002; 34:354–62.
109. Lawrence B, Perez-Atayde A, Hibbard MK, Rubin BP, Dal Cin P, Pinkus JL, Pinkus GS, Xiao S, Yi ES, Fletcher CD, Fletcher JA. TPM3-ALK and TPM4-ALK oncogenes in inflammatory myofibroblastic tumors. Am J Pathol. 2000;157:377–84.
110. Bridge JA, Kanamori M, Ma Z, Pickering D, Hill DA, Lydiatt W, Lui MY, Colleoni GW, Antonescu CR, Ladanyi M, Morris SW. Fusion of the ALK gene to the clathrin heavy chain gene, CLTC, in inflammatory myofibroblastic tumor. Am J Pathol. 2001; 159:411–5.
111. Ma Z, Hill DA, Collins MH, Morris SW, Sumegi J, Zhou M, Zuppan C, Bridge JA. Fusion of ALK to the Ran-binding protein 2 (RANBP2) gene in inflammatory myofibroblastic tumor. Genes Chromosomes Cancer. 2003;37:98–105.
112. Panagopoulos I, Nilsson T, Domanski HA, Isaksson M, Lindblom P, Mertens F, Mandahl N. Fusion of the SEC31L1 and ALK genes in an inflammatory myofibroblastic tumor. Int J Cancer. 2006; 118:1181–6.
113. Tavora F, Shilo K, Ozbudak IH, Przybocki JM, Wang G, Travis WD, Franks TJ. Absence of human herpesvirus-8 in pulmonary inflammatory myofibroblastic tumor: immunohistochemical and molecular analysis of 20 cases. Mod Pathol. 2007; 20:995–9.
114. Zen Y, Kitagawa S, Minato H, Kurumaya H, Katayanagi K, Masuda S, Niwa H, Fujimura M, Nakanuma Y. IgG4-Positive plasma cells in inflammatory pseudotumor (plasma cell granuloma) of the lung. Hum Pathol. 2005;36:710–7.
115. Malhotra V, Tatke M, Malik R, Gondal R, Beohar PC, Kumar S, Puri V. An unusual case of plasma cell granuloma involving lung and brain. Indian J Cancer. 1991;28:223–7.
116. Petridis AK, Hempelmann RG, Hugo HH, Eichmann T, Mehdorn HM. Metastatic low-grade inflammatory myofibroblastic tumor (IMT) in the central nervous system of a 29-year-old male patient. Clin Neuropathol. 2004;23:158–66.
117. Cerfolio RJ, Allen MS, Nascimento AG, Deschamps C, Trastek VF, Miller DL, Pairolero PC. Inflammatory pseudotumors of the lung. Ann Thorac Surg. 1999;67:933–6.

11 Malignant Lymphomas Involving Lung and Pleura

Francisco Vega

Introduction

Primary malignant lymphomas of the lung are traditionally defined as lymphomas presenting as pulmonary lesions, affecting one or both lungs, in a patient with no evidence of lymphoma elsewhere in the past, at present, or for 3 months after presentation [1]. Primary pulmonary lymphomas are rare and represent only 0.4 % of all malignant lymphomas, 3.6 % of extranodal lymphomas [2], and only 0.5 % of all primary neoplasms of the lung [3]. By contrast, secondary involvement of the lung in patients with systemic lymphoma is common and occurs by hematogenous dissemination and/or by contiguous invasion from a nodal or mediastinal lymphoma. It is important to recognize that the assessment between primary and secondary lymphomas is impossible to make on histologic grounds alone, because both processes share similar histopathologic and immunophenotypic features.

Most of the lymphomas involving the lung are B-cell neoplasms. About 80 % of the primary lung lymphomas are extranodal marginal zone lymphoma of mucosa-associated lymphoid tissue (MALT lymphomas), often in the past considered as "pseudotumors" because of its indolent clinical course. The second most frequent lymphoma of the lung is diffuse large B-cell lymphoma (DLBCL) (~20 %); some of them representing large cell transformation of a previous MALT lymphoma. Other types of B-cell lymphomas are distinctly uncommon. Lymphomatoid granulomatosis and intravascular large cell lymphoma (IVLBCL) are rare B-cell lymphomas that characteristically involve the lung. Very rare cases of primary lung plasmacytoma and primary lung classical Hodgkin's lymphoma (HL) have been described. Follicular lymphoma, chronic lymphocytic leukemia/small lymphocytic lymphoma, mantle cell lymphoma, and lymphoplasmacytic lymphoma may involve the lung but they represent, in virtually all the cases, secondary involvement by a systemic lymphoma.

Primary T- and NK-cell lymphomas seem to present very rarely as primary tumors in the lung. Peripheral T-cell lymphomas, NOS, and anaplastic large cell lymphoma (ALCL) are T-cell lymphomas that may present with predominant lung involvement [4, 5]. Mycosis fungoides frequently involves the lung after visceral and systemic dissemination (the lung is the second most involved extracutaneous site after lymph nodes). Angioimmunoblastic T-cell lymphoma is another systemic T-cell lymphoma that frequently involves the lungs.

Secondary involvement of the pleura in patients with systemic lymphoma is very common. However, primary pleural lymphomas are rare. Two distinct clinicopathologic malignancies will be reviewed at the end of this chapter: primary effusion lymphomas (PEL) and DLBCL associated with chronic inflammation, also known as pyothorax-associated lymphoma (PAL). PEL are seen in human immunodeficiency virus (HIV) patients and associated with infection by human herpes virus 8 (HHV-8).

B-Cell Lymphomas

Extranodal Marginal Zone Lymphoma: MALT Lymphoma

Extranodal marginal zone lymphoma of mucosa-associated lymphoid tissue, also known as MALT lymphoma, arises in extranodal sites and is the most frequent lymphoma involving the lung (80 % of the all primary lung lymphomas). Other common sites are stomach, skin, ocular adnexa, salivary glands, and thyroid gland, but virtually any extranodal site can be involved [6].

MALT lymphoma is the prototype for antigen-driven B-cell lymphoma. Most extranodal sites involved by MALT

F. Vega, M.D., Ph.D.
Department of Hematopathology, Unit 72,
The University of Texas MD Anderson Cancer Center,
1515 Holcombe Blvd., Houston, TX 77030, USA
e-mail: fvegava@mdanderson.org

A. Weissferdt, C.A. Moran, *Diagnostic Pathology of Pleuropulmonary Neoplasia*,
DOI 10.1007/978-1-4419-0787-5_11, © Springer Science+Business Media New York 2013

lymphoma such as stomach, salivary gland, lung, thyroid, and ocular adnexa normally lack lymphoid tissue. Chronic antigenic stimulation results in these sites acquiring lymphoid tissue, within which MALT lymphomas can arise. Antigens involved in lymphomagenesis result from either chronic infection (e.g., *Helicobacter pylori* in stomach, *Borrelia burgdorferi* in skin, *Chlamydophila psittaci* in conjunctiva) or autoimmune diseases (e.g., Hashimoto thyroiditis in thyroid, Sjogren's syndrome in salivary glands). Lung MALT lymphomas are thought to be a consequence of long-term exposure to a variety of antigenic stimuli—including smoking, inflammatory disorders, or autoimmune diseases. Acquired MALT (also named in the lung as BALT for bronchus-associated lymphoid tissue) is not present in normal lung. Acquired MALT/BALT has been found more common in smokers than in nonsmokers, and there is experimental evidence that rats exposed to cigarette smoke have enlarged BALT [7, 8]. BALT has also been identified in fetal and neonatal lung from infants with pulmonary infections of an undetermined nature [9]. Patients with interstitial lung diseases, rheumatoid arthritis, Sjogren's syndrome, and systemic sclerosis have inducible BALT (condition also named follicular bronchiolitis) [10, 11].

BALT consists of B-cell lymphoid follicles containing follicular dendritic cell networks and germinal center B- and T-cells. T-cells also surround the lymphoid follicles and may form distinct interfollicular zones [12, 13]. It is believed that some degree of lymphoid hyperplasia is a necessary precondition to the development of MALT lymphoma and explains the finding of reactive germinal centers in MALT lymphomas. This single observation had also led to erroneous diagnoses of MALT lymphomas as "pseudolymphomas" for many years [14, 15].

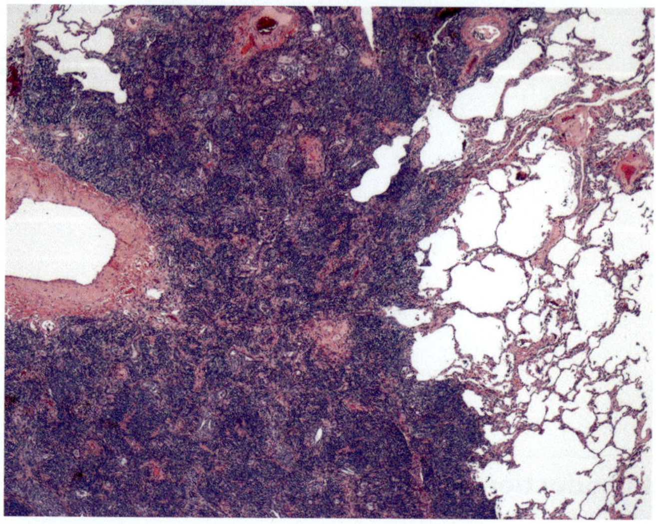

Fig. 11.1 Primary lung MALT lymphoma. The neoplastic lymphoid infiltrate forms a mass lesion that effaces the lung architecture and consolidates the airspaces

Clinical and Radiological Features

Patients range in age from the second to the ninth decades, with an average of 60 years [16]. The incidence in men and women is approximately equal. Up to 40–50 % of the patients have radiological abnormalities without respiratory or B-cell symptoms. Dry cough and mild dyspnea are the most frequent respiratory symptoms [17]. Chest X-ray may show a small mass, usually less than 5 cm, with blurred or well-defined contours frequently associated with air bronchogram [18–20]. Computed tomography (CT) scan, which is more sensitive than standard chest X-rays, usually shows bronchocentric lesions that usually are bilateral (up to 70 %) and multiple (up to 80 % of the cases) [21, 22]. A solitary nodule is seen in less than 10 % of the cases [17]. Less than 10 % of the patients present with diffuse reticulonodular opacities, atelectasis, or pleural effusion [21, 22]. Necrosis and hemorrhage are not seen. An 18F-2-fluoro-2-deoxy-D-glucose (FDG) positron emission tomography (PET) scan usually shows mild uptake in most of the cases [17]. Up to 35 % of the patients have concomitant involvement of other extranodal sites (extrapulmonary lymphoma) [17, 23, 24]. Systematic gastric endoscopy biopsies in patients with pulmonary MALT lymphomas show gastric lymphoma in ~40 % of the patients. Approximately, 20 % of the patients have also bone marrow involvement [17, 24].

Histopathologic Features

Three histological findings are usually present in MALT lymphomas: a tumor population of small- to medium-sized lymphoma cells, lymphoepithelial lesions, and reactive lymphoid follicles. At low magnification, the neoplasm may have different growth patterns. The neoplasm may present as a dense and relatively monotonous lymphoid infiltrate that effaces and destroys the lung architecture and consolidates the air spaces (Fig. 11.1). It can also present as small multiple scattered nodules or may manifest as ill-defined infiltrates along bronchovascular bundles and interlobular septa. In some cases, the neoplasm may also resemble nodular lymphoid hyperplasia. One striking low-magnification feature is the presence of lymphoid follicles with reactive germinal centers. In the early stages of disease, the tumor cells infiltrate around reactive B-cell follicles, external to a preserved mantle zone, in a marginal zone distribution; however, eventually the tumor cells overrun some or most of the follicles (follicular colonization). Follicular colonization may result in a vaguely nodular pattern of the neoplasm. Invasion of the bronchial cartilage and visceral pleura can also be seen (Fig. 11.2). Hyaline sclerosis and/or hyalinized small vessels are frequently seen. Amyloid deposition can be seen; this seems to be more frequent in MALT lymphomas involving the lung than in those involving other sites.

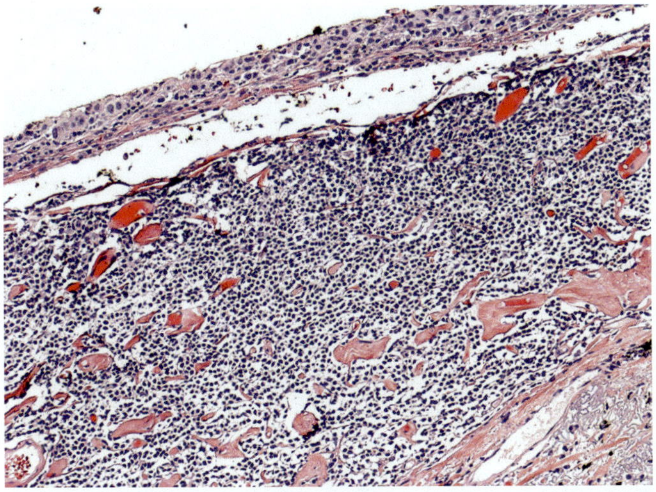

Fig. 11.2 MALT lymphoma invading the visceral pleura. The tumor cells are small in size. Note the presence of hyalinization of some of the vessel walls. The pleura shows mild mesothelial hyperplasia

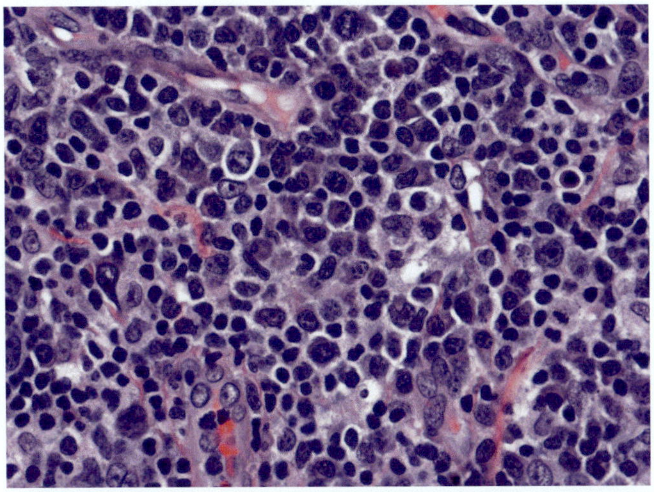

Fig. 11.4 MALT lymphoma involving the lung with marked plasmacytic differentiation. Scattered centroblasts and immunoblasts are also seen

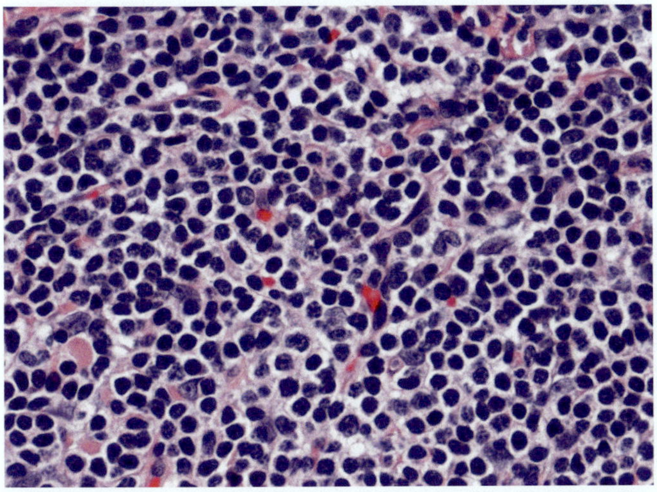

Fig. 11.3 MALT lymphoma involving the lung. The tumor cells are predominantly small with scant cytoplasm. Occasional tumor cells with irregular-shaped nuclei are also noted

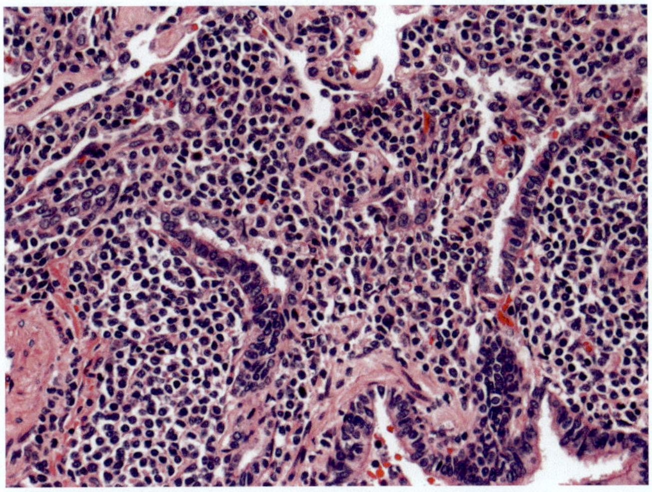

Fig. 11.5 MALT lymphoma involving the lung. Note the presence of numerous lymphoepithelial lesions associated with destruction of the bronchiolar epithelium

The most characteristic tumor cells are small- to medium-sized with slightly irregular nuclei and inconspicuous nucleoli, resembling centrocytes, (Fig. 11.3). Isaacson designated these cells as "centrocyte-like" because their resemblance to germinal center centrocytes (small cleaved cells). The accumulation of more pale-staining cytoplasm may lead to a monocytoid appearance of the lymphoma cells. Scattered large cells resembling centroblasts or immunoblasts are usually present, but they do not form confluent clusters or sheets. If solid or sheet-like proliferations of these large lymphoid cells are present, the presence of a DLBCL component should be mentioned. This large cell transformation may or may not result in complete overgrowth of the preceding MALT lymphoma. Plasma cell differentiation is common (Fig. 11.4), and the plasmacytoid lymphocytes may have Russell (eosinophilic cytoplasmic inclusions) or Dutcher bodies (eosinophilic intranuclear pseudoinclusions of cytoplasm). The presence of frequent Dutcher bodies appears to correlate more often with malignant than reactive processes. As seen in other MALT lymphomas involving other sites, the plasmacytic cells may be compartmentalized beneath the bronchiolar epithelium.

The neoplastic cells of MALT lymphoma have a marked tendency to invade mucosal epithelium, usually forming lymphoepithelial lesions, each seen as a cluster of cells within the bronchiolar epithelium (Fig. 11.5). However, in neoplasms with extensive lung involvement, lymphoepithelial lesions may be difficult to recognize because most of the bronchiolar epithelium is destroyed. In those cases,

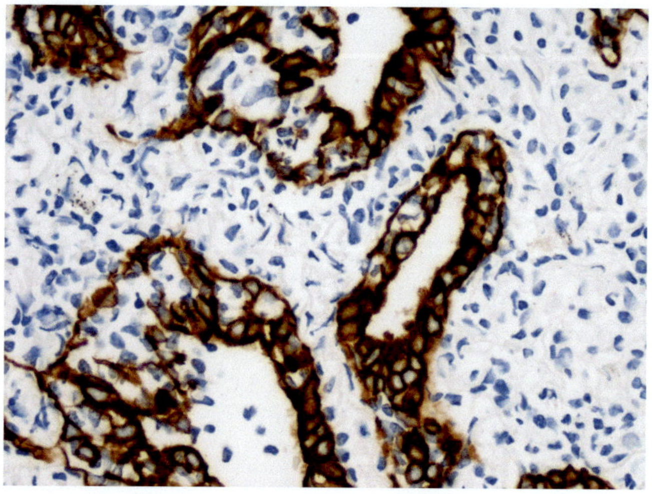

Fig. 11.6 The presence of lymphoepithelial lesions is easily demonstrated using immunostains against cytokeratins

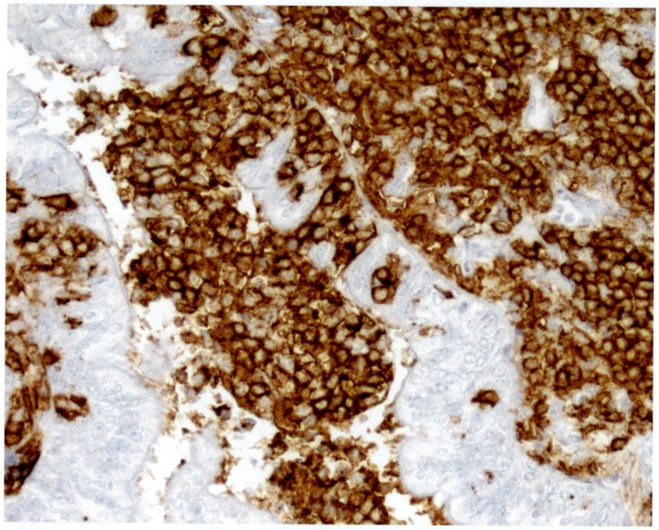

Fig. 11.8 MALT lymphoma involving the lung. A CD20 immunostain highlights the presence of lymphoepithelial lesions

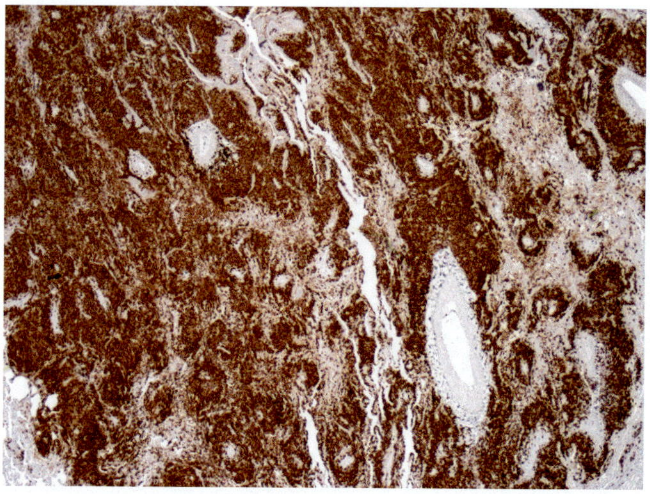

Fig. 11.7 The CD20 immunohistochemical stain highlights numerous B-cells in this case of MALT lymphoma involving the lung. A perivascular distribution of the B-cells is noted

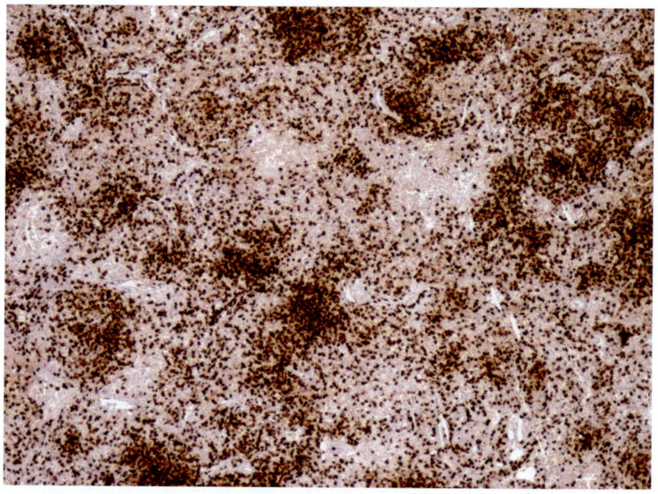

Fig. 11.9 MALT lymphoma involving the lung. Numerous small CD3+ T-cells are present. This is a characteristic feature of MALT lymphomas

immunostains for keratin can be helpful in identifying residual epithelium surrounded by tumor cells (Fig. 11.6).

Secondary morphologic findings that can be seen in pulmonary MALT lymphomas include foci of organizing pneumonia, multinucleated giant cells, sarcoid-like granulomas, and cholesterol cleft granulomas.

Immunohistochemical Features

The tumor cells are B-cells positive for common pan B-cell markers (CD19, CD20, CD22, and CD79a), PAX-5, BCL-2, and CD45/LCA, and usually are negative for CD5, CD10, CD23, and IgD (Figs. 11.7 and 11.8). Few cases can be positive for CD5. CD43 expression by the B-cells is indicative of a neoplastic phenotype and is found in ~50 % of cases. A significant intratumoral population of CD3+, predominantly CD4+ T cells is characteristic (Fig. 11.9). Follicular colonization is not always apparent on H&E stains, but it is easily demonstrated with immunostains for follicular dendritic cells (Fig. 11.10) such as CD21, CD23, or CD35, or with immunostains for follicular germinal center B-cells such as CD10 or BCL-6 (follicular germinal center B-cells will be positive for CD10 and BCL-6 and negative for BCL-2). The demonstration of immunoglobulin (Ig) light chain restriction using antibodies (Fig. 11.11) or by in situ hybridization assays is important in the differential diagnosis with benign lymphoid infiltrates, in particular for those cases resembling nodular lymphoid hyperplasia. In MALT lymphomas, the tumor proliferation index, as measured by MIB-1 (Ki-67), is usually low (Fig. 11.12).

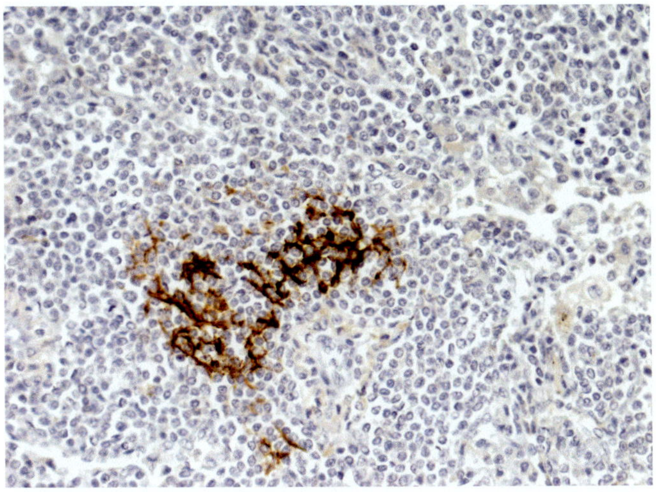

Fig. 11.10 MALT lymphoma involving the lung. Residual networks of follicular dendritic cells are frequently seen using markers such as CD23. They indicate the presence of follicular colonization by the tumor cells and support the diagnosis of MALT lymphoma

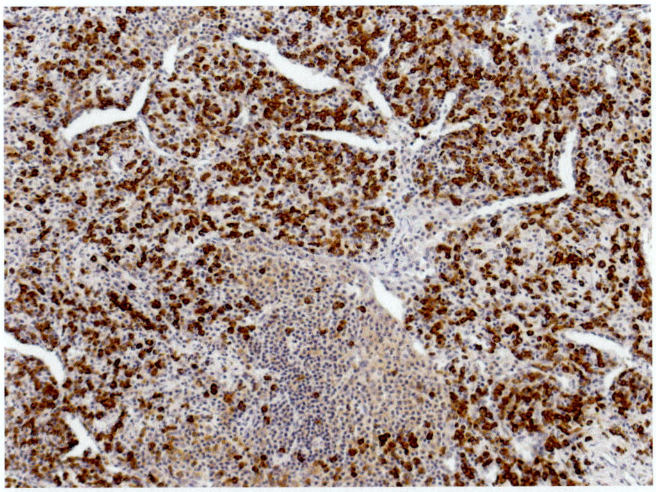

Fig. 11.11 A monotypic population of plasma cells and lymphoplasmacytoid B-cells, in this case kappa light chain restricted, is frequently demonstrated in MALT lymphomas

Genetics and Molecular Findings

Molecular studies typically reveal *Ig* heavy and light chain gene rearrangements. The presence of ongoing mutations has been reported indicating direct antigenic stimulation of the neoplastic clone, resulting in clonal evolution [25]. Because of the difficulty in distinguishing between acquired benign MALT and low-grade MALT lymphoma, particularly in small endoscopic biopsy specimens, there has been a tendency to rely on molecular evidence of monoclonality detected by polymerase chain reaction (PCR) for the diagnosis of lymphoma. However, it is important to know that this technique may fail to detect monoclonality (false-negative results) in up to 40 % of cases of overt lymphoma and vice versa; monoclonality may be detected by PCR in

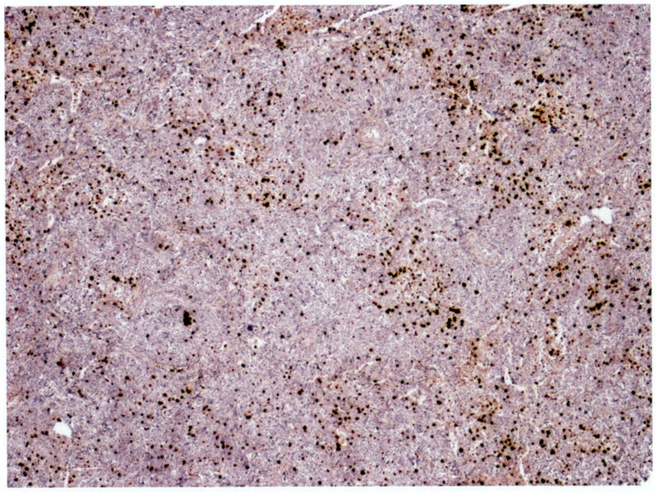

Fig. 11.12 Primary lung MALT lymphomas usually show a low proliferation index (less than 10 %) as detected using the immunomarker MIB1 (Ki-67). Note the presence of small clusters of positive cells, indicating the presence of residual nonneoplastic germinal center cells of almost completed colonized germinal centers

nonneoplastic conditions (false positive results). The relatively high percentage of false-negative rate is attributable to the frequent presence of somatic mutations of the *IgH* variable (V) region genes in this lymphoma type that may disturb the annealing of the primers with the V region [26]. In addition, small monoclonal B-cell populations may be present in lesions that histologically and immunohistochemically do not meet the criteria for a malignant process. These findings emphasize that the diagnosis of MALT lymphoma should not rely exclusively in the clonality studies by PCR.

Chromosomal translocations, usually resulting in oncogene activation, occur in many types of lymphoma, and their detection is helpful for establishing the diagnosis of lymphoma and monitoring the disease after therapy. In MALT lymphomas, a total of 10 chromosomal translocations have been reported, of which four are well characterized and implicated in pathogenesis, with six more recently described and variably defined [6, 27]. The most common is t(11;18)(q21;q21), which is identified in up to one-third of cases, and results in a chimeric *api2-malt1* gene. The t(14,18)(q32;q21)/*IgH-malt1*, t(3,14)(p14.1;q32)/*IgH-foxp1*, and t(1,14)(p22;q32)/*IgH-bcl10* have been identified in approximately 10–20, 10, and 1–2 % of MALT lymphomas, respectively, and result in overexpression of *malt1*, *foxp1*, and *bcl10* genes. These translocations are mutually exclusive in an individual MALT lymphoma and correlate with site of disease [28]. MALT lymphomas associated with t(11;18) arise most often in the lung (40 %) and stomach (30 %). In contrast, MALT lymphomas associated with t(14;18) arise commonly in skin, ocular adnexa, salivary glands, and liver. MALT lymphomas associated with t(3;14) tend to occur in the thyroid gland, skin, and the ocular adnexa, while MALT lymphomas associated with t(1;14) may have a predilection for the intestines. The heterogeneity of MALT lymphomas, in their site of origin, associated diseases, and translocations, suggests that MALT lymphoma is actually a number of different, but related, diseases. The t(11;18) can be detected in paraffin-embedded tissue by reverse transcription PCR and by fluorescence in situ hybridization (FISH).

Differential Diagnosis

The distinction between a reactive lymphoid infiltrate and MALT lymphoma can be difficult in particular with cases of follicular bronchiolitis, nodular hyperplasia of the bronchial lymphoid tissue, and lymphocytic interstitial pneumonitis (LIP) (Fig. 11.13) [29]. In general, the larger the infiltrate, the greater the likelihood of lymphoma. Clear evidence of cytological atypia, lymphoplasmacytoid cells, and Dutcher bodies, if numerous, support lymphoma. Areas of cartilage invasion and plaque-like invasion of the pleura also support lymphoma. A relatively monotonous lymphoid population is also more likely to be lymphoma. The interstitial infiltrate in LIP consists predominantly of T-cells [30].

However, this distinction may be not possible in some cases without ancillary studies in particular in cases of nodular lymphoid hyperplasia. Coexpression of CD43 by the B-cells is a useful hint that the B-cell population is neoplastic. MALT lymphoma is also generally accepted if a monotypic B-cell (lymphoplasmacytoid) or plasma cell population is detected using immunophenotypic or in situ hybridization methods. However, as previously mentioned, the presence of monoclonal *Ig* gene rearrangements without immunophenotypic evidence of clonality is more controversial [31, 32].

It is also important to differentiate MALT lymphoma from the other small B-cell lymphomas that may present or involve the lungs. These include mantle cell lymphoma, chronic lymphocytic leukemia/small lymphocytic lymphoma, follicular lymphoma, and lymphoplasmacytic lymphoma. Classical mantle cell lymphoma may show diffuse or vaguely nodular patterns and is composed of small- to medium-sized lymphoid cells with slightly irregular nuclear contours resembling centrocytes as MALT lymphoma. However, the tumor cells in mantle cell lymphoma are positive for CD5, IgD, and cyclin D1—a consequence of the translocation t(11;14). Chronic lymphocytic leukemia/small lymphocytic lymphoma is composed of a relatively monomorphic population of small and round lymphocytes and may show, at low power, characteristic pale areas corresponding to proliferation centers that are diagnostic of this lymphoma type. Expression of CD5, CD23, and IgD without cyclin D1 provides further distinction from MALT lymphoma. Follicular lymphoma, which can arise extranodally, can be difficult to distinguish from MALT lymphoma with

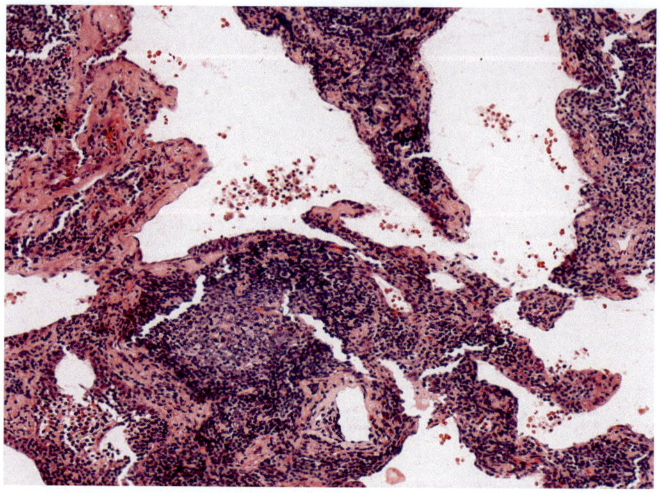

Fig. 11.13 High-power view of diffuse hyperplasia of the bronchus-associated lymphoid tissue (BAL, lymphoid interstitial pneumonia) showing small lymphoid follicles with reactive germinal centers and an interstitial lymphoid infiltrate composed of T-cells as demonstrated by immunohistochemistry (not shown)

follicular colonization. The tumor cells in follicular lymphoma are positive for germinal center cell markers such as CD10, BCL-6, and LMO2 and are negative for CD5 and CD43. The presence of reactive germinal centers and a marginal zone growth pattern with lymphoepithelial lesions will help in distinguish MALT lymphomas with plasmacytic differentiation from lymphoplasmacytic lymphoma and primary lung plasmacytoma.

Treatment and Prognosis

MALT lymphomas are among the most indolent of all lymphomas and have a good prognosis, regardless of clinical stage. The outcome is favorable with a 5-year survival rate of >80 % and a median survival time of >10 years [17]. In the largest series of pulmonary MALT lymphoma (63 cases), Borie and associates [17] found that 44 % of patients had a disseminated disease at diagnosis, which appears greater than the 10–34 % previously published in nongastric MALT lymphomas [24, 33, 34]. However, extrapulmonary location of lymphoma was not a prognostic factor of overall survival or for progression-free survival. Transformation to DLBCL results in a significantly lower survival of approximately 50 % at 5 years.

Current treatment options are surgery, chemotherapy, and radiotherapy as well as "watch and wait" (abstention from therapy). The management of these lymphomas has not been clearly determined. Surgical resection is commonly preferred for localized tumors. Chemo- and immunotherapy is generally used for patients with bilateral and extensive extrapulmonary involvement, relapse, or tumor progression.

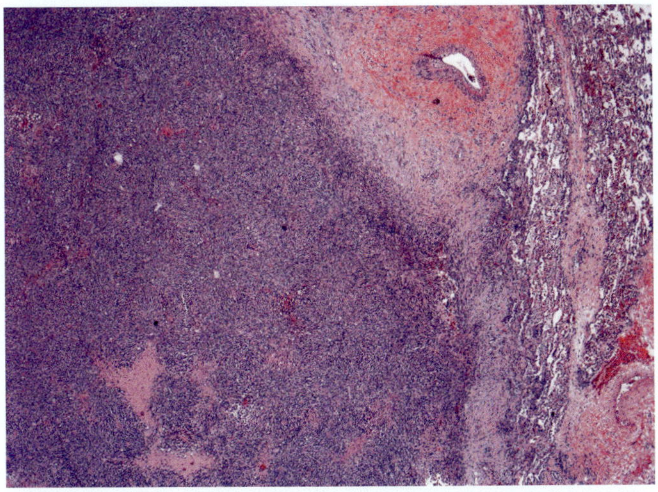

Fig. 11.14 Low-power view of a DLBCL involving the lung. The neoplasm has a diffuse growth pattern and effaces the lung architecture. Focal areas of necrosis are seen

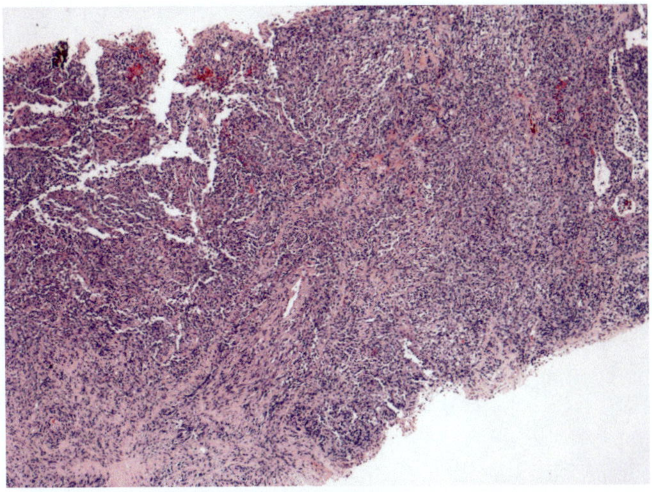

Fig. 11.15 CT-guided 20-gauge core needle biopsy specimen showing DLBCL involving the lung. The neoplasm is diffuse and effaces the lunch architecture

Diffuse Large B-Cell Lymphoma

Diffuse large B-cell lymphoma (DLBCL) is the next most common type of primary pulmonary lymphoma, accounting for approximately 10–30 % of cases [5, 35]. Some of these lymphomas may arise from the transformation of a previous MALT lymphoma (50 % of the cases) or occur in individuals with an underlying immunodeficiency disorder (HIV, organ transplantation, etc.) [35, 36]. However, most of the DLBCLs involving lung and/or pleura represent a manifestation of systemic disease, and most of the patients have evidence of involvement of other anatomic sites at the same time.

Clinical and Radiological Features

Most patients are adults, but there is a wide range of age, including children. Excluding HIV-infected patients, mean age at onset is ~60 years [20, 37–39]. In contrast to patients with MALT lymphomas, most patients with DLBCL present with shortness of breath, fever, chest pain, weight loss, and hemoptysis, as well as paraneoplastic syndromes. Up to 40 % of the patients may be asymptomatic [35].

Chest X-rays reveal solitary nodules and infiltrates that may involve one or more lobes, mass or masses, and consolidations [5, 35]. Cavitation and pleural effusions are commonly seen. Regional lymph nodes are frequently enlarged.

Histopathologic Features

Morphologically these lymphomas are identical to the nodal DLBCL. The diagnosis is based on the presence of a diffuse proliferation of large- or medium-sized lymphoid cells (nuclear size greater than or equal to that of a histiocyte nucleus or more than twice the size of a small lymphocyte) that diffusely efface the lung architecture (Figs. 11.14 and 11.15).

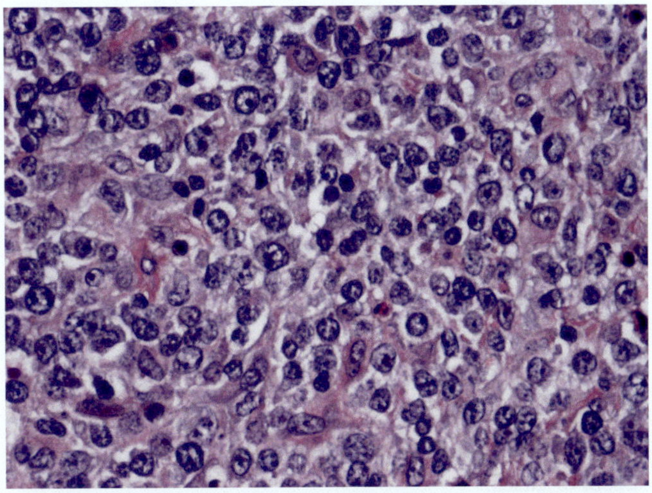

Fig. 11.16 High-power view of an open lung biopsy showing DLBCL. The neoplasm is composed of intermediate to large atypical lymphoid cells with features of immunoblasts and centroblasts

DLBCL can have centroblastic and/or immunoblastic cytologic features (Fig. 11.16). By definition, in the centroblastic variant at least 10 % of the cells are centroblasts (2–3 nucleoli with 1 central and 1 or 2 apposed to the nuclear membrane), and in the immunoblastic variant, immunoblasts (centrally located nucleolus and moderate basophilic cytoplasm) must be >90 % of all cells. The immunoblasts may exhibit plasmacytoid features, with eccentrically located nuclei and a paranuclear hof. Some studies identified the immunoblastic variant as being more clinically aggressive than centroblastic variant. Nonetheless, the lymphoma cells

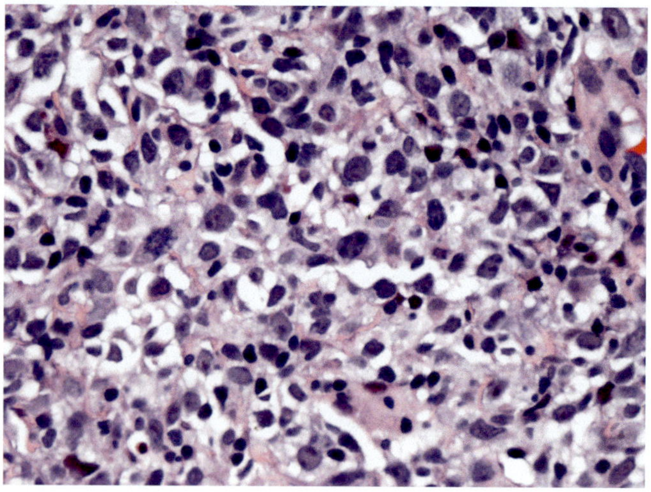

Fig. 11.17 High-power view of a CT-guided 20-gauge core needle lung biopsy specimen showing DLBCL. The tumor cells are intermediate to large, some with irregular nuclear contours and frequent mitoses

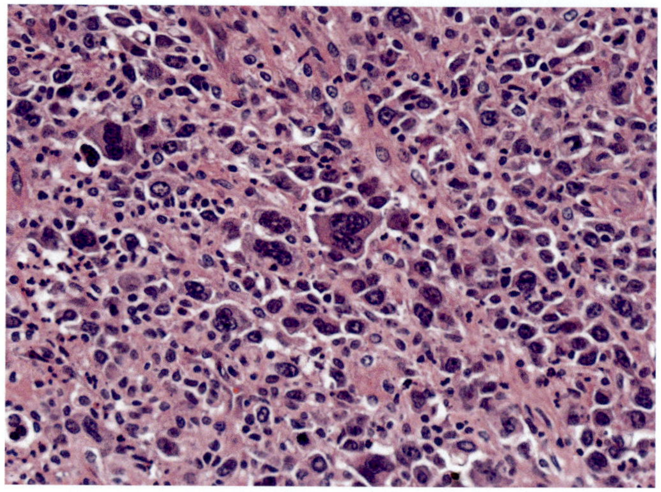

Fig. 11.18 High-power view of a DLBCL anaplastic variant involving the lung. Note the presence of pleomorphic multinucleated neoplastic cells with irregular nuclei contours

may not conform to these classic cell types, exhibiting hybrid features of centroblasts and immunoblasts and frequently is difficult to decide whether a lymphoma cell is a centroblast or an immunoblast (Fig. 11.17). The anaplastic variant comprises cells with bizarre pleomorphic nuclei, often with multinucleated forms (Fig. 11.18). In this variant, the tumor cells may form deceptively cohesive nodules mimicking carcinoma, and some of the tumor cells can express CD30.

In DLBCL, there can be a variable number of reactive cells, such as small lymphocytes, plasma cells, and histiocytes. There may be a "starry sky" appearance imparted by interspersed histiocytes with phagocytosed cell debris. Sclerosis and necrosis may be present. As mentioned before, an underlying MALT lymphoma may be recognized in a subset of cases.

Immunohistochemical Features

The tumor cells are B-cells positive for common pan B-cell markers (CD19, CD20, CD22, and CD79a), PAX-5, and CD45/LCA (Fig. 11.19a, b). CD10 and BCL-6 are expressed in variable proportion of cases. Cases with plasmacytoid differentiation usually have dim expression of CD20 and expression of MUM1/IRF-4. The proliferation fraction, as detected by MIB-1 antibody (Ki-67), is usually high (usually more than 30 %). The tumor cells are usually negative for T-cell antigens, although CD3 can be very rarely coexpressed. Association with Epstein-Barr virus (EBV) is uncommon in nonimmunocompromised patients.

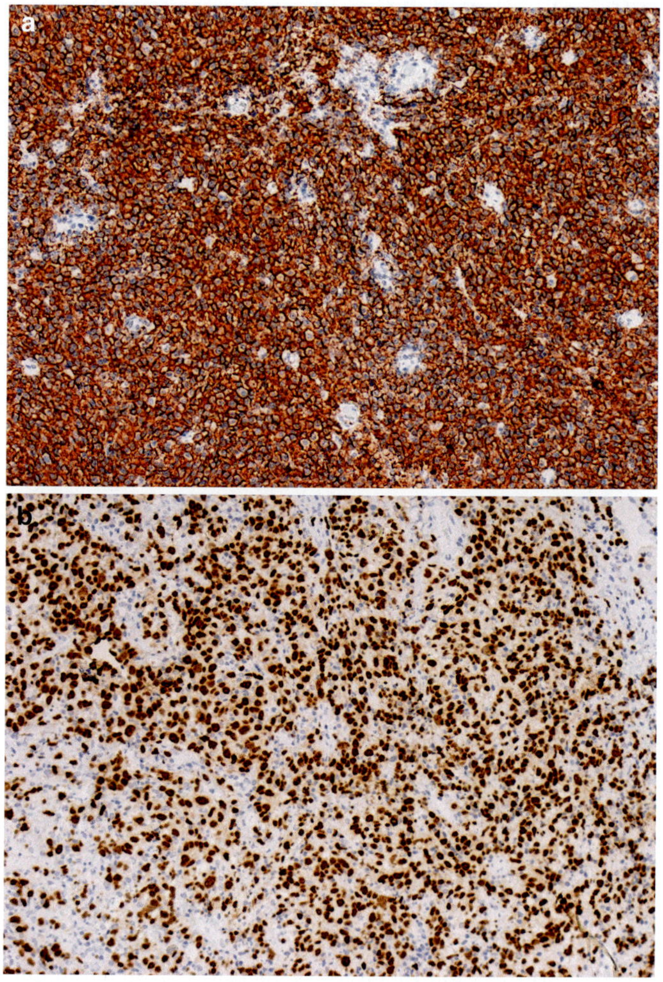

Fig. 11.19 Primary DLBCL involving the lung. The tumor cells are uniform and strongly positive for (**a**) CD20 and (**b**) PAX-5. PAX-5 is particularly useful to demonstrate a B-cell phenotype in relapsed tumors in patients previously treated with rituximab

Genetics and Molecular Findings

Molecular studies typically reveal *Ig* heavy- and light-chain gene rearrangements and germ line T-cell receptor genes. Approximately, 20 % of cases show *bcl-2* rearrangements due to the t(14;18)(q32;q21) and 30 % show *bcl-6* (at 3q27)

gene rearrangements [40–42]. Chromosomal translocations involving *myc* (at 8q24), a molecular hallmark of Burkitt's lymphoma, are reported up to 10 % of DLBCL, more frequently in HIV-infected patients [43–45]. Gene rearrangements of *myc* frequently occur as part of complex genetic alterations and indicate clonal evolution [46]. Approximately 20 % of cases with *myc* gene rearrangements are associated with the presence of translocation involving *bcl-2* and/or *bcl-6*. These "double- or triple-hit lymphomas" can be de novo or follow follicular lymphoma. These lymphomas usually have a high proliferation rate, blastic appearance, systemic involvement (including peripheral blood, leukemic expression), and a very poor prognosis with poor response to current chemotherapy protocols [47].

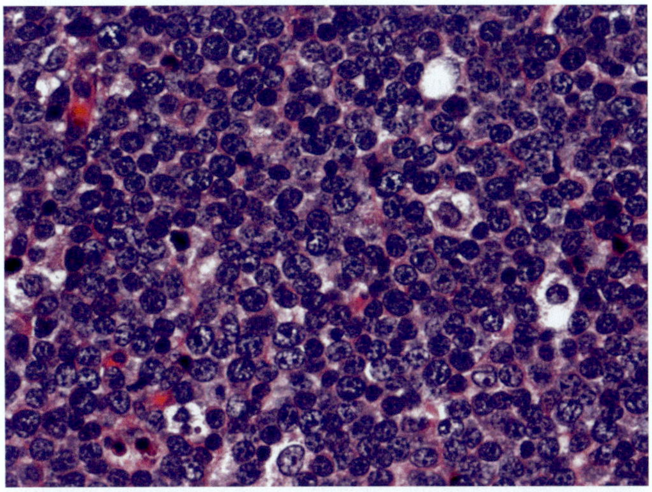

Fig. 11.20 High-power view of a B-cell lymphoma, unclassified with features intermediate between DLBCL and Burkitt's lymphoma (*BL*). The neoplasm is composed of intermediate to large cells. The variability in the nuclear size and the prominent nucleoli in numerous tumor cells are not typical features of BL. A starry sky pattern can be appreciated (tingible body macrophages represent the "stars" in the starry sky pattern)

Differential Diagnosis

Undifferentiated primary or metastatic carcinomas are important differential diagnoses. The use of a broad panel of immunohistochemical studies, including keratins, epithelial membrane antigen (EMA), CD45/LCA, and CD20, should help to obtain an accurate diagnosis. However, rare DLBCL can be focally positive for EMA and/or keratins; in particular, cases of DLBCL with plasmacytic differentiation may have weak and focal positivity for keratins [48].

T-cell lymphomas comprising large neoplastic lymphoid cells may be morphologically indistinguishable from DLBCL, but the distinction can be easily made by immunohistochemistry or flow cytometry immunophenotyping.

Burkitt's lymphoma (BL) is an important differential diagnosis with therapeutic implications. In BL, the tumor cells are intermediate in size with squared-off cytoplasmic borders and multiple (2–4) nucleoli. In addition, BL has characteristic immunophenotypic and genetic features; the tumor cells are positive for CD10, CD20, BCL-6 (uniform and strong), and Ki-67 (virtually 100 % of the tumor cells) and are negative for BCL-2. Chromosomal translocations involving *myc* gene are detected in most of the cases. A new diagnostic category recognized by the 2008 World Health Organization (WHO) lymphoma classification is B-cell lymphoma, unclassifiable, with features intermediate between DLBCL and BL. In this neoplasm, the tumor cells have morphologic and/or immunophenotypic features that are atypical for BL (Fig. 11.20). Other B-cell lymphoma that can be confused with DLBCL is the pleomorphic variant of mantle cell lymphoma (Fig. 11.21). In this lymphoma, the tumor cells are positive for CD5 and cyclin D1.

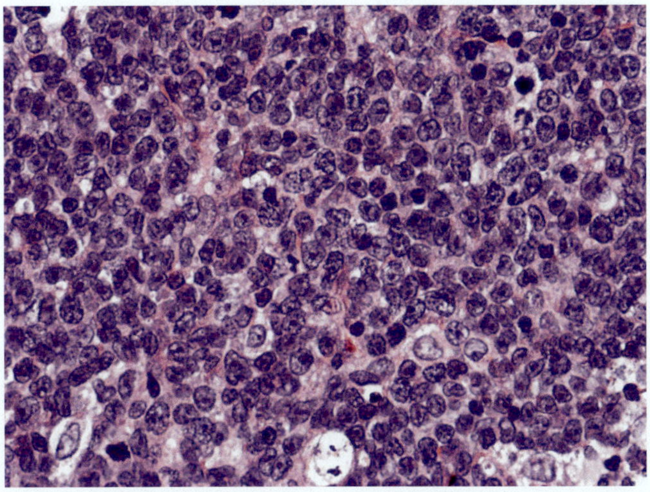

Fig. 11.21 High-power view of pleomorphic mantle cell lymphoma. Note the mixture of intermediate and large lymphoid cells with vesicular nuclear chromatin, numerous mitoses, and few tingible body macrophages. The tumor cells were strongly positive for cyclin D1

Treatment and Prognosis

The 5-year overall survival for patients with DLBCL is 40–70 %, depending on prognostic factors present at diagnosis. The prognosis and evolution are the same as for DLBCL involving other sites. The conventional treatment is R-CHOP (rituximab + cyclophosphamide, doxorubicin, vincristine, prednisone). The addition of rituximab has improved overall survival by 20 % especially in elderly patients and those DLBCL positive for BCL-2 [49]. Those "double- or triple-hit lymphomas" with translocations involving *myc* and *bcl-2* and/or *bcl-6* have a rapidly progressive clinical course, refractory disease, and short survival (usually <1 year) despite aggressive therapy [47, 50]. Proper identification of these cases using ancillary studies is important. All the DLBCLs with high-grade feature (high proliferation rate, apoptosis/necrosis, and starry sky pattern) are candidates for cytogenetic or FISH studies to assess the presence of *myc*, *bcl-2* and/or *bcl-6* gene rearrangements.

Lymphomatoid Granulomatosis

Lymphomatoid granulomatosis (LyG) is an extranodal EBV-positive B-cell lymphoproliferative disorder that characteristically presents with multifocal angiocentric and angiodestructive lesions and is composed predominantly of reactive T-cells and variable number of neoplastic EBV-positive B-cells.

Our understanding of the pathogenesis of LyG has evolved since its first description in 1972 by Liebow and colleagues [51], when it was unclear whether it was neoplastic or inflammatory in nature. In 1979, Katzenstein and associates [52] published the largest series of patients with LyG to date, 152 cases, that highlighted several important clinicopathologic features of this disease, i.e., the prognosis of LyG inversely correlated with the number of large atypical lymphoid cells, the association between LyG and immunosuppression, and the absence of features of Wegener's granulomatosis such as giant cells and palisading epitheliod cells. However, these authors did not solve the question of whether LyG is a variant of Wegener's granulomatosis or whether it is a form of malignant lymphoma. Later, LyG was thought to be a form of T-cell lymphoma and considered part of the spectrum of angiocentric immunoproliferative lesions (AIL)/angiocentric lymphomas (also known as polymorphic reticulosis, midline malignant reticulosis) that are now recognized to be extranodal NK/T-cell lymphomas [53–55]. LyG was thought to be a T-cell lymphoma because of the predominance of CD4-positive helper cells, aggressive clinical course, and the failure to detect B-cell gene rearrangements in these lesions [54]. The failure to detect B-cell gene rearrangements at that time could be explained by the use of less sensitive techniques (Southern blot) and also the scarcity of neoplastic cells within the lesions. Alternatively, in some LyG cases, the EBV-infected B-cells may be polyclonal [56].

The nature of LyG has been largely resolved in more recent years. As initially suggested by Liebow and associates, LyG has been demonstrated to be associated with EBV [57]. Later, Guinee and associates, using in situ hybridization, demonstrated the presence of EBV within B-cells and the presence of monoclonal *IgH* gene rearrangements by PCR analysis in a subset of cases [58]. This and other recent studies have helped to characterize LyG as a type of EBV-positive B-cell lymphoproliferative disease with a prominent T-cell reaction and vasculitis with many similarities to post-transplant lymphoproliferative disorder [58–60].

Clinical Features

LyG is a rare neoplasm, ~600 cases reported in the literature, most in the form of case reports and small series. Patients of all ages can be affected, although most cases occur in young adults (30–50 years). Children also can be affected. Males seem to be more susceptible than females (approximately 2:1). No clear geographical or ethnic susceptibility has been found. There is no increase in Asians, in contrast to EBV+ T-cell and NK-cell lymphomas [61].

LyG is a multisystem disease, and the lung is the most frequent organ involved, and virtually all patients will have pulmonary disease at some point during the course of the disease. Patients usually present with signs and symptoms related to the respiratory tract such as cough, dyspnea, and chest pain [51, 52]. Constitutional symptoms are common, including fever, malaise, weight loss, night sweats, arthralgias, myalgias, and gastrointestinal symptoms [62, 63]. Other organs involved in LyG include skin (second most frequent organ involved), kidneys, central nervous system (CNS), adrenal glands, and gastrointestinal tract. Lymphadenopathies and splenomegaly are uncommon [52]. Moreover, the presence of lymph node involvement should raise questions regarding the diagnosis.

The skin is the extrapulmonary organ most commonly involved in LyG, occurring in 25–50 % of the patients [52, 63]. Most of the patients (55 %) exhibit disseminated cutaneous nodules with or without ulceration, multiple papules, and or plaques frequently located on lower extremities, trunk, and head and neck [63]. Lesions are typically painless but may be pruritic. Cutaneous lesions are the initial manifestations of LyG in up to one-third of patients, and the skin is a common site of recurrence [52]. The central nervous system is involved in one-third of patients, and peripheral nerve involvement has been reported in 7 % of patients [52]. The most common radiological abnormalities, encountered in at least 50 % of the patients, are brain masses as well as multiple focal intraparenchymal lesions, which exhibit T2 prolongation and commonly punctate and/or linear enhancement [64, 65]. This type of enhancement has been shown that correlates with the histopathology findings of perivascular and vascular wall infiltration as seen in LyG involving the CNS [64–66].

A striking clinical feature of LyG is the sparing of lymphoid tissues. Involvement of the spleen is seen in few patients and lymphadenopathies are unusual early in the disease course [52]. However, up to 25 % of patients develop DLBCL EBV positive and histologic progression may be associated with lymph node involvement. Usually, LyG does not involve bone marrow. Some patients may develop a hemophagocytic syndrome, secondary to systemic EBV infection with fever, splenomegaly, adenopathies, pancytopenia, and rapidly progressive course.

LyG is associated with both congenital and acquired immunodeficiencies, such as those related to the X-linked lymphoproliferative syndrome, Wiskott-Aldrich syndrome, HIV infection, and after chemotherapy and/or organ transplant. Even in patients who do not have a known

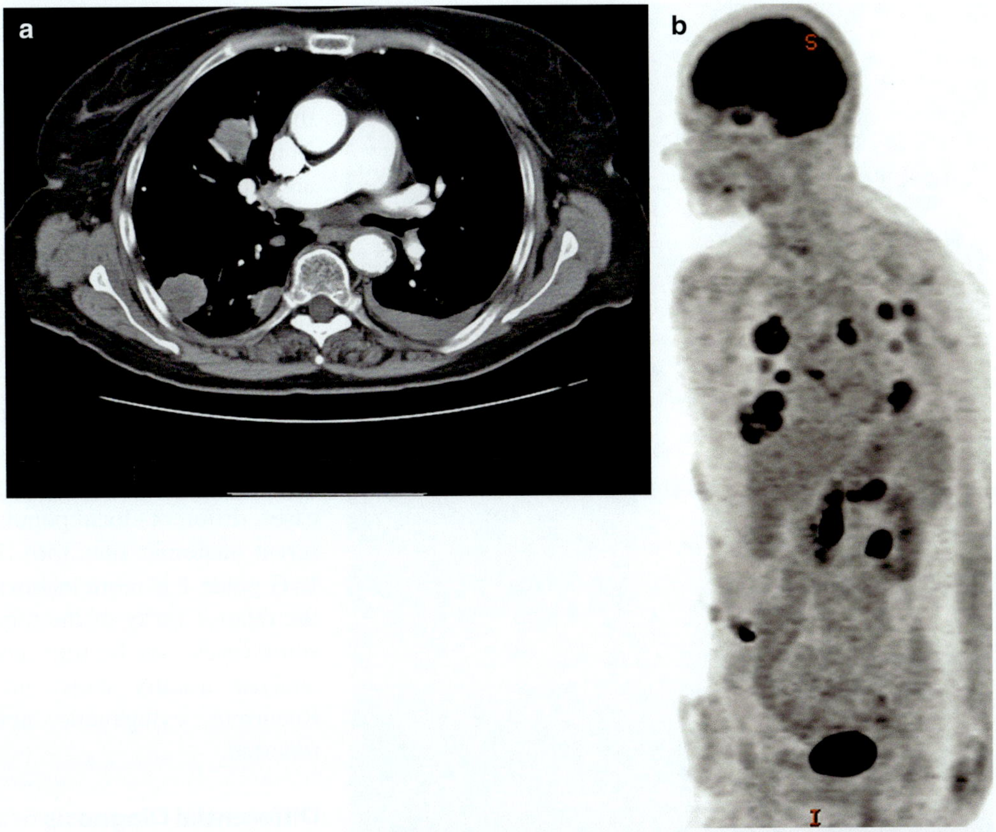

Fig. 11.22 (**a**) CT scan shows bilateral pulmonary masses that are larger and confluent in the right lung. A small left pleural effusion is also noted. The left lung masses are not shown in the figure. (**b**) PET/CT scan of the same patient shows, in addition of the bilateral hypermetabolic pulmonary masses, a 3.5-cm left adrenal mass is also noted. Fluorodeoxyglucose uptake in the liver and spleen appears normal. There are no hypermetabolic abdominal lymph nodes

immunodeficiency disorder, testing of the immune system may reveal abnormalities. This association between LyG and immunosuppression implicates abnormal immune system regulation in the context of an expanding EBV-infected B-cell population [58].

Radiological Features

Imaging studies of the lung usually reveal multiple small to large nodules (80 % of the cases) (Fig. 11.22a, b) with cavitation in up to 25 % [62]. The tumors are most often bilateral and characteristically involve the middle and lower lung fields [51, 52]. Several reports have described spontaneous regression of some of the nodules with growth of other nodules in different sites [67, 68]. Cases presenting as interstitial pneumonitis have been also described [69, 70].

Histopathologic Features

LyG is characterized by an angiocentric and angiodestructive polymorphic infiltrate of small lymphocytes, plasma cells, histiocytes, variable number of scattered large atypical cells, and necrosis (Figs. 11.23 and 11.24). The EBV+ B-cells, hallmark of LyG, vary in size and may resemble immunoblasts and Reed-Sternberg cells. Neutrophils, eosinophils, well-formed granulomas, and multinucleated giant cells are usually absent. The majority of the small lymphocytes are T-cells. Reactive lymphoid follicles are generally absent. The necrosis is infarct-like (coagulative) and appears to be due to both vascular occlusion by the lymphoid infiltrate or vascular necrosis mediated by EBV-induced chemokines.

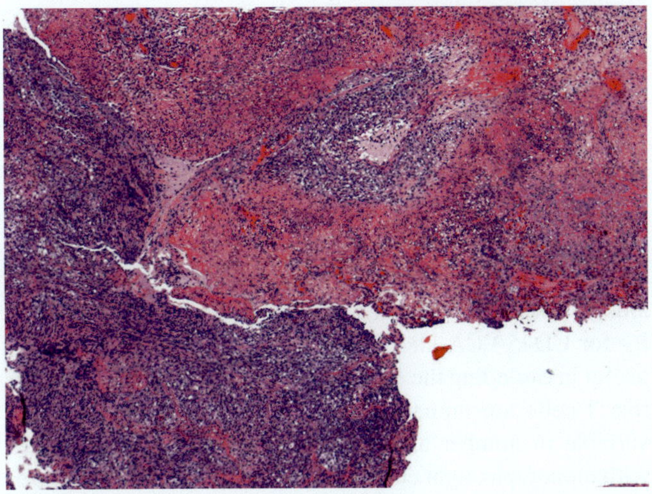

Fig. 11.23 Open lung biopsy of a 29-year-old man with pulmonary LyG grade 3. There are large areas of geographic necrosis as well as a dense lymphohistiocytic infiltrate. The infiltrate is diffuse in some areas but maintained an angiocentric pattern in others

Immunohistochemical Features

The large atypical tumor cells are B-cells positive for common pan B-cell markers (CD19, CD20, CD22, and CD79a),

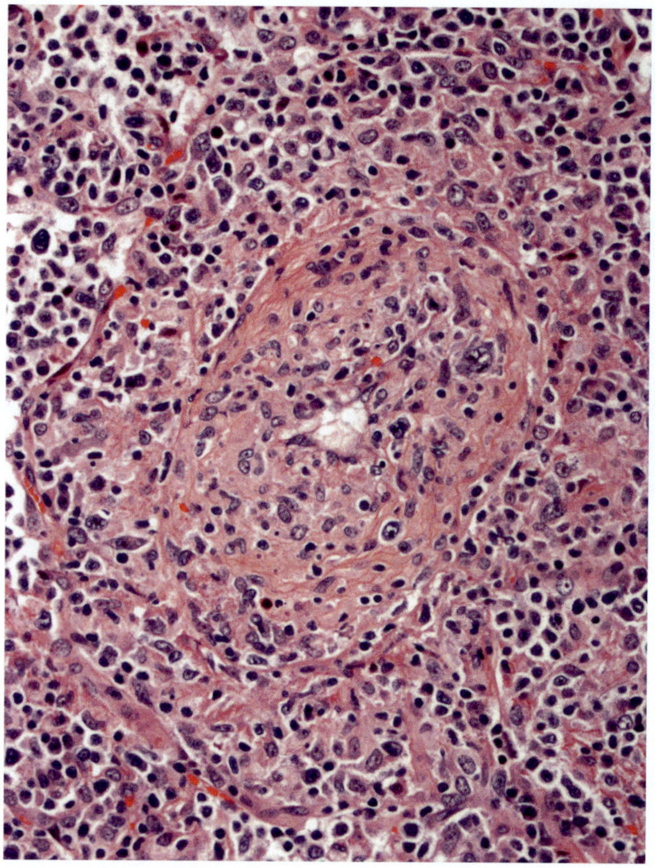

Fig. 11.24 The morphologic hallmark of LyG is the presence of vessel walls with a transmural infiltrate of small lymphocytes and variable number of large atypical lymphoid cells with angiodestruction

PAX-5, and CD45/LCA (Fig. 11.25a). They are usually positive for CD30 but negative for CD15. LMP1 is usually positive. In situ hybridization for EBV-encoded RNA (EBER) is positive in a variable number of the large neoplastic B-cells. The number of EBV+ neoplastic B-cells varies among cases and correlated with the prognosis. The positivity for CD45/LCA and CD79a and negativity for CD15 is useful in excluding the diagnosis of classical HL. Small reactive T-cells are numerous (Fig. 11.25b). Plasma cells are variable in number and usually polyclonal, but rare cases with monotypic, light chain-restricted plasma cells have been described [56].

Grading

This neoplasm is graded on the basis of the number of EBER positive B-cells and extent of the necrosis [71]. LyG grade 1 shows less than five EBER positive cells per high-power field. LyG grade 1 is usually characterized by a polymorphic lymphoid infiltrate with few scattered large atypical cells (better appreciated by immunohistochemistry) and usually small and focal areas of necrosis. LyG grade 2 shows between 5 and 20 EBER positive cells per high-power field (Fig. 11.25c). The number of large atypical cells is more prominent, and necrosis is common. Small clusters of large atypical cells can be seen, especially highlighted using immunostains for B-cell markers. LyG grade 3 shows more than 20 EBER positive cells per high-power field (Fig. 11.26). In these cases, large atypical cells forming large aggregates are seen, and there is extensive necrosis. The end point of the spectrum is a monomorphic EBV+ large B-cell lymphoma. A uniform population of large, atypical EBV+ B-cells without a polymorphic background should be classified as DLBCL and is beyond the spectrum of LyG as currently defined.

Genetics and Molecular Findings

In most cases of LyG grades 2 and 3, clonality of the *IgH* genes can be demonstrated by PCR methods [58]. In some cases, different clonal populations may be identified in different anatomic sites [56]. Demonstration of clonality in LyG grade 1 is more inconsistent. This could be related to the relative rarity of the tumor cells in these cases or that some cases may be truly polyclonal. T-cell receptor gene analysis usually shows no evidence of clonality [72]. Recurrent cytogenetic abnormalities have not been reported.

Differential Diagnosis

The clinical presentation of LyG and Wegener's granulomatosis may be very similar. Wegener's granulomatosis is a systemic necrotizing vasculitis that primarily involves the upper and lower respiratory tracts and kidneys. Wegener's granulomatosis shows the following hallmark histologic features: geographic-shaped liquefactive and/or coagulative necrosis, variable number of eosinophils, multinucleated giant cells without forming well-defined granulomas, and destructive leukocytolytic angiitis involving arteries and veins (Fig. 11.27a). In Wegener's granulomatosis, the multinucleated giant cells contain elastic fibers, and the destructive character of the leukocytolytic angiitis is outlined by the disruption of the network of elastic fibers of the vessel wall (Fig. 11.27b). Elastophagocytosis, multinucleated giant cells, and disruption of the networks of elastic fibers of the vessel wall are not seen in LyG. In addition, the upper respiratory tract is rarely involved in LyG.

The exact relationship between LyG and posttransplant lymphoproliferative disorders (PTLD) is not clear. Both are observed in immunodeficient patients and are EBV driven. These disorders are, however, considered distinct based on clinical presentation, histopathologic features, and the immune response elicited; LyG is extranodal, with angiocentric and angiodestructive lesions, and rich in T-cells (T-cell rich B-cell EBV lymphoproliferative disease). PTLD can be nodal and/or extranodal with diffuse effacement of the architecture and are T-cell poor with plasmacytoid B-cells (T-cell poor B-cell EBV lymphoproliferative

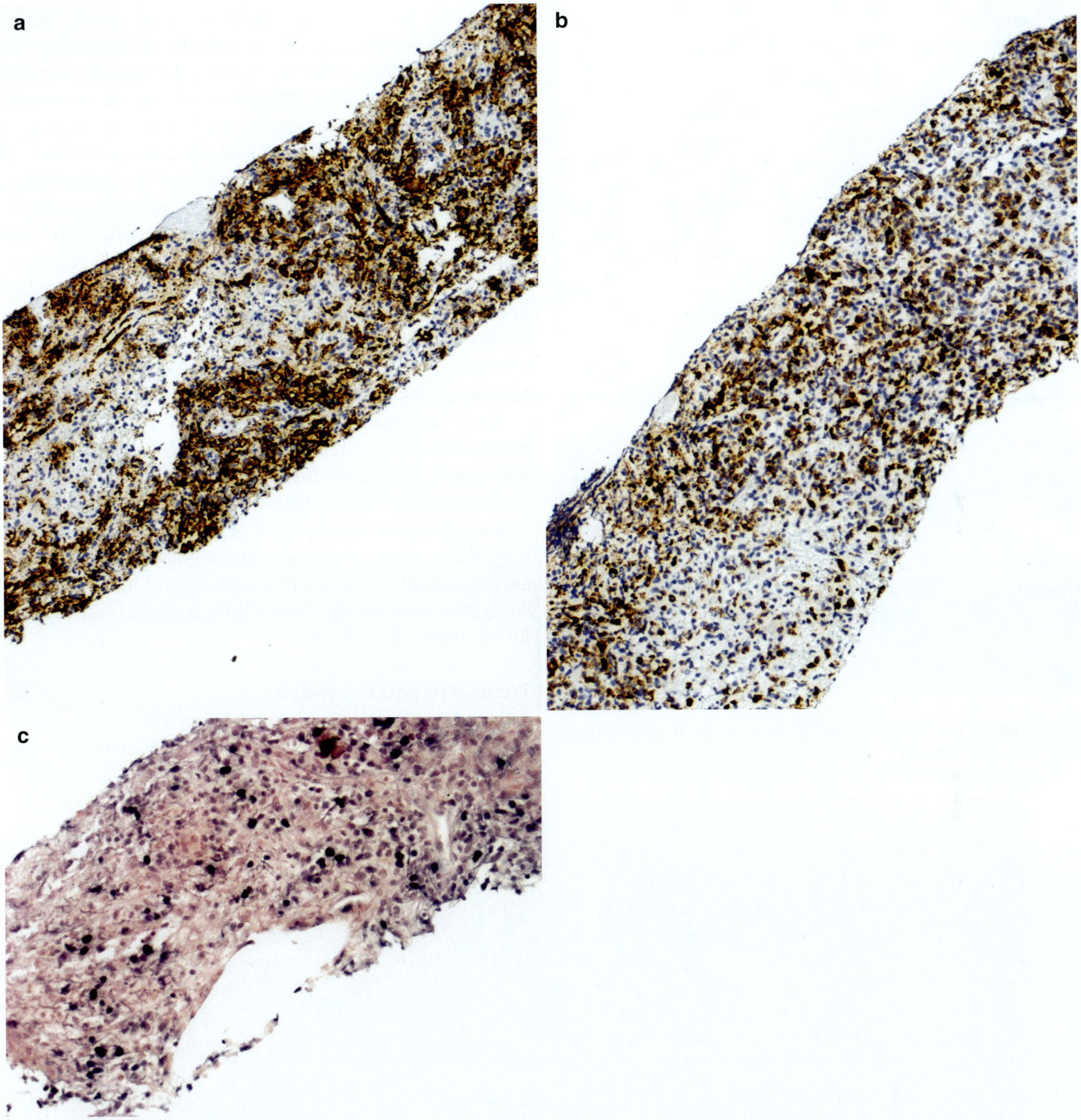

Fig. 11.25 (**a**) CT-guided 19-gauge core needle biopsy specimen showing LyG involving the lung. There are clusters of large atypical cells that are positive for CD20. Although an angiocentric pattern was not recognized in the H&E slide, this pattern was highlighted with CD20 immunostain. (**b**) Numerous CD3+ T-cells were associated with the neoplasm. (**c**) This case of LyG involving lung shows less than ten large cells positive for EBER per high-power field (LyG grade 2)

disease) [56]. Cases of PTLD demonstrating histopathologic features of LyG have been described [73, 74].

LyG also shares some similarities with extranodal NK/T-cell lymphoma, nasal type. Both diseases are extranodal, EBV associated, and show necrosis with vascular invasion and destruction. Immunohistochemical studies differentiate both diseases, with variable number of large cells positive for EBER and CD20 in LyG and atypical cells positive for CD2, CD56, TIA-1, and cytoplasmic CD3ε(epsilon), and negative for β(beta)F1 and surface CD3 in NK/T-cell lymphoma. Clinically, there are also important differences. Nearly all patients with extranodal NK/T-cell lymphoma present with

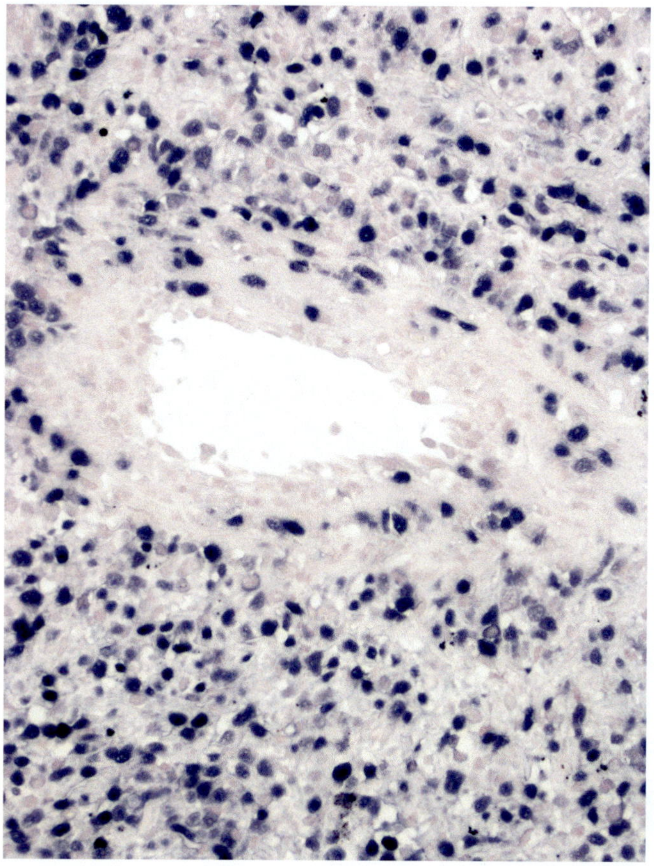

Fig. 11.26 In this case of LyG, EBER shows numerous positive tumor cells. This case is grade 3

disease in the upper aerodigestive tract (nasal cavity, nasopharynx, paranasal sinuses, and palate), and pulmonary involvement is rare, whereas, in LyG, the opposite distribution of disease is seen. In addition, clonal *IgH* gene rearrangements are not usually detected in NK/T-cell lymphomas.

Histologically, LyG can be similar to classical HL, as both have a polymorphic cellular composition and pleomorphic atypical large EBV-positive cells. The tumor cells in classical HL are positive for CD30, usually positive for CD15 and usually negative for CD20 and CD45/LCA. The large cells in LyG are usually strongly positive for CD20, CD45/LCA, and negative for CD15. In LyG, the EBV-positive cells usually exhibit a range of sizes and nuclear features, whereas in EBV-positive classical HL, only the Hodgkin and Reed-Sternberg cells are positive for EBV.

Some aggressive DLBCL or T-cell lymphomas may invade and destroy blood vessels. However, most of these tumors will be negative for EBER.

Similarities between the pathology features of acute pulmonary histoplasmosis to LyG grade 1 have been reported [75]. The presence of tiny necrotizing granulomas and multinucleated giant cells support the diagnosis of histoplasmosis. Grocott's methenamine silver (GMS) stain also will be helpful to confirm the diagnosis.

Treatment and Prognosis

Although some patients follow a waxing and waning clinical course with rare spontaneous remissions without therapy, in

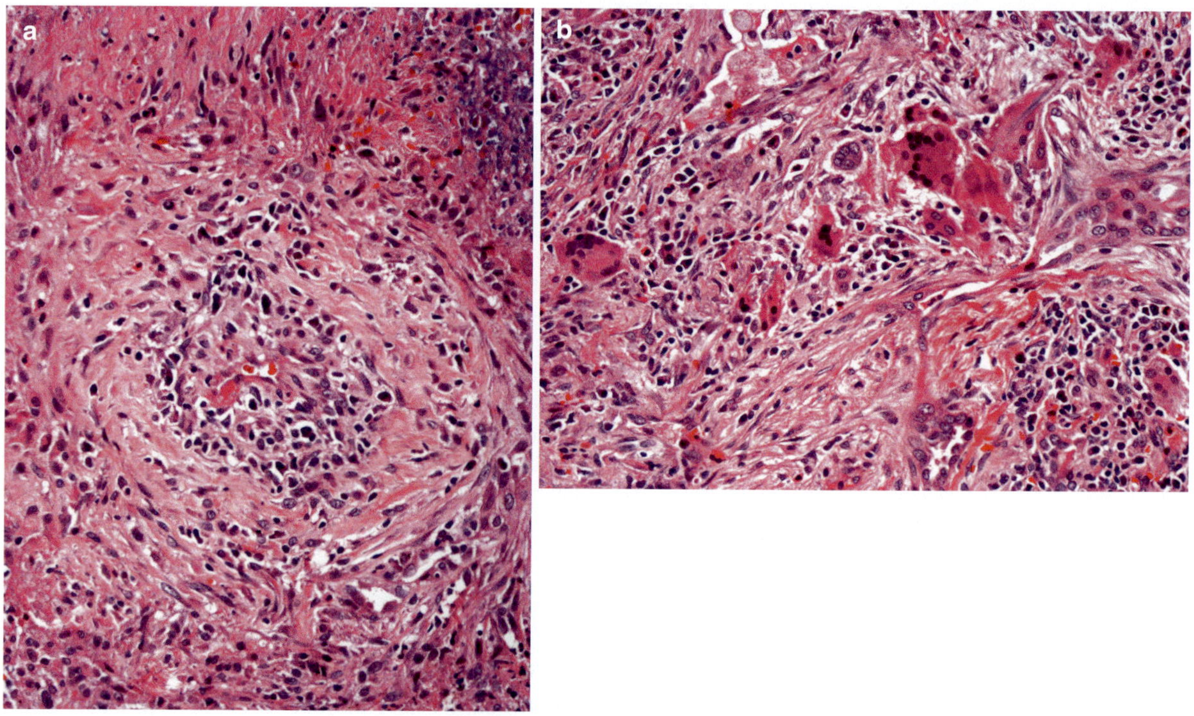

Fig. 11.27 (**a**) Wegener's granulomatosis involving the lung showing leukocytolytic angiitis. There are scattered large lymphoid cells admixed with small lymphocytes and plasma cells infiltrating the vessels wall. (**b**) Clusters of multinucleated giant cells are also seen. Some multinucleated giant cells contain elastic fibers (elastophagocytosis). Well-defined granulomas are not a characteristic of Wegener's granulomatosis

most patients, the disease is aggressive with a median survival of less than 2 years. In the largest series reported, more than 60 % of patients died, most within a year of diagnosis, and the overall median survival was 14 months [52]. LyG grades 1 and 2 are considered a B-cell lymphoproliferative disorder of uncertain malignant potential. LyG grade 3 is equivalent to DLBCL. Corticosteroids, interferon-alfa-2b, chemotherapy, rituximab, and autologous hematopoietic stem cell transplantation are commonly used for the treatment of LyG [76].

Intravascular Large B-Cell Lymphoma

Intravascular large B-cell lymphoma (IVLBCL) is a systemic large B-cell lymphoma characterized by selective intravascular growth [77]. This preferential intravascular growth is a *conditio sine qua non* for diagnosing IVLBCL, although a minimal extravascular location of neoplastic cells, usually surrounding involved vessels, can be seen [78]. The disease was first reported in 1959 by Pfleger and Tappeiner in Germany and was described as "angioendotheliomatosis proliferans systemisata" [79]. The remarkable restriction of malignant cells to the intraluminal space led the authors to believe that the neoplastic cells derived from the endothelium.

Clinical and Radiological Features

This lymphoma is most frequent in middle-aged or elderly patients; median age 67 years. The incidence in men and women is approximately 1.3:1. IVLBCL can involve any organ (most common CNS, skin, kidney, lung, adrenal gland and liver), and the symptoms are usually nonspecific and heterogeneous (fever of unknown origin, general fatigue, and deterioration in performance status). The most common clinical manifestations involve the skin and CNS. The diagnosis can be clinically difficult, and some cases are diagnosed postmortem. A variant associated with hemophagocytic syndrome has been reported mostly in Japan [80–82].

Autopsy studies revealed that lung involvement is common but predominant lung presentation of this neoplasm is rare [83]. Dyspnea, hypoxemia, and pulmonary arterial hypertension have been reported associated with IVLBCL. Imaging studies of the lung may reveal diffuse interstitial infiltrates, pleural effusion, signs of pulmonary hypertension, multifocal ground-glass opacities, and diffuse narrowing of the pulmonary veins throughout the lung [36, 84–87]. It has been shown that FDG-PET provides a high-sensitivity method to detect IVLBCL involving the lungs [88, 89].

Histopathologic Features

Diagnosis of IVLBCL can be made by random transbronchial lung biopsies [87, 89–91]. Lymphoma cells are mainly located in the lumina of small vessels, arterioles, and capillaries (Fig. 11.28a, b). The tumor cells are usually large, with vesicular nuclear chromatin with distinct nucleoli (Fig. 11.28c). In some cases, the tumor cells have coarse nuclear chromatin, irregular or indented nuclei, and are smaller than usual. Mitoses are frequently seen. Some cases may have a small extravascular component.

Immunohistochemical Features

The tumor cells are B-cells positive for pan B-cell markers (CD19, CD20, CD22, and CD79a), PAX-5, and CD45/LCA (Fig. 11.29a, b). They are usually positive for BCL-2 and MUM1/IRF-4. CD5 is positive in 30 % of the cases, CD10 in 10 %, and BCL-6 in 25 %. Ki-67 usually reveals a high proliferative activity (Fig. 11.29c). Rare cases of intravascular lymphoma are of T-cell or NK-cell lineage (peripheral T- or NK-cell lymphomas with intravascular pattern). These rare lymphomas are not recognized as diagnostic categories in the 2008 WHO lymphoma classification.

Molecular Biology and Cytogenetics

Pathognomonic cytogenetic abnormalities have not been reported. Monoclonal rearrangements of the *IgH* gene can be detected by PCR. Chromosomal translocations involving *bcl-2* gene are not detected, and *TCR* genes are in germ line configuration. EBV association is uncommon, but it has been reported in HIV patients [92, 93].

Differential Diagnosis

Rare cases of T-cell or NK-cell lymphomas can be intravascular. As mentioned, these rare lymphomas do not exist as diagnostic categories in the 2008 WHO lymphoma classification. Some of the T-cell lymphomas with an intravascular phenotype are gamma/delta T-cell lymphomas or hepatosplenic T-cell lymphomas [94, 95]. Hepatosplenic T-cell lymphomas are positive for T-cell markers, CD2, CD3, and TIA-1, and are negative for granzyme B and perforin (inactive cytotoxic phenotype). Isochromosome 7q is present in most cases of hepatosplenic T-cell lymphoma. Cases of DLBCL can relapse with the outlook of IVLBCL [96]. In patients with carcinomatosis, clusters of carcinoma cells may be lodged in small lymphovascular channels. Carcinoma cells are generally cohesive, and they are positive for cytokeratin and are negative for CD20 and CD45/LCA.

Treatment and Prognosis

IVLBCL is frequently a fatal disease characterized by an aggressive clinical course. However, this poor prognosis is in part related to the failure to make an early diagnosis. Complete remission and long-term survival can be achieved in patients treated early with aggressive combination chemotherapy [97]. Prognostic factors that are useful for risk stratification are not established. The patients are usually treated with rituximab-containing chemotherapy plus CNS-oriented therapy (R-CHOP plus high-dose methotrexate or cytarabine).

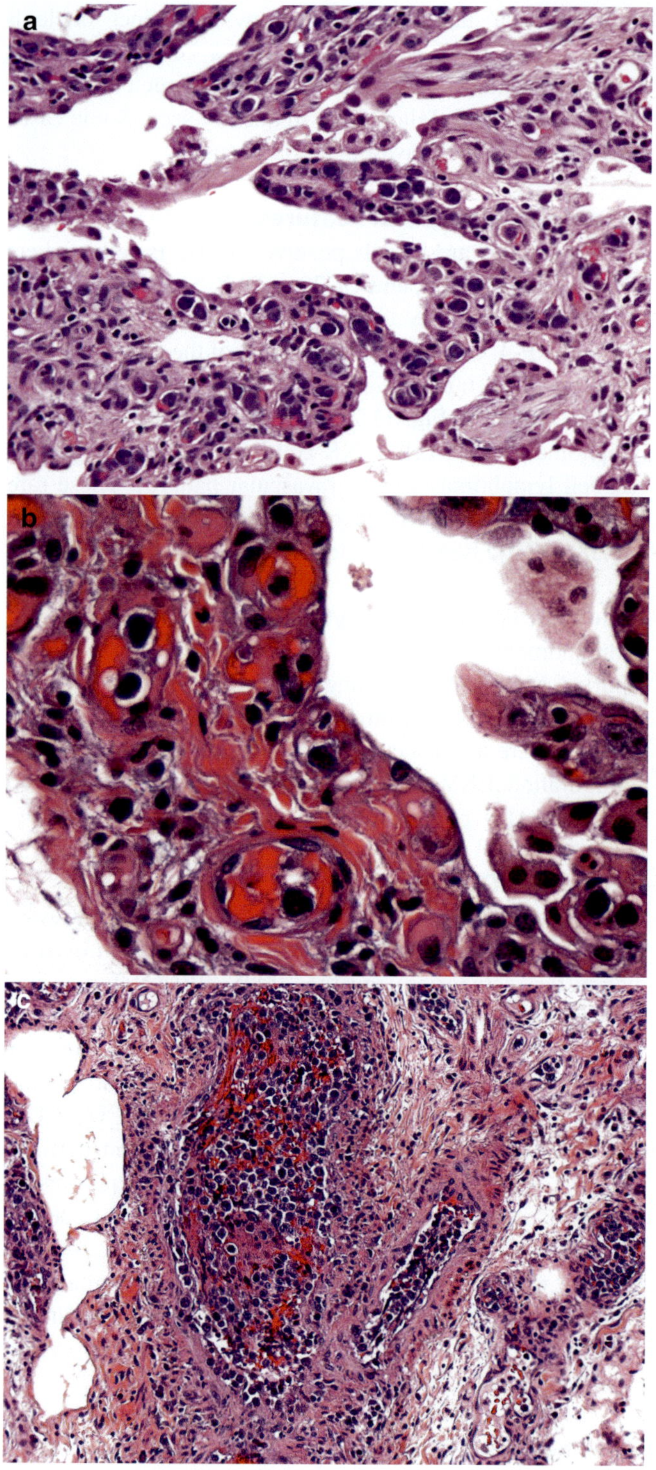

Fig. 11.28 (**a**, **b**) IVLBCL involving a lung biopsy specimen. The tumor cells are large, compared with the reactive lymphocytes, and located within the alveolar capillaries. (**c**) Tumor cells present within middle size vessels are also noted

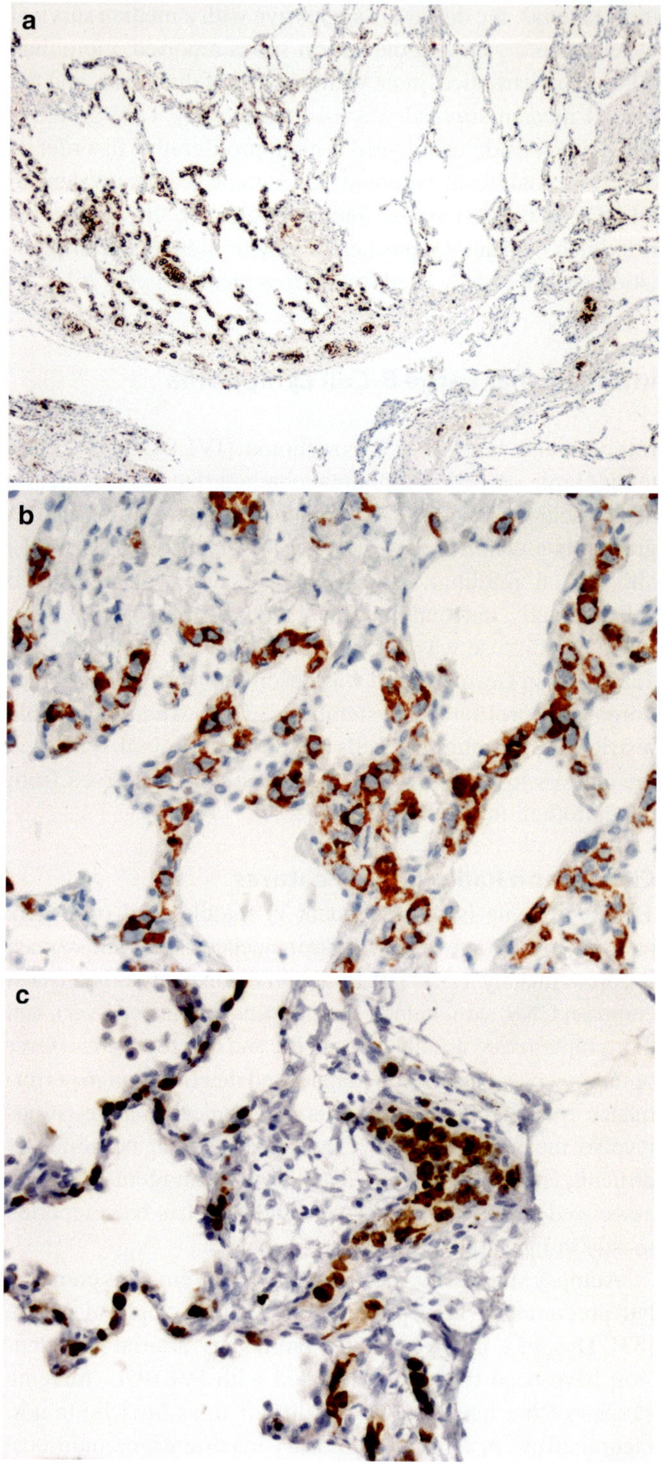

Fig. 11.29 (**a**, **b**) The intravascular neoplastic infiltrate is easy to recognized using immunostains specific for B-cell markers, such as CD20. (**c**) IVLBCL is usually characterized by a high proliferation rate as shown by reactivity with the Ki-67 (MIB-1) antibody. Note that virtually all the tumor cells are positive for this proliferation marker

Primary Lung Plasmacytoma

Extramedullary plasmacytoma is a neoplasm composed of monoclonal plasma cells that involved tissues other than bone. By definition, there is no evidence of bone marrow involvement, no clinical features of plasma cell myeloma, and small or absent M-component in urine or serum.

Although extramedullary plasmacytoma can arise in almost any organ, by far the commonest site of presentation is the mucosa/submucosa of the upper respiratory tract (nasopharynx, sinuses, and tonsils), and the second most common site is the gastrointestinal tract [98, 99]. Few cases of primary lung plasmacytoma have been described in the literature [100–105]. Extramedullary plasmacytoma can arise in immunosuppressed and in immunocompetent patients.

Clinical and Radiological Features

The median age of occurrence is between 40 and 60 years with exceptional cases in childhood and without gender predominance [103, 104]. They present as a perihilar mass, solitary lung nodule, peribronchial lesions, and less commonly as lobar consolidation [100, 101]. The right and left lungs are equally affected, with the upper lobes being more commonly involved. The patients are usually asymptomatic or may present with cough, dyspnea, and/or hemoptysis. Rarely, a peripheral blood monoclonal gammopathy is detected, which should disappear after surgical resection of the tumor.

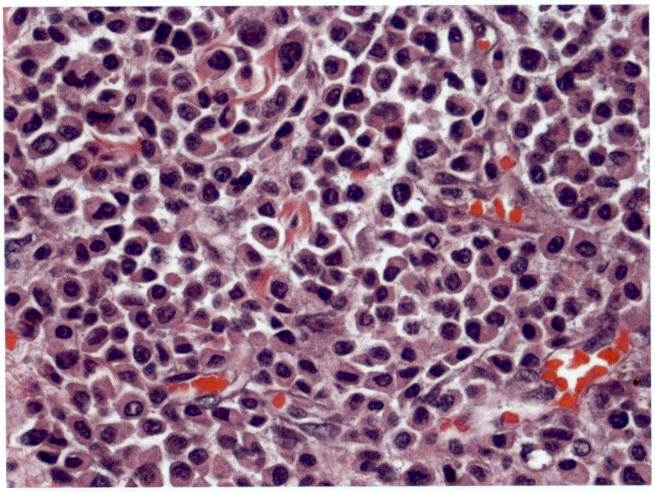

Fig. 11.30 Plasmacytoma involving the lung. Sheets of well-differentiated plasma cells are replacing the lung architecture. Note that the plasma cells have atypical morphologic features; enlarged nuclei, with irregular nuclear contours, and distinct nucleoli

Histopathologic Features

The infiltrate comprises a diffuse infiltrate of plasma cells (Fig. 11.30). The infiltrate is frequently peribronchial or involved the bronchial wall directly [103]. The neoplastic plasma cells may show a spectrum of maturation from mature to immature (pleomorphic nuclei, fine nuclear chromatin, and distinct nucleoli) and plasmablasts (large nuclei with vesicular nuclear chromatin and centrally located nucleoli; immunoblast-like). Crystal-like inclusions can be found in the tumor cells or in histiocytes and amyloid deposits may be observed [103]. Extension to peribronchial or mediastinal lymph nodes can occur.

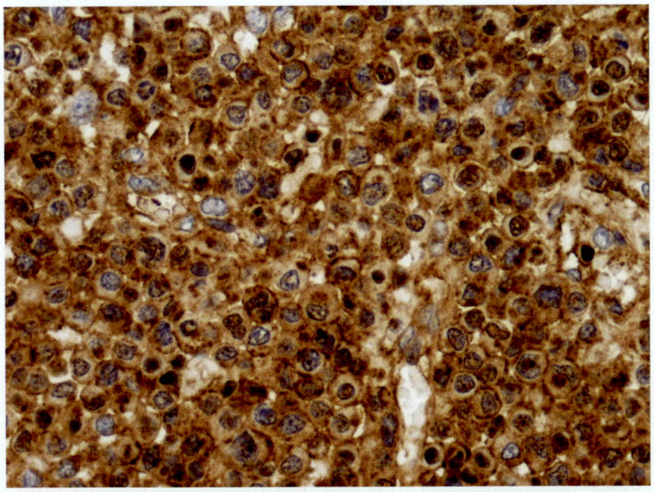

Fig. 11.31 Plasmacytoma involving the lung. The tumor cells are strongly positive for CD138

Immunohistochemical Features

Plasmacytoma shows an immunophenotype similar to plasma cell myeloma. The tumor cells are positive for CD138 (Fig. 11.31), CD38, MUM1/IRF-4, CD79a, and EMA, and are cytoplasmic light chain restricted. They are usually positive for IgG or IgA. They are usually negative for CD19 and CD45/LCA. Cyclin D1 may be positive in a small subset of cases due to amplifications of *ccnd1* gene [106]. EBER is usually negative; however, those cases associated with immunosuppression can be EBER+.

Molecular Biology and Cytogenetics

In general, plasmacytoma shows cytogenetic abnormalities similar to plasma cell myeloma [107]. The t(11;14) (*ccnd1/IgH*) is not present, but amplifications of *ccnd1* gene have been described [106, 107]. Chromosomal translocations involving *myc* are common in cases of plasma cell myeloma with extramedullary spread but uncommon in extramedullary plasmacytoma. Loss of 13q (40 %), as well as chromosomal gains (82 %), are common, and the t(4;14) (*fgfr3/IgH*) may occur (~15 %) [107].

Differential Diagnosis

It is difficult to distinguish primary lung plasmacytoma from MALT lymphoma with marked plasmacytic differentiation. The presence of a B-cell lymphoid infiltrate supports the diagnosis of MALT lymphoma. In MALT lymphoma, the B-cells are monoclonal and usually positive for IgM and may coexpress CD20 and CD43. In addition, the presence of one of MALT lymphoma related translocations support the diagnosis of MALT lymphoma, t(11;18)(q21:q21)/*malt1-iap2*, t(1;14)(p22;q32)/*bcl10-IgH*, and t(14;18)(q32;q21)/*malt1-IgH*.

However, some cases of extramedullary plasmacytoma may in fact be MALT lymphoma with extreme plasmacytic differentiation. There are clinical data that supports this idea; some patients presenting with MALT lymphoma recur as extramedullary plasmacytoma and, some patients presenting with extramedullary plasmacytoma recur as MALT lymphoma.

Another differential diagnosis is plasma cell granuloma or inflammatory pseudotumor of the lung. These lesions usually show a polymorphic inflammatory infiltrate in addition to plasma cells. These lesions are frequently seen in children and constitute the most common isolated primary lesions of the lung in patients under 16 years of age. In these lesions the plasma cells lack of cytologic atypia and are polytypic.

Treatment and Prognosis

Patients are mostly treated with surgery and radiotherapy. This lung neoplasm is too rare to comment on the prognosis. Two patients have been reported to survive for 9 years, and two patients have been reported to survive for >20 years [103]. The prognosis for extramedullary plasmacytoma involving other body sites is relatively good, ~75 % of the patients are alive for more than 10 years, and only ~15 % will progress to plasma cell myeloma.

Primary Anaplastic Large Cell Lymphoma (ALCL) of the Lung

Primary anaplastic lymphoma kinase (ALK)-positive and negative ALCL of the lung are very rare malignancies, with very few cases reported in the literature [4, 5]. However, lung involvement by systemic ALK-positive and negative ALCL is relatively frequent. ALK-negative ALCL is currently defined as a lymphoma morphologically and immunophenotypically within the spectrum of ALK-positive ALCL but lacking expression of ALK protein [4, 108]. Importantly, in most of the cases of primary pulmonary ALCL published in the literature, ALK expression has not been determined.

Clinical and Radiological Features

These tumors affect both male and female patients and may occur in any age group. Clinical signs and symptoms may include cough, chest pain, dyspnea, fever, night sweats, and weight loss. The involvement can be unilateral or bilateral. By definition, clinical and radiological staging shows no evidence of mediastinal or extrathoracic disease.

Histopathologic Features

Histologically, primary pulmonary ALCL is characterized by a diffuse infiltrate of small to large atypical cells with bizarre, often polylobated, nuclei. This variability in the cytologic features of the tumor cells is helpful in distinguishing ALCL from classical HL. "Hallmark" cells (large cells with eccentric horseshoe- or kidney-shaped nuclei with a prominent paranuclear eosinophilic Golgi region) are characteristic. Multinucleated giant cells, some with Reed-Sternberg-like features, are frequently seen. Variable number of reactive small lymphocytes is frequently admixed with the tumor cells (feature also frequently seen in systemic ALCL). Some tumors are described to have intraluminal polypoid masses that partially occluded large airways [108].

Immunohistochemical Features

In ALK-positive ALCL the tumor cells will be strongly and uniformly positive for CD30 and ALK. ALCL can be of T- or null cell lineage; in cases of T-cell lineage, an aberrant T-cell immunophenotype is common; most tumors do not express CD3, CD5, or T-cell receptors. CD2 and CD43 are the most frequent expressed T-cell markers. EMA may be positive in a subset of cases [109]. The type of ALK immunostaining correlates with the type of underlying genetic abnormality. Cytoplasmic and nuclear positivity for ALK indicates the presence of the t(2;5); cytoplasmic, not coarsely granular, indicates a variant translocation except t(2;X) and t(2;17); cytoplasmic, coarsely granular, indicates t(2;17), and a membranous staining indicates t(2;X).

Molecular Biology and Cytogenetics

ALK-positive ALCL is characterized by chromosomal translocations involving *alk* gene being the t(2;5)(p23;q35) the most frequent, ~80 % of the cases [110]. The t(2;5) fuses the nucleophosmin (*npm*) gene, at 5q35 with the *alk* gene, at 2p23. The fusion gene encodes an oncogenic 80-kd chimeric protein [111]. In other variants translocations, *alk* gene is rearranged with other genes including *tropomyosin 3*, *TRK-fused gene*, *ATIC*, *moesin*, *clathrin heavy chain*, *tropomyosin 4*, *alo17*, and *myh9* [112].

Differential Diagnosis

Classical HL and pleomorphic carcinomas (primary or metastatic) are important differential diagnoses. The tumor cells in classical HL are usually positive for PAX-5 (characteristically weak) and CD15 and are negative for EMA, CD45/LCA, and ALK. Carcinomas are usually positive for cytokeratins and EMA and are negative for CD45/LCA and negative for CD30. Remember that some cases of ALCL can be positive for EMA and negative for CD45/LCA and that CD30 may be positive in carcinomas and other tumors (however, when positive is usually focal and weak).

Distinction between ALK-positive and ALK-negative ALCL is important. ALK-positive ALCL has a better prognosis and responds better to therapy than ALK-negative ALCL [113]. ALK-positive ALCL is consistently negative for EBV: however, a subset of cases of ALK-negative ALCL is EBV positive.

DLBCL can also express ALK and carry either the t(2;5) or t(2;17) [114]. These lymphomas usually have plasmablastic morphology, express CD138, CD4, and often IgA, and are mostly negative for B-cell markers and CD30. ALK protein may also be expressed in tumors other than lymphoid neoplasms. Expression of ALK has been documented in several types of primary solid cancers including lung carcinomas [115].

Treatment and Prognosis

The overall 5-year survival rate in systemic ALK-positive ALCL is 80 % (when the pediatric patients are included in this analysis). These tumors are sensitive to anthracycline-based therapies. Relapses are not uncommon (30–40 %) but often remain sensitive to chemotherapy. The clinical outcome of ALK-negative ALCL is clearly poorer than that of ALK-positive ALCL. The overall 5-year survival of patients with ALK-negative ALCL is only 49 % [116]. Furthermore, peripheral T-cell lymphoma, NOS with CD30 expression, which can be difficult to differentiate histologically from ALK-negative ALCL, has a poorer prognosis and a 5-year overall survival of 19 %.

Primary Pulmonary Classical Hodgkin's Lymphoma (HL)

Classical HL is characterized by a heterogeneous cellularity comprising, in most of the cases, a minority of neoplastic cells—the Hodgkin cells and the Reed-Stenberg cells—in a variable background of reactive nonneoplastic cells.

Although classical HL is almost always a node-based lymphoma, practically any site and organ can be involved during the course of the disease. Classical HL frequently involves the lung; more than 13 % of patients with classical HL have lung involvement at presentation [115]. Fifty percent have relapses in the lung, and almost 60 % are found to have pulmonary involvement at autopsy [117]. However, primary pulmonary classical HL is very rare but apparently well documented [118–121].

Clinical and Radiological Features

Primary pulmonary classical HL shows the usual bimodal age distribution of systemic classical HL. Symptoms include cough, dyspnea, hemoptysis, and chest pain. B symptoms are observed in one-third of the patients [120]. Chest radiographs and CT scans usually demonstrate multiple nodular lesions, solitary nodules, and pneumonic consolidation with and without air bronchograms [120, 122]. Upper lobe involvement is twice as common as lower lobe disease, and cavitation is found in nearly one-third of cases [122].

Histopathologic Features

The most common subtypes of classical HL involving the lung are nodular sclerosis (Fig. 11.32) and mixed cellularity. In general, nodular sclerosis HL is the type most frequently associated with mediastinal involvement, and mixed cellularity is the most common type in patients with HIV/AIDS. Yousem and colleagues [119] documented several different growth patterns of classical HL involving the lungs, including nodular, diffuse, involving lymphatic routes, pneumonic, endobronchial, and subpleural. Bronchial involvement can result in a polypoid endobronchial mass, mural permeation, and destruction of the cartilage.

The cellular infiltrates are identical to those seen in nodal classical HL (Fig. 11.33) and can be associated with variable

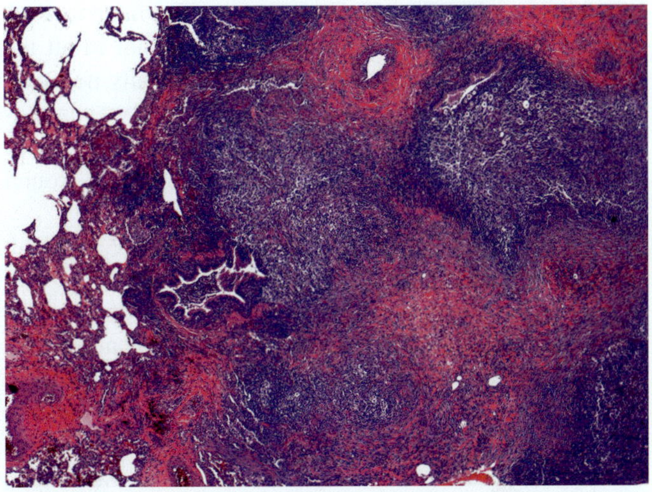

Fig. 11.32 Nodular sclerosis classical Hodgkin's lymphoma involving the lung. The neoplasm is nodular and surrounded by collagen bands. Note that some of the tumoral nodules are in close proximity to bronchial walls

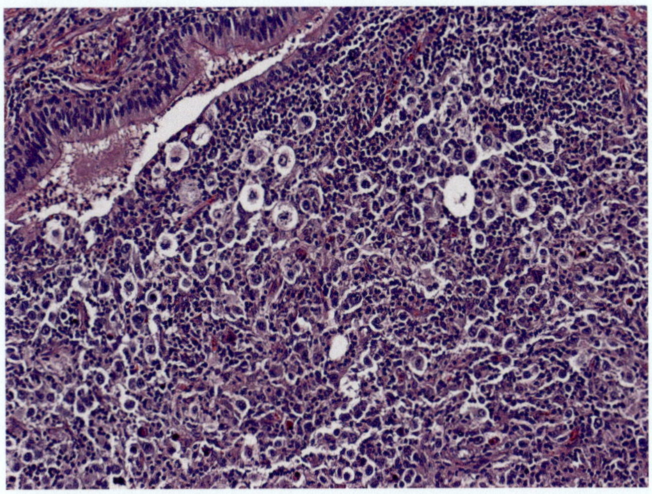

Fig. 11.33 Nodular sclerosis HL involving the lung. The neoplasm partially destroyed a bronchial wall. Note the presence of clusters of lacunar cells in a polymorphic inflammatory background

granulomatous inflammation and necrosis. Reed-Sternberg cells are considered the morphologic feature of classical HL. However, the tumor cells (Hodgkin and Reed-Sternberg cells) show great morphologic variability, and cells of striking similarity can be observed in several benign conditions such as infectious mononucleosis, toxoplasmosis, and in various unrelated neoplasms.

Immunohistochemical Features

Despite the morphologic variability of classical HL, the immunophenotype of the neoplastic cells is quite constant. The tumor cells are characteristic positive for CD15 (75 %), CD30 (membranous and cytoplasmic with frequent dot-like perinuclear accentuation), and PAX-5 (expressed weaker than in reactive B-cells) (Fig. 11.34a, b) and are negative for CD45/LCA and CD79a. CD20 may be positive in up to 40 % of cases, although usually weak and usually not in all the tumor cells. ALK is negative, and EMA is usually negative. The background population of reactive lymphocytes is generally composed of numerous T-cells with a CD4-positive (helper) phenotype; these cells often form rosettes around Reed-Sternberg cells.

Molecular Biology and Cytogenetics

In general, molecular and cytogenetic studies of classical HL have yielded variable results because the neoplastic cells in most cases represent only a very small amount of the tissue analyzed. In bulk tissue extracts of classical HL, detection of B-cell clonality by PCR is successful in only a minority of cases and usually yields weak clonal bands, reflecting the paucity of neoplastic cells [123]. Cases of classical HL selected for the presence of numerous tumor cells have shown clonal rearrangements for the *IgH* gene and no rearrangements for the *TCR* gene [124]. The genetic lesions most frequently found so far in Reed-Sternberg cells involve members of two signaling pathways: Janus kinase (Jak)-Stat and nuclear factor-kB (NF-kB). There are frequent genomic gains of *jak2*, and the suppressor of cytokine signaling 1 (*socs1*) gene, a negative regulator of Jak-Stat signaling, is frequently mutated and inactivated in classical HL [125, 126]. The *rel* gene, on 2p16, that encodes one component of NK-kB pathway shows gains or amplifications in 50 % of the cases [127]. Inactivating mutations of one NF-kB inhibitor IkBα are seen in 20 % of the cases [128]. Mutations of *p53* are demonstrated by PCR analysis in ~10 % of the cases [129].

Differential Diagnosis

The differential diagnosis includes inflammatory/infectious processes, sarcoidosis, and malignant neoplasms such as pleomorphic giant cell carcinoma, LyG, ALCL, and other B-cell lymphomas. Immunohistochemical studies are helpful to confirm the diagnosis of classical HL and to exclude other non-Hodgkin's lymphomas. The expression of CD15 is useful for differentiating Reed-Sternberg of Hodgkin cells from CD30+ reactive immunoblasts, which are usually CD15 negative. However, cytomegalovirus-infected cells are positive for CD15 and CD30 and may simulate Hodgkin cells by virtue of their eosinophilic nuclear inclusions [130]. In neoplastic lesions, other than classical HL, coexpression of CD15 and CD30 is infrequent [131, 132].

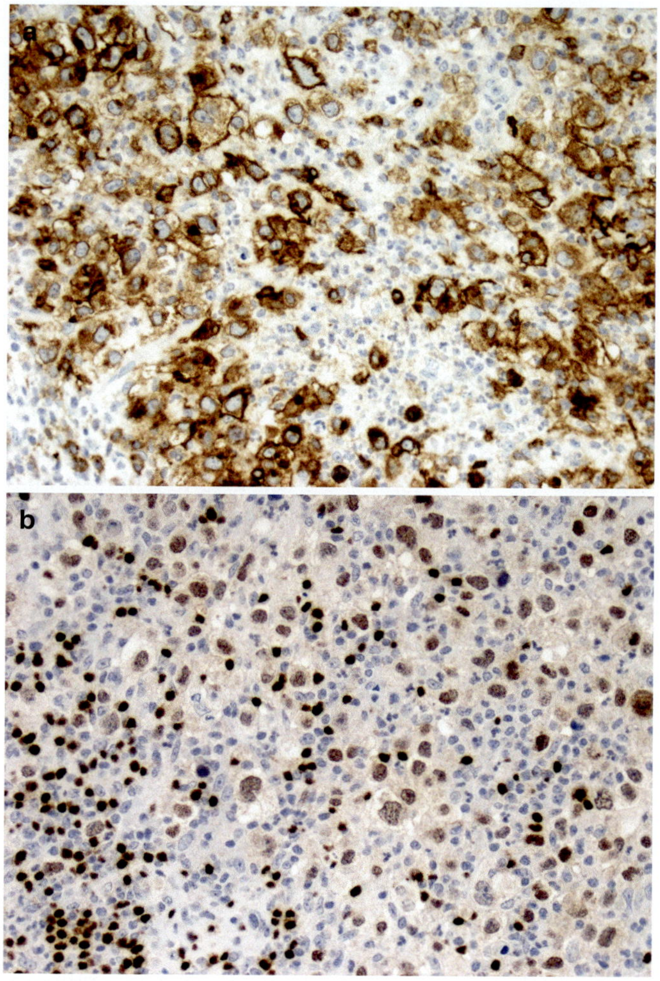

Fig. 11.34 Classical HL involving the lung. (**a**) The Hodgkin and Reed-Sternberg cells are uniformly and strongly positive for CD30 and (**b**) weakly positive for PAX-5 as compared with reactive small B-cells

Treatment and Prognosis

The number of cases of primary pulmonary classical HL published is very small, so it is difficult to draw meaningful conclusions regarding the prognosis of this neoplasm. In general, early stage classical HL has a very good prognosis with a 5-year and 10-year survivals of 98 and 97 %, respectively [133]. Classical HL is a neoplasm that usually responds very well to chemotherapy and radiotherapy.

Lymphomas Involving the Pleura

Primary Effusion Lymphoma (PEL)

Primary effusion lymphoma (PEL), also known as body cavity-based lymphoma, is a human herpes virus 8 (HHV-8)-associated large B-cell neoplasm that most often involves body cavities (pleural, pericardial, or peritoneal cavity) causing effusions without identifiable tumor masses [134]. HHV-8-positive lymphomas indistinguishable from PEL rarely present as solid tumor mass and are designated as extracavitary or solid variants of PEL. PEL arises from HHV-8-infected B-cells that are frequently coinfected (>90 %) by EBV [135].

HHV-8 virus, also known as Kaposi's sarcoma-associated herpes virus, is an oncogenic γ (gamma) herpes double-stranded DNA lymphotropic virus. It is endemic in sub-Saharan Africa (seroprevalence of 50–70 %) and the Mediterranean region (seroprevalence of 20–30 %), while North America exhibits only a 1–3 % infection rate among asymptomatic blood donors [136]. In addition to PEL, HHV-8 is associated with Kaposi's sarcoma, multicenter Castleman disease (MCD), and MCD-associated plasmablastic lymphoma [137–139].

Clinical and Radiological Features

PEL is a rare lymphoma seen frequently in HIV-infected patients; it represents about 4 % of all acquired immune deficiency syndrome (AIDS)-related lymphomas and 0.3 % of all aggressive lymphomas in HIV-negative patients [134, 140]. PEL can occasionally occur in HIV-negative patients, especially in the setting of other forms of immunosuppression. PEL not related to an overt immunodeficiency has been reported, in particular, in older individuals and from HHV-8 endemic geographical areas (same risk population for HIV-negative classical Kaposi's sarcoma) [141, 142].

The patients usually presents with B symptoms and bilateral or unilateral pleural effusion associated with slight thickening of parietal pleura in the absence of solid tumor masses, parenchymal abnormalities, or mediastinal enlargement [143]. Dyspnea is common and results from massive malignant pleural and/or pericardial effusions. The patients usually have clinical and laboratory findings of severe immunosuppression and marked depletion of T-cells (T-cell counts <100/mm^3). A significant portion of patients has preexisting Kaposi's sarcoma or MCD, reflecting the other known manifestations of HHV-8 infection. Rare cases of PEL are associated with hepatitis C and/or B.

Histopathologic Features

The diagnosis is usually made on cytological preparations of involved effusion fluid. The tumor cells are large with abundant basophilic cytoplasm sometimes with vacuoles, irregular nuclear contours, and prominent nucleoli (Figs. 11.35 and 11.36). Cytomorphologic appearances range from immunoblastic (round nuclei with centrally located nucleoli) to anaplastic (large with bizarre nuclei, multinucleated, and Reed-Sternberg-like). The tumor cells exhibit frequent plasmablastic differentiation (eccentric nuclei with abundant cytoplasm, sometimes with perinuclear hof). Biopsy specimens of the pleura may show small number of large neoplastic cells adherent to the mesothelial surface and/or embedded in fibrin. Occasionally, there is underlying invasion of the pleural

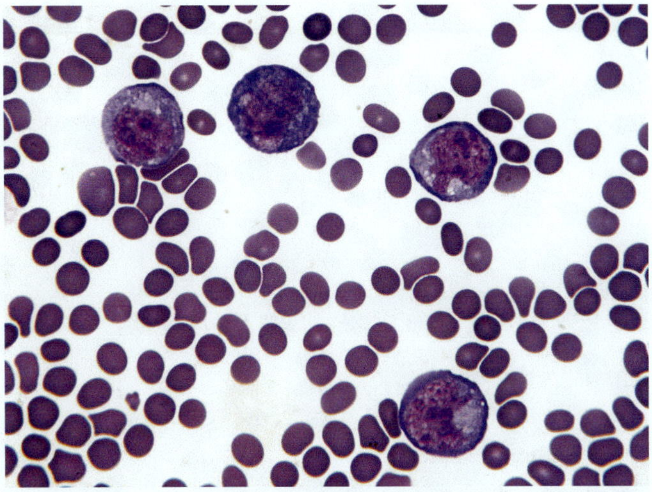

Fig. 11.35 Cytologic specimen of pleural fluid showing PEL. The tumor cells are medium- to large-sized lymphoid cells with abundant finely vacuolated cytoplasm and irregular nuclei (Courtesy of W. Chen, MD)

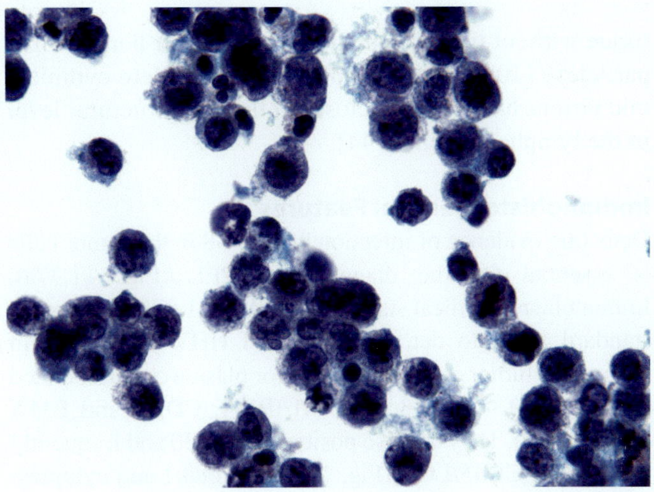

Fig. 11.36 Cytologic specimen of pleural fluid showing PEL. In this case, PEL cells are medium to large in size with oval to markedly irregular nuclear contours, slightly open chromatin, and relatively abundant and slightly vacuolated cytoplasms. Apoptotic cells are also seen

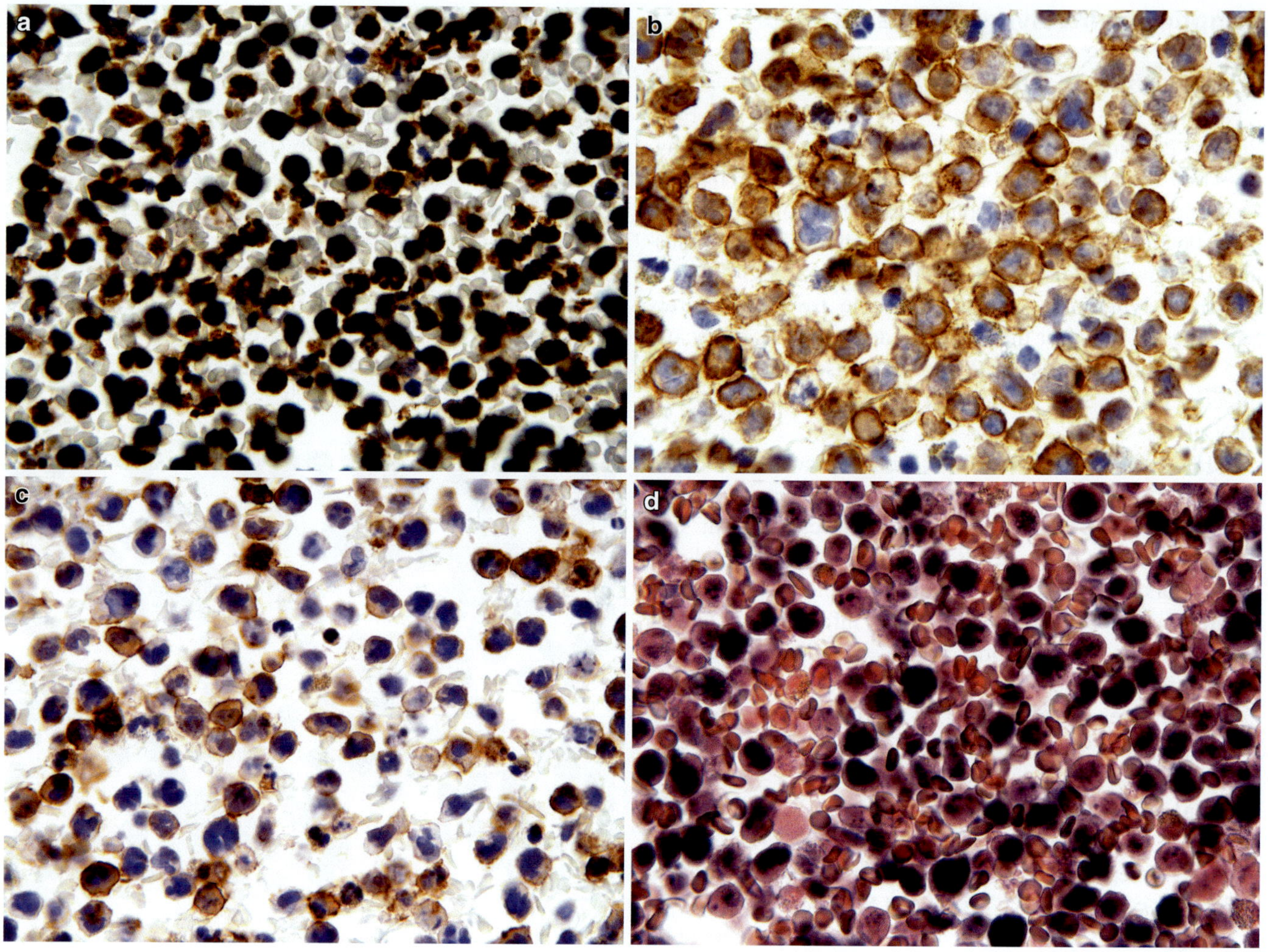

Fig. 11.37 (**a**) Cell block of PEL that shows that the neoplastic cells are strongly positive for HHV-8, (**b**) positive for CD38, (**c**) weakly and variable positive for CD45/LCA, and (**d**) positive for EBER

tissue without tumor formation. Intranuclear herpes virus particles (110-nm nucleocapsids) and complete cytoplasmic virions have been disclosed at the ultrastructural level in the lymphoma cells [144].

Immunohistochemical Features

Detecting evidence of infection by HHV-8 in the tumor cells is essential for the diagnosis of PEL (Fig. 11.37a). Immunohistochemical staining for LANA-1 (ORF-73) is the standard assay to detect evidence of HHV-8 infection in tissue. The tumor cells are positive for plasma cell-associated markers CD138, VS38c, MUM1/IRF-4, CD38, and EMA (Fig. 11.37b). They are also positive for CD30 and frequently positive for CD45/LCA (Fig. 11.37c), Notch1 and cytoplasmic Ig λ (lambda) light chain restricted [145]. They are negative for CD19, CD20, CD79a, PAX-5, CD15, CD10, BCL6, and surface immunoglobulin. A subset of cases may express some T-cell markers such as CD45RO (~90 %), CD7 (~30 %), CD4 (~20 %), and cytoplasmic CD3 [146, 147]. EBER is positive in 80–90 % of cases (Fig. 11.37d). Immunohistochemical staining for EBV latent membrane protein (LMP-1) is negative.

Molecular Biology and Cytogenetics

In most of the cases, PCR methods detect the presence of monoclonal *IgH* gene rearrangements with frequent somatic hypermutations of the *IgH* variable regions. Aberrant clonal rearrangements of the TCR gene have been reported [148]. Cytogenetic studies usually reveal a complex karyotype but failed to disclose recurrent chromosomal abnormalities. Gains of chromosomes 7q (58 %), 8q (63 %), 12 (61 %) and loss of 14q32 (63 %) have been described by comparative genomic hybridization (CGH) array [149]. The HHV-8 genome contains potential oncogenes, including a viral cyclin homologue, viral IL-6, and a gene homologous to a G-protein-coupled receptor (GPCR) [150].

Differential Diagnosis

Many aggressive lymphomas and carcinomas can present with neoplastic pleural effusion. A lymphoma should not be classified as PEL without evidence of HHV-8 infection and supportive morphological and immunophenotypical criteria. HIV patients may have Burkitt's lymphoma with plasmacytoid differentiation that rarely presents as a lymphomatous effusion; such cases may show morphologic overlap with PEL but will have chromosomal translocations involving *myc* gene and will be negative for HHV-8 infection.

Because of similar morphology, ALCL may also be confused with PEL; immunohistochemical staining for ALK and negativity for plasma cell-associated markers will help to confirm the diagnosis. PAL is another differential diagnosis. This lymphoma is more common in Japan and usually arises in elderly men without HIV but with a history of pulmonary tuberculosis or tuberculous pleuritis treated with pneumothorax. PAL is usually a large cell lymphoma of B-cell lineage expressing B-cell markers, positive for LMP-1 and EBER and negative for HHV-8 [151].

Treatment and Prognosis

The prognosis is usually poor; median survival <6 months with very few long-term survivors [152, 153]. The use of highly active antiretroviral therapy (HAART) improves prognosis, suggesting a role for immune reconstitution in control of this aggressive lymphoma. Much like other lymphomas, combination traditional chemotherapy (usually cyclophosphamide, doxorubicin, vincristine, and prednisone) forms the backbone of therapy for PEL. Novel approaches include intracavitary cidofovir (antiviral agent that inhibits replication of HHV-8) [154], bortezomib (proteasome inhibitor that inhibits NK-kB pathway) [155], antivirals such as valganciclovir or foscarnet [156]. Rituximab does not play a role in PEL therapy because the tumor cells are usually CD20 negative.

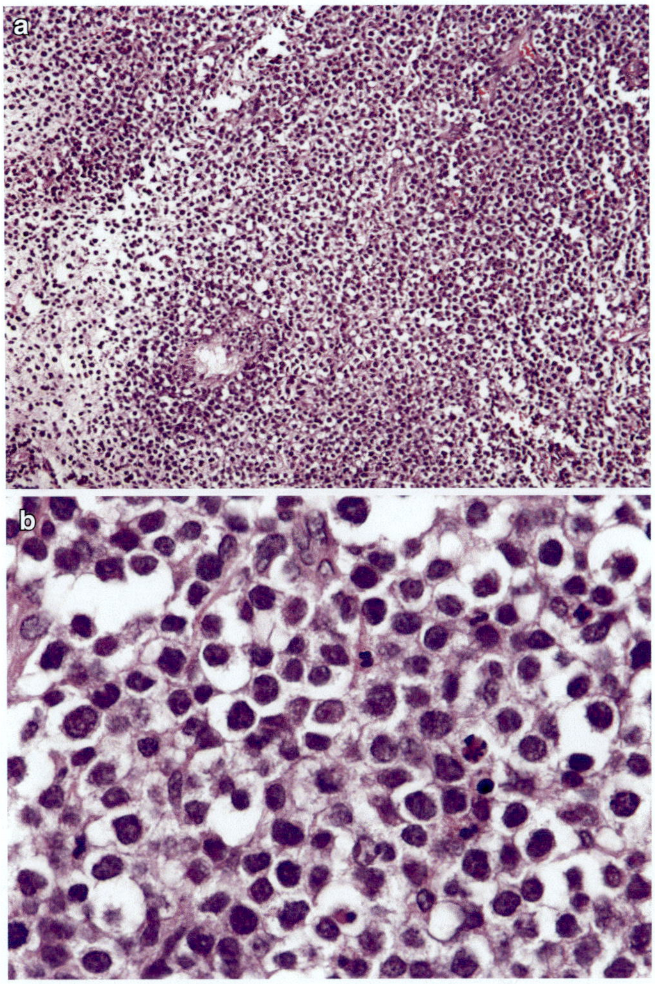

Fig. 11.38 (**a**) DLBCL associated with chronic inflammation of PAL type. The neoplasm is diffuse and shows large areas with apoptosis and/or necrosis. (**b**) The cells are large with relatively abundant retracted cytoplasm due to fixation artifact or poor preservation

Diffuse Large B-Cell Lymphoma Associated with Chronic Inflammation (Pyothorax-Associated Lymphoma; PAL)

PAL is another type of large B-cell lymphoma occurring primary in the pleura in patients with long-standing pleural inflammation [157]. The chronic inflammation may result from therapeutic artificial pneumothorax or from tuberculous pleuritis and is associated with latent EBV infection but without HHV-8 infection [157, 158]. Artificial pneumothorax is the most significant risk factor for development of PAL. Most cases are reported in Japan and are exceedingly rare in Western countries. The higher incidence in Japan is explained by the more popular use of artificial pneumothorax for the treatment of pulmonary tuberculosis in the past.

Clinical and Radiological Features

Patients are commonly in the seventh decade of life (median age of 63 years) and are mostly male (male-to-female ratio 12:1) [151, 159]. The patients have a long history of chronic pyothorax and usually complain of chest or shoulder pain, dyspnea, and constitutional symptoms, such as fever or weight loss. Almost half of the patients present with a tumor or swelling in the chest wall. Chest radiography and CT scan revealed frequently a large tumor mass (located at the pleura, 80 %; pleura and lung, 10 %; and lung near the pleura, 7 %) as well as irregular pleural thickening. Direct invasion of adjacent structures (ribs, spinal cord) and organs is frequent; patients presenting with paralysis of the lower extremities caused by tumor invasion of the spinal cord have been reported [151].

Histopathologic Features

The neoplasm is composed of large atypical lymphoid cells usually with immunoblastic morphology and plasmacytoid differentiation (Figs. 11.38a, b and 11.39). Rare Reed-Sternberg-like cells can be observed. An angiocentricity growth pattern with focal vascular wall destruction has been

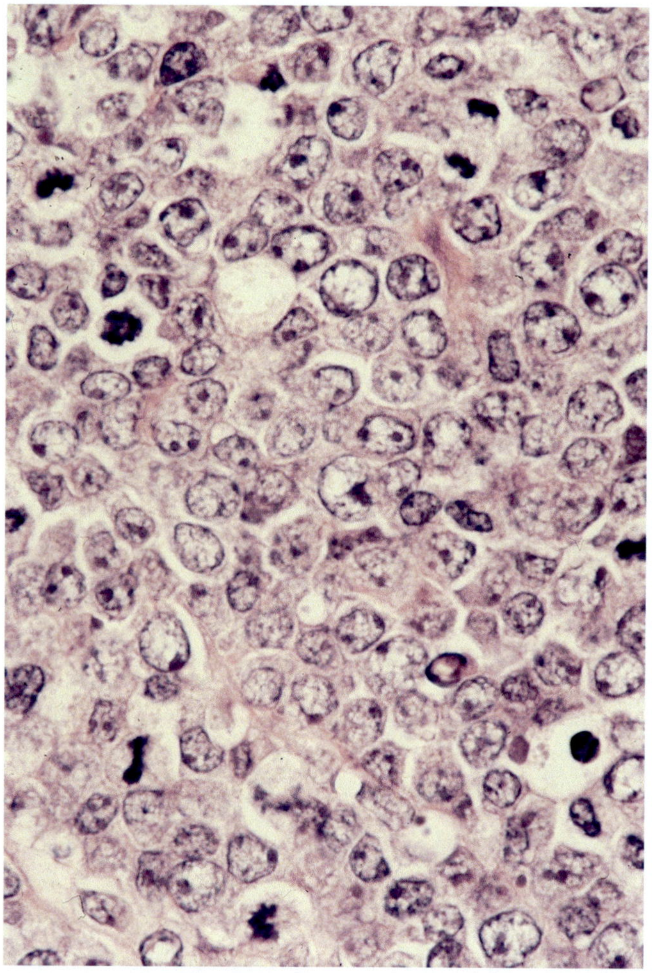

Fig. 11.39 In this case of DLBCL associated with chronic inflammation of PAL type, the tumor cells are a mixture of centroblasts and immunoblasts. Note the presence of numerous mitoses (Courtesy of Dr. Shigeo Nakamura)

described [160]. Cytologic examination of the pleural effusion fluid also shows large atypical cells with the morphology of immunoblasts, plasmablasts, anaplastic large cells, or even giant cells similar to those seen in PEL.

Immunohistochemical Features

The tumor cells are usually positive for CD20, CD79a, and CD45/LCA. Intracytoplasmic monotypic immunoglobulin expression is frequently detected. A subset of cases with plasmacytoid differentiation may be negative for CD20 and CD79a but positive for MUM1/IRF-4 or CD138 (similar to PEL). EBER is positive, EBNA2 (Fig. 11.40) and LMP1 are often positive, but HHV-8 is negative. A subset of cases may express some T-cell markers such as CD2, CD3, and CD4 in addition to pan-B markers [160]. PAL of a T-cell phenotype has also been reported rarely [151].

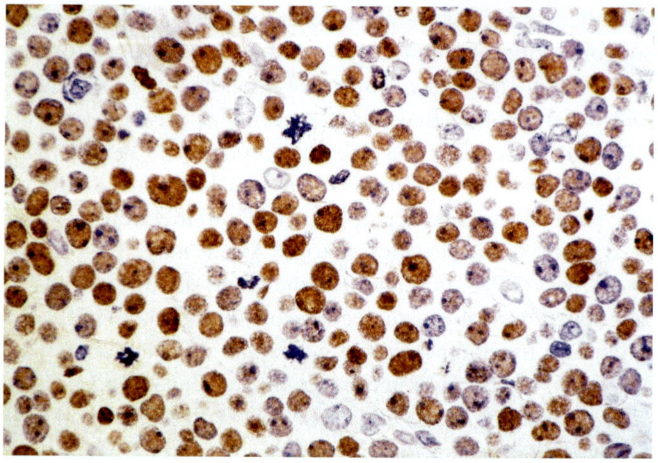

Fig. 11.40 DLBCL associated with chronic inflammation of PAL type. The tumor cells are positive for EBNA2. This supports a type III latency pattern of EBV infection

Molecular Biology and Cytogenetics

In most of the cases, PCR methods detect the presence of monoclonal *IgH* gene rearrangements with frequent somatic hypermutations of the *IgH* variable regions but do not show ongoing somatic mutations. Mutations of *p53* are detected in 71 % of the cases, and *myc* amplification is found in 80 % [161].

Differential Diagnosis

One important differential diagnosis is PEL. The most important criteria to rule out PEL is the absence of infection by HHV-8. In addition, patients with PAL will be HIV negative, will have a long clinical history of pleural or pleuropulmonary inflammation (tuberculosis) and presence of tumor masses.

Plasmacytoma arising from ribs or vertebra may involve the pleura or the lung. The plasmablastic form of plasmacytoma can mimic PAL. Features favoring the diagnostic of plasmacytoma include history of plasma cell myeloma and the presence of a background of smaller neoplastic plasma cells. Cases of PAL with plasmacytoid differentiation may have a similar immunophenotype to plasmablastic plasmacytoma.

Carcinoma and malignant mesothelioma may show diffuse growth simulating PAL. Demonstration of positivity for CD20 or CD45/LCA and negativity for cytokeratin will help excluding these diagnoses.

Treatment and Prognosis

PAL is responsive to chemotherapy and radiotherapy, but the overall prognosis is poor, with a 5-year survival of 35 % [162]. Underlying chronic pyothorax, respiratory failure, and other comorbidities frequently seen in these patients are additional obstacles to the successful treatment of this lymphoma.

Pleural Involvement by Systemic Lymphomas

Patients with lymphoma may present with or subsequently develop pleural involvement during course of disease. Approximately 16 % of patients with non-Hodgkin lymphoma present with or subsequently develop pleural involvement [163]. Pleural involvement can be unilateral or bilateral; unilateral involvement is more common on left side [163]. Most patients are symptomatic, presenting mainly with dyspnea, cough, or chest pain. Most of the patients have evidence of involvement of other anatomic site at the same time they have pleural involvement [164].

Any systemic lymphoma may involve pleural cavity; the most frequent type is DLBCL (60 %) followed by follicular lymphoma (20 %) [164]. Very few cases of classical HL involving the pleura have been described [165, 166]. For those cases of DLBCL involving pleura, the immunophenotype is similar to DLBCL elsewhere, and they are HHV-8 negative.

References

1. Papaioannou AN, Watson WL. Primary lymphoma of the lung: an appraisal of its natural history and a comparison with other localized lymphomas. J Thorac Cardiovasc Surg. 1965;49:373–87.
2. Berkman N, Breuer R, Kramer MR, Polliack A. Pulmonary involvement in lymphoma. Leuk Lymphoma. 1996;20(3–4):229–37.
3. L'Hoste Jr RJ, Filippa DA, Lieberman PH, Bretsky S. Primary pulmonary lymphomas. A clinicopathologic analysis of 36 cases. Cancer. 1984;54(7):1397–406.
4. Yang HB, Li J, Shen T. Primary anaplastic large cell lymphoma of the lung. Report of two cases and literature review. Acta Haematol. 2007;118(3):188–91.
5. Kim JH, Lee SH, Park J, Kim HY, Lee SI, Park JO, et al. Primary pulmonary non-Hodgkin's lymphoma. Jpn J Clin Oncol. 2004;34(9): 510–4.
6. Sagaert X, De Wolf-Peeters C, Noels H, Baens M. The pathogenesis of MALT lymphomas: where do we stand? Leukemia. 2007;21(3):389–96.
7. Richmond I, Pritchard GE, Ashcroft T, Avery A, Corris PA, Walters EH. Bronchus associated lymphoid tissue (BALT) in human lung: its distribution in smokers and non-smokers. Thorax. 1993; 48(11):1130–4.
8. Escolar Castellon JD, Escolar Castellon A, Roche Roche PA, Minana Amada C. Bronchial-associated lymphoid tissue (BALT) response to airway challenge with cigarette smoke, bovine antigen and anti-pulmonary serum. Histol Histopathol. 1992;7(3): 321–8.
9. Gould SJ, Isaacson PG. Bronchus-associated lymphoid tissue (BALT) in human fetal and infant lung. J Pathol. 1993;169(2): 229–34.
10. Rangel-Moreno J, Hartson L, Navarro C, Gaxiola M, Selman M, Randall TD. Inducible bronchus-associated lymphoid tissue (iBALT) in patients with pulmonary complications of rheumatoid arthritis. J Clin Invest. 2006;116(12):3183–94.
11. Tashiro K, Ohshima K, Suzumiya J, Yoneda S, Yahiro M, Sugihara M, et al. Clonality of primary pulmonary lymphoproliferative disorders; using in situ hybridization and polymerase chain reaction for immunoglobulin. Leuk Lymphoma. 1999;36(1–2):157–67.
12. Pabst R, Gehrke I. Is the bronchus-associated lymphoid tissue (BALT) an integral structure of the lung in normal mammals, including humans? Am J Respir Cell Mol Biol. 1990;3(2):131–5.
13. Moyron-Quiroz JE, Rangel-Moreno J, Kusser K, Hartson L, Sprague F, Goodrich S, et al. Role of inducible bronchus associated lymphoid tissue (iBALT) in respiratory immunity. Nat Med. 2004;10(9):927–34.
14. Addis BJ, Hyjek E, Isaacson PG. Primary pulmonary lymphoma: a re-appraisal of its histogenesis and its relationship to pseudolymphoma and lymphoid interstitial pneumonia. Histopathology. 1988;13(1):1–17.
15. Isaacson P, Wright DH. Extranodal malignant lymphoma arising from mucosa-associated lymphoid tissue. Cancer. 1984;53(11):2515–24.
16. Oh SY, Kim WS, Kim JS, Kim SJ, Kwon HC, Lee DH, et al. Pulmonary marginal zone B-cell lymphoma of MALT type – what is a prognostic factor and which is the optimal treatment, operation, or chemotherapy? Consortium for Improving Survival of Lymphoma (CISL) study. Ann Hematol. 2010;89(6):563–8.
17. Borie R, Wislez M, Thabut G, Antoine M, Rabbat A, Couderc LJ, et al. Clinical characteristics and prognostic factors of pulmonary MALT lymphoma. Eur Respir J. 2009;34(6):1408–16.
18. Herbert A, Wright DH, Isaacson PG, Smith JL. Primary malignant lymphoma of the lung: histopathologic and immunologic evaluation of nine cases. Hum Pathol. 1984;15(5):415–22.
19. Le Tourneau A, Audouin J, Garbe L, Capron F, Servais B, Monges G, et al. Primary pulmonary malignant lymphoma, clinical and pathological findings, immunocytochemical and ultrastructural studies in 15 cases. Hematol Oncol. 1983;1(1):49–60.
20. Cordier JF, Chailleux E, Lauque D, Reynaud-Gaubert M, Dietemann-Molard A, Dalphin JC, et al. Primary pulmonary lymphomas. A clinical study of 70 cases in nonimmunocompromised patients. Chest. 1993;103(1):201–8.
21. Lee DK, Im JG, Lee KS, Lee JS, Seo JB, Goo JM, et al. B-cell lymphoma of bronchus-associated lymphoid tissue (BALT): CT features in 10 patients. J Comput Assist Tomogr. 2000;24(1):30–4.
22. Wislez M, Cadranel J, Antoine M, Milleron B, Bazot M, Mayaud C, et al. Lymphoma of pulmonary mucosa-associated lymphoid tissue: CT scan findings and pathological correlations. Eur Respir J. 1999;14(2):423–9.
23. Raderer M, Vorbeck F, Formanek M, Osterreicher C, Valencak J, Penz M, et al. Importance of extensive staging in patients with mucosa-associated lymphoid tissue (MALT)-type lymphoma. Br J Cancer. 2000;83(4):454–7.
24. Thieblemont C, Berger F, Dumontet C, Moullet I, Bouafia F, Felman P, et al. Mucosa-associated lymphoid tissue lymphoma is a disseminated disease in one third of 158 patients analyzed. Blood. 2000; 95(3):802–6.
25. Du M, Diss TC, Xu C, Peng H, Isaacson PG, Pan L. Ongoing mutation in MALT lymphoma immunoglobulin gene suggests that antigen stimulation plays a role in the clonal expansion. Leukemia. 1996;10(7):1190–7.
26. Tierens A, Delabie J, Pittaluga S, Driessen A, DeWolf-Peeters C. Mutation analysis of the rearranged immunoglobulin heavy chain genes of marginal zone cell lymphomas indicates an origin from different marginal zone B lymphocyte subsets. Blood. 1998;91(7):2381–6.
27. Vinatzer U, Gollinger M, Mullauer L, Raderer M, Chott A, Streubel B. Mucosa-associated lymphoid tissue lymphoma: novel translocations including rearrangements of ODZ2, JMJD2C, and CNN3. Clin Cancer Res. 2008;14(20):6426–31.
28. Streubel B, Simonitsch-Klupp I, Mullauer L, Lamprecht A, Huber D, Siebert R, et al. Variable frequencies of MALT lymphoma-associated genetic aberrations in MALT lymphomas of different sites. Leukemia. 2004;18(10):1722–6.
29. Begueret H, Vergier B, Parrens M, Lehours P, Laurent F, Vernejoux JM, et al. Primary lung small B-cell lymphoma versus lymphoid

hyperplasia: evaluation of diagnostic criteria in 26 cases. Am J Surg Pathol. 2002;26(1):76–81.
30. Nicholson AG, Wotherspoon AC, Diss TC, Hansell DM, Du Bois R, Sheppard MN, et al. Reactive pulmonary lymphoid disorders. Histopathology. 1995;26(5):405–12.
31. Fishleder A, Tubbs R, Hesse B, Levine H. Uniform detection of immunoglobulin-gene rearrangement in benign lymphoepithelial lesions. N Engl J Med. 1987;316(18):1118–21.
32. Collins RD. Is clonality equivalent to malignancy: specifically, is immunoglobulin gene rearrangement diagnostic of malignant lymphoma? Hum Pathol. 1997;28(7):757–9.
33. Zucca E, Conconi A, Pedrinis E, Cortelazzo S, Motta T, Gospodarowicz MK, et al. Nongastric marginal zone B-cell lymphoma of mucosa-associated lymphoid tissue. Blood. 2003;101(7): 2489–95.
34. de Boer JP, Hiddink RF, Raderer M, Antonini N, Aleman BM, Boot H, et al. Dissemination patterns in non-gastric MALT lymphoma. Haematologica. 2008;93(2):201–6.
35. Ferraro P, Trastek VF, Adlakha H, Deschamps C, Allen MS, Pairolero PC. Primary non-Hodgkin's lymphoma of the lung. Ann Thorac Surg. 2000;69(4):993–7.
36. Cadranel J, Wislez M, Antoine M. Primary pulmonary lymphoma. Eur Respir J. 2002;20(3):750–62.
37. Kennedy JL, Nathwani BN, Burke JS, Hill LR, Rappaport H. Pulmonary lymphomas and other pulmonary lymphoid lesions. A clinicopathologic and immunologic study of 64 patients. Cancer. 1985;56(3):539–52.
38. Koss MN, Hochholzer L, Nichols PW, Wehunt WD, Lazarus AA. Primary non-Hodgkin's lymphoma and pseudolymphoma of lung: a study of 161 patients. Hum Pathol. 1983;14(12):1024–38.
39. Li G, Hansmann ML, Zwingers T, Lennert K. Primary lymphomas of the lung: morphological, immunohistochemical and clinical features. Histopathology. 1990;16(6):519–31.
40. Gascoyne RD. Pathologic prognostic factors in diffuse aggressive non-Hodgkin's lymphoma. Hematol Oncol Clin North Am. 1997; 11(5):847–62.
41. Lo Coco F, Ye BH, Lista F, Corradini P, Offit K, Knowles DM, et al. Rearrangements of the BCL6 gene in diffuse large cell non-Hodgkin's lymphoma. Blood. 1994;83(7):1757–9.
42. Otsuki T, Yano T, Clark HM, Bastard C, Kerckaert JP, Jaffe ES, et al. Analysis of LAZ3 (BCL-6) status in B-cell non-Hodgkin's lymphomas: results of rearrangement and gene expression studies and a mutational analysis of coding region sequences. Blood. 1995;85(10):2877–84.
43. Ladanyi M, Offit K, Jhanwar SC, Filippa DA, Chaganti RS. MYC rearrangement and translocations involving band 8q24 in diffuse large cell lymphomas. Blood. 1991;77(5):1057–63.
44. Kramer MH, Hermans J, Wijburg E, Philippo K, Geelen E, van Krieken JH, et al. Clinical relevance of BCL2, BCL6, and MYC rearrangements in diffuse large B-cell lymphoma. Blood. 1998; 92(9):3152–62.
45. Kawasaki C, Ohshim K, Suzumiya J, Kanda M, Tsuchiya T, Tamura K, et al. Rearrangements of bcl-1, bcl-2, bcl-6, and c-myc in diffuse large B-cell lymphomas. Leuk Lymphoma. 2001;42(5):1099–106.
46. Hummel M, Bentink S, Berger H, Klapper W, Wessendorf S, Barth TF, et al. A biologic definition of Burkitt's lymphoma from transcriptional and genomic profiling. N Engl J Med. 2006;354(23): 2419–30.
47. Lin P, Medeiros LJ. High-grade B-cell lymphoma/leukemia associated with t(14;18) and 8q24/MYC rearrangement: a neoplasm of germinal center immunophenotype with poor prognosis. Haematologica. 2007;92(10):1297–301.
48. de Mascarel A, Merlio JP, Coindre JM, Goussot JF, Broustet A. Gastric large cell lymphoma expressing cytokeratin but no leukocyte common antigen. A diagnostic dilemma. Am J Clin Pathol. 1989;91(4):478–81.
49. Mounier N, Briere J, Gisselbrecht C, Emile JF, Lederlin P, Sebban C, et al. Rituximab plus CHOP (R-CHOP) overcomes bcl-2–associated resistance to chemotherapy in elderly patients with diffuse large B-cell lymphoma (DLBCL). Blood. 2003;101(11):4279–84.
50. Le Gouill S, Talmant P, Touzeau C, Moreau A, Garand R, Juge-Morineau N, et al. The clinical presentation and prognosis of diffuse large B-cell lymphoma with t(14;18) and 8q24/c-MYC rearrangement. Haematologica. 2007;92(10):1335–42.
51. Liebow AA, Carrington CR, Friedman PJ. Lymphomatoid granulomatosis. Hum Pathol. 1972;3(4):457–558.
52. Katzenstein AL, Carrington CB, Liebow AA. Lymphomatoid granulomatosis: a clinicopathologic study of 152 cases. Cancer. 1979; 43(1):360–73.
53. Nichols PW, Koss M, Levine AM, Lukes RJ. Lymphomatoid granulomatosis: a T-cell disorder? Am J Med. 1982;72(3):467–71.
54. Lipford Jr EH, Margolick JB, Longo DL, Fauci AS, Jaffe ES. Angiocentric immunoproliferative lesions: a clinicopathologic spectrum of post-thymic T-cell proliferations. Blood. 1988;72(5): 1674–81.
55. DeRemee RA, Weiland LH, McDonald TJ. Polymorphic reticulosis, lymphomatoid granulomatosis. Two diseases or one? Mayo Clin Proc. 1978;53(10):634–40.
56. Wilson WH, Kingma DW, Raffeld M, Wittes RE, Jaffe ES. Association of lymphomatoid granulomatosis with Epstein-Barr viral infection of B lymphocytes and response to interferon-alpha 2b. Blood. 1996;87(11):4531–7.
57. Katzenstein AL, Peiper SC. Detection of Epstein-Barr virus genomes in lymphomatoid granulomatosis: analysis of 29 cases by the polymerase chain reaction technique. Mod Pathol. 1990;3(4):435–41.
58. Guinee Jr D, Jaffe E, Kingma D, Fishback N, Wallberg K, Krishnan J, et al. Pulmonary lymphomatoid granulomatosis. Evidence for a proliferation of Epstein-Barr virus infected B-lymphocytes with a prominent T-cell component and vasculitis. Am J Surg Pathol. 1994;18(8):753–64.
59. Myers JL, Kurtin PJ, Katzenstein AL, Tazelaar HD, Colby TV, Strickler JG, et al. Lymphomatoid granulomatosis. Evidence of immunophenotypic diversity and relationship to Epstein-Barr virus infection. Am J Surg Pathol. 1995;19(11):1300–12.
60. Haque AK, Myers JL, Hudnall SD, Gelman BB, Lloyd RV, Payne D, et al. Pulmonary lymphomatoid granulomatosis in acquired immunodeficiency syndrome: lesions with Epstein-Barr virus infection. Mod Pathol. 1998;11(4):347–56.
61. Jaffe ES, Chan JK, Su IJ, Frizzera G, Mori S, Feller AC, et al. Report of the Workshop on Nasal and Related Extranodal Angiocentric T/Natural Killer Cell Lymphomas. Definitions, differential diagnosis, and epidemiology. Am J Surg Pathol. 1996;20(1):103–11.
62. Koss MN, Hochholzer L, Langloss JM, Wehunt WD, Lazarus AA, Nichols PW. Lymphomatoid granulomatosis: a clinicopathologic study of 42 patients. Pathology. 1986;18(3):283–8.
63. Beaty MW, Toro J, Sorbara L, Stern JB, Pittaluga S, Raffeld M, et al. Cutaneous lymphomatoid granulomatosis: correlation of clinical and biologic features. Am J Surg Pathol. 2001;25(9):1111–20.
64. Patsalides AD, Atac G, Hedge U, Janik J, Grant N, Jaffe ES, et al. Lymphomatoid granulomatosis: abnormalities of the brain at MR imaging. Radiology. 2005;237(1):265–73.
65. Tateishi U, Terae S, Ogata A, Sawamura Y, Suzuki Y, Abe S, et al. MR imaging of the brain in lymphomatoid granulomatosis. AJNR Am J Neuroradiol. 2001;22(7):1283–90.
66. Kapila A, Gupta KL, Garcia JH. CT and MR of lymphomatoid granulomatosis of the CNS: report of four cases and review of the literature. AJNR Am J Neuroradiol. 1988;9(6):1139–43.
67. Bolaman Z, Kadikoylu G, Polatli M, Barutca S, Culhaci N, Senturk T. Migratory nodules in the lung: lymphomatoid granulomatosis. Leuk Lymphoma. 2003;44(1):197–200.
68. Sheehy N, Bird B, O'Briain DS, Daly P, Wilson G. Synchronous regression and progression of pulmonary nodules on chest CT in

untreated lymphomatoid granulomatosis. Clin Radiol. 2004; 59(5):451–4.
69. Braham E, Ayadi-Kaddour A, Smati B, Ben Mrad S, Besbes M, El Mezni F. Lymphomatoid granulomatosis mimicking interstitial lung disease. Respirology. 2008;13(7):1085–7.
70. Makol A, Kosuri K, Tamkus D, de M Calaca W, Chang HT. Lymphomatoid granulomatosis masquerading as interstitial pneumonia in a 66-year-old man: a case report and review of literature. J Hematol Oncol. 2009;2:39.
71. Guinee Jr DG, Perkins SL, Travis WD, Holden JA, Tripp SR, Koss MN. Proliferation and cellular phenotype in lymphomatoid granulomatosis: implications of a higher proliferation index in B cells. Am J Surg Pathol. 1998;22(9):1093–100.
72. Medeiros LJ, Peiper SC, Elwood L, Yano T, Raffeld M, Jaffe ES. Angiocentric immunoproliferative lesions: a molecular analysis of eight cases. Hum Pathol. 1991;22(11):1150–7.
73. Kwon EJ, Katz KA, Draft KS, Seykora JT, Rook AH, Wasik MA, et al. Posttransplantation lymphoproliferative disease with features of lymphomatoid granulomatosis in a lung transplant patient. J Am Acad Dermatol. 2006;54(4):657–63.
74. Saxena A, Dyker KM, Angel S, Moshynska O, Dharampaul S, Cockroft DW. Posttransplant diffuse large B-cell lymphoma of "lymphomatoid granulomatosis" type. Virchows Arch. 2002; 441(6):622–8.
75. Mukhopadhyay S, Katzenstein AL. Biopsy findings in acute pulmonary histoplasmosis: unusual histologic features in 4 cases mimicking lymphomatoid granulomatosis. Am J Surg Pathol. 2010; 34(4):541–6.
76. Rao R, Vugman G, Leslie WT, Loew J, Venugopal P. Lymphomatoid granulomatosis treated with rituximab and chemotherapy. Clin Adv Hematol Oncol. 2003;1(11):658–60; discussion 60.
77. Ponzoni M, Ferreri AJ, Campo E, Facchetti F, Mazzucchelli L, Yoshino T, et al. Definition, diagnosis, and management of intravascular large B-cell lymphoma: proposals and perspectives from an international consensus meeting. J Clin Oncol. 2007;25(21):3168–73.
78. Ponzoni M, Arrigoni G, Gould VE, Del Curto B, Maggioni M, Scapinello A, et al. Lack of CD 29 (beta1 integrin) and CD 54 (ICAM-1) adhesion molecules in intravascular lymphomatosis. Hum Pathol. 2000;31(2):220–6.
79. Pfleger L, Tappeiner J. On the recognition of systematized endotheliomatosis of the cutaneous blood vessels (reticuloendotheliosis? Hautarzt. 1959;10:359–63.
80. Murase T, Nakamura S, Tashiro K, Suchi T, Hiraga J, Hayasaki N, et al. Malignant histiocytosis-like B-cell lymphoma, a distinct pathologic variant of intravascular lymphomatosis: a report of five cases and review of the literature. Br J Haematol. 1997; 99(3):656–64.
81. Murase T, Nakamura S, Kawauchi K, Matsuzaki H, Sakai C, Inaba T, et al. An Asian variant of intravascular large B-cell lymphoma: clinical, pathological and cytogenetic approaches to diffuse large B-cell lymphoma associated with haemophagocytic syndrome. Br J Haematol. 2000;111(3):826–34.
82. Ohno T, Miyake N, Hada S, Hirose Y, Imura A, Hori T, et al. Hemophagocytic syndrome in five patients with Epstein-Barr virus negative B-cell lymphoma. Cancer. 1998;82(10):1963–72.
83. Snyder LS, Harmon KR, Estensen RD. Intravascular lymphomatosis (malignant angioendotheliomatosis) presenting as pulmonary hypertension. Chest. 1989;96(5):1199–200.
84. Chim CS, Choy C, Ooi GC, Chung LP, Wong KK, Liang R. Two unusual lymphomas. Case 2: pulmonary intravascular lymphomatosis. J Clin Oncol. 2000;18(21):3733–5.
85. Jang HJ, Lee KS, Han J. Intravascular lymphomatosis of the lung: radiologic findings. J Comput Assist Tomogr. 1998;22(3):427–9.
86. Nambu A, Kurihara Y, Ichikawa T, Ohkubo S, Onoue M, Oyama T, et al. Lung involvement in angiotropic lymphoma: CT findings. AJR Am J Roentgenol. 1998;170(4):940–2.
87. Walls JG, Hong YG, Cox JE, McCabe KM, O'Brien KE, Allerton JP, et al. Pulmonary intravascular lymphomatosis: presentation with dyspnea and air trapping. Chest. 1999;115(4):1207–10.
88. Kitanaka A, Kubota Y, Imataki O, Ohnishi H, Fukumoto T, Kurokohchi K, et al. Intravascular large B-cell lymphoma with FDG accumulation in the lung lacking CT/(67)gallium scintigraphy abnormality. Hematol Oncol. 2009;27(1):46–9.
89. Kotake T, Kosugi S, Takimoto T, Nakata S, Shiga J, Nagate Y, et al. Intravascular large B-cell lymphoma presenting pulmonary arterial hypertension as an initial manifestation. Intern Med. 2010; 49(1):51–4.
90. Takamura K, Nasuhara Y, Mishina T, Matsuda T, Nishimura M, Kawakami Y, et al. Intravascular lymphomatosis diagnosed by transbronchial lung biopsy. Eur Respir J. 1997;10(4):955–7.
91. Demirer T, Dail DH, Aboulafia DM. Four varied cases of intravascular lymphomatosis and a literature review. Cancer. 1994; 73(6):1738–45.
92. Yegappan S, Coupland R, Arber DA, Wang N, Miocinovic R, Tubbs RR, et al. Angiotropic lymphoma: an immunophenotypically and clinically heterogeneous lymphoma. Mod Pathol. 2001; 14(11):1147–56.
93. Hsiao CH, Su IJ, Hsieh SW, Huang SF, Tsai TF, Chen MY, et al. Epstein-Barr virus-associated intravascular lymphomatosis within Kaposi's sarcoma in an AIDS patient. Am J Surg Pathol. 1999; 23(4):482–7.
94. Vega F, Medeiros LJ, Bueso-Ramos C, Jones D, Lai R, Luthra R, et al. Hepatosplenic gamma/delta T-cell lymphoma in bone marrow. A sinusoidal neoplasm with blastic cytologic features. Am J Clin Pathol. 2001;116(3):410–9.
95. Vega F, Medeiros LJ, Gaulard P. Hepatosplenic and other gammadelta T-cell lymphomas. Am J Clin Pathol. 2007;127(6):869–80.
96. Zhao XF, Sands AM, Ostrow PT, Halbiger R, Conway JT, Bagg A. Recurrence of nodal diffuse large B-cell lymphoma as intravascular large B-cell lymphoma: is an intravascular component at initial diagnosis predictive? Arch Pathol Lab Med. 2005;129(3):391–4.
97. Ferreri AJ, Campo E, Seymour JF, Willemze R, Ilariucci F, Ambrosetti A, et al. Intravascular lymphoma: clinical presentation, natural history, management and prognostic factors in a series of 38 cases, with special emphasis on the "cutaneous variant". Br J Haematol. 2004;127(2):173–83.
98. Wiltshaw E. The natural history of extramedullary plasmacytoma and its relation to solitary myeloma of bone and myelomatosis. Medicine (Baltimore). 1976;55(3):217–38.
99. Dimopoulos MA, Kiamouris C, Moulopoulos LA. Solitary plasmacytoma of bone and extramedullary plasmacytoma. Hematol Oncol Clin North Am. 1999;13(6):1249–57.
100. Shaikh G, Sehgal R, Mehrishi A, Karnik A. Primary pulmonary plasmacytoma. J Clin Oncol. 2008;26(18):3089–91.
101. Edelstein E, Gal AA, Mann KP, Miller Jr JI, Mansour KA. Primary solitary endobronchial plasmacytoma. Ann Thorac Surg. 2004; 78(4):1448–9.
102. Chang CC, Chang YL, Lee LN, Lee YC. Primary pulmonary plasmacytoma with immunoglobulin G/lambda light chain monoclonal gammopathy. J Thorac Cardiovasc Surg. 2006;132(4): 984–5.
103. Koss MN, Hochholzer L, Moran CA, Frizzera G. Pulmonary plasmacytomas: a clinicopathologic and immunohistochemical study of five cases. Ann Diagn Pathol. 1998;2(1):1–11.
104. Joseph G, Pandit M, Korfhage L. Primary pulmonary plasmacytoma. Cancer. 1993;71(3):721–4.
105. Wise JN, Schaefer RF, Read RC. Primary pulmonary plasmacytoma: a case report. Chest. 2001;120(4):1405–7.
106. Kojima M, Motoori T, Tamaki Y, Igarashi T, Matsumoto M, Shimizu K, et al. Cyclin D1 protein overexpression in extramedullary plasmacytoma: a clinicopathologic study of 11 cases. J Clin Exp Hematop. 2009;49(1):53–6.

107. Bink K, Haralambieva E, Kremer M, Ott G, Beham-Schmid C, de Leval L, et al. Primary extramedullary plasmacytoma: similarities with and differences from multiple myeloma revealed by interphase cytogenetics. Haematologica. 2008;93(4):623–6.
108. Rush WL, Andriko JA, Taubenberger JK, Nelson AM, Abbondanzo SL, Travis WD, et al. Primary anaplastic large cell lymphoma of the lung: a clinicopathologic study of five patients. Mod Pathol. 2000;13(12):1285–92.
109. Delsol G, Al Saati T, Gatter KC, Gerdes J, Schwarting R, Caveriviere P, et al. Coexpression of epithelial membrane antigen (EMA), Ki-1, and interleukin-2 receptor by anaplastic large cell lymphomas. Diagnostic value in so-called malignant histiocytosis. Am J Pathol. 1988;130(1):59–70.
110. Morris SW, Kirstein MN, Valentine MB, Dittmer KG, Shapiro DN, Saltman DL, et al. Fusion of a kinase gene, ALK, to a nucleolar protein gene, NPM, in non-Hodgkin's lymphoma. Science. 1994;263(5151):1281–4.
111. Morris SW, Naeve C, Mathew P, James PL, Kirstein MN, Cui X, et al. ALK, the chromosome 2 gene locus altered by the t(2;5) in non-Hodgkin's lymphoma, encodes a novel neural receptor tyrosine kinase that is highly related to leukocyte tyrosine kinase (LTK). Oncogene. 1997;14(18):2175–88.
112. Vega F, Medeiros LJ. Chromosomal translocations involved in non-Hodgkin lymphomas. Arch Pathol Lab Med. 2003;127(9):1148–60.
113. Falini B, Pileri S, Zinzani PL, Carbone A, Zagonel V, Wolf-Peeters C, et al. ALK+ lymphoma: clinico-pathological findings and outcome. Blood. 1999;93(8):2697–706.
114. Onciu M, Behm FG, Downing JR, Shurtleff SA, Raimondi SC, Ma Z, et al. ALK-positive plasmablastic B-cell lymphoma with expression of the NPM-ALK fusion transcript: report of 2 cases. Blood. 2003;102(7):2642–4.
115. Soda M, Choi YL, Enomoto M, Takada S, Yamashita Y, Ishikawa S, et al. Identification of the transforming EML4-ALK fusion gene in non-small-cell lung cancer. Nature. 2007;448(7153):561–6.
116. Savage KJ, Harris NL, Vose JM, Ullrich F, Jaffe ES, Connors JM, et al. ALK- anaplastic large-cell lymphoma is clinically and immunophenotypically different from both ALK+ ALCL and peripheral T-cell lymphoma, not otherwise specified: report from the International Peripheral T-Cell Lymphoma Project. Blood. 2008;111(12):5496–504.
117. Colby TV, Hoppe RT, Warnke RA. Hodgkin's disease at autopsy: 1972–1977. Cancer. 1981;47(7):1852–62.
118. Kern WH, Crepeau AG, Jones JC. Primary Hodgkin's disease of the lung. Report of 4 cases and review of the literature. Cancer. 1961;14:1151–65.
119. Yousem SA, Weiss LM, Colby TV. Primary pulmonary Hodgkin's disease. A clinicopathologic study of 15 cases. Cancer. 1986;57(6):1217–24.
120. Radin AI. Primary pulmonary Hodgkin's disease. Cancer. 1990;65(3):550–63.
121. Kumar R, Sidhu H, Mistry R, Shet T. Primary pulmonary Hodgkin's lymphoma: a rare pitfall in transthoracic fine needle aspiration cytology. Diagn Cytopathol. 2008;36(9):666–9.
122. Cartier Y, Johkoh T, Honda O, Muller NL. Primary pulmonary Hodgkin's disease: CT findings in three patients. Clin Radiol. 1999;54(3):182–4.
123. Weiss LM, Chang KL. Molecular biologic studies of Hodgkin's disease. Semin Diagn Pathol. 1992;9(4):272–8.
124. Brinker MG, Poppema S, Buys CH, Timens W, Osinga J, Visser L. Clonal immunoglobulin gene rearrangements in tissues involved by Hodgkin's disease. Blood. 1987;70(1):186–91.
125. Joos S, Kupper M, Ohl S, von Bonin F, Mechtersheimer G, Bentz M, et al. Genomic imbalances including amplification of the tyrosine kinase gene JAK2 in CD30+ Hodgkin cells. Cancer Res. 2000;60(3):549–52.
126. Mottok A, Renne C, Willenbrock K, Hansmann ML, Brauninger A. Somatic hypermutation of SOCS1 in lymphocyte-predominant Hodgkin lymphoma is accompanied by high JAK2 expression and activation of STAT6. Blood. 2007;110(9):3387–90.
127. Martin-Subero JI, Gesk S, Harder L, Sonoki T, Tucker PW, Schlegelberger B, et al. Recurrent involvement of the REL and BCL11A loci in classical Hodgkin lymphoma. Blood. 2002;99(4):1474–7.
128. Cabannes E, Khan G, Aillet F, Jarrett RF, Hay RT. Mutations in the IkBa gene in Hodgkin's disease suggest a tumour suppressor role for IkappaBalpha. Oncogene. 1999;18(20):3063–70.
129. Trumper LH, Brady G, Bagg A, Gray D, Loke SL, Griesser H, et al. Single-cell analysis of Hodgkin and Reed-Sternberg cells: molecular heterogeneity of gene expression and p53 mutations. Blood. 1993;81(11):3097–115.
130. Rushin JM, Riordan GP, Heaton RB, Sharpe RW, Cotelingam JD, Jaffe ES. Cytomegalovirus-infected cells express Leu-M1 antigen. A potential source of diagnostic error. Am J Pathol. 1990;136(5):989–95.
131. Sheibani K, Battifora H, Burke JS, Rappaport H. Leu-M1 antigen in human neoplasms. An immunohistologic study of 400 cases. Am J Surg Pathol. 1986;10(4):227–36.
132. Wieczorek R, Burke JS, Knowles 2nd DM. Leu-M1 antigen expression in T-cell neoplasia. Am J Pathol. 1985;121(3):374–80.
133. Ferme C, Eghbali H, Meerwaldt JH, Rieux C, Bosq J, Berger F, et al. Chemotherapy plus involved-field radiation in early-stage Hodgkin's disease. N Engl J Med. 2007;357(19):1916–27.
134. Nador RG, Cesarman E, Chadburn A, Dawson DB, Ansari MQ, Sald J, et al. Primary effusion lymphoma: a distinct clinicopathologic entity associated with the Kaposi's sarcoma-associated herpes virus. Blood. 1996;88(2):645–56.
135. Horenstein MG, Nador RG, Chadburn A, Hyjek EM, Inghirami G, Knowles DM, et al. Epstein-Barr virus latent gene expression in primary effusion lymphomas containing Kaposi's sarcoma-associated herpesvirus/human herpesvirus-8. Blood. 1997;90(3):1186–91.
136. Dukers NH, Rezza G. Human herpesvirus 8 epidemiology: what we do and do not know. AIDS. 2003;17(12):1717–30.
137. Cesarman E, Chang Y, Moore PS, Said JW, Knowles DM. Kaposi's sarcoma-associated herpesvirus-like DNA sequences in AIDS-related body-cavity-based lymphomas. N Engl J Med. 1995;332(18):1186–91.
138. Soulier J, Grollet L, Oksenhendler E, Cacoub P, Cazals-Hatem D, Babinet P, et al. Kaposi's sarcoma-associated herpesvirus-like DNA sequences in multicentric Castleman's disease. Blood. 1995;86(4):1276–80.
139. Dupin N, Diss TL, Kellam P, Tulliez M, Du MQ, Sicard D, et al. HHV-8 is associated with a plasmablastic variant of Castleman disease that is linked to HHV-8-positive plasmablastic lymphoma. Blood. 2000;95(4):1406–12.
140. Knowles DM, Inghirami G, Ubriaco A, Dalla-Favera R. Molecular genetic analysis of three AIDS-associated neoplasms of uncertain lineage demonstrates their B-cell derivation and the possible pathogenetic role of the Epstein-Barr virus. Blood. 1989;73(3):792–9.
141. Carbone A, Gaidano G. HHV-8-positive body-cavity-based lymphoma: a novel lymphoma entity. Br J Haematol. 1997;97(3):515–22.
142. Schulz TF. Epidemiology of Kaposi's sarcoma-associated herpesvirus/human herpesvirus 8. Adv Cancer Res. 1999;76:121–60.
143. Morassut S, Vaccher E, Balestreri L, Gloghini A, Gaidano G, Volpe R, et al. HIV-associated human herpesvirus 8-positive primary lymphomatous effusions: radiologic findings in six patients. Radiology. 1997;205(2):459–63.

144. Said W, Chien K, Takeuchi S, Tasaka T, Asou H, Cho SK, et al. Kaposi's sarcoma-associated herpesvirus (KSHV or HHV8) in primary effusion lymphoma: ultrastructural demonstration of herpesvirus in lymphoma cells. Blood. 1996;87(12):4937–43.
145. Wang HY, Fuda FS, Chen W, Karandikar NJ. Notch1 in primary effusion lymphoma: a clinicopathological study. Mod Pathol. 2010;23(6):773–80.
146. Said JW, Shintaku IP, Asou H, de Vos S, Baker J, Hanson G, et al. Herpesvirus 8 inclusions in primary effusion lymphoma: report of a unique case with T-cell phenotype. Arch Pathol Lab Med. 1999;123(3):257–60.
147. Beaty MW, Kumar S, Sorbara L, Miller K, Raffeld M, Jaffe ES. A biophenotypic human herpesvirus 8 – associated primary bowel lymphoma. Am J Surg Pathol. 1999;23(8):992–4.
148. Ansari MQ, Dawson DB, Nador R, Rutherford C, Schneider NR, Latimer MJ, et al. Primary body cavity-based AIDS-related lymphomas. Am J Clin Pathol. 1996;105(2):221–9.
149. Luan SL, Boulanger E, Ye H, Chanudet E, Johnson N, Hamoudi RA, et al. Primary effusion lymphoma: genomic profiling revealed amplification of SELPLG and CORO1C encoding for proteins important for cell migration. J Pathol. 2010;222(2):166–79.
150. Cesarman E, Mesri EA, Gershengorn MC. Viral G protein-coupled receptor and Kaposi's sarcoma: a model of paracrine neoplasia? J Exp Med. 2000;191(3):417–22.
151. Nakatsuka S, Yao M, Hoshida Y, Yamamoto S, Iuchi K, Aozasa K. Pyothorax-associated lymphoma: a review of 106 cases. J Clin Oncol. 2002;20(20):4255–60.
152. Simonelli C, Spina M, Cinelli R, Talamini R, Tedeschi R, Gloghini A, et al. Clinical features and outcome of primary effusion lymphoma in HIV-infected patients: a single-institution study. J Clin Oncol. 2003;21(21):3948–54.
153. Boulanger E, Gerard L, Gabarre J, Molina JM, Rapp C, Abino JF, et al. Prognostic factors and outcome of human herpesvirus 8-associated primary effusion lymphoma in patients with AIDS. J Clin Oncol. 2005;23(19):4372–80.
154. Halfdanarson TR, Markovic SN, Kalokhe U, Luppi M. A non-chemotherapy treatment of a primary effusion lymphoma: durable remission after intracavitary cidofovir in HIV negative PEL refractory to chemotherapy. Ann Oncol. 2006;17(12):1849–50.
155. An J, Sun Y, Fisher M, Rettig MB. Antitumor effects of bortezomib (PS-341) on primary effusion lymphomas. Leukemia. 2004;18(10):1699–704.
156. Klass CM, Krug LT, Pozharskaya VP, Offermann MK. The targeting of primary effusion lymphoma cells for apoptosis by inducing lytic replication of human herpesvirus 8 while blocking virus production. Blood. 2005;105(10):4028–34.
157. Iuchi K, Ichimiya A, Akashi A, Mizuta T, Lee YE, Tada H, et al. Non-Hodgkin's lymphoma of the pleural cavity developing from long-standing pyothorax. Cancer. 1987;60(8):1771–5.
158. Fukayama M, Ibuka T, Hayashi Y, Ooba T, Koike M, Mizutani S. Epstein-Barr virus in pyothorax-associated pleural lymphoma. Am J Pathol. 1993;143(4):1044–9.
159. Martin A, Capron F, Liguory-Brunaud MD, De Frejacques C, Pluot M, Diebold J. Epstein-Barr virus-associated primary malignant lymphomas of the pleural cavity occurring in longstanding pleural chronic inflammation. Hum Pathol. 1994;25(12):1314–8.
160. Androulaki A, Drakos E, Hatzianastassiou D, Vgenopoulou S, Gazouli M, Korkolopoulou P, et al. Pyothorax-associated lymphoma (PAL): a western case with marked angiocentricity and review of the literature. Histopathology. 2004;44(1):69–76.
161. Yamato H, Ohshima K, Suzumiya J, Kikuchi M. Evidence for local immunosuppression and demonstration of c-myc amplification in pyothorax-associated lymphoma. Histopathology. 2001;39(2):163–71.
162. Narimatsu H, Ota Y, Kami M, Takeuchi K, Suzuki R, Matsuo K, et al. Clinicopathological features of pyothorax-associated lymphoma; a retrospective survey involving 98 patients. Ann Oncol. 2007;18(1):122–8.
163. Das DK, Gupta SK, Ayyagari S, Bambery PK, Datta BN, Datta U. Pleural effusions in non-Hodgkin's lymphoma. A cytomorphologic, cytochemical and immunologic study. Acta Cytol. 1987;31(2):119–24.
164. Vega F, Padula A, Valbuena JR, Stancu M, Jones D, Medeiros LJ. Lymphomas involving the pleura: a clinicopathologic study of 34 cases diagnosed by pleural biopsy. Arch Pathol Lab Med. 2006;130(10):1497–502.
165. Olson PR, Silverman JF, Powers CN. Pleural fluid cytology of Hodgkin's disease: cytomorphologic features and the value of immunohistochemical studies. Diagn Cytopathol. 2000;22(1):21–4.
166. Bernardeschi P, Bonechi I, Urbano U. Recurrent pleural effusion as manifesting feature of primitive chest wall Hodgkin's disease. Chest. 1988;94(2):424–6.

12 Tumors of the Pleura

The Pleura

The gamut of neoplastic and pseudoneoplastic conditions that may seed the pleural surface is extensive and can be divided into primary and metastatic neoplasms. In addition, the pleura may be the site for tumors of different lineage including epithelial, mesenchymal, neural, and neuroectodermal, as well as lymphoid neoplasms. However, in order to properly assess the origin of lesions seeding the pleural surface, it is important to properly correlate findings with imaging studies, which can be of important aid in addressing issues such as extent of disease and possible origin. In this chapter, the emphasis will be on primary pleural lesions leaving the issue of metastatic disease in the context of differential diagnosis.

Epithelial Tumors

Mesothelioma is by far the most popular tumor of the pleural surface and is one that poses the most diagnostic problems. However, it is important to highlight that epithelial tumors of the pleura may be as varied as they are in other anatomic sites. Some of the most common epithelial tumors that can present as primary pleural tumors include:

- Malignant mesothelioma
- Pseudomesotheliomatous adenocarcinoma
- Mucoepidermoid carcinoma
- Thymoma
- Adenomatoid tumor
- Endometriosis

Malignant Mesothelioma

Even though pleural mesotheliomas in practice are uncommon tumors, due to their legal implications, they appear to dominate pleural pathology. For the same reason plenty of resources in terms of immunohistochemical and ultrastructural analysis have been devoted to properly address and support the diagnosis of mesothelioma. It has been estimated that their incidence in the USA is approximately three to seven cases per million persons per year, with a tendency to increase in more recent years [1, 2]. Even though mesotheliomas have been associated to asbestos fiber exposure, approximately 50 % of individuals affected by mesotheliomas do not disclose such history, leading to believe that their etiology may be a multifactorial one and not one limited to the exposure of asbestos fibers [1–5].

Careful analysis of the radiological studies with the appropriate material for histopathological evaluation should lead both clinicians and pathologists to a more specific diagnosis. It is not uncommon to observe that many times the clinical and radiological aspects of the cases are clear, but the available material for histopathological examination is not adequate. In such circumstances, one should not make a definitive diagnosis but rather raise the level of suspicion and request additional material if clinically indicated. Part of this rationale is the fact that the surgical treatment for cases of mesothelioma can be radical. Thus, it is imperative for a pathologist to be absolutely certain about the diagnosis. Furthermore, it is well known that there are other pleural conditions of an inflammatory nature that may mimic malignant mesothelioma. Therefore, one should carefully evaluate the clinical and radiological information and use it as an aid to guide decision making in terms of the use of immunohistochemistry and/or electron microscopy. Ultimately the diagnosis of mesothelioma is a pathological one and requires histopathological assessment.

Historical Perspective

Wagner is credited for having described this tumor in the pleura in 1870 [6]. However, in the following years and into the nineteenth century, there was great controversy around

A. Weissferdt, C.A. Moran, *Diagnostic Pathology of Pleuropulmonary Neoplasia*,
DOI 10.1007/978-1-4419-0787-5_12, © Springer Science+Business Media New York 2013

tumors with diffuse pleural involvement. Thus, many of these tumors were classified under different designations, which included endothelial carcinoma, sarcoma, lymphangitis proliferans, sarcocarcinoma, and endothelioma [7, 8]. It was not until 1920 that Dubray and Rosson proposed the term mesothelioma [9], a name that is commonly used now. Even though there was some resistance to accept the notion of primary tumors of the pleura, in time well-documented cases were reported [8, 10]. In 1931, Klemperer and Rabin [8] essentially divided pleural tumors by their macroscopic appearance into those affecting the pleura in a localized fashion and those affecting the pleura in a diffuse manner. This division of pleural tumors gave rise to what is now known as diffuse pleural mesothelioma and solitary fibrous tumors of the pleura.

Wagner et al. [11] in 1960 described 33 patients with mesothelioma and suggested their association with asbestos fibers. According to the authors, all patients with only one exception had probable exposure to asbestos. Later, Hirsch et al. [12] described 28 cases in which the authors established asbestos exposure in 17 cases. Other authors reported larger series of cases with more emphasis on the association of mesothelioma and asbestos exposure [4, 5], while some others stated the histopathological variability of mesotheliomas [13]. Although in the past, the diagnosis was essentially established using conventional histology and histochemical stains such as periodic acid-Schiff (PAS) with and without diastase and mucicarmine, new modalities such as electron microscopy and immunohistochemistry have shifted the emphasis in the study of mesotheliomas. In general, the numerous clinicopathological correlations on mesotheliomas have provided valuable information in the understanding of this tumor [14–22].

Clinical Features

The evaluation of clinical and radiological information is crucial in the diagnosis of mesothelioma. Every effort should be made to properly correlate the histological findings with the clinical and radiological ones. In general terms, mesotheliomas are more common in adult individuals over 50 years of age. However, mesotheliomas may also occur in children [23, 24]. History of long-standing exposure to asbestos, whether factual or not, should lead to a careful analysis of the biopsy material available for diagnosis. It is important to recognize that mesotheliomas, as stated before, can occur in the setting of a negative history of asbestos exposure, and examples of it are the cases that have been described in children and women (housewives). Other possible etiopathologic causes that have been mentioned in the development of mesothelioma include radiation, chronic inflammation, viral infections, and diethylstilbestrol [25].

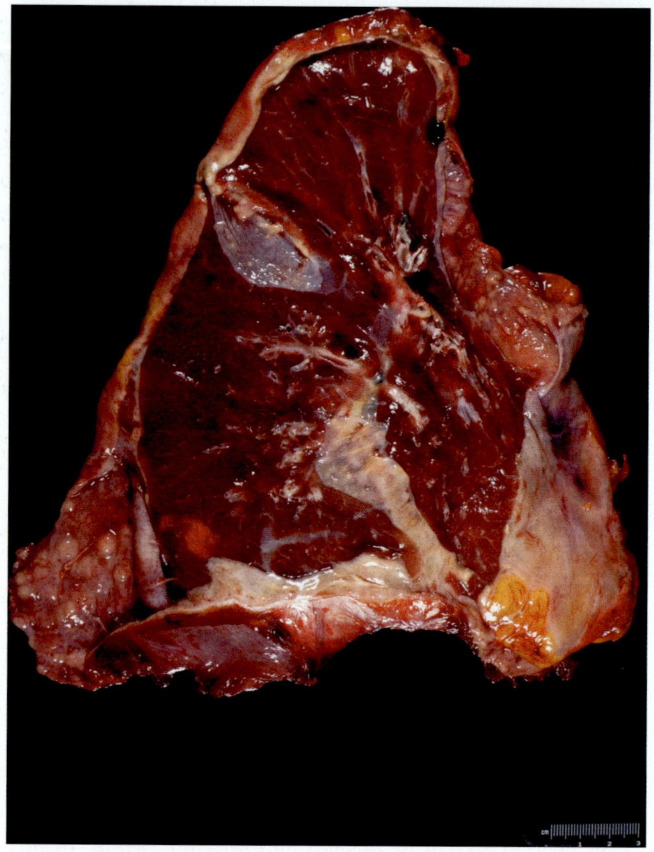

Fig. 12.1 Extrapleural pneumonectomy specimen; note the thickening of the pleural surface and the encasement of the lung parenchyma

In the evaluation of a potential case of mesothelioma, one should emphasize the following aspects:

- Diffuse involvement of the pleura
- Intraparenchymal tumor nodules or masses (peripheral)
- Diffuse thickening of the pleura
- Encasement of the lung
- Unilateral or bilateral pleural involvement
- Pleural-based tumor mass

Clinically patients with mesothelioma may present with nonspecific symptoms such as chest pain, dyspnea, cough, weight loss, and pleural effusions. Similar symptoms may also be present in other types of pathology.

Gross Features

The tumor will show diffuse pleural involvement with thickening of the pleural lining encasing the entire lung (Fig. 12.1). In some cases, the tumor follows the intrapulmonary septa, and in rare instances, the tumor may involve the lung parenchyma. Therefore, the gross appearance of mesothelioma rarely poses problems with its diagnosis. However, the presence of a well-defined tumor mass in the periphery of the lung, even if the tumor also shows diffuse pleural involvement, should alert the pathologist to the possibility of an adenocarcinoma with diffuse

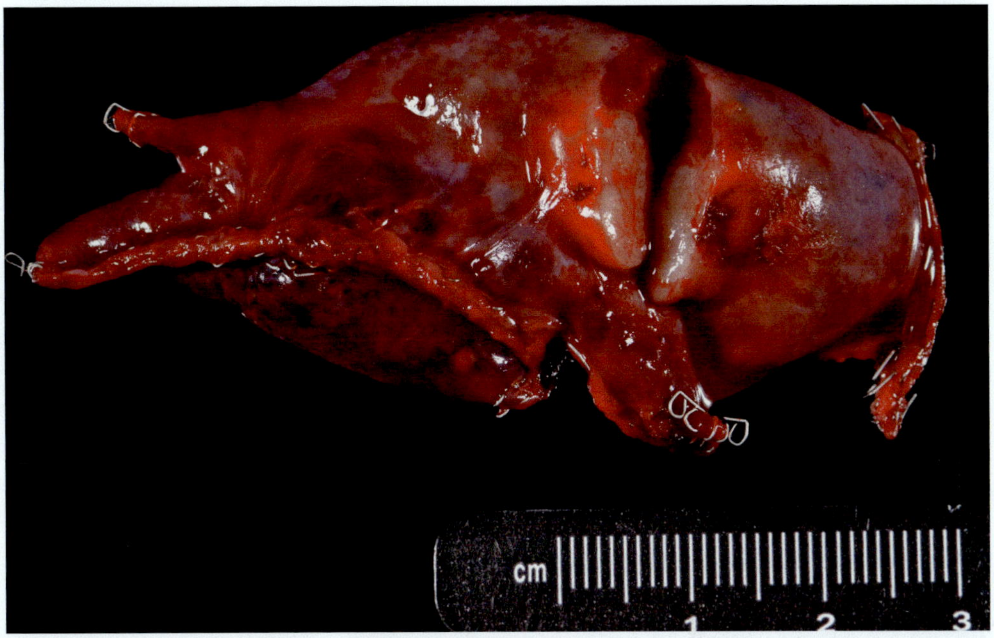

Fig. 12.2 Localized malignant mesothelioma; contrary to the conventional and more common form of diffuse pleural thickening the localized form is rather uncommon

pleural involvement. Even though those previously described gross findings occur in the great majority of cases, in some unusual cases, mesotheliomas may present as an intrapulmonary mass involving the pleural surface [26] (Fig. 12.2). Crotty et al. [26] described six patients, in whom the tumor presented a as localized tumor mass within the lung parenchyma, ranging in size from 2.8 to 10 cm. Based on their experience, the authors stated that it is possible that mesotheliomas presenting in this manner may not be as aggressive as the diffuse form of the tumor. In such situations, careful histopathological and immunohistochemical analysis is of utmost importance in order to arrive at the correct interpretation. In addition, such finding is important to mention, as those patients are most likely not candidates for extrapleural pneumonectomy.

Histopathologic Features

Mesotheliomas may show an extensive spectrum of histopathological growth patterns. However, traditionally mesotheliomas have been divided into three distinct growth patterns:

- Epithelioid
- Sarcomatoid
- Biphasic (combination of epithelioid and sarcomatoid)

Epithelioid Mesothelioma

Epithelioid mesothelioma represents the most common of the three variants. It has been estimated that it accounts for about 70 % of all mesotheliomas. Several distinct histopathological growth patterns of epithelioid malignant mesothelioma have been described. Some of those growth patterns in cases with limited tissue for diagnosis may pose a diagnostic challenge [27–31]. Among the variants that have been recognized are:

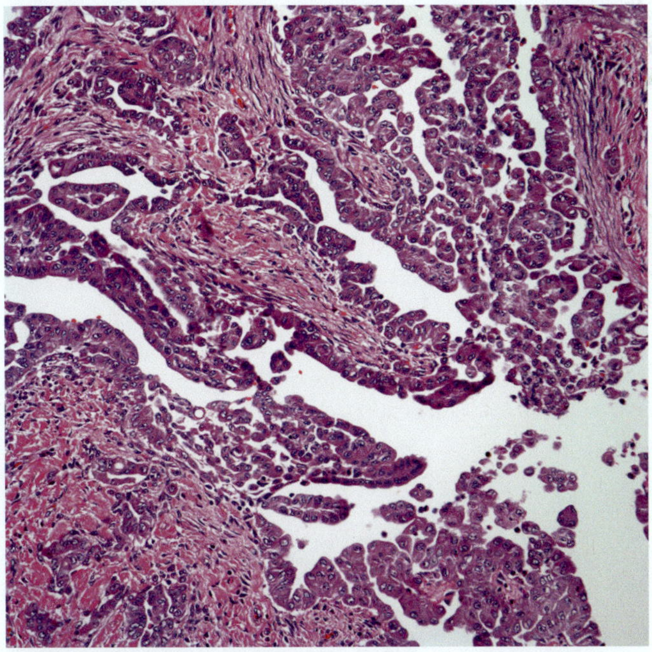

Fig. 12.3 Low power view of an epithelioid mesothelioma showing a papillary growth pattern

- *Tubulopapillary* (Figs. 12.3, 12.4, 12.5, 12.6, 12.7, 12.8, and 12.9): This is likely the most common growth pattern encountered in epithelioid mesotheliomas. The tumor may show the characteristic papillary growth pattern composed of medium-size, round to oval cells, with moderate amounts of eosinophilic cytoplasm, round nuclei, and conspicuous nucleoli. In other areas, this cellular

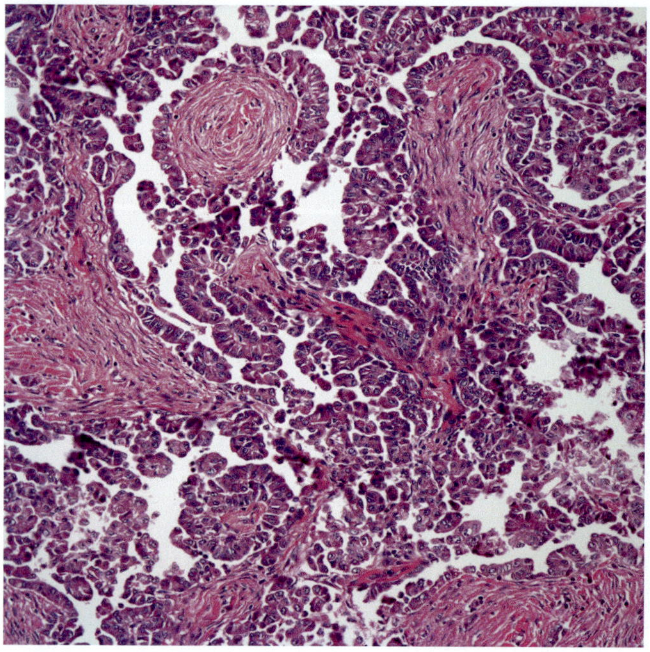

Fig. 12.4 Epithelioid mesothelioma showing prominent papillary features

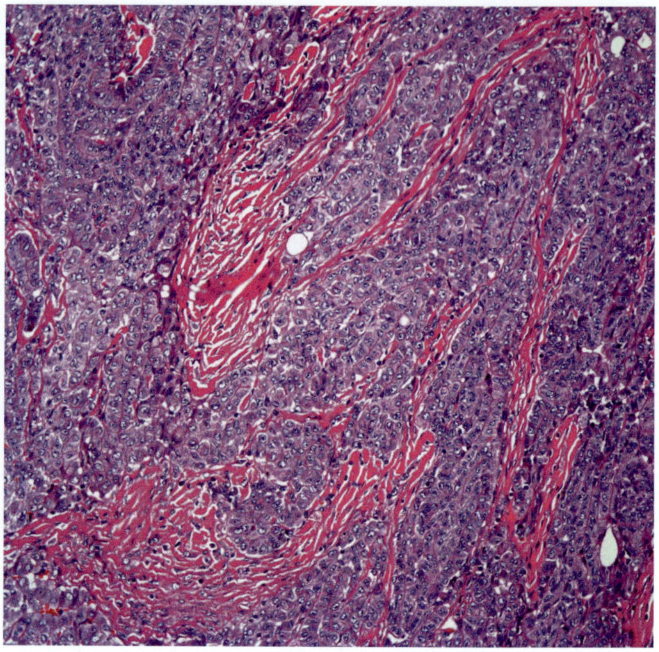

Fig. 12.6 Epithelioid mesothelioma dissecting fibroconnective tissue

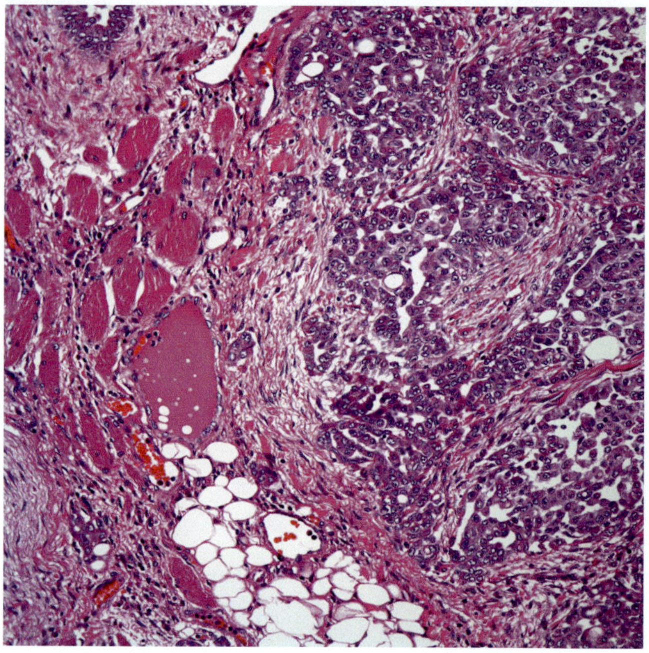

Fig. 12.5 Epithelioid mesothelioma infiltrating into adipose tissue and skeletal muscle

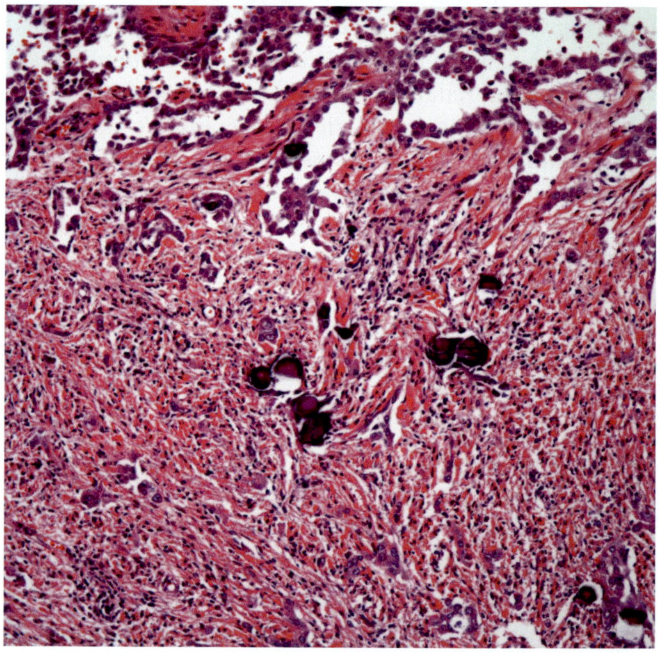

Fig. 12.7 Epithelioid mesothelioma showing numerous psammoma bodies (calcifications)

proliferation may show elongated tubular structures that appear to anastomose with each other. The tumor characteristically is fairly uniform with very mild nuclear atypia and low mitotic activity. Areas of necrosis and/or hemorrhage are not commonly seen with this growth pattern.

- *Clear cell* (Figs. 12.10, 12.11, 12.12, and 12.13): The tumor is characterized by a cellular proliferation composed of medium-size, round to oval cells with round nuclei, conspicuous nucleoli and clear cytoplasm. The tumor shows a diffuse cellular proliferation dissecting fibroconnective tissue. Mitotic activity although present is

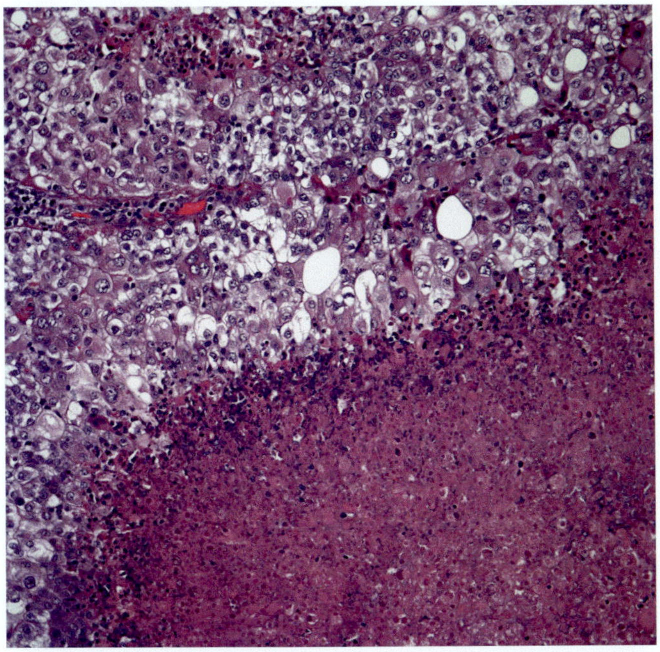

Fig. 12.8 Epithelioid mesothelioma showing areas of necrosis

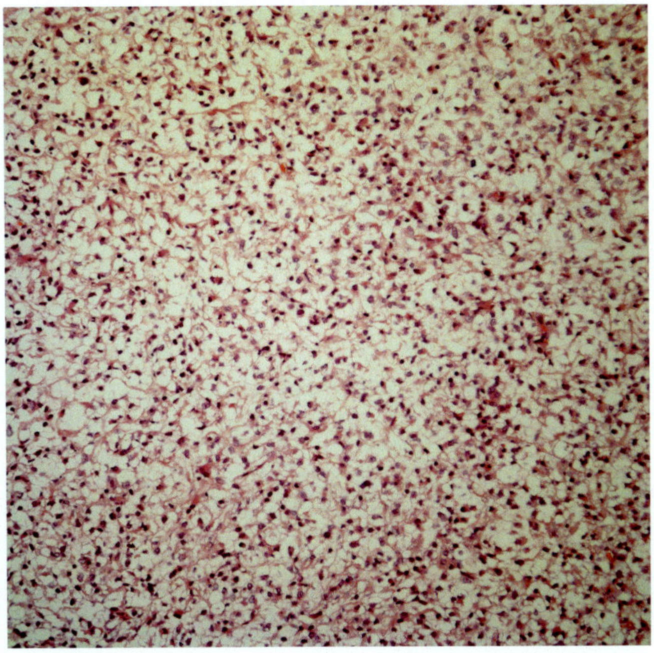

Fig. 12.10 Epithelioid mesothelioma with prominent clear cell features

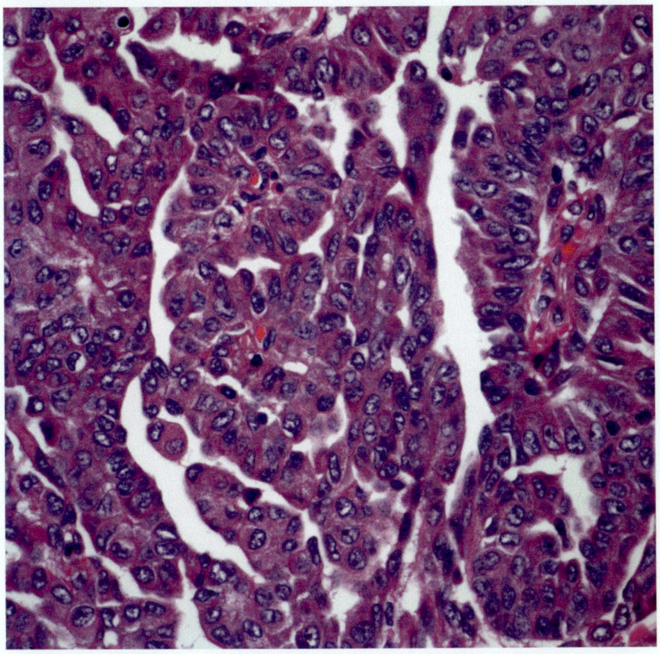

Fig. 12.9 Higher magnification of an epithelioid mesothelioma. Note the absence of prominent nuclear atypia or increased mitotic activity

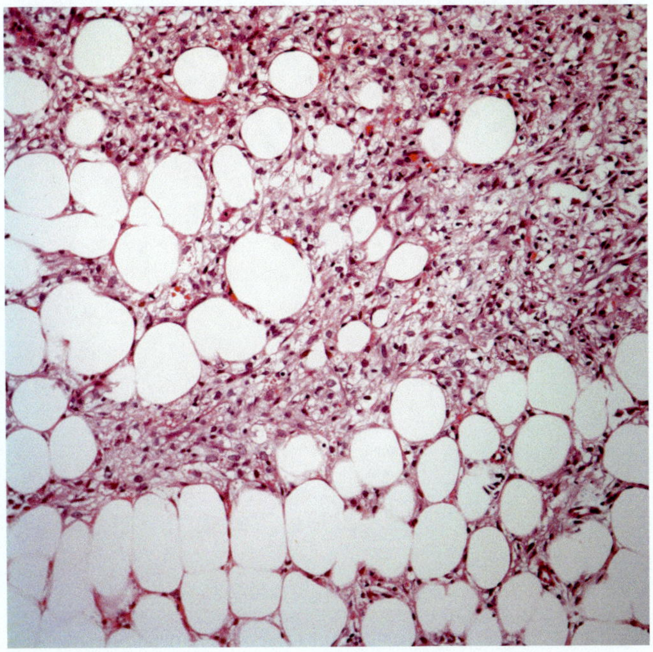

Fig. 12.11 Clear cell mesothelioma infiltrating into adipose tissue

not prominent, and focal areas of necrosis may be seen. This growth pattern mimics clear cell carcinoma of renal origin.

- *Glandular* (Figs. 12.14a, b and 12.15): The tumor is characterized by the presence of well-formed glands similar to those seen in cases of adenocarcinoma. The glandular proliferation appears to dissect fibroconnective tissue, and in some cases, there may be a desmoplastic reaction with an inflammatory infiltrate. This growth pattern closely resembles adenocarcinoma.
- *Myxoid/Mucoid* (Figs. 12.16 and 12.17a, b): The neoplastic cellular proliferation is embedded in a myxoid or mucoid

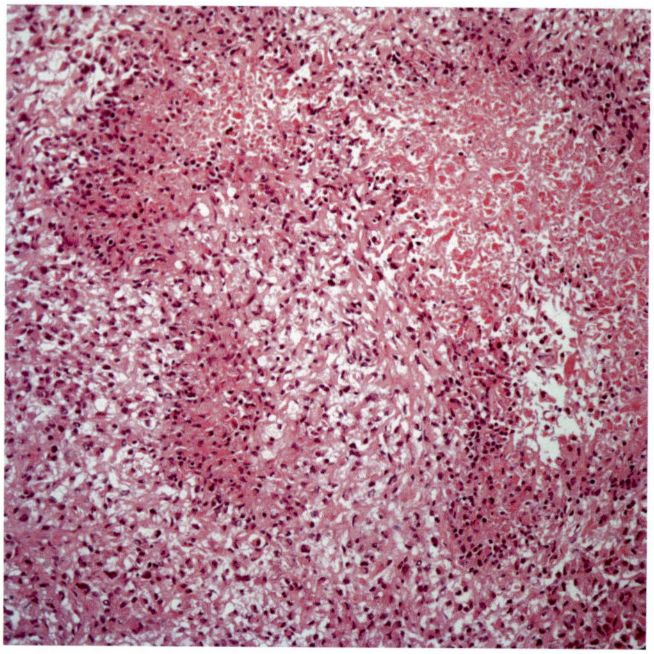

Fig. 12.12 Clear cell mesothelioma with focal areas of necrosis

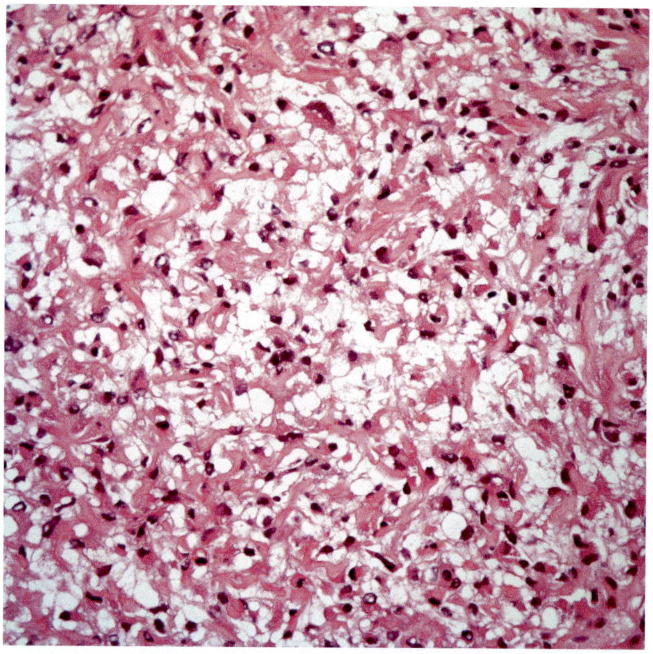

Fig. 12.13 Higher magnification of a clear cell mesothelioma showing moderate nuclear atypia but lack of mitotic activity

background. The tumor may display glandular differentiation, which can be easily confused for adenocarcinoma, or the tumor may show the conventional tubulopapillary growth pattern. In some cases, the tumor can show such abundant mucoid material, that it can be confused with a mucinous adenocarcinoma. However, in these cases, a mucicarmine stain does not show intracellular mucin production.

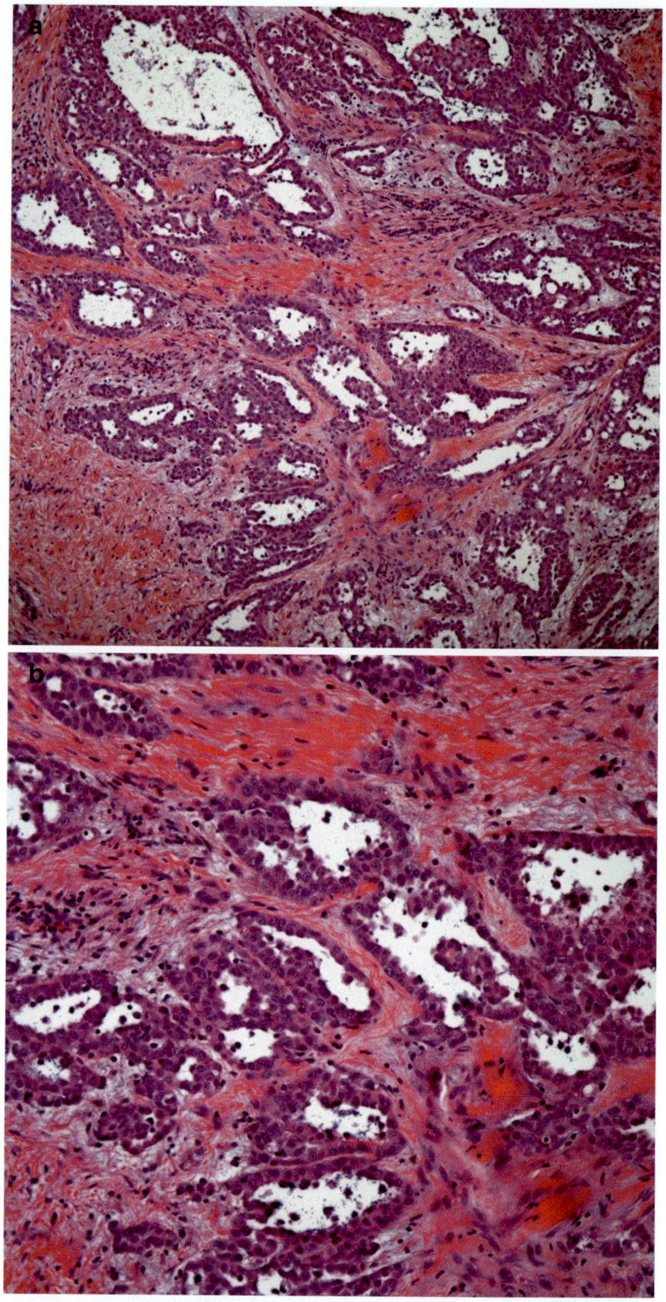

Fig. 12.14 (**a**) Epithelioid mesothelioma showing a prominent glandular growth pattern. (**b**) In some areas the gland-like structures are embedded in fibroconnective tissue

- *Adenomatoid* (Figs. 12.18, 12.19, and 12.20): This growth pattern closely resembles that of the conventional adenomatoid tumor. Cords of medium-size cells with clear cytoplasm and displacement of the nuclei toward the periphery of the cells characterize the tumors. Nuclear atypia, mitotic activity, necrosis, and/or hemorrhage is not common.
- *Deciduoid* (Figs. 12.21, 12.22, and 12.23): This tumor is characterized by the presence of a cellular proliferation

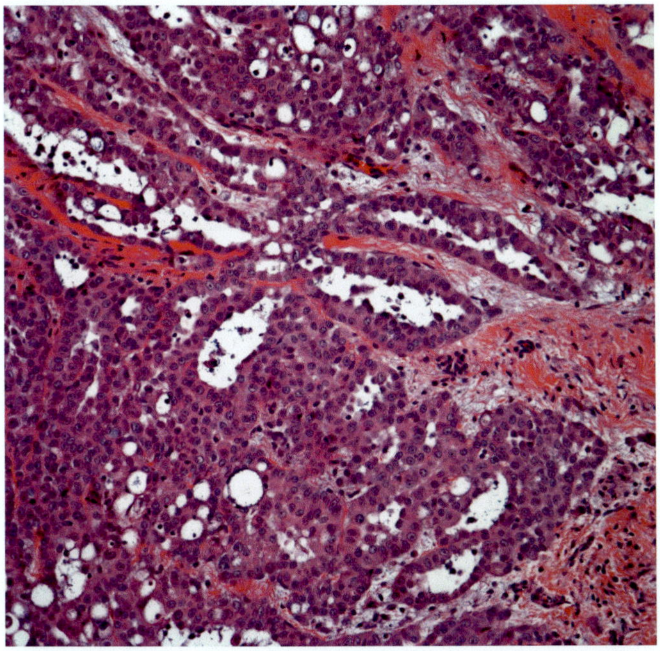

Fig. 12.15 Epithelioid mesothelioma showing areas of glandular and solid growth patterns

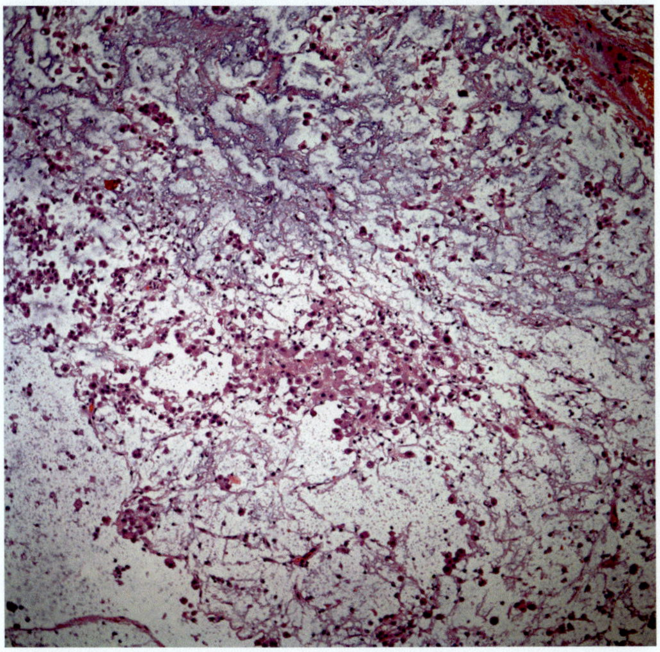

Fig. 12.16 Epithelioid mesothelioma showing mesothelial cells embedded in a mucoid stroma

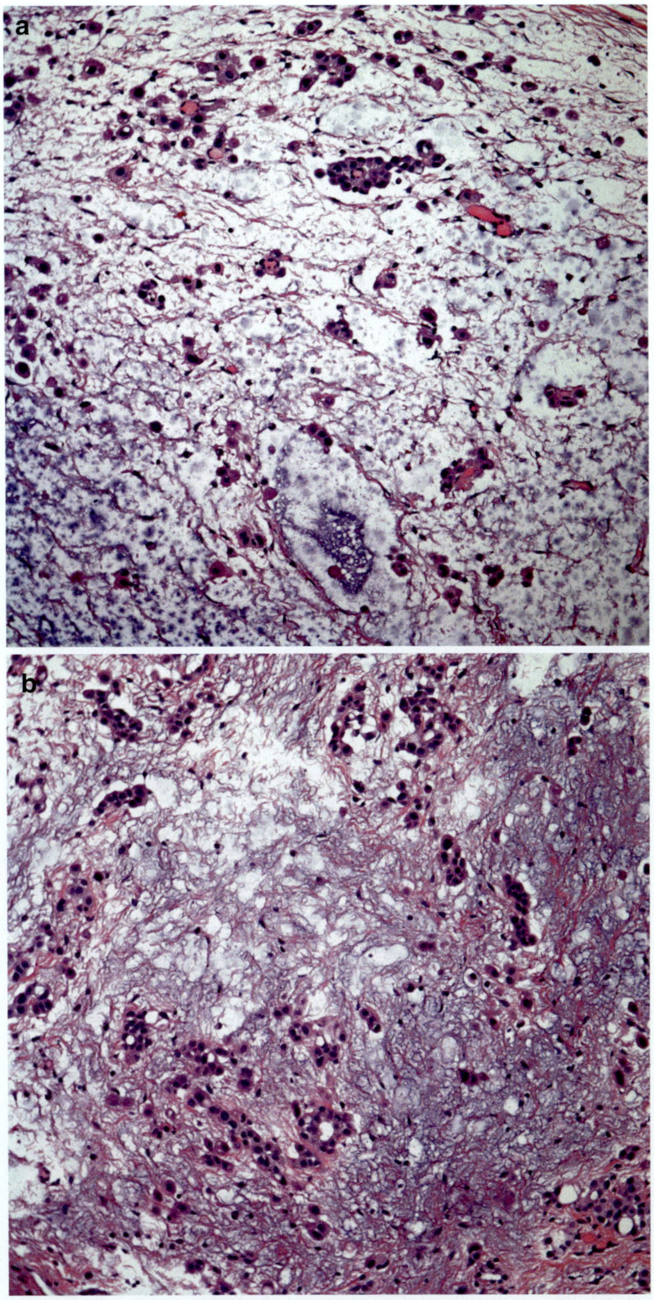

Fig. 12.17 (**a**) Cluster of malignant cells and single cells embedded in a mucoid stroma. (**b**) In some other areas the cellularity is higher and the stroma has a mucoid/chondroid-like appearance

composed of medium-size cells with eosinophilic cytoplasm displaying a "deciduoid" appearance similar to that seen in the gravid uterus.

- *Cartilaginous and osseous metaplasia* (Fig. 12.24): This variant of mesothelioma represents a highly unusual growth pattern and may pose serious diagnostic problems. The tumor characteristically shows areas of "osteoid" formation or immature cartilage that may be confused with a primary bone or cartilage tumor. However, dispersed among the cartilaginous or osseous changes, there is cellular proliferation composed of medium-size cells with round to oval nuclei and conspicuous nucleoli. In some areas, the cellular proliferation may show spindle cell features or a mixture of spindle and epithelioid cells.

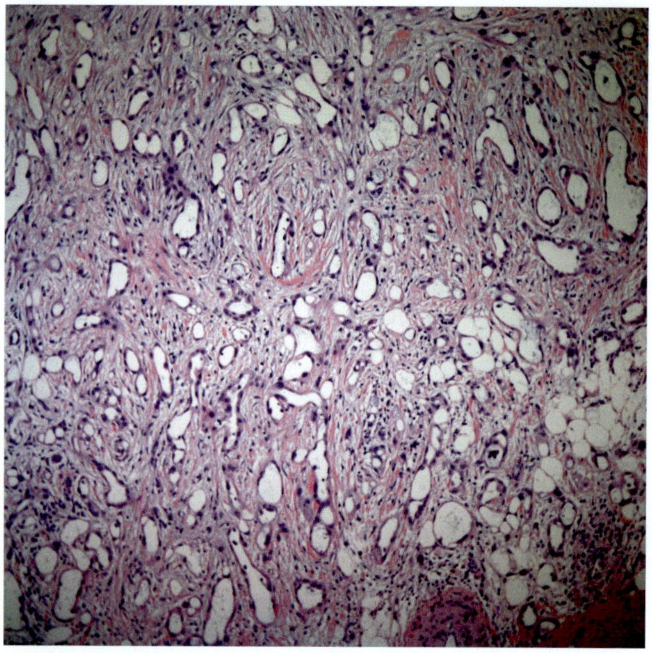

Fig. 12.18 Epithelioid mesothelioma showing prominent "adenomatoid" features

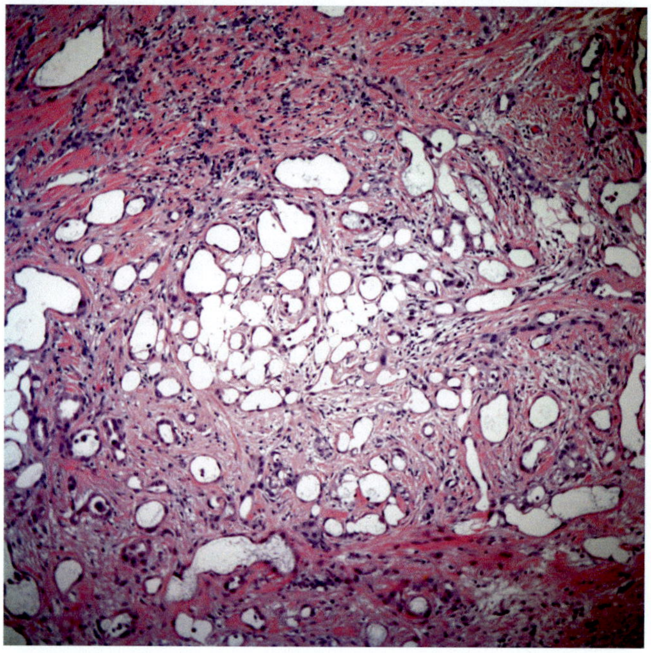

Fig. 12.19 Adenomatoid mesothelioma infiltrating into fibroconnective tissue

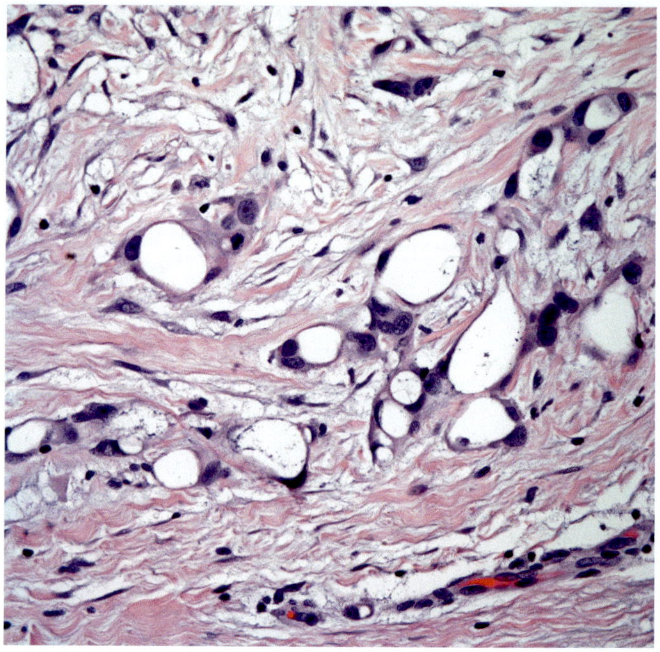

Fig. 12.20 Higher magnification of an adenomatoid mesothelioma showing areas mimicking signet ring cell-like features

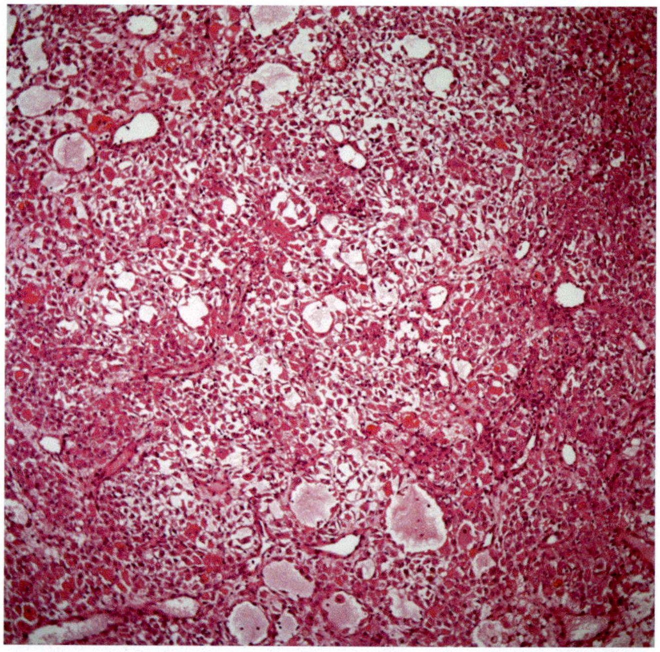

Fig. 12.21 Deciduoid mesothelioma composed of sheets of neoplastic cells

It is comforting to know, however, that among the described histopathological growth patterns, the tubulopapillary is the most common one and the one easiest to recognize. However, it is very important to be familiar at least in theory with the other growth patterns in order to properly assess a possible differential diagnosis. Regardless of the growth pattern, whether the tumor shows clear cell change, myxoid areas, glandular differentiation, or an adenomatoid pattern, one cannot overlook the fact that radiologically the tumor characteristically involves the pleura in a diffuse manner. This latter fact should always alert the pathologist to the possibility of mesothelioma. It is also important to note that in the great majority of cases, only a small biopsy is available to render a diagnosis. Recently, Arrossi et al. [32] evaluated

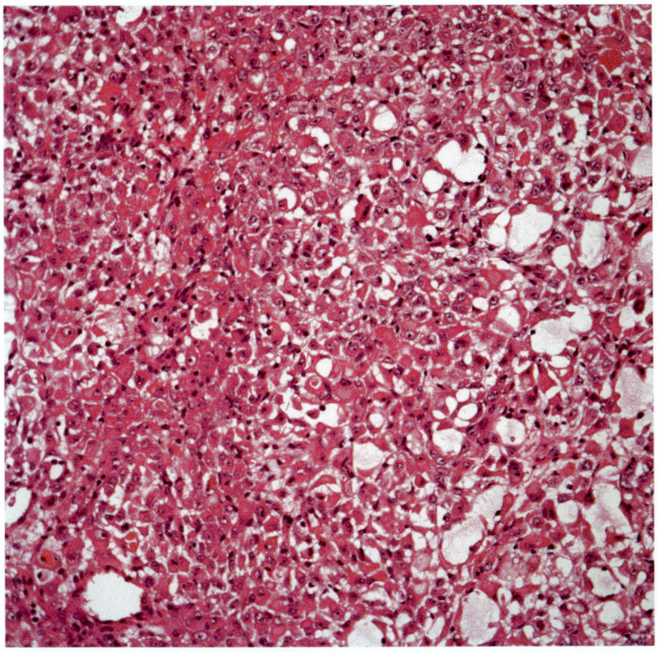

Fig. 12.22 Deciduoid mesothelioma showing a fairly homogeneous neoplastic cellular proliferation. Note the absence of necrosis or prominent nuclear atypia

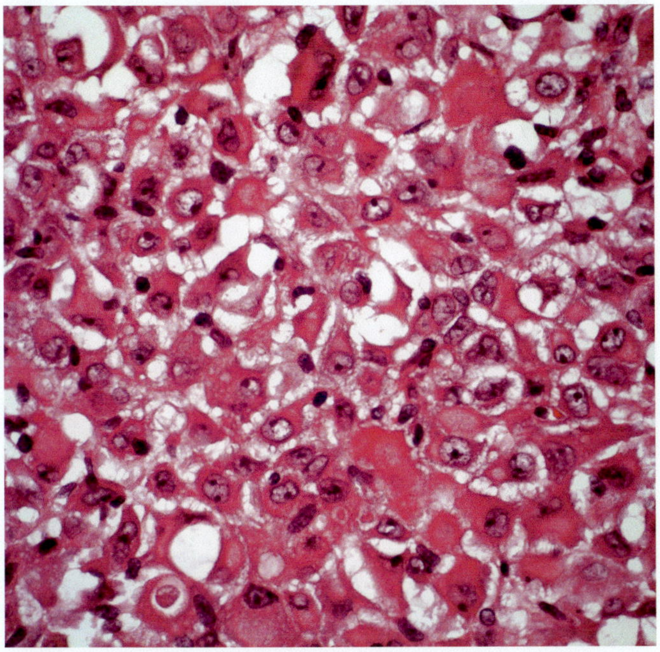

Fig. 12.23 Higher magnification of a deciduoid mesothelioma showing relatively large cells with round to oval nuclei and ample eosinophilic cytoplasm. Mitotic activity is not present

56 cases of extrapleural pneumonectomy to correlate the original subtype of mesothelioma on biopsy specimen versus the resected specimen. The authors found that in many cases, mesotheliomas need further reclassification after more complete histologoical evaluation is possible.

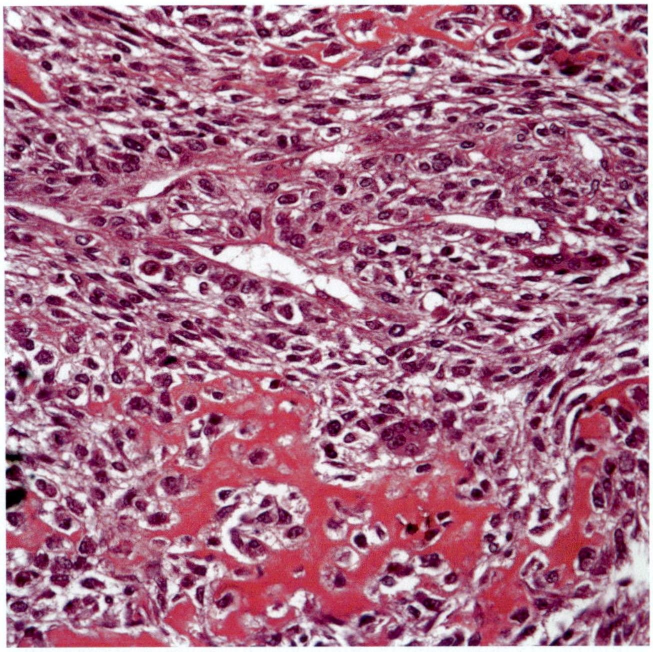

Fig. 12.24 Epithelioid mesothelioma showing areas of osteoid differentiation

Histochemical Features

Traditionally and before the widespread use of immunohistochemistry, histochemical stains played an important role in the diagnosis of mesothelioma. Currently, these stains can still help solve the problem easily in the more banal cases. The use of PAS with and without diastase digestion and mucicarmine on one hand or, hyaluronic acid with and without diastase digestion on the other has been used in the past with some success. Although either histochemical technique is very good, one should primarily evaluate the technique that one is more familiar with, and only one of these techniques should suffice in order to evaluate a particular lesion. It is important to state that although a positive finding of intracellular mucin is a strong indicator of adenocarcinoma, this finding has also been reported in up to 5 % of the cases of mesothelioma. It is also important to note that some mesotheliomas will show abundant extracellular mucin; however, they lack intracellular mucin. However, in current practice, the use of histochemical techniques many times is bypassed for the use of immunohistochemical stains often due to the fact that only a small biopsy is submitted for evaluation.

Immunohistochemical Features

The use of immunohistochemical studies in the evaluation of mesotheliomas has been the subject of numerous well-designed studies, which have brought considerable knowledge to the diagnosis of this tumor. Recent attempts to define the application and limitation of these studies have been reviewed in order to provide important practical information

Table 12.1 Practical immunohistochemical approach to the diagnosis of mesothelioma versus adenocarcinoma

Stain	Mesothelioma	Adenocarcinoma
TTF-1	Negative	Positive
MOC-31	Negative[a]	Positive
Pan-Keratin	Positive	Positive
Keratin 5/6	Positive	Negative
Calretinin	Positive	Negative[b]
CD15	Negative	Positive
B72.3	Negative	Positive
D2-40	Positive	Negative

[a]MOC-31 may show some focal positive staining in some cases of mesothelioma

[b]Calretinin is usually negative in lung adenocarcinomas but has been shown positive in other carcinomas of non-pulmonary origin

in the evaluation of mesotheliomas [33–35]. Numerous studies attempting to positively identify mesothelioma markers have been published, some of them with relative usefulness, while others have merely attempted to identify adenocarcinomatous epitopes in order to properly rule out the presence of mesothelioma. Consequently, in the past, the diagnosis of mesothelioma has been considered one of exclusion. Although there is essentially a wide spectrum of immunohistochemical markers that have been stated to be helpful in the diagnosis of these tumors, only a few are used in practice. A practical approach to the use of immunohistochemical stains in the diagnosis of mesothelioma is presented in Table 12.1.

For practical purposes we can separate these markers into positive and negative markers for mesothelioma. The positive markers for mesothelioma would include keratin 5/6 (Fig. 12.25), calretinin (Fig. 12.26), Wilms' tumor susceptibility gene (WT1), HBME-1, thrombomodulin, and mesothelin.

Keratin 5/6 labels epithelioid mesotheliomas in approximately 90 % of cases. It is considered a valuable marker for mesothelioma [36–39]; however, this antibody may also be seen positive in carcinomas of extra-thoracic origin [36, 40] and also in cases of squamous cell carcinoma of the lung. Therefore, its value depends largely on the setting in which this antibody is used. Calretinin is a member of a large family of cytoplasmic calcium-binding proteins and labels approximately 85 % of cases of mesothelioma of the epithelioid type. Of the three antibodies in the family of calcium-binding proteins, only calretinin labels mesothelioma and nonneoplastic mesothelium [41–43]. WT1 is the product of the Wilms' tumor gene, a tumor suppressor located on 11p13 in mesangial cells of the kidney. WT1 shows strong positive reaction in mesotheliomas; however, WT1 may also show positive reaction in tumor cells of other neoplasms including ovarian and peritoneal serous carcinomas, malignant melanoma, and renal cell carcinoma. Therefore, care must be used in the interpretation of this antibody [44–50]. HBME-1

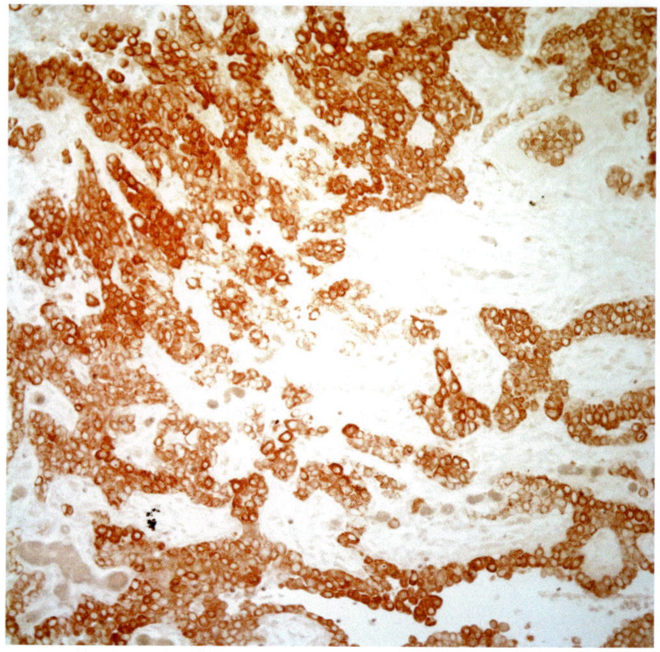

Fig. 12.25 Immunohistochemical stains for keratin 5/6 showing positive staining in tumor cells

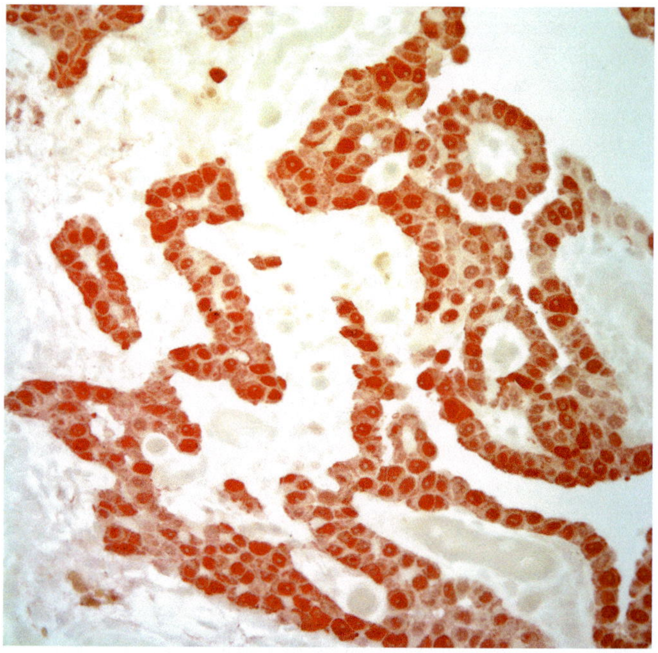

Fig. 12.26 Immunohistochemical stain for calretinin showing positive nuclear and cytoplasmic staining in tumor cells

was generated from a human cell line derived from a patient with malignant mesothelioma. This antibody decorates the membrane of mesothelial cells as opposed to cytoplasmic staining in adenocarcinomas [51]. However, because of this caveat, HMBE-1 may not be a highly reliable marker of mesothelioma since a good percentage of adenocarcinomas and serous tumors of the ovary may also show positive staining [51, 52]. Thrombomodulin (CD141) is a glycoprotein expressed in endothelial cells and in a variety of other cell types, including mesothelial cells. Several reports have been presented in the literature with different claims ranging from 60 to 100 % staining in malignant mesotheliomas. Thrombomodulin may also show positive staining in about 75 % of adenocarcinomas, therefore limiting its usefulness [53–55]. Mesothelin is a surface protein that is expressed in the membrane of neoplastic cells in mesotheliomas and in nonneoplastic mesothelial cells. Mesothelin may also show positive staining in serous carcinomas of the ovary, pancreatic adenocarcinomas, cholangiocarcinoma, colonic adenocarcinoma, and pulmonary adenocarcinoma [56–59]. More recently D2-40, which is a marker of lymphatics, has also shown to be helpful in the diagnosis of mesothelioma as it stains mesothelial cells.

On the contrary, there are a wide variety of markers that have been used in the diagnosis of mesothelioma but mainly in the context of ruling out adenocarcinoma. The most common markers used in this scenario include carcinoembryonic antigen (CEA), MOC-31, thyroid transcription factor-1 (TTF-1), CD15, and B72.3; other markers include Ber-EP4 and BG-8. Clearly the goal is to have a positive marker that may exclude the possibility of mesothelioma.

CEA is a highly reliable marker to distinguish adenocarcinoma from mesothelioma since the vast majority of mesotheliomas are negative for this antibody. Although up to 5% of mesotheliomas have been claimed to be positive for this marker, some studies have suggested that this staining is due to the use of an unabsorbed heteroantiserum to CEA labelling unrelated epitopes. In this setting, the use of monoclonal antibodies to specific CEA epitopes is more reliable [60–67]. MOC-31 has been reported in several studies as an important marker in the separation between mesothelioma and adenocarcinoma, as this marker is purportedly seen positive in adenocarcinoma [68–70]. However, in our experience, some cases of mesothelioma may show focal and spotty positive staining for MOC-31. TTF-1 is expressed in normal lung and thyroid epithelial cells. TTF-1 shows high specificity for lung adenocarcinoma, and so far it has been reported to be negative in mesotheliomas. The use of TTF-1 may prove useful in cases in which the tumor in question is an adenocarcinoma of lung origin [71–73]. However, it is also important to keep in mind that not all pulmonary adenocarcinomas are positive for this marker. CD15 has a high level of specificity for adenocarcinoma; however, some mesotheliomas, namely, peritoneal mesotheliomas may also show positive staining in tumor cells [74, 75]. B72.3 is a generic epithelial determinant (tumor-associated glycoprotein-72), which is a high molecular weight cell membrane glycoprotein. Although a good marker for adenocarcinoma, some cases of mesotheliomas may also show focal positive staining [66, 76]. As previously stated, the number of antibodies used in the diagnosis of mesothelioma goes beyond the scope of this chapter; some of these markers have been presented in the literature as very specific for the distinction between adenocarcinoma and mesothelioma. However, as they are tested against other tumors, these antibodies have shown unreliability for such a distinction. One of those antibodies is Ber-EP4, which was originally presented as specific for adenocarcinoma; however, it has shown to cross-react with mesotheliomas in more than 20 % of the cases [75]. BG-8 is another antibody that may react strongly in cases of adenocarcinoma; however, some cases of mesotheliomas may also show positive staining [77].

Electron Microscopy

Ultrastructural analysis in cases of mesothelioma is very important due to the specific features that these tumors show. The use of ultrastructural studies in many cases is limited by the lack of material when it is needed the most. In the majority of cases, the initial biopsy, which is the one in which one needs to establish the diagnosis, is the only material available for diagnosis, thus, limiting its use. On the other hand, the use of electron microscopic features is helpful in the better differentiated tumors, while in those cases in which the tumor is poorly differentiated, the ultrastructural findings are rarely helpful. It is not uncommon to see that in most cases in which immunohistochemistry has failed to provide a clear interpretation of the tumor electron microscopy will also be questionable. Nevertheless, it can be very helpful and one should make every effort to obtain a sample for such studies. The finding of long, slender microvilli is a classical feature for mesothelioma. More recently, Ordonez [78] described nine cases of pleural mesotheliomas in which the author demonstrated the presence of crystalloid structures, which in turn can also be used as another identifiable feature of mesothelioma.

Differential Diagnosis

The most important conditions to rule out in the differential diagnosis of mesothelioma are either pulmonary adenocarcinoma that has extended into the pleura, a metastatic epithelial tumor of other origin, or more importantly atypical mesothelial hyperplasia. If one has concluded that the cellular proliferation in question is malignant, then the use of immunohistochemical studies, namely, the use of carcinomatous epitopes, as previously mentioned in the section on immunohistochemistry, will be the next step and needed to rule out either metastatic adenocarcinoma from the lung or elsewhere. The interpretation can be more difficult in cases of mesothelial hyperplasia. In this setting, there is no immunohistochemical stain, which can separate a neoplastic cellular proliferation from a hyperplastic one. Therefore, it is imperative not only to correlate the histology with the clinical and radiological features but also to properly interpret the results of the immunohistochemical studies. As a matter of fact, even electron microscopic studies would fail to separate such cellular proliferations. Such diagnosis becomes a morphologic one and requires careful attention to specific histopathological features such as invasion into adipose tissue or skeletal muscle, which are features associated with malignant mesothelioma.

Sarcomatoid Mesothelioma

Although a well-recognized growth pattern, sarcomatoid mesothelioma is less common than its counterpart the epithelioid type and accounts for approximately 10–15 % of tumors in its pure form. The tumor characteristically has a growth pattern of spindle cells with elongated nuclei and inconspicuous nucleoli in a manner resembling a sarcoma of soft tissues. Carter and Otis [79] in a study of spindle cell tumors of the pleura concluded that there are three types of these tumors that may range from low grade (possibly benign) to high grade tumors and separated them into fibroma (keratin-negative tumor), sarcomatoid mesothelioma (keratin-positive tumor), and sarcoma (malignant spindle cell tumor—keratin negative). Due to a possible overlap in histopathological features, the use of immunohistochemical stains were proposed to play an important role in this context.

Sarcomatoid mesotheliomas of the pleura can be further subdivided into three distinct categories based on their growth pattern:

- *Spindle cell type* (*fibrosarcoma-like or MFH-like*) (Figs. 12.27, 12.28, 12.29, 12.30, 12.31, 12.32, and 12.33): The diagnosis of either one of these variants is rather straightforward. In the fibrosarcoma-like pattern, the tumor is composed of a spindle cellular proliferation that may show the so-called herringbone pattern with intersecting fascicles of spindle cells showing indistinguishable cell membranes, moderate amounts of light eosinophilic cytoplasm, elongated nuclei, and inconspicuous nucleoli. Nuclear atypia is present and mitotic activity is easily encountered. In the MFH-like pattern, the tumor displays features of a high grade sarcoma with a fascicular growth pattern composed of spindle and/or oval cells with elongated or round nuclei and conspicuous nucleoli. In addition, the tumor may also show the presence of multinucleated malignant giant cells intermixed with the spindle cell proliferation. Nuclear atypia is prominent and mitotic activity is easily encountered.
- *Desmoplastic mesothelioma* (Figs. 12.34, 12.35, 12.36, 12.37, 12.38, and 12.39): The diagnosis of desmoplastic mesothelioma may pose a serious challenge in diagnosis mainly when only a limited biopsy material is available for interpretation. Initially described by Kannerstein and Churg [80] in 1980, this variant has been further analyzed in different reports. Cantin et al. [81] reported 27 cases in which the authors concluded that the clinical course was often rapid and that the mean survival for

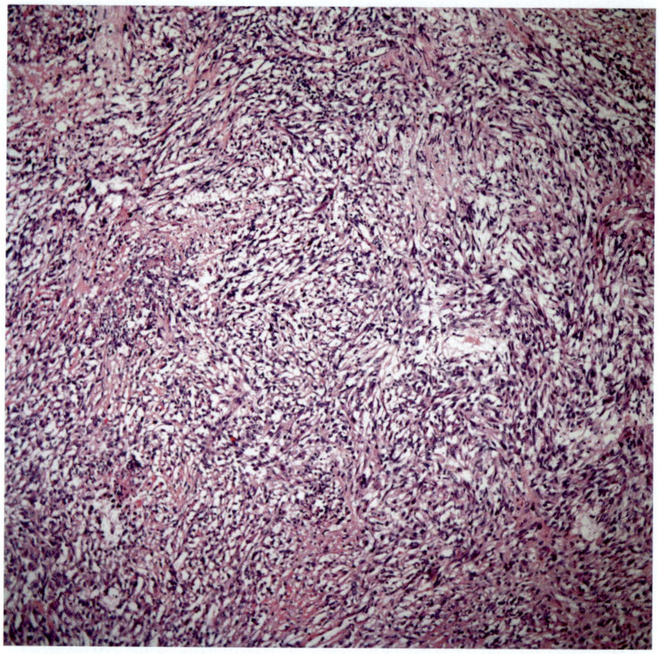

Fig. 12.27 Low power view of a sarcomatoid mesothelioma. Note the prominent spindle cell features

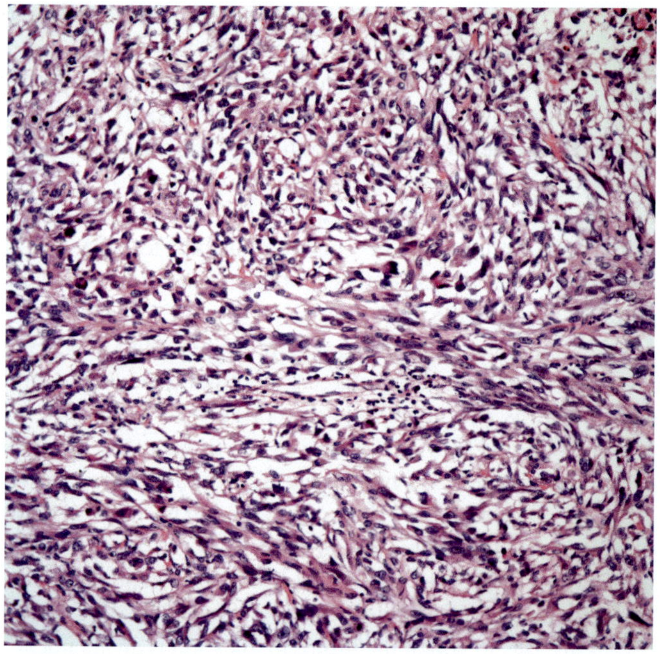

Fig. 12.28 Closer view of the malignant spindle cell proliferation arranged in a subtle storiform pattern

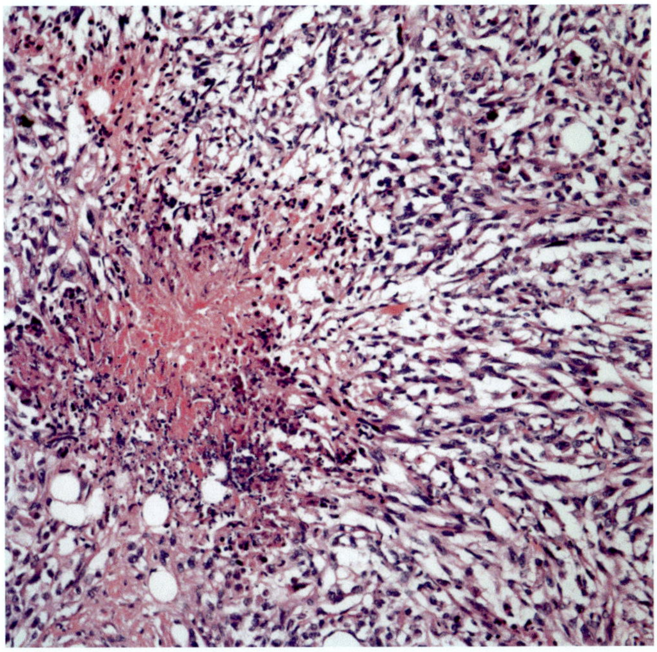

Fig. 12.29 Areas of necrosis are sometimes encountered, even though they may not be apparent in biopsy specimens

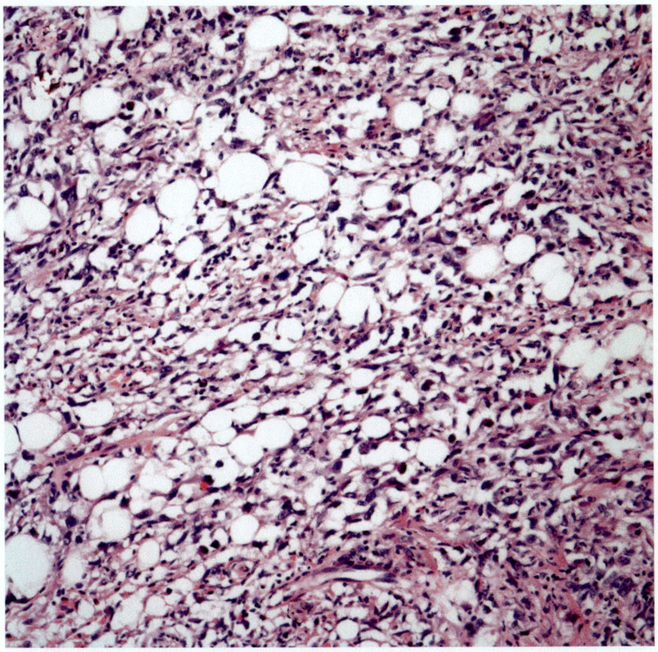

Fig. 12.30 Malignant spindle cell invading into adipose tissue

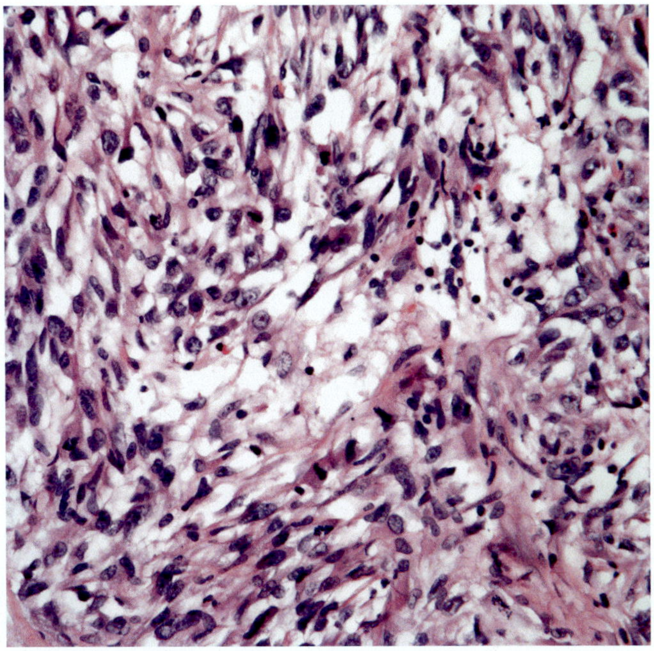

Fig. 12.31 Numerous mitotic figures are present in this sarcomatoid mesothelioma

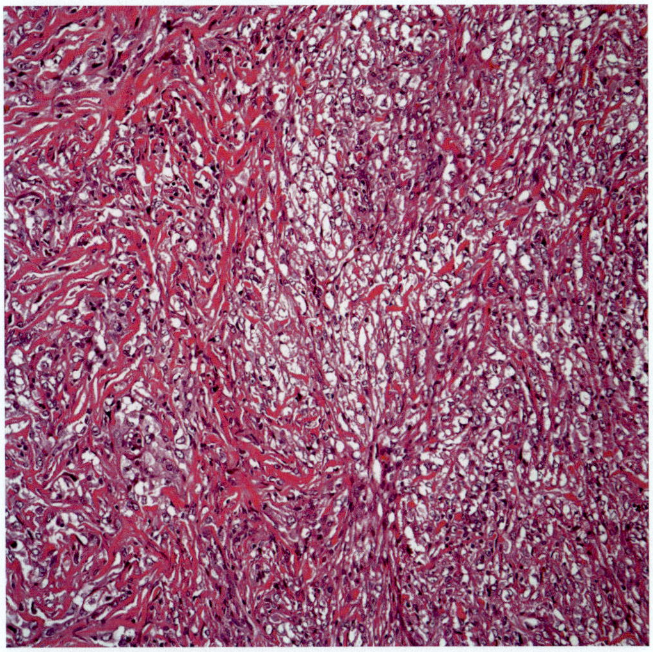

Fig. 12.32 Malignant spindle cells dissecting into fibrocollagenous tissue

cases in which there was pure sarcomatoid tumor was about 6.18 months. In their experience, desmoplastic mesothelioma also shows more tendency toward metastatic disease with 60 % compared to 40 % of the non-desmoplastic variant. Also Mangano et al. [82] reported a series of 31 cases in which the emphasis was to separate desmoplastic mesotheliomas from fibrous pleurisy. The authors reported the presence of p53 in these two conditions and concluded that it can be positive in both conditions and although more commonly seen in

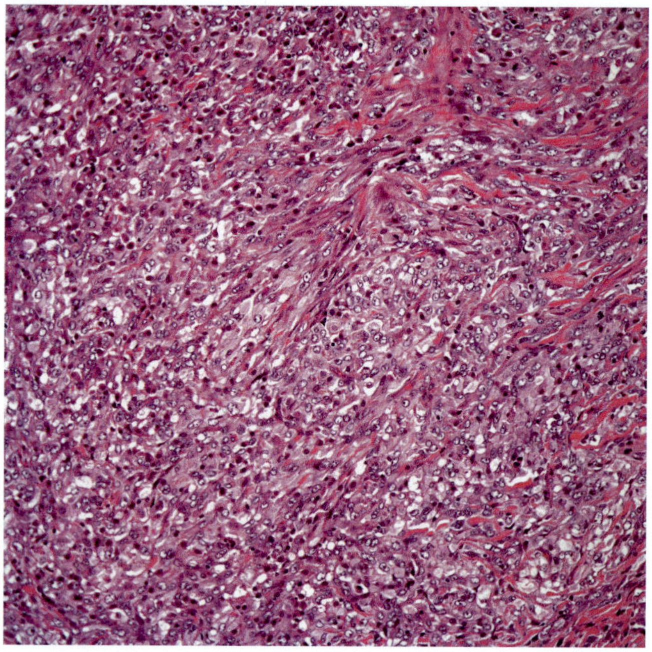

Fig. 12.33 Closer view of the spindle cells with more fibroblastic-like appearance

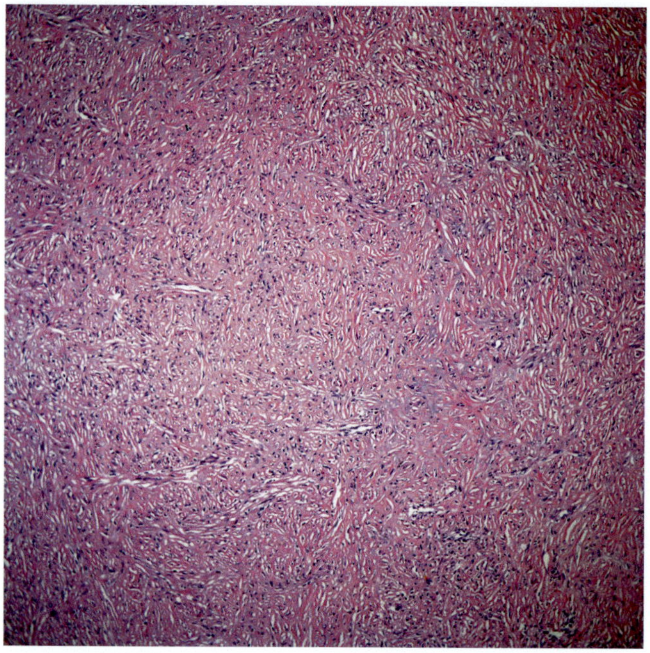

Fig. 12.34 Low power view of a desmoplastic mesothelioma. Note the lack of prominent cellularity

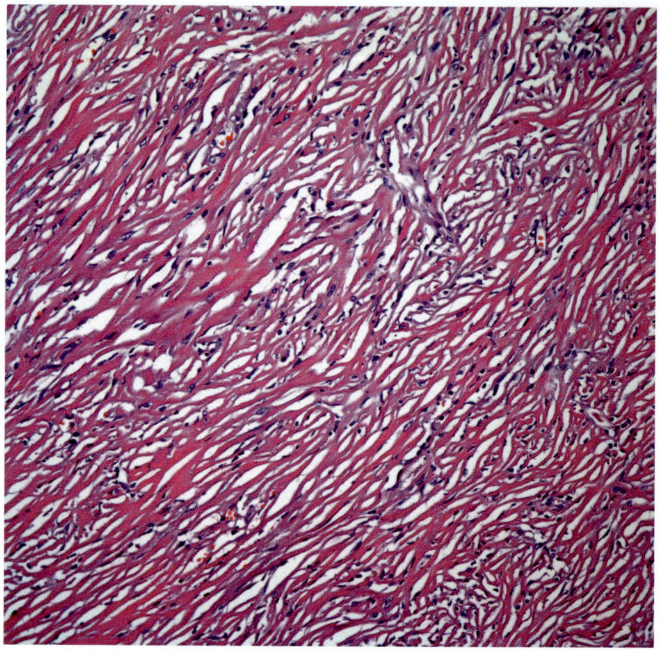

Fig. 12.35 Desmoplastic mesothelioma with extensive collagenization

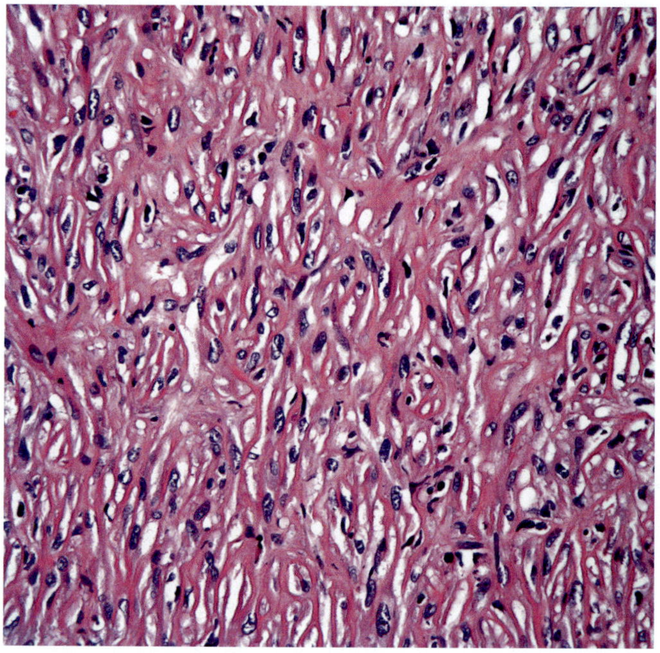

Fig. 12.36 Higher magnification of desmoplastic mesothelioma showing spindle cells dissecting fibrocollagen

desmoplastic mesothelioma, the difference in staining was not statistically significant. Histologically, these tumors may show extensive areas of collagenization with a very discrete spindle cell proliferation, which may be missed in a cursory review of the histological sections. The most salient histopathological features [82, 83] that have been associated with the diagnosis of desmoplastic mesothelioma include:

– Invasion of chest wall or lung
– Foci of bland necrosis
– Frank sarcomatoid foci
– Distant metastasis

It is obvious that the aforementioned criteria apply to resected specimens, pleural peeling, or a very generous pleural biopsy. Otherwise, in a small sample, such diagnosis may prove to be very difficult if not impossible. To that

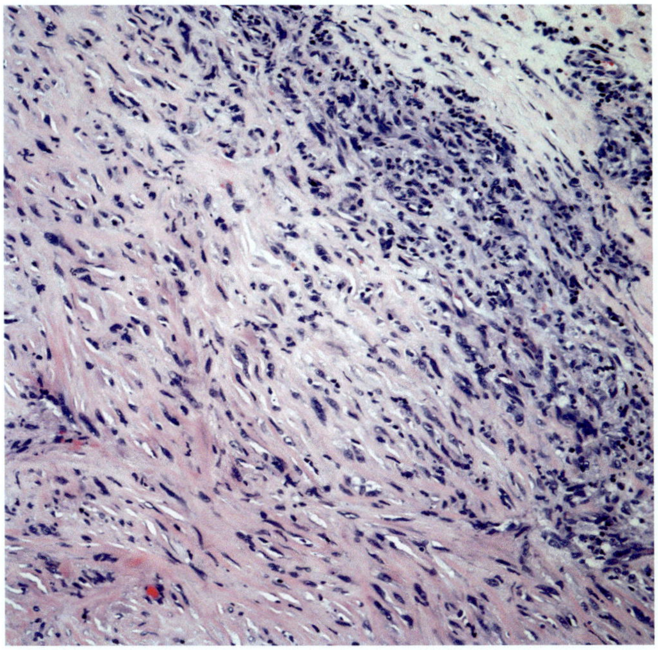

Fig. 12.37 Desmoplastic mesothelioma with focal areas of inflammatory cells

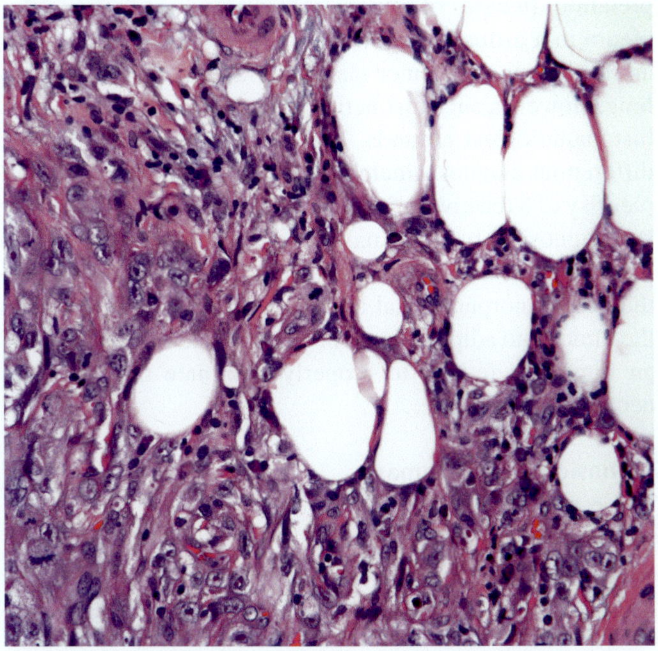

Fig. 12.38 Desmoplastic mesothelioma infiltrating adipose tissue

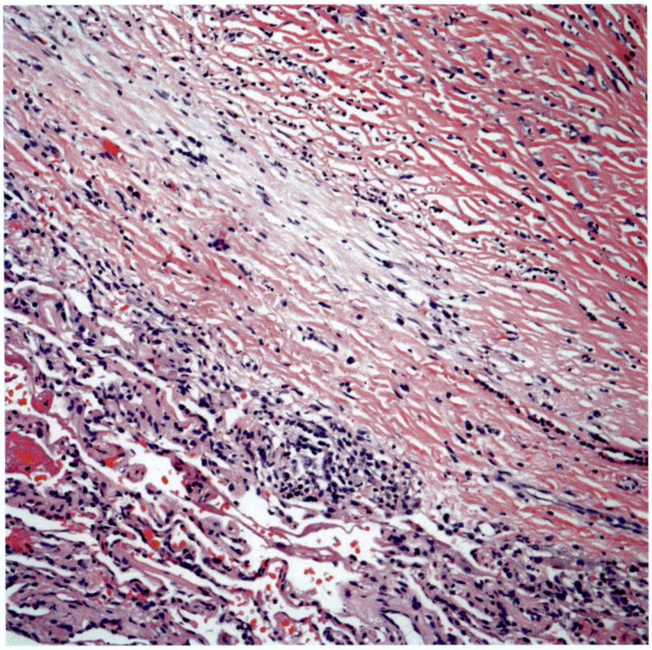

Fig. 12.39 Desmoplastic mesothelioma infiltrating lung parenchyma

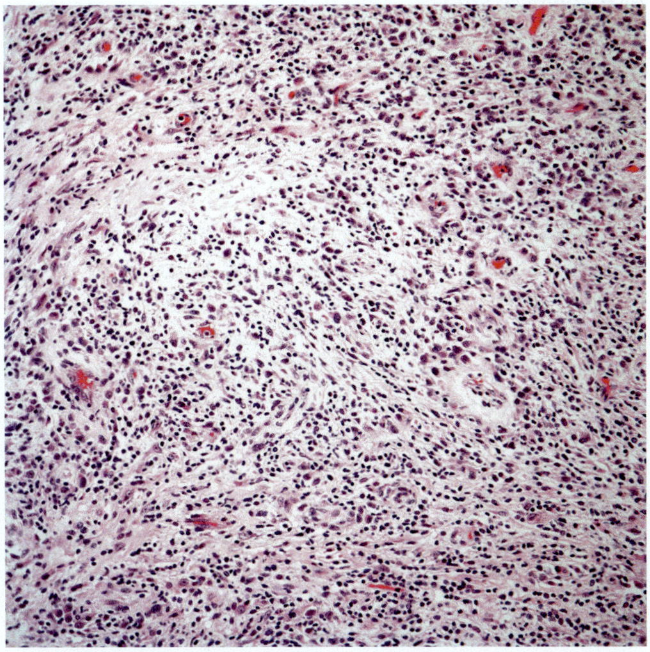

Fig. 12.40 Low power view of a lymphohistiocytic mesothelioma showing a mixture of spindle cells and lymphocytes

extent, Colby [83] has warned about the care that must be exercised when making such a diagnosis and has stated that since there is not a proven therapy for desmoplastic mesothelioma, underdiagnosis is preferable to overdiagnosis. This latter statement cannot be emphasized enough given the current tendency of performing extrapleural pneumonectomies for the treatment of mesothelioma.

- *Lymphohistiocytoid* variant (Figs. 12.40, 12.41, and 12.42): This type of mesothelioma is included in the subcategory of sarcomatoid mesotheliomas [84], although in some cases the tumor may not be formed by spindle cells but rather by oval cells. This subtype of mesothelioma is unusual and it is characterized by the presence of a prominent lymphoid component admixed with a cellular proliferation composed of epithelial cells with a "histiocytoid appearance".

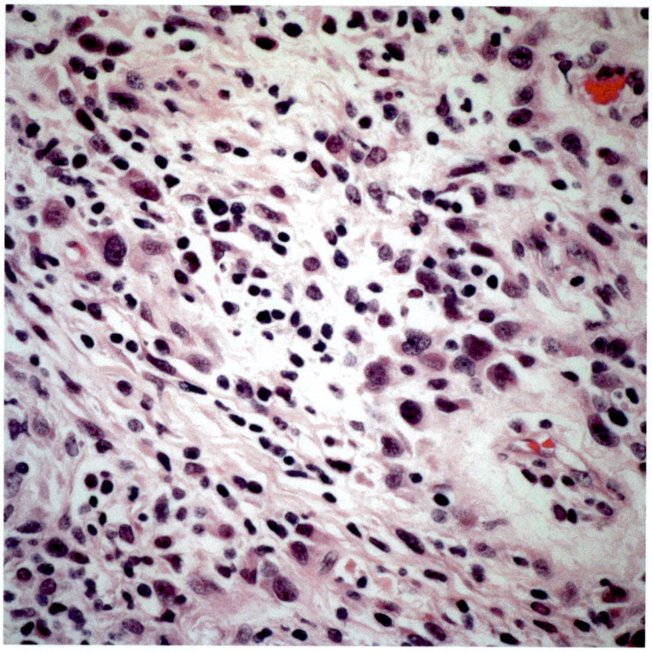

Fig. 12.41 Higher magnification showing an atypical cellular proliferation admixed with lymphocytes

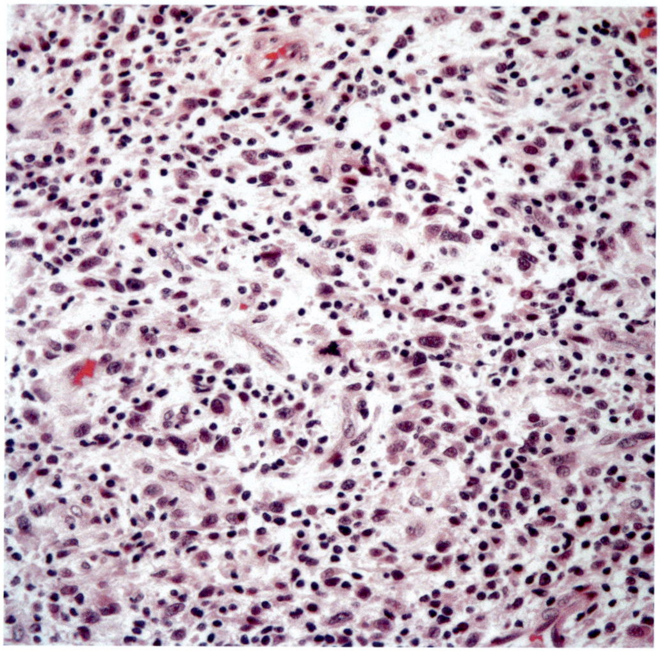

Fig. 12.42 Lymphohistiocytoid mesothelioma showing atypical mitotic figures

Histochemical Studies

The use of histochemical studies such as PAS with and without diastase, mucicarmine, and/or hyaluronic acid with and without diastase digestion has no role in the diagnosis of these tumors.

Immunohistochemical Studies

In the setting of a spindle cell mesothelioma, whether the tumor is desmoplastic or not, the role of immunohistochemistry is relatively limited. Most of the antibodies used in conventional epithelioid mesotheliomas have no practical use in sarcomatoid mesotheliomas. The use of broad-spectrum keratin is by far the most important while all other carcinomatous epitopes are known not to react with sarcomatoid tumors. The use of calretinin and keratin 5/6 is also limited since its positivity may vary and negative results do not rule out a diagnosis of mesothelioma. Because of the lack of more specificity from immunohistochemical markers, the issue of fibrous pleurisy and desmoplastic mesothelioma cannot be solved by immunohistochemistry since both lesions may cross-react with keratin antibodies. In short, the use of immunohistochemistry is primarily limited to rule out other spindle cell tumors of different cell lineage including muscle or fibrous differentiation or other mesenchymal tumors.

Differential Diagnosis

The most important differential diagnosis includes another spindle cell neoplasm of mesenchymal origin. In this setting, the use of proper immunohistochemical studies and/or electron microscopy will lead to a more appropriate interpretation. In cases of sarcomatoid carcinoma involving the pleura in a diffuse manner, tradiographic demonstration of an intrapulmonary tumor mass will favor carcinoma of the lung. However, such distinction may prove to be difficult on histopathological grounds. The most relevant and difficult differential diagnosis includes fibrinous pleuritis or fibrous pleurisy of a reactive or inflammatory nature. In these cases, the diagnosis is based on morphologic grounds since immunohistochemistry cannot solve the problem. To this extent, the use of morphological landmarks such as infiltration of the tumor into adipose tissue or skeletal muscle will become an important feature to properly designate the lesion as neoplastic or reactive.

Biphasic Mesotheliomas

These tumors are composed of a mixture of epithelial and sarcomatoid areas (Figs. 12.43, 12.44, and 12.45). As a rule unequivocal sarcomatoid and epithelioid areas have to be identified in order to classify these tumors as biphasic. The designation of these cases as biphasic mesotheliomas may change from the initial biopsy to the final resected specimen. In a more recent study on the issue of biopsy and resection, a considerable number of cases in which the biphasic nature of the specimen was not easily determined in the original biopsy material [32] were identified. One important differential diagnosis for biphasic mesotheliomas includes primary synovial sarcomas of the pleura. However, in the latter setting the tumor is a pleural-based mass without diffuse pleural involvement. Close clinical and radiological correlation is highly advised in that setting.

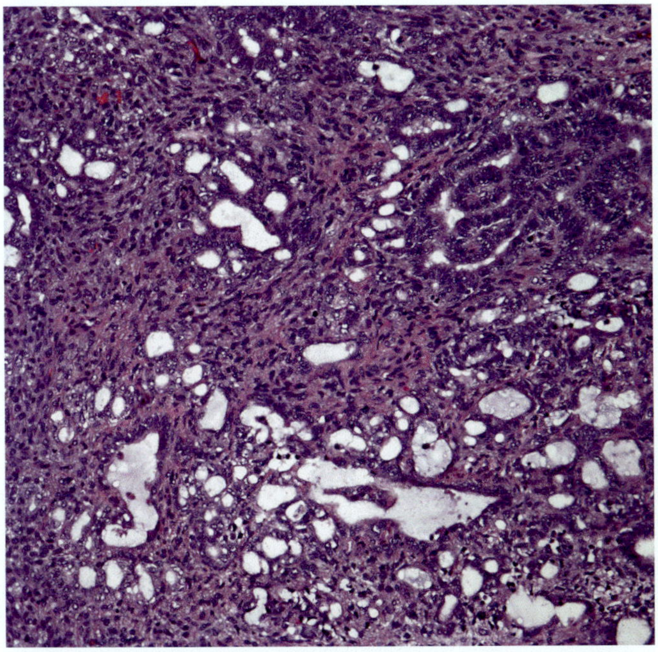

Fig. 12.43 Biphasic mesothelioma showing a mixture of glands and spindle cells

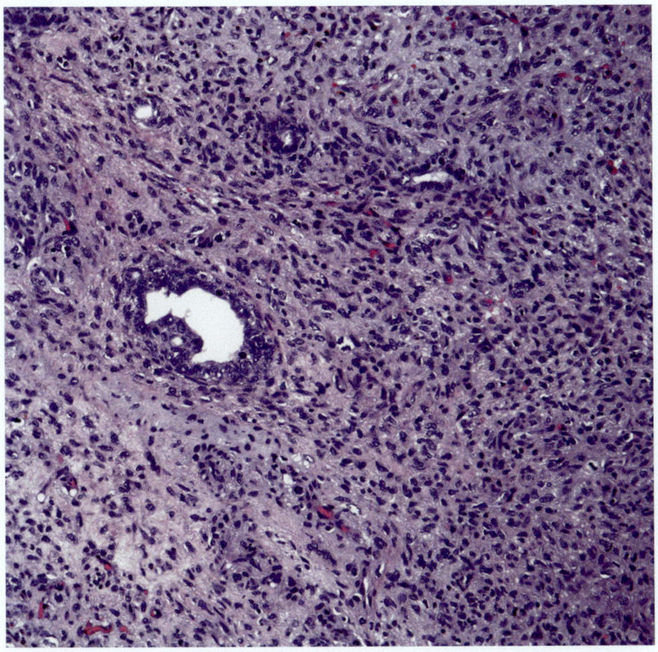

Fig. 12.44 Biphasic mesothelioma showing a predominantly sarcomatoid component

Treatment and Prognosis

The use of extrapleural pneumonectomy as a treatment modality for mesothelioma has become more popular in recent years. Rice [85] recently reviewed this subject and stated that despite improvements in the operative mortality, surgery alone is associated with high rates of local failure. The use of neoadjuvant treatment modalities, which includes radiation, and chemotherapy, appears to be an accepted protocol for these patients. Nevertheless, in the majority of cases, the prognosis is still poor, with survival rates of no more than 12 and 18 months after initial diagnosis. Due to the widespread acceptance of these modalities in the treatment of mesothelioma, it is imperative to develop close correlations among the clinical, radiological, histological, and immunohistochemical features of these patients.

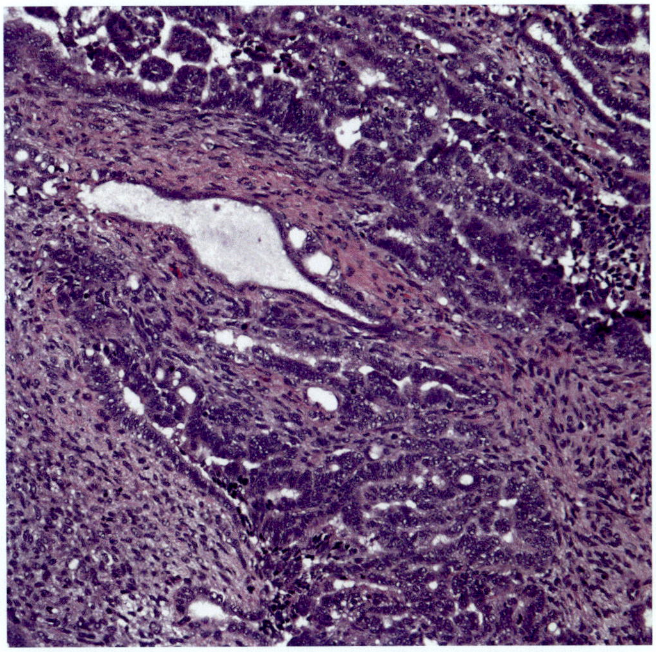

Fig. 12.45 Biphasic mesothelioma showing a predominantly epithelial component

Practical Approach

A conceptual and more practical approach has been suggested for these tumors. Such an approach may be of aid mainly when there are doubts about the diagnosis. Important issues to consider are the following:

- Detailed clinical history
- Detailed radiological information
- Adequate biopsy material (preferably containing adipose tissue or skeletal muscle in order to evaluate invasion)
- Immunohistochemical studies
- Electron microscopy

Clinical Setting

- If the tumor is epithelioid, then the use of a battery of immunohistochemical studies is in order, and these may include keratin 5/6, calretinin, CEA, CD15, B72.3, MOC-31, and TTF-1 and WT1.

- If the tumor is sarcomatoid, then the immunohistochemical studies can be limited to broad-spectrum keratin. Keratin 5/6 and calretinin can be added; however, it is well known that those antibodies may be negative in sarcomatoid mesotheliomas. Other immunohistochemical studies to rule out other mesenchymal neoplasms may be included depending on the degree of suspicion.
- In cases in which the differential diagnosis is between mesothelioma and mesothelial hyperplasia, the diagnosis is essentially based on histopathological grounds by determining invasion, and the use of immunohistochemical studies is not reliable.
- In cases in which the differential diagnosis is between sarcomatoid mesothelioma and fibrous pleurisy, the use of immunohistochemical stains is not reliable, and the diagnosis is based on histopathological grounds by demonstrating invasion.

Pseudomesotheliomatous Adenocarcinoma

The existence of peripheral pulmonary adenocarcinomas growing along the pleural surface is rather uncommon. However, when it occurs it may pose considerable problems in separating this tumor from pleural mesothelioma; therefore, there is a need for the extensive use of immunohistochemical stains. In 1976, Harwood et al. [86] described six cases of pulmonary carcinomas of the lung, which were characterized by diffuse pleural thickening in a manner similar to that described in malignant mesothelioma. The author stated that due to the gross and microscopic characteristics of the tumor, this particular variant of lung carcinoma should be recognized as specific variant and one that the authors named pseudomesotheliomatous carcinoma. Over the last 25 years, several series of cases have been described paying special attention not only to the similarities of this tumor in comparison to malignant mesothelioma but also to provide the necessary tools to separate both conditions due to the treatment implications of both these tumors [87–93].

Clinical Features

There are no specific clinical features to differentiate pseudomesotheliomatous adenocarcinoma of the pleura and malignant mesothelioma. The majority of patients are men over 50 years of age, with a history of tobacco use. Some of these tumors have been reported in patients exposed to asbestos, iron, and stone dust. The most common symptoms include weight loss, dyspnea, cough, chest pain, and pleural effusion. By imaging, the pleura may appear thickened while at thoracotomy extensive thickening of the pleura or the presence of multiple pleural nodules studding the pleural surface may be seen.

Macroscopic Features

The gross features associated with pseudomesotheliomatous adenocarcinoma may mimic those seen in pleural mesotheliomas, namely, the presence of extensive pleural thickening that may encase the entire lung and extend into the pulmonary septa. In some cases, a small peripheral intrapulmonary nodule may be seen, but this feature may not be easily identified. The tumor may also extend to involve the diaphragm or pericardium.

Histological Features

Pseudomesotheliomatous adenocarcinoma closely mimics the epithelioid variant of malignant mesothelioma. It shows areas of glandular, tubular, and/or papillary features embedded in a collagenous stroma (Figs. 12.46a–c and 12.47a, b). The neoplastic cellular proliferation is often haphazardly embedded in a background of collagenous stroma. This stroma may, in some cases, show a desmoplastic reaction, mimicking a biphasic mesothelioma. In some cases, this desmoplastic-like reaction may also contain prominent inflammatory changes.

Histochemical and Immunohistochemical Features

The use of histochemical stains like PAS with and without diastase digestion as well as mucicarmine may be helpful, as the presence of intracellular mucin will lead to a diagnosis of adenocarcinoma. However, such findings may not be present in all cases; therefore, the use of immunohistochemical stains may be necessary. In this setting, the use of carcinomatous epitopes in the evaluation of mesotheliomas may be of help. These carcinomatous epitopes include CEA, B72.3, MOC-31, and TTF-1. Although there is a wider variety of antibodies that can be used, those previously mentioned are part of the practical evaluation of mesothelioma versus adenocarcinoma.

Treatment and Prognosis

Patients with pseudomesotheliomatous adenocarcinomas of the pleura are not candidates for extrapleural pneumonectomy. Therefore, it is important to establish the correct diagnosis and separate pseudomesotheliomatous adenocarcinoma from mesotheliomas. Pseudomesotheliomatous adenocarcinomas are adenocarcinomas in advanced stage (IIIb). Most likely these patients will be treated with chemotherapy. The prognosis is rather poor as the reported survival in larger series is less than 18 months.

Mucoepidermoid Carcinoma

The existence of salivary gland-type tumors in the lung is well known. In the great majority of cases, these tumors occur in a bronchial location. When it comes to the presence of similar tumors on the pleural surface, although rare, their occurrence has been documented. So far, two cases of mucoepidermoid carcinoma presenting as pleural tumors have been described [94]. These two cases presented in adult individuals with no previous

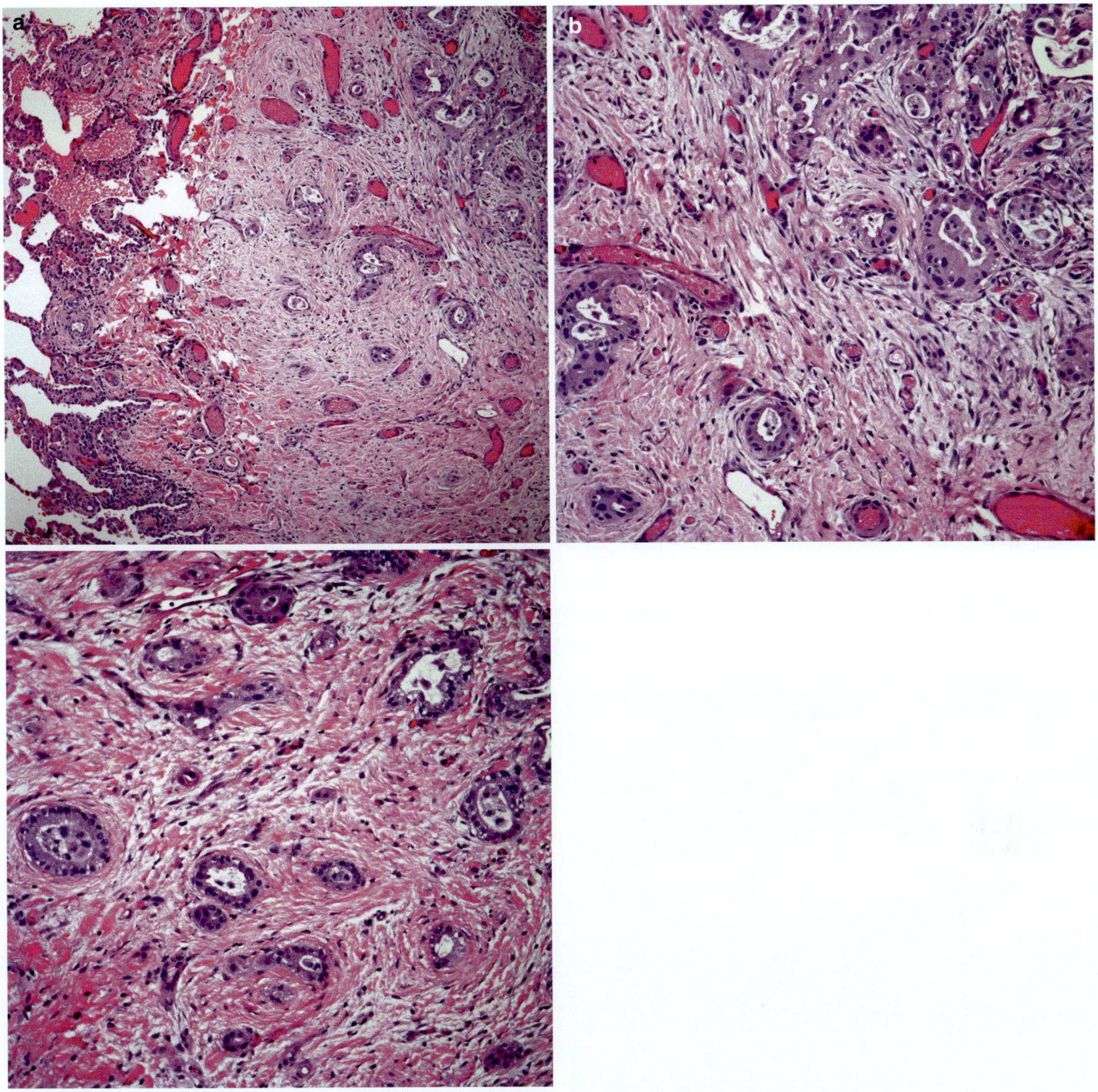

Fig. 12.46 (**a**) Low power view of a pseudomesotheliomatous adenocarcinoma, note the pleural thickening. (**b**) Well-formed glands are embedded in a collagenous stroma. (**c**) Glands are dissecting collagenous stroma with a minimal inflammatory reaction

history of a head and neck neoplasm. Both patients had symptoms of chest pain and shortness of breath. Radiologically, the two tumors were described as pleural-based tumors.

Histopathological Features

The histopathological features of these tumors described are similar to those described for lesions arising in the salivary glands. The tumor exhibits an epithelial cellular proliferation composed of medium-size cells with eosinophilic cytoplasm, round nuclei, and in some cases prominent nucleoli. The cellular proliferation has epidermoid features; however, keratinization is not present. In addition, the presence of mucus-secreting cells admixed with intermediate cells and epidermoid cells is the hallmark of these tumors (Figs. 12.48 and 12.49a–c). Areas of fibrinous pleuritis may also be seen in these cases. In addition, the tumors may show sclerotic areas composed of a spindle fibroblastic cellular proliferation with islands of cells in which the tumor shows the classical elements of intermediate or epidermoid cells admixed with mucus-secreting cells (mucocytes). This so-called sclerosing mucoepidermoid carcinoma has also been described in the pleura (Fig. 12.50a–c).

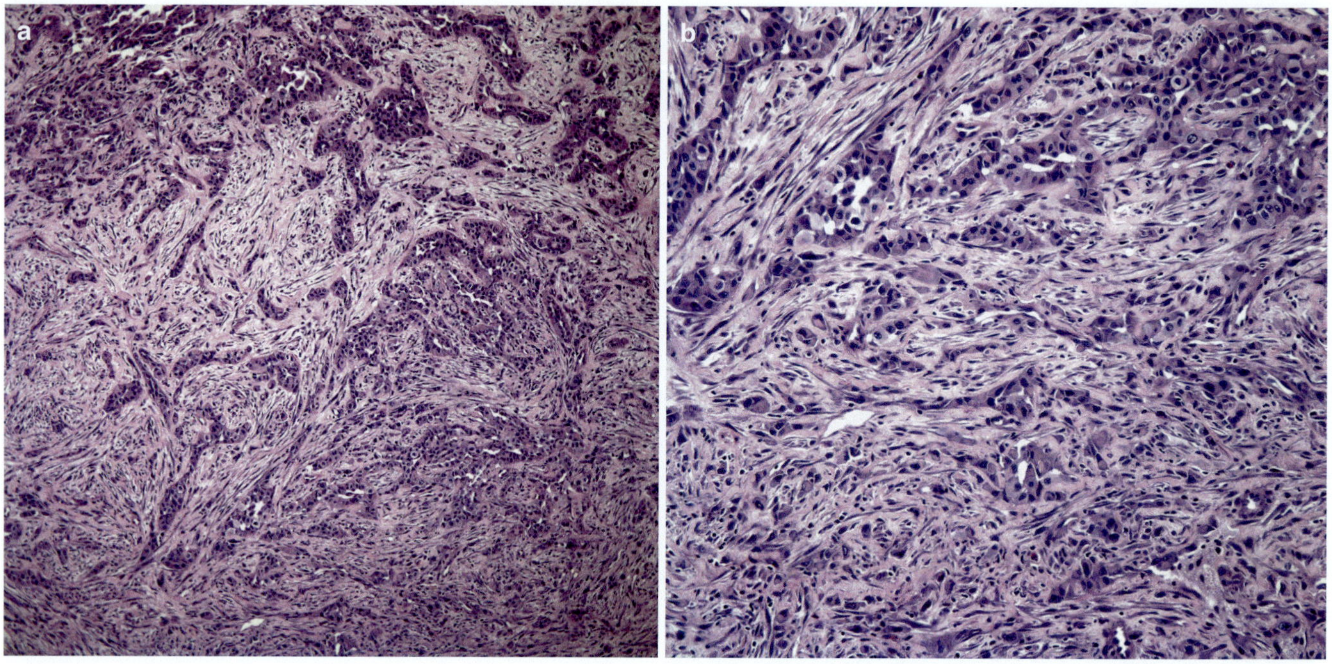

Fig. 12.47 (**a**) Cords of neoplastic and irregular glands are embedded in a reactive stroma. (**b**) Pseudomesotheliomatous adenocarcinoma mimicking biphasic mesothelioma. Note the atypia in the glandular component

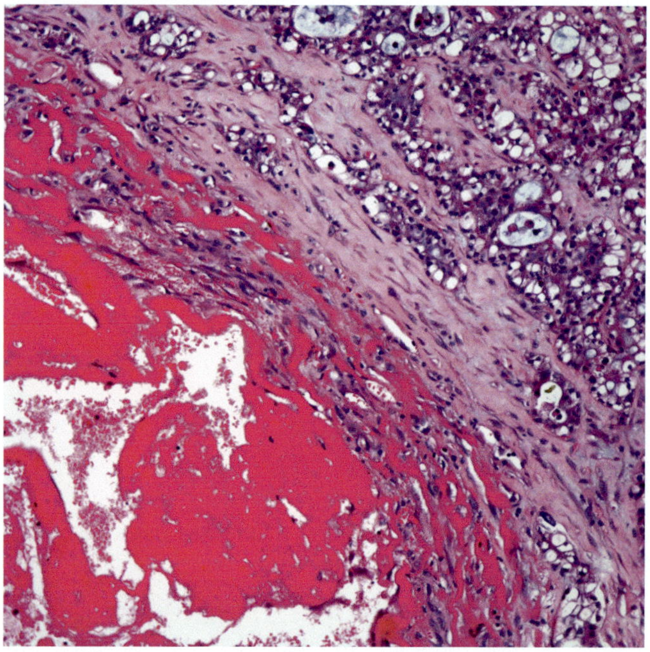

Fig. 12.48 Pleural mucoepidermoid carcinoma showing a gland-like proliferation admixed with areas of fibrinous pleuritis

Immunohistochemical Features

The diagnosis of mucoepidermoid carcinoma does not require immunohistochemical analysis. However, the tumor may show positive staining for keratin 5/6, p63, CEA, keratin, and epithelial membrane antigen. However, it is important to note that this immunophenotype may be seen in either primary or metastatic mucoepidermoid tumors of the pleura.

Treatment and Prognosis

The treatment of choice is complete surgical resection of the tumor. Due to the rarity of this tumor in the pleura, it is difficult to determine its true biological behavior. However, the cases described corresponded to the low grade category of these tumors; thus, it is possible that complete surgical resection may be the only treatment needed and that the behavior is that of an indolent neoplasm.

Pleural Thymomas

Thymomas are epithelial tumors more commonly seen in the anterior mediastinum. However, as stated elsewhere in this text, this tumor may occur ectopically in different sites including the head and neck, trachea, thyroid, and lung, and in usual circumstances the tumor may present as a diffuse process involving the pleural surface in a manner similar to that seen in mesothelioma [95–99]. However, it is important to understand that anterior mediastinal thymomas commonly invade the pleura. Therefore, it is imperative to exclude such possibility before rendering a diagnosis of primary ectopic pleural thymoma. Thymomas growing along the pleural surface in a manner mimicking mesothelioma have been reported sporadically [100, 101]. However, in the recent past, more attention

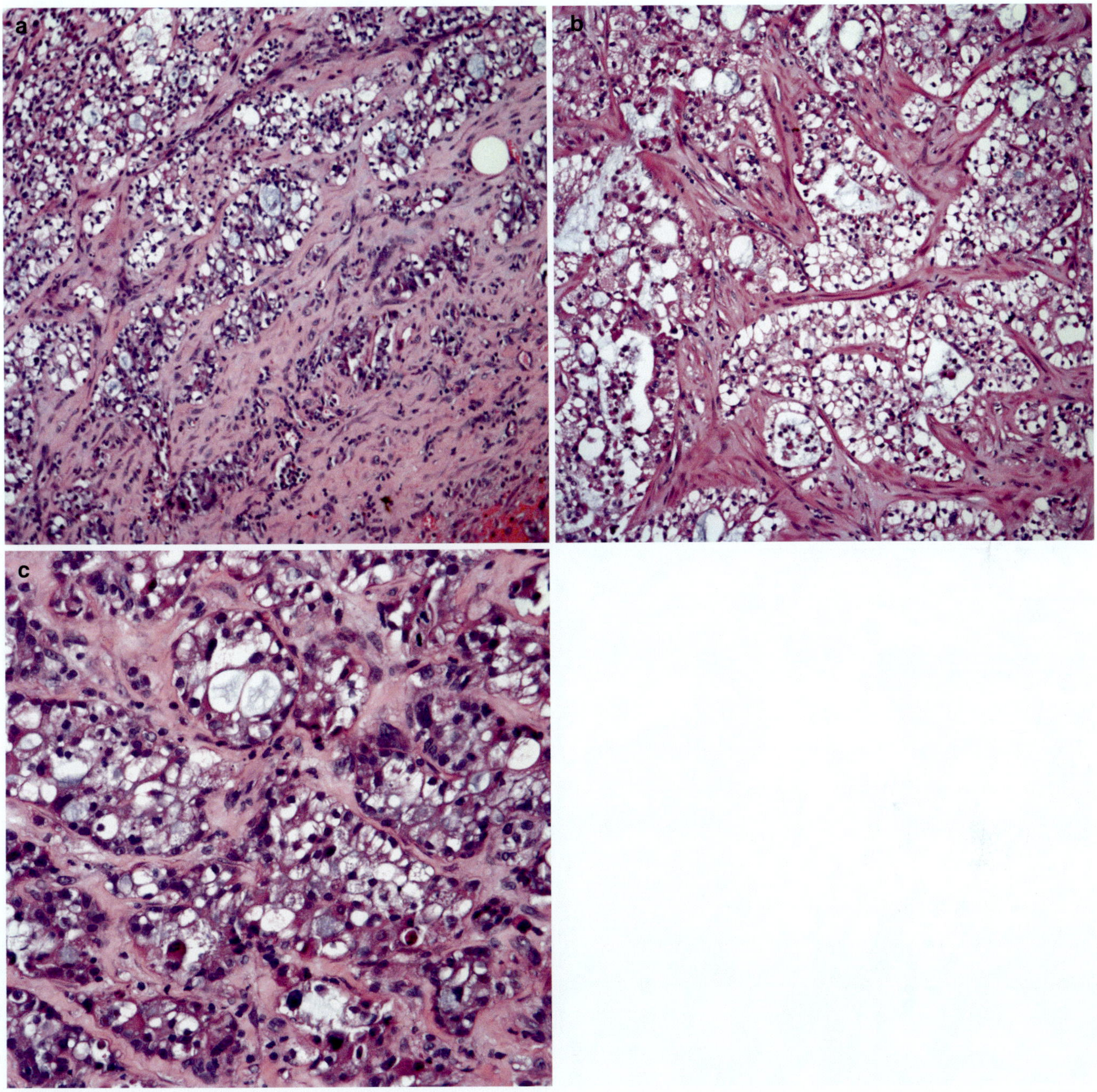

Fig. 12.49 (**a**) Pleural mucoepidermoid carcinoma composed of a gland-like proliferation embedded in a fibrocollagenous stroma. (**b**) Prominent clear cell appearance. (**c**) Clear cells admixed with mucus-producing cells (mucocytes)

has been given to this unusual presentation of thymoma [102–109].

Clinical Features

Pleural thymomas appear to affect adult individuals with a mean age of 54 years and without predilection for any particular gender. The patients may present with symptoms of cough, chest pain, fever, shortness of breath, or, more unusual, myasthenia gravis or be completely asymptomatic. Radiographically, the tumors appear either as a pleural-based mass or as diffuse pleural thickening in a manner similar to that seen in malignant mesothelioma.

Macroscopic Features

The gross appearance of pleural thymomas will depend on the anatomic distribution of the tumor. Tumors that present as pleural-based lesions, are often attached to the pleura in a broad based fashion. The tumors are well circumscribed, solid, and light tan in color. The cut surface of the tumor may show a slight nodular or lobulated surface. Areas of

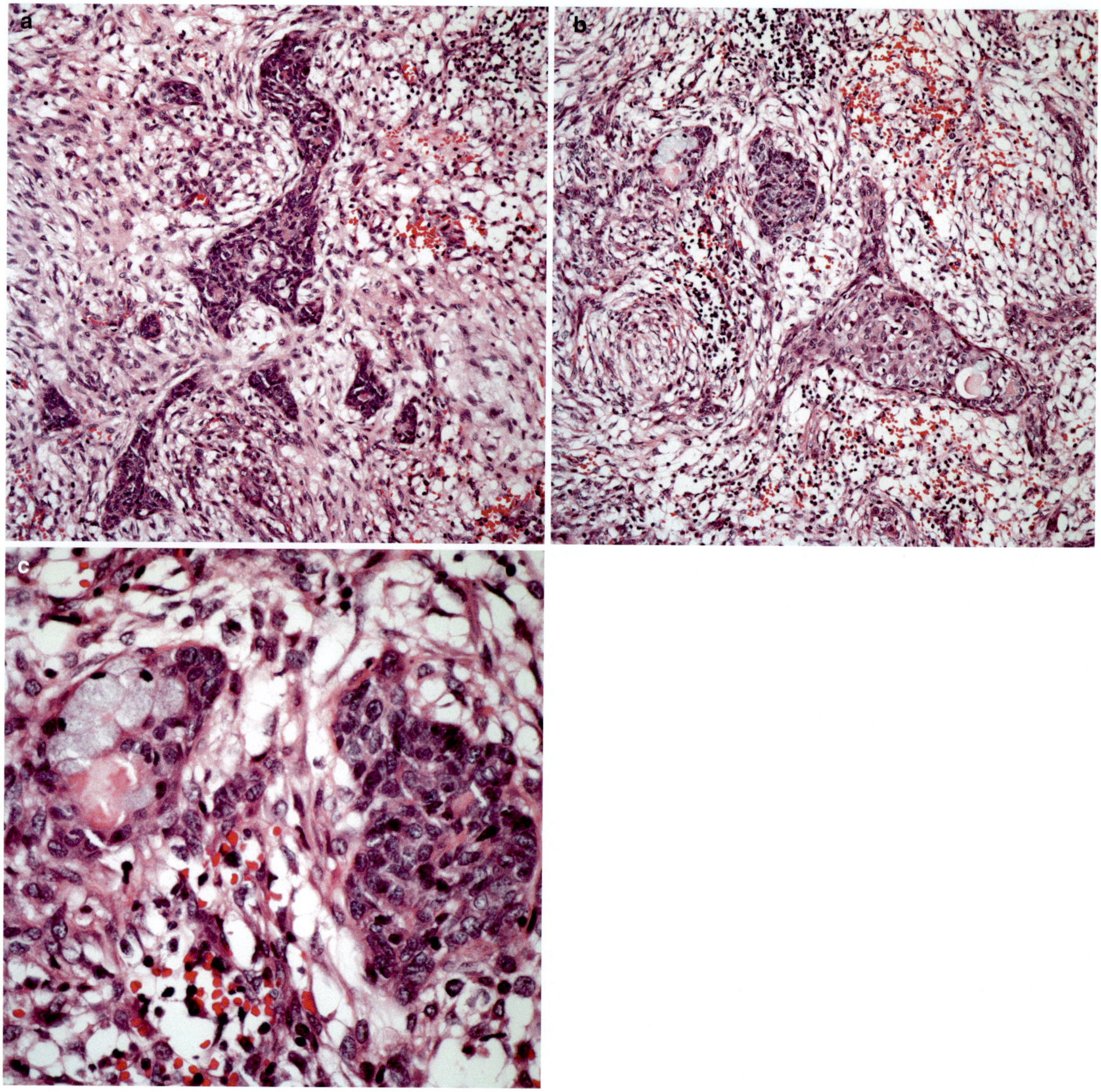

Fig. 12.50 (**a**) Sclerosing mucoepidermoid carcinoma of the pleura; note the islands of epidermoid cells embedded in spindle cell stromal tissue. (**b**) The islands of epidermoid cells show focal areas of mucus-producing cells. (**c**) Higher magnification of the mucus-producing cells

hemorrhage and/or necrosis are not common. When the tumor involves the pleura in a diffuse manner, it spreads along the pleural surface causing pleural thickening.

Histopathological Features

The histological features of pleural thymomas are essentially the same as those seen in anterior mediastinal tumors, namely, an admixture of epithelial cells and lymphocytes (Fig. 12.51a, b), in various proportions (Fig. 12.52). The tumor may also show prominent lobulation. The tumor lobules are separated by fibrous bands and perivascular spaces are also present. In the spindle cell growth pattern, the tumors are composed of a spindle cellular proliferation with a hemangiopericytoma-like growth pattern. However, in none of the different thymoma types, nuclear atypia or mitotic activity is identified.

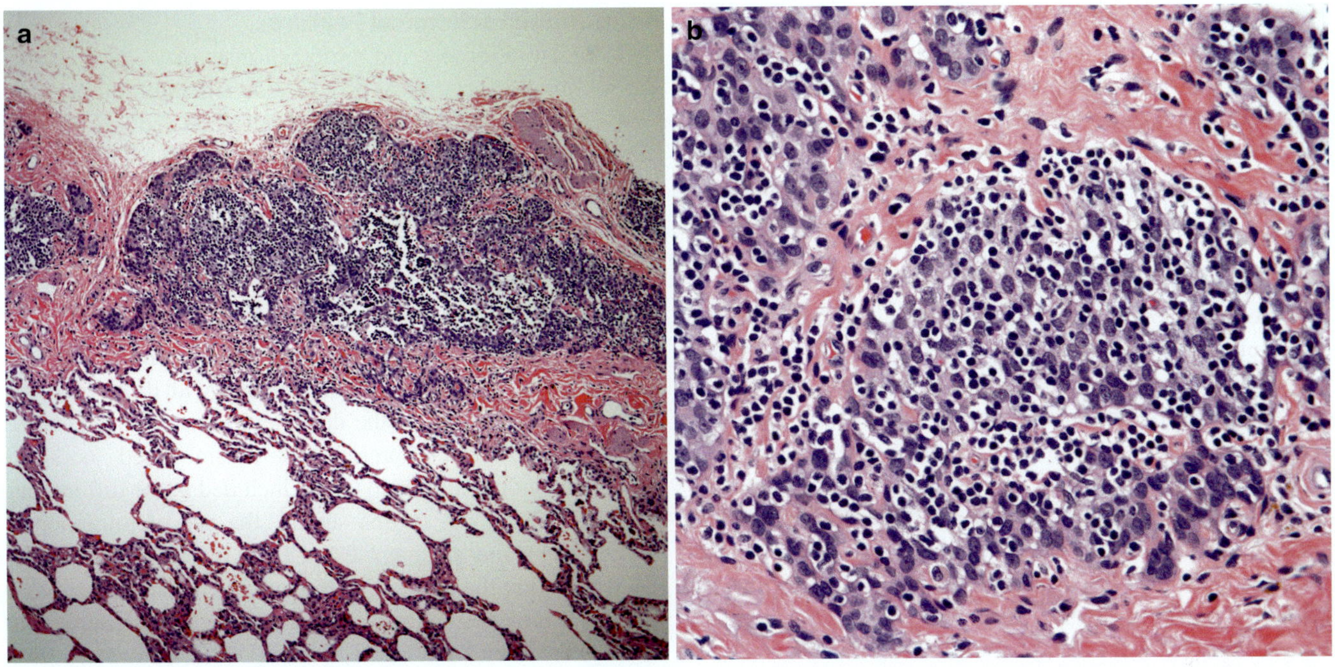

Fig. 12.51 (**a**) Pleural thymoma with the characteristic cellular composition. (**b**) Higher magnification showing the admixture of epithelial cells and lymphocytes

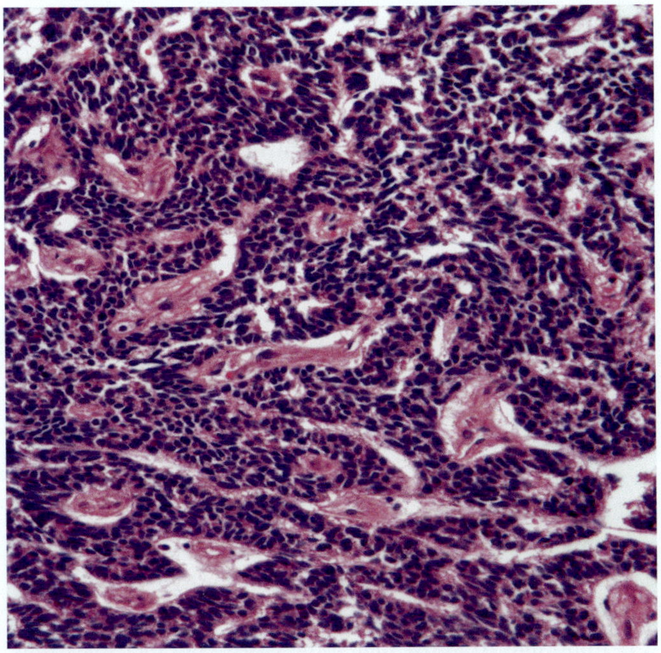

Fig. 12.52 Pleural thymoma with spindle cell features

Immunohistochemical Features

The immunophenotype of thymomas—whether in the anterior mediastinum, lung, pleura, or neck—is similar. The tumors will display positive staining in the epithelial component with keratin antibodies, most commonly pan keratin, low molecular weight keratin (CAM 5.2), and keratin 5/6, while the lymphocytic component shows positive staining for lymphoid markers including B- and T-cell markers. In addition, the tumors may occasionally display positive staining in the epithelial component with calretinin. Interestingly, epithelial membrane antigen in thymomas may show either only focal weak staining or be entirely negative in the epithelial cells. More recently, Pax8 has been demonstrated to show positive staining in thymomas as well as thymic carcinomas.

Differential Diagnosis

The most important differential diagnosis of pleural thymomas is either mesothelioma or metastatic carcinoma to the pleura. In both cases the presence of a biphasic cellular proliferation composed of lymphocytes and epithelial cells may lead to the correct interpretation. However, one of the histopathological variants of mesothelioma, the lymphohistiocytoid type, may pose a more difficult diagnostic problem. In this setting, staining with calretinin and keratin 5/6 can overlap with cases of thymoma. Also, from a histopathological point of view, most of the cases of lymphohistiocytoid mesothelioma display a spindle cell proliferation embedded in a lymphoid stroma, which would be unusual for a spindle cell thymoma, which characteristically shows very little lymphoid cells. In cases of carcinoma, the absence of marked nuclear atypia and/or mitotic activity and negative findings of a pulmonary mass may lead to a more correct interpretation.

Lymphomas involving the pleura may also enter in the differential diagnosis; however, the use of keratin antibodies will be of help in this setting. Important to mention is the fact that in cases in which flow cytometry is performed, it is likely that the results will point to an immature T-cell proliferation, which should not be misinterpreted as a T-cell neoplasm, since immature T-cells are a normal component of thymomas.

Treatment and Prognosis

The treatment of pleural thymomas is essentially surgical resection of the tumor. However, the extent of the surgical procedure will be determined by the extent of disease. In cases in which the tumor is a pleural-based mass, the tumor is more amenable to a more conservative surgical approach. However, in cases in which there is diffuse pleural involvement, the procedure may require a more radical procedure such as pneumonectomy. The prognosis of these patients will also not only depend on the extent of disease and but also the resectability of the tumor.

Adenomatoid Tumor

Adenomatoid tumors can be interpreted as benign mesothelial lesions, which often occur in the male and female genital tract. In the thoracic cavity, the tumor may arise in the mediastinal compartment or in the pleural surface [110–112]. However, these tumors are of unusual occurrence in the thoracic cavity.

Clinical Features

The few cases described so far of this particular entity have been in adult individuals who have been followed for different conditions. In the two cases described by Kaplan et al. [112], one patient had an adenocarcinoma of the lung, while the other patient had histoplasmosis. The pleural tumors were found incidentally during surgery, and the two cases were described as pleural nodules varying in size from 0.5 to 2.5 cm in greatest diameter.

Histopathological Features

Like adenomatoid tumors elsewhere, the lesions are characterized by the presence of cords or sheets of medium-size cells with vacuolated cytoplasm and nuclei that are displaced to the periphery of the cell almost mimicking a signet ring cell appearance. In other areas, the tumor may show sheets of medium-size cells with light eosinophilic cytoplasm and round nuclei, and in some cells nucleoli may be seen. The cellular proliferation is essentially embedded in a fibrous stroma, and the cords of cells may be separated by thin fibrocollagenous tissue (Fig. 12.53a–d). The tumor does not show nuclear pleomorphism or increased mitotic activity. Areas of hemorrhage and/or necrosis are not commonly observed.

Immunohistochemical Features

Adenomatoid tumors and mesotheliomas may share a similar immunohistochemical profile. Adenomatoid tumors may show positive staining for keratin, calretinin and CK5/6. The tumor is negative for CEA, CD15, B72.3, and MOC-31.

Differential Diagnosis

Adenomatoid tumors should not pose a big diagnostic problem. However, it is important to recognize that malignant mesotheliomas may show adenomatoid-like areas; therefore, it is important to properly assess the extent of disease. Malignant mesothelioma usually presents with diffuse pleural involvement contrary to the documented cases of adenomatoid tumors, which present as pleural-based nodules. Adenocarcinoma also needs to be included in the differential diagnosis; however, in this setting, the use of immunohistochemical stains such as CEA, CD15, B72.3, and/or MOC-31 will lead to the correct interpretation. One last differential diagnosis includes epithelioid hemangioendothelioma; in this setting, the use of markers such as CD34, CD31, and factor VIII may lead to the correct diagnosis as adenomatoid tumors are negative for vascular markers. Also ultrastructurally, the presence of Weibel-Palade bodies is a feature of vascular tumors but not adenomatoid tumor.

Treatment and Prognosis

The treatment of choice for these tumors is complete surgical resection. Since the tumor is considered a benign lesion, complete surgical resection is curative. Metastatic disease or recurrence have not been documented.

Pleuropulmonary Endometriosis

Although pleuropulmonary endometriosis is not a neoplastic condition, its presence in this location can easily mimic a tumoral process and will therefore be discussed here. Endometrial tissue ectopically occuring in the thoracic cavity, although rare, has been reported in the literature. The pleural surface is most commonly affected. Even though in a good number of cases, this finding of ectopic endometrial tissue may be an incidental finding, in some cases, the endometrial tissue may appear as a pleural-based tumor. However, it is important to know that some cases endometriosis may also primarily involve the lung parenchyma [113–117].

Clinical Features

Endometriosis predominantly affects women in reproductive age; however, cases of pleuropulmonary endometriosis have been seen in older women. In the cases described by Flieder et al. [113], the age range was between 27 and 74 years. Therefore, one cannot completely rule out the possibility of endometriosis in older women. The most common symptoms

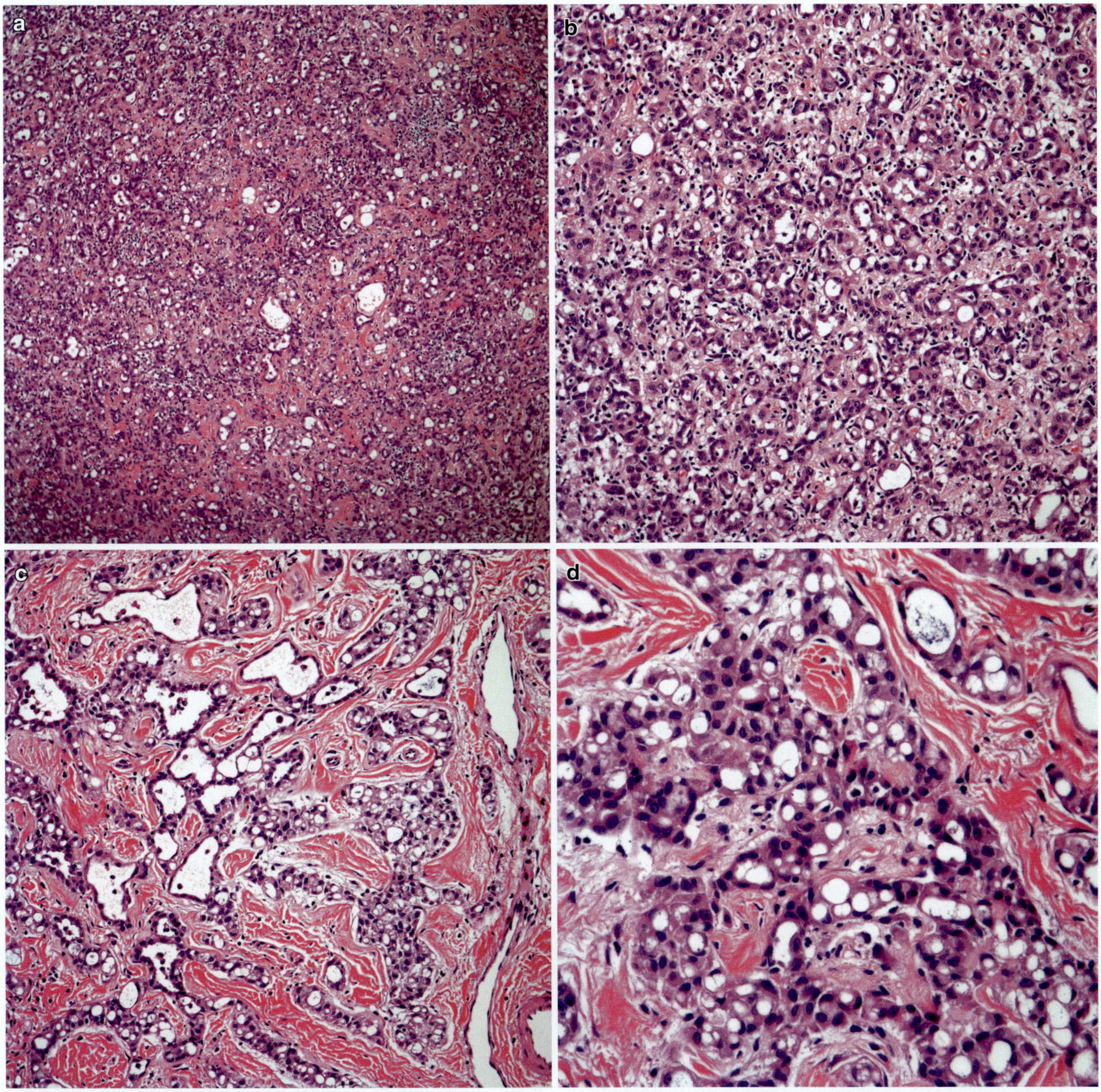

Fig. 12.53 (**a**) Low power view of an adenomatoid tumor showing a small acinar-like type of cellular proliferation. (**b**) Adenomatoid tumor showing gland-like structures. (**c**) Cords of cells dissecting into fibrocollagenous tissue. (**d**) Higher magnification showing cells with a signet ring cell-like appearance, note the absence of nuclear atypia or mitotic activity

for those women with pleuropulmonary endometriosis include shortness of breath, cough, pleuritic chest pain, and/or hemoptysis. Interestingly, the finding of pleuropulmonary endometriosis may be the only site affected without involvement of pelvic endometriosis. Also, some of these women have no previous history of pregnancy or gynecologic surgery, but in some patients, the use of hormonal therapy could be elicited. Radiologically, the patients may present with pneumothorax, pulmonary infiltrates, or the presence of distinct pleural nodules. Lesions within the pulmonary parenchyma most likely will demonstrate intraparenchymal tumor nodules.

Macroscopic Features

The gross features of pulmonary endometriosis may vary from strips of hemorrhagic tissue to well-formed small tumors that may range in size from under 1 cm to 3 cm in greatest diameter.

However, cases in which the clinical presentation has been that of large pulmonary mass have also been described [117]. In general, the lesions may appear cystic, hemorrhagic and well circumscribed but not encapsulated.

Histopathological Features

The histology of pleuropulmonary endometriosis is that of a proliferative type of endometrium composed of glands lined by columnar, cuboidal, or pseudostratified epithelium with oval nuclei, inconspicuous nucleoli, and scant eosinophilic or clear cytoplasm. Periglandular myxoid changes may be seen in some areas while mitotic activity is invariably present. The stromal tissue is characterized by areas of fibrocollagenous tissue with inflammatory cells, namely, plasma cells, lymphocytes, eosinophils, and hemosiderin-laden macrophages (Fig. 12.54a–c). The pleural nodules may display a broad based attachment to the visceral pleura without involvement of the underlying lung parenchyma. Stromal proliferation of vessels may or may not be seen in these cases.

Immunohistochemical Features

The use of immunohistochemical stains may help in the diagnosis of endometriosis mainly in cases in which the tissue available for evaluation is a small biopsy. The glandular and/or stromal component may show positive staining for estrogen and progesterone receptors, broad-spectrum keratin, CK7, and WT1. In some cases, the glands may also show positive staining for CEA and for HER2/neu. However, other carcinomatous epitopes like CD15, B72.3, and neuroendocrine markers appear to be negative.

Differential Diagnosis

The differential diagnosis depends largely on the material available for evaluation and also on the location of the lesion. In limited biopsy material, the diagnosis may pose considerable challenge as endometriosis may be confused with a neoplastic glandular proliferation. In this setting, the use of immunohistochemical markers may be of help; however, it is important to take into consideration that some markers may actually show overlap between carcinoma and endometriosis. When the lesions are in the pleura, the differential diagnosis will also include biphasic mesothelioma, especially in cases in which there is a marked stromal reaction. However, the finding of a small pleural based nodule would be most unusual for a case of mesothelioma. In addition, immunohistochemical stains may be of help. Although most cases of endometriosis occur in adult females, one last possible condition to be considered in the differential diagnosis is pleuropulmonary blastoma (PPB). Some cases of endometriosis may present with prominent cystic changes and stromal growth, which can be confused with PPB. However, the presence of glands more akin to the proliferative phase of endometrium and the presence of inflammatory cells, namely, plasma cell in the stroma, are important features in cases of endometriosis. Needless to say, the occurrence of PPB in an adult female patient would be very unusual. In addition, positive staining for estrogen and progesterone receptors as well as WT1 would be most unusual for PPB.

Neuroendocrine Tumors

Although the vast majority of neuroendocrine tumors occur predominantly in an intrapulmonary location, in certain unusual circumstances, carcinoid tumorlets may present as single or multiple pleural nodules (Fig. 12.55a–c). It is important to properly evaluate such lesions, namely, primarily to assess whether there is an intrapulmonary mass with metastasis to the pleura. Otherwise, the diagnostic criteria for carcinoid tumorlets are similar to those for an intrapulmonary location, basically tumor lesions up to no more than 0.5 cm in greatest diameter. However, if radiologically identified, the clinical differential diagnosis may be more challenging and include primary tumors of the pleura or metastatic disease to the pleura. Nevertheless, the size of the lesions in addition to their immunohistochemical profile will lead to a more accurate diagnostic interpretation.

Non-epithelial Tumors of the Pleura

Non-epithelial tumors of the pleura are uncommon but their presence is well recognized. It encompasses tumors of different etiologies and wide spectrum of differentiation. Their diagnosis may require not only familiarity with the histological features of the particular tumors but also some degree of suspicion since most of these tumors are rarely seen as primary pleural neoplasms. Therefore, it is important to be aware of their existence and to consider them in the differential diagnosis of tumors of the pleura. Because this group of tumors is more commonly seen in extrathoracic sites, it is highly important to properly exclude the possibility of metastatic disease. This group of tumors includes vascular, muscle, fibrous, neural, and neuroectodermal tumors among others.

Fibroblastic Tumors

This group of tumors may represent the most common among the non-epithelial tumors of the pleura. Not surprisingly, solitary fibrous tumor is the most commonly encountered. Basically, the three most important tumors include:

- Solitary fibrous tumor (SFT)
- Calcifying fibrous pseudotumor (CFPT)
- Desmoid tumor

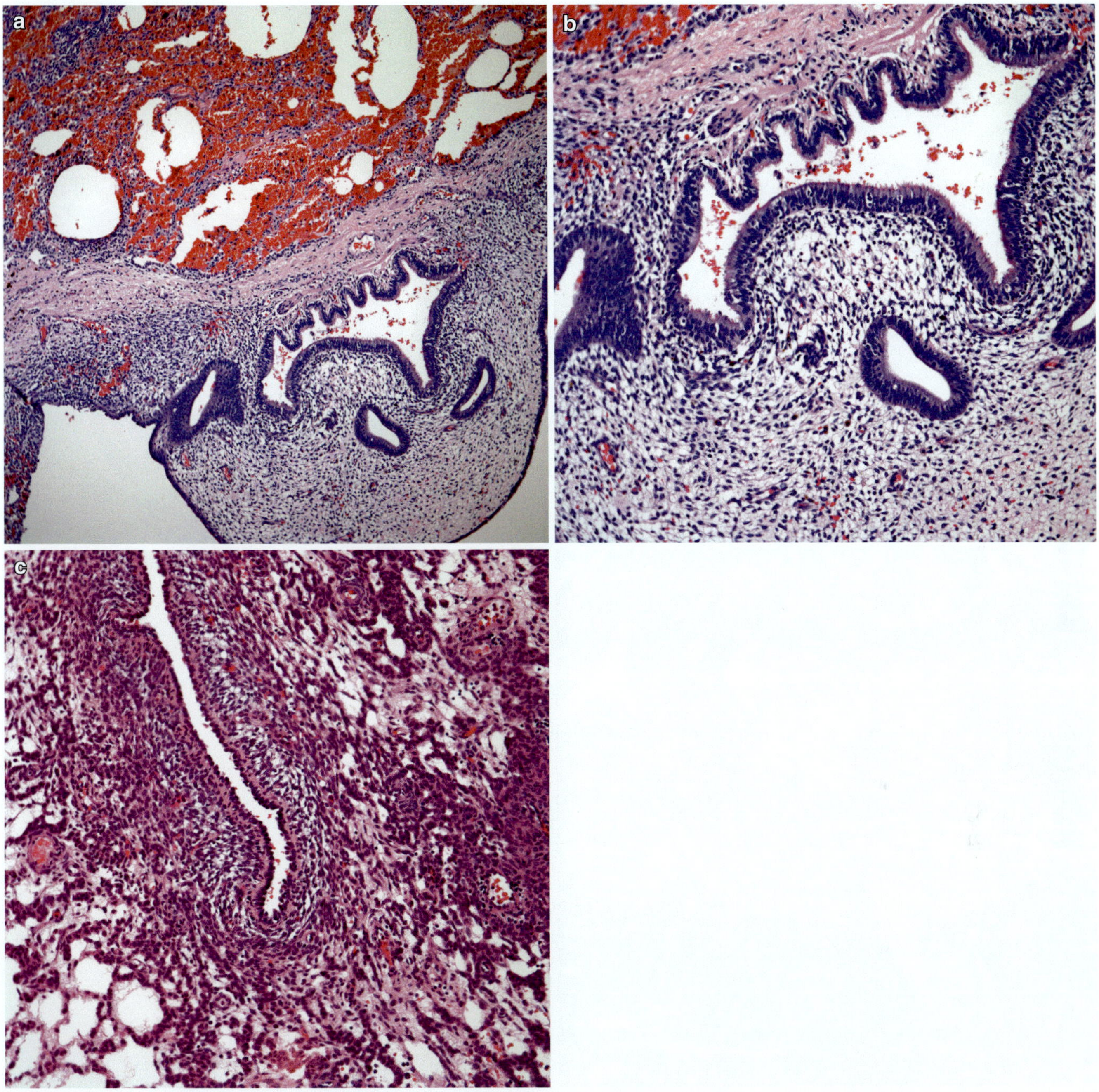

Fig. 12.54 (**a**) Low power view of pleural endometriosis showing the classic presentation of glands embedded in a cellular stroma. (**b**) Closer view showing dilated glands of different sizes. (**c**) Pleural endometriosis in which the stroma is more prominent with only small residual gland-like structures

Solitary Fibrous Tumor (SFT)

SFT is a tumor most commonly encountered on the serosal surfaces; however, it has been described in diverse anatomic areas including the lung, head and neck, soft tissue, and viscera [118–121]. Throughout the history of this neoplasm, many different names have been coined to designate this tumor including localized fibrous mesothelioma, submesothelial fibroma, and fibrous mesothelioma. Klemperer and Ravin [8] should be credited for recognizing this tumor as a different clinicopathological entity in the pleura. The authors separated SFT from the conventional diffuse pleural tumors and stated that their behavior was also different from tumors involving the pleura in a diffuse manner. Although there has been some debate regarding the histogenesis of these tumors, ultrastructural studies have not supported the notion of a mesothelial origin and have suggested a fibroblastic origin. Currently the tumor is well

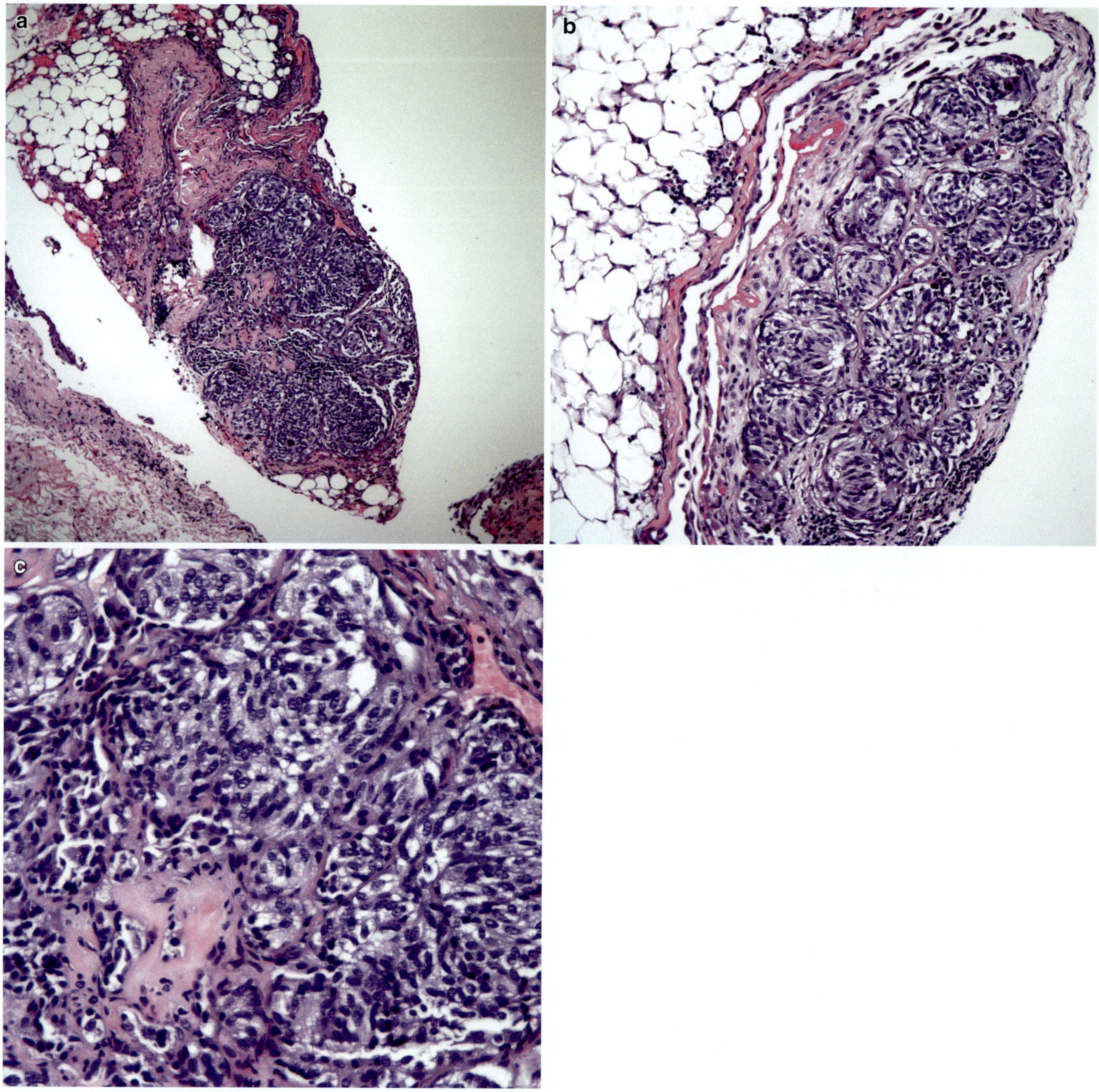

Fig. 12.55 (**a**) Low power view of a "carcinoid tumorlet" on the pleural surface. (**b**) The carcinoid tumorlet does not invade into adipose tissue. (**c**) Higher magnification showing a cellular proliferation similar to that seen in conventional carcinoid tumors

recognized as a distinct clinicopathological entity; however, there are only a few large series documenting the different clinical, histopathological, immunohistochemical, and behavioral features of this neoplasm [122–129].

Clinical Features

The tumor does not have any predilection for any particular gender, and it has been described in a wide range of ages, from pediatric patients under 10 years of age to older patients of more than 80 years. The tumor appears to be most common in the sixth decade of life. Clinically, the patients may present with symptoms of cough, chest pain, pleural effusion, shortness of breath, hemoptysis, and general malaise. One important clinical finding in patients with SFT is hypoglycemia that may be present in about 10 % of the cases. About 25 % of patients present with no symptoms at all, and their tumors are discovered during a routine radiographic examination. By diagnostic imaging, SFT is a pleural-based tumor that may arise from the visceral or less often from the parietal pleura.

Macroscopic Features

The majority of tumors are described as sharply circumscribed and/or encapsulated, polypoid tumors attached to the pleura by a short pedicle. The size of these tumors may vary from 1 to more than 25 cm in greatest diameter. The cut surface of the tumor is tan white, whorled, and rubbery with fibrotic areas. Necrosis, hemorrhage, and cystic changes may be present in some cases. Those macroscopic features are important to document, as they have been associated with malignant tumors. Some tumors are not attached to the pleura by a pedicle but rather involve the pleura in a broad based, while other tumors are described to have an inward growth with compression and displacement of the lung.

Histopathological Features

The microscopic features of SFT are rather wide and in a good proportion of cases, more than one pattern may be observed in these tumors. Essentially, this tumor has been separated into two main growth patterns: the solid spindle type and the diffuse sclerosing type. Of those two patterns, the solid spindle type is the most versatile, as the tumors may show a wide range of microscopic features that are commonly observed in other mesenchymal neoplasms. These features include short storiform (so-called patternless pattern) (Fig. 12.56a, b), angiofibroma-like (Fig. 12.57), hemangiopericytoma-like (Fig. 12.58a–c), fibrosarcoma-like (herringbone) (Fig. 12.59), monophasic synovial sarcoma-like (Fig. 12.60a, b), and neural-like patterns (Fig. 12.61) [129]. On the other hand tumors can show extensive collagenization, which often has a rope-like appearance (Fig. 12.62a–c). Based on these histopathological growth patterns, the finding of a tumor showing hypo- and hypercellular areas, presence of ectatic blood vessels, spindle cells, which can mimic any known spindle cell sarcoma, and areas of extensive collagenization can lead to the correct interpretation of SFT. These different histopathological patterns become more apparent in complete surgical resections rather than in small limited biopsies. In some cases, the tumor may infiltrate into peripheral lung parenchyma or mediastinal structures.

In a study by England et al. [125], the authors divided SFT into histologically benign and malignant tumors based on the presence of mitotic activity (more than four mitotic figures per ten high-power fields), high cellularity, pleomorphism, hemorrhage, and necrosis. Of the 223 cases presented in this study, 141 were classified as benign, while 82 were classified as malignant. Other parameters such as size of the tumor and clinical findings may not completely correlate with clinical behavior. However, it is logical to assume that the larger the tumor, the more likely it will infiltrate adjacent structures, thus, being less amenable for complete surgical resection.

Immunohistochemical Features

The most consistent positive immunohistochemical stains in SFT include vimentin, CD34, and Bcl-2. Other stains that may reveal weak or scattered positive cells include smooth muscle actin and desmin. Immunohistochemical stains for keratin, EMA, S100 protein, factor VIII, and CD31 are generally negative. In some cases in which the tumor infiltrates the periphery of the lung, entrapped lung parenchyma will show positive staining for keratin antibodies.

Differential Diagnosis

The histopathological features of SFT may mimic several mesenchymal neoplasms including synovial sarcoma, angiofibroma, or neural tumors. However, the presence of more than one growth pattern in the same tumor, the use of immunohistochemical markers, especially CD34 and Bcl-2, and negative staining for S100 protein, epithelial, and/or vascular markers should lead to the correct interpretation. However, it is important to point out that some of the markers used to support a diagnosis of SFT may also show positivity in other tumors of mesenchymal origin. Thus, the interpretation of the immunophenotype should always be in conjunction with the morphology of the tumor. In limited biopsies, the diagnosis may not be readily recognizable due to sampling limitations. Therefore, extensive evaluation is recommended in these tumors in order to properly appreciate the different growth patterns.

Treatment and Prognosis

The treatment of choice for SFT is complete surgical resection. The clinical behavior of these tumors may be determined in great part not only by the histological features of the tumor but also by its resectability. Tumors that are attached to the pleura by a pedicle, despite possible worrisome histology, may not follow an aggressive behavior. In 45 % of the cases designated as malignant by England et al. [125], these patients were apparently cured by complete surgical resection. This group of patients was described as having pedunculated, well-circumscribed tumors. On the other hand, the other 55% of patients followed a fatal course with recurrences and metastasis. The authors concluded that resectability is the single most important indicator of clinical behavior. Briselli et al. [124] also arrived at a similar conclusion and stated that nuclear pleomorphism and high mitotic rate do not necessarily indicate poor prognosis if the tumor is circumscribed.

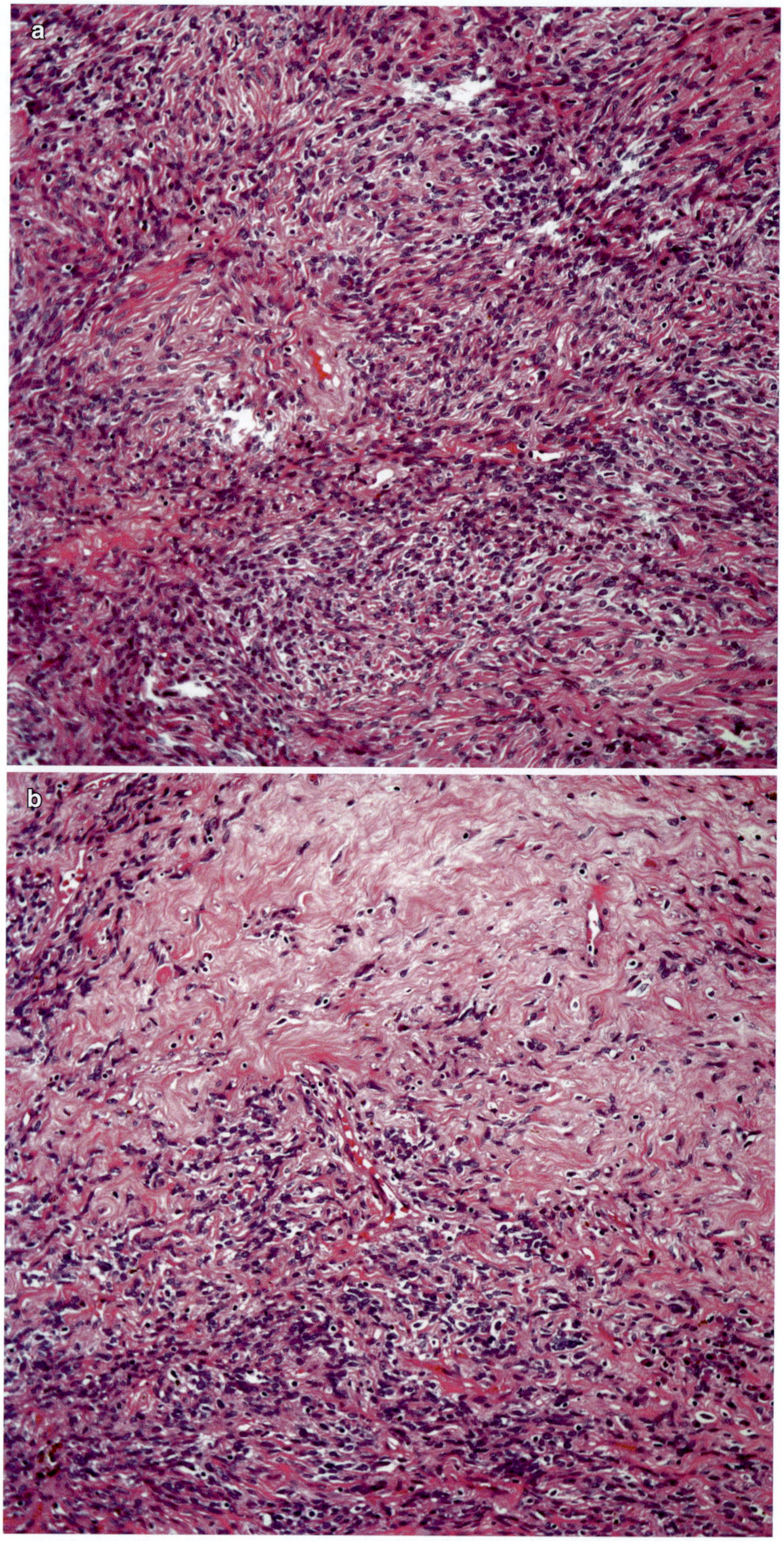

Fig. 12.56 (**a**) Solitary fibrous tumors composed of a spindle cell proliferation (so-called patternless pattern). (**b**) Higher magnification showing hypo- and hypercellular areas

Desmoid Tumor

Fibromatosis or desmoid tumors are neoplasms of ubiquitous distribution that are commonly seen in an intra-abdominal location or that involve the musculature of the shoulder, chest wall, or back [130, 131]. Those tumors in the chest wall are usually in an extrathoracic location and the patients present with a palpable mass. Also desmoid tumors of the chest wall with pleural involvement have been reported [132]. However, desmoid tumors occurring primarily as pleural tumors are rather rare and have been recorded in the literature only sparsely [133, 134].

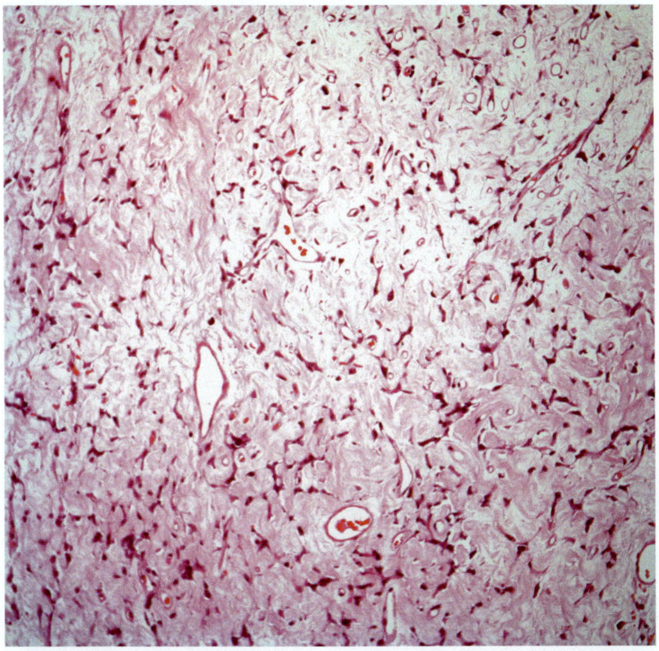

Fig. 12.57 Solitary fibrous tumor with angiofibroma-like appearance

Clinical Features

The tumor appears to affect individuals ranging in age from 16 to 66 years of age without gender predilection. Clinically, patients may present with symptoms of chest pain, shortness of breath, and cough. In some cases, a history of trauma has been obtained. By diagnostic imaging, the tumors appear as pleural based neoplasms that may involve either the visceral or the parietal pleura.

Macroscopic Features

The tumors have been described as well demarcated, not pedunculated, and with a glistening surface. The tumors vary in size from 5 to more than 15 cm in greatest dimension. At cut surface, the tumor shows a firm, white-grayish, and bosselated appearance; areas of necrosis and hemorrhage are not common (Fig. 12.63a–c).

Histopathological Features

The histological features of desmoid tumors of the pleura are essentially the same as those described for desmoid tumors in other locations. The tumor characteristically shows intersecting fascicles of spindle cells with tapered, wavy to

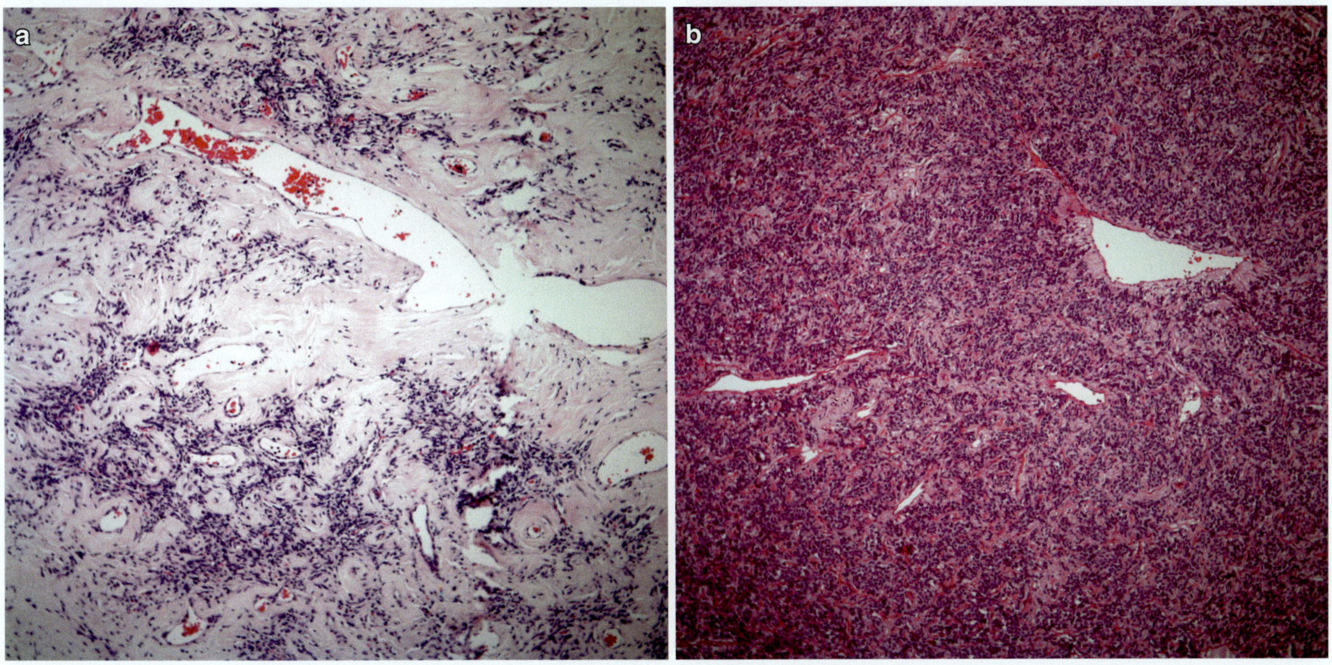

Fig. 12.58 (**a**) Solitary fibrous tumor with a hemangiopericytic growth pattern showing ectatic blood vessels and adjacent spindle cell proliferation. (**b**) More dense spindle cell proliferation around ectatic blood vessels. (**c**) Monotonous spindle cell proliferation and prominent vasculature

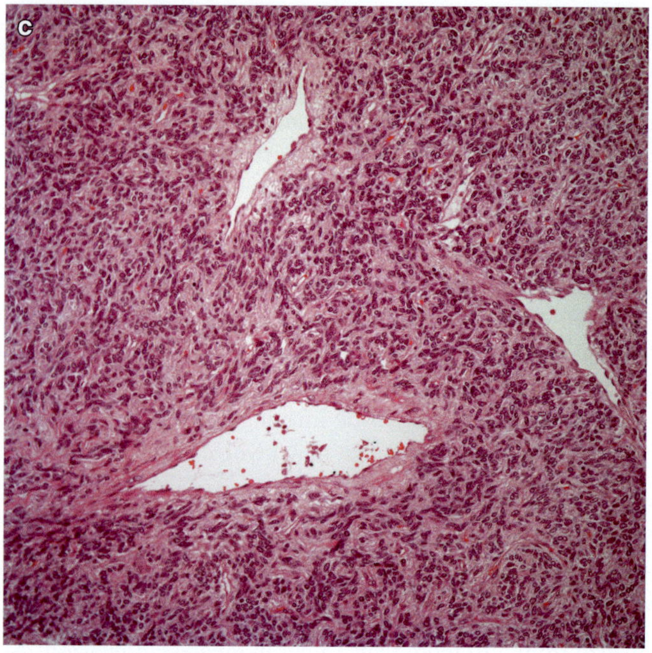

Fig. 12.58 (continued)

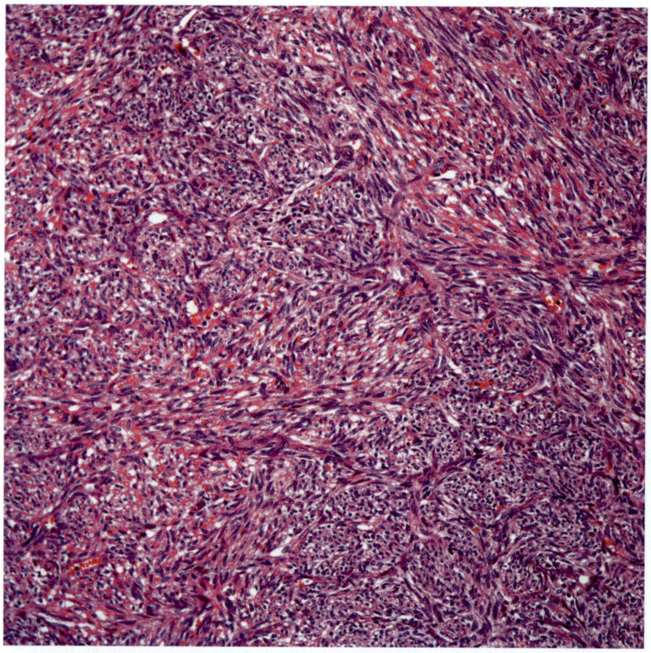

Fig. 12.59 Solitary fibrous tumor with fibrosarcoma-like growth pattern

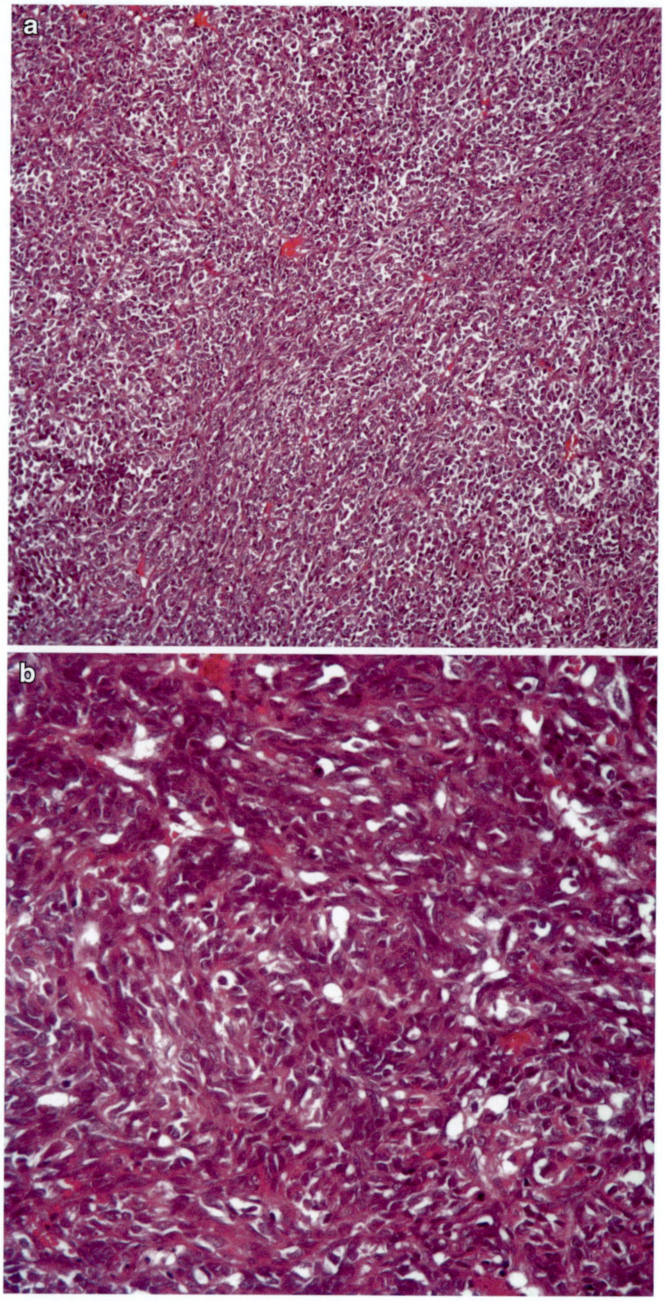

Fig. 12.60 (**a**) Solitary fibrous tumor with a monophasic synovial sarcoma-like growth pattern. (**b**) Higher magnification of the epithelial-like cellular proliferation

elongated nuclei without nuclear atypia. The cells appear to be present in a background of a collagenous or finely fibrillary matrix. Numerous blood vessels with either thin or thick walls are invariably present. The tumors appear to have infiltrative borders; however, the tumor usually does not show prominent nuclear atypia, mitotic activity, hemorrhage and/or necrosis.

Immunohistochemical Features

The immunohistochemical profile for tumors arising on the pleural surface are the same than for any other site. Those tumors present in the pleura are positive for vimentin and actin; they may show focal positive staining for desmin. In addition, these tumors are positive for beta-catenin and cytoplasmic staining for cyclin D1. However, in general,

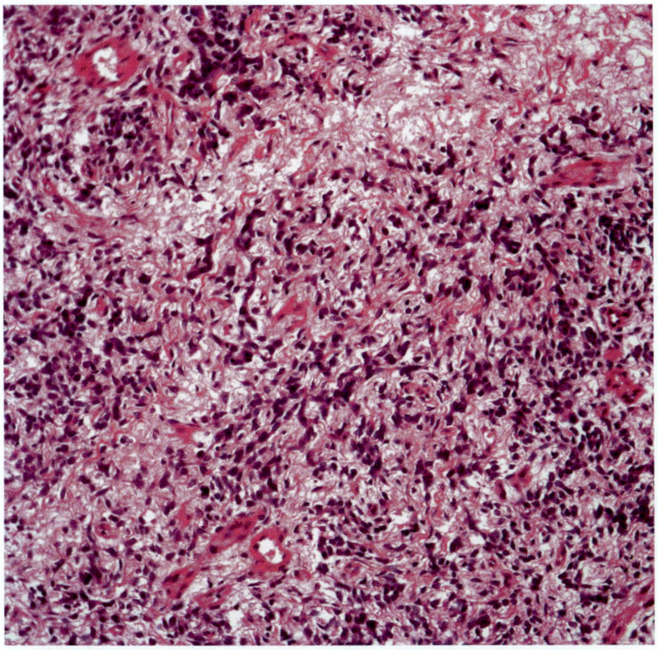

Fig. 12.61 Solitary fibrous tumor with a neural-like growth pattern

desmoid tumors are negative for epithelial markers, CD34, and S100 protein.

Differential Diagnosis

Solitary fibrous tumor is the most difficult and important differential diagnosis to consider in the evaluation of desmoid tumors. In this setting the use of immunohistochemical studies may prove beneficial, as desmoid tumors are generally negative for CD34 and Bcl-2, while SFT are positive with these markers. Although SFT may show positive staining for actin, it is usually focal in contrast to desmoid tumors, which usually show a stronger positive reaction. Equally important would be the use of beta-catenin as this is commonly seen positive in desmoid tumor and negative in SFT.

Treatment and Prognosis

The treatment of choice is surgical treatment with negative margins. Therefore, complete surgical resection is the most important parameter in the evaluation of clinical behavior. Those patients with tumors that are not amenable to complete resection are at risk to develop recurrence of the tumor.

Calcifying Fibrous Pseudotumor (CFPT)

Fetsch et al. [135] should be credited for the initial description of calcifying fibrous pseudotumors. The authors described CFPT as a tumor of the soft tissues with distinct morphologic features characterized by abundant hyalinized collagen with psammomatous or dystrophic calcifications and a lymphoplasmacytic infiltrate. The authors stated that this tumoral condition is most likely fibroinflammatory or reactive in nature. Some authors [136] have suggested that this neoplasm is a late sclerosing stage of inflammatory myofibroblastic tumor in at least some cases, while others have not found convincing evidence to support an association between calcifying fibrous pseudotumor and inflammatory myofibroblastic tumor and have suggested that this tumor should be designated as calcifying fibrous tumor [137].

CFPT originating in the thoracic cavity are extremely rare and have been described in the chest wall and the lung [138–140]. Pinkard et al. [141] are credited for the description of these tumors in the pleura. The authors described three cases with similar characteristics as those described in the soft tissues. Single case reports have followed that initial description [142–148].

Clinical Features

The tumors appear not to have any particular gender predilection, and have been described in a wide range of ages from 23 to 55 years. Clinically, symptoms of chest pain, shortness of breath, and cough, have been described while some patients are entirely asymptomatic. Use of diagnostic imaging shows well-marginated, pleural tumors, which on CT demonstrate common calcifications [149].

Macroscopic Features

The tumors can be solitary or multiple lesions on the pleural surface. They are well circumscribed, firm, tan, and lobulated, which on cut surface may show a gritty consistency. The tumors vary in size from 1 to more than 10 cm in greatest diameter.

Histopathological Features

The tumors in the pleura are solitary to those described in soft tissues. The hallmark of these tumors is extensive hyalinization with a discrete spindle cell proliferation, numerous calcifications of different sizes and a subtle lymphoplasmacytic infiltrate (Fig. 12.64a–c). The tumor does not show necrosis and/or hemorrhage nor does it show areas of cellular atypia or mitotic activity.

Immunohistochemical Features

Since only few cases of pleural CFPT have been reported, there is limited information about immunohistochemical studies. However, calcifying fibrous pseudotumors have been found to react with CD34 and are negative for epithelial markers.

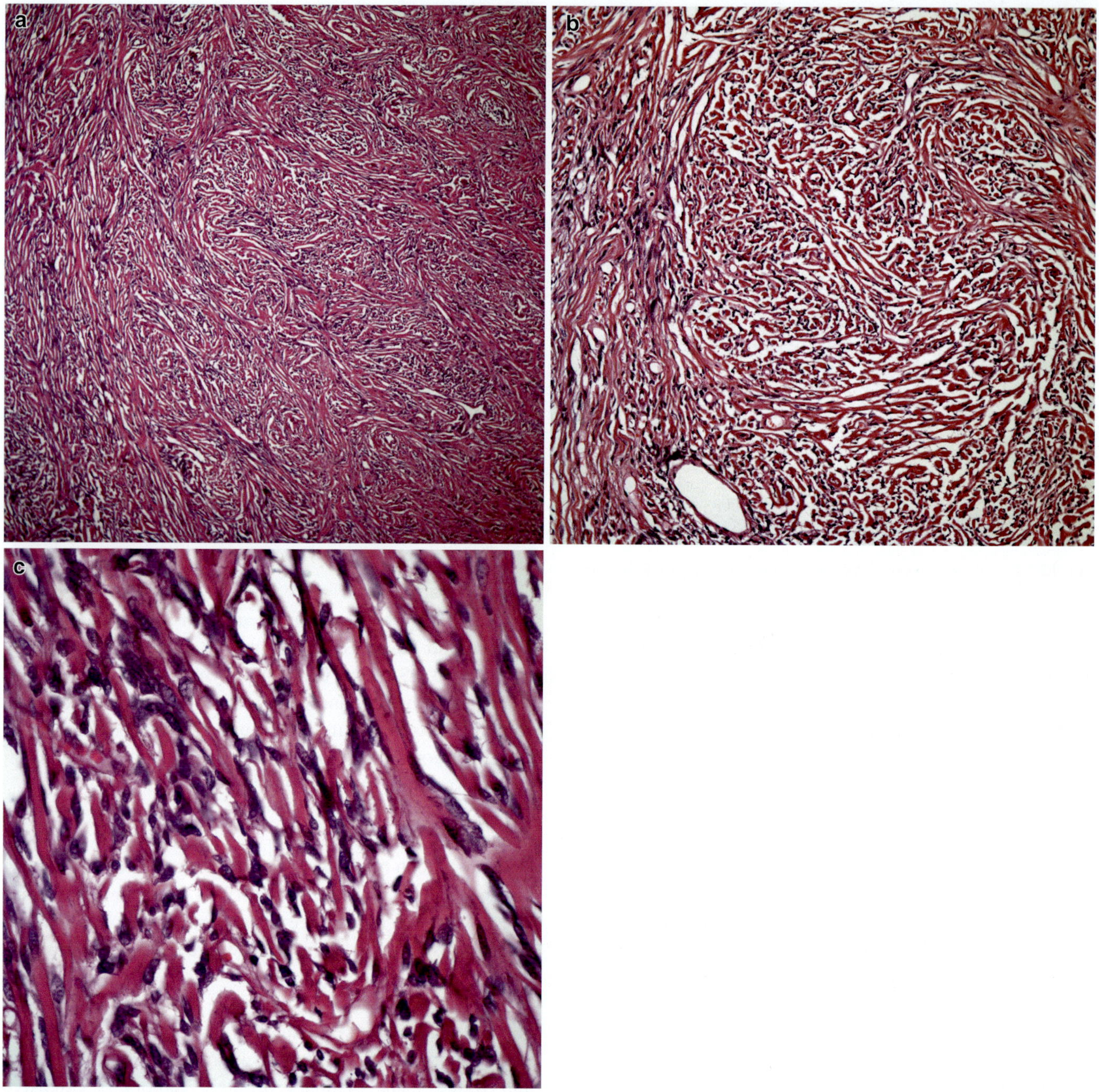

Fig. 12.62 (**a**) Solitary fibrous tumor with prominent fibroblastic component. (**b**) Classic rope-like collagen. (**c**) Higher magnification of a bland spindle cell proliferation admixed with collagen

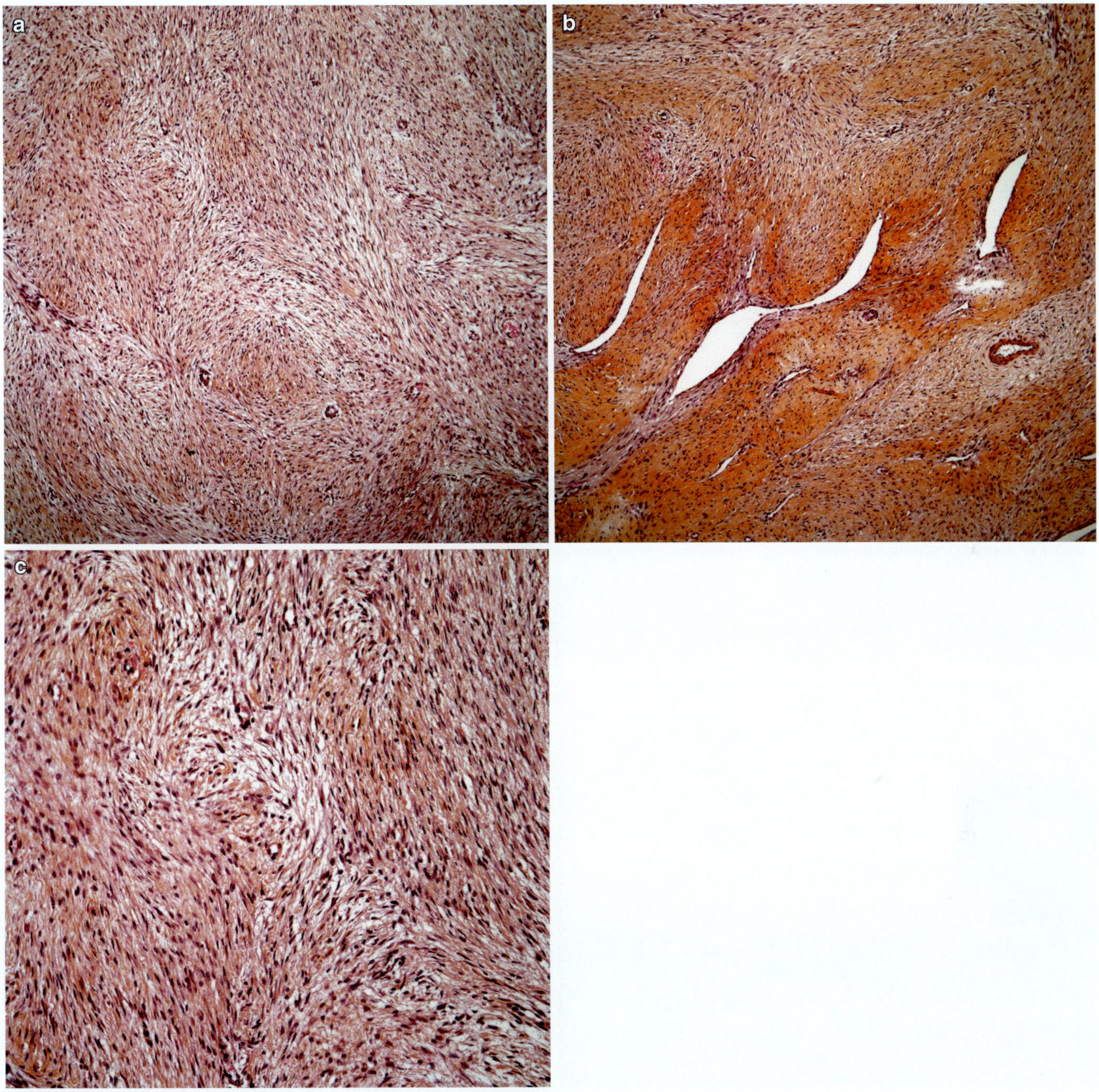

Fig. 12.63 (**a**) Spindle cell proliferation in a background of fibrillary-like matrix. (**b**) Spindle cell proliferation with numerous dilated blood vessels. (**c**) Interlacing fascicles of spindle cells. Note the absence of necrosis or increased mitotic activity

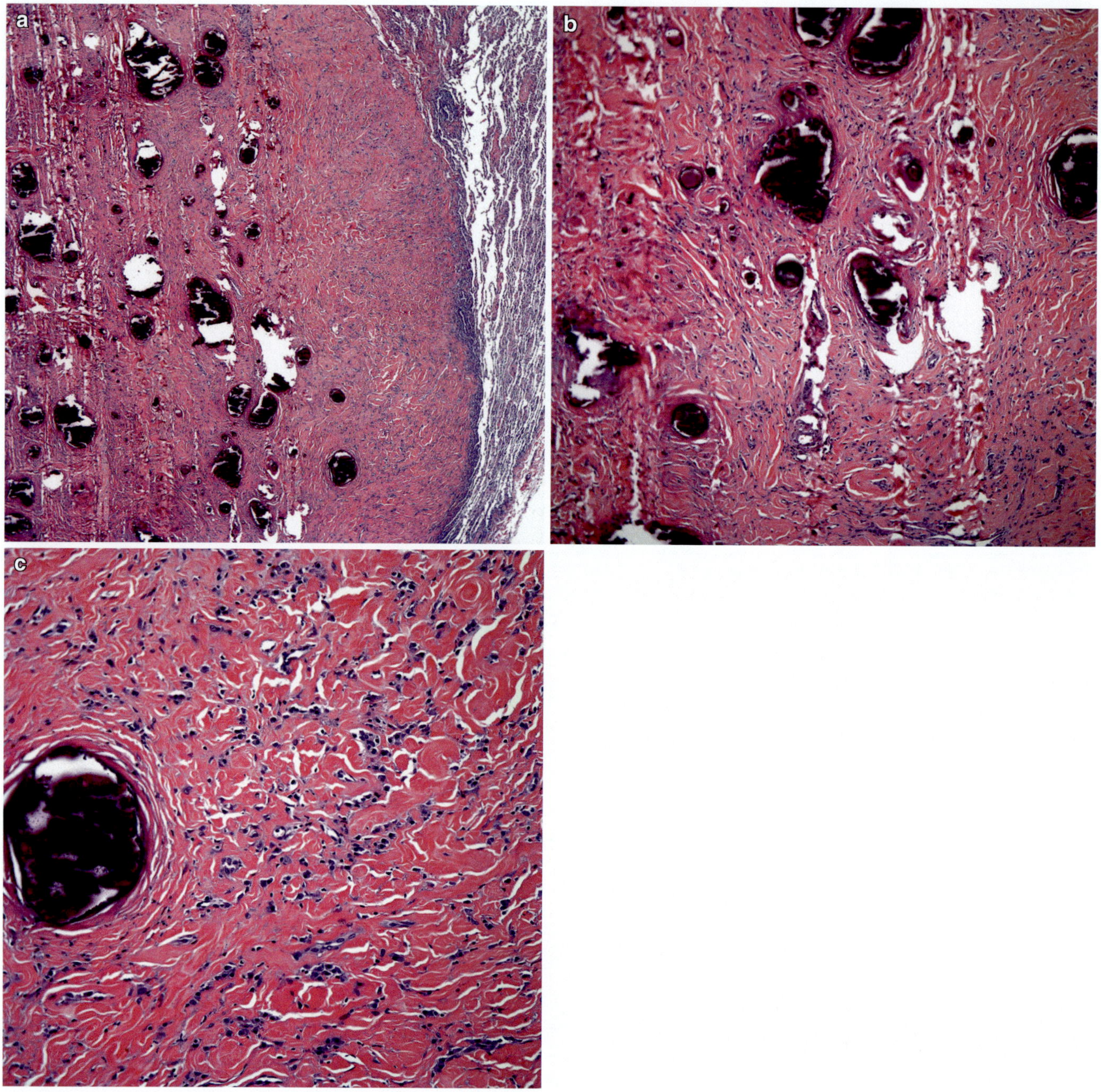

Fig. 12.64 (**a**) Low power view of a calcifying fibrous pseudotumor of the pleura; note the numerous calcifications present. (**b**) The calcifications are embedded in a collagenous matrix. (**c**) The collagenous matrix shows the presence of a plasmacytic inflammatory component

Differential Diagnosis

Solitary fibrous tumor is the most important differential diagnosis, and its separation from CFPT may be difficult, if not impossible, on biopsy material. In resected material, the presence of psammomatous of dystrophic calcifications in a tumor with abundant collagen and lymphoplasmacytic infiltrate should lead to the correct diagnosis. Contrary to solitary fibrous tumor, which may show different patterns of growth in the same tumor, CFPT is rather uniform and does not show the variability that solitary fibrous tumor shows. Both of these tumors may show CD34 positive staining [150]. The immunohistochemical reaction for Bcl-2 in CFPT is unknown so far.

Treatment and Prognosis

Complete surgical resection is the treatment of choice. However, in those cases in which there are multiple pleural tumors, complications of complete surgical resection may be high. When the tumor occurs in soft tissues, local recurrences have been described in a few cases. Thus, one might expect similar behavior for pleural CFPT.

Amyloid Tumor

Even though amyloid does not represent a neoplastic condition, it is important to highlight that in unusual conditions amyloid may involve the pleura in a manner that may mimic mesothelioma [151]. However, the most important aspect is the fact that a pleural biopsy may a collection of amorphous material that may be confused with the dense collagen present in calcifying fibrous pseudotumor of the pleura or solitary fibrous tumor. Therefore, it is important to keep amyloid tumor in the differential diagnosis of pleural lesions.

Smooth Muscle and Biphasic Mesenchymal Tumors

Primary pleural neoplasms showing smooth muscle differentiation are exceedingly rare. Similarly, biphasic neoplastic processes arising in the pleural surface other than biphasic mesotheliomas are very rare. However, the existence of primary leiomyosarcomas and primary synovial sarcomas of the pleura has been well recognized in the literature.

Smooth Muscle Tumors

These tumors are among the most unusual primary pleural neoplasms. In a series of five cases [152], the patients were three women and two men ranging in age from 21 to 69 years. Clinically, the patients presented with symptoms of chest pain and empyema, while one patient was asymptomatic. In four of these patients, the tumor presented as a solitary pleural based mass, while in one patient the tumor appears to encase the lung in a manner similar to malignant mesothelioma. The tumors varied in size from 10 to 18 cm in greatest diameter. All patients underwent surgical resection; however, in two patients the surgical removal of the tumor was incomplete. Unfortunately, the follow-up provided (2–12 months) was not long enough to provide more meaningful behavior of these tumors. Therefore, the clinical behavior of these tumors is uncertain [152].

Histopathological Features

The tumors described span from smooth muscle tumors of uncertain malignant potential to leiomyosarcomas of low, intermediate, and high grade histology (Fig. 12.65a–f). The tumors of low grade histology were characterized by interlacing fascicles of elongated cells intersecting at right angles. The cytology of the cellular proliferation was that of spindle cells with cigar-shaped nuclei and moderate amounts of eosinophilic cytoplasm. No areas of hemorrhage and/or necrosis were present and nuclear atypia was mild with only rare mitotic figures found. In the tumors of intermediate and high grade histology, the basic arrangement of the neoplastic cellular proliferation was similar to that seen in low grade tumors; however, the areas of necrosis and hemorrhage were present. In addition, nuclear atypia and mitotic figures were easily identified and were numerous.

Immunohistochemical Features

Smooth muscle actin and desmin are of help as these tumors generally exhibit positive staining in tumor cells for these antibodies. However, it is of interest to note that in some cases of smooth muscle tumors of the pleura, keratin may also be positive. Therefore, it is important to perform a wider panel of antibodies in cases in which the suspicion is high for a smooth muscle neoplasm.

Differential Diagnosis

The most important differential diagnosis includes either malignant mesothelioma or a metastatic smooth muscle tumor. In the former, the use of immunohistochemical stains—namely, keratin, CK5/6 and calretinin—may lead to the correct interpretation. However, some cases of pleural smooth muscle tumors may react positively for keratin antibodies. Nevertheless, it would be unusual for a mesothelioma to show a strong positive reaction for smooth muscle actin and/or desmin. In the latter, a good clinical history and radiological evaluation play the most important role.

Biphasic Synovial Sarcoma

Because this tumor is more common in the soft tissues, it is highly important to properly exclude the possibility of metastatic disease. Nevertheless, synovial sarcoma may rarely present as primary pleural based tumor. Gaertner et al. [153] reported five cases: three females and two males between the ages of 9 and 50 years. Clinically, the patients presented with symptoms of dysphagia, chest pain, fever, and/or pneumothorax. In four patients the findings were those of a pleural mass; however, in one of the patients described, the radiological findings also showde pleural thickening. The tumors varied in size from 5 to more than 20 cm in greatest diameter. All the patients were treated with surgery and at least three additional patients received chemoradiation. According to this report, four patients followed a fatal outcome with death within a period of 12–30 months. Only one patient in this series was alive with disease 8 years after the initial diagnosis.

Histopathological Features

The histological features of these tumors are the same as those described for biphasic synovial sarcomas of the soft tissues. The tumors typically show a spindle cell proliferation of tightly arranged fascicles of neoplastic cells with fusiform nuclei and inconspicuous nucleoli; mitotic figures are easily identifiable. This spindle cell proliferation may assume a fibrosarcomatous or hemangiopericytic growth pattern. Admixed with this spindle cell proliferation, is a glandular epithelial component composed of acinar structures lined by either low cuboidal or tall columnar epithelium, which may show intraluminal secretion and papillary arrangement. Mitotic activity in the glandular component is not readily identifiable. In addition, the tumor may

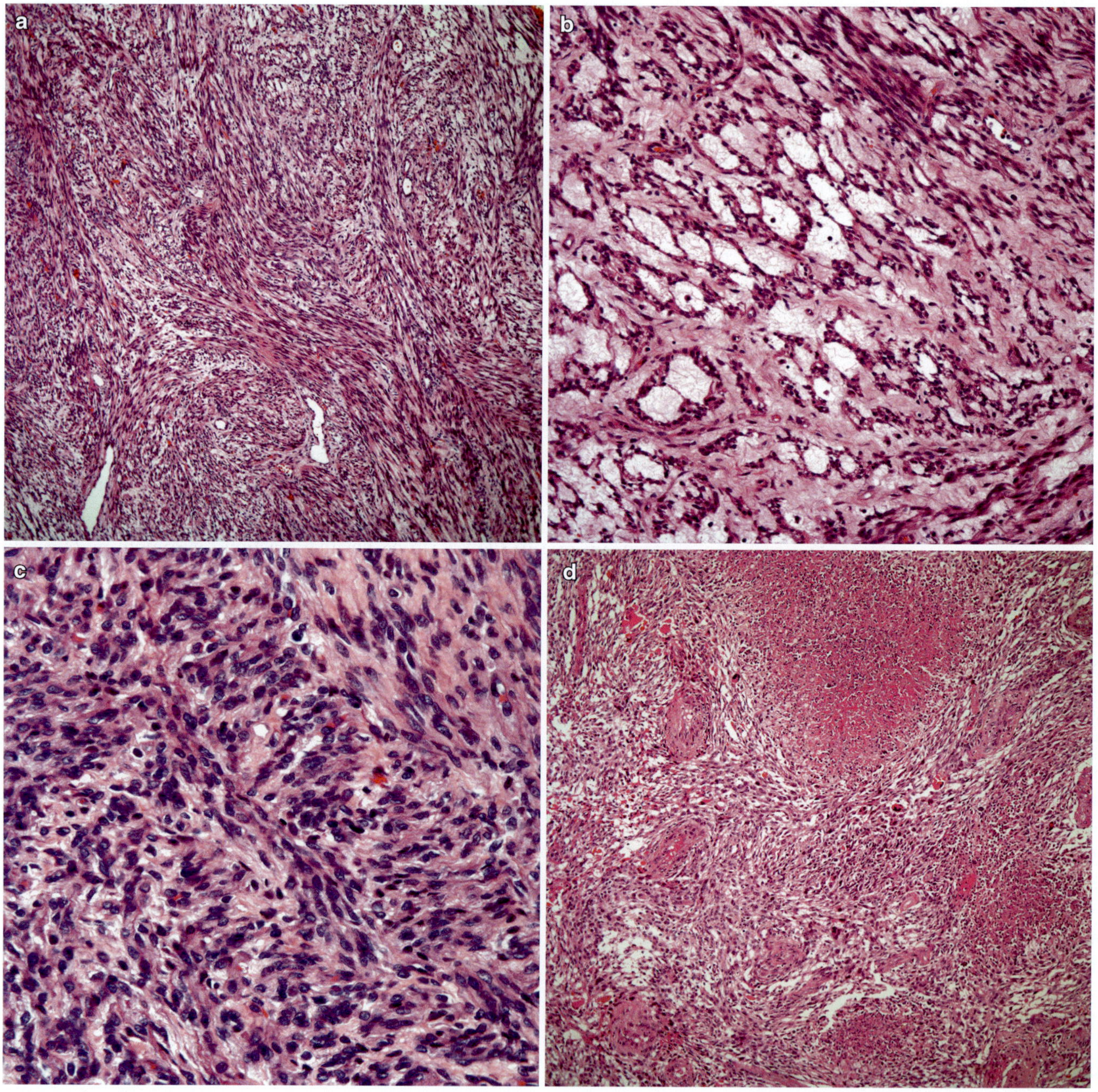

Fig. 12.65 (**a**) Low grade leiomyosarcoma showing the classical spindle cell proliferation of interlacing fascicles of cells. (**b**) Low grade leiomyosarcoma showing epithelioid features. (**c**) High power view of a low grade leiomyosarcoma showing mild nuclear atypia and low mitotic activity. (**d**) Low power view of a high grade leiomyosarcoma showing areas of necrosis. (**e**) High grade leiomyosarcoma with prominent cellular atypia. (**f**) High power view of a high grade leiomyosarcoma showing mitotic activity

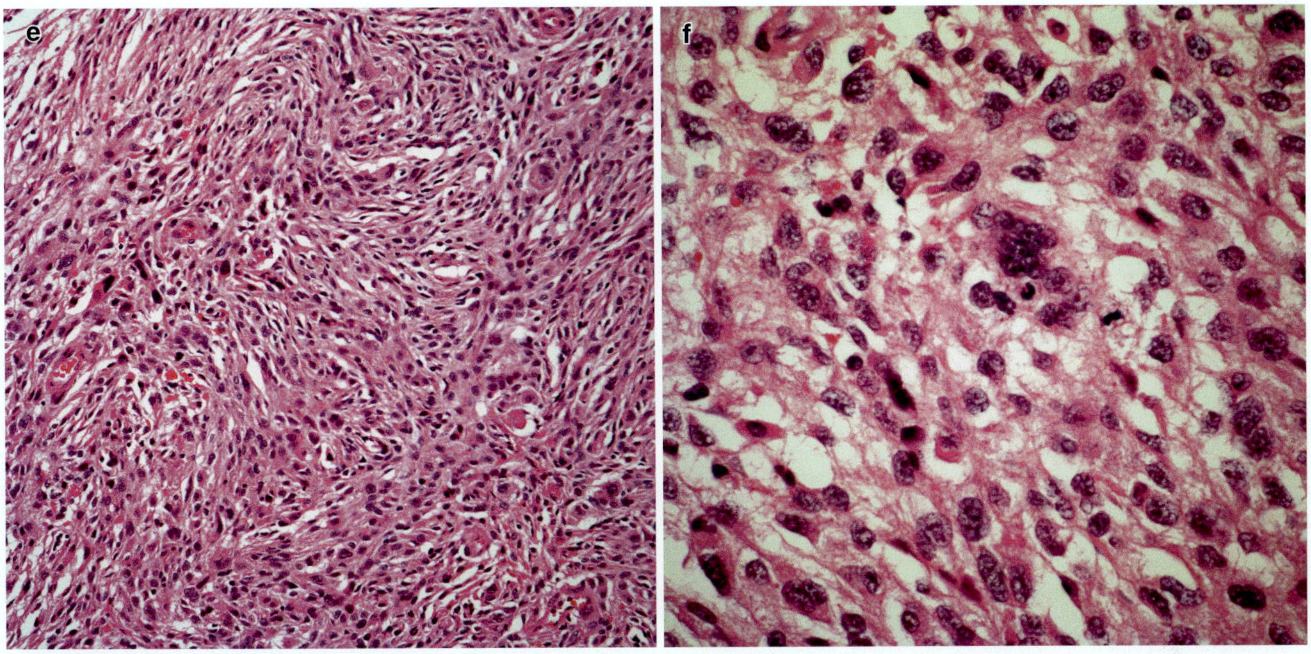

Fig.12.65 (continued)

show an inflammatory infiltrate composed of mast cells, lymphocytes and/or plasma cells, metaplastic bone formation, or calcifications (Fig. 12.66a–d).

Histochemical and Immunohistochemical Features

The use of periodic acid-Schiff (PAS) with and without diastase and mucicarmine may help show positive staining for mucin, mainly in the glandular component of the tumor. Immunohistochemical studies may show the presence of positive staining for the epithelial markers keratin and EMA as well as CEA in the glandular component. On the other hand, keratin and EMA may show focal staining in the spindle cell component. S100 protein and Bcl-2 may also show a positive reaction in the spindle cell component of the tumor.

Differential Diagnosis

Because of the biphasic nature of these tumors, the most important differential diagnosis includes biphasic malignant mesothelioma. Although rare, a few cases of malignant mesothelioma have been described presenting as a pleural mass. However, the use of immunohistochemical stains, mainly CEA positivity in the glandular component of the tumor, would be highly unusual for mesothelioma. In addition, a positive reaction of the tumor cells for epithelial markers, namely, keratin and EMA is, rather focal in synovial sarcomas contrary to the more global strong positive reaction in cases of mesothelioma. The other important differential diagnosis includes metastatic synovial sarcoma of soft tissue origin. In this setting a complete clinical history and radiological evaluation would be the best parameters to arrive at a more definitive diagnosis.

Neural and Neuroectodermal Neoplasms

Although neural and neuroectodermal neoplasms are mainly represented by the so-called small round cell tumors of the thoracopulmonary region, in essence primitive neuroectodermal tumor (PNET), in some unusual circumstances, the authors have also seen primary meningiomas arising from the pleural surface. Important to highlight is the fact that small round cell tumors may also be present as metastatic disease; therefore, it is important to properly exclude that possibility. Similarly, metastatic meningiomas to the pleura are by far more common and as such have been presented in the literature.

Primitive Neuroectodermal Tumor

Extraosseous small round cell tumors bearing features similar to those described in the bone under the name of Ewing's sarcoma and occurring in the thoracopulmonary region, are rare. Over the years, these tumors have been known by a variety of names including extraskeletal Ewing's sarcoma, malignant small cell tumor of the thoracopulmonary region, Askin's tumor, paravertebral round cell tumor, and PNET. Currently, most of those tumors have been grouped into a single family of PNET [154–163].

Angerval and Enzinger [154] described 39 cases, some of them occurring in the thoracic area. They were characterized by small round cells with scant cytoplasm, moderate amounts of nuclear chromatin inconspicuous nucleoli,

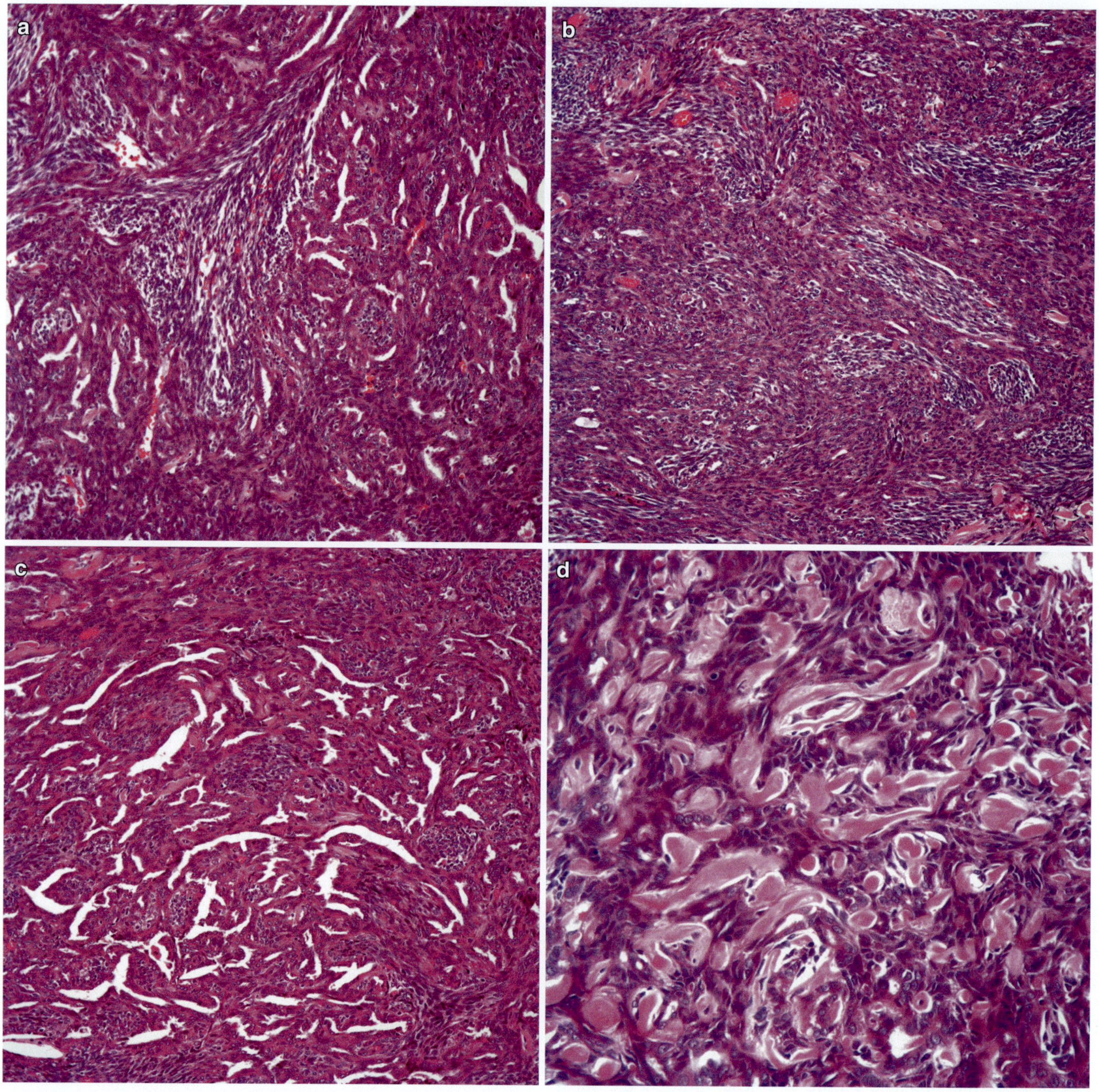

Fig. 12.66 (**a**) Low power view of pleural biphasic synovial sarcoma showing the classical epithelioid (glandular) and spindle cell component. (**b**) Synovial sarcoma with a prominent spindle cell component. (**c**) Synovial sarcoma with a prominent glandular component. (**d**) High power view of a pleural synovial sarcoma showing the neoplastic cells admixed with collagenous material

mitoses, rosettes, hemorrhage, and necrosis. In addition, intracellular glycogen was identified. Traditionally, the latter had been considered to be a characteristic feature observed in extraskeletal Ewing's sarcoma but not in the other neoplasms of this group including neuroblastoma and Askin's tumor. However, it is well known that some neuroblastomas may also contain glycogen in their cytoplasm [164]. Thus, the finding of glycogen alone does not indicate a particular neoplasm. Askin et al. [155] is credited for the description of these tumors in the thoracopulmonary region. The authors described 20 cases designated under the name of malignant small cell tumors of the thoracopulmonary region. Interestingly, none of the cases described contained glycogen in the cytoplasm of the cells, but histologically the tumors showed high similarity to the cases previously described by Angerval and Enzinger as extraskeletal Ewing's sarcoma. However, the absence of glycogen was one of the parameters used to separate these two previously mentioned entities. Electron microscopic studies have also been controversial stating that the features of extraskeletal Ewing's sarcoma are distinctive enough to allow separation from other small cell tumors [165], while others stated that the ultrastructure of these tumors is broad and shows some overlapping features [166].

Clinical Features

Younger patients appear to be more commonly affected by these tumors, presenting with symptoms of chest pain, shortness of breath, and/or pneumothorax. By imaging, the tumor is often restricted to one hemithorax involving pleura and/or chest wall. However, it is important to note that PNETs have also been described as tumors arising within the lung parenchyma as primary lung neoplasm [167–170].

Macroscopic Features

These tumors may vary in size from 2 to more than 10 cm in greatest dimension. They are tan white, firm, and have a homogeneous cut surface. Areas of hemorrhage and/or necrosis may be present. Calcifications have also been reported. Even though PNET may have a pleural origin, the tumor may also invade the lung and/or the ribs. In some cases the tumor may be at the hilum of the lung, paraspinal region, or chest wall.

Histopathological Features

The low magnification of these tumors shows a neoplastic cellular proliferation, which can be separated in lobules by thin fibroconnective tissue, while in other areas the cellular proliferation is distributed in sheets of neoplastic cells, cords, or nests. Cystic areas filled with blood and pools of blood may also be seen. At higher magnification, the neoplastic cellular population is rather homogenous composed of round cells with indistinct cell borders, scant cytoplasm, round to elongated nuclei, and inconspicuous small nucleoli. In some areas, the tumor cells have a tendency to be distributed around vessels. Mitotic activity can be brisk, and necrosis and hemorrhage are invariably present. In better differentiated tumors, the presence of rosettes helps in the diagnosis; however, rosettes are not always present in these tumors (Fig. 12.67a–d). In some cases, necrosis and/or hemorrhage can be so prominent that the tumor cells are difficult to visualize. In other tumors, the so-called Azzopardi phenomenon may be seen.

Histochemical and Immunohistochemical Features

Periodic acid-Schiff (PAS) may aid in the diagnosis; however, not only may this histochemical stain be negative but also positive staining may also be seen in other types of neoplasms in this particular anatomic location.

On the other hand, the use of immunohistochemistry has shaped to some extent our views regarding these tumors. Initially, the use of neuron-specific enolase (NSE) was considered specific for the neural derivation of these tumors; however, that notion has changed after NSE has been observed to show positive staining in several other tumors, which were not necessarily of neural origin [171, 172]. An additional marker that has been used with partial results in the evaluation of these tumors is S100 protein; however, the results obtained have been controversial [157, 173]. More recently, the use of CD99 (HBA-71 or the MIC2 gene product) has been viewed as an important immunohistochemical tool for the diagnosis of these tumors; however, CD99 may also show positive staining in other tumors of epithelial and mesenchymal origin. One other immunohistochemical markers that can be of help in the proper clinical setting is synaptophysin, which is more widely used as a neuroendocrine marker. This latter immunohistochemical marker appears to be consistent in the staining of these tumors [174]. Other markers that have been used with some success in small round cell tumors include WT1, which has been stated to reliably differentiate desmoplastic small round cell tumor from Ewing's sarcoma/PNET [175]. In addition, NB84 also appears to show positive staining in some cases of PNET. However, this antibody is more commonly seen positive in neuroblastomas [176].

Molecular Biology Features

Molecular techniques have established a closer relationship between Ewing's sarcoma and PNET. The current view of these tumors is that they are closely related. Chromosome translocations t(11; 22)(q24; q12) and t(21; 22)(q22; 1q12) and their oncoproteins are frequently found in cases of Ewing's sarcoma/PNET [177–179].

Differential Diagnosis

Since there are other types of sarcoma and/or neural tumors that can occur more commonly within this location and because of the rarity of PNET in this location the diagnosis may not be as straightforward as in other anatomic areas. By far the most important differential diagnostic considerations include rhabdomyosarcoma, neuroblastoma, lymphoma/leukemia, and more unusually metastatic small cell carcinoma or metastatic sarcoma from an osseous primary. The two latter conditions can be dealt with by careful clinical history and radiological evaluation. However, with the former ones, careful histological and immunohistochemical analysis is required. In cases of rhabdomyosarcoma, the presence of rhabdomyoblasts in better differentiated tumors may be diagnostic. In cases in which the histology is not so characteristic, the use of a panel of immunohistochemical studies including muscle markers (desmin, calponin, myoglobin) can help with this problem. Neuroblastomas can be more difficult to rule out since these tumor vary in their immunohistochemical profile. NSE and S100 protein may

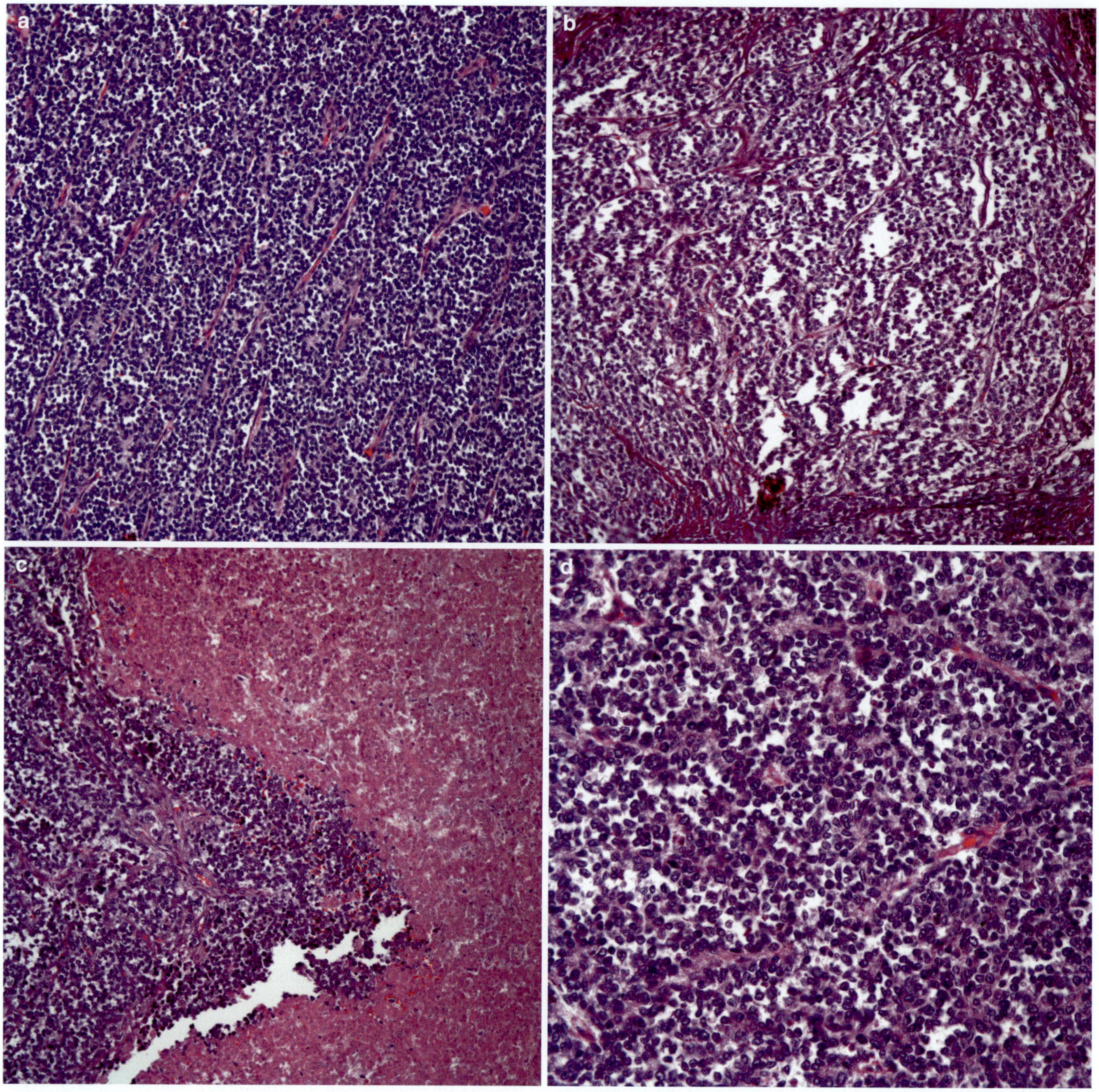

Fig. 12.67 (**a**) Low power view of a small round cell tumor so-called Askin's tumor. (**b**) PNET showing subtle nested growth pattern. (**c**) PNET with extensive necrosis. (**d**) Higher magnification showing an attempt to rosette formation

show positive staining in both tumors; however, the presence of synaptophysin and CD99 positivity coupled with tumor histology will bias toward a PNET. In cases of lymphoma or leukemia, the histological features and the presence of positive staining in tumor cells with LCA and B- or T-cell markers should lead to a correct interpretation.

Treatment and Prognosis

The treatment of choice for PNET is chemotherapy; however, the prognosis is relatively poor for these patients. In a study of 30 cases by Contesso et al. [180], the overall survival was 38 % at 2 years and 14 % at 6 years.

Pleural Meningioma

As stated earlier, the majority of reports on the occurrence of meningiomas involving the pleural surface have centered on metastatic meningiomas from a CNS primary. It is important to note that these tumors can occur within the lung parenchyma, but to our knowledge no report of pleural involvement by primary pulmonary meningiomas has been reported.

We recently analyzed a case of primary meningioma arising from the pleural surface and involving extensive areas of the pleura.[1] The tumor showed unusual histological features including rosettes, palisading of the nuclei, papillary features, nuclear atypia, and mitotic activity (Fig. 12.68a–f). Based on those findings the tumor was regarded as an anaplastic (malignant) meningioma. However, it is important to highlight that before rendering a diagnosis of primary pleural meningioma, a complete evaluation is performed to rule the possibility of a present or past meningioma of CNS origin.

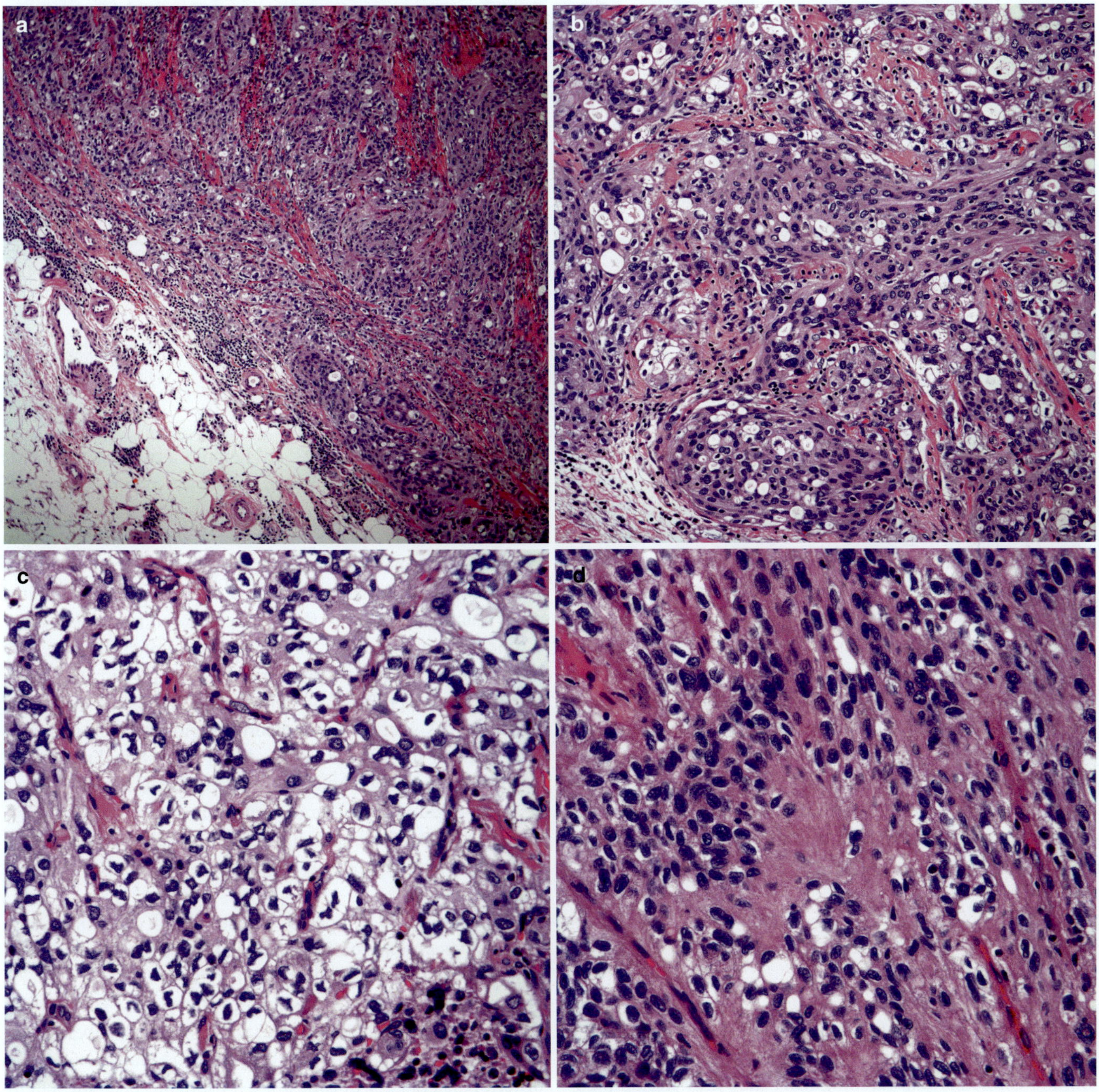

Fig. 12.68 (**a**) Low power view of a primary pleural meningioma. Note the tumor infiltrating into adipose tissue. (**b**) Higher magnification showing more conventional cellular characteristics. (**c**) Areas of clear cells. (**d**) Areas in which the cells appear to be embedded in a neurofibrillary matrix. (**e**) Ependymal-like rosettes. (**f**) Presence of mitotic activity

[1] Own observations. Unreported data.

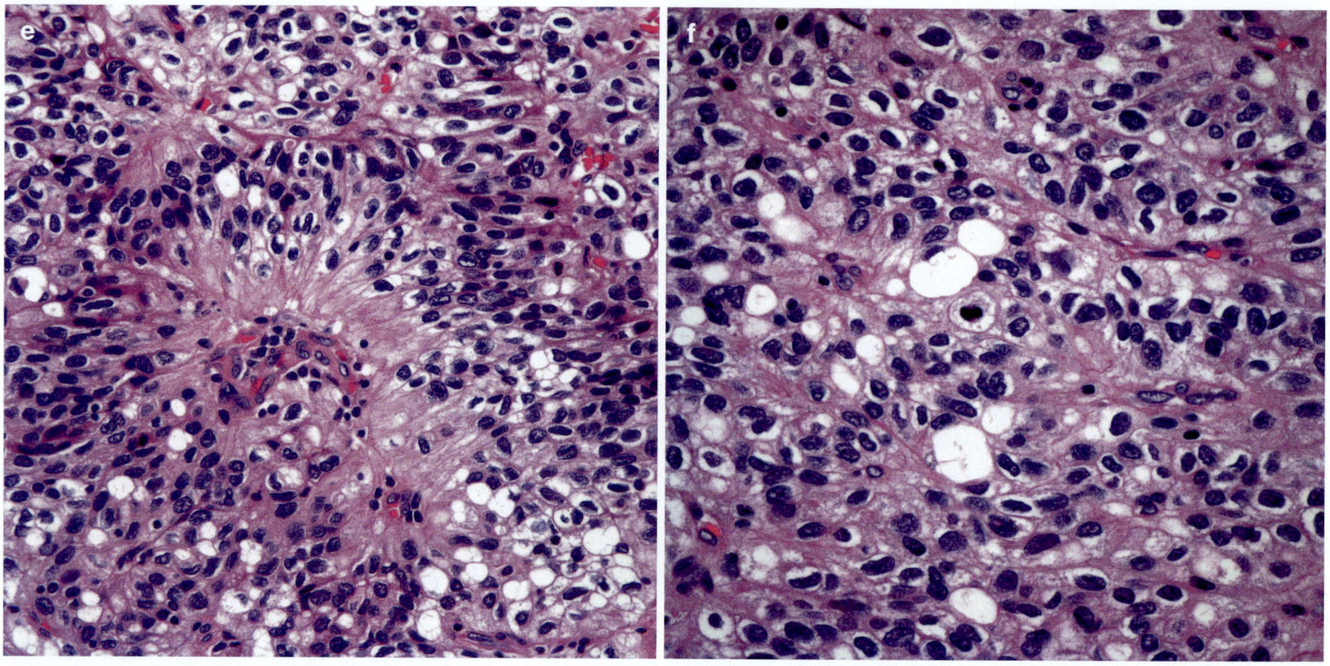

Fig 12.68 (continued)

Vascular Tumors

Primary vascular tumors arising on the pleural surface are very rare. More interesting is the fact that most of the reports of tumors of vascular origin have dealt essentially with malignant tumors or at least tumors of low grade malignancy. Therefore, the two most often encountered tumors in this location are epithelioid hemangioendothelioma and angiosarcoma. It is important to point out that in some authors' views, these two tumors may represent the same entity when they are present in the pleura, and often the designation of a low grade angiosarcoma is applied even for tumors that others would have called epithelioid hemangioendothelioma. Nevertheless, both tumors are unusual and metastatic disease to the pleura needs to be excluded before a diagnosis of primary vascular neoplasm can be rendered since the histological features for both are identical.

Pleural Angiosarcoma

Angiosarcomas are commonly seen as primary tumors of the soft tissue but they are exceedingly rare as primary pleural tumors. Clinically and radiologically they may mimic pleural mesothelioma. Therefore, a histopathological assessment including immunohistochemical studies and possibly electron microscopic analysis is needed in order to arrive at this particular diagnosis.

In 1997, Falconieri et al. [181] reported two autopsy cases of what the authors described as diffuse pleuropulmonary angiosarcoma simulating mesothelioma. The tumors grew along the serosal surface and were characterized by thick rinds of tissue encasing the lung. Thus, the authors concluded that, although rare, angiosarcomas might involve the pleura in a manner similar to that described for mesotheliomas. Clinically, patients with pleural angiosarcoma may present with hemothorax, chest pain, cough, hemoptysis, and shortness of breath [182–187]. Tuberculous pyothorax has been found in association with pleural angiosarcomas in cases described in the Japanese literature [188, 189]. Frate et al. [190] reported a case with CT and PET features of circumferential right-sided pleural thickening. In addition, a PET scan performed for staging purposes showed the presence of multiple lobulated areas of increased uptake similar to those seen on CT scan.

Zhang et al. [191] reported a series of five cases of epithelioid angiosarcomas of the pleura and stated that these tumors appear to affect adult individuals ranging from 22 and 79 years of age with a male-to-female ratio of 9:1. The authors found that in Western cases, no history of tuberculous pyothorax was present contrary to the Japanese cases described. A history of asbestos exposure has been present in some cases. The authors also raised some questions about cases that had been classified as pleural epithelioid hemangioendothelioma and noted that some if not all of those cases may represent cases of epithelioid angiosarcoma.

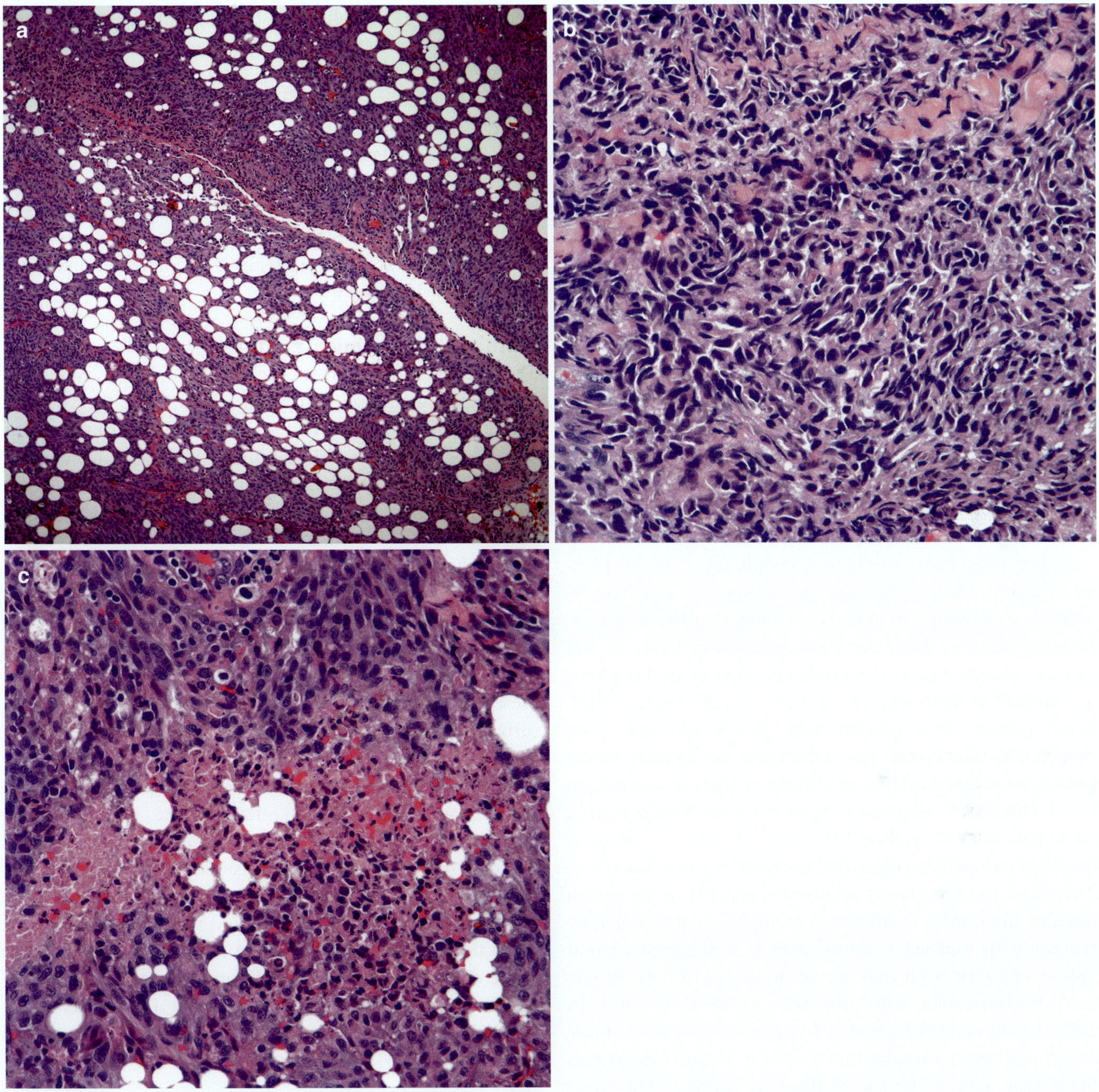

Fig. 12.69 (**a**) Pleural angiosarcoma infiltrating adipose tissue. (**b**) Spindle cell proliferation with marked cellular atypia. (**c**) Areas of necrosis and mitotic activity are present

Histopathological Features

Pleural angiosarcomas are similar to those described in the soft tissues. The tumors may be formed by sheets, strands, or cords of epithelioid cells embedded in a collagenous or hyalinized stroma. The neoplastic cellular proliferation is composed of round to oval cells with moderate amounts of light eosinophilic cytoplasm, round nuclei, and small nucleoli. The cells appear to be plump given the appearance of a histiocytic or epithelioid cellular proliferation. Necrosis and/or areas of hemorrhage may be present. Mitotic figures are easily encountered and nuclear atypia is commonly seen. The neoplastic cellular proliferation may also be seen infiltrating adjacent adipose tissue (Fig. 12.69a–c).

Immunohistochemical Features

Vascular markers including CD31, CD34, and factor VIII are usually positive in tumors cells. However, cytokeratin and CEA may also show focal or weak positive staining [191]. Therefore, the use of a complete panel including vascular and epithelial markers is indicated in tumors in which there is a suspicion of pleural angiosarcoma.

Treatment and Prognosis

The prognosis of patients with pleural angiosarcomas is poor. Surgical resection and chemotherapy have been attempted as treatment options for these patients. Metastatic disease to distant organs including the brain has been documented in some cases.

Pleural Epithelioid Hemangioendothelioma (EH)

Epithelioid hemangioendothelioma (EH) in the thoracic cavity is more commonly seen in the lung in which the tumor characteristically presents as multiple bilateral pulmonary nodules. In unusual circumstances, EH may affect the pleura in a manner closely resembling that of mesothelioma. Clinically, EH appears to affect men and women over 45 years of age who may present with varied symptomatology including chest pain, weight loss, cough, fever, and/or pleural effusion. These symptoms are nonspecific and may be seen in a diversity of tumors of lung or pleural origin. Imaging features that have been reported in cases of EH include unilateral pleural fluid and nodular pleural thickening similar to that seen in cases of mesothelioma [192]. Some patients may present with pleural effusion, even though the tumor may not necessarily be located in the pleura but rather in adjacent structures such as diaphragm [193]. History of asbestos exposure has been documented in some patients with pleural EH [194]. However, no ferruginous bodies have been identified in any of the cases described. Therefore, the association of asbestos and EH of the pleura remains unclear. It is important to highlight that EH may present with unusual features such as a bilateral pleural tumor with extension into the peritoneum [195] or as primary pleural tumor with metastasis to the skin [196]. In 1996, Lin et al. [197] reported 14 cases of what the authors called malignant vascular tumors of the serous membranes mimicking mesothelioma; of these 14 cases, eight cases were in the pleura. The mean age of these patients was 52 years and all patients were males except for two female patients with peritoneal tumors. The patients with pleural tumors had diffuse pleural thickening and pleural effusion; in one of these patients a 1.5-cm solitary subpleural tumor was also identified, while one patient had a previous history of bone EH now presenting with pleural involvement in a manner mimicking mesothelioma. It is worth mentioning that at least two patients had a history of asbestos exposure, which could not be proven by histological means.

Histological Features

The tumor is composed of strands, cords, or solid areas of epithelioid cells composed of round to oval or spindle cells with a myxoid or hyalinized stromal component. The cells may show a nucleus displaced toward the cell periphery strongly resembling signet ring cells; mitotic activity is not high and nuclear pleomorphism is mild. In some cases, areas forming intracellular lumina containing red cells may be seen. A case of pleural EH with prominent rhabdoid features has been described [198]. The cellular proliferation appears to be embedded in a collagenous background, and in some cases the tumor may extend into adjacent adipose tissue in manner similar to that seen in cases of epithelioid mesotheliomas (Fig. 12.70a–c).

Immunohistochemical Features

The use of vascular markers such as CD34, CD31, and factor VIII is important and will aid in determining the vascular nature of the tumor. However, it is important to recognize that in some cases of EH, the tumor cells may also express focal or weak positive staining for epithelial markers such as keratin. Therefore, it is crucial that if one is suspecting the possibility of EH, vascular markers as those previously mentioned should be part of a panel of immunohistochemical studies. In addition, EH appears to show a strong positive reaction for vimentin.

Differential Diagnosis

Mesotheliomas or adenocarcinomas involving the pleural surface are by far more common and are tumors that need to be carefully excluded. In this setting, the use of immunohistochemical studies including vascular and epithelial markers should lead to the correct interpretation. As one would expect, the diagnosis may be more challenging in small biopsies in which the characteristic histopathological features of EH may not be apparent. In this setting immunohistochemical markers to include epithelial and vascular markers may prove useful. One other condition that may present a diagnostic challenge is adenomatoid tumor. However, adenomatoid tumor may show positive staining for markers like calretinin and keratin and negative staining for vascular markers like CD31, CD34, and factor VIII.

Treatment and Prognosis

The treatment of choice for these tumors is surgical resection. However, the issue may be more complicated in cases in which there is extensive involvement of the pleura with encasement of the lung, which may require an extrapleural pneumonectomy or medical treatment with chemotherapy. Such decisions are based on medical and radiological grounds. The prognosis of these tumors will be defined by the extension of the tumor. In cases in which there is a pleural based nodule or mass that is amenable to complete surgical resection, the prognosis may be better than in cases with extensive involvement of the pleura. In the cases reported by Lin et al. [197], the majority of the patients had a fatal outcome.

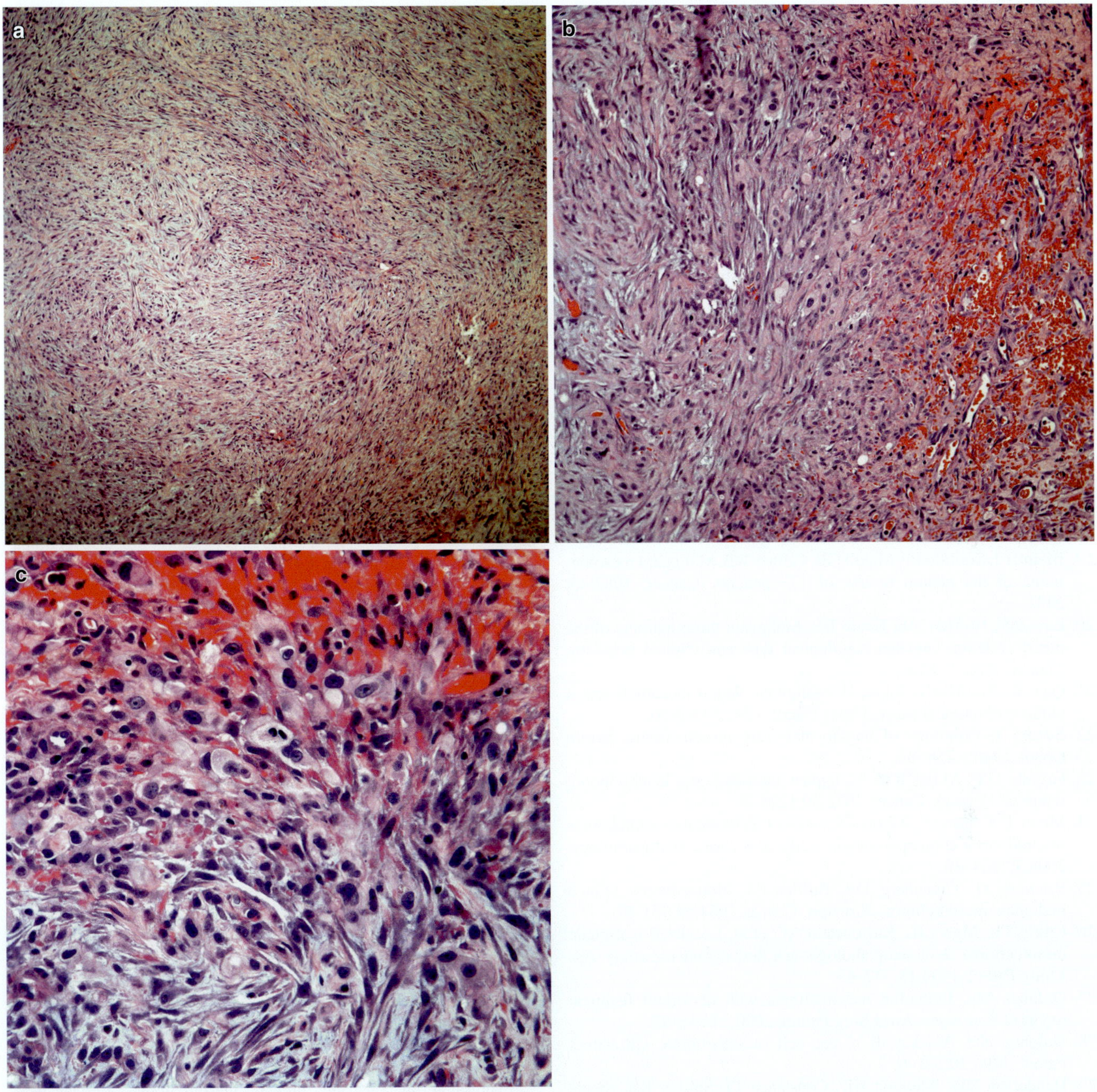

Fig. 12.70 (**a**) Pleural epithelioid hemangioendothelioma showing a spindle cellular proliferation with subtle myxoid changes. (**b**) Spindle cell proliferation admixed with numerous red cells. (**c**) Higher magnification showing a spindle cellular proliferation lacking mitotic activity

References

1. Hinds MW. Mesothelioma in the United States: incidence in the 1970s. J Occup Med. 1978;20:469–71.
2. National Cancer Institute. SEER Cancer Statistics Review 1975–2003. http://seer.cancer.gov/csr/1975_2003/results_merged/sect_17mesothelioma.pdf. Accessed 3 Jan 2012.
3. Craighead JE. The epidemiology and pathogenesis of malignant mesothelioma. Chest. 1989;96:92–3.
4. Wright WE, Sherwin RP. Histological types of malignant mesothelioma and asbestos exposure. Br J Ind Med. 1984;41:514–7.
5. Borow M, Conston A, Livornese L, et al. Mesothelioma following exposure to asbestos: a review of 72 cases. Chest. 1973;64:641–6.
6. Wagner E. Das tuberkelähnliche Lymphadenom. Arch F Heilk. 1870;11:497–525.
7. Robertson HE. Endothelioma of the pleura. J Cancer Res. 1923–1924;8:317.
8. Klemperer P, Rabin CB. Primary neoplasms of the pleura. Arch Pathol. 1931;11:385–412.
9. DuBray ES, Rosson FB. Primary mesothelioma of the pleura: a clinical and pathological contribution to the pleural malignancy, with report of a case. Arch Intern Med. 1920;26:715–37.

10. Godwin MC. Diffuse mesotheliomas: with comment on their relation to localized fibrous mesotheliomas. Cancer. 1957;10: 298–319.
11. Wagner JC, Sleggs CA, Marchand P. Diffuse pleural mesothelioma and asbestos exposure in the North Western Cape Town province. Br J Ind Med. 1960;17:260–71.
12. Hirsch A, Brochard P, Cremoux H, et al. Features of asbestos-exposed and unexposed mesothelioma. Am J Ind Med. 1982;3:413–22.
13. McCaughey WTE. Criteria for the diagnosis of diffuse mesothelial tumors. Ann N Y Acad Sci. 1965;132:603–13.
14. Huncharek M, Kelsey K, Mark EJ, et al. Treatment and survival in diffuse malignant pleural mesothelioma: a study of 83 cases from Massachusetts General Hospital. Anticancer Res. 1996;16:1265–8.
15. Aaisner J, Wiernik PH. Malignant mesothelioma: current status and future prospects. Chest. 1978;74:438–44.
16. Gardner MJ, Acheson ED, Winter PD. Mortality from mesothelioma of the pleura during 1968–78 in England and Wales. Br J Cancer. 1982;46:81–8.
17. Oels HC, Harrison EG, Carr DT, Bernatz PE. Diffuse malignant mesothelioma of the pleura: a review of 37 cases. Chest. 1971;60:564–70.
18. Chahinian AP, Pajak TF, Holland JF, et al. Diffuse malignant mesothelioma: prospective evaluation of 69 patients. Ann Intern Med. 1982;96:746–55.
19. Brenner J, Sordillo PP, Magill GB, Golbey RB. Malignant mesothelioma of the pleura: review of 123 patients. Cancer. 1982;49: 2431–5.
20. Law MR, Hodson ME, Heard BE. Malignant mesothelioma of the pleura: relation between histological type and clinical behavior. Thorax. 1982;37:810–5.
21. Qua JC, Rao UMN, Takita H. Malignant pleural mesothelioma: a clinicopathological study. J Surg Oncol. 1993;54:47–50.
22. Suzuki Y. Pathology of human malignant mesothelioma. Semin Oncol. 1980;8:268–82.
23. Grundy GW, Miller RW. Malignant mesothelioma in childhood: report of 13 cases. Cancer. 1972;30:1216–8.
24. Moran CA, Suster S, Albores-Saavedra J. Peritoneal mesotheliomas in children: a clinicopathologic study of 8 cases. Histopathology. 2008;52:824–30.
25. Peterson JT, Greenberg DS, Buffler PA. Non-asbestos related malignant mesothelioma. A review. Cancer. 1984;54:951–60.
26. Crotty TB, Myers JL, Katzenstein AL, et al. Localized malignant mesothelioma. A clinicopathologic and flow cytometric study. Am J Surg Pathol. 1994;18:357–63.
27. Ordoñez NG. Epithelial mesothelioma with deciduoid features: report of four cases. Am J Surg Pathol. 2000;24:816–23.
28. Ordoñez NG, Mackay B. Clear cell mesothelioma. Ultrastruct Pathol. 1996;20:331–6.
29. Henderson DW, Attwood HD, Constance TJ, Shilkin KB, Steele RH. Lymphohistiocytoid mesothelioma: a rare lymphomatoid variant of predominantly sarcomatoid mesothelioma. Ultrastruct Pathol. 1988;12:367–84.
30. Yousem SA, Hochholzer L. Malignant mesothelioma with osseous and cartilaginous differentiation. Arch Pathol Lab Med. 1987;111:62–6.
31. Weissferdt A, Kalhor N, Suster S. Malignant mesothelioma with prominent adenomatoid features: a clinicopathological and immunohistochemical study of 10 cases. Ann Diagn Pathol. 2011;15:25–9.
32. Arrossi AV, Lin E, Rice D, Moran CA. Histologic assessment and prognostic factors of malignant pleural mesothelioma treated with extrapleural pneumonectomy. Am J Clin Pathol. 2008;130:754–64.
33. Moran CA, Wick MR, Suster S. The role of immunohistochemistry in the diagnosis of malignant mesothelioma. Semin Diagn Pathol. 2000;17:178–83.
34. Suster S, Moran CA. Applications and limitations of immunohistochemistry in the diagnosis of malignant mesothelioma. Adv Anat Pathol. 2006;13:316–29.
35. Wick MR, Moran CA, Mills SE, Suster S. Immunohistochemical differential diagnosis of pleural effusions with emphasis on malignant mesothelioma. Curr Opin Pulm Med. 2001;7:187–92.
36. Ordonez NG. Valued of cytokeratin 5/6 immunostain in distinguishing epithelial mesothelioma of the pleura from lung adenocarcinoma. Am J Surg Pathol. 1998;22:1215–21.
37. Ordonez NG. In search for a positive immunohistochemical marker for mesothelioma: an update. Adv Anat Pathol. 1998;5:53–60.
38. Moll R, Dhouailly D, Sun TT. Expression of keratin 5 as a distinctive feature of epithelial and biphasic mesotheliomas: an immunohistochemical study using monoclonal antibody AE14. Virchows Arch B Cell Pathol Incl Mol Pathol. 1989;58:129–45.
39. Clover J, Oates J, Edwards C. Anti-cytokeratin 5/6: a potential marker for epithelioid mesothelioma. Histopathology. 1997;31: 140–3.
40. Chu PG, Weiss LM. Expression of cytokeratin 5/6 in epithelial neoplasms: an immunohistochemical study of 509 cases. Mod Pathol. 2002;15:6–10.
41. Gotzos V, Vogt P, Celio MR. The calcium binding protein calretinin is a selective marker for malignant mesothelial proliferation using formalin-fixed paraffin sections. J Pathol. 1992;192:137–47.
42. Dogliioni C, dei Tos AP, Laurino L, et al. Calretinin: a novel immunocytochemical marker for mesothelioma. Am J Surg Pathol. 1996;20:1037–46.
43. Dei Tos AP, Doglioni C. Calretinin: a novel tool for diagnostic immunohistochemistry. Adv Anat Pathol. 1998;5:61–6.
44. Oates J, Edwards C. HBME-1, MOC31, WT1 and calretinin: an assessment of recently described markers for mesothelioma and adenocarcinoma. Histopathology. 2000;36:341–7.
45. Foster MR, Johnson JE, Olson SJ, et al. Immunohistochemical analysis of nuclear versus cytoplasmic staining of WT1 in malignant mesothelioma and primary pulmonary adenocarcinoma. Arch Pathol Lab Med. 2001;125:1316–20.
46. Kuman-Sing S, Segers K, Rodeck U, et al. WT1 mutation in malignant mesothelioma and WT1 immunoreactivity in relation to p53 and growth factor receptor expression, cell type transition and prognosis. J Pathol. 1997;181:67–74.
47. Yazjii H, Battifora H, Barry TS, et al. Evaluation of 12 antibodies for distinguishing epithelioid mesothelioma from adenocarcinoma: identification of a three antibody immunohistochemical panel with maximal sensitivity and specificity. Mod Pathol. 2006;19:514–23.
48. Amin KM, Litzky LA, Smythe RW, et al. Wilm's tumor −1 susceptibility (WT1) gene products are selectively expressed in malignant mesothelioma. Am J Pathol. 1995;146:344–56.
49. Walker C, Rutten F, Yuan X, et al. Wilms' tumor suppressor gene expression in rat and human mesothelioma. Cancer Res. 1994;54:3101–6.
50. Ordonez NG. The value of thyroid transcription factor-1, E-cadherin, BG8, WT1, and CD44S immunostaining in distinguishing epithelial pleural mesothelioma from pulmonary and nonpulmonary adenocarcinoma. Am J Surg Pathol. 2000;24:598–606.
51. Miettinen M, Kovatich AJ. HMBE-1 – a monoclonal antibody useful in the differential diagnosis of mesothelioma, adenocarcinoma, and soft tissue and bone tumors. Appl Immunohistochem. 1995;3:115–22.
52. Kennedy AD, King G, Kerr KM. HBME-1 and antithrombomodulin in the differential diagnosis of malignant mesothelioma of the pleura. J Clin Pathol. 1997;50:859–62.
53. Attanoos RL, Goddard H, Gibbs AR. Mesothelioma-binding antibodies: thrombomodulin, OV632, and HBME-1 and their use for the diagnosis of malignant mesothelioma. Histopathology. 1996;29:209–15.

54. Collins CL, Ordonez SG, Schaefer R, et al. Thrombomodulin expression in malignant pleural mesothelioma and pulmonary adenocarcinoma. Am J Pathol. 1992;141:827–33.
55. Ascoli V, Scalso CC, Taccogna S, et al. the diagnostic value of thrombomodulin immunolocalization in serous effusions. Arch Pathol Lab Med. 1995;119:1136–40.
56. Argani P, Iacobuziio-Donahue C, Ryu B, et al. Mesothelin is overexpressed in the vast majority of ductal adenocarcinomas of the pancreas: identification of a new pancreatic cancer marker by serial analysis of gene expression. Clin Cancer Res. 2001;7:3862–8.
57. Ordonez NG. Application of mesothelin immunostaining in tumor diagnosis. Am J Surg Pathol. 2003;27:1418–28.
58. Hassan R, Kreitman RJ, Pastan I, et al. Localization of mesothelin in epithelial ovarian cancer. Appl Immunohistochem Mol Morphol. 2005;13:243–7.
59. Cao D, Ji H, Ronnett BM. Expression of mesothelin, fascin, prostate stem cell antigen in primary ovarian mucinous tumors and their utility in differentiating primary ovarian mucinous tumors from metastatic pancreatic mucinous carcinomas in the ovary. Int J Gynecol Pathol. 2005;24:67–72.
60. Comin CE, Novelli L, Boddi V, et al. Calretinin, thrombomodulin, CEA, and CD-15: a useful combination of immunohistochemical markers for differentiating pleural epithelial mesothelioma from peripheral pulmonary adenocarcinoma. Hum Pathol. 2001;32:529–36.
61. Garcia-Prats MD, Ballestin C, Sotelo T, et al. A comparative evaluation of immunohistochemical markers for the differential diagnosis of malignant pleural tumors. Histopathology. 1998;32:462–72.
62. Roberts F, Harper CM, Downie I, et al. Immunohistochemical analysis still has a limited role in the diagnosis of malignant mesothelioma: a study of thirteen antibodies. Am J Clin Pathol. 2001;116:253–62.
63. Leosli H, Hurliman J. Immunohistochemical study of malignant diffuse mesothelioma of the pleura. Histopathology. 1984;8:793–803.
64. Battifora H, Kopinsky M. Distinction of mesothelioma from adenocarcinoma. An immunohistochemical approach. Cancer. 1985;55:1679–85.
65. Pfaltz M, Odermatt B, Christen B, et al. Immunohistochemistry in the diagnosis of malignant mesothelioma. Virchows Arch. 1987;411:387–93.
66. Otis CN, Carter D, Cole S, et al. Immunnohistochemical evaluation of pleural mesothelioma and pulmonary adenocarcinoma. Am J Surg Pathol. 1987;11:445–56.
67. Wharhol MJ. The ultrastructural localization of keratin proteins and carcinoembryonic antigen in malignant mesothelioma. Am J Pathol. 1984;116:385–90.
68. Sosolik RC, McGauhy VR, De Young BR. Anti-MOC31: a potential addition to the pulmonary adenocarcinoma versus mesothelioma immunohistochemistry panel. Mod Pathol. 1997;10:716–9.
69. Ordonez NG. The value of MOC31 monoclonal antibody in differentiating epithelial pleural mesothelioma from lung adenocarcinoma. Hum Pathol. 1998;29:166–9.
70. Gonzalez-Lois C, Ballentin C, Sotelo M, et al. Combined use of novel epithelial (MOC31) and mesothelial (HBME-1) immunohistochemical markers for optimal first line diagnostic distinction between mesothelioma and metastatic carcinoma in pleura. Histopathology. 2001;38:528–34.
71. Di Loreto C, Pubglisi F, Di Lauro V, et al. TTF-1 protein expression in pleural malignant mesotheliomas and adenocarcinomas of the lung. Cancer Lett. 1998;13:73–8.
72. Bakir K, Kocer NE, Deniz H, et al. TTF-1 and surfactant-B as co-adjuvants in the diagnosis of adenocarcinoma and pleural mesothelioma. Ann Diagn Pathol. 2004;8:337–41.
73. Khoor A, Whitset JA, Stahlman MT, et al. Utility of surfactant protein B precursor and thyroid transcription factor-1 in differentiating adenocarcinoma of the lung from malignant mesothelioma. Hum Pathol. 1999;30:695–700.
74. Skov BG, Lauritzen AF, Hirsch FR, et al. Differentiation of adenocarcinoma of the lung and malignant mesothelioma: predictive value and reproducibility of immunoreactive antibodies. Histopathology. 1993;25:431–7.
75. Moch H, Oberholzer M, Christen H, et al. Diagnostic tools for differentiating pleural mesothelioma from lung adenocarcinoma in paraffin embedded tissue. Part II. Virchows Arch A. 1993;423:493–6.
76. Brown RW, Clark GM, Tandon AK, et al. Multiple-marker immunohistochemical phenotypes distinguishing malignant pleural mesothelioma from pulmonary adenocarcinoma. Hum Pathol. 1993;24:347–54.
77. Jordon D, Jagirdar J, Kaneko M. Blood group antigens, Lewis and Lewis, in the diagnostic discrimination of malignant mesothelioma versus adenocarcinoma. Am J Pathol. 1989;135:931–7.
78. Ordonez NG. Mesotheliomas with crystalloid structures: report of nine cases, including one with oncocytic features. Mod Pathol. 2012;25:272–81.
79. Carter D, Otis CN. Three types of spindle cell tumors of the pleura. Fibroma, sarcoma, and sarcomatoid mesothelioma. Am J Surg Pathol. 1988;12:747–53.
80. Kannerstein M, Churg J. Desmoplastic diffuse malignant mesothelioma. In: Fenoglio CM, Wolff M, editors. Progress in surgical pathology, vol. 11. New York: Masson Publishing; 1980. p. 19–29.
81. Cantin R, al-Jabi M, McCaughey WTE. Desmoplastic diffuse mesothelioma. Am J Surg Pathol. 1982;6:215–22.
82. Mangano WE, Cagle PT, Churg A, Vollmer RT, Roggli VL. The diagnosis of desmoplastic malignant mesothelioma and its distinction from fibrous pleurisy. Am J Clin Pathol. 1998;110:191–9.
83. Colby TV. The diagnosis of desmoplastic malignant mesothelioma. Am J Clin Pathol. 1998;110:135–6.
84. Henderson DW. Lymphohistiocytoid mesothelioma: a rare lymphomatoid variant of predominantly sarcomatoid mesothelioma. Ultrastruct Pathol. 1988;12:367–84.
85. Rice D. Surgery for malignant pleural mesothelioma. Ann Diagn Pathol. 2009;13(1):65–72.
86. Harwood TR, Gracey DR, Yokoo H. Pseudomesotheliomatous carcinoma of the lung: a variant of peripheral lung cancer. Am J Clin Pathol. 1976;65:159–67.
87. KossMN,TravisW,MoranC,HochholzerL.Pseudomesotheliomatous adenocarcinoma: a reappraisal. Semin Diagn Pathol. 1992;9:117–23.
88. Nishimoto Y, Ohno T, Saito K. Pseudomesotheliomatous carcinoma of the lung with histochemical and immunohistochemical study. Acta Pathol Jpn. 1983;33:415–23.
89. Dessy E, Pietra G. Pseudomesotheliomatous carcinoma of the lung: an immunohistochemical and ultrastructural study of three cases. Cancer. 1991;68:1747–53.
90. Shah I, Salvatore JR, Kummet T, et al. Pseudomesotheliomatous carcinoma involving pleura and peritoneum: a clinicopathological and immunohistochemical study of three cases. Ann Diagn Pathol. 1999;3:148–59.
91. Attanos RL, Gibbs AR. Pseudomesotheliomatous carcinomas of the pleura: a 10-year analysis of cases from the environmental lung disease research group, Cardiff. Histopathology. 2003;43:444–52.
92. Koss MN, Fleming M, Pzygodski RM, et al. Adenocarcinoma simulating mesothelioma: a clinicopathological and immunohistochemical study of 29 cases. Ann Diagn Pathol. 1999;3:148–59.

93. Pardo J, Torres W, Martinez-Penuela A, et al. Pseudomesotheliomatous carcinoma of the lung with distinct morphology, immunohistochemistry, and comparative genomic hybridization profile. Ann Diagn Pathol. 2007;11:241–51.
94. Moran CA, Suster S. Primary mucoepidermoid carcinoma of the pleura: a clinicopathological study of two cases. Am J Surg Pathol. 2003;120:381–5.
95. Asa SL, Dardick I, Van Nostrand PAW, et al. Primary thyroid thymoma: a distinct clinicopathologic entity. Hum Pathol. 1988;19:1463–6.
96. Martin JME, Randhawa G, Temple WJ. Cervical thymoma. Arch Pathol Lab Med. 1986;110:354–7.
97. Yamashita H, Murakami N, Noguchi S, et al. Cervical thymoma. Acta Pathol Jpn. 1983;33:189–94.
98. Wadon A. Thymoma intratracheal. Am J Pathol. 1934;60:308–12.
99. Moran CA, Suster S, Fishback NF, Koss MN. Intrapulmonary thymoma: a clinicopathologic correlation of eight cases. Am J Surg Pathol. 1995;19:304–12.
100. Payne CB, Mornigstar WA, Chester EH. Thymoma of the pleura masquerading as diffuse mesothelioma. Am Rev Respir Dis. 1960;94:441–6.
101. Honma K, Shimada K. Metastasizing ectopic thymoma arising in the right thoracic cavity and mimicking diffuse pleural mesothelioma. An autopsy study of a case with review of the literature. Wien Klin Wochenschr. 1986;98:14–20.
102. Moran CA, Travis WD, de-Christenson M, Koss MN, Rosai J. Thymomas presenting as pleural tumors: report of eight cases. Am J Surg Pathol. 1992;16:138–44.
103. Vural M, Abali H, Oksuzog B, Akbulut M. An atypical presentation of thymoma with diffuse pleural dissemination mimicking mesothelioma. Cancer Invest. 2006;24:615–20.
104. Qing G, Ionescu DN, Colby TV, Leslie KO. A 75-year-old man with an asymptomatic pleural-based mass discovered on routine chest radiographs. Primary pleural thymoma. Arch Pathol Lab Med. 2006;130:e62–5.
105. Kim HS, Lee HJ, Cho SY, et al. Myasthenia gravis in ectopic thymoma presenting as pleural masses. Lung Cancer. 2007;57:115–57.
106. Yamazaki K, Yoshino I, Oba T, et al. Ectopic pleural thymoma presenting as a giant mass in the thoracic cavity. Ann Thorac Surg. 2007;83:315–7.
107. Shin DF, Wang JS, Tseng HH, Tiao VM. Primary pleural thymoma. Arch Pathol Lab Med. 1997;1221:79–82.
108. Higasiyama M, Doi O, Kodama K, et al. Ectopic primary thymoma: report of a case. Surg Today. 1996;26:747–50.
109. Fushimi H, Tanio Y, Koth K. Ectopic thymoma mimicking diffuse pleural mesothelioma: a case report. Hum Pathol. 1998;29:409–10.
110. Plaza JA, Dominguez F, Suster S. Cystic adenomatoid tumor of the mediastinum. Am J Surg Pathol. 2004;28:132–8.
111. Ikuta N, Tano M, Iwata M, et al. A case of adenomatoid mesothelioma of the pleura. Jpn J Thorac Dis. 1989;27:1540–4.
112. Kaplan MA, Tazelaar HD, Hayashi T, et al. Adenomatoid tumors of the pleura. Am J Surg Pathol. 1996;20:1219–23.
113. Flieder D, Moran CA, Travis WD, et al. Pleuro-pulmonary endometriosis and pulmonary ectopic deciduosis: a clinicopathologic and immunohistochemical study of 10 cases with emphasis in diagnostic pitfalls. Hum Pathol. 1998;12:1495–503.
114. Karpel JP, Appel D, Merav A. Pulmonary endometriosis. Lung. 1985;163:151–9.
115. Lattes R, Shepard F, Tovell H, et al. A clinical and pathological study of endometriosis of the lung. Surg Gynecol Obstet. 1956;103:552–8.
116. Foster DC, Stern JL, Buscema J, et al. Pleural and parenchyma pulmonary endometriosis. Obstet Gynecol. 1981;58:552–6.
117. Austin MB, Frierson HF, Fechner RE, et al. Endometrioma of the lung presenting as hemoptysis and a large pulmonary mass. Surg Pathol. 1988;1:165–9.
118. Witkin GB, Rosai J. Solitary fibrous tumor of the mediastinum. Report of 14 cases. Am J Surg Pathol. 1989;13:547–57.
119. Goodlad JR, Fletcher CDM. Solitary fibrous tumor arising at unusual sites: analysis of a series. Histopathology. 1991;19:512–22.
120. Dorfman DM, To K, Dickersin GR, et al. Solitary fibrous tumor of the orbit. Am J Surg Pathol. 1994;18:281–7.
121. Suster S, Nascimiento AG, Miettinen M, et al. Solitary fibrous tumor of soft tissue. A clinicopathologic and immunohistochemical study of 12 cases. Am J Surg Pathol. 1995;19:1257–66.
122. Scharifker D, Kaneko M. Localized fibrous "mesothelioma" of pleura (submesothelial fibroma): a clinicopathologic study of 18 cases. Cancer. 1979;43:627–35.
123. Dalton WT, Zolliker AS, McCaughey WTE, et al. Localized primary tumors of the pleura. An analysis of 40 cases. Cancer. 1979;44:1465–75.
124. Briselli M, Mark EJ, Dickersin R. Solitary fibrous tumor of the pleura. Eight new cases and review of 360 cases in the literature. Cancer. 1981;47:2678–89.
125. England DM, Hochholzer L, McCarthy MJ. Localized benign and malignant fibrous tumors of the pleura: a clinicopathologic review of 223 cases. Am J Surg Pathol. 1989;13:640–58.
126. Westra WH, Gerald WL, Rosai J. Solitary fibrous tumor: consistent CD34 immunoreactivity and occurrence in the orbit. Am J Surg Pathol. 1994;18:992–8.
127. Chilosi M, Facchetti F, Dei Tos AP, et al. bcl-2 expression in pleural and extrapleural solitary fibrous tumours. J Pathol. 1997;181:362–7.
128. Said JW, Nash G, Banks-Schlegel S, et al. Localized fibrous mesothelioma: an immunohistochemical and electron microscopic study. Hum Pathol. 1984;15:440–3.
129. Moran CA, Suster S, Koss MN. The spectrum of histopathologic growth patterns in benign and malignant fibrous tumors of the pleura. Semin Diagn Pathol. 1992;9:169–80.
130. McDougall A, McGarrity G. Extra-abdominal desmoid tumors. J Bone Joint Surg Br. 1979;61:373–7.
131. Brodsky JT, Gordon MS, Hajdu SI, et al. Desmoid tumors of the chest wall: a locally recurrent problem. J Thorac Cardiovasc Surg. 1992;104:900–3.
132. Varghese TK, Gupta R, Yeldandi AV, et al. Desmoid tumor of the chest wall with pleural involvement. Ann Thorac Surg. 2003;76:937–9.
133. Andino L, Cagle PT, Murer B, et al. Pleuropulmonary desmoid tumors: immunohistochemical comparison with solitary fibrous tumors and assessment of B-catenin and cyclin D1 expression. Arch Pathol Lab Med. 2006;130:1503–9.
134. Wilson RW, Gallateau-Salle F, Moran CA. Desmoid tumors of the pleura: a clinicopathologic mimic of localized fibrous tumor. Mod Pathol. 1999;12:9–14.
135. Fetsch JF, Montgomery EA, Meis JM. Calcifying fibrous pseudotumor. Am J Surg Pathol. 1993;17:502–8.
136. Van Dorpe J, Ectors N, Geboes K, et al. Is calcifying fibrous tumor pseudotumor a late sclerosing stage of inflammatory myofibroblastic tumor? Am J Surg Pathol. 1999;23:329–35.
137. Nascimiento AF, Ruiz R, Hornick JL, et al. Calcifying fibrous "pseudotumor" clinicopathologic study of 15 cases and analysis of its relationship to inflammatory myofibroblastic tumor. Int J Surg Pathol. 2002;10:189–96.
138. Reed MK, Margraf LR, Nikaidoh H, et al. Calcifying fibrous pseudotumor of the chest wall. Ann Thorac Surg. 1996;62:873–4.
139. Maeda T, Hirose T, Furuya K, Kameoka K. Calcifying fibrous pseudotumor: an ultrastructural study. Ultrastruct Pathol. 1999;23:189–92.

140. Soyer T, Ciftci AO, Gucer S, et al. Calcifying fibrous pseudotumor of the lung: a previously unreported entity. J Pediatr Surg. 2004;39: 1729–30.
141. Pinkard NB, Wilson RW, Lawless N, et al. Calcifying fibrous pseudotumor of the pleura: a report of three cases of a newly described entity involving the pleura. Am J Clin Pathol. 1996;105: 189–94.
142. Hainaut P, Lesage V, Weynand B, et al. Calcifying fibrous pseudotumor (CFPT): a patient presenting with multiple pleural lesions. Acta Clin Belg. 1999;54:162–4.
143. Mito K, Kashima K, Daa T, et al. Multiple calcifying fibrous tumor of the pleura. Virchows Arch. 2005;446:78–81.
144. Ammar A, El Hammami S, Horchani H, et al. Calcifying fibrous pseudotumor of the pleura: a rare location. Ann Thorac Surg. 2003;76:2081–2.
145. Jang KS, Oh YH, Han HX, et al. Calcifying fibrous pseudotumor of the pleura. Ann Thorac Surg. 2004;78:87–8.
146. Kawahara K, Yasukawa M, Nakagawa K, et al. Multiple calcifying fibrous tumor of the pleura. Virchows Arch. 2005;447: 1007–8.
147. Shibata K, Yuki D, Sakata K. Multiple calcifying fibrous pseudotumors disseminated in the pleura. Ann Thorac Surg. 2008;85:3–5.
148. Suh JH, Shin OR, Kim YH. Multiple calcifying fibrous pseudotumor of the pleura. J Thorac Oncol. 2008;3:1356–8.
149. Erasmus JJ, McAdams P, Patz EF, et al. Calcifying fibrous pseudotumor of pleura: radiologic features in three cases. J Comput Assist tomogr. 1996;20:763–5.
150. Zamecnik M, Michal M, Boudova L, Sulc M. CD34 expression in calcifying fibrous pseudotumours. Histopathology. 2000;36: 182–91.
151. Adams AL, Castro CY, Singh P, Moran CA. Primary amyloidosis of the pleura mimicking mesothelioma. Ann Diagn Pathol. 2001;5:229–32.
152. Moran CA, Suster S, Koss MN. Smooth muscle tumours presenting as pleural neoplasms. Histopathology. 1995;27:227–34.
153. Gaertner E, Zeren EH, Fleming MV, et al. Biphasic synovial sarcomas arising in the pleural cavity. A clinicopathologic study of five cases. Am J Surg Pathol. 1996;20:36–45.
154. Angerval L, Enzinger FM. Extra skeletal neoplasms resembling Ewing's sarcoma. Cancer. 1977;101:446–9.
155. Askin FB, Rosai J, Sibley R, Dehner LP, et al. Malignant small cell tumors of the thoracopulmonary region in children. Cancer. 1979;43:2438–51.
156. Gould V, Jannson D, Warren W. Primitive neuroectodermal tumors (PNET) of the chest wall in adults. Mod Pathol. 1991;4:115A (Abstract 681).
157. Hashimoto H, Enjoji M, Nakajima T, et al. Malignant neuroepithelioma (peripheral neuroblastoma). Am J Surg Pathol. 1983;7: 309–18.
158. Lane S, Ironside JW. Extraskeletal Ewing's sarcoma of the nasal fossa. J Laryngol Otol. 1990;104:570–3.
159. Soule EH, Newton W, Moon TE, et al. Extraskeletal Ewing's sarcoma. A preliminary review of 26 cases encountered in the intergroup rhabdomyosarcoma study. Cancer. 1978;42: 259–64.
160. Suster S, Ronnen M, Huczar M. Extraskeletal Ewing's sarcoma of the scalp. Pediatr Dermatol. 1988;5:126–8.
161. Tefft M, Vawter GF, Metus A. Paravertebral "round cell" tumors in children. Radiology. 1969;92:1501–9.
162. Wigger JH, Salazar G, Blanc WA. Extraskeletal Ewing's sarcoma. Arch Pathol Lab Med. 1977;101:446–9.
163. Fujii Y, Hongo T, Nakagawa Y, et al. Cell culture of small round cell tumor originating in the thoracopulmonary region, evidence for derivation from a primitive pluripotent cell. Cancer. 1989;64:43–51.
164. Yunis EJ, Agostini RM, Walpusk JA, et al. Glycogen in neuroblastomas. Am J Surg Pathol. 1979;3:199–208.
165. Guillespie JJ, Roth LM, Wills ER, et al. Extraskeletal Ewing's sarcoma. Am J Surg Pathol. 1979;3:99–108.
166. Schmidt D, Mackay B, Ayala A. Ewing's sarcoma with neuroblastoma like features. Ultrastruct Pathol. 1982;3:99–108.
167. Tsuji S, Hisaoka M, Morimitsu Y, et al. Peripheral primitive neuroectodermal tumour of the lung: report of two cases. Histopathology. 1998;33:369–74.
168. Kahn AG, Avagnina A, Nazar J, et al. Primitive neuroectodermal tumor of the lung. Arch Pathol Lab Med. 2001;125: 397–9.
169. Mikami Y, Nakajima M, Hashimoto H, et al. Primary pulmonary primitive neuroectodermal tumor (PNET): a case report. Pathol Res Pract. 2001;197:113–9.
170. Imamura F, Funakoshi T, Nakamura S, et al. Primary primitive neuroectodermal tumor of the lung. Report of two cases. Lung Cancer. 2000;27:55–60.
171. Linnoila RI, Tsokos M, Triche TJ, et al. Evidence for neural origin and PAS-positive variants of the malignant small cell tumor of thoracopulmonary region ("Askin's tumor"). Am J Surg Pathol. 1986;10:124–33.
172. Tsokos M, Linnoila RI, Chandra RS, et al. Neuron-specific enolase in the diagnosis of neuroblastoma and other small, round cell tumors in children. Hum Pathol. 1984;15:575–84.
173. Gonzales-Crussi F, Wolfson SL, Misugi K, et al. Peripheral neuroectodermal tumors of the chest wall in childhood. Cancer. 1984;54:2519–27.
174. Ordonez NG. Application of immunohistochemistry in the diagnosis of soft tissue sarcomas: a review and update. Adv Anat Pathol. 1998;5(2):67–85.
175. Hill DA, Pfeifer JD, Marley EF, et al. WT1 staining reliability differentiates desmoplastic small round cell tumor from Ewing sarcoma/primitive neuroectodermal tumor: an immunohistochemical and molecular diagnostic study. Am J Clin Pathol. 2000;114: 345–53.
176. Miettinen M, Chatten J, Paetau A, Stevenson A. Monoclonal antibody NB84 in the differential diagnosis of neuroblastoma and other small round cell tumors. Am J Surg Pathol. 1998;22: 327–32.
177. Batsakis JG, El-Nagar A. Ewing's sarcoma and primitive neuroectodermal tumors: cytogenetic cynosures seeking a common histogenesis. Adv Anat Pathol. 1997;4(4):207–20.
178. Brown NP, Reid MM, Malcolm AJ, et al. Cytogenetic abnormalities of small round cell tumours. Med Pediatr Oncol. 1994;23:124–9.
179. Peng JW, Triche TJ, Knutsen T, et al. Cytogenetic characterization of selected small round cell tumors of childhood. Cancer Genet Cytogenet. 1986;21:185–208.
180. Contesso G, Llombart-Bosch A, Terrier P, et al. Does malignant small round cell tumor of the thoracopulmonary region (Askin tumor) constitute a clinicopathologic entity? An analysis of 30 cases with immunohistochemical and electron-microcopy support treated at the Institute Gustave Roussy. Cancer. 1992;69: 1012–20.
181. Falconieri G, Bussani R, Mirra M, Zanella M. Pseudomesotheliomatous angiosarcoma: a pleuropulmonary lesion simulating malignant pleural mesothelioma. Histopathology. 1997; 30:419–24.
182. Chen L, Shih HJ, Seguerra E, Lin JH. Pathologic quiz case: a 39-year-old man with diffuse pleural thickening and massive hemothorax. Arch Pathol Lab Med. 2004;128:1299–300.
183. Pramesh CS, Madur BP, Raina S, et al. Angiosarcoma of the pleura. Ann Thorac Cardiovasc Surg. 2004;10:187–90.
184. Maglaras GC, Katsenos S, Kakadelis J, et al. Primary angiosarcoma of the lung and pleura. Monaldi Arch Chest Dis. 2004;61: 234–6.

185. Liu SF, Hsieh MJ. Massive hemoptysis and hemothorax caused by pleuropulmonary angiosarcoma. Am J Emerg Med. 2002;20:374–5.
186. Alexiou C, Clelland CA, Robinson D, Morgan WE. Primary angiosarcomas of the chest wall and pleura. Eur J Cardiothorac Surg. 1998;14:523–6.
187. Roh MS, Seo JY, Hong SH. Epithelioid angiosarcoma of the pleura: a case report. J Korean Med Sci. 2001;16:792–5.
188. Kimura M, Ito H, Furuta T, et al. Pyothorax-associated angiosarcoma of the pleura with metastasis to the brain. Pathol Int. 2003;53:547–51.
189. Aozasa K, Naka N, Tomita Y, et al. Angiosarcoma developing from chronic pyothorax. Mod Pathol. 1994;7:906–11.
190. Del Frate C, Mortele K, Zanardi R, et al. Pseudomesotheliomatous angiosarcoma of the chest wall and pleura. J Thorac Imaging. 2003;18:200–3.
191. Zhang PJ, Livolvsi VA, Brooks JJ. Malignant epithelioid vascular tumors of the pleura: report of a series and literature review. Hum Pathol. 2000;31:29–34.
192. Crotty EJ, McAdams HP, Erasmus JJ, et al. Epithelioid hemangioendothelioma of the pleura: clinical and radiological features. AJR Am J Roentgenol. 2000;175:1545–9.
193. Bevelaqua FA, Valensi Q, Hulnick D. Epithelioid hemangioendothelioma: a rare tumor with variable prognosis presenting as a pleural effusion. Chest. 1988;93:665–6.
194. Attanos RL, Suvarna SK, Rhead E, et al. Malignant tumours of the pleura in “asbestos” workers and endothelial differentiation in malignant mesothelioma. Thorax. 2000;55: 860–3.
195. Pinet C, Magnan A, Garbe L, et al. Aggressive form of pleural epithelioid hemangioendothelioma: complete response after chemotherapy. Eur Respir J. 1999;14:237–8.
196. Al-Shraim M, Mahboub B, Nelligan PC, et al. Primary pleural epithelioid hemangioendothelioma with metastases to the skin. A case report and literature review. J Clin Pathol. 2005;58: 107–9.
197. Lin BTY, Colby T, Gown AM, et al. Malignant vascular tumors of the serous membranes mimicking mesothelioma: a report of 14 cases. Am J Surg Pathol. 1996;20:1431–9.
198. Saqi A, Nisbet L, Gagneja P, Leslie KO. Primary pleural epithelioid hemangioendothelioma with rhabdoid phenotype: report and review of the literature. Diagn Cytopathol. 2007;35: 203–8.

13 Tumor-like Conditions and Benign Tumors of the Lung

Introduction

Technically speaking any shadow or abnormality in the lung parenchyma can be considered a tumor-like lesion. However, in this chapter, we will concentrate only on all those lesions that, although unusual, represent true pathological processes. Nevertheless, it is impossible and to some extent impractical to be too inclusive; therefore, we will limit ourselves to discuss those lesions that not only represent a challenge in diagnosis but also may be encountered in daily practice. It is important to note that these lesions by themselves do not have any relationship among them and truly represent miscellaneous conditions. In order to facilitate their study, we have arbitrarily divided them into histiocytic and non-histiocytic lesions.

Histiocytic Lesions

The family of histiocytic proliferations that may present as pulmonary tumor or tumor-like lesions is rather extensive and encompasses processes of different etiologies including infectious, metabolic, environmental ones, and those of unknown histogenesis among others. Herein, we will present lesions that may present either as a pulmonary mass or pulmonary nodules. However, even with this subgrouping, it is impossible to cover the wide spectrum of pathological conditions that may be present in that form. For instance, it is well known that systemic conditions such as storage diseases like Fabry's disease [1], infantile GM1-gangliosidosis [2], Gaucher's disease [3, 4], and Niemann-Pick disease [5, 6] may involve the lung. It is very likely, however, that in those conditions a previous diagnosis has already been established and the lung is involved secondarily. Other systemic conditions such as Whipple disease may in some cases involve the lung and also show a histiocytic proliferation within the lung parenchyma [7, 8]. Even though those previously mentioned conditions may be part of the spectrum of histiocytic lesions, they will not be covered in this chapter as they represent systemic diseases with only secondary pulmonary involvement. The selected group of lesions, which may share similar histopathological and immunohistochemical (see Table 13.1) features, included in this chapter are:

- Rosai-Dorfman disease
- Erdheim-Chester disease
- Langerhans cell histiocytosis
- Juvenile xanthogranuloma
- Crystal-storing histiocytosis
- Malacoplakia
- Pulmonary xanthoma
- Unclassified xanthomatous lesions

Rosai-Dorfman Disease

Rosai-Dorfman disease, also known as sinus histiocytosis with massive lymphadenopathy (SHML), is a process of ubiquitous distribution. This histiocytosis has been described virtually everywhere in the body [9–15]. Although the etiology of this condition is still unknown, different theories to explain its occurrence have been presented, including an immunologic response or an infectious origin. Paulli et al. [14] evaluated two cases in which the authors used the human androgen receptor assay (HUMARA), with the result that the histiocytic proliferation was polyclonal. Initially, this condition was described more commonly in lymph nodes with a common occurrence in young adults. However, it has been stated that Rosai-Dorfman disease may involve extranodal site in about 20 % of the cases. However, the respiratory system, namely, the lung and pleura, is among the most unusual sites of occurrence. In some of the cases described involving lung parenchyma, the lung and lymph nodes have been involved simultaneously making the original site of occurrence difficult to assess. Therefore, the

A. Weissferdt, C.A. Moran, *Diagnostic Pathology of Pleuropulmonary Neoplasia*,
DOI 10.1007/978-1-4419-0787-5_13, © Springer Science+Business Media New York 2013

Table 13.1 Commonly used immunohistochemical stains in the diagnosis of histiocytic lesions

Lesion	S100 protein	CD68	CD1a	Factor XIIIa	Keratin
Rosai-Dorfman	pos	pos	neg	neg	neg
Erdheim-Chester	neg/pos	pos	neg	pos	neg
PLCH	pos	pos	pos	neg	neg
PJXG	pos	pos	neg	pos	neg
Xanthoma	neg	neg/pos	neg	neg	neg

pos positive, *neg* negative, PLCH pulmonary Langerhans cell histiocytosis, PJXG pulmonary juvenile xanthogranuloma

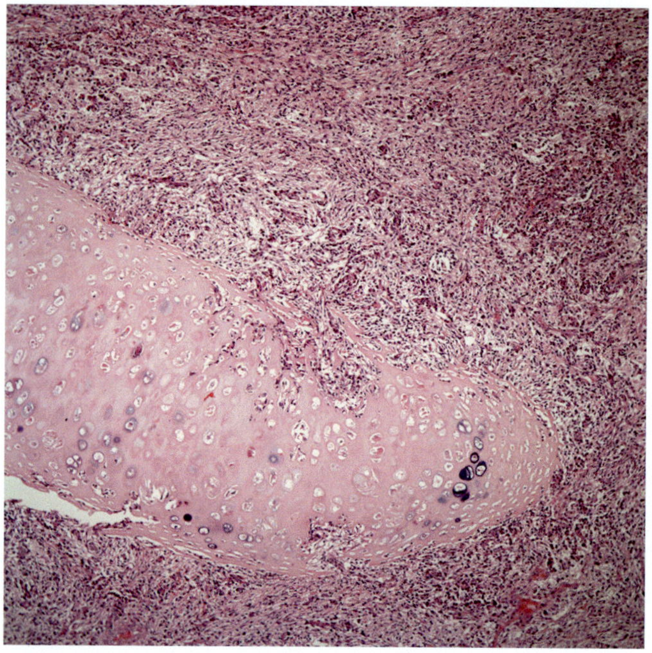

Fig. 13.1 Low power view of Rosai-Dorfman disease involving the lung. Note the presence of bronchial cartilage and the marked inflammatory reaction

presence of Rosai-Dorfman disease occurring solely and primarily in the lung parenchyma and/or pleura is exceedingly rare. When this condition affects the lung parenchyma, the patient may present with an intrapulmonary mass, which may be indistinguishable clinically or radiologically from other neoplastic processes. Therefore, the best approach to arrive at a more specific diagnosis is tissue diagnosis. However, in a small biopsy, a definitive diagnosis may be challenging. On complete surgical resection of the tumor mass, the diagnosis may become more apparent.

Histopathological Features

The histological features of Rosai-Dorfman disease in the lung are similar to those described for other anatomic sites. The main histologic hallmark of the process is a proliferation of large histiocytes, which may have one or more nuclei and ample pale cytoplasm (Figs. 13.1, 13.2, 13.3, 13.4, 13.5, 13.6, and 13.7). Some of these lymphocytes may show the presence of lymphophagocytosis or emperipolesis; however, such findings may not be readily apparent in some cases. The histiocytic proliferation is usually present in a background of a prominent inflammatory response composed predominantly of plasma cells and lymphocytes. In general, the two most important cellular components of Rosai-Dorfman disease are the presence of large histiocytes and plasma cells. The pulmonary parenchyma is clearly replaced by the process, and the adjacent uninvolved lung parenchyma may show features of interstitial lung disease.

Immunohistochemical studies may aid in the diagnosis of this lesion as the histiocytes show positive staining for S100 protein, CD68, CD15, CD163, and α-1-antichymotrypsin, while the histiocytes are negative for CD1a and factor XIIIa.

Treatment and Prognosis

In the lung, complete surgical resection of the lesion is the conventional approach. However, there is no specific treatment for this condition, and the prognosis may be related to the extent of the process at the time of diagnosis. In cases with limited disease to the lung, surgical resection of the mass may be accomplished followed by observation; while in cases with more systemic involvement, surgical resection followed by medical therapy could be attempted. However, the use of chemotherapy has not provided meaningful benefits. Foucar et al. [9] followed 238 patients and found that 21 patients had died; four of them secondary to the histiocytic process, 13 with the process, and four without the process. On the other hand, 49 patients were alive without disease after 1 year, while 36 had persistent disease. Whether lung involvement plays a role in the survival rate of these patients is difficult to determine due to the rare occurrence of this process in the lung.

Erdheim-Chester Disease (ECD)

This type of histiocytosis is rare, and only a few series of cases have been presented in the literature [16–21]. William Chester and Jacob Erdheim described this condition in 1930 as a form of lipoid granulomatosis different from other lipidosis [16]. The authors described two autopsy cases in which the process was present in bone and viscera. Jaffe [17] in 1973 reported an additional case and created the term Erdheim-Chester disease.

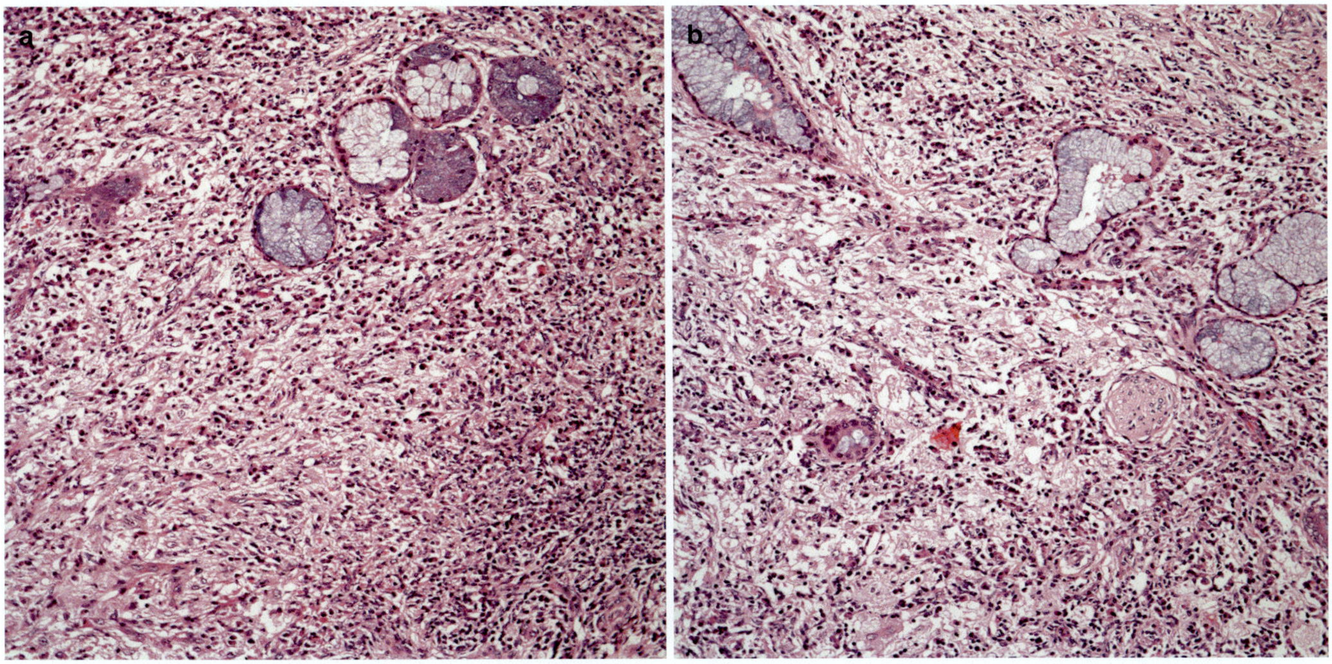

Fig. 13.2 (**a**) Rosai-Dorfman disease involving lung parenchyma and dissecting normal bronchial glands. (**b**) Closer view at the prominent histiocytic proliferation admixed with inflammatory cells, mainly plasma cells

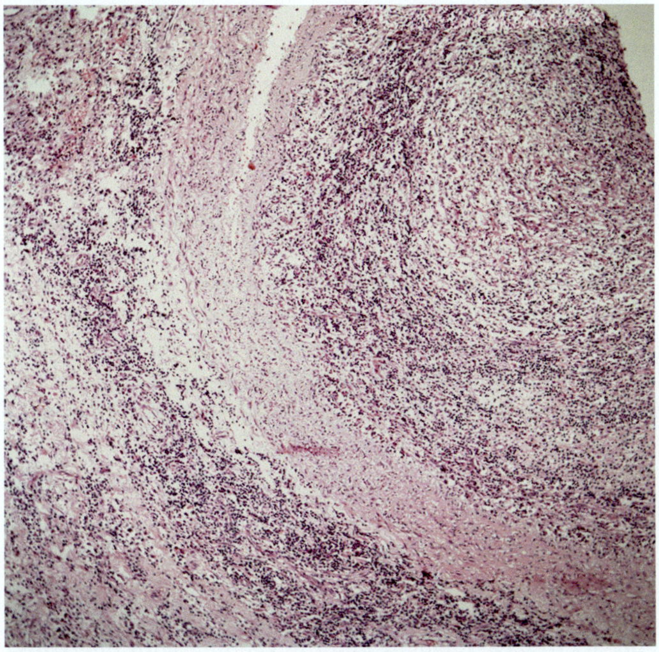

Fig. 13.3 The histiocytic process in Rosai-Dorfman disease occluding a pulmonary vessel

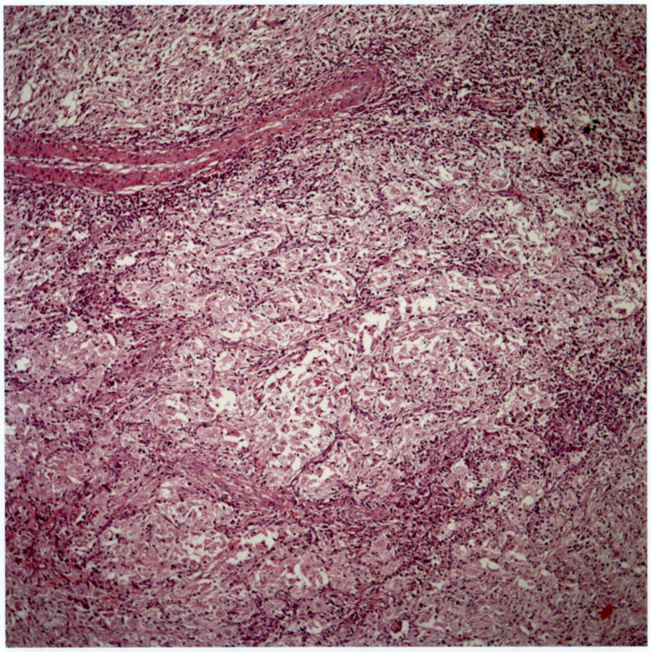

Fig. 13.4 Rosai-Dorfman disease destroying normal lung parenchyma. Note the prominent histiocytic process admixed with inflammatory cells

Clinical Features

Clinically, patients with Erdheim-Chester disease may vary considerably depending of the organs involved. Even though the emphasis here will be on the involvement of this condition in the respiratory tract, it is important to recognize that although patients with this condition may present with pulmonary symptoms, that does not necessarily mean that the lung is the only site involved, and a search for other involved organs is highly recommended. Therefore, it is important to keep in mind that Erdheim-Chester disease is usually a systemic process that may involve different anatomic sites at the same time. One of the most common presentations is that of skeletal abnormalities including expansile lesions

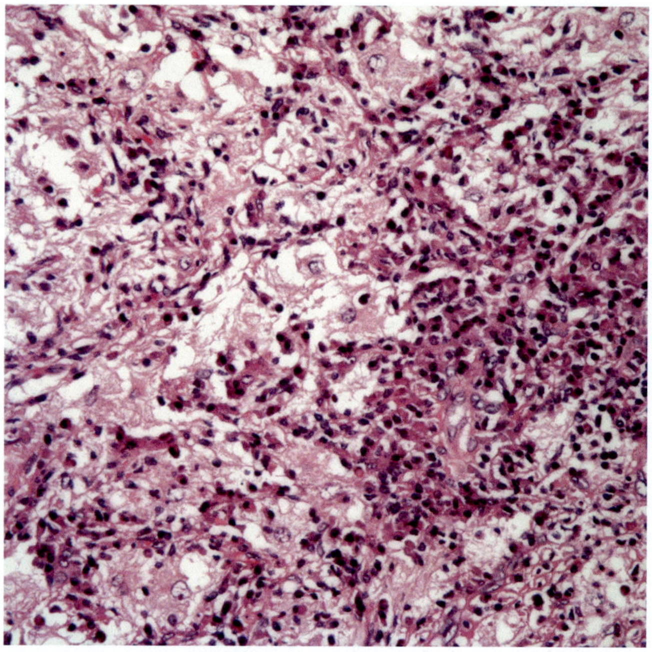

Fig. 13.5 The histiocytic process is commonly admixed with plasma cells. Note the large size of the histiocytes

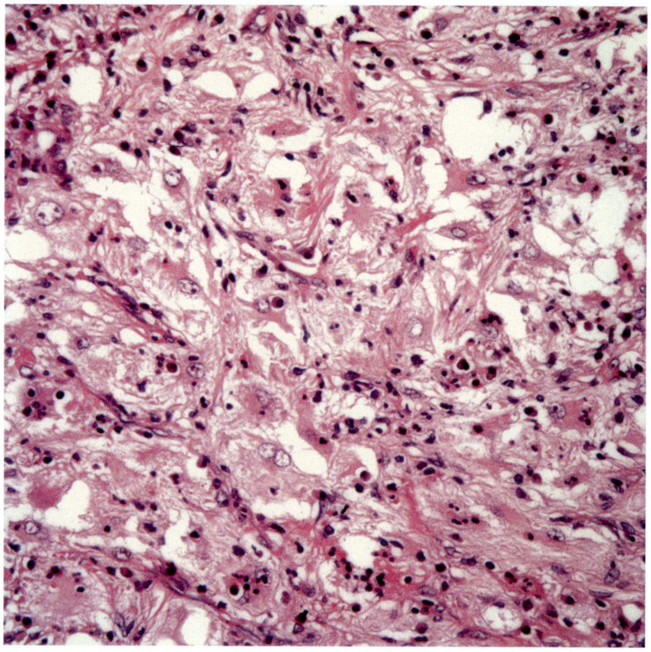

Fig. 13.6 In some areas, the inflammatory cells is less conspicuous; however, the histiocytic process is obvious

of the ribs, symmetrical patchy sclerosis and thickening of metaphyses of long tubular bones, and/or patchy sclerosis of the calcaneus. Other extraskeletal symptoms may include dyspnea, pulmonary infiltrates and pleural effusion, pulmonary fibrosis, congenital megacalyces, hydronephrosis, hydroureter, chronic lipogranulomatous pyelonephritis, retroperitoneal xanthogranulomas, ophthalmic abnormalities,

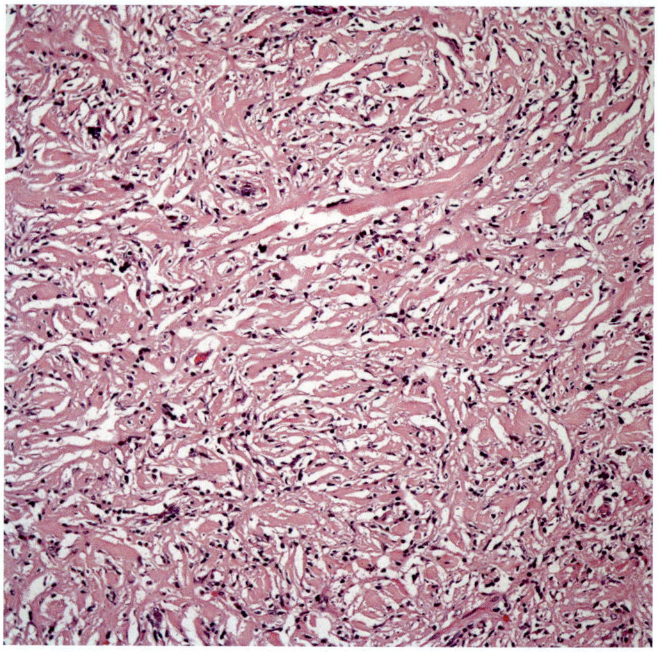

Fig. 13.7 Large areas of lung parenchyma may be destroyed and replaced by collagenous material; however, histiocytes may still be present

and hyperlipidemia. The best way to diagnose lung involvement is by performing an open lung biopsy in patients with pulmonary symptoms.

Histopathological Features

The histopathological features of this process in the lung are rather characteristic (Figs. 13.8, 13.9, 13.10, 13.11, 13.12, 13.13, and 13.14). The low power view is that of a pathologic process involving the pleura and pulmonary septa. In some cases, the involvement is more extensive with pleural, septal, and parenchymal involvement. The histiocytic proliferation is composed of small to medium sized histiocytes with foamy or finely granular cytoplasm. The nuclei do not show the grooving typically seen in cases of pulmonary Langerhans cell histiocytosis (PLCH). In addition, Granulomatous changes are not characteristic of this process. The histiocytic infiltrate usually involves the pleura and pulmonary septa, while the lung parenchyma appears to have changes more in keeping with interstitial lung disease and/or emphysematous changes. The histiocytic proliferation may be accompanied by a discrete inflammatory infiltrate composed of lymphocytes and plasma cells. The presence of eosinophils is not marked, and when present, eosinophils are not present in increased numbers.

Immunohistochemical studies of the histiocytic proliferation show positive staining for CD68 and factor XIIIa, while CD1a is negative. On the other hand, S100 protein may show variable staining, and reported cases of both negative and positive staining have been documented.

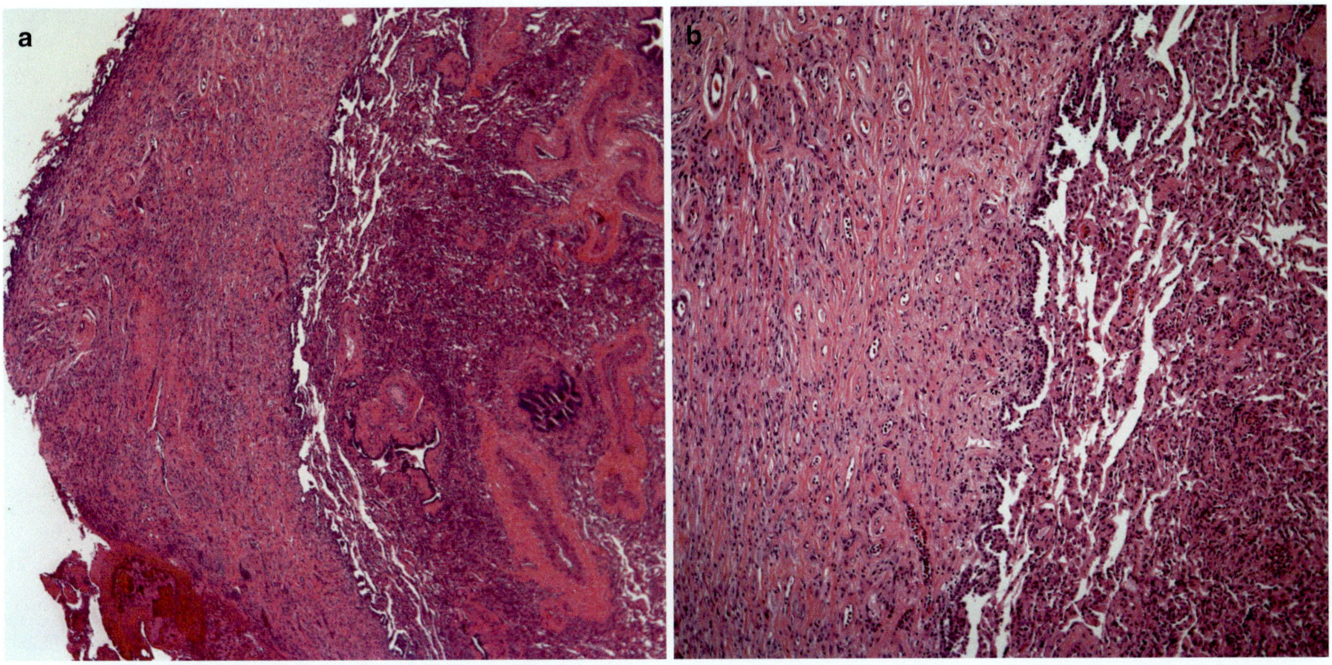

Fig. 13.8 (**a**) Erdheim-Chester disease involving the lung; note the predominant involvement of the pleura, which shows marked thickening. (**b**) Higher magnification showing a histiocytic proliferation in a markedly thickened pleura

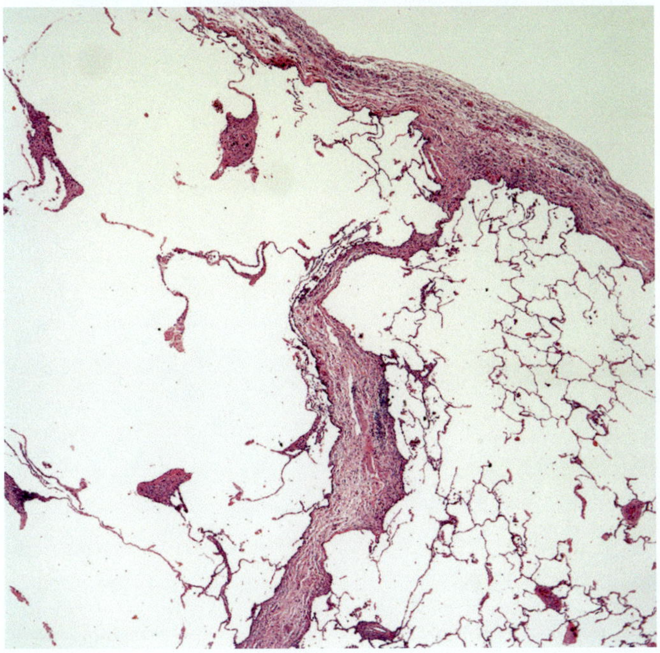

Fig. 13.9 Erdheim-Chester disease involving predominantly the pleura and the pulmonary septa. These features are commonly seen in Erdheim-Chester disease

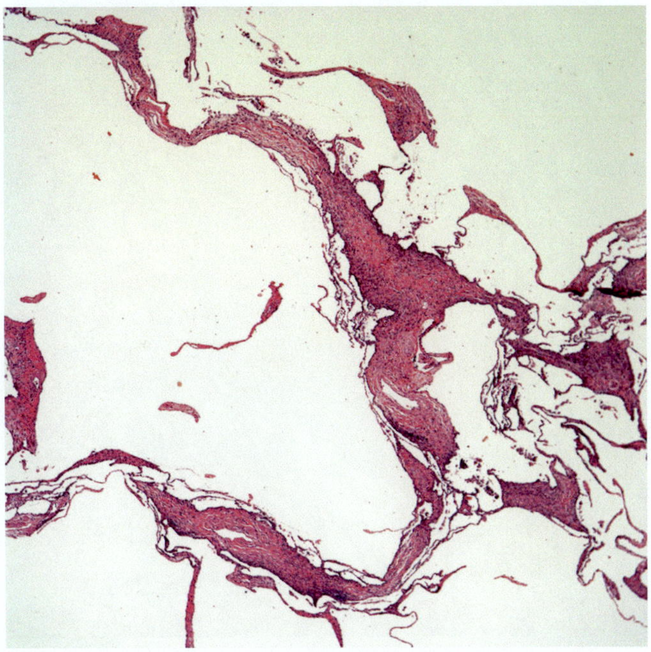

Fig. 13.10 Lung parenchyma showing cystic and emphysematous changes in Erdheim-Chester disease involving lung

Treatment and Prognosis

There is no specific treatment for this condition, and different treatment approaches have been attempted including corticosteroids, interferon-α-2a, surgical debulking, and/or chemotherapy; however, the prognosis for patients with Erdheim-Chester disease and pulmonary involvement is rather poor as those patients often follow a fatal course with respiratory failure.

Pulmonary Langerhans Cell Histiocytosis (PLCH)

PLCH has also been known by other names including primary pulmonary histiocytosis X, eosinophilic granuloma of the lung, and Langerhans cell granulomatosis. This type of histiocytosis may involve the lung in two different patterns: either as a solitary lung process or secondarily as part of a

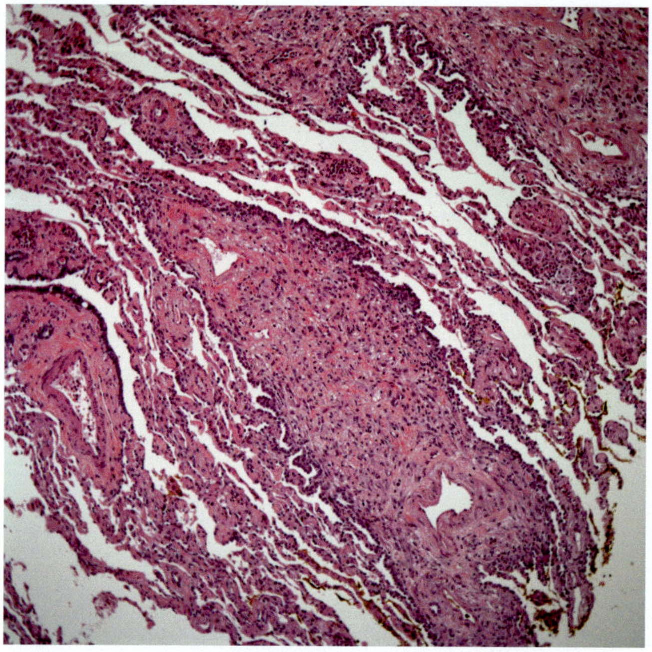

Fig. 13.11 In some cases of Erdheim-Chester disease, it is possible to observe small subpleural nodules involving lung parenchyma

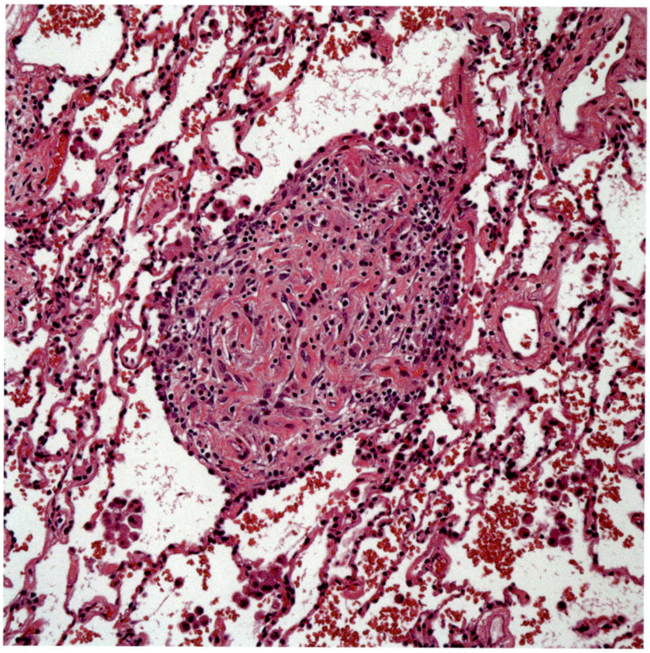

Fig. 13.12 Although Erdheim-Chester disease can involve large portions of lung parenchyma, in some cases, small nodules may also be present scattered in the lung parenchyma

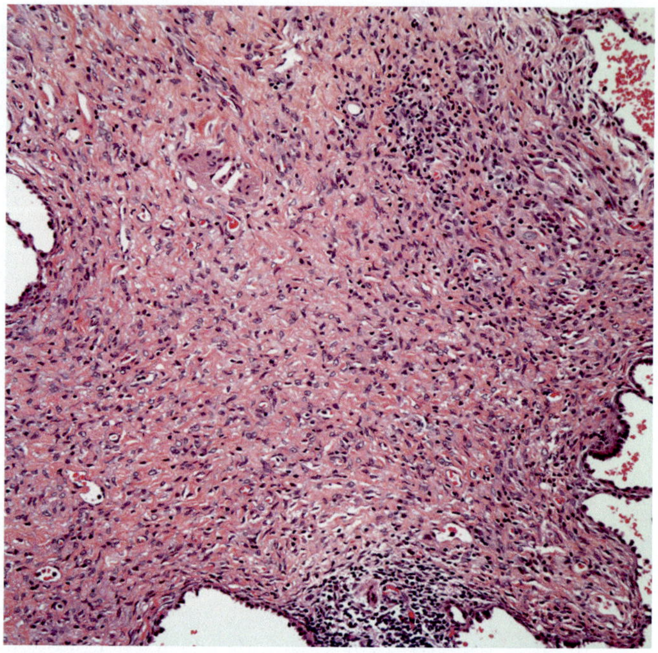

Fig. 13.13 Closer view at Erdheim-Chester disease showing a histiocytic proliferation with minimal inflammatory changes

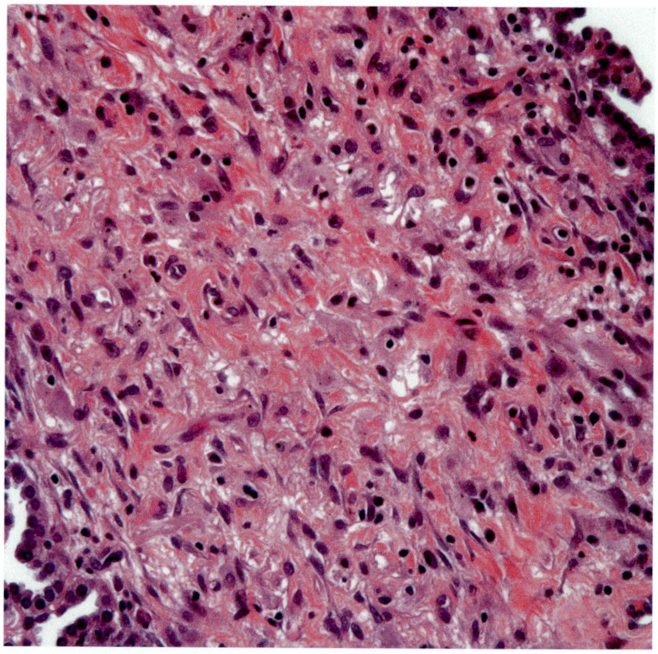

Fig. 13.14 Higher power view showing the presence of a proliferation of medium-sized histiocytes without the presence of other inflammatory cells

systemic process. This section will cover the single organ involvement, namely, that occurring in the lung.

Although numerous reviews and case series have been reported [22–40], the incidence of PLCH is difficult to determine, and there is no hard data on its prevalence. In a study of 502 patients who had a lung biopsy, 17 patients (3.4 %) were diagnosed with PLCH [41]. However, others have estimated that about 25 % of the cases are initially identified during routine chest radiographs, which may disclose pulmonary abnormalities. Although the exact pathogenesis of PLCH is unknown, Soler et al. [22] suggested an immune -related reaction. Nevertheless, it is important to highlight that clonality has been determined in cases of Langerhans cell histiocytosis [32–35]. Willman et al. [35] studied ten cases of Langerhans cell histiocytosis—none of them in the lung—using a HUMARA assay and identified clonality in nine of ten cases studied. Yu et al. [33] in a different study also documented clonality. Yousem et al. [32] also using HUMARA studied 24 nodules of 13 patients, with result that 29 % of cases showed clonality and 71 % of cases were non-clonal. The authors concluded that PLCH is primarily a reactive process.

Clinical Features

PLCH occurs more often in adult patients in their third of fourth decade of life. However, PLCH has also been described in children [38]. This histiocytosis is more common in the white than in the black population. Regarding gender, different studies have determined equal incidence in both genders, higher incidence in men, and higher incidence in women. However, one consistent association is with cigarette smoking, which can be seen in about 80 % of patients. Patients with PLCH may present with respiratory symptoms including cough, chest pain, dyspnea, hemoptysis, and/or pneumothorax. Approximately 20 % of the patients may be completely asymptomatic, and the process is first evident during a routine chest radiograph. Radiologically, the characteristic feature is that of a reticulonodular bilateral pulmonary infiltrate. However, it has also been stated that in some cases the radiographic findings may be nonspecific. Although the diagnosis is more often made on an open lung biopsy, in some studies, a few cases have been diagnosed on transbronchial biopsy.

PLCH has also been associated with neoplastic conditions including non-Hodgkin's lymphoma, Hodgkin's lymphoma, and carcinoma [27–29]. Therefore, close clinical, radiological, and histopathological correlation is required in order to properly address such associations.

Macroscopic Features

In open lung biopsies or wedge resections, PLCH shows multiple parenchymal nodules of different sizes, which may vary from under 1 cm to more than 3 cm in diameter. These nodules are whitish, firm, and well circumscribed but not encapsulated. Areas of necrosis and/or hemorrhage are not common but may occasionally be seen.

Histopathological Features

The low power magnification is that of multiple parenchymal nodules of different sizes obliterating the normal lung parenchyma (Figs. 13.15, 13.16, 13.17, 13.18, 13.19, 13.20, 13.21, 13.22, and 13.23). These nodules have a stellate shape some times resulting in the so-called Medusa's head; however, other nodules do not show this feature but rather have more rounded contours. Necrosis and/or cavitations may be seen in about 20–25 % of the cases. High power magnification shows the presence of a proliferation of histiocytes admixed with inflammatory cells, which in the majority of cases will characteristically contain numerous eosinophils. However, some nodules show more fibrotic changes and only a subtle inflammatory infiltrate containing only scattered eosinophils. The presence of eosinophils although helpful in the diagnosis is not required. The histiocytes characteristically show indented or grooved nuclei. The process may also extend into the alveolar walls, blood vessels, and airways. Another important feature to mention includes the changes that may be observed in the non-involved lung parenchyma. These changes may include a desquamative interstitial pneumonitis (DIP)-like reaction, which is characterized by an accumulation of pigmented laden macrophages within alveolar spaces and mild interstitial fibrosis.

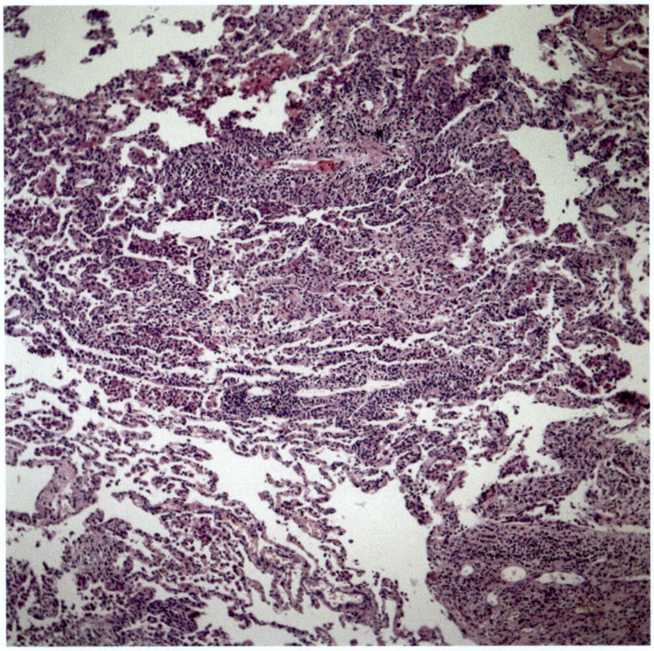

Fig. 13.15 LCH involving lung parenchyma. Note the presence of a well demarcated nodule destroying normal lung parenchyma

Immunohistochemically, PLCH shows positive staining for S100 protein, CD1a (Fig. 13.24a, b), HLA-DR, langerin, and E-cadherin. Ultrastructurally, Langerhans cells contain characteristic Birbeck granules cytoplasmic organelles with a typical tennis racket-like appearance.

Differential Diagnosis

Although PLCH is a rather straightforward diagnosis, in some cases the characteristic features are not readily apparent and other conditions may be considered in the differential diagnosis including Erdheim-Chester disease, malignant lymphoma, and/or eosinophilic pneumonia [39]. In any of these settings, the use of immunohistochemical studies and correlation with radiographic findings may help in arriving at the correct diagnosis.

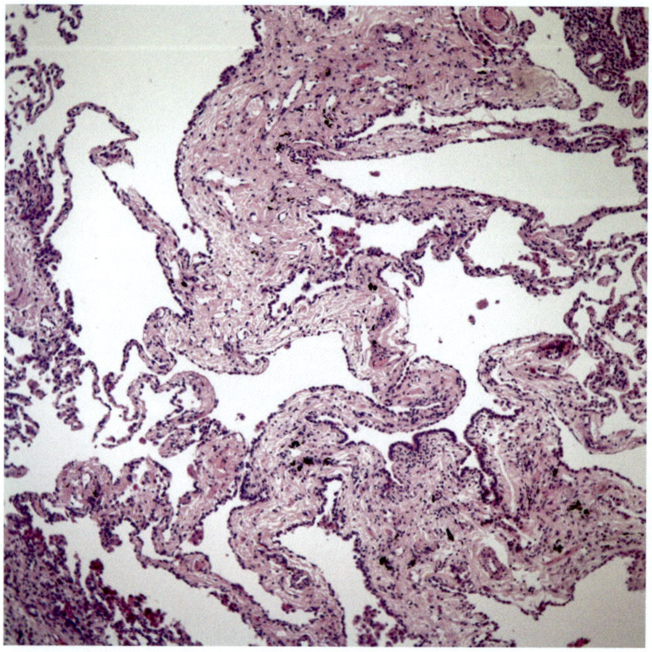

Fig. 13.16 Pulmonary scarring and widening of the interstitium may also be present when LCH involves the lung parenchyma

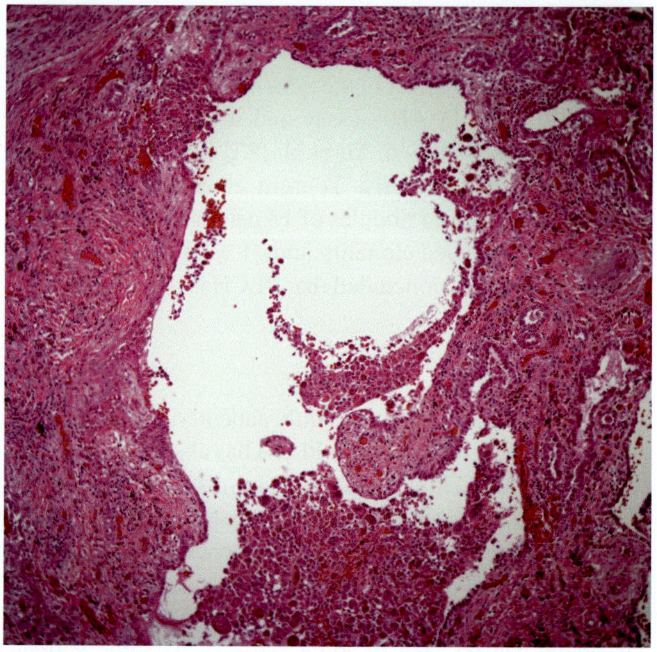

Fig. 13.18 Cystic areas, which can be extensive, may be present in cases of LCH involving the lung

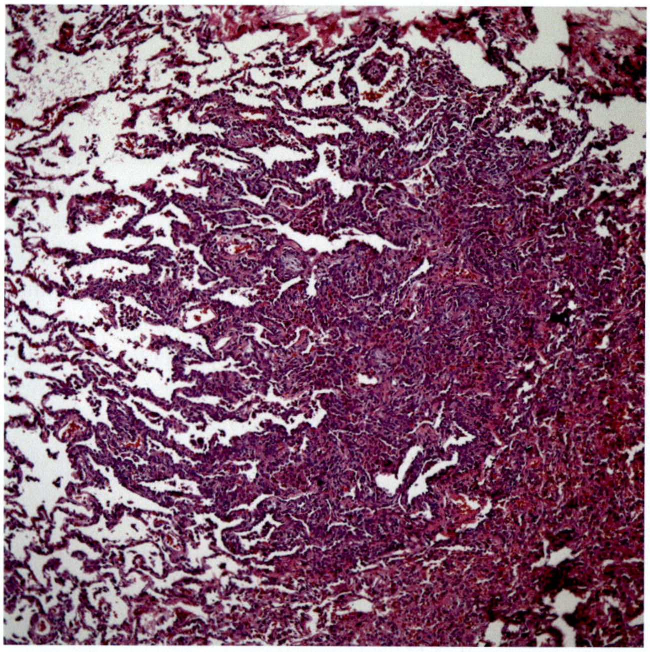

Fig. 13.17 LCH involving lung parenchyma. Note the presence of a pulmonary nodule, which discretely expands to involve other pulmonary areas, the so-called Medusa's head

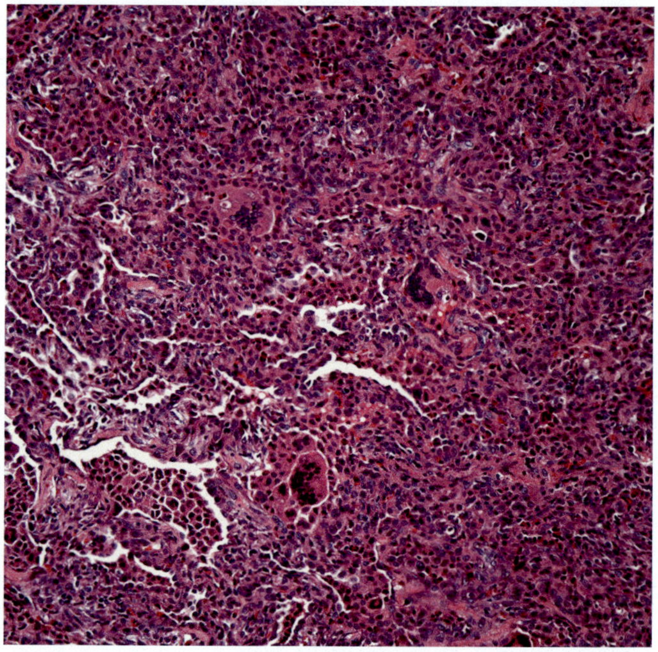

Fig. 13.19 Pulmonary LCH showing the presence of multinucleated giant cells

Treatment and Prognosis

Different treatment approaches may be undertaken in the treatment of PLCH including cessation of smoking, steroid therapy, steroid therapy, chemotherapy, or lung transplantation. This latter form of treatment (lung transplantation) is reserved for patients with severe compromised lung function. However, it is important to keep in mind that recurrences of PLCH have been documented in the transplanted lung. Each one of these treatment modalities will depend largely on an individual basis and on the respiratory function of the an individual. Smoking cessation appears to be very important in the treatment of these patients. Although many studies have suggested a good prognosis, some patients have gone on to develop respiratory insufficiency and died as a consequence of PLCH. Vassallo et al. [37] reviewed 102 adults with PLCH who were followed up for a period of 0–23 years (median: 4 years). In this study the authors found 33 deaths, 15 of those deaths were attributed to respiratory failure with an overall median survival of 12.5 years. The authors also found six patients with malignant lymphoproliferative disorders and five patients with lung carcinoma. The authors concluded that the survival of adults with PLCH is shorter than that of the general population.

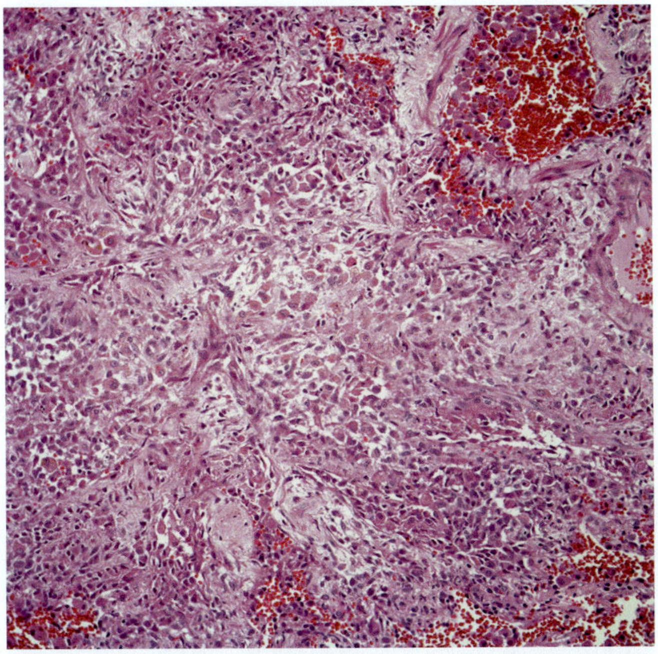

Fig. 13.20 Higher magnification of a nodule of pulmonary LCH showing a histiocytic proliferation; note the absence of other inflammatory cells

Pulmonary Juvenile Xanthogranuloma (PJXG)

PJXG belongs to the group of histiocytoses classified under the term non-Langerhans cell histiocytosis. This is an unusual condition of rare occurrence in the lung parenchyma, and only a few cases have been reported in the literature [42–48]. Contrary to Langerhans cell histiocytosis in which the cell of origin is basically known, in PJXG the putative cell of origin is proposed to be the dermal dendrocyte; however, this theory would not explain those lesions that occur primarily in deep-seated tissues or in the viscera. Therefore, some authors have speculated on the possibility of a plasmacytoid monocyte as the cell of origin [44]. Nevertheless, such theories remain speculative.

PJXG is more common in children and young adults. However, the lung parenchyma is rarely affected. When the lung is involved, the lesion may be bilateral, unilateral, multiple, or solitary. Rarely will the lesion be solitary or the cause of the main presenting symptom; however, this has been reported in sporadic cases. Often, the patients have dermal involvement and/or involvement of other viscera.

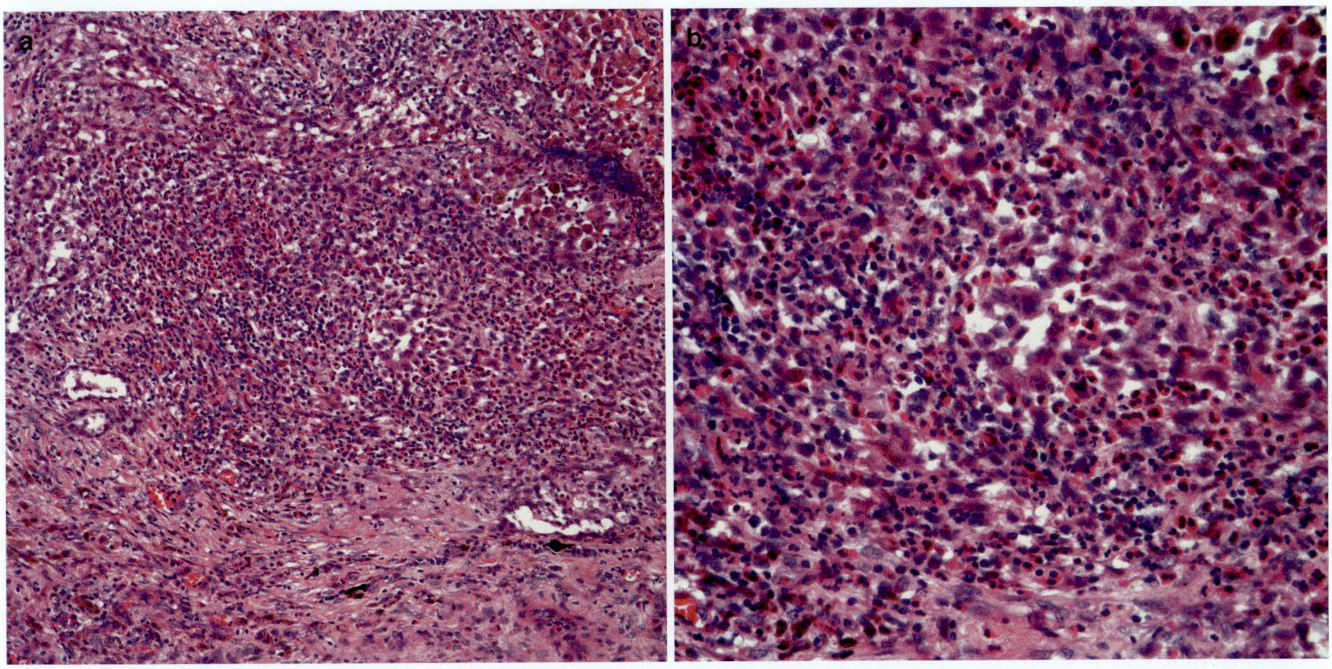

Fig. 13.21 (**a**) Pulmonary LCH in which the histiocytic proliferation is admixed with a marked number of eosinophils. (**b**) Higher magnification of histiocytes admixed with eosinophils

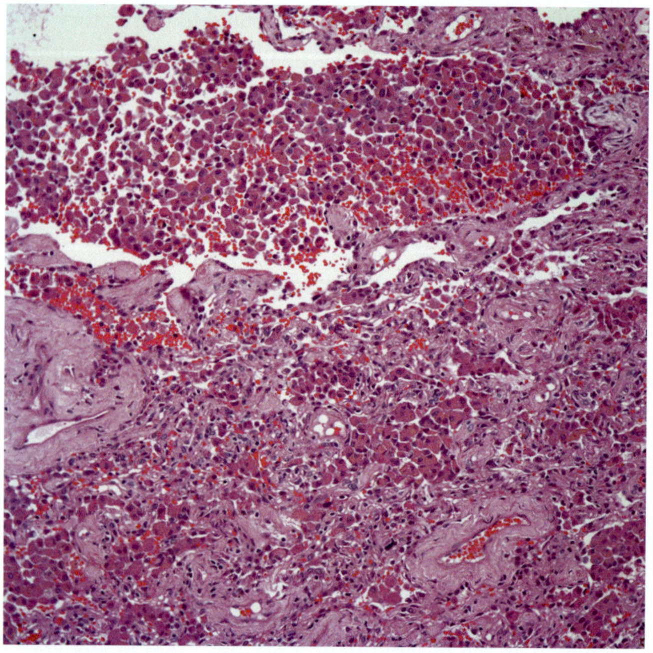

Fig. 13.22 Adjacent lung parenchyma in pulmonary LCH shows a desquamative interstitial pneumonitis (*DIP*)-like reaction

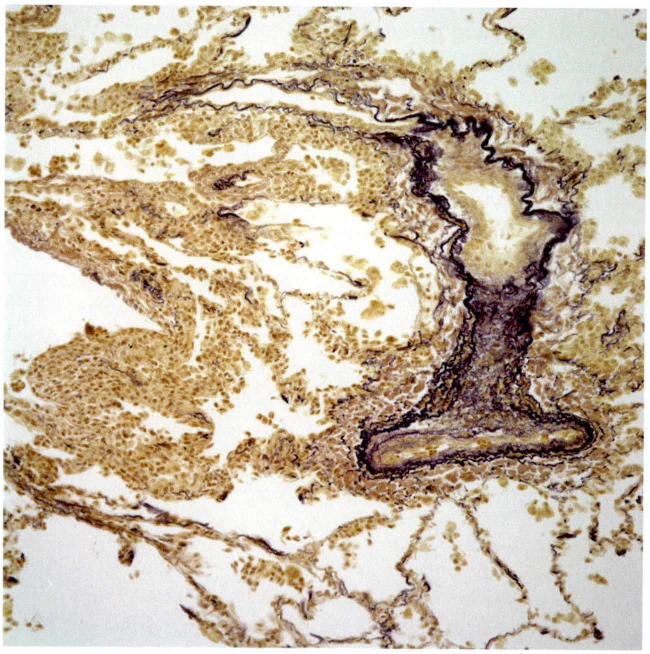

Fig. 13.23 Elastic-Van-Gieson stain showing medial hypertrophy and intimal fibrosis in pulmonary LCH

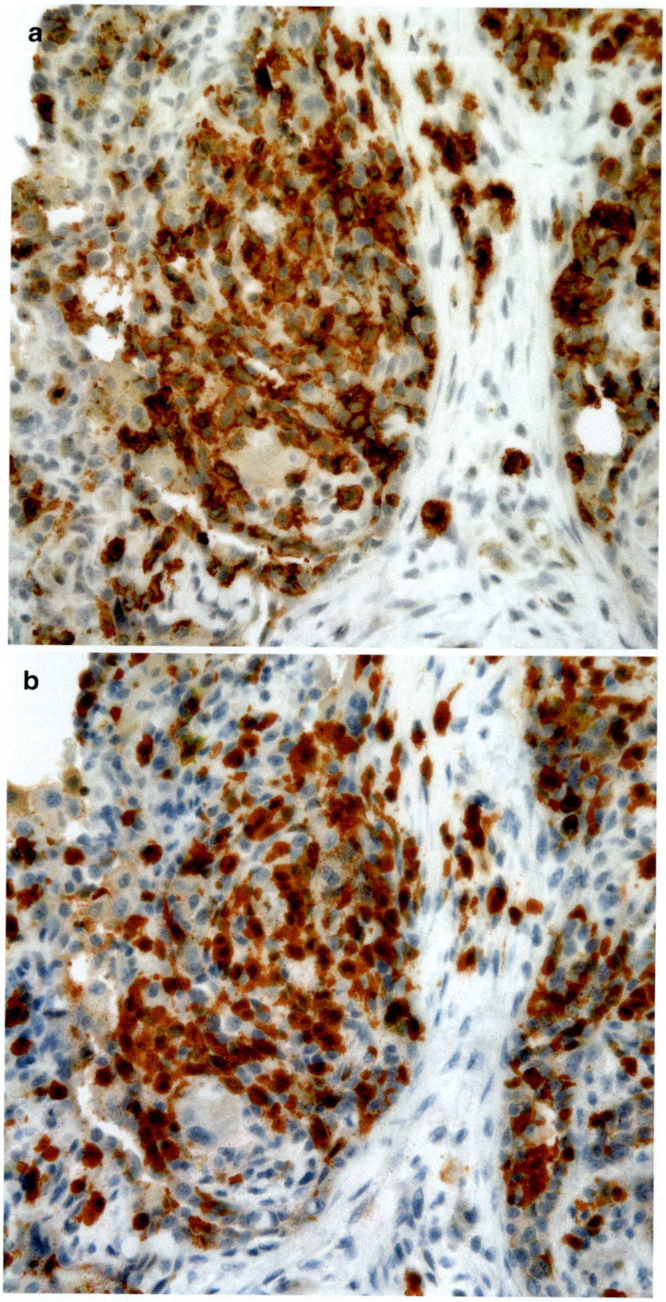

Fig. 13.24 (**a**) Immunohistochemical stain for CD1a showing positive staining in histiocytes. (**b**) Immunohistochemical stain for S100 protein showing positive staining in histiocytes

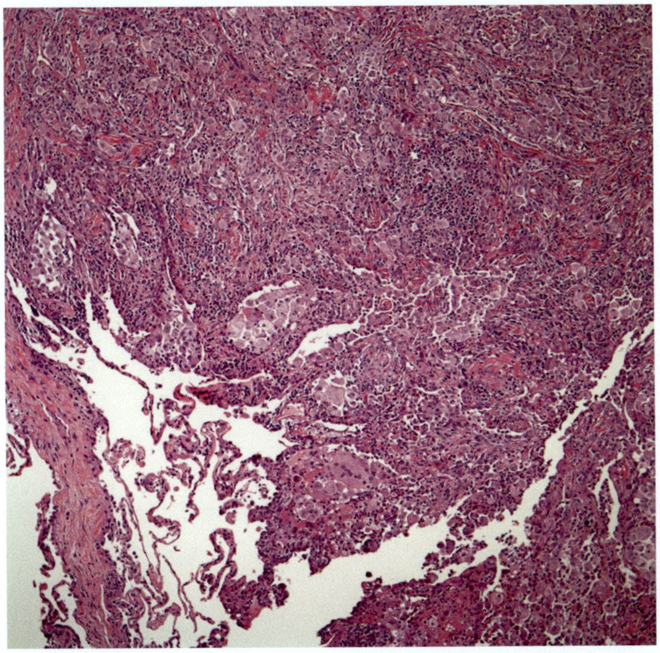

Fig. 13.25 Low power view of PJXG involving lung parenchyma; the lesion has ill-defined borders and shows a histiocytic proliferation

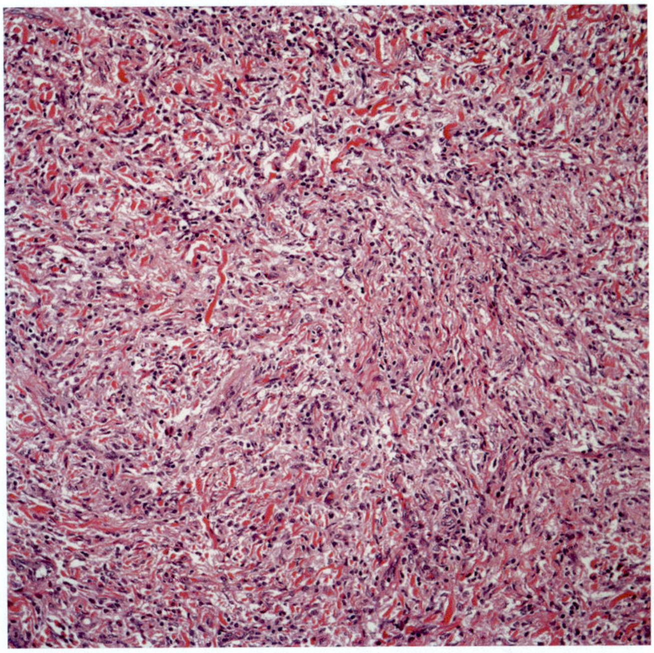

Fig. 13.26 Normal lung parenchyma obliterated by a histiocytic proliferation in a background of collagenous stroma

Pathological Features

Grossly, this lesions often appear as a solitary lung nodule or mass of varying size, which may range from under 1 cm to more than 3 cm in greatest dimension. The lesions are soft and yellowish, well demarcated but not encapsulated.

Histologically, the low power view is that of a well circumscribed but unencapsulated mass destroying normal lung parenchyma (Figs. 13.25, 13.26, 13.27, 13.28, 13.29, 13.30, and 13.31). Higher magnification shows a proliferation of histiocytes, which may range from small to medium sized with or without prominent nuclei. The histiocytic proliferation may be accompanied by an inflammatory infiltrate composed of lymphocytes and plasma cells. In some areas, nodular collections of lymphocytes may be seen. Also in focal areas, admixed with the histiocytic proliferation, scattered multinucleated giant cells may be seen. These giant cells are difficult to find, and in many cases, are absent. Nuclear atypia, mitotic activity, necrosis, and/or hemorrhage are not common in this process.

Immunohistochemical studies of dermal JXG have shown positive staining of histiocytes for CD68, factor XIIIa, HLA-DR, LCA, CD4, and S100 protein. However, the tumor is negative for CD1a, CD3, CD21, CD34, and CD35. In addition, ultrastructural studies are negative for the presence of Birbeck granules.

Treatment and Prognosis

The rarity of this lesion in the lung parenchyma precludes from unequivocally stating whether there is an impact on the survival of these patients. Most likely, it is the extent of the disease at the time of diagnosis what determines the outcome of these patients. Surgical resection of the pulmonary lesions appears to be a logical approach in cases in which such procedure can be accomplished.

Crystal-Storing Histiocytoma or Histiocytosis

This is an unusual process that can present with or without an association with lymphoproliferative disorders [49–65]. The most common lymphoproliferative process involved is multiple myeloma. Crystal-storing histiocytoma has been suggested as a term when this process is unassociated with a lymphoproliferative disorder. It is believed that this condition is reactive in nature in contrast to the form associated with a lymphoproliferative disorder. On the other hand, if the process is associated with a lymphoproliferative disorder, the more generic name of crystal-storing histiocytosis should be used. This lesion has been identified in several organ systems including the gastrointestinal, genitourinary, hematopoietic, and respiratory systems. Three different storing components have been identified: (1) crystallized immunoglobulins, (2) phagocytosed clofazimine in patients receiving treatment for leprosy, and (3) Charcot-Leyden crystals. However, regardless of the material accumulated, the basic histology is similar, namely, the presence of a histiocytic proliferation containing crystalline material.

Pathologic Features

In crystal-storing histiocytosis, the lung parenchyma appears to keep its basic architecture; however, the alveoli are filled with an eosinophilic material that in some areas

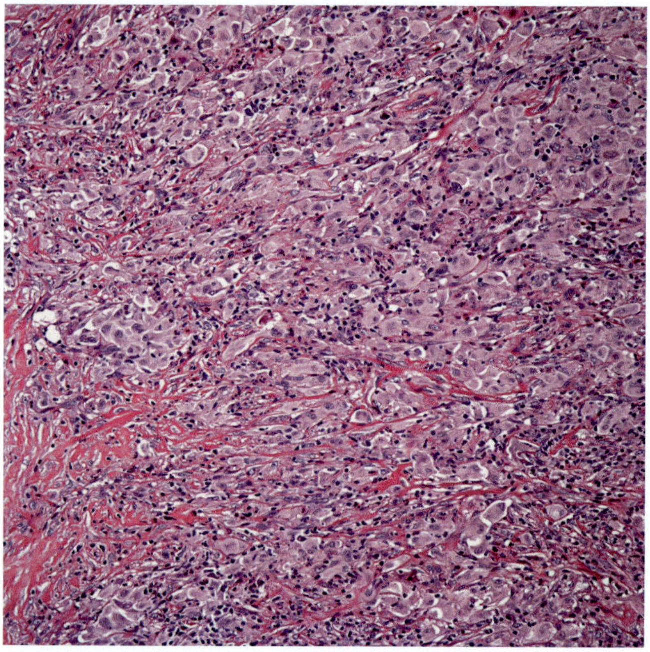

Fig. 13.27 PJXG showing a prominent histiocytic proliferation with minimal presence of other inflammatory cells

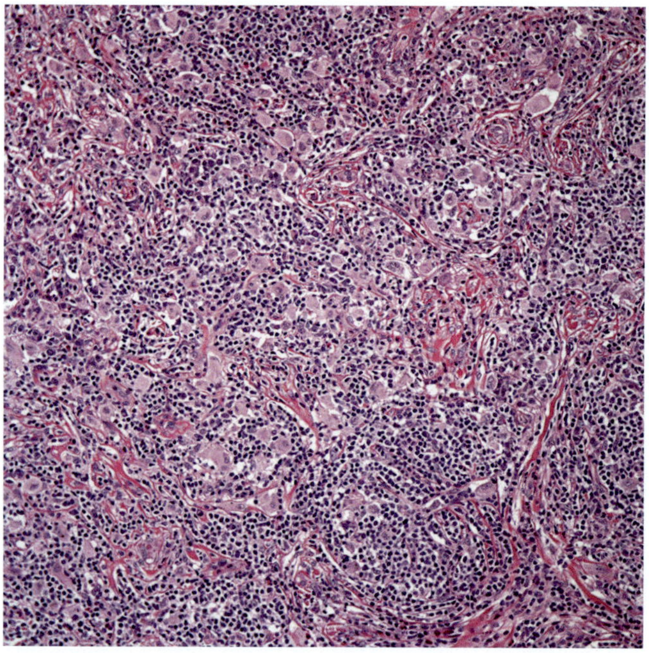

Fig. 13.28 PJXG showing a histiocytic proliferation admixed with inflammatory cells, predominantly lymphocytes

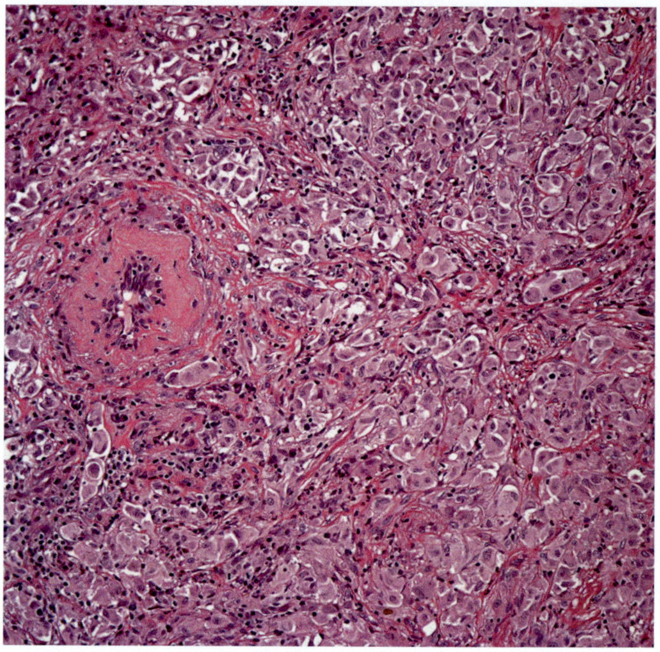

Fig. 13.29 Histiocytic proliferation of PJXG compressing vascular structures without causing vasculitis

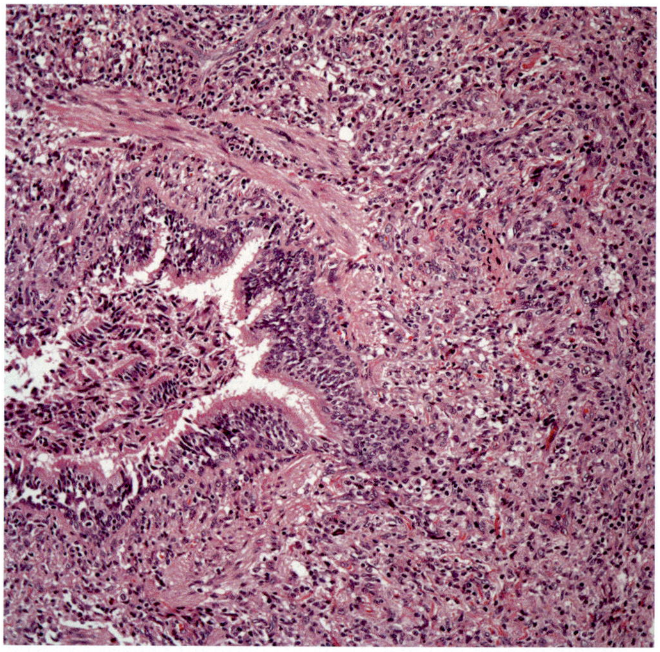

Fig. 13.30 PJXG with a predominantly histiocytic proliferation around an airway without obstructing the airway lumen

can spill into the interstitium mimicking fibrinous exudates (Figs. 13.32, 13.33, 13.34, 13.35, 13.36, 13.37, and 13.38). At higher magnification, the material filling the alveoli is characterized by the presence of large histiocytes with ample cytoplasm and small round nuclei. The cytoplasm of the histiocytes is filled with crystalloid material representing crystallized immunoglobulins. On the other hand, crystal-storing histiocytoma presents as a pulmonary mass or nodule replacing the normal lung parenchyma. In some cases, the appearance of the histiocytes may suggest muscle differentiation mimicking those cells seen in rhabdomyomas. In other cases, the histiocytes appear to contain a rather granular type of material, probably non-crystalline immunoglobulin.

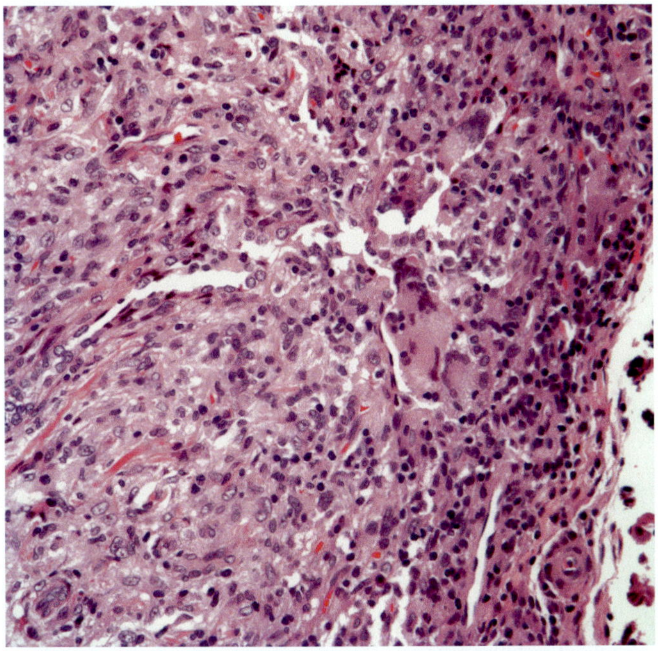

Fig. 13.31 PJXG showing a prominent histiocytic proliferation and scattered giant cells in the periphery of the lesion

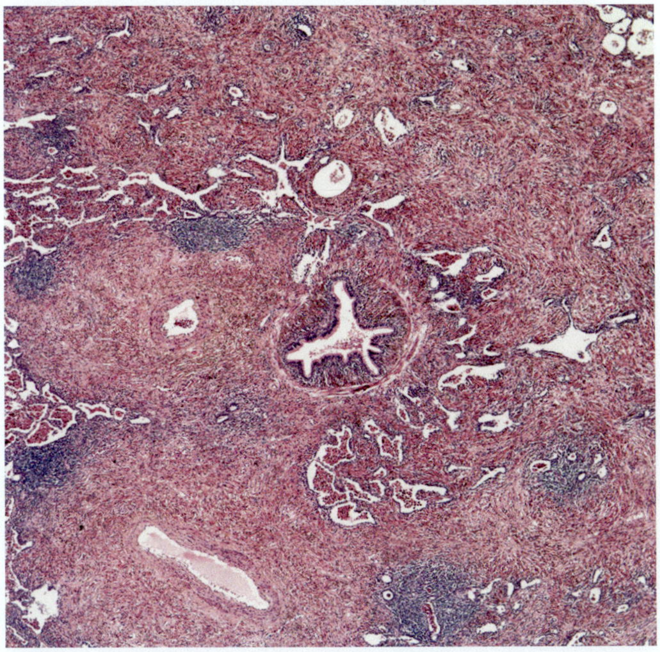

Fig. 13.32 Crystal-storing histiocytosis showing a cellular proliferation with bright eosinophilic cytoplasm. Note the residual airway structure

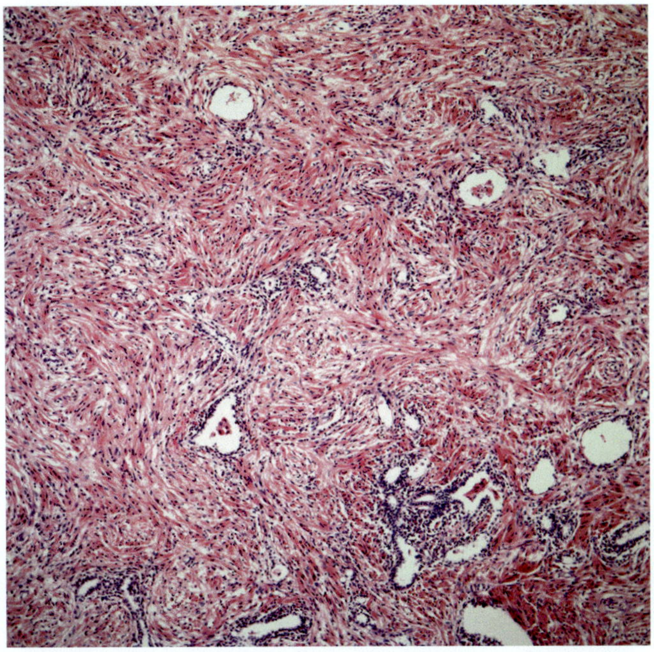

Fig. 13.33 Lung parenchyma replaced by a histiocytic proliferation mimicking smooth muscle

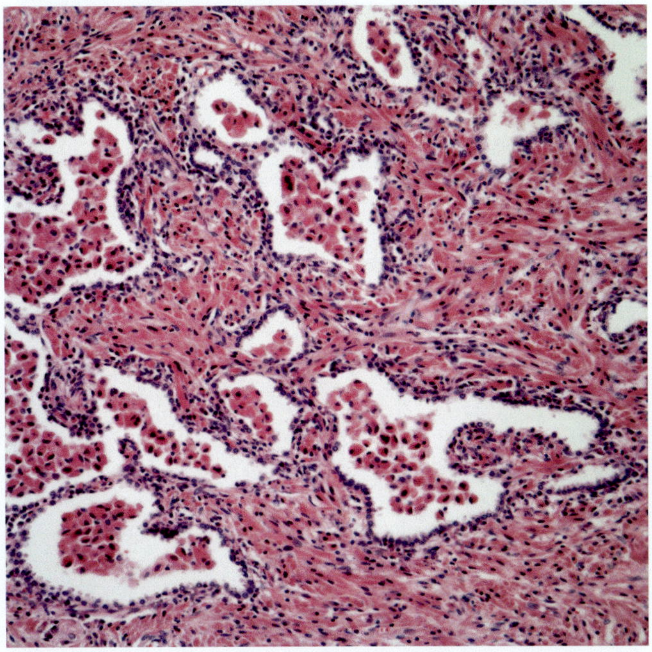

Fig. 13.34 Residual alveolar structures containing numerous histiocytes. Note the presence of the histiocytic proliferation around the alveolar structures

Immunohistochemical studies may help in determining histiocytic differentiation as the cells also show positive staining for CD68 and may show a monoclonal arrangement of immunoglobulin using kappa or lambda stains. The histiocytes are negative for CD1a and Factor XIIIa. Electron microscopy evaluation will ultimately determine the type of crystalline material present in the cytoplasm of these histiocytes.

Treatment and Prognosis

Surgical resection appears to be the treatment of choice. However, recurrences have been documented. The prognosis of

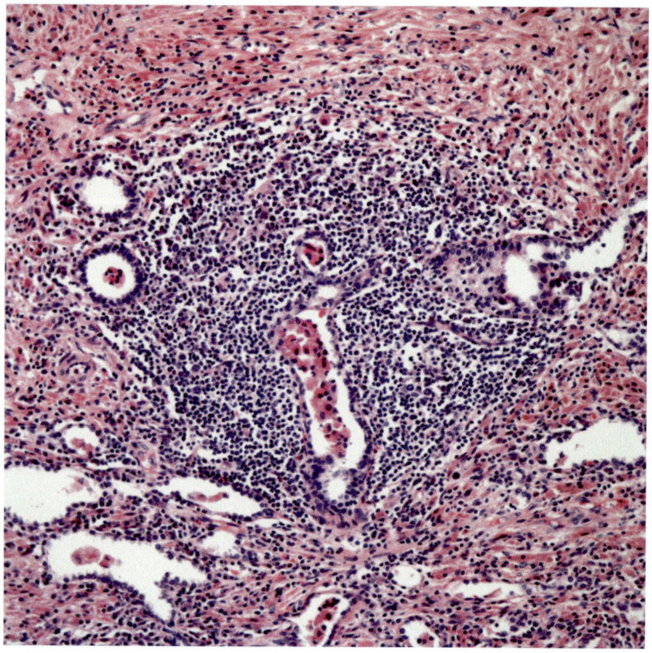

Fig. 13.35 Lymphoid aggregates are commonly seen in crystal-storing histiocytosis

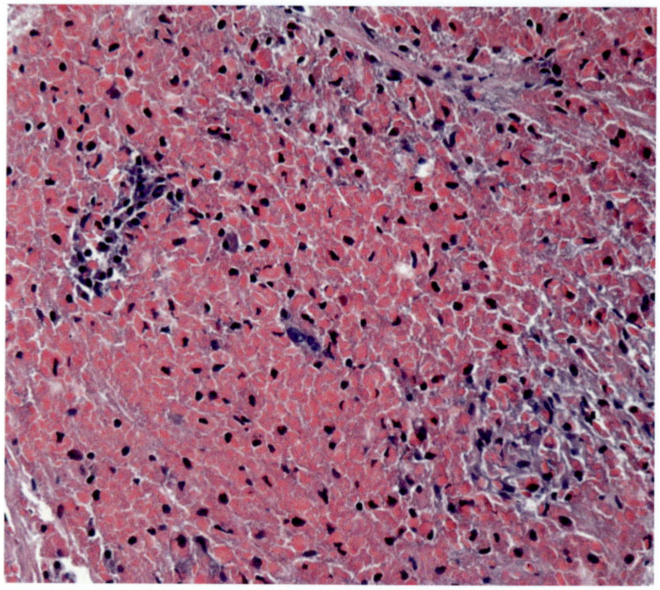

Fig. 13.37 High power magnification showing histiocytes filled with crystalloid granular material

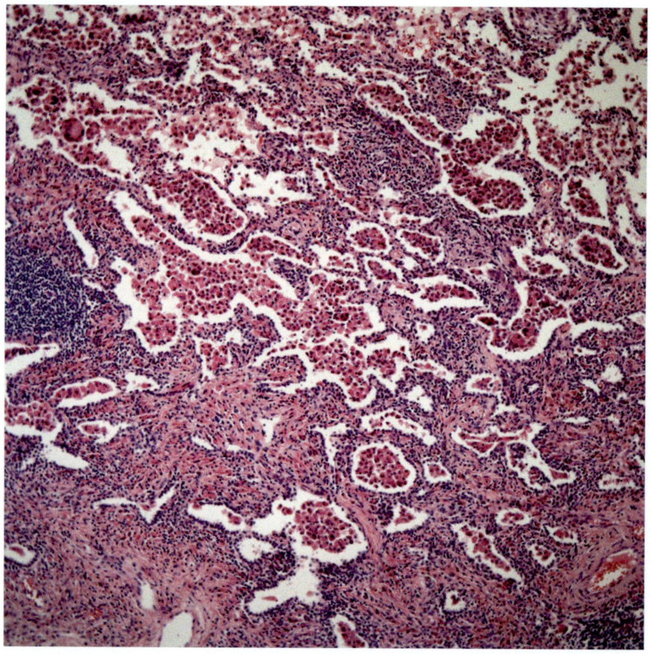

Fig. 13.36 Interphase between solid areas of crystal-storing histiocytosis and presence of similar histiocytes filling alveolar spaces

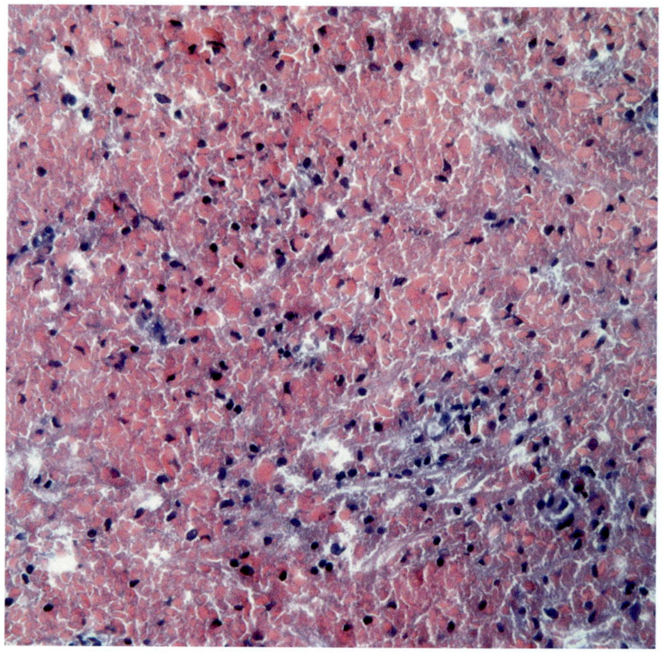

Fig. 13.38 Higher magnification showing histiocytes with crystalloid material of different shapes

this process will be determined by the presence of any associated condition. It is imperative that in cases limited to the pulmonary parenchyma and without an obvious lymphoproliferative process, a complete clinical evaluation should be undertaken in order to evaluate the patient for any occult neoplasm.

Pulmonary Malacoplakia

Even though pulmonary malacoplakia may contain a histiocytic proliferation, this condition does not represent a bona fide histiocytic process. It is rather an infectious process, which may elicit a histiocytic response. This lesion is discussed among this group of histiocytic lesions in order to complement these unusual processes.

Malacoplakia is a process of ubiquitous distribution that has been described in many organ systems including the genitourinary, central nervous, and gastrointestinal systems. Although some authors have suggested that the process is secondary to an infection with *E. coli*, in the lung, it has been commonly associated with the acquired immunodeficiency syndrome (AIDS) or in patients with other immunosuppressive states [66–70]. Other infectious agents commonly seen in association with pulmonary malacoplakia include *Rhodococcus equi* and *Pasteurella*. Clinical and radiological features of patients with pulmonary malacoplakia are rather nonspecific. Tissue histological evaluation is required for final diagnosis.

Pathologic Features

Malacoplakia in the lung can present as an endobronchial nodule or as an intraparenchymal pulmonary mass with destruction of the lung parenchyma and necrosis indistinguishable from any pulmonary neoplasm.

The lung parenchyma may contain one or more pulmonary nodules of different sizes (Figs. 13.39, 13.40, 13.41, and 13.42). These nodules are composed of a histiocytic proliferation admixed with plasma cells and scattered Michaelis-Gutmann bodies, which is the pathognomonic feature of malacoplakia. However, in some instances, malacoplakia in the lung may mimic the low power appearance of bronchiolitis obliterans organizing pneumonia (BOOP) by showing a spindle cell fibroblastic proliferation admixed with lymphocytes and plasma cells admixed with numerous Michaelis-Gutmann bodies. This type of pattern may be easily confused with BOOP or inflammatory pseudotumor of the lung. The use of special histochemical stains for iron or a Von-Kossa stain can be helpful in the identification of the Michaelis-Gutmann bodies. Ultrastructural studies of Michaelis-Gutmann bodies may show the presence of a fingerprint-like pattern in some cases of malacoplakia.

Treatment and Prognosis

If the lesion is forming a pulmonary nodule, complete surgical resection is curative. If there is any particular infection associated with this process, then treatment for that specific infection should be started. Although this process is benign, the underlying condition is the one that will determine the outcome in these patients.

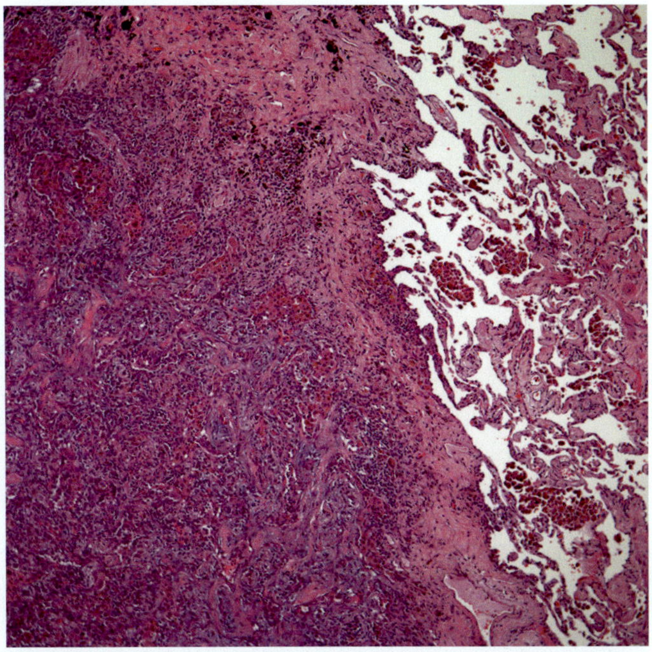

Fig. 13.39 Pulmonary malacoplakia showing a well demarcated tumor nodule replacing normal lung parenchyma

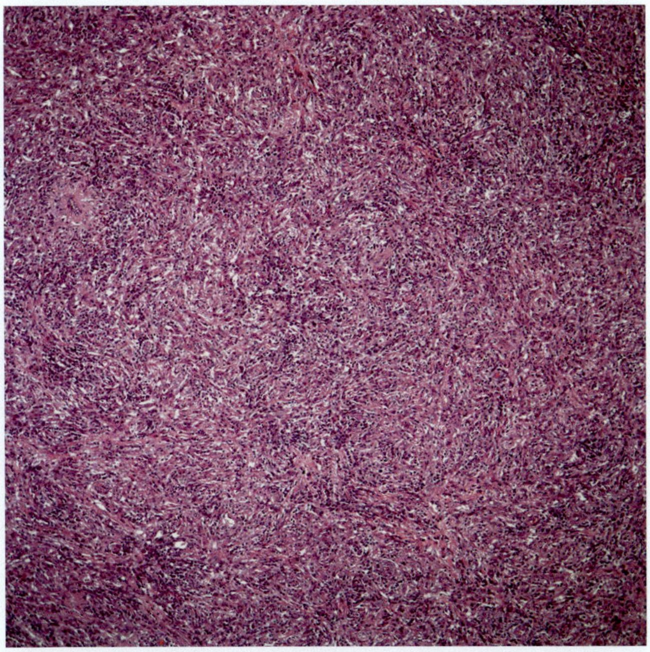

Fig. 13.40 Histiocytic proliferation admixed with scattered inflammatory cells replacing lung parenchyma

Pulmonary Xanthoma

Andrianopooulos et al. [71] described the only case of pulmonary xanthoma reported in the literature today. The patient was a 32-year-old asymptomatic man without any pertinent clinical history. During a routine chest radiograph, the patient was found to have the presence of a solitary pulmonary mass of 4 cm in greatest dimension. Immunohistochemically, the tumor was reported to be negative for epithelial membrane antigen, keratin, S100 protein, chromogranin, periodic acid-Schiff (PAS) and diastase-resistant PAS (D-PAS),

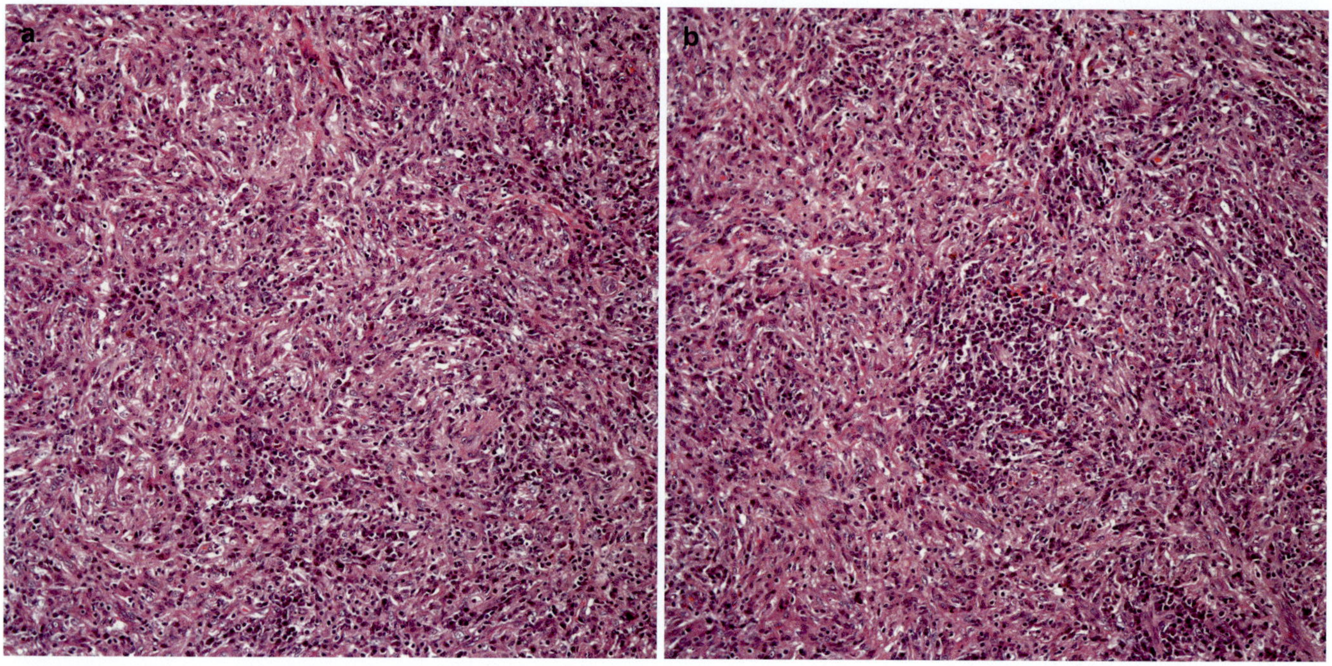

Fig. 13.41 (**a**) The presence of an inflammatory component may not be as marked in some areas. (**b**) Clusters of plasma cell may be present. Plasma cells are commonly encountered in pulmonary malacoplakia

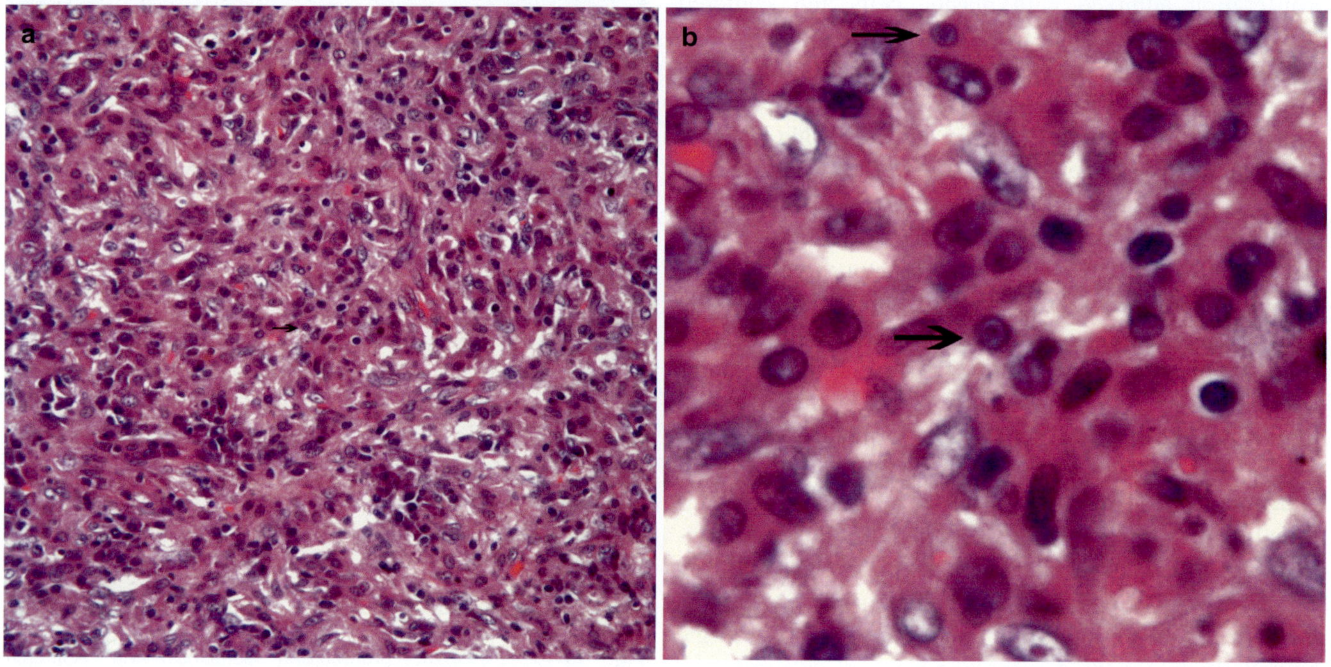

Fig. 13.42 (**a**) High power magnification of the histiocytic proliferation in which the presence of Michaelis-Gutmann bodies is identified (*arrow*). (**b**) Higher magnification showing the presence of Michaelis-Gutmann bodies (see *arrows*)

mucicarmine, and oil-red-O. Electron microscopic studies were nonspecific, and the DNA histogram showed the presence of a diploid cell population. Although this is the only such case described in the literature, it is possible that similar cases exist but have not been reported in the literature.

Histopathological Features

Low power view of this lesion shows a well-circumscribed but unencapsulated subpleural process that replaces the normal lung parenchyma and is composed of a homogenous cellular proliferation composed of medium-sized cells with ample clear or pale cytoplasm and nuclei displaced toward the periphery of the cells (Figs. 13.43, 13.44, and 13.45). Higher magnification shows that this cellular proliferation shows no mitotic activity, nuclear atypia, necrosis, and/or hemorrhage. Admixed with the xanthomatous component, are scattered inflammatory cells, namely, lymphocytes and plasma cells.

Immunohistochemical studies show the process to be negative for epithelial, neuroendocrine, and neural markers. However, it is possible that CD68 may show positive staining.

The treatment of choice for this process is complete surgical resection that may be accomplished by wedge resection or segmentectomy. Surgical resection appears to be curative.

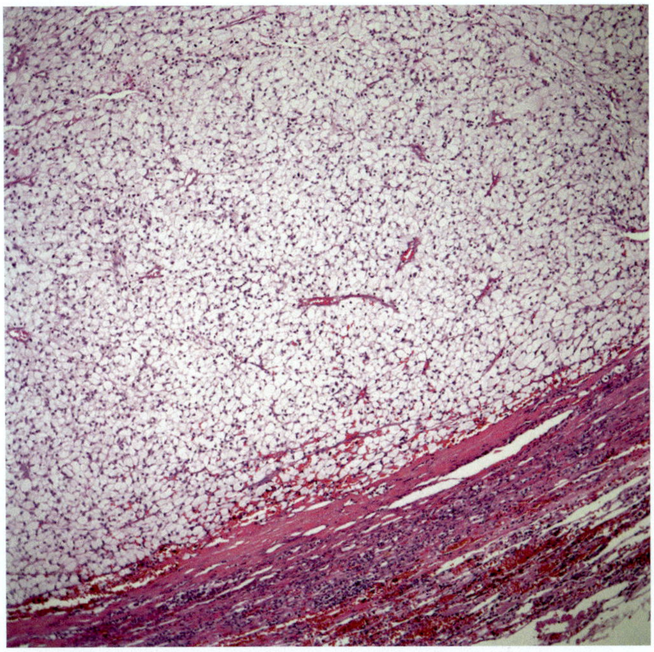

Fig. 13.43 Primary xanthoma of the lung characterized by sheets of xanthoma cells replacing lung parenchyma. Note the rim of pulmonary parenchyma still present

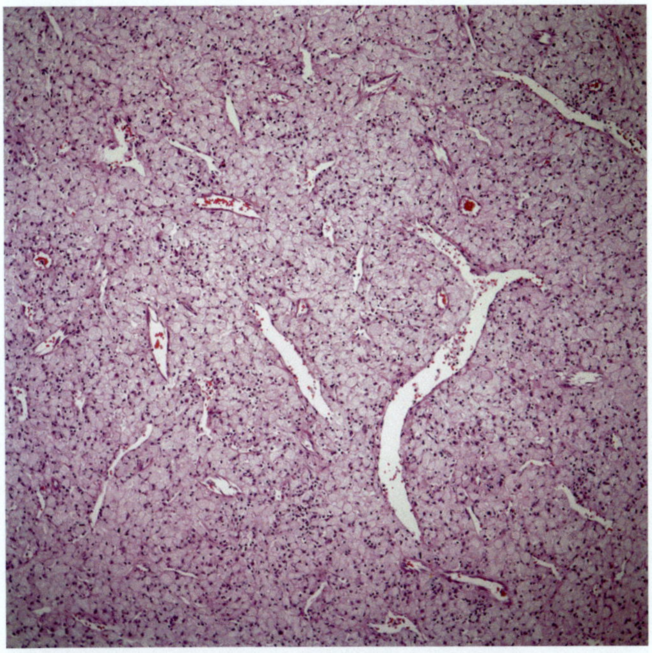

Fig. 13.44 Pulmonary xanthoma showing prominent dilated vascular structures mimicking a vascular tumor

Unclassified Xanthomatous Lesions

In general practice, there is a group of lesions characterized by the presence of "xanthomatous" cells that does not quite fit the previously described entities. However, this group of lesions may share some immunohistochemical features with previously described entities. The authors have encountered a few of these proliferations that clinically have been thought to represent a neoplastic condition but that histologically are characterized by a proliferation of xanthomatous cells. The approach to these lesions is to group them under the term "xanthoma" or "xanthomatous lesion not otherwise specified." It is possible that these lesions per se may represent variants of other already well known histiocytic proliferations.

Benign Tumors of Non-histiocytic Origin

This group of lesions comprises rare entities in thoracic pathology; however, because of their unusual occurrence, they can easily be confused with malignant neoplasms. It is important to highlight that these lesions per se do not share any relationship among each other and clearly have a completely different origin. Therefore, even though they are grouped together in this chapter, this is done primarily to facilitate their study and to become familiar with their presentation, histological, and immunohistochemical characteristics. The group of unusual benign tumoral conditions that will be discussed in this chapter include:

- Pulmonary metastatic calcification
- Pulmonary alveolar microlithiasis
- Placental transmogrification

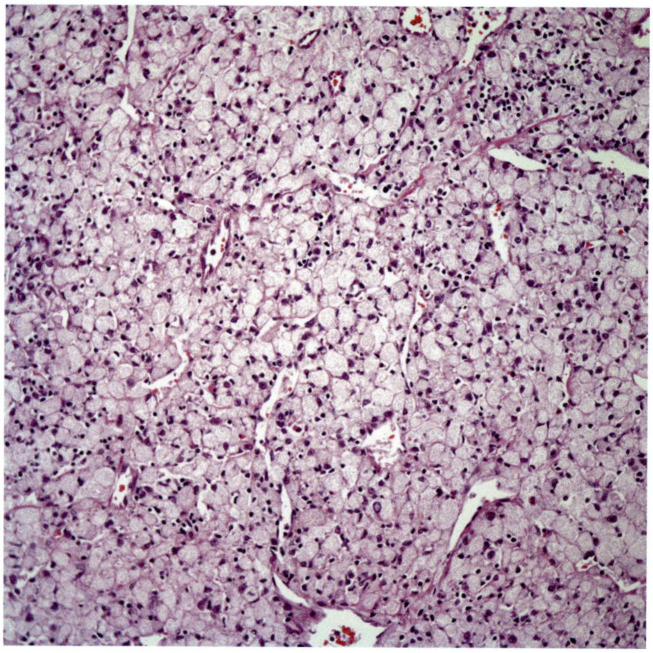

Fig. 13.45 High power magnification showing a homogenous cellular proliferation with ample cytoplasm and peripheral nuclei. Note the absence of nuclear atypia or mitotic activity

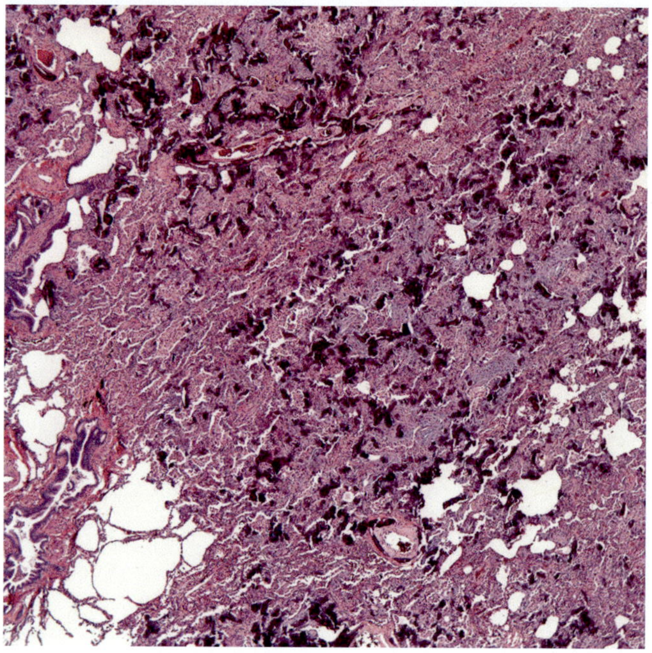

Fig. 13.46 Dendritic calcification showing deposits of calcium predominantly in alveolar walls and interstitium

- Pulmonary lymphangioleiomyomatosis
- Alveolar proteinosis
- Pulmonary amyloid tumor
- Mucous gland adenoma
- Alveolar adenoma
- Pulmonary dirofilariasis

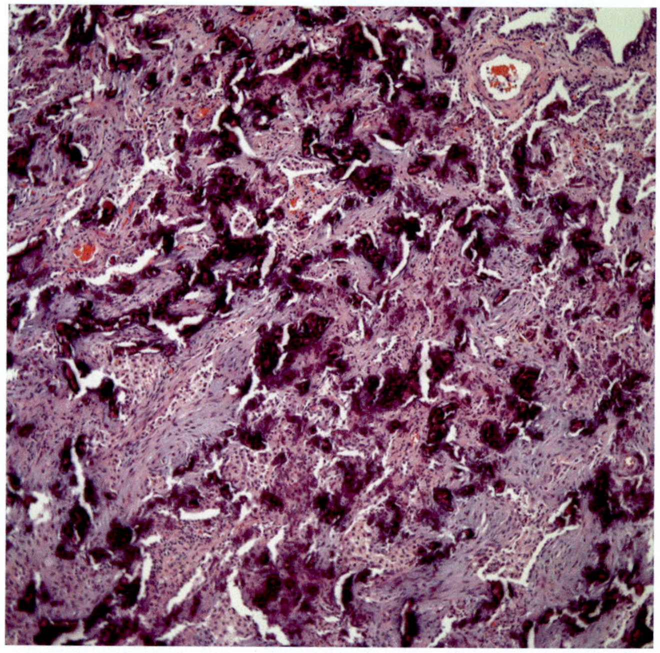

Fig. 13.47 Prominent deposits of calcifying material without forming a well defined mass

Pulmonary Metastatic Calcification

This is an unusual phenomenon that may present a problem for the clinician since the clinical presentation may mimic a neoplastic process. Metastatic calcification presents in different clinical settings, for instance patients treated for malignancies, such as parathyroid carcinoma, lymphoproliferative disorders, transplant patients, or patients with abnormal renal function [72–80]. Based on the clinical background, metastatic calcification can be seen at any age in any patient. Radiologically, conventional chest radiographs may not be as accurate as CT scan. In any case, the process is bilateral, dense, and asymmetric [81, 82]. Some authors have suggested the use of dual-energy digital radiography as a more sensitive tool than conventional chest radiography for the diagnosis of metastatic calcification. The exact mechanism for this process is not known. However, it has been stated that metastatic calcification may be influenced by serum calcium and phosphate concentrations, alkaline phosphatase activity, and local physicochemical conditions such as pH [83]. Contrary to what happens in dystrophic calcification in which there is prior tissue injury, metastatic calcification does not require such a background [80].

Histopathological Features

Grossly, the lungs appear congested and have a gritty cut surface. Contrary to the features seen in alveolar microlithiasis in which the calcospherites fill the alveolar spaces metastatic calcification follows a more haphazard pattern in which the calcified material is deposited in the interstitium, bronchial wall, and airways

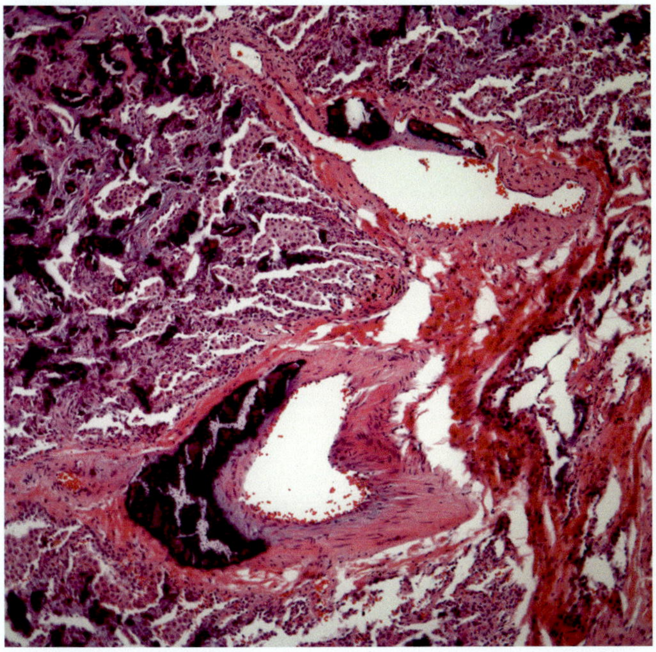

Fig. 13.48 Calcification of the wall of the vessels may be observed in dendritic calcification

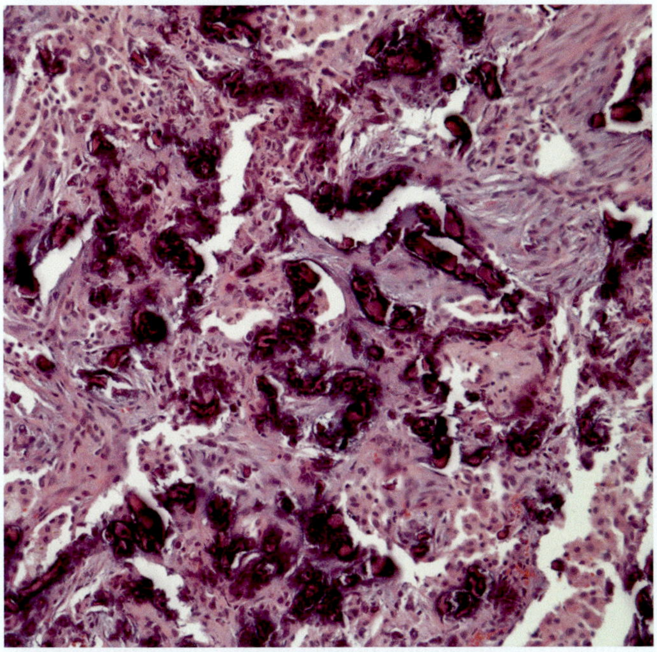

Fig. 13.49 Higher magnification showing calcifications following to some extent the outlines of the alveolar walls

(Figs. 13.46, 13.47, 13.48, and 13.49). In many cases, the pattern of calcification follows the outlines of the alveoli.

Treatment and Prognosis

The treatment and prognosis of metastatic calcification will be determined by the underlying condition. In some patients, the process may lead to respiratory failure and death.

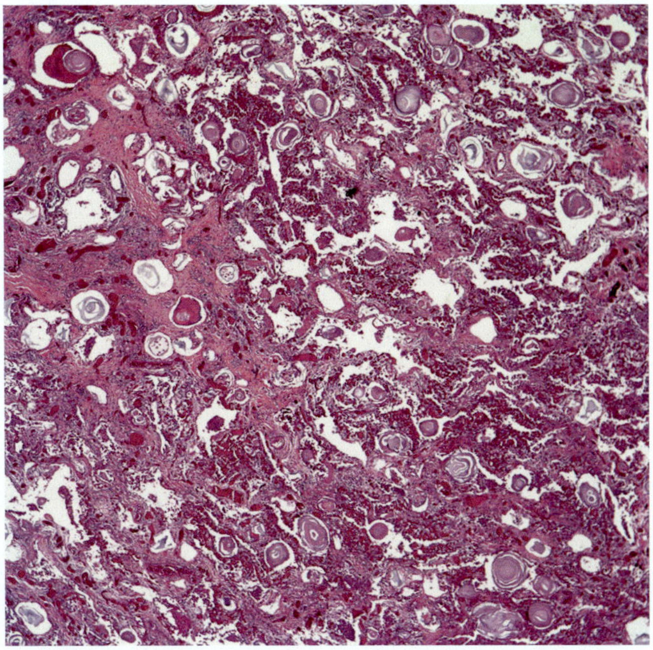

Fig. 13.50 Pulmonary alveolar microlithiasis showing the characteristic pattern of calcospherites filling alveolar spaces

Pulmonary Alveolar Microlithiasis

This condition represents an unusual process in the lung of unknown etiology, and although the composition of the microliths seem to point to a chemical imbalance, clinically none of the patients were reported as having a metabolic abnormality as their primary clinical presentation. The process does not seem to have special predilection for any gender and may follow a protracted clinical course. Due to the rarity of this condition, most of what is known in the literature is based on multiple case reports and only a couple of short series [84, 85].

Clinical Features

Based on the published literature, there is no sex predilection and the condition can affect virtually any patient at any age. Alveolar microlithiasis has been documented in small children and older individuals. A familial pattern has been observed in about half of the cases described [85]. Clinically, patients may present with shortness of breath or gradual decrease of respiratory function [84]. Radiographically, there is a diffuse bilateral pulmonary infiltrate that has been described as a "sandstorm pattern". Even though chemical analysis of the microliths shows that they are composed of calcium and phosphorus salts [84], no metabolic abnormality related to disturbances of phosphorus or calcium is associated with this condition. Macroscopically, the lung may show features mimicking pulmonary fibrosis.

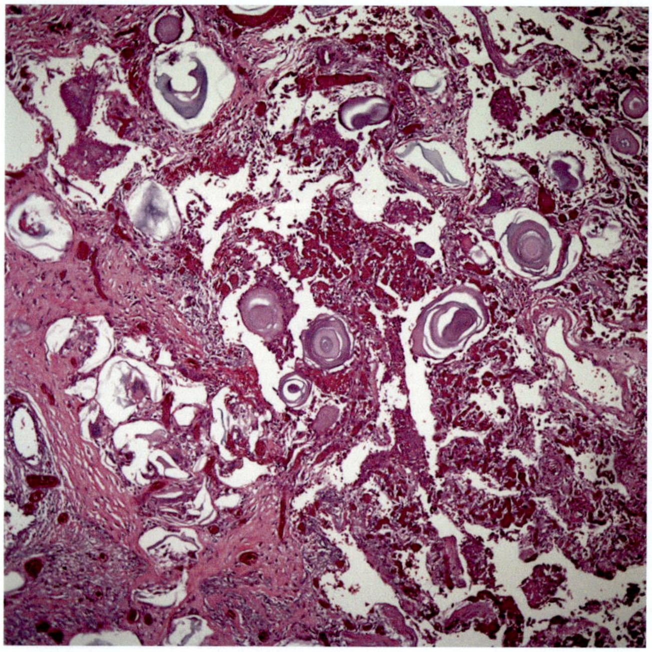

Fig. 13.51 Pulmonary alveoli filled with calcifications. Most of the normal lung architecture has been destroyed

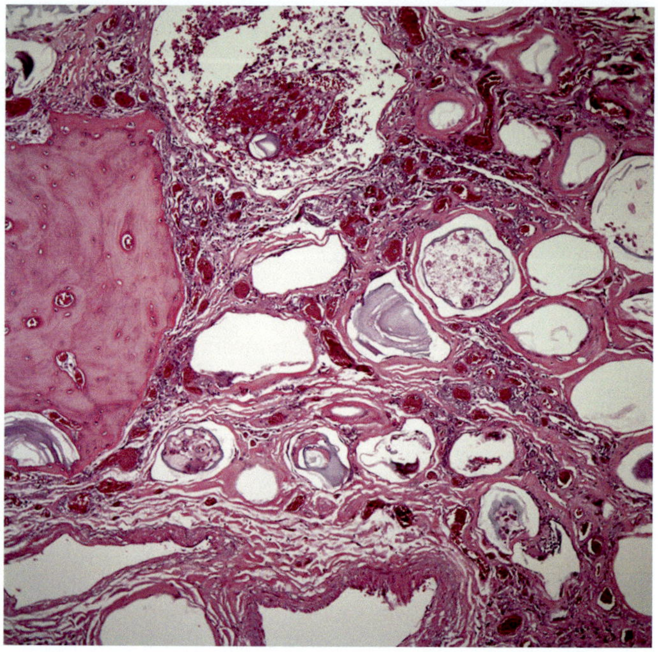

Fig. 13.53 The presence of ossification may also be present, which is in contrast with the alveolar microliths

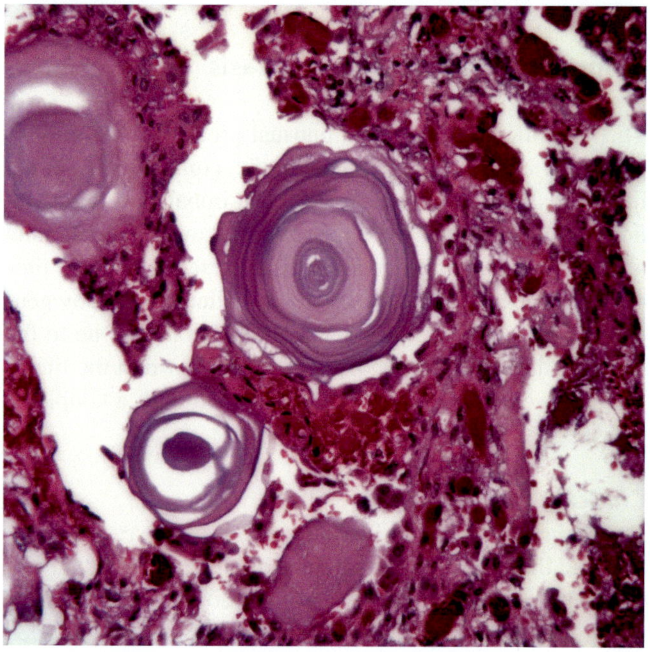

Fig. 13.52 Higher magnification of a calcospherite showing the characteristic "onion skin" pattern

Histological Features

Typically, alveolar microlithiasis is characterized by the presence of numerous spherical bodies filling the alveolar spaces (Figs. 13.50, 13.51, 13.52, and 13.53). Each of these calcospherites measures approximately 250–750 μm in diameter. Morphologically, they appear as laminated bodies with an onionskin-like appearance. In some cases, focal ossification may be present.

Differential Diagnosis

The histopathological features of pulmonary alveolar microlithiasis are fairly straightforward; therefore, there are only few lesions that may enter the differential diagnosis. Pulmonary "blue bodies" may have similar shape and composition; however, they are not filling the alveolar spaces, and they are few in number. In addition, these blue bodies are commonly associated with inflammatory lesions, pneumoconiosis, or interstitial pneumonitis [86]. Diffuse pulmonary ossification or heterotopic ossification may also enter the differential diagnosis [87, 88]. In both of these conditions, the process is characterized by lamellar bone formation and the distribution is interstitial. In addition, the light microscopy of the round-shaped calcospherites is in sharp contrast with the irregular bone formation present in pulmonary ossification. In some cases in which multiple corpora amylacea are present, the round shape on the corpora amylacea may be confused with the round shape of microliths. However, it would be highly unusual to have diffuse corpora amylacea filling alveolar spaces.

Treatment and Prognosis

There is no specific treatment for this condition, and the process may follow a protracted clinical course, but eventually most patients succumb to respiratory failure. Some of these patients may live with this condition for up to 40 years [84].

Pulmonary Placental Transmogrification

The term *transmogrification* (origin obscure) means "to change into a different form or shape, especially one that is fantastic or bizarre". This definition clearly denotes the grotesque nature of the process that takes place within the lung parenchyma. Since the original description by McChesney [89] in abstract form, only a few additional cases have been presented in the literature, using different names or describing variants of this condition [90–92]. It is possible that all those previous descriptions of variants of this process represent the same condition with a spectrum of histopathological features. Mark et al. [91] described this condition under the designation of "placentoid bullous lesion of the lung" in four adult patients with "unilateral multicystic lung disease". Two of the patients had a history of repeated childhood pneumonias. Almost simultaneously, Fidler et al. [90] reported three patients aged 24 to 33 years with cystic lesions of the lung. The authors' interpretation of this process was variant of giant bullous emphysema. An additional case report of this condition [92] was interpreted as pulmonary lipomatosis in an adult patient with a history of bronchopneumonia and a cystic intrapulmonary lesion. Based on this, it is evident that these reports correspond to the same lesion demonstrating different histopathological patterns. Although these lesions are exceedingly rare, the preferred terminology is that of "placental transmogrification of the lung".

Clinical Features

Placental transmogrification appears to affect a wide spectrum of adult individuals or young adults commonly with a history of a pneumonic process. Tobacco use could be elicited in some of these patients. Radiographic features on all the cases described have been that of a unilateral intrapulmonary cystic lesion, which may appear as a bulla or enlarging cystic lesion.

Macroscopic Features

Invariably the gross descriptions of the resected lesions of this process are similar, namely, the presence of a degenerated intrapulmonary lesions with cystic degeneration, papillary-like areas, or grape-like structures resembling molar placental tissue. The normal lung parenchyma appears collapsed with total destruction of the normal macroscopic appearance of the lung.

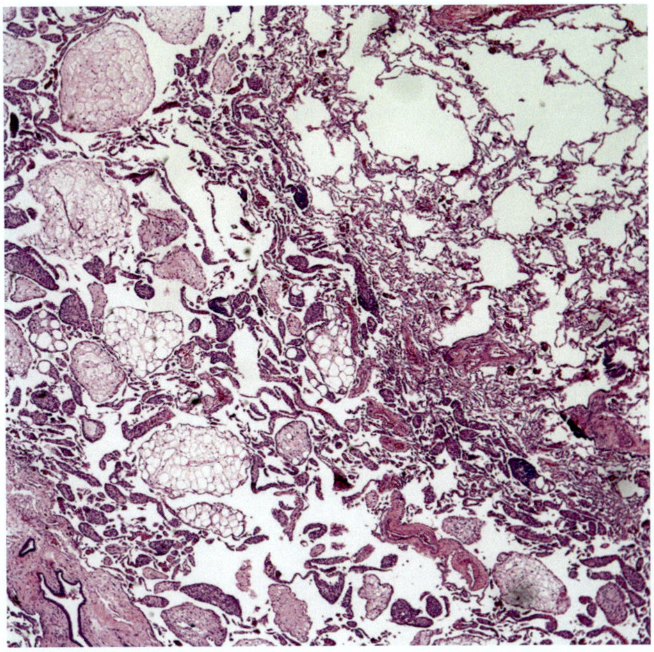

Fig. 13.54 Placental transmogrification showing a transition between normal lung parenchyma and replaced lung parenchyma

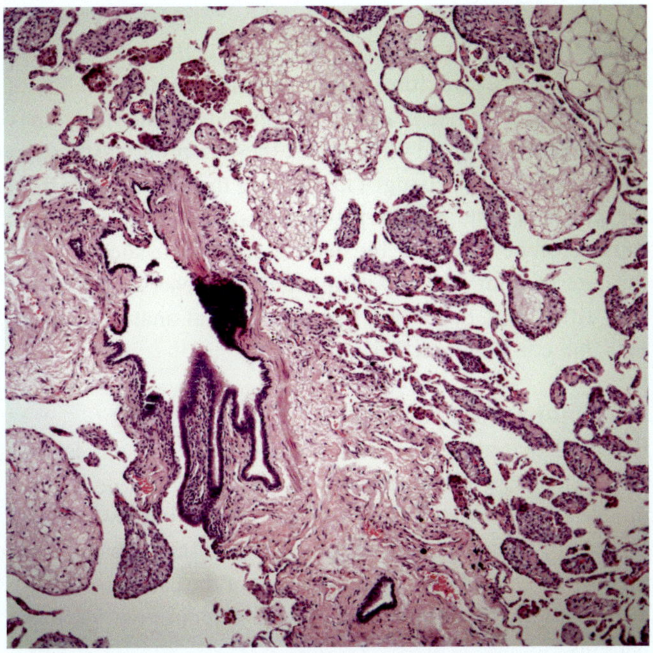

Fig. 13.55 Placental transmogrification usually involves alveolated lung parenchyma. Note the presence of an uninvolved airway

Histopathological Features

The spectrum of histopathological features encountered in placental transmogrification of the lung is varied (Figs. 13.54, 13.55, 13.56, and 13.57). Essentially, the lung parenchyma is replaced by a proliferation of papillary-like

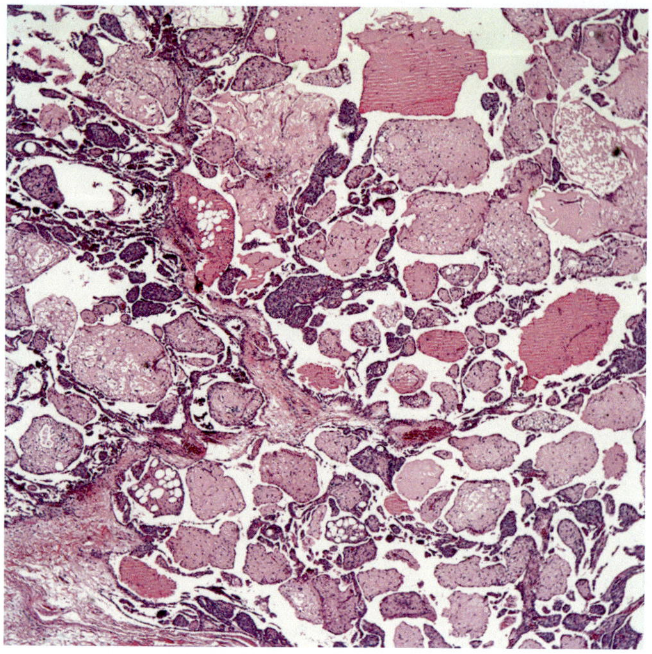

Fig. 13.56 Typical features of placental transmogrification showing structures mimicking placental tissue

structures lined by cuboidal epithelial cells. The cores of these papillary structures may contain variable amounts of inflammatory cells, namely, lymphocytes, and they may appear edematous. In other areas, these papillary structures show degenerated changes mimicking the chorionic villi of the placenta. The papillary structures may contain smooth muscle or be replaced by mature adipose tissue or show mixture of both. In focal areas, there is preservation of airway structures, this being the only normal anatomic structure that can be identified.

Treatment and Prognosis

For final diagnosis and treatment of these unusual lesions complete surgical resection is required, and was performed in all cases described. Diagnosis on limited biopsy material or cytology may be difficult, and is of limited value. No recurrences have been reported in any of the cases described. Thus, surgical resection appears to be curative in these patients.

Pulmonary Lymphangioleiomyomatosis (LAM)

Pulmonary lymphangioleiomyomatosis (LAM) is an unusual disorder of unknown etiology that predominantly affects premenopausal women. However, in unusual cases, LAM has also been described in children, men, and postmenopausal women [93–97]. This disorder may occur without evidence of another disease process or in association with tuberous sclerosis complex (TSC). LAM occurs in approximately one to two cases per million women; however, LAM may be underreported. Even though the pathogenesis of LAM is still unknown, it appears that LAM and TSC may share a genetic relationship. The TSC2 tumor suppressor gene located on chromosome 16p13 has been implicated in the pathogenesis of LAM. This genetic abnormality has also been identified in about half the cases of renal angiomyolipomas in patients with LAM or tuberous sclerosis. It is also important to highlight that LAM and tuberous sclerosis are two different disorders; however, the separation of LAM from pulmonary involvement of TSC, which may occur in less than 5 % of these patients, may pose great difficulty not only histologically but also clinically and radiologically. Furthermore, contrary to the female predominance of LAM, TSC affects both genders. In the past, some authors have argued that tuberous sclerosis has a relative higher frequency among relatives while LAM does not and have suggested that based on this LAM and tuberous sclerosis may represent two different disorders [98, 99]. Tuberous sclerosis has an autosomal dominant pattern of inheritance and is characterized by the presence of neurological and cutaneous manifestations [100]. On the other hand, it's been suggested that pulmonary lymphangioleiomyomatosis and Bourneville's tuberous sclerosis may represent two forms of the same process [101].

Clinical Features

The clinical manifestations of patients affected by LAM include recurrent pneumothorax, chylous effusion, dyspnea, cough, and hemoptysis. Radiologically, the a CT scan shows the presence of multiple bilateral nodular and cystic changes in the lung parenchyma [102]. However, cases of unilateral pulmonary involvement have been described [103]. The mean age of the onset of symptoms has been estimated at 32 years of age [104]. Although, in the past, an open lung biopsy was the procedure of choice to establish the diagnosis of LAM, currently the use of transbronchial biopsies has yielded some satisfactory results [105–109].

Pathological Features

Grossly, the lungs with LAM are characterized by the presence of multiple cysts with a honeycomb appearance. The cyst walls are of different size and varying thickness. Microscopically, the low power view shows numerous cysts, which may resemble emphysematous changes; some of these cysts may be filled with pools of blood or pigmented macrophages. At higher magnification, it is possible to identify the presence of a cellular proliferation composed of spindle cells with elongated nuclei, inconspicuous nucleoli and scant

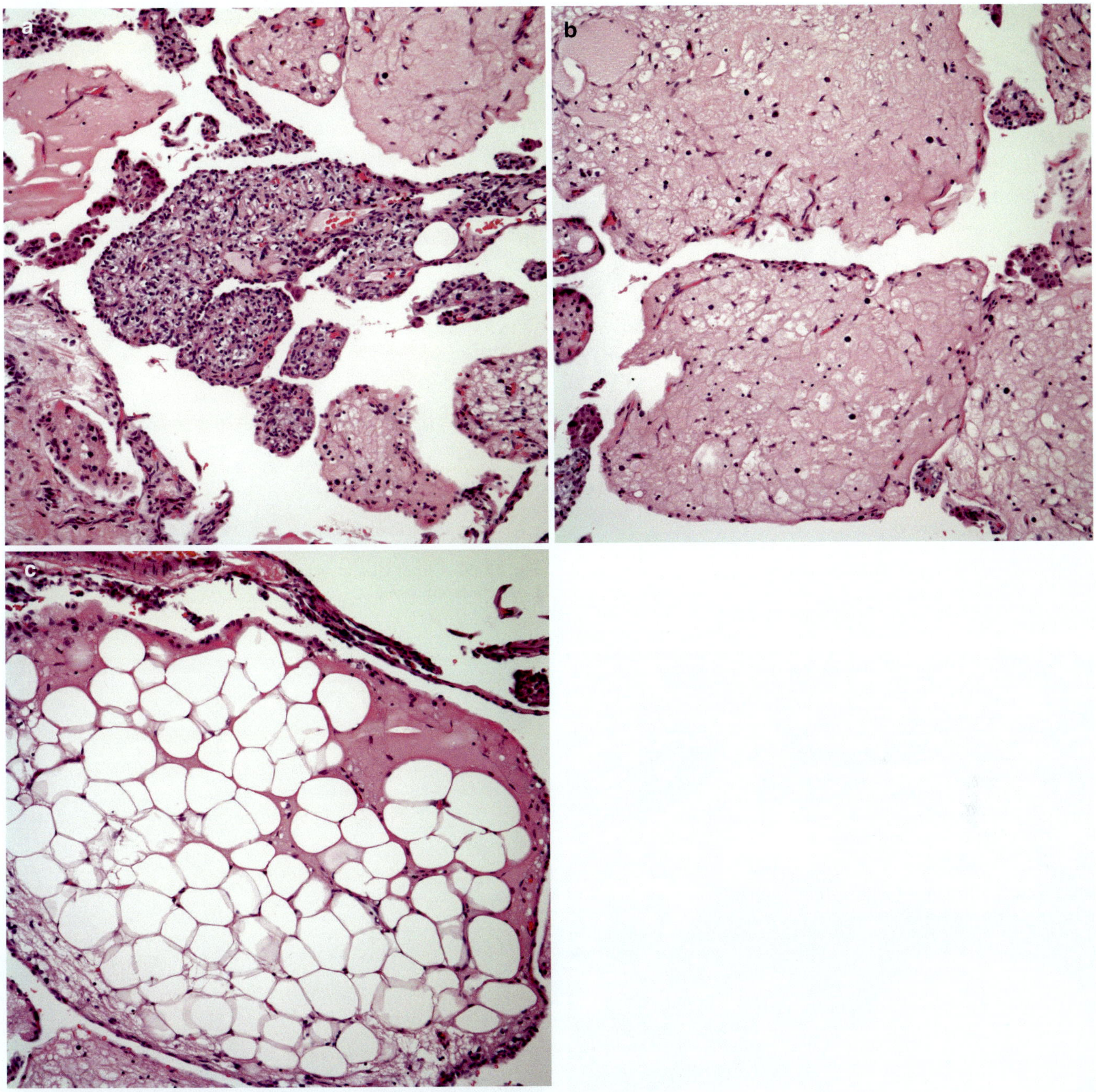

Fig. 13.57 (**a**) Cellular type of placenta-like structures. (**b**) Myxoid type. (**c**) Adipose tissue type

cytoplasm. In some areas more oval cells with clear cytoplasm are apparent. This cellular proliferation appears to be partially lining some of the cystic structures, while in other areas the process involves the interstitium of the lung parenchyma (Figs. 13.58, 13.59, 13.60, 13.61, 13.62, 13.63, 13.64, 13.65, and 13.66). The cellular proliferation does not show evidence of nuclear atypia or mitotic activity. In adjacent areas, hyperplasia of type II pneumocytes, which may be arranged in a micronodular pattern may be seen. Some authors have divided LAM into two separate histological groups—predominantly cystic and predominantly muscular—and have argued that such a separation has prognostic importance [110].

Immunohistochemically, LAM shows positive staining for muscle markers including smooth muscle actin and desmin. In addition, positive staining has been reported with estrogen and progesterone receptors, HMB45 [111], insulin-like growth factor (IGF), and matrix metalloproteinases (MMPs).

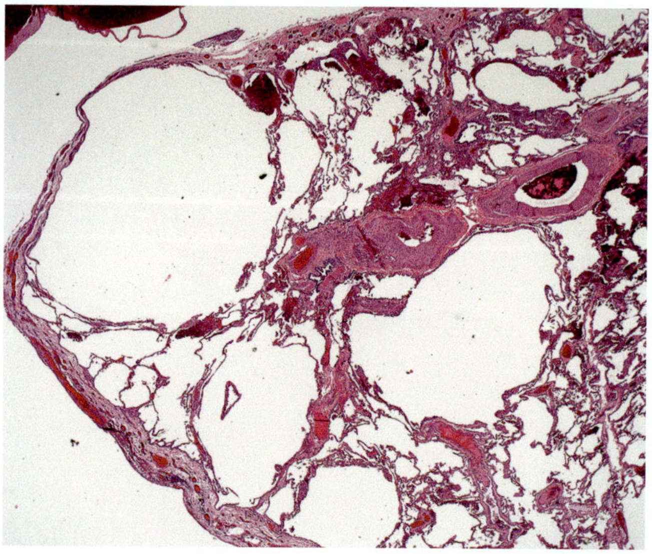

Fig. 13.58 Low power view of lung parenchyma showing marked cystic changes in LAM

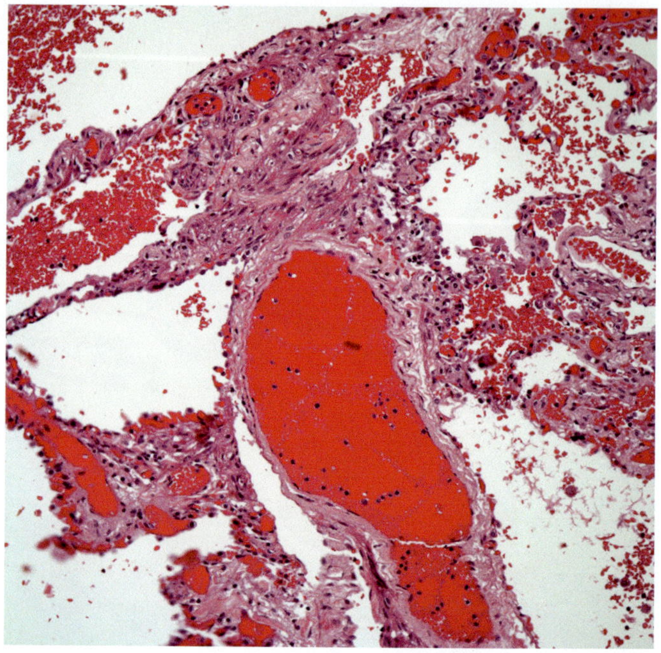

Fig. 13.60 Closer view at an area with vascular congestion adjacent to a muscle proliferation

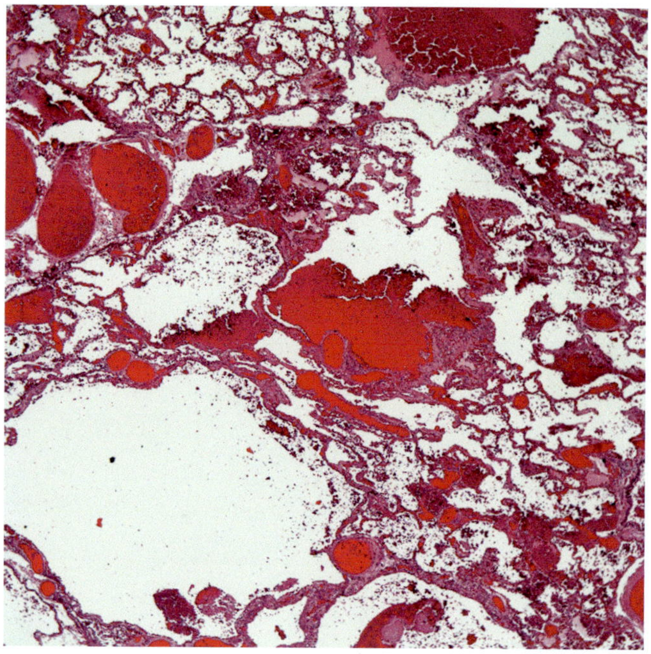

Fig. 13.59 Areas of congestion and cystic changes in LAM. The congested changes may at times obscure the diagnosis

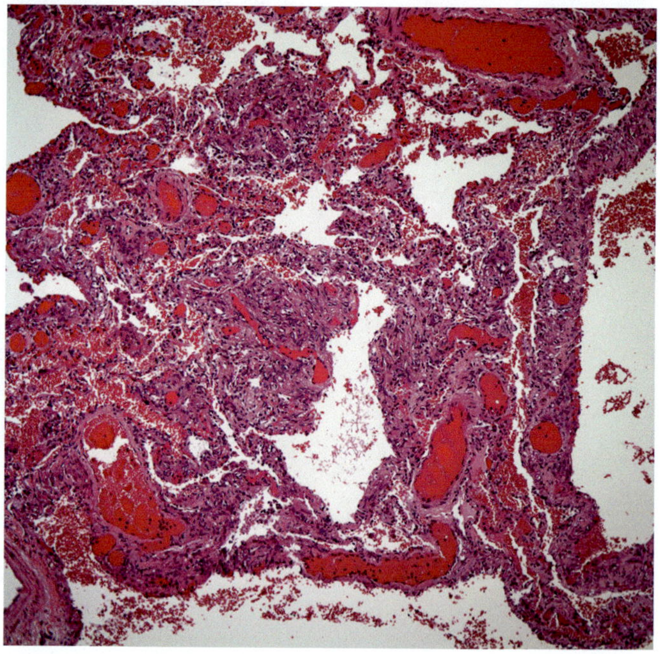

Fig. 13.61 In other areas, the presence of muscle is more obvious despite the parenchymal congestion

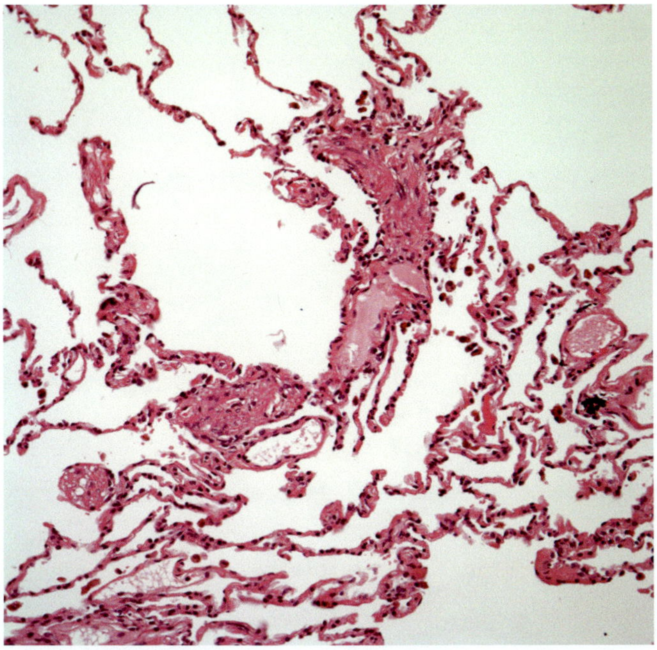

Fig. 13.62 LAM with a more discrete presence of muscle involving alveolar walls

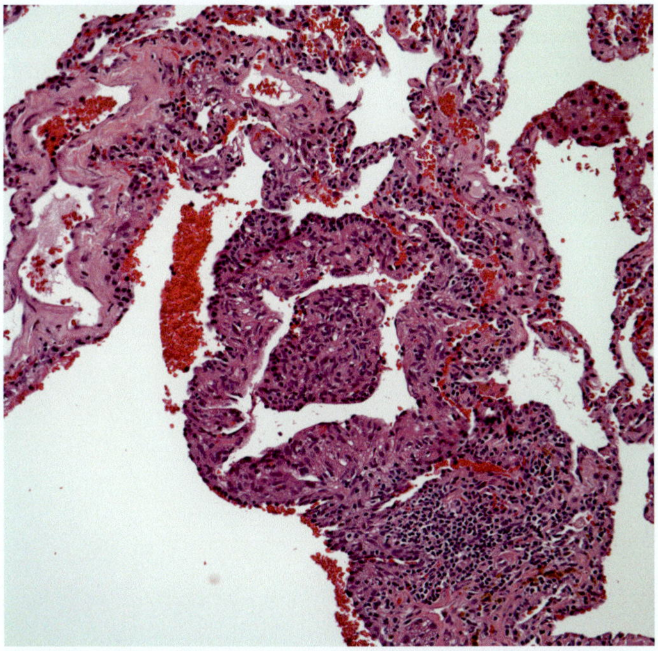

Fig. 13.63 The presence of muscle is obvious as it closely follows the alveolar wall

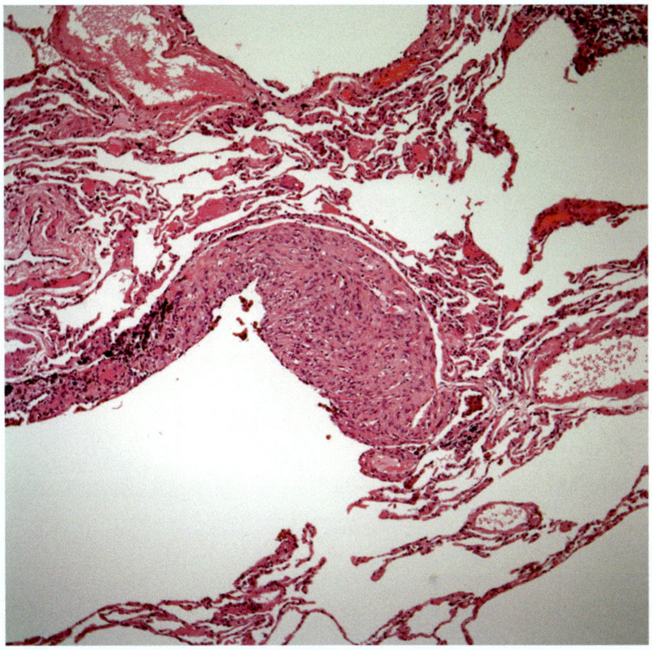

Fig. 13.64 The presence of muscle may be seen only focally while other areas of lung parenchyma appear within normal limits

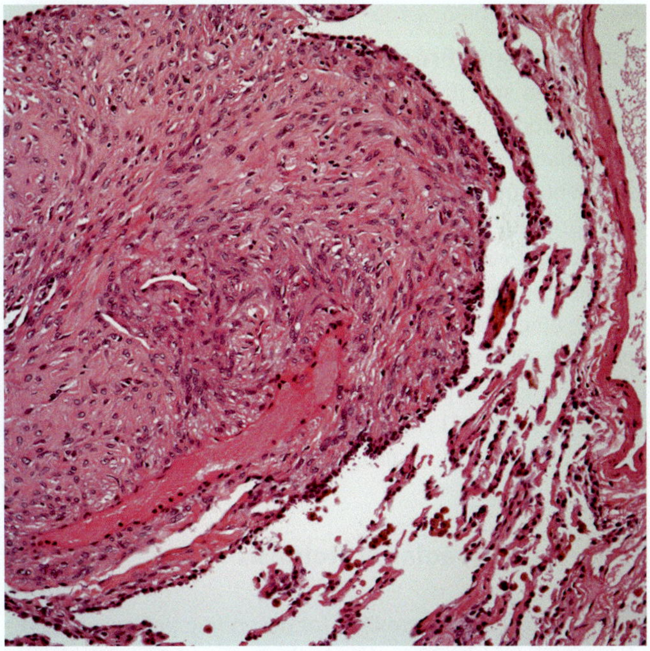

Fig. 13.65 Closer view at the muscle proliferation showing the conventional spindle cell pattern

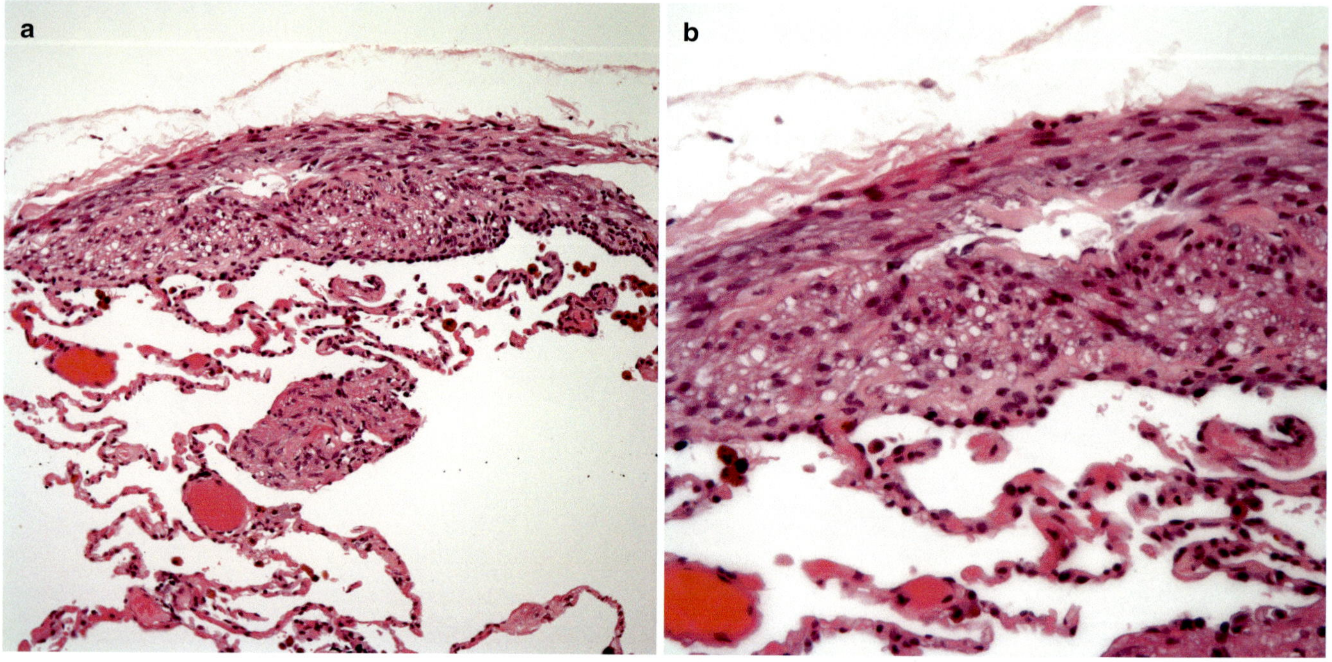

Fig. 13.66 (**a**) Discrete subpleural muscle proliferation. (**b**) High magnification showing a spindle cell proliferation with clear cell changes

Treatment and Prognosis

There is no specific treatment for LAM. However, the current methods of treatment these patients include hormonal manipulation with antiestrogen therapy or with progesterone treatment, oophorectomy, or lung transplantation with varying degrees of success [112–114]. A correlation of histological findings with prognosis has disclosed that those lesions with predominant cystic changes have poor prognosis [110]. On the other hand, a scoring of combined features—cystic and solid—has estimated that the survival from tissue diagnosis to lung transplant or death is about 85 % at 5 years and 71 % at 10 years [115]. The cause of death in these patients is due to respiratory insufficiency.

Pulmonary Alveolar Proteinosis

Rosen et al. [116] are credited for describing pulmonary alveolar proteinosis in 27 patients who suffered from a process that deposited PAS-positive proteinaceous material rich in lipid in the alveolar spaces. The authors speculated that this material was produced by the alveolar lining cells, which slough into the lumen, ultimately becoming necrotic and yield granules and variable laminated bodies to the alveolar content. In addition, the authors acknowledged the resemblance of this condition with *Pneumocystis jiroveci* infection of the lung. Interestingly, alveolar proteinosis is can also be seen in patients with immunosuppressed systems. Bedrossian et al. [117] reported eight cases of alveolar proteinosis associated with hematologic malignancies and acknowledged that all the cases reported in the literature were either associated with infectious processes and/or hematologic malignancies. Radiologically, three patterns of involvement have been described for this

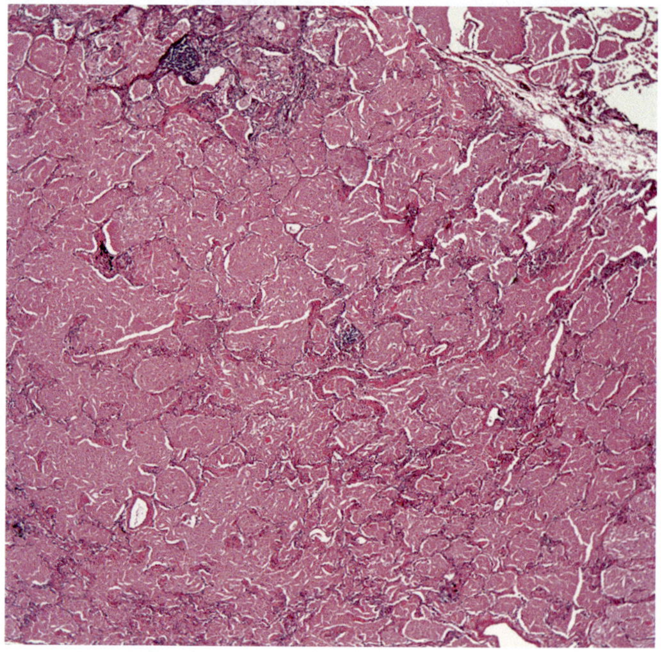

Fig. 13.67 Lung parenchyma filled with proteinaceous material typical of alveolar proteinosis

condition: the reticulonodular pattern; small acinar nodules mimicking miliary disease and coalescence of various-sized acinar nodules leading to focal consolidation [118]. Clinically, the majority of patients will present with symptoms of cough, dyspnea, chest pain, and/or fever [119].

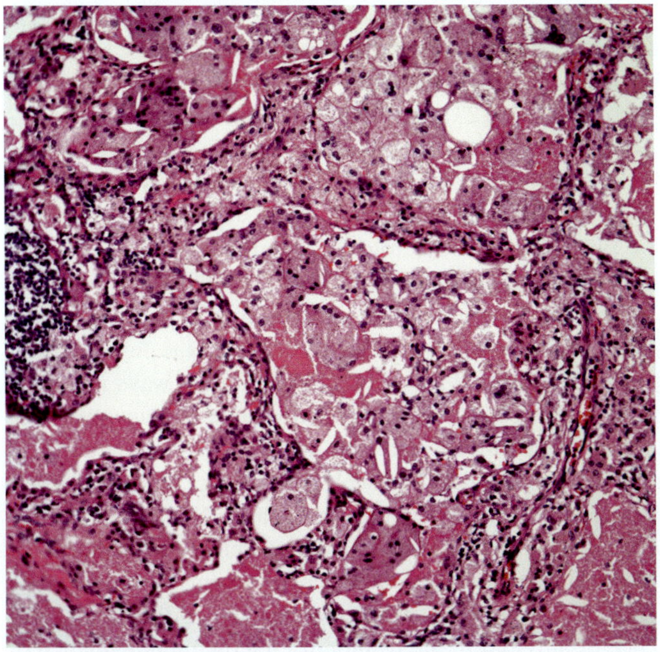

Fig. 13.68 In some areas of alveolar proteinosis, it is possible to observe the presence of histiocytic aggregates

Histopathological Features

The hallmark of alveolar proteinosis is the filling of alveoli by a proteinaceous acellular material (Figs. 13.67, 13.68, 13.69, 13.70, and 13.71), which characteristically stains positively using the periodic acid-Schiff (PAS) histochemical stain. The pulmonary architecture is preserved with only minimal changes in the interstitium. By electron microscopy, annular inclusions, lamellar osmiophilic inclusions, dense granules, and myeloid bodies have been identified.

Differential Diagnosis

The most important differential diagnosis is *Pneumocystis jiroveci* pneumonia. Given the fact that both of these processes may affect immunocompromised individuals, the use of PAS or silver stains (Grocott's methenamine silver [GMS]) may help in confirming the diagnosis as alveolar proteinosis will show positive staining for PAS and negative staining with silver stains, contrary to *Pneumocystis jiroveci* pneumonia. One other condition that has to be excluded is pulmonary edema; however, the use of a PAS stain will lead to the correct interpretation.

Treatment and Prognosis

Pulmonary lavage has been use with some success in these patients. Kariman et al. [120] studied 28 patients with alveolar proteinosis and divided them into two groups depending on the course of their disease. One group, 24 % of the

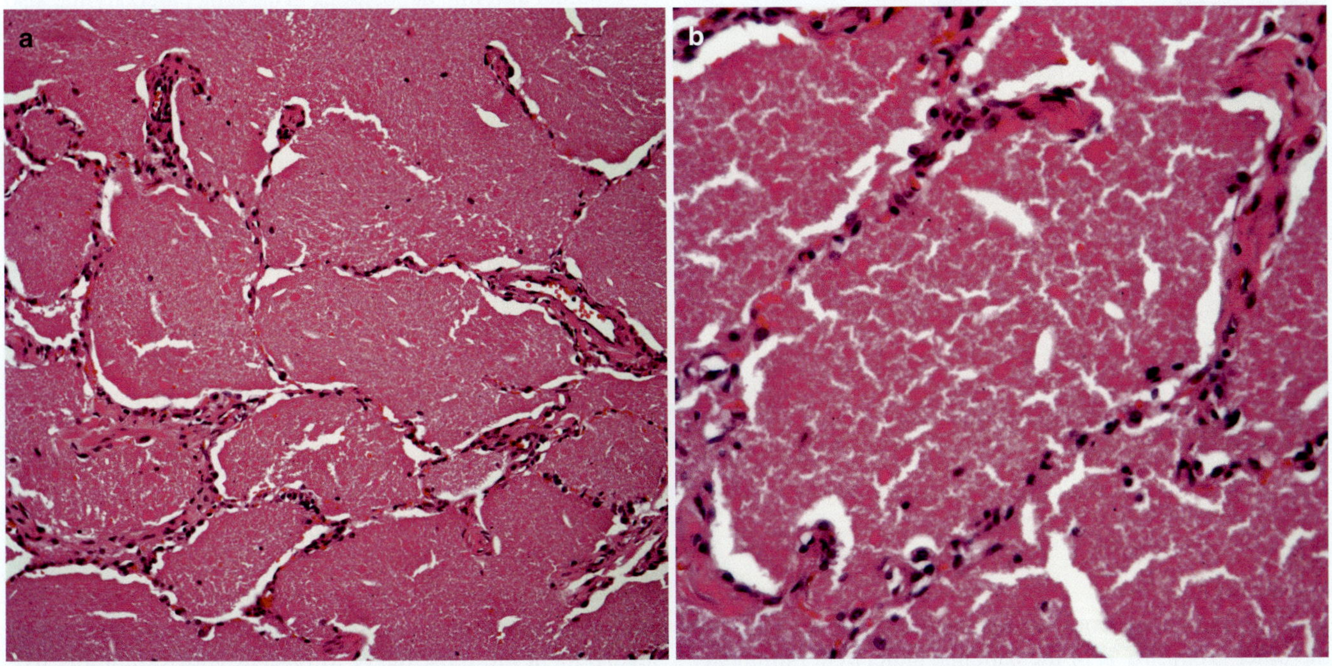

Fig. 13.69 (**a**) Acellular proteinaceous material filling alveolar spaces. Note the preservation of the alveolar outlines. (**b**) Higher magnification showing a rather granular proteinaceous material

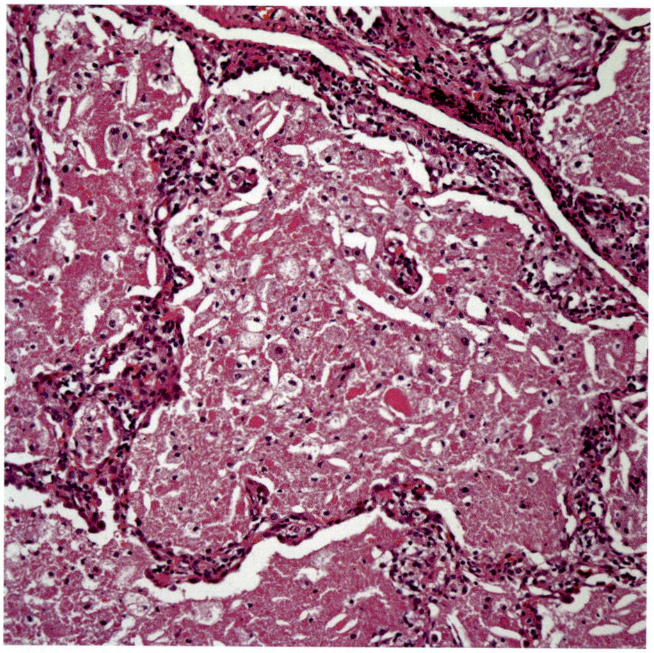

Fig. 13.70 In some areas, the proteinaceous material is also admixed with some histiocytes

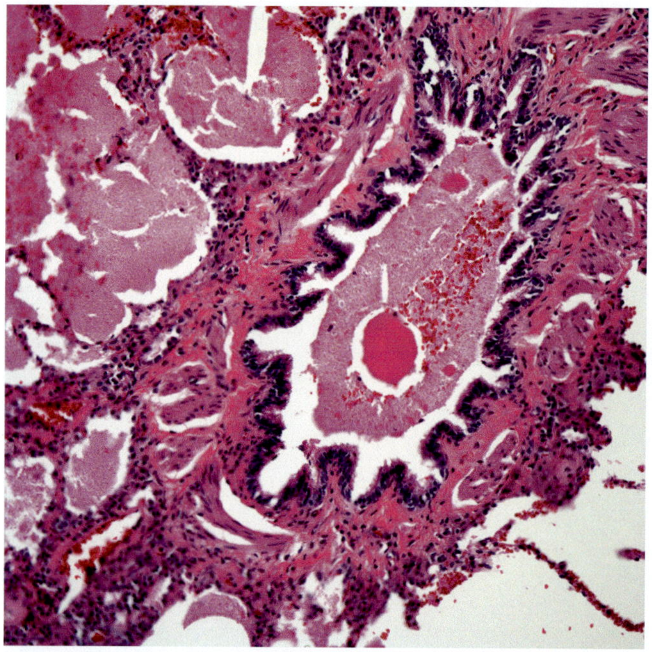

Fig. 13.71 The proteinaceous material may not only be present in alveolar spaces but also in the airways

patients, had spontaneous remission with no treatment, while the other group, 76 % of the patients, underwent pulmonary lavage. Interestingly in the latter group 21 % of the patients did not respond to treatment.

Pulmonary Amyloid Tumor (Amyloidoma)

Amyloid deposition within the lung parenchyma is a well-known pathological process that has been recognized for many decades. However, it is important to realize that amyloid in the lung may be identified secondarily due to systemic amyloidosis or to other conditions. Several studies analyzing the presence of amyloid in the respiratory tract including the tracheobronchial area and lung parenchyma have been reported [121–123]. Celli et al. [122] published a study of 22 autopsy cases of patients with systemic amyloidosis that were categorized as 12 patients with primary systemic amyloidosis, 3 patients with amyloidosis secondary to myeloma or Waldenström's macroglobulinemia, and 7 patients with secondary amyloidosis. Also Cordier et al. [123] reported 21 patients with systemic amyloidosis involving the lower respiratory tract. In these two series of cases, the lung and tracheobronchial tree was involved in different ways including diffuse, nodular, interstitial, and plaque-like involvement. The authors emphasized that the lung may show amyloid deposition in conditions such as myeloma, Waldenström's macroglobulinemia, familial neuropathy, Niemann-Pick disease, or Gaucher's disease, as well as senile cardiac forms of amyloid. Although secondary involvement of the lungs by amyloid is important, herein, we will only address the presence of amyloid in the respiratory tract without evidence of systemic disease, as in some cases, the pulmonary nodules of primary pulmonary amyloidosis may raise the clinical possibility of a pulmonary malignancy.

Nodular amyloid depositions in the lung parenchyma, also known as amyloidomas, are well known to occur. Possible etiologic factors include light chain immunoglobulin deposition or the presence of abundant plasma cells often seen adjacent to amyloid tumors although, these possibilities remain speculative. Potassium permanganate oxidation technique which can separate type AA amyloid from other forms of amyloid has provided results which may support immunoglobulin derived amyloid deposition by excluding AA type amyloid. However, the exact etiology is still unknown. In some cases, amyloid tumor has been associated with other conditions such as Sjögren's syndrome [124, 125] and MALT type pulmonary lymphoma; [126]; other cases have been characterized by extensive lung involvement [127] or a solitary nodules [128]. In 1986, Hui et al. [129] presented 48 cases of amyloidosis restricted to the lower respiratory tract. The authors encountered 14 cases involving the tracheobronchial tree, 24 cases with solitary or multiple pulmonary nodules, and 6 cases with diffuse interstitial involvement. The authors concluded that those patients with tracheobronchial involvement are most likely to present with symptoms like dyspnea, while those with nodular parenchymal involvement are most likely asymptomatic.

Macroscopic Findings

Pulmonary amyloid may present in different forms. Tracheobronchial involvement may happen in a diffuse or localized form, while parenchymal involvement may be in the form of single or multiple nodules, which may vary in size from 1 cm to more than 10 cm in diameter. The tumors may be unilateral or bilateral. The tumors have been described as soft, well circumscribed, and gray in color, while those in the tracheobronchial tree are often plaque-like or polypoid.

Histopathological Features

The low power view of nodular amyloidosis (amyloidoma) is that of a well circumscribed but unencapsulated amorphous eosinophilic tumor nodule replacing the normal lung parenchyma (Figs. 13.72, 13.73, 13.74, and 13.75). Higher magnification shows that this nodule is composed of acellular amorphous material; however, in the periphery of the nodule, an inflammatory infiltrate rich in plasma cells and with numerous multinucleated giant cells can be identified. In some cases, the process is diffuse with some preservation of the normal architecture in which the amyloid is deposited in an interstitial pattern with widening of the interstitial spaces and involvement of the pulmonary vasculature. In this pattern, the inflammatory infiltrate is not as prominent as in the nodular pattern, and multinucleated giant cells are less common or absent.

Special Studies

Even though the morphologic presence of amyloid is rather characteristic, the use of a Congo red histochemical stain may be of help in small biopsies or in cases in which the presence of amyloid is subtle. A congo red stain displays the presence of birefringent apple-green material under polarized light microscopy. In addition, amyloid may also show λ (lambda) light chains by immunohistochemical stains and serum amyloid P. In addition, Immunohistochemical studies in the plasma cells associated with amyloid tumors have shown a polyclonal cellular proliferation. Rodriguez et al. [130] performed spectrometric studies in proteinaceous deposits in neural tissue and concluded that liquid chromatography-electrospray tandem mass spectrometry represents a novel application for characterization of proteinaceous deposits including amyloid.

Differential Diagnosis

One important non-neoplastic condition that may be confused with amyloid tumor is the so-called hyalinizing granuloma of the lung. As its name implies, in hyalinizing granuloma of the lung, there are extensive areas of hyalinization with an associated inflammatory reaction closely mimicking amyloid. Hyalinizing granuloma of the lung is a rare condition, probably related to sclerosing mediastinitis, retroperitoneal fibrosis, sclerosing cholangitis, and other similar lesions. It usually occurs in adult individuals and may

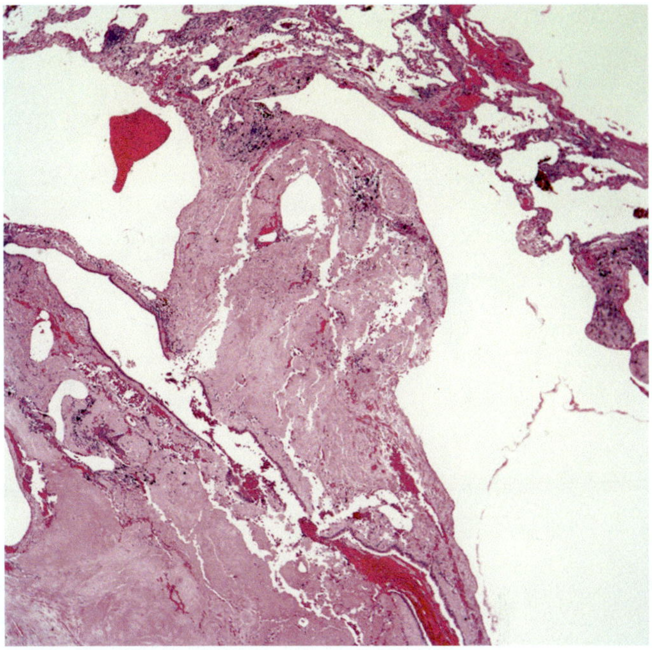

Fig. 13.72 Lung parenchyma replaced by amorphous acellular material

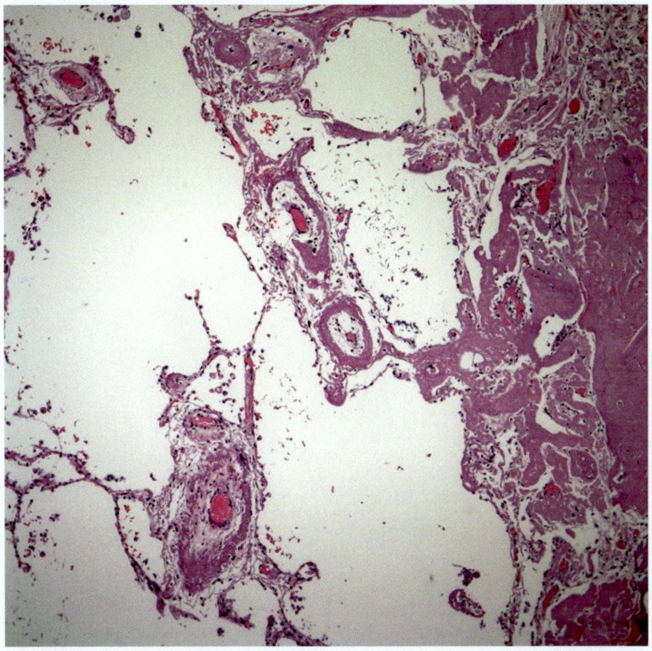

Fig. 13.73 Extensive deposition of amyloid replacing normal lung parenchyma and involving vascular structures

present as a pulmonary mass, which may produce symptoms of pulmonary obstruction. Histologically this lesion shows a well-demarcated lesion with extensive fibrosis and thick collagen bundles admixed with an inflammatory cell infiltrate. However, a histochemical stain for Congo red is negative in those cases. One other possible differential diagnosis

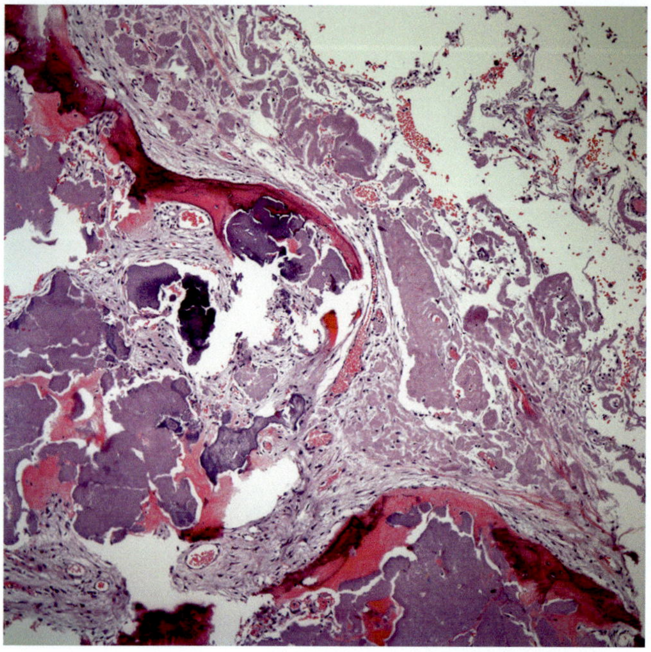

Fig. 13.74 Pulmonary amyloid tumor showing bone formation

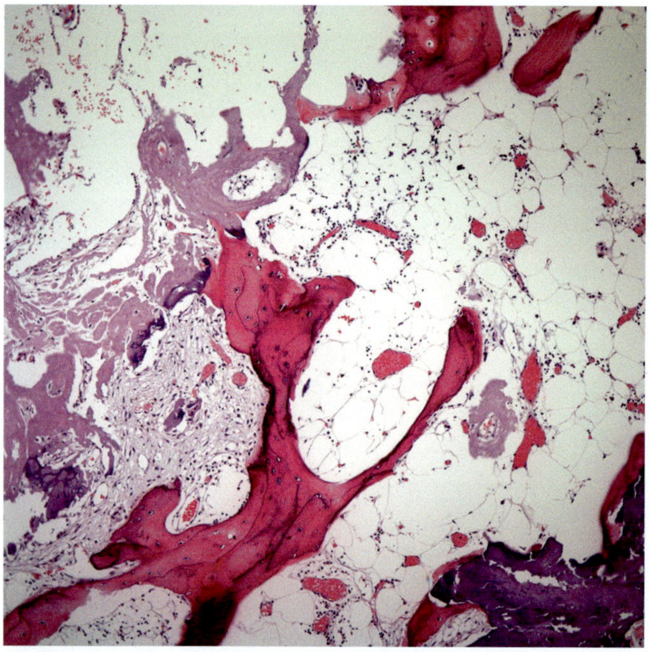

Fig. 13.75 Extensive ossification with marrow elements may be present in some cases of pulmonary amyloid tumor

includes intrapulmonary solitary fibrous tumor, namely, when the tumors shows extensive areas of collagenization. Application of congo red or immunohistochemical studies for CD34 and Bcl-2 should lead to the correct diagnosis.

Treatment and Prognosis

Complete surgical resection appears to be the treatment of choice when amyloid presents as a pulmonary mass. In these cases, the prognosis appears to be good in comparison to patients in whom there is diffuse pulmonary involvement making surgical resection impossible. Diffuse pulmonary involvement appears to lead to death due to respiratory insufficiency.

Mucous Gland Adenoma

Mucous gland adenomas are unusual benign tumors that may pose diagnostic problems [131–139]. Unfortunately in the past, these tumors have been lumped with other so-called adenomas that corresponded to different tumor types. Thus, it is difficult to determine their exact incidence. Mucous gland adenoma has been suggested to originate from the submucosal seromucous glands and ducts of the proximal airways and probably represent some form of overdilatation of the normal glandular structures. In some publications, these tumors have been grouped with salivary gland-type tumors of the lung. England and Hochholzer in 1995 [140] presented 10 cases of this entity and summarized the different previous names for this tumor and found only 41 cases of this rare benign tumor.

Clinical Features

Mucous gland adenoma appears to affect men and women without any particular predilection, and the tumor has been recorded in adult individuals between the ages of 25 and 67 years. The patients may be asymptomatic however, because of the central location of the tumor, symptoms of bronchial obstruction such as cough, dyspnea, chest pain, and/or hemoptysis may occur.

Macroscopic Features

The tumors often present as polypoid, exophytic endobronchial tumors obstructing the pulmonary lumen. The size of the tumors varies from tumor under 1 cm to more than 5 cm in greatest diameter. They have been described as well circumscribed, soft, and mucoid neoplasms with cystic changes. Areas of hemorrhage and necrosis are not common in these tumors.

Histopathological Features

The hallmark feature of mucous gland adenoma is its growht limitation by the bronchial cartilaginous plate (Figs. 13.76, 13.77, 13.78, 13.79, 13.80, 13.81, 13.82, 13.83, and 13.84). Thus, the tumor is circumscribed and fails to invade into adjacent lung parenchyma or beyond the bronchial cartilage. The low power magnification shows an exuberant dilation of the normal submucosal seromucinous glands of the lung with areas of an inflammatory reaction and mucoid material filling the dilated glandular structures. The tumors tumor may show a prominent papillary growth pattern. Closer view of the tumor shows a gamut of histopathological changes

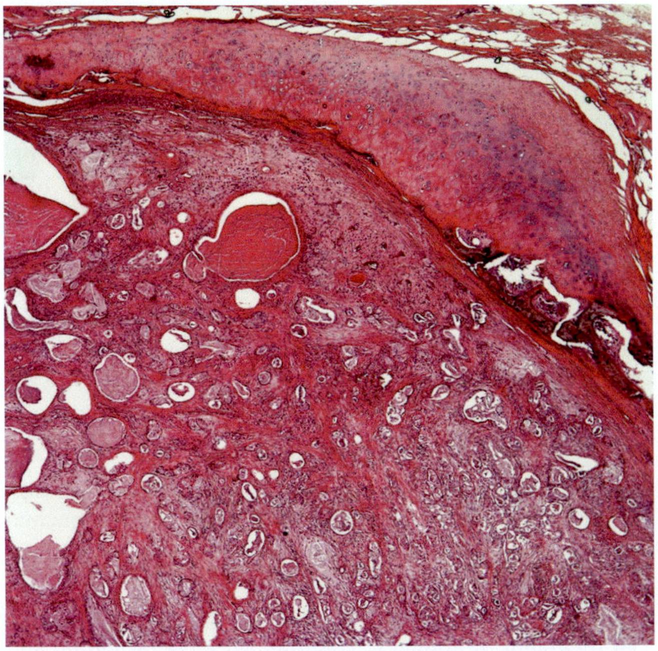

Fig. 13.76 Bronchial glandular proliferation. Note the bronchial cartilage and confinement of the tumor

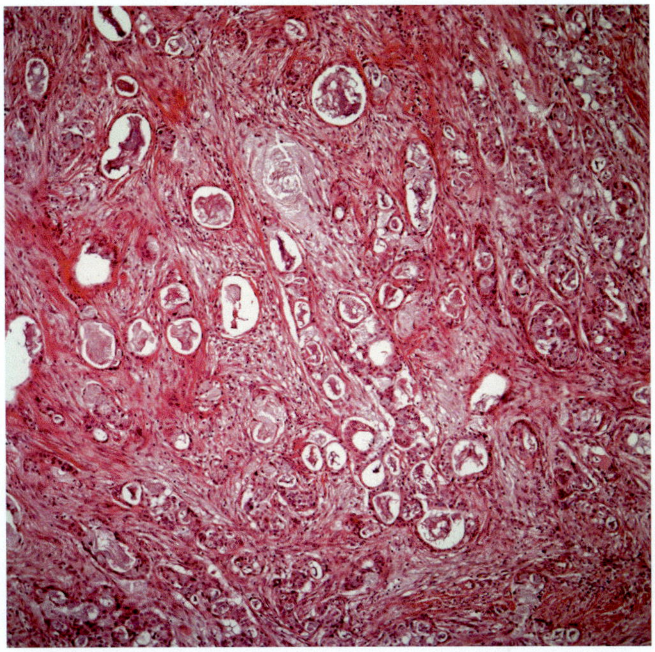

Fig. 13.78 Small glandular proliferation in a background of fibrosis

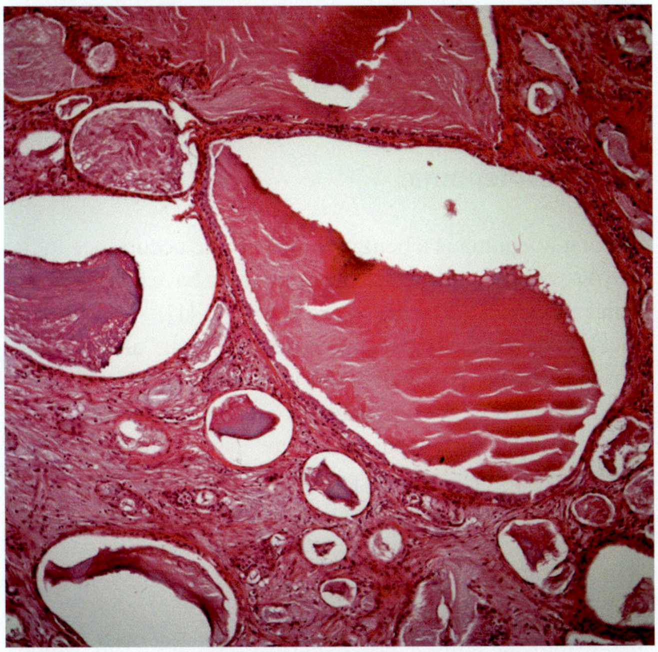

Fig. 13.77 Mucous gland adenoma showing a mixture of cystically dilated glands containing mucus and smaller glands some of which concontain mucous material

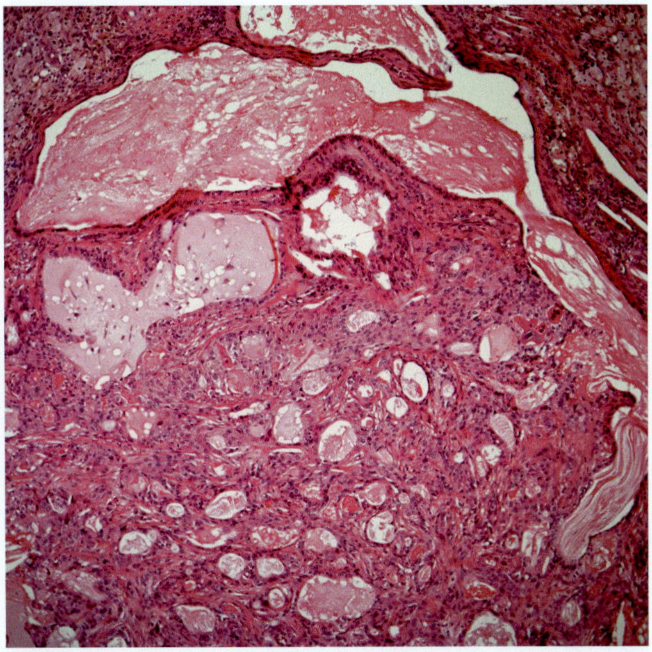

Fig. 13.79 Mucous gland adenoma showing dilated glands and more solid areas

that ranges from the presence of a glandular component with a mucinous type of epithelium with little intervening stromal tissue to a compact a glandular proliferation of seromucinous glands. In other areas, the tumor may show cystically dilated glands of different sizes lined by squamous epithelium and separated by fibrocollagenous stroma. In most cases, it is possible to identify an admixture of patterns that vary from cystic to solid. Areas of cholesterol cleft granulomas, an inflammatory reaction predominantly composed of plasma cells, and areas of squamous metaplasia are commonly seen. The most important feature is that the glandular proliferation does not involve the adjacent lung parenchyma.

Although the diagnosis of mucous gland adenoma is essentially a morphologic one, immunohistochemical stud-

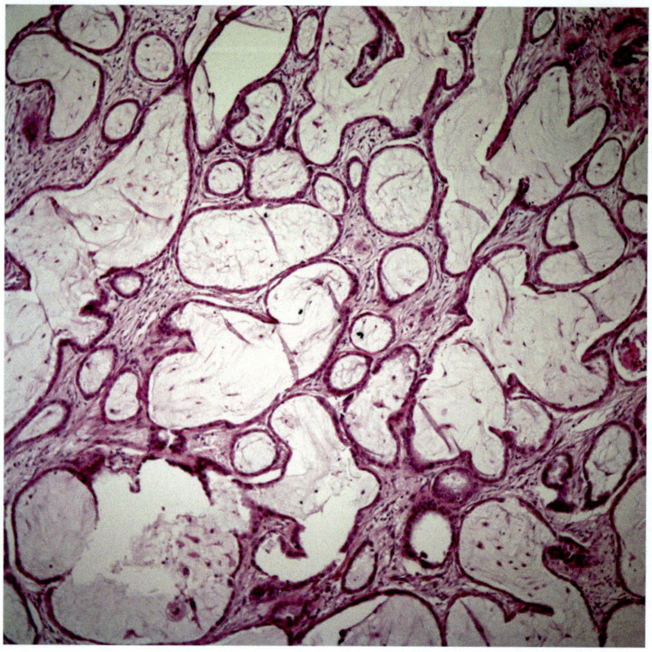

Fig. 13.80 The glandular proliferation can be lined by different types of epithelium—in this case, low cuboidal epithelium

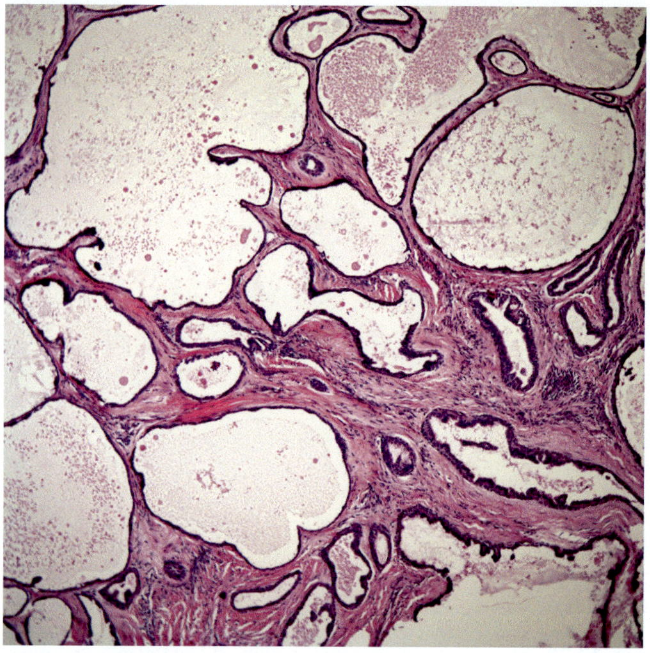

Fig. 13.81 Glands lined by either low cuboidal or squamous epithelium may be seen

ies have been performed in some of these cases. As expected, the tumor shows positive staining for epithelial markers including keratins, epithelial membrane antigen (EMA), and carcinoembryonic antigen (CEA). Proliferative markers such as Ki-67 will label only scattered cells.

Differential Diagnosis

The most important differential diagnosis includes low grade mucoepidermoid carcinoma and adenocarcinoma. In small biopsies, an unequivocal diagnosis may prove to be difficult. However, the presence of an exuberant dilatation of normal endobronchial glands should alert to the possibility of a mucous gland adenoma. However, if the biopsy is from an area of glandular proliferation, the diagnosis may be very difficult to impossible. On the other hand, in a resected specimen, a glandular proliferation limited to the space between the surface respiratory epithelium and the bronchial cartilage should alert to the possibility of an adenoma rather than a mucoepidermoid carcinoma. Contrary to the bland features of mucus gland adenoma, adenocarcinomas are characterized by an atypical glandular proliferation with nuclear atypia and mitotic activity and growth beyond the bronchial cartilage.

Treatment and Prognosis

The treatment of choice is complete surgical resection, and the prognosis is excellent. However, surgical treatment of mucous gland adenoma may vary depending on the anatomic distribution of the tumor, level of confidence of the initial biopsy results, and radiological findings. Therefore, even though the tumor is completely benign, the treatment may include a more radical procedure such as lobectomy.

Alveolar Adenoma

Alveolar adenoma is a benign tumor of rare occurrence in the lung parenchyma. Although the tumor may have been reported earlier under a different designation [141], Yousem and Hochholzer are the ones who coined the term "alveolar adenoma", reporting six cases of this unusual tumor. The authors' report included four women and two men between the ages of 45 and 74 years. All patients were asymptomatic or with symptoms unrelated to their pulmonary tumors. All the lesions were solitary pulmonary nodules, and all the patients underwent surgical resection of their tumors.

Pathological Features

Grossly, these tumors are generally solitary coin lesions within the lung parenchyma. The size varies from 1 to 3 cm in greatest diameter; the tumors may be cystic and hemorrhagic.

Histologically, at low magnification, the tumors appear to be well circumscribed with prominent large cystic spaces containing clear acellular fluid within the cyst lumina. At the periphery of the lesion, the tumor appears to be more cellular and glandular with a microcystic pattern. Higher magnification shows the presence of a discrete inflammatory infiltrate composed of lymphocytes and plasma cells in the

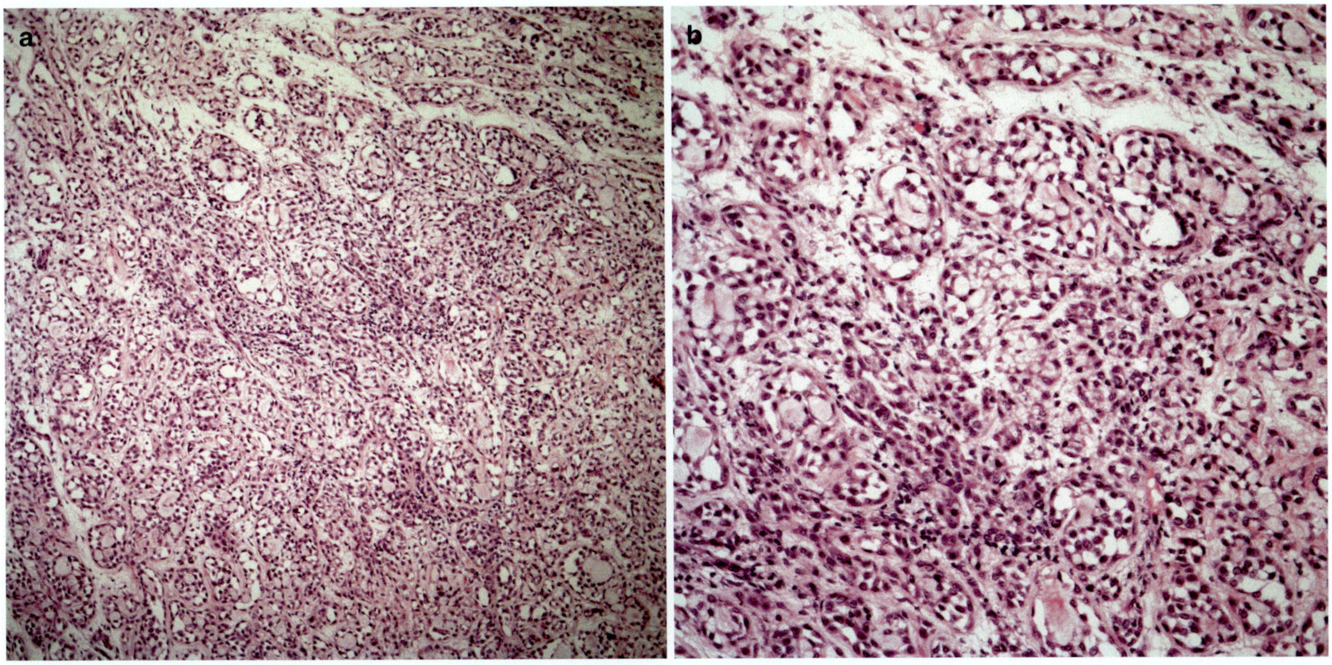

Fig. 13.82 (**a**) Tightly packed small glandular proliferation. (**b**) Small glands some of them showing focal signet ring cell appearance

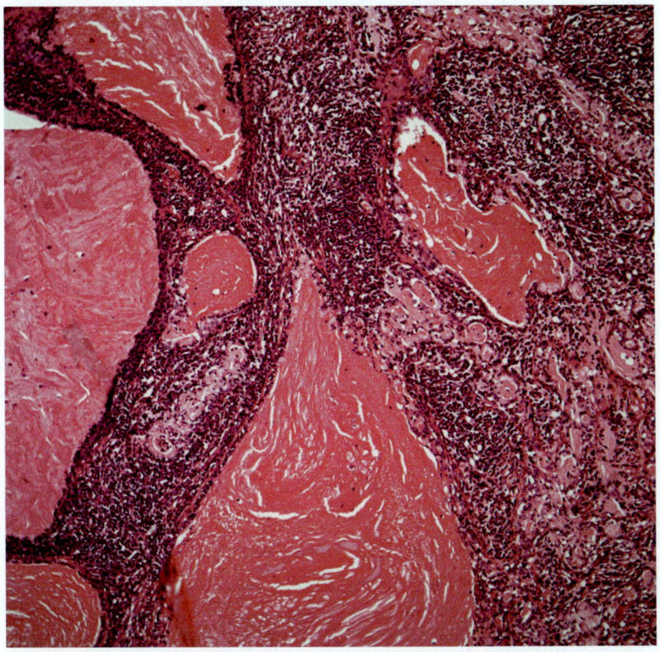

Fig. 13.83 Cystically dilated glands containing mucus embedded in a heavy inflammatory reaction, namely, plasma cells

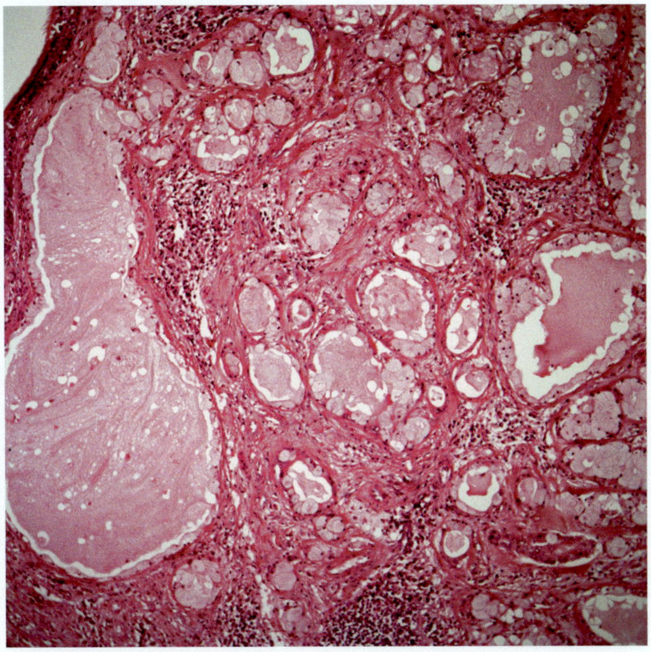

Fig. 13.84 Glandular proliferation composed predominantly of glands lined by mucinous epithelium

septa separating the cystic from the glandular areas (Figs. 13.85, 13.86, 13.87, and 13.88). The cystic spaces are lined by medium-sized cuboidal cells with a hobnail appearance resembling pneumocytes, while the peripheral areas with a more glandular appearance are composed of type II pneumocytes. Mitotic activity is rare or non-existent in these lesions, and necrosis is not a feature of alveolar adenomas. A PAS histochemical stain shows positive staining in the fluid contained in the cystic spaces.

Immunohistochemical studies have been performed in these lesions, demonstrating that, epithelial markers such as keratin and EMA are positive as is surfactant protein alpha

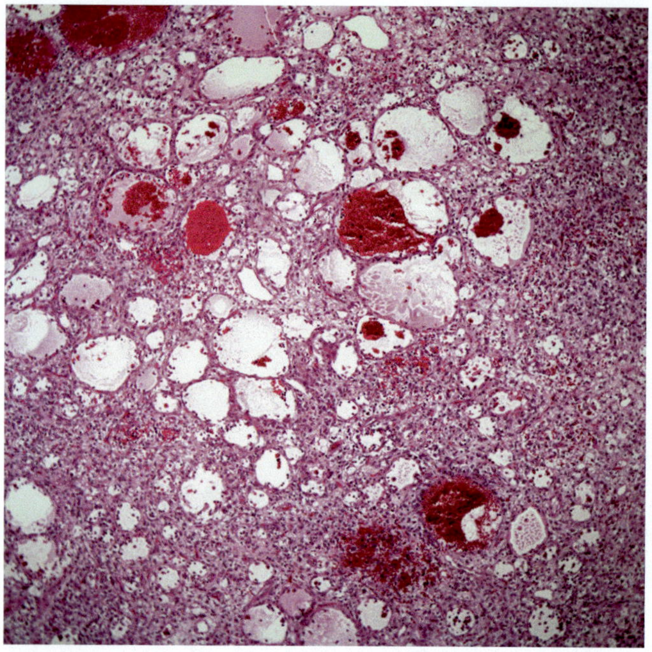

Fig. 13.85 Alveolar adenoma with the characteristic cystic and solid growth patterns

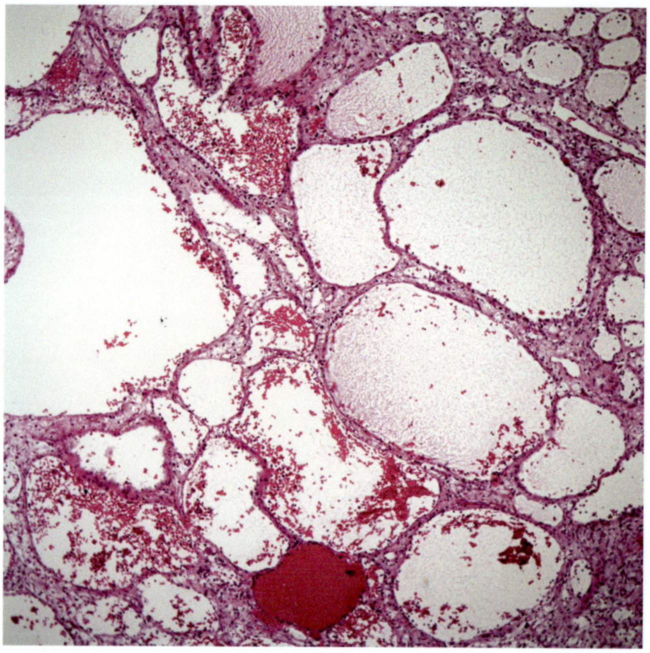

Fig. 13.86 Alveolar adenomas may be predominantly cystic and present as distended alveolar structures

[142, 143]. The tumor is negative for vascular markers including CD31, CD34, and Factor VIII.

Differential Diagnosis

Because of the glandular proliferation the most important differential diagnosis includes adenocarcinoma with a bronchioloalveolar pattern. Both of these conditions may show positive staining for the conventional immunomarkers including TTF-1, surfactant protein alpha, and epithelial immunomarkers. Thus, there is no real way in making an unequivocal diagnosis of alveolar adenoma in a small biopsy. As such, the diagnosis can only be accomplished after complete resection of the tumor. Because of the large cystic spaces present in these lesions, another differential diagnostic possibility is lymphangioma. However, an epithelial lining of type II pneumocytes and the negative staining for vascular markers will aid at arriving at the correct diagnosis.

Treatment and Prognosis

Surgical resection is the treatment of choice for alveolar adenomas, and is curative. Although in some of the cases the treatment has ranged from wedge resection to lobectomy, it is possible that a more conservative approach is warranted in these cases. However, the problem may be in assessing the true nature of this tumor on a small biopsy. In the cases described the available follow up has indicated an indolent benign process.

Pulmonary Dirofilariasis

This parasitic infectious process is produced by *Dirofilaria immitis*, a helminth common in dogs with man as an accidental host. Pulmonary dirofilariasis usually presents as a coin nodule or nodules affecting patients from childhood to adulthood. Because of the clinical and radiological presentation, it is often thought to represent a neoplastic process, and the diagnosis is accomplished by tissue examination. Initially described by Dashiell [144] and Goodman [145], numerous reports of this entity have been presented, namely, in the form of case reports or short series of cases [146–150]. In humans, similar to what happens in dogs, the worms may also lodge in the heart; however, they may die before reaching maturity, and then pass into the pulmonary arteries. However, this infectious process is rather rare, and it may account for only a very small percentage of cases that may present with a granulomatous reaction in the lung. Ulbright and Katzenstein [151] studied 86 cases of solitary pulmonary granulomas in the lung and determined that in 60 of their cases fungal or acid-fast organisms were identified, in 25 cases an infectious etiology could not be determined, and in only 1 case, fragments of a helminth were identified. Microbiological cultures were found to be less productive than direct tissue examination. Thus, it is logical to assume that in actual practice, the presence of pulmonary dirofilariasis is an unusual occurrence. The largest series of cases presenting with pulmonary dirofilariasis is the one analyzed by Flieder et al. [152] who studied 41 lesions from 39 patients and summarized the entire spectrum of histopathological changes associated with this infection.

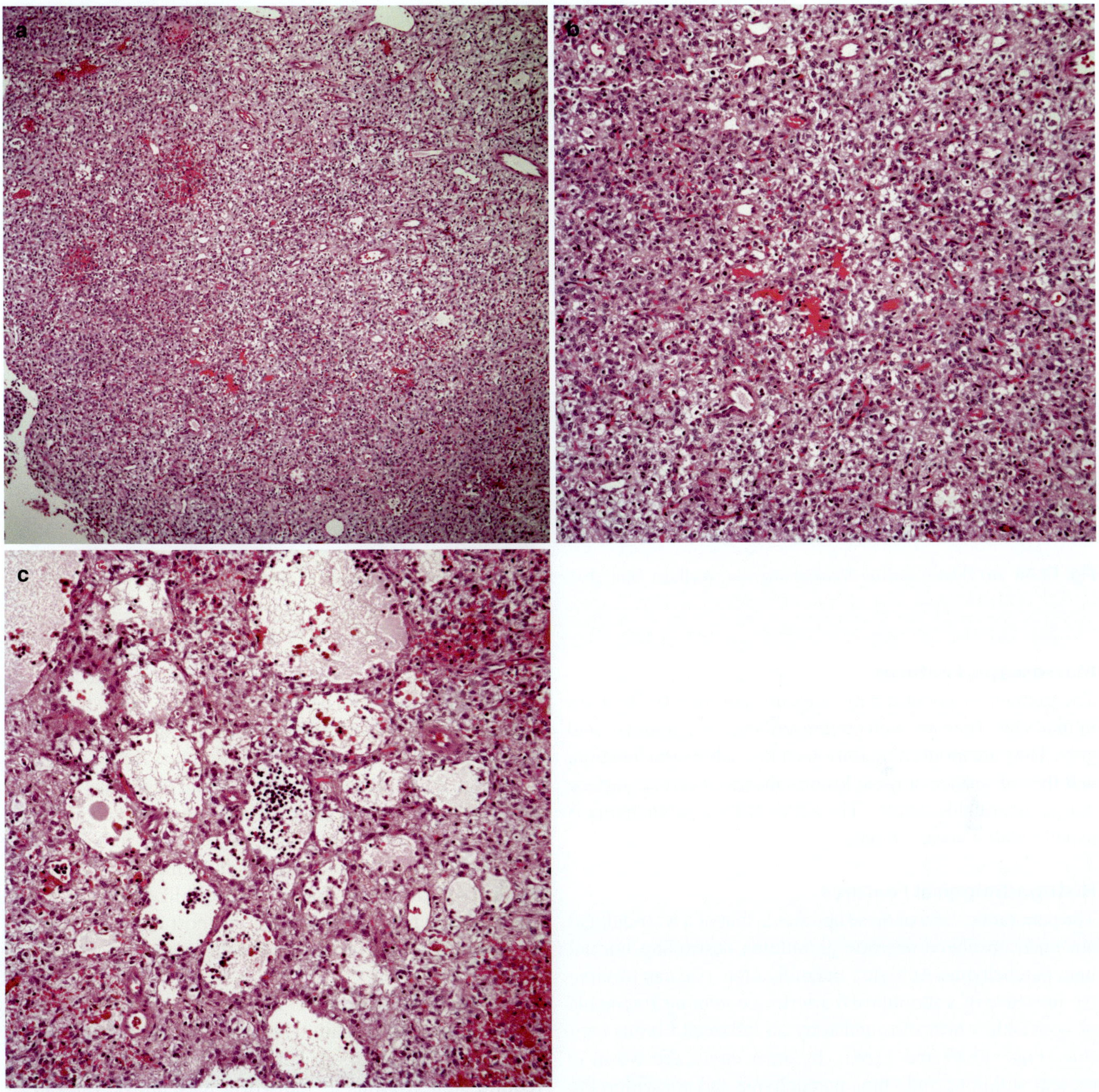

Fig. 13.87 (**a**) Alveolar adenoma showing a predominantly solid component. (**b**) Higher magnification shows a homogeneous cellular proliferation without nuclear atypia or mitotic activity. (**c**) Alveolar adenoma with mixed cystic and solid components

Clinical Features

Pulmonary dirofilariasis is an infectious process that may be seen in patients ranging from 8 to 80 years of age with a median age of 58 years. The infection appears to be more common in men than women, and it is not necessarily associated with immunosuppression. However, in some cases, there may be a history of previous malignancies. At least half of the patients are asymptomatic, and their pulmonary nodule is discovered during a routine chest radiograph. For those patients who are symptomatic, cough, dyspnea, chest pain, fever, and wheezing are common symptoms, while hemoptysis is rare. Eosinophilia may be present in up to 15 % of these patients. Radiologically, dirofilariasis presents more commonly as a solitary pulmonary nodule; however, in some cases, multiple nodules may be seen. The right lung appears to be more commonly affected than the left, and although these nodules may be more common in the periphery of the lung, central lesions may also occur.

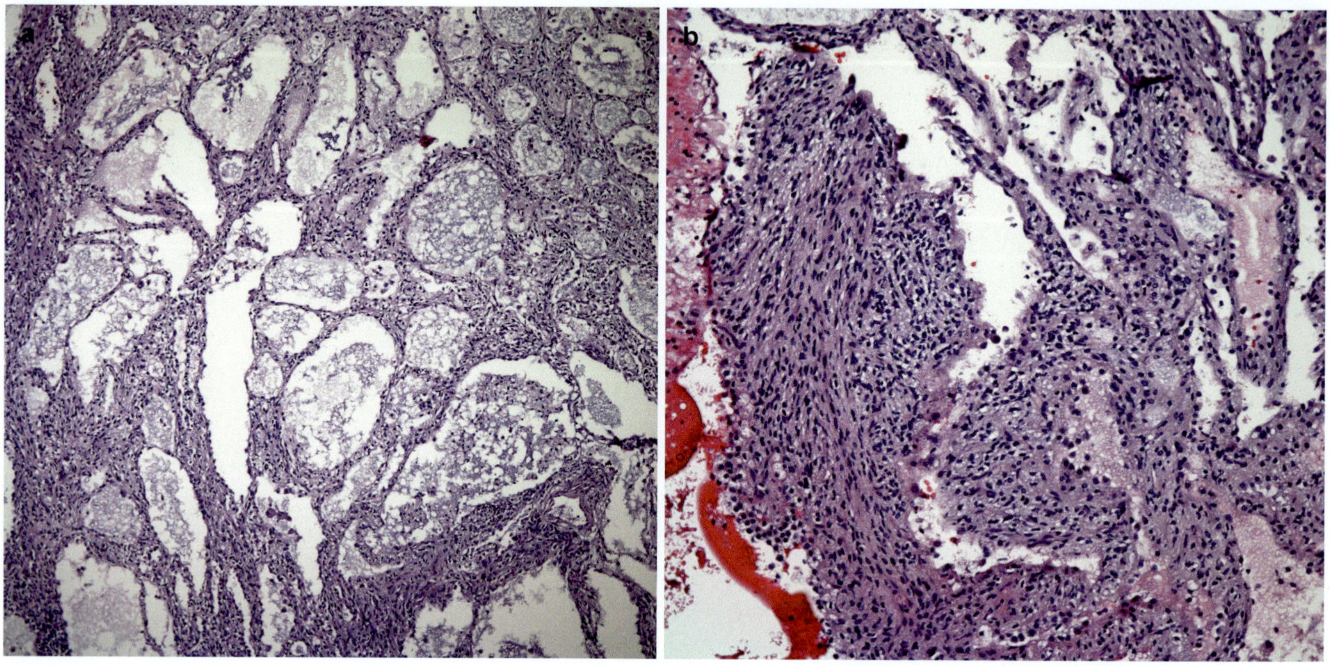

Fig. 13.88 (**a**) Dilated structures containing clear acellular fluid. (**b**) In focal areas, alveolar adenomas may show a spindle cell component

Macroscopic Features

The pulmonary nodules may range in size from 0.5 to 4 cm in diameter. They are well circumscribed, soft, granular, and gray. They are more commonly seen in a subpleural location, and the cut surface of these lesions shows a necrotic surface but no identifiable worms. The adjacent lung parenchyma is usually within normal limits.

Histopathological Features

The panoramic view of these nodules is that of a well-defined but unencapsulated necrotic granuloma destroying normal lung parenchyma. At higher magnification, one can observe the presence of a thrombosed arteries containing fragments of nonviable worm surrounded by an inflamed fibrous capsule (Figs. 13.89 and 13.90). In some cases, the worm is present within necrotic lung parenchyma and not within the vascular spaces. The worms are usually immature and do not contain ova, measuring approximately 125–250 μm, while the cuticle thickness varies from 5 to 25 μm. These parasites may be highlighted by using histochemical stains for PAS and/or Movat. In Flieder's account [152] of the histopathological changes of dirofilaria, the authors encountered that the granulomatous reaction may have round, geographic, or wedge-shaped forms in about one-third of the cases, while caseous necrosis was present in 41 % of the cases, and Charcot-Leyden crystals were present in 27 % of the lesions. In most of the cases, the nodules have a rim of dense hyalinized tissue with an inflammatory reaction composed of lymphocytes, plasma cells, and histiocytes. Langhans type giant cells, neutrophils, and non-necrotizing granulomas may also be present. On the other hand, the adjacent lung parenchyma may show features of desquamative interstitial pneumonitis (DIP)-like areas, follicular bronchiolitis, and/or organizing pneumonia. Focal areas showing vasculitis and capillaritis may also be observed in some cases. Other features that may be observed in association with pulmonary dirofilariasis include microcalcifications, cholesterol cleft granulomas, amyloid-like stromal areas, and fibrinous pleuritis. However, the most important issue in the diagnosis is the recognition of the worm.

Differential Diagnosis

The most important feature in the diagnosis of dirofilariasis is the identification of helminth fragments. This may require step sections as the worm may not be present in the initial superficial sections. On the other hand, in cases in which there is limited material for evaluation, the differential diagnosis will include any other infectious process caused by fungal or acid-fast bacilli, Wegener's granulomatosis, Churg-Strauss syndrome, and possibly pulmonary lymphoma. However, depending on the setting, the use of special stains or tissue culture will rule out those possibilities. On the other hand, if the material available for evaluation is from areas adjacent to the granulomatous reaction, other entities such as bronchiolitis obliterans, organizing pneumonia, extrinsic allergic alveolitis, or DIP may be considered in the differential diagnosis.

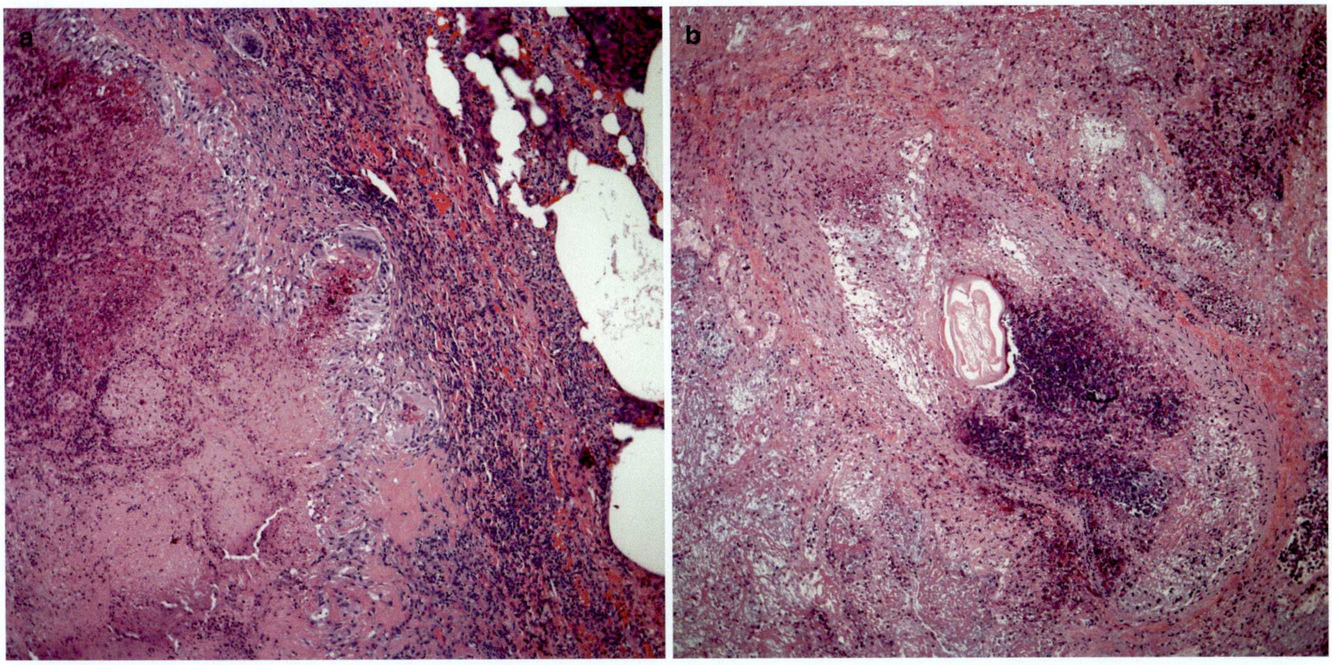

Fig. 13.89 (**a**) Necrotizing granuloma replacing normal lung parenchyma. (**b**) Adjacent areas showing vascular structures containing worms compatible with dirofilaria immitis

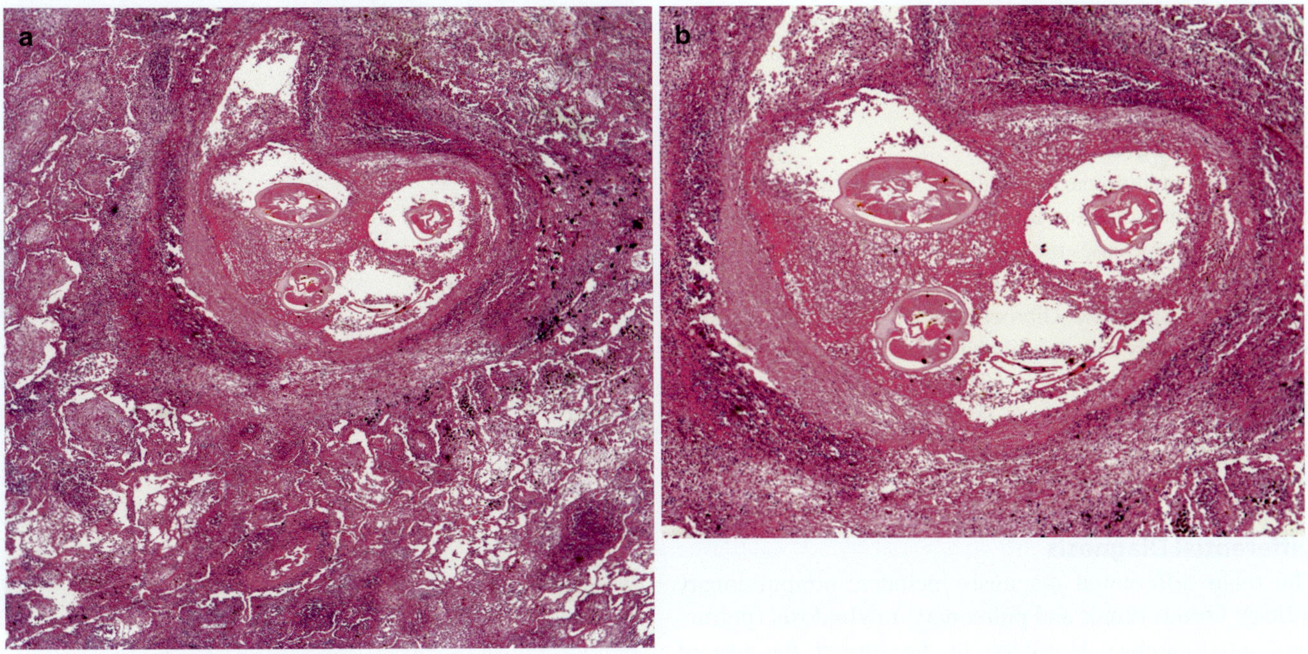

Fig. 13.90 (**a**) In some cases, the presence of worms is easily identified and may be present in areas with acute inflammatory changes. (**b**) Higher magnification of dirofilaria immitis

Treatment and Prognosis

Surgical excision of these nodules is curative for these patients. However, it is advisable that in cases in which there are multiple nodules, all of those nodules be sampled as in some cases dirofilariasis may be associated with other processes including primary carcinomas of the lung.

Hyalinizing Granuloma of Lung

Hyalinizing granuloma of the lung represents an unusual condition of unknown etiology. However, some authors have suggested an autoimmune origin for this process. Its presence in the lung may also be associated with other conditions including retroperitoneal fibrosis and sclerosing mediastinitis. Hyalinizing granuloma can occur at any age and does not appear to have a specific gender predilection; however, it appears to be more common in adult individuals [153–155].

Clinical Features

Just like any other mass in the lung, patients may present with symptoms related to pulmonary obstruction such as cough, dyspnea, and fever. However, patients may also be asymptomatic, and the lesion may be discovered during a routine radiographic study. It has been reported that patients with hyalinizing granuloma may show positive serum antinuclear antibodies, rheumatoid factor, or suffer from Coombs-positive hemolytic anemia.

Histopathological Features

Hyalinizing granuloma is usually a solitary intrapulmonary nodule that may measure up to 10 cm in greatest dimension. However, in some cases more than one nodule may be present. Microscopically, the lesions are characterized by the presence of a tumor with prominent fibrocollagenous deposition admixed with inflammatory cells, mainly lymphocytes and plasma cells. Distended vascular structures may also be present as well as calcifications (Figs. 13.91, 13.92, 13.93, 13.94, and 13.95). The use of immunohistochemical studies is not helpful unless one is trying to rule out other tumoral conditions.

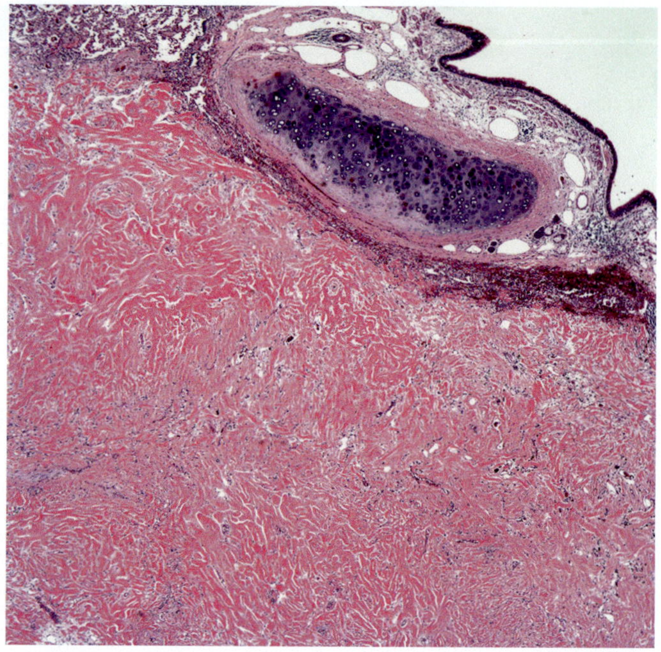

Fig. 13.91 Hyalinizing granuloma showing a dense fibrocollagenous matrix. Note the presence of uninvolved cartilage and respiratory epithelium

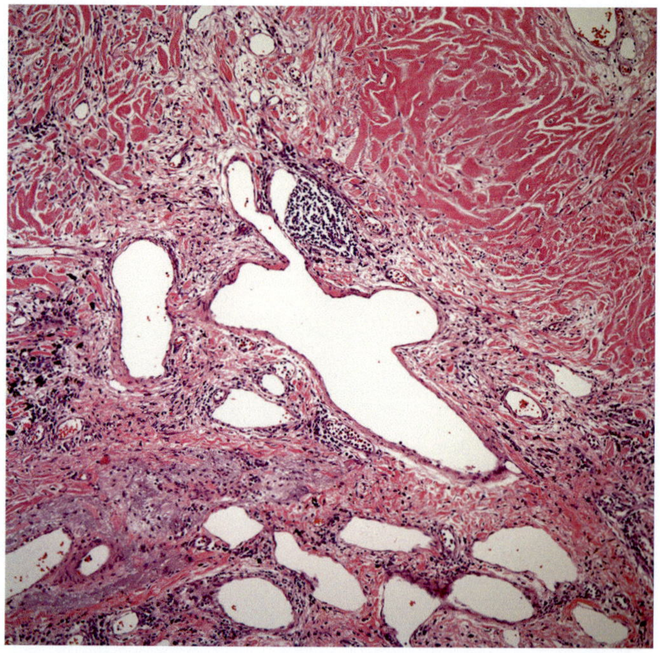

Fig. 13.92 The dense fibrocollagenous matrix may be admixed with dilated vascular structures

Differential Diagnosis

The main differential diagnosis includes intrapulmonary solitary fibrous tumor and pulmonary amyloidosis (pulmonary amyloidoma). However, in the former the use of immunohistochemical stains, mainly CD34 and Bcl-2, may prove helpful; hyalinizing granuloma will be negative for both of those antibodies. In the latter, the use of a histochemical stain for Congo red will be helpful as under polarized light the characteristic apple-green refringency will be absent in cases of hyalinizing granuloma. One other possibility that has to be considered is the question whether the lesion is not an extension of sclerosing mediastinitis. The presence of a mediastinal mass either by radiographic means or direct inspection should lead to the correct interpretation.

Treatment and Prognosis

The treatment of choice is surgical resection of the mass. If the tumor is resected completely, the prognosis is favorable.

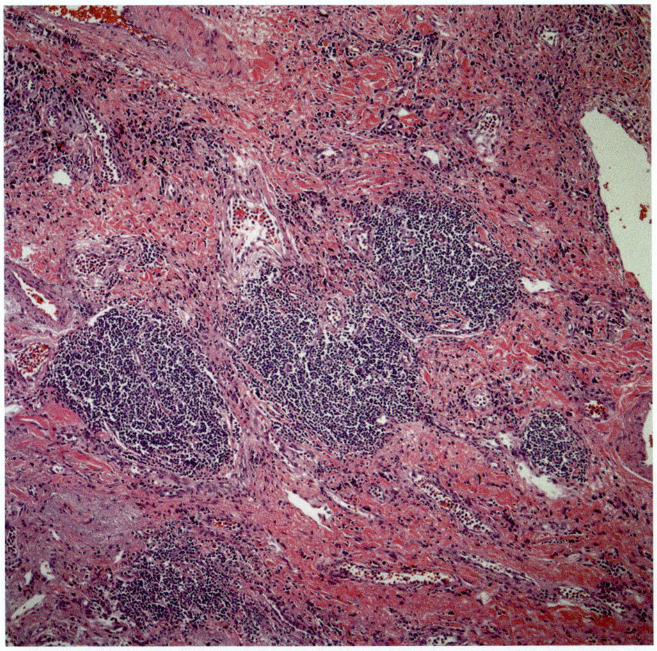

Fig. 13.93 In other areas, the dense fibrocollagenous matrix may contain collections of lymphocytes

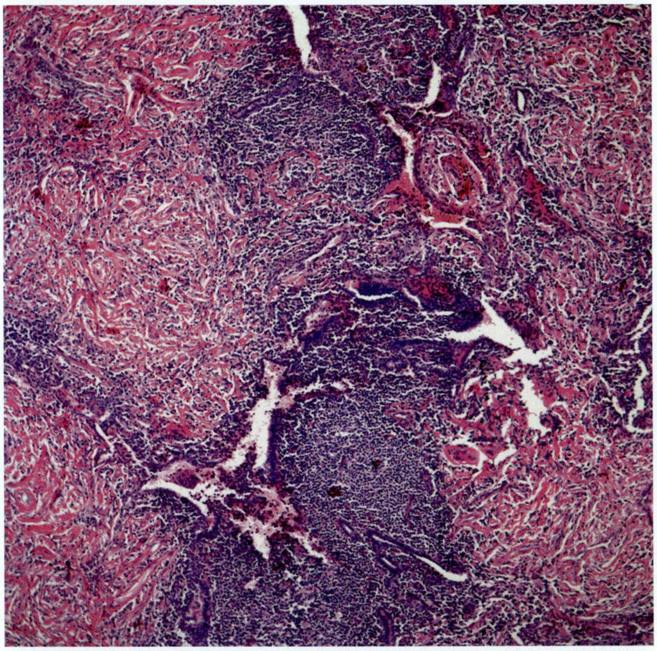

Fig. 13.94 Lymphoid aggregates and airway structures are surrounded by a fibrocollagenous matrix

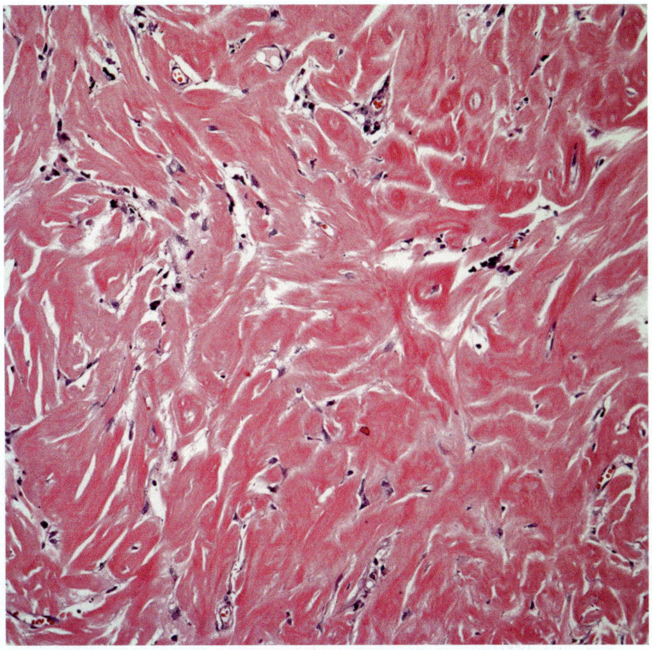

Fig. 13.95 High power magnification of dense acellular collagenous matrix

References

1. Brown LK, Miller A, Bhuptani A, et al. Pulmonary involvement in Fabry disease. Am J Respir Crit Care Med. 1997;155:1004–10.
2. Matsumoto T, Matsumori H, Taki T, et al. Infantile GM1-gangliosidosis with marked manifestations of lungs. Acta Pathol Jpn. 1979;29:269–76.
3. Amir G, Ron N. Pulmonary pathology in Gaucher's disease. Hum Pathol. 1999;30:666–70.
4. Miller A, Brown LK, Pastores GM, Desnick RJ. Pulmonary involvement in type 1 Gaucher disease: functional and exercise findings in patients with and without clinical interstitial lung disease. Clin Genet. 2003;63:368–76.
5. Minai OA, Sullivan EJ, Stoller JK. Pulmonary involvement in Niemann-Pick disease: case report and literature review. Respir Med. 2000;94:1241–51.
6. Nicholson AG, Florio R, Hansell DM, et al. Pulmonary involvement by Niemann-Pick disease. A report of six cases. Histopathology. 2006;48:596–603.
7. Muir-Padilla J, Myers JB. Whipple disease: a case report and review of the literature. Arch Pathol Lab Med. 2005;129:933–6.
8. Kelly CA, Egan M, Rawinson J. Whipple's disease presenting with lung involvement. Thorax. 1996;51:343–4.
9. Foucar E, Rosai J, Dorfman R. Sinus histocytosis with massive lymphadenopathy (Rosai-Dorfman Disease): review of the entity. Semin Diagn Pathol. 1990;7:19–73.
10. Wright DH, Richards DB. Sinus histiocytosis with massive lymphadenopathy (Rosai Dorfman disease): report of a case with widespread nodal and extranodal dissemination. Histopathology. 1981;5:697–709.
11. Huang Q, Change KL, Weiss LM. Extranodal Rosai-Dorfman disease involving the bone marrow: a case report. Am J Surg Pathol. 2006;30:1189–92.
12. Ben Ghorbel I, Naffati H, Khanfir M, et al. Disseminated for of Rosai-Dorfman disease: a case report. Rev Med Interne. 2005;26:415–9.
13. Ohori P, Yu J, Landreneau RJ. Rosai-Dorfman disease of the pleura: a rare extranodal presentation. Hum Pathol. 2003;34:1210–1.
14. Paulli M, Bergamaschi G, Tonon L, et al. Evidence of polyclonal nature of the cell infiltrate in sinus histiocytosis with massive lymphadenopathy (Rosai-Dorfman disease). Br J Haematol. 1995;91:415–8.
15. Bonetti F, Chilosi M, Menestrina F, et al. Immunohistological analysis of Rosai-Dorfman histiocytosis: a disease of S-100+CD1a – histiocytes. Virchows Arch A. 1987;411:129–35.
16. Chester WD. Uber lipoidgranulomatose. Virchows Arch Pathol Anat. 1930;279:561–602.

17. Jaffe HL. Lipid (cholesterol) granulomatosis. In: Metabolic, degenerative, and inflammatory disease of bone. Philadelphia: Lea & Febiger; 1972. p. 535–41.
18. Veyssier-Belot C, Cacoub P, Caparros-Lefebvre D, et al. Erdheim-Chester disease: clinical and radiological characteristics of 59 cases. Medicine. 1996;75:157–69.
19. Shamburek RD, Brewer B, Gochuico BR. Erdheim-Chester disease: a rare multisystem histiocytic disorder associated with interstitial lung disease. Am J Med Sci. 2001;321:66–75.
20. Egan AJ, Boardman LA, Tazelaar HD, et al. Erdheim-Chester disease: clinical, radiologic, and histopathologic findings in five patients with interstitial lung disease. Am J Surg Pathol. 1999;23:17–26.
21. Rush WL, Andriko JA, Galateau-Salle F, et al. Pulmonary pathology of Erdheim-Chester disease. Mod Pathol. 2000;13:747–54.
22. Soler P, Kambouchner M, Valeyre D, Hance AJ. Pulmonary Langerhans cell granulomatosis. Annu Rev Med. 1992;43:105–15.
23. Marcy TW, Reynolds HY. Pulmonary histiocytosis X. Lung. 1985;163:129–50.
24. Vassallo RV, Ryu JH, Colby TV, et al. Pulmonary Langerhans cell histiocytosis. N Engl J Med. 2000;342:1969–78.
25. Colby TV, Lombard C. Histiocytosis X in the lung. Hum Pathol. 1983;14:847–56.
26. Allen TC. Pulmonary Langerhans cell histiocytosis and other pulmonary histiocytic diseases. Arch Pathol Lab Med. 2008;132: 1171–81.
27. Lombard CM, Medeiros J, Colby TV. Pulmonary histiocytosis X and carcinoma. Arch Pathol Lab Med. 1987;111:339–41.
28. Neumann MP, Frizzera G. The coexistence of Langerhans cell granulomatosis and malignant lymphoma may take different forms: report of seven cases with a review of the literature. Hum Pathol. 1986;17:1060–5.
29. Sajjad SM, Luna MA. Primary pulmonary histiocytosis X in two patients with Hodgkin's disease. Thorax. 1982;37:110–3.
30. O'Donnel AE, Tsou E, Awh C, et al. Endobronchial eosinophilic granuloma: a rare cause of total lung atelectasis. Am Rev Respir Dis. 1987;136:1478–80.
31. Meier B, Rhyner K, Medici TC, Kistler G. Eosinophilic granuloma of the skeleton with involvement of the lung: a report of three cases. Eur J Respir Dis. 1983;64:551–6.
32. Yousem SA, Colby TV, Chen YY, et al. Pulmonary Langerhans cell histiocytosis: molecular analysis of clonality. Am J Surg Pathol. 2001;25:630–6.
33. Yu RC, Chu C, Buluwela L, Chu AC. Clonal proliferation of Langerhans cells in Langerhans cell histiocytosis. Lancet. 1994;343: 767–8.
34. Willman CL. Detection of conal histiocytosis in Langerhans cell histiocytosis: biology and clinical significance. Br J Cancer. 1994;70:S29–33.
35. Willman CL, Busque L, Griffith BB, et al. Langerhans cell histiocytosis (Histiocytosis X) – a clonal proliferative disease. N Engl J Med. 1994;331:154–60.
36. Travis WD, Borok Z, Roum JH, et al. Pulmonary Langerhans cell granulomatosis (Histiocytosis X): a clinicopathologic study of 48 cases. Am J Surg Pathol. 1993;17:971–86.
37. Vassallo R, Ryu JH, Schroeder DR, et al. Clinical outcomes of pulmonary Langerhans cell histiocytosis in adults. N Engl J Med. 2002;346:484–90.
38. McDowell HP, Macfarlane PI, Martin J. Isolated pulmonary histiocytosis. Arch Dis Child. 1988;63:423–6.
39. Pomeranz SJ, Proto AV. Histiocytosis X: unusual confusing features of eosinophilic granuloma. Chest. 1986;89:88–92.
40. Friedman PJ, Lievow AA, Sokoloff J. Eosinophilic granuloma of lung: clinical aspects of primary histiocytosis in the adult. Medicine. 1981;60:385–96.
41. Gaenler EA, Carrington CB. Open biopsy for chronic diffuse infiltrative lung disease: clinical, roentgenographic, and physiologic correlations in 502 patients. Ann Thorac Surg. 1980;30:411–26.
42. Bakir B, Unuvar E, Terzibasioglu E, Guven K. Atypical lung involvement in a patient with systemic juvenile xanthogranuloma. Pediatr Radiol. 2007;37:325–7.
43. Matcham NJ, Andronikou S, Sibson K, et al. Systemic juvenile xanthogranulomatosis imitating a malignant abdominal wall tumor with lung metastases. J Pediatr Hematol Oncol. 2007;29:72–3.
44. Kraus MD, Haley JC, Ruiz R, et al. Juvenile xanthogranuloma: an immunophenotype study with a reappraisal of histogenesis. Am J Dermatopathol. 2001;23(2):104–11.
45. Guthrie JA, Arthur RJ. Juvenile xanthogranuloma with pulmonary, subcutaneous, and hepatic involvement. Clin Radiol. 1994;49:498–500.
46. Lottsfeldt FI, Good RA. Juvenile xanthogranuloma with pulmonary lesions. A case report. Pediatrics. 1964;33:233–8.
47. Kourilsky S, Pieron R, Renault P, et al. Isolated round intrapulmonary mass in a young person: xanthogranuloma. J Fr Med Chir Thorac. 1965;19:307–19.
48. Diard F, Cadier L, Billaud C, et al. Neonatal juvenile xanthogranulomatosis with pulmonary, extrapleural and hepatic involvement. One case report. Ann Radiol (Paris). 1982;25:113–8.
49. Ionescu DN, Pierson DM, Qing G, et al. Pulmonary crystal-storing histiocytoma. Arch Pathol Lab Med. 2005;129:1159–63.
50. Jones D, Renshaw AA. Recurrent crystal-storing histiocytosis of the lung in a patient without a clonal lymphoproliferative disorder. Arch Pathol Lab Med. 1996;120:978–80.
51. Pais AV, Pereira S, Garg I, et al. Intra-abdominal, crystal histiocytosis due to clofazimine in a patient with lepromatous leprosy and concurrent carcinoma of the colon. Lepr Rev. 2004;75:171–6.
52. Lewis JT, Candelora JN, Hogan RB, et al. Crystal-storing histiocytosis due to massive accumulation of charcot-leyden crystals: a unique association producing colonic polyposis in a 78-year-old woman with eosinophilic colitis. Am J Surg Pathol. 2007;31:481–5.
53. Pitman SD, Wang J, Serros E, Zuppan C. A 70-year-old woman with acute renal failure. Arch Pathol Lab Med. 2006;130:1077–8.
54. Joo M, Kwak JE, Chang SH, et al. Localized gastric crystal-storing histiocytosis. Histopathology. 2007;51:116–9.
55. Keane C, Gill D. Multi-organ involvement with crystal-storing histiocytosis. Br J Haematol. 2008;141:750.
56. Prassad ML, Charney DA, Sarlin J, Keller SM. Pulmonary immunocytoma with massive crystal storing histiocytosis: a case report with review of literature. Am J Surg Pathol. 1998;22:1148–53.
57. Kusakabe T, Watanabe K, Mori T, et al. Crystal-storing histiocytosis associated with MALT lymphoma of the adnexa: a case report with review of literature. Virchows Arch. 2007;450:103–8.
58. Pock L, Stuchlik D, Hercogova J. Crystal storing histiocytosis of the skin associated with multiple myeloma. Int J Dermatol. 2006;45:1408–11.
59. Chantranuwat C. Noncrystallized form of immunoglobulin-storing histiocytosis as a cause of chronic lung infiltration in multiple myeloma. Ann Diagn Pathol. 2007;11:220–2.
60. Fairweather PM, Williamson R, Tsikleas G. Pulmonary extranodal marginal zone lymphoma with massive crystal storing histiocytosis. Am J Surg Pathol. 2006;30:262–7.
61. Papla B, Spolnik P, Rzenno E, et al. Generalized crystal-storing histiocytosis as a presentation of multiple myeloma: a case with a possible pro-aggregation defect in the immunoglobulin heavy chain. Virchows Arch. 2004;445:83–9.
62. Sun Y, Tawfiqul B, Valderrama E, et al. Pulmonary crystal-storing histiocytosis and extranodal marginal zone B-cell lymphoma associated with a fibroleiomyomatous hamartoma. Ann Diagn Pathol. 2003;7:47–53.
63. Zioni F, Giovanardi P, Bozzoli M, et al. Massive bone marrow crystal-storing histiocytosis in a patient with IgA-lambda multiple myeloma and extensive extramedullary disease: a case report. Tumori. 2004;90:348–51.
64. Galed-Placed I. Immunoglobulin crystal-storing histiocytosis in a pleural effusion from a woman with Iga κ multiple myeloma. Acta Cytol. 2006;50:539–41.

65. Stokes MB, Aronoff B, Siegel D, D'Agati VD. Dysproteinemia-related nephropathy associated with crystal-storing histiocytosis. Kidney Int. 2006;70:597–602.
66. Guerrero MF, Ramos JM, Renedo G, et al. Pulmonary malacoplakia associated with *Rhodococcus equi* infection in patients with AIDS: case reports and review. Clin Infect Dis. 1999;28: 1334–6.
67. Hodder RV, Hyslop PG, Chalvardjian A, et al. Pulmonary malakoplakia. Thorax. 1984;39:70–1.
68. Bastas A, Markou N, Botsi C, et al. Malakoplakia of the lung caused by *Pasteurella multocida* in a patient with AIDS. Scand J Infect Dis. 2002;34:53–538.
69. Shin MS, Allen J, Cooper D, et al. Pulmonary malacoplakia associated with *Rhodococcus equi* infection in a patient with AIDS. Chest. 1999;115:889–92.
70. Colby TV, Hunt S, Pelzmann K, Carrington DB. Malakoplakia of the lung: a report of two cases. Respiration. 1980;39:295–9.
71. Andrianpoulos E, Lautides G, Kormas P, et al. Pulmonary xanthoma: a case report with immunohistologic study and DNA-image analysis. Eur J Cardiothorac Surg. 1995;9:534–6.
72. Nakamura M, Ohishi A, Watanabe R, Kaneko K, Sakauchi M, Tokuhira M, Aosaki N, Sugiura H, Miyoshi Y, Saruta T. Adult T-cell leukemia with hypercalcemia-induced metastatic calcification in the lungs due to production of parathyroid hormone-related protein. Intern Med. 2001;40(5):409–13.
73. Liou JH, Cho LC, Hsu YH. Paraneoplastic hypercalcemia with metastatic calcification. Kaohsiung J Med Sci. 2006;22:85–8.
74. Valdivielso P, Lopez-Sanchez J, Garrido A, Sanchez-Carrillo JJ. Metastatic calcifications and severe hypercalcemia in a patient with parathyroid carcinoma. J Endocrinol Invest. 2006;29:641–4.
75. Alfrey AC. The role of abnormal phosphorus metabolism in the progression of chronic kidney disease and metastatic calcification. Kidney Int. 2004;66(suppl):s13–7.
76. Lingam RK, The J, Sharma A, Friedman E. Metastatic pulmonary calcification in renal failure: a new HRCT pattern. Br J Radiol. 2002;75:74–7.
77. Cherng SC, Cheng CY, Chen CY, Hsu HH, Chu P. Metastatic pulmonary calcification in renal failure mimicking pulmonary embolism on lung scan. Clin Nucl Med. 2005;30(5):322–3.
78. Kobayashi T, Satoh K, Nakano S, Toyama Y, Ohakawa M. A case of metastatic pulmonary calcification after transient acute renal failure. Radiat Med. 2005;23:435–8.
79. Ullmer E, Borer H, Sandoz P, Mayr M, Dalquen P, Soler M. Diffuse pulmonary nodular infiltrates in a renal transplant recipient. Chest. 2001;120:1394–8.
80. Eggert C, Albright RC. Metastatic pulmonary calcification in a dialysis patient. Hemodial Int. 2006;10:551–5.
81. Guermazi A, Esperou H, Selimi F, Gluckman E. Imaging of diffuse metastatic and dystrophic pulmonary calcification in children after haematopoietic stem cell transplantation. Br J Radiol. 2005;78: 708–13.
82. Marchiori E, Muller NL, Soares A, Escuissato DL, Gasparetto EL, Cerqueira EM. Unusual clinicalmanifestations of metastatic pulmonary calcification. J Thorac Imaging. 2005;20:66–70.
83. Chan ED, Morales DV, Welsh CH, McDermott MT, Schwarz MI. Calcium deposition with or without bone formation in the lung. Am J Respir Crit Care Med. 2002;165:1654–69.
84. Moran CA, Hocholzer L, Hasleton PS, Johnson FB, Koss MN. Pulmonary clinical microlithiasis: a clinicopathological and chemical analysis of seven cases. Arch Pathol Lab Med. 1997;121: 607–11.
85. Prakash UBS, Barham SS, Rosenow EC, Brown ML, Payne WS. Pulmonary alveolar microlithiasis: a review including ultrastructural and pulmonary function studies. Mayo Clin Proc. 1983;58: 290–300.
86. Koss MN, Johnson FB, Hocholzer L. Pulmonary blue bodies. Hum Pathol. 1981;12(3):258–66.
87. Kanne JP, Godwin D, Takasugi JE, Schmidt RA, Stern EJ. Diffuse pulmonary ossification. J Thorac Imaging. 2004;19(2):98–102.
88. Bossche LV, Vanderstraeten G. Heterotopic ossification: a review. J Rehabil Med. 2005;37:129–36.
89. McChesney T. Placental transmogrification of the lung: a unique case with remarkable histopathologic features. Lab Investig. 1979;40:245–6.
90. Fidler ME, Koomen M, Sebek B, Greco MA, Rizk CC, Askin FB. Placental transmogrification of the lung. A histologic variant of giant bullous emphysema. Am J Surg Pathol. 1995;19(5):563–70.
91. Mark EJ, Muller KM, McChesney T, Dong-Hwan S, Honig C, Mark MA. Placentoid bullous lesion of the lung. Hum Pathol. 1995;26:74–9.
92. Hochholzer L, Moran CA, Koss MN. Pulmonary lipomatosis: a variant of placental transmogrification. Mod Pathol. 1997;10(8): 846–9.
93. Kelly J, Moss J. Lymphangioleiomyomatosis. Am J Med Sci. 2001;321:17–25.
94. Ferrans VJ, Yu ZX, Nelson WK, et al. Lymphangioleiomyomatosis (LAM): a review of clinical and morphological features. J Nippon Med Sch. 2000;67:311–29.
95. Hohman DW, Noghrehkar D, Ratnayake S. Lymphangioleiomyomatosis: a review. Eur J Intern Med. 2008;19:319–24.
96. Kalassian KG, Doyle R, Kao P, et al. Lymphangioleiomyomatosis: new insights. Am J Respir Crit Care Med. 1997;155:1183–6.
97. Schiavina M, Di Scioscio V, Contini P, et al. Pulmonary lymphangioleiomyomatosis in a karyotypically normal man without tuberous sclerosis complex. Am J Respir Crit Care Med. 2007;176:96–8.
98. Basset F, Soler P, Marsac J, Corrin B. Pulmonary lymphangiomyomatosis: three new cases studied with electron microscopy. Cancer. 1976;38:2357–66.
99. Stovin PGI, Lum LC, Flower DR, et al. The lungs in lymphangioleiomyomatosis and in tuberous sclerosis. Thorax. 1975;30: 497–509.
100. Urban T, Lazor R, Lacronique J, et al. Pulmonary lymphangioleiomyomatosis: a study of 69 patients. Medicine. 1999;78: 321–37.
101. Capron F, Ameille J, Leclerc P, et al. Pulmonary lymphangioleiomyomatosis and Bourneville's tuberous sclerosis with pulmonary involvement: the same disease? Cancer. 1983;52:851–5.
102. McCormack F, Brody A, Meyer C, et al. Pulmonary cysts consistent with lymphangioleiomyomatosis are common in women with tuberous sclerosis. Chest. 2002;121:61S.
103. Wenaden AE, Copley SJ. Unilateral lymphangioleiomyomatosis. J Thorac Imaging. 2005;20:226–8.
104. Oh YM, Mo EK, Jang SH, et al. Pulmonary lymphangioleiomyomatosis in Korea. Thorax. 1999;54:618–21.
105. Delgrange E, Delgrange B, Wallon J, Rosoux P. Diagnostic approach to pulmonary lymphangioleiomyomatosis. J Intern Med. 1994;236:461–4.
106. Bonetti F, Chiodera PL, Pea M, et al. Transbronchial biopsy in lymphangiomyomatosis of the lung: HMB45 for diagnosis. Am J Surg Pathol. 1993;17:1092–102.
107. Guinee DG, Feuerstein I, Koss MN, et al. Pulmonary lymphangioleiomyomatosis: diagnosis based on results of transbronchial biopsy and immunohistochemical studies and correlation with high-resolution computed tomography findings. Arch Pathol Lab Med. 1994;118:846–9.
108. Matsui K, Riemenschneider WK, Hilbert SL, et al. Hyperplasia of type II pneumocytes in pulmonary lymphangioleiomyomatosis: immunohistochemical and electron microscopic study. Arch Pathol Lab Med. 2000;124:1642–8.
109. Maruyama H, Seyama K, Sobajima J, et al. Multifocal micronodular pneumocyte hyperplasia and lymphangioleiomyomatosis in tuberous sclerosis with TSC2 gene. Mod Pathol. 2001;14: 609–14.

110. Kitaichi M, Nishimura K, Itoh H, Izumi T. Pulmonary lymphangioleiomyomatosis: a report of 46 patients including a clinicopathologic study of prognostic factors. Am J Respir Crit Care Med. 1995;151:527–33.
111. Tanaka H, Imada A, Morikawa T, et al. Diagnosis of pulmonary lymphangioleiomyomatosis by HMB45 in surgically treated spontaneous pneumothorax. Eur Repir J. 1995;8:1879–82.
112. Bittmann I, Dose TB, Muller C, et al. Lymphangioleiomyomatosis: recurrence after single lung transplantation. Hum Pathol. 1997;26:1420–3.
113. Dishner W, Cordasco EM, Blackburn J, et al. Pulmonary lymphangiomyomatosis. Chest. 1984;85:796–9.
114. El-Allaf D, Borlee G, Hadjoudj H, et al. Pulmonary lymphangiomyomatosis. Eur J Respir Dis. 1984;65:147–52.
115. Beasly MB, Matsui K, Yu ZX, et al. Histologic predictors of survival in 101 cases of pulmonary lymphangioleiomyomatosis (LAM): prognostic significance of histology score. Am J Respir Crit Care Med. 2000;161:A15.
116. Rosen SH, Castleman B, Liebow AA. Pulmonary alveolar proteinosis. N Engl J Med. 1958;258:1123–42.
117. Bedrossian CWM, Luna M, Conklin RH, Miller WC. Alveolar proteinosis as a consequence of immunosuppression. Hum Pathol. 1980;11:527–35.
118. McCook TA, Kirks DR, Merten DF, et al. Pulmonary alveolar proteinosis in children. Am J Radiol. 1981;137:1023–7.
119. Prakash UBS, Barham SS, Carpenter HA, et al. Pulmonary alveolar phospholipoproteinosis: experience with 34 cases and a review. Mayo Clin Proc. 1987;62:499–518.
120. Kariman K, Kylstra JA, Spock A. Pulmonary alveolar proteinosis: prospective clinical experience with 23 patients for 15 years. Lung. 1984;162:223–31.
121. Attwood HD, Price CG, Riddell RJ. Primary diffuse tracheobronchial amyloidosis. Thorax. 1972;27:620–4.
122. Celli BR, Rubinow A, Cohen AS, Brody JS. Patterns of pulmonary involvement in systemic amyloidosis. Chest. 1978;74: 543–7.
123. Cordier JF, Loire R, Brune J. Amyloidosis of the lower respiratory tract: clinical and pathologic features in a series of 221 patients. Chest. 1986;90:827–31.
124. Bonner H, Ennis RS, Geelhoed GW, Tarpley TM. Lymphoid infiltration and amyloidosis of lung in Sjögren's syndrome. Arch Pathol. 1973;95:42–4.
125. Kobayashi H, Matsuoka R, Kitamura S, et al. Sjögren's syndrome with multiple bullae and pulmonary nodular amyloidosis. Chest. 1988;94:438–40.
126. Lantuejoul S, Moulai N, Quetant S, et al. Unusual cystic presentation of pulmonary nodular amyloidosis associated with MALT-type lymphoma. Eur Respir J. 2007;30:589–92.
127. Laden SA, Cohen ML, Harley RA. Nodular pulmonary amyloidosis with extrapulmonary involvement. Hum Pathol. 1984;15: 594–7.
128. Chaudhuri MR, Parker DJ. A solitary amyloid nodule in the lung. Thorax. 1970;25:382–6.
129. Hui AN, Koss MN, Hocholzer L, Wehunt WD. Amyloidosis presenting in the lower respiratory tract. Arch Pathol Lab Med. 1986;110:212–8.
130. Rodriguez FJ, Gamez JD, Vrana JA, et al. Immunoglobulin derived depositions in the nervous system: novel mass spectrometry application for protein characterization in formalin-fixed tissues. Lab Invest. 2008;88:1024–37.
131. Weinberger MA, Katz S, Davis EW. Peripheral bronchial adenoma of mucous gland type: clinical and pathologic aspects. J Thorac Surg. 1955;29:626–35.
132. Ramsey JH, Reimann DL. Bronchial adenomas arising in mucous glands: illustrative case. Am J Pathol. 1953;29:339–45.
133. Pritchtett PS, Key BM. Mucous gland adenoma of the bronchus: ultrastructural and histochemical studies. Ala J Med Sci. 1978;15:44–8.
134. Allen MS, Marsh WL, Geissinger WT. Mucous gland adenoma of the bronchus. J Thorac Cardiovasc Surg. 1974;67: 966–8.
135. Edwards CW, Mattthews HR. Mucous gland adenoma of the bronchus. Thorax. 1981;36:147–8.
136. Emory WB, Mitchell WT, Hatch HB. Mucous gland adenoma of the bronchus. Am Rev Respir Dis. 1973;108: 1407–10.
137. Gilman RA, Klassen KP, Scarpelli DG. Mucus gland adenoma of bronchus. Am J Clin Pathol. 1956;26:131–54.
138. Heard BE, Corrin B, Dewar A. Pathology of seven mucous cell adenomas of the bronchial glands with particular reference to ultrastructure. Histopathology. 1985;9:687–701.
139. Kroe DJ, Pitcock JA. Benign mucous gland adenoma of the bronchus. Arch Pathol. 1967;84:539–42.
140. England DM, Hochholzer L. Truly benign "bronchial adenoma:" report of 10 cases of mucous gland adenoma with immunohistochemical and ultrastructural findings. Am J Surg Pathol. 1995;19:887–99.
141. Wada A, Tateishi R, Terazawa T, et al. Lymphangioma of the lung. Arch Pathol Lab Med. 1974;98:211.
142. Yousem SA, Hochholzer L. Alveolar adenoma. Hum Pathol. 1986;17:1066–71.
143. Burke LM, Rush WI, Khoor A, et al. Alveolar adenoma: a histochemical, immunohistochemical, and ultrastructural analysis of 17 cases. Hum Pathol. 1999;30:158–67.
144. Dashiel GF. A case of dirofilariasis involving the lung. Am J Trop Med Hyg. 1961;10:37–8.
145. Goodman ML, Gore I. Pulmonary infarct secondary to *Dirofilaria larva*. Arch Intern Med. 1964;113:702–5.
146. Asimacopoulos PJ, Katras A, Christie B. Pulmonary dirofilariasis. The largest single-hospital experience. Chest. 1992;102:851–5.
147. Melanez de Campos JR, Barbas CS, Filomeno LT, et al. Human pulmonary dirofilariasis: analysis of 24 cases from Sao Paulo, Brazil. Chest. 1997;112:729–33.
148. Ro JY, Tsakalakis PJ, White VA, et al. Pulmonary dirofilariasis: the great imitator of primary or metastatic lung tumor. A clinicopathologic analysis of seven cases and a review of the literature. Hum Pathol. 1989;20:69–76.
149. Kahn FW, Wester SM, Agger WA. Pulmonary dirofilariasis and transitional cell carcinoma: benign lung nodules mimicking metastatic malignant neoplasms. Arch Intern Med. 1983;143:1259–60.
150. Neafie RC, Piggott J. Human pulmonary dirofilariasis. Arch Pathol. 1971;92:342–9.
151. Ulbright TM, Katzenstein ALA. Solitary necrotizing granulomas of the lung. Differentiating features and etiology. Am J Surg Pathol. 1980;4:13–28.
152. Flieder DB, Moran CA. Pulmonary dirofilariasis: a clinicopathologic study of 41 lesions in 39 patients. Hum Pathol. 1999;30:251–6.
153. Yousem SA, et al. Pulmonary hyalinizing granuloma. Am J Clin Pathol. 1987;87:1–6.
154. Young AS, et al. Pulmonary hyalinizing granuloma and retroperitoneal fibrosis in an adolescent. Pediatr Radiol. 2007;37:91–5.
155. Engleman P, et al. Pulmonary hyalinizing granuloma. Am Rev Respir Dis. 1977;115:997–1008.

Molecular Pathology of Lung Cancer

14

Luisa M. Solis and Ignacio I. Wistuba

Introduction

Lung cancer continues to be the most common and deadly malignancy in the USA and worldwide [1]. Current standard therapies include surgical resection, platinum-based doublet chemotherapy, and radiation therapy alone or in combination [2]. However, most lung cancers present at an advanced stage and are not amenable to curative surgery or radiotherapy [3]. The main challenge to improve the poor survival rate (5-year survival, 15 %) of this disease is to develop strategies to better stratify high-risk population for early diagnosis and to select the adequate treatment for different lung cancer subsets [4].

Lung tumors are the result of a multistep and complex process in which normal lung cells accumulate genetic and epigenetic abnormalities and evolve into cells with malignant biological capabilities, which represent the "hallmark of cancer" [5]. These biological capabilities include sustaining proliferative signaling, evading growth suppressors, resisting cell death, enabling replicative immortality, inducing angiogenesis, and activating invasion and metastasis [5]. The identification of an oncogene, or other specific products required by the tumor cells for sustained growth ("oncogene addiction"), followed by administration of a specific inhibitor to the target, is the basis of personalized cancer treatment [6]. Recent advances in understanding the complex biology of lung cancer, particularly "oncogene addictions," have provided new treatment targets and allowed the identification of subsets of tumors with unique molecular profiles that can predict response to therapy in this disease [3, 7].

The successful development of personalized therapy depends on the identification of a specific molecular target that drives cancer growth, subsequent validation of a clinically applicable biomarker, and development of a clinically sound and rational endpoint, coupled with understanding of the molecular mechanisms associated to tumor's resistance [8]. In this process, the analysis of molecular changes is becoming increasingly important and poses multiple challenges to adequately integrate both routine histopathology analysis and molecular testing into the clinical pathology diagnosis for selection of therapy.

In this chapter, we will describe the molecular abnormalities associated to the most common histological types of lung cancer. We will discuss the current state of molecular studies applied in clinical tissue samples for targeted therapy selection and some areas of active investigation in this field. We will describe the advantages and disadvantages of the currently available molecular pathology methodologies and the future research directions of lung cancer molecular pathology in the new era of targeted therapy and personalized medicine approaches.

Molecular Abnormalities of Lung Cancer by Histology Subtypes

Traditionally, lung cancer is classified in two major histological types, non-small cell lung carcinoma (NSCLC) and small-cell lung carcinoma (SCLC) [9]. Both tumor types have different clinical behavior, response to treatment, biology, and molecular characteristics. NSCLC grows and spreads much slower than SCLC and often is refractory to chemotherapy [10]. Depending on the stage of the disease, surgical-based approaches result in longer disease-free survival and potential cure of ~30 % of resected patients [11]. Although

L.M. Solis, M.D.
Department of Pathology, Unit 85, The University of Texas MD Anderson Cancer Center, 1515 Holcombe Boulevard, Houston, TX 77030, USA

I.I. Wistuba, M.D. (✉)
Department of Pathology and Thoracic/Head and Neck Medical Oncology, Unit 85, The University of Texas MD Anderson Cancer Center, 1515 Holcombe Boulevard, Houston, TX 77030, USA
e-mail: iiwistuba@mdanderson.org

A. Weissferdt, C.A. Moran, *Diagnostic Pathology of Pleuropulmonary Neoplasia*,
DOI 10.1007/978-1-4419-0787-5_14, © Springer Science+Business Media New York 2013

Table 14.1 Summary of molecular abnormalities associated with the lung adenocarcinoma and squamous cell carcinoma histologies

Gene	Molecular change	Adenocarcinoma (%)	Squamous cell carcinoma (%)
EGFR	Mutation	10–40	Very rare
	Amplification/CNG	15	40
	IHC overexpression	15–39	~58
KRAS	Mutation	10–30	Very rare
BRAF	Mutation	2	3
EML4-ALK	Translocation	3–9	Very rare
LKB1	Mutation	8–30	0–5
HER2	Mutation	2–3	Very rare
	Amplification	8	2
	IHC overexpression	35	1
TP53	LOH and mutations	50–70	60–70
FGFR1	Amplification	1–3	8–22
PIK3CA	Amplification/CNG	2–6	33–35
	Mutation	2	2

CNG copy number gain, *IHC* immunohistochemistry, *LOH* loss of heterozygosity

most NSCLC are associated with smoking, a significant proportion of them (10–15 %) occur also in never-smoker patients, mostly with adenocarcinoma tumor histology. Importantly, these tumors harbor targetable genetic abnormalities such as mutations of epidermal growth factor receptor gene (*EGFR)* and translocation of the echinoderm microtubule-associated protein-like 4 and anaplastic lymphoma kinase (*EML4-ALK*) genes [12, 13]. Recently, specific targetable genetic abnormalities have been also described in smoking-related squamous cell carcinoma (SCC) of the lung, including the fibroblast growth factor receptor-1 (*FGFR1*) gene amplification [14] and the discoidin domain-containing receptor-2 (*DDR2*) gene mutation [15].

On the other hand, SCLC has a unique natural history with earlier development of widespread metastases, a uniform initial response to chemotherapy and radiation, and a poor 5-year survival rate of ~5 %, especially due to the almost certain recurrence after chemotherapy [16]. SCLCs are invariably associated to tobacco smoking, have a neuroendocrine phenotype, and are characterized for frequent inactivation of the tumor suppressor genes (TSG) *TP53* and *retinoblastoma* (*RB*) and activation of *MYC* oncogene [17–19]. However, there are no specific novel molecular targets recently described in SCLC.

Non-small Cell Lung Carcinoma

NSCLCs are histologically classified in adenocarcinomas, SCC, adenosquamous cell carcinoma, large cell carcinoma, and sarcomatoid carcinomas [9]. Both adenocarcinoma (40 %) and SCC (30 %) are the most common histological subtypes [9]. We will discuss recent advances on the molecular abnormalities associated to the pathogenesis of both adenocarcinoma and SCC histologies, with special emphasis on targetable genes, proteins, and pathways (Table 14.1 and Fig. 14.1).

Adenocarcinoma

Lung adenocarcinomas are histologically and biologically heterogeneous tumors [9, 20]. Most adenocarcinomas (~90 %) have mixed histological growth patterns, and the attempts to establish correlations between histological features and molecular abnormalities have been unsuccessful [9, 21]. Recently, the International Association for the Study of Lung Cancer (IASLC) proposed a new working classification of lung adenocarcinoma to be used to potentially improve correlations with clinical, radiological, and molecular features of this tumor type [21].

The preneoplastic lesion suggested to precede at least subset of adenocarcinomas, particularly those with lepidic or bronchioloalveolar (BAC) features, is the atypical adenomatous hyperplasia (AAH) [22, 23]. The molecular abnormalities described in AAH include deletions or loss of heterozygocity (LOH) in regions containing TSGs (chromosomes/genes 3p/*FUS-1*, 18 %; 9p/$p16^{INK4a}$, 13 %, 9q/*TSC1*, 53 %; 16p/*TSC2*, 6 %; and 17p/*TP53*, 6 %), *KRAS* mutation (codon 12, 39 %), upregulation of telomerase activity (27–78 %), loss of expression of LKB1 protein, and overexpression of cyclin D1 (70 %), p53 (10–58 %), survivin (48 %), and HER-2/Neu (7 %) proteins [24–26]. The respiratory structures and the specific epithelial cell types involved in the origin of most lung adenocarcinomas are unknown, and candidates include Clara cells, alveolar type II cells, and an epithelial cell located at the junction between the terminal bronchiole and alveolus, termed bronchioloalveolar stem cell [25]. In addition, lung adenocarcinoma may arise from

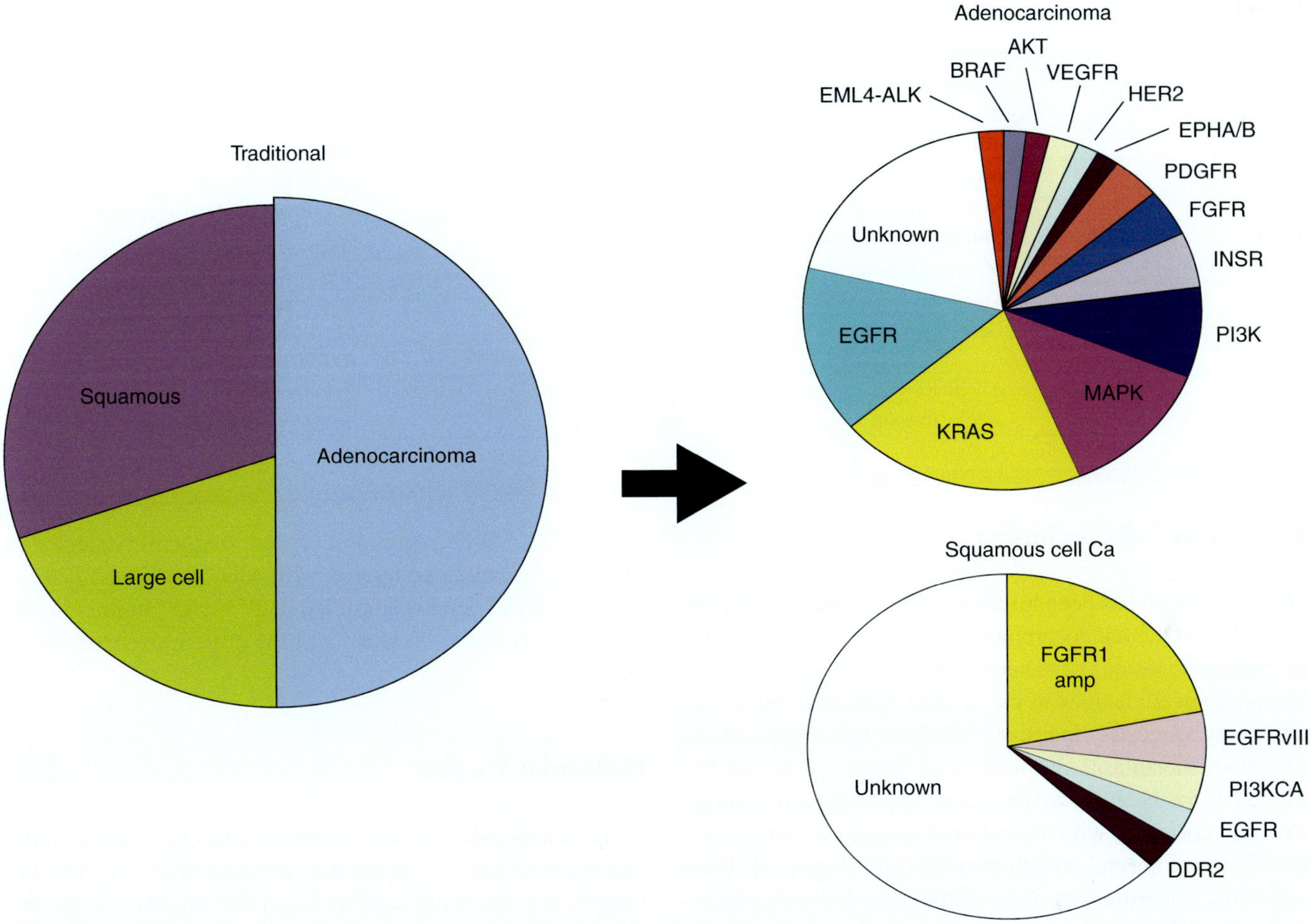

Fig. 14.1 Paradigm changes in the classification of NSCLC. Targetable abnormalities of multiple oncogenes, particularly mutations, translocations, and gene amplifications, have been recently discovered in both adenocarcinoma and squamous cell carcinoma histologies. All abnormalities are referred to gene mutations, except *EML4-ALK* rearrangement and *FGFR1* amplification (*amp*)

bronchial or bronchiolar epithelia since *EGFR* activating mutation has been found in normal bronchial epithelium adjacent to *EGFR*-mutant adenocarcinomas in 43 % of the patients [25].

Most (70–80 %) lung adenocarcinomas express the thyroid transcription factor-1 (TTF-1) protein encoded by the gene *TITF-1*, also termed *NKX2-1* [27, 28]. TTF-1 is a homeodomain-containing transcription factor expressed at the onset of lung morphogenesis in epithelial cells and throughout fetal lung development and plays an important role in lung morphogenesis including the formation of the lung parenchyma and the subsequent differentiation of the respiratory epithelial cells [29, 30]. In the postnatal lung, TTF-1 expression is restricted primarily to alveolar type II cells and subsets of non-ciliated bronchiolar epithelial cells [31]. The *TITF-1* gene has been suggested to be a lineage-specific oncogene, and gene amplification has been detected in ~11 % of lung adenocarcinomas, which correlated with poor survival rates in surgically resected tumors [28, 32, 33]. However, conversely to the putative oncogene properties, high level of TTF-1 protein expression in adenocarcinomas has been correlated with smaller tumor size, lower pathologic tumor-nodes-metastasis (TNM) stage, and better survival rates [28, 32].

At least two different pathways have been identified in the pathogenesis of lung adenocarcinoma, a smoking-associated activation of the *KRAS* signaling, and non-smoking-associated activation of the *EGFR* signaling [12] (Table 14.2). Lung adenocarcinomas arising in never-smokers are characterized by significantly higher frequencies of *EGFR* (54 %) and *HER2* (3 %) tyrosine kinase domain activating mutations and *EML4-ALK* translocations (9 %). In addition, these tumors demonstrated certain specific types of *KRAS* (G-to-A transition; GGT12GAT) and *TP53* (G-to-A transitions) mutations and higher expression of certain microRNAs (miR), including miR-21 and miR-38 [12, 34–36]. Lung adenocarcinomas arising in ever-smokers are characterized, among others, by significantly higher frequencies of *KRAS* (up to 30 %; mostly G-to-T or G-to-C transversions), *TP53* (70 %; mostly G-to-T transversions and A-to-G transitions), and *LKB1* mutations (14 %) [12, 37–40].

Table 14.2 Molecular characteristics in lung adenocarcinoma arising in never-smokers and smokers

Gene	Molecular change	Never-smokers	Smokers
EGFR	Mutations	25–60 %	5–10 %
ERBB2	Mutations	~3 %	~1 %
EML4-ALK	Translocation	~6 %	Rare
KRAS	Mutations	5–15 %	20–30 %
	Mutation pattern	G→A transitions	G→T or G→C transversions
TP53	Mutations	50 %	70 %
	Mutation pattern	G→A transitions	G→T transversions**
LKB1	Mutations	Rare	Frequent
Tumor suppressor genes	Genes methylated	Relatively low	Relatively high; e.g., *p16* and *RASSF1A*
	Allelic loss	Relatively low	Relatively high
	Allelic loss sites	9p, 12p, 19q	3p, 6q, 9p, 16p, 17p, 19p

Squamous Cell Carcinoma

SCC of the lung has been histologically and molecularly less studied than the adenocarcinoma histology. However, SCC preneoplastic lesions have been better characterized [22, 41]. Morphological changes in the normal bronchial epithelium that may precede invasive SCC include hyperplasia, squamous metaplasia, dysplasia, and carcinoma in situ [25, 41, 42]. It has been shown that these sequential morphologic changes correlate with cumulative genetic abnormalities, which start at normal bronchial epithelium stage [25]. These molecular abnormalities are usually extensive and multifocally distributed throughout the bronchial tree of NSCLC patients and smokers, who are individuals at high risk of developing lung cancer [42–44]. The molecular abnormalities associated with the early pathogenesis of SCC include allelic losses at multiple regions of chromosome 3p and 9p21 ($p16^{INK4a}$), subsequent losses of chromosome regions 8p21–23, 13q14 (*RB*), and 17p13 (*TP53*). Additionally, it has been shown that $p16^{INK4a}$ methylation increases during the progression of SCC preneoplastic lesions [25, 42].

Invasive SCC frequently harbors multiple genetic abnormalities, including activation of several oncogenes (e.g., *SOX2*, *FGFR1*, *PIK3CA*, *EGFR*, and *DDR2*) and inactivation of TSGs (e.g., *TP53* and $p16^{INK4a}$). Recently, the sex determining region Y-box 2 (*SOX2*) gene has been suggested to be a lineage-survival oncogene in lung SCC [45]. SOX2 is a transcription factor coded by a gene located at 3q26.33. SOX2 protein is implicated in the maintenance of embryonic stem cells and the induction of pluripotent stem cells from various different cell types and plays important roles in multiple developmental processes, including lung branching [31]. This protein is selectively expressed in conducting airway epithelial cells, where it regulates basal, ciliated, and secretory cell differentiation [31]. In the lung, SOX2 is expressed in normal bronchial epithelium, alveolar bronchiolization changes, and preneoplastic squamous lesions [46]. In NSCLC, SOX2 expression is more frequently detected in SCC (90 %) when compared with adenocarcinoma (20 %) [46, 47]. *SOX2* gene is amplified in 20 % SCC tumors in cell lung cancers and correlates with the protein overexpression [45, 46, 48].

Molecular Targets

In the last decade, significant progress has been made in the characterization of molecular abnormalities in NSCLC tumors that are being used as molecular targets and predictive biomarkers for patients' selection for targeted therapy (Fig. 14.1). Some of these molecular changes occur preferentially in adenocarcinoma or SCC and others in both NSCLC histologies.

Epidermal Growth Factor Receptor (EGFR)

This protein, member of the receptor tyrosine kinase (RTK) family, is a cell-surface receptor protein that responds to signals conveyed by extracellular growth factors [49, 50]. Following binding of these growth factor ligands, EGFR homo- or heterodimerizes with other RTKs and triggers the activation of two major pathways: PI3K/AKT/mTOR and RAS/RAF/MEK/MAPK [49, 50]. These signaling pathways are important in the tumorigenic process, including proliferation, apoptosis, angiogenesis, and invasion [50–52].

EGFR molecular abnormalities are common events in NSCLC and include gene activating mutation, gene copy number gain and amplification, and overexpression of the protein and its ligands [50]. Mutations of *EGFR* occur in ~24 % of NSCLCs and are limited to the first four exons of the tyrosine kinase (TK) domain (exons 18–21) (Fig. 14.2). The most frequent mutations are in-frame deletions in exon 19 (44 % of all mutations) and missense mutations in exon 21 (41 % of all mutations) [35, 53]. In addition, in-frame duplications/insertions occurring in exon 20 have been

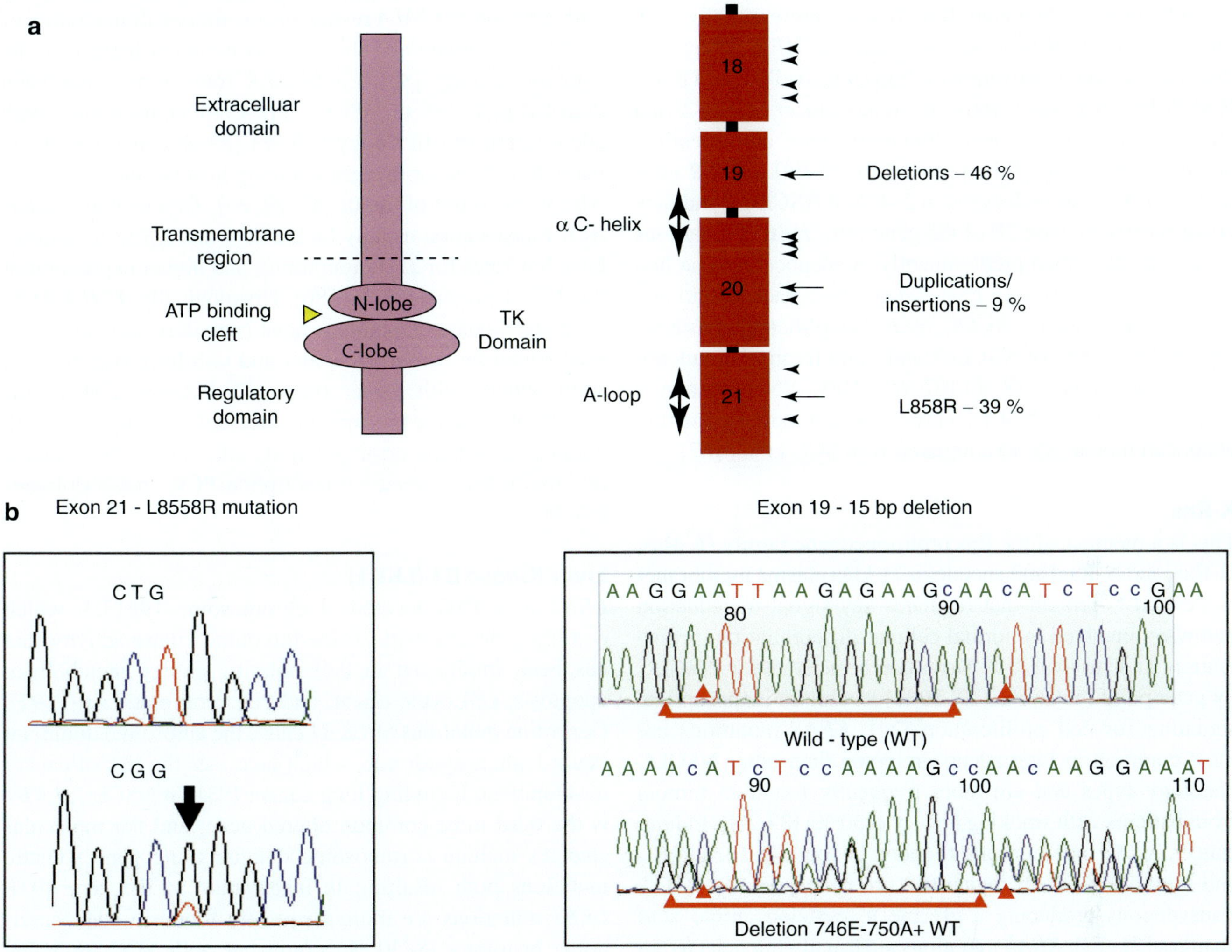

Fig. 14.2 *EGFR* mutations in lung adenocarcinomas. *Panel* **a**: location and frequency of most frequent activating *EGFR* mutations occurring in lung adenocarcinomas affecting exons 18–21, which encode the tyrosine kinase (*TK*) domain portion of the protein. *Panel* **b**: representative examples of PCR-based Sanger sequencing illustrating L858R point mutation at exon 21 and a 15-base pair (bp) deletion at exon 21 in lung adenocarcinoma tumors

described in about 5 % of the mutant cases, and rare missense mutations occur in multiple sites [35]. *EGFR* mutations occur predominantly in adenocarcinoma (~20–48 % versus other NSCLC histologies ~2 %) and are more frequent in never-smokers (54 % versus ever-smokers 16 %) and female patients (49 % versus male patients 19 %) [35]. Activating *EGFR* mutations strongly correlate with clinical response to tyrosine kinase inhibitors (TKIs) and currently are the most important criterion to select patients for EGFR TKI therapy in lung cancer [8, 35, 53, 54].

EGFR gene copy number gain (CNG), high polysomy and gene amplification, has been detected in 22–54 % of NSCLCs by fluorescence in situ hybridization (FISH), being more frequently detected in SCCs (CNG, 29 %; gene amplification, 11 %) than adenocarcinomas (CNG, 11 %; gene amplification, 4 %) [55]. *EGFR* CNG is more frequently detected in more advanced, stages III/IV, tumors (up to 54 %) [56–61]. Although some studies showed that CNG may be a predictor of EGFR TKI treatment, these data have not be confirmed, and this marker is currently not used clinically [62]. Overexpression of EGFR protein has been reported in ~46 % NSCLCs [63] and is higher in SCC (~58 %) compared with adenocarcinoma (15–39 %) [63]. In a subset of NSCLCs, the canonical EGFR ligands, particularly epidermal growth factor (EGF), transforming growth factor--α(alpha) (TGF-α) and amphiregulin, are overexpressed in tumor cells, leading to EGFR activation through an autocrine loop [64, 65].

HER-2/Neu

This is a transmembrane receptor and member of the RTK family that drives and regulates cell proliferation [66]. The HER-2/Neu receptor does not have a known ligand and is putatively activated by homodimerization with other HER-2/

Neu receptors or by heterodimerization, preferentially with either EGFR or HER-3 [66]. Activation of HER-2/Neu produces downstream activation of PI3K/AKT/mTOR and RAS/RAF/MEK pathways [66]. In lung cancer, HER-2/Neu abnormalities include gene mutation, gene amplification, and overexpression of the protein [36, 67–69]. *HER-2* gene mutations have been detected in 2–4 % of NSCLCs, and they occur mostly in exon 20 of the gene [36]. *HER-2* mutations have been described predominantly in adenocarcinoma histology and patients with East-Asian ethnic background and never-smoker history [36, 68]. *HER-2* amplification has been reported in 4–5 % of NSCLCs and more frequent in adenocarcinoma histology (8 %) [67, 69]. HER-2/Neu protein is highly expressed in NSCLCs (16 %), being more frequent in adenocarcinoma (35 %) compared with SCC (1 %) [67].

K-Ras

This is a member of the Ras proto-oncogene family (K-Ras, H-Ras, and N-Ras) and encodes a 21-kDa plasma membrane-associated G-protein that regulates key signal transduction pathways involved in normal cellular differentiation, proliferation, and survival [70]. K-ras can be activated in NSCLC by gene point mutations (10–30 %) leading to inappropriate signaling for cell proliferation [24]. *KRAS* mutations are most common in lung adenocarcinoma than other NSCLC histology types and are more frequently found in tumors from patients with smoking history (~30 %) [37, 38]. In lung cancer, *KRAS* mutations are found in codons 12, 13, and 61, and they (42 % of all mutations) are mainly GGT to TGT transversions producing a glycine to cysteine amino acid changes [71–73]. *KRAS* mutations are usually not detected in *EGFR*-mutant tumors and have been associated to low response rates to EGFR TKI therapies [73–75]. Ras is considered a not targetable molecule; therefore, recent studies have evaluated the activation of the Ras downstream pathway, RAS/RAF/MEK, as a potential target for therapy in lung cancer [76, 77].

Echinoderm Microtubule-Associated Protein-Like 4 and Anaplastic Lymphoma Kinase (EML4-ALK) Fusion Protein

ALK is a RTK belonging to the insulin receptor superfamily [78]. Over the last decade, a variety of mechanisms leading to aberrant *ALK* activation have been identified in hematologic and solid tumors [79–81]. In lung cancer, aberrant *ALK* expression has been identified in a subset of NSCLC, and this abnormality consists in the formation of a fusion transcript with cell transforming activity, which is the product of a translocation of *EML4* gene located at chromosome 2p21 and the *ALK* gene located at 2p23 [82] (Fig. 14.3). The encoded protein contains the N-terminal part of *EML4* and the intracellular catalytic domain of *ALK* [82]. Replacement of the extracellular and transmembrane domain of ALK protein with a region of EML4 results in constitutive dimerization of the kinase domain and thereby a consequent increase in its catalytic activity [82]. *EML4-ALK* translocation has been detected in 1–7 % of NSCLCs, predominantly tumors with adenocarcinoma histology (13 %) [82–86], particularly in patients with never or light smoking history, and associated with young onset of tumor [83, 84, 86]. Tumors with *EML4-ALK* translocation usually lack *EGFR* and *KRAS* mutations, have low rates for *TP53* mutations, and higher expression of the TTF-1 protein [83, 84, 86]. Histologically, *EML4-ALK*-rearranged adenocarcinomas have been described to have a predominantly combined acinar and cribiform patterns or a solid pattern with signet ring cells [82–87]. *EML4-ALK* translocations have multiple distinct isoforms (up to 9) with demonstrated transforming activity and that can be detected by multiplex reverse transcription-PCR methodologies [88–90].

Liver Kinase B1 (LKB1)

LKB1 is a TSG located at chromosome 19p13.3, which codifies a protein with serine-threonine kinase activity that has been implicated in cell polarity, energy metabolism, apoptosis, cell cycle arrest, and cell proliferation [91, 92]. Germ-line mutations of *LKB1* cause the autosomal dominant Peutz-Jeghers syndrome, which increases the risk of cancer development, including lung cancer [93]. In NSCLC, *LKB1* is the third most common altered gene, and the molecular changes include chromosome deletions and gene somatic mutations both resulting in inactivation of the gene [93]. *LKB1* mutations are more frequently found in adenocarcinoma histology (8–30 %) compared with SCC (0–5 %). These mutations have been more frequently detected in smoker patients (14 %) compared with never-smokers (3 %) and in patients with a Western (17 %) compared with patients with East-Asian (5 %) origins [39, 40]. The most frequent *LKB1* mutation is G to T transversion and occurs at multiple sites of the gene, without hot spots [40]. *LKB1* mutations overlap with alterations at other genes, including *KRAS*, $p16^{INK4a}$, *TP53*, *MYC*, and *PIK3CA* [40, 93, 94].

Fibroblast Growth Factor Receptor-1 (FGFR1)

This is a transmembrane TK and member of the FGFR TK that comprises four kinases, FGFR-1 to 4 [95, 96]. FGFRs and their ligands, the fibroblast growth factors (FGFs), constitute a robust signaling system orchestrating many important signaling pathways and biological responses [97]. FGFRs play important roles in human development and cell proliferation, differentiation, survival, and migration [98]. FGF/FGFR signaling modulates distinct downstream pathways including RAS/MAPK and PI3K/AKT and stimulates proliferation and cell migration and acts as pro-survival/anti-apoptotic signals in many cell types [97]. In addition, FGF/FGFR signaling plays a role in angiogenesis by influencing

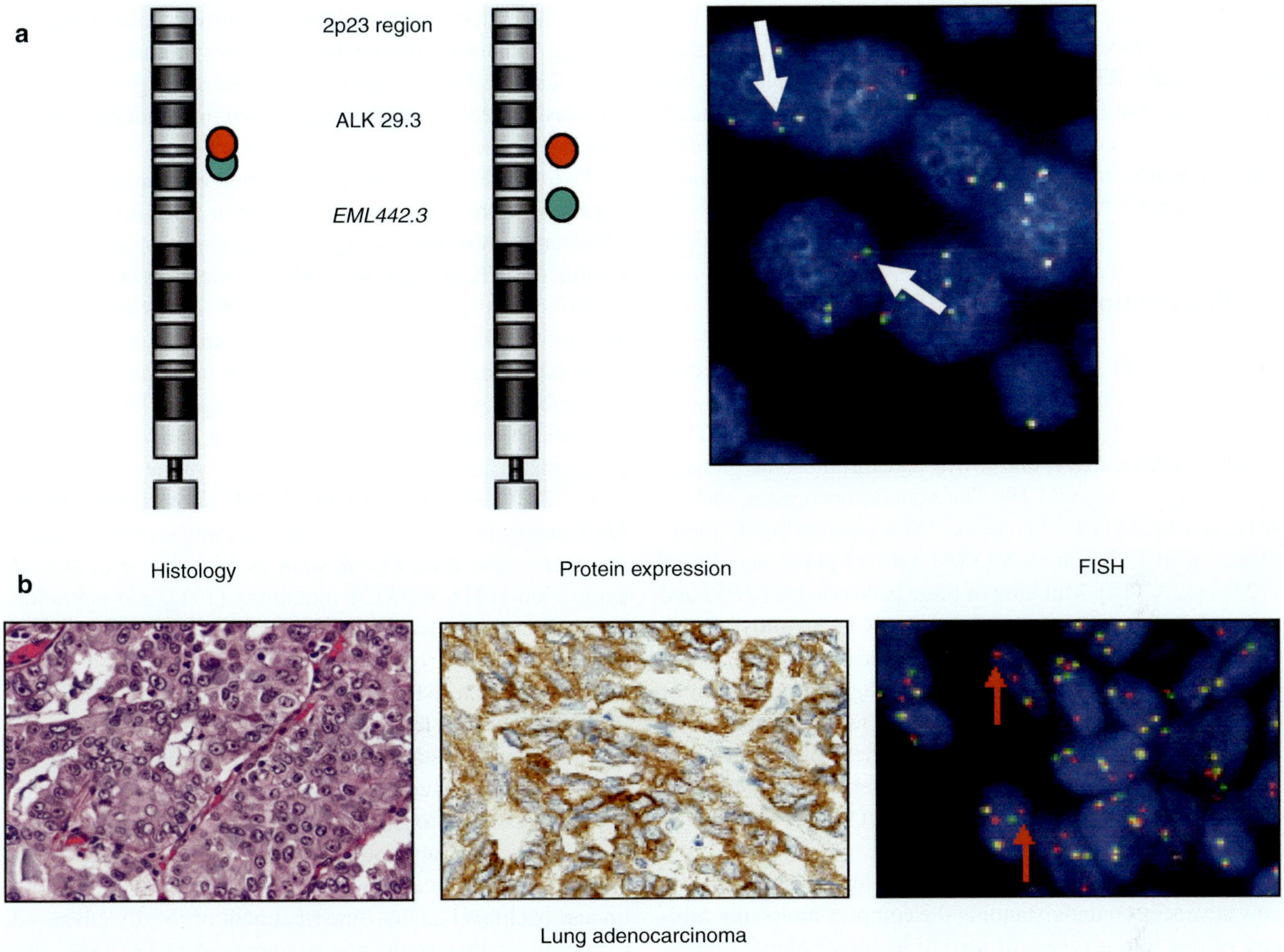

Fig. 14.3 *EML4-ALK* rearrangement in lung adenocarcinomas. *Panel* **a**: representation of the translocation of *EML4* (*green signal*) and *ALK* (*red signal*) genes in the chromosome 2p23 region and a representative example of the fluorescence in situ hybridization (*FISH*) "break-apart" test showing separation of the two signals (*white arrows*) in a nucleus of a lung cancer cell line harboring the *EML4-ALK* rearrangement. *Panel* **b**: representative microphotographies of histology (H&E staining), ALK protein expression by immunohistochemistry (*IHC*), and FISH "break-apart" assay in a tissue specimen of lung adenocarcinomas with the *EML4-ALK* rearrangement. The histology shows malignant cells with intracellular mucus accumulation; the IHC depicts brown staining corresponding to ALK expression in malignant cells, and the FISH test shows nucleus of cells with "break-apart" signal (*red arrows*)

other key signaling molecules such as hepatocyte growth factor (HGF) and vascular endothelial growth factor (VEGF) [96, 97]. In solid and hematological malignancies, deregulation of the FGF/FGFR is the result of *FGFR* genes activating mutations, chromosomal translocation, aberrant transcriptional regulation, and amplification [96, 97]. In lung cancer, amplification of *FGFR1* (chromosome 8p11–12) is a driver event in NSCLC, predominantly in SCC histology subtype (8–22 %) compared with adenocarcinomas (1–3 %) [14]. In vitro and in vivo studies have shown that *FGFR1*-amplified cell lines are sensitive to pan-FGFR1 inhibitors, while non-amplified cell lines are resistant to those agents [98]. Targeting *FGFR1* function may represent a promising therapeutic target in SCC of the lung [96, 99].

Phosphoinositide-3-Kinase Catalytic Alpha (PIK3CA)

This gene codes for the catalytic subunit p110 of class IA phosphatidylinositol 3-kinases (PI3Ks). PI3Ks are lipid kinases that regulate several cellular processes such as proliferation, growth, apoptosis, and cytoskeletal rearrangement [100]. Molecular abnormalities of the p110 subunit *PIK3CA* can lead to the activation of the PI3K pathway [101, 102]. In NSCLC, copy number gain (>3 copies per cell) of *PIK3CA* is a common abnormality, predominantly in SCCs (33–35 %) compared to adenocarcinomas (2–6 %) [103, 104]. Mutations in the helical or kinase domain of *PIK3CA* have been reported in very low frequencies (2–6 %) in NSCLC [101, 104–106]. Recently it has been shown that the acquired *PIK3CA* mutations lead to resistance to treatment with EGFR TKIs [107]. In addition, the PI3K pathway can be activated by the activation of oncogenic RTKs acting upstream or phosphatase and tensin homolog (*PTEN*) gene loss [108, 109]. PI3K and its downstream effectors, PTEN, mTOR, and AKT, are potential therapeutic targets for NSCLC therapy and are evaluated in clinical trials for lung cancer [109, 110].

Small-Cell Lung Carcinoma (SCLC)

SCLC is one of the most genetically complex human cancers. SCLC has recurrent deletions in chromosomes 3p, 5q, 13q, and 17p that contain important TSGs such as *TP53, RASSF1, FUS1, FHIT, and RARB* and chromosome gains of 1p, 2p, 3q, 5p, 8q, and 19p that contain oncogenes such as *MYC* and *KRAS* [19, 111]. Some TSGs are also highly methylated in SCLC such as *RASSF1* (90 %) [112] and *RARB* (72 %) [113, 114]. Mutation of these genes such as *TP53* and retinoblastoma (*RB*) occurs in most SCLCs (~90 %) [19, 115, 116]. SCLCs have higher frequencies of overexpression of the *MYC* oncogene (18–31 %) through amplification or transcriptional deregulation; the *MYC* family functions as transcription factors for genes in a variety of cellular processes including cell growth, cell proliferation, and apoptosis. Upregulation of anti-apoptotic BCL2 is present in approximately 75–95 % of SCLC [117].

For SCLC, the targeted treatment options are limited, and new advances on understanding the complex molecular biology of this tumor type will help to identify potential therapeutic targets and predictive markers of treatment benefit [18, 118]. Currently, there are several clinical trials targeting pathways activated in SCLC such as the PI3K/AKT/mTOR pathway, VEGF/VEGFR, HGF/HGFR, IGF-1R, and the hedgehog signaling pathway [118].

Molecular Studies in Lung Cancer Clinical Samples

Clinical Applications

Current treatments of most lung cancers rely on the precise histological and molecular characterization of the tumors. The recent advances in NSCLC targeted therapy require the identification of a panel of molecular abnormalities of tumor specimens [7] (Fig. 14.4). It has been shown in advanced lung cancer that cisplatin/gemcitabine offered a significantly longer survival compared to cisplatin/pemetrexed in patients with SCC [119]. These findings prompted restriction of the pemetrexed, an antifolate drug, to patients with NSCLC with "non-squamous" histology only [120]. Pemetrexed is a potent inhibitor of thymidylate synthase and other folate-dependent enzymes, including dihydrofolate reductase and glycinamide ribonucleotide formyltransferase [121, 122]. The mechanisms involved in the varying outcomes of patients treated with pemetrexed based on tumor histological type are unknown.

Two EGFR inhibitors, gefitinib and erlotinib, have been approved in the USA for second-line or third-line treatment of advanced NSCLC [54, 123]. These compounds reversibly inhibit the TK activity of EGFR. Patients with activating mutation of the TK domain of *EGFR* are associated with sensitivity to EGFR TKIs [124]. Unfortunately, some patients with activating *EGFR* mutations that respond initially to erlotinib and gefitinib subsequently relapse [125–127]. This resistance appears to occur through a range of different mechanisms, including a second *EGFR* mutation (50 %) in exon 20 (*T790M* and *D761Y*) [128], amplification of the *MET* oncogene (21 %) [129, 130], activation of RTK family members other than *EGFR* such as high levels of IGF-IR expression [131], *PI3KCA* mutations [107], and epithelial-to-mesenchymal transition phenomenon (EMT) [132], although the underlying biological processes linking these events to drug resistance have not all been fully elucidated [52]. Interestingly, lung tumors with *EGFR* activating mutation and adenocarcinoma histology have demonstrated SCLC features when tissue has been examined after the tumor became resistance to EGFR TKI therapy [107].

A monoclonal antibody directed against VEGF, bevacizumab, is currently approved in combination with carboplatin and paclitaxel as first-line treatment of locally advanced, recurrent, or metastatic non-squamous NSCLC [54]. This drug is only administered to patients whose tumors have non-squamous histology because of the association with fatal hemorrhagic events in this tumor type after cavitation and is not recommended for patients with hemorrhage or recent hemoptysis [119]. The VEGF signaling is a critical mediator in the angiogenesis process, which is a necessary step in tumor growth, metastasis, and malignancy [133, 134]. In lung cancer, overexpression of VEGF and higher microvascular density are associated to poor prognosis [133, 134]. Recently VEGFR-2 gene (*KDR*) copy number gain (>4 gene copies/cell by quantitative PCR) has been found to be a common event in both SCCs (35 %) and adenocarcinomas (31 %), and it was associated to resistance to platinum-based adjuvant therapy [135]. However, there are no data available that *KDR* CNG could be associated to response to VEGF/VEGFR targeted therapies.

A phase I clinical trial using crizotinib, an oral inhibitor of the ALK and MET TKs, showed that this drug is effective against advanced NSCLC carrying activated *EML4-ALK* translocation assessed by a fluorescence in situ hybridization (FISH) utilizing an *ALK* "break-apart" probe [136]. The cut-off criteria for positive *ALK* "break-apart" FISH test is the presence of >15 % tumor cells having split *ALK* 5′ and 3′

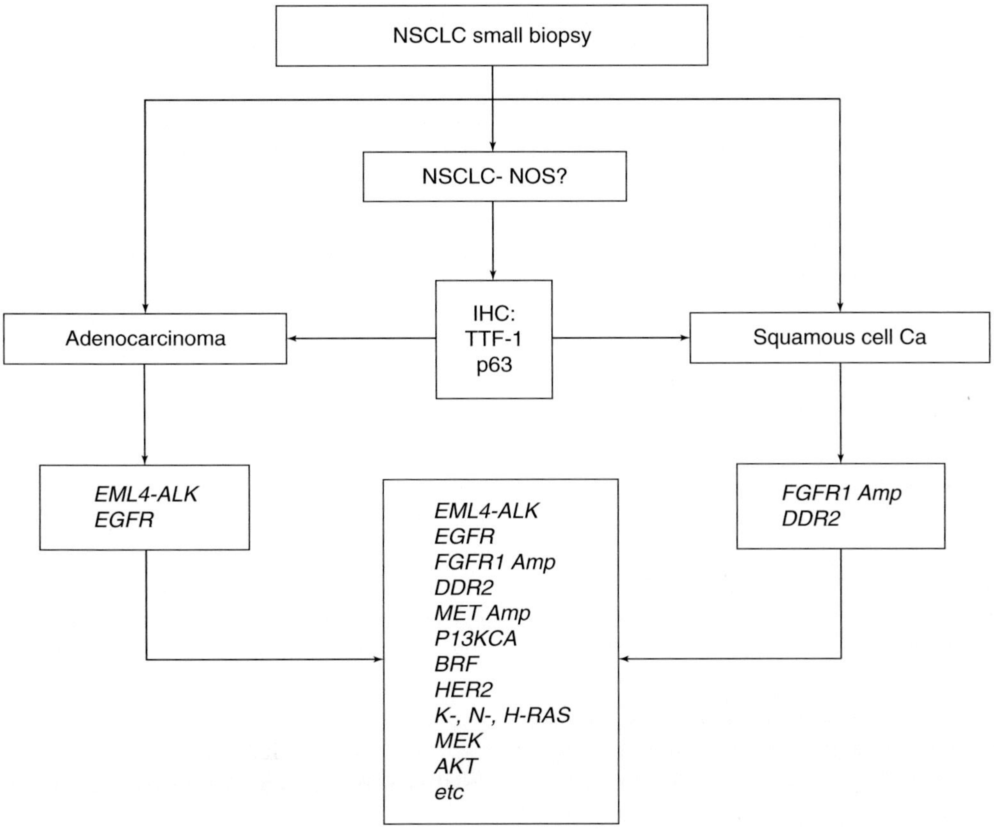

Fig. 14.4 Suggested algorithm for molecular testing of small diagnostic NSCLC biopsies. If the histology diagnosis is adenocarcinomas or squamous cell carcinoma, testing of a limited panel of targetable molecular abnormalities in standard of care or clinical trial settings is recommended. However, if the diagnosis of NSCLC no otherwise specified (NOS) is made, a limited panel of immunohistochemical (*IHC*) markers is available to better define the histology. However, the utilization of multiplexed methodologies (SNaPshot Sequenom) or next-generation of sequencing for testing multiple mutations with a small amount of DNA make possible that a comprehensive panel of actionable mutations can be tested in all samples regardless of the NSCLC subtype. All genetic abnormalities are referred to gene mutations, except *EML4-ALK* rearrangement and *FGFR1* and *MET* amplifications (*Amp*)

probe signals or had isolated 3′ signals [136]. The overall partial and complete tumor response rate observed in patients with NSCLC tumors with positive FISH test and treated with crizotinib was of 57 %, and the rate of stable disease was 33 % [136]. It has been shown that patients with NSCLC *EML4-ALK* rearrangement treated with ALK inhibitors developed resistance [137]. The genetic alterations associated with documented acquired resistance to crizotinib are amplification of the *EML4-ALK* gene followed by secondary mutations within the kinase domain of *EML4-ALK* (*L1196M*, *C1156Y*, and *F1174L*) [137–139]. However, second-generation ALK TKIs or Hsp90 inhibitors may be effective in treating crizotinib-resistant tumors harboring secondary mutations [138].

Translational Research

Most biomarkers discovered and used in clinical applications to date consist of a single genetic mutation ("driver-mutation"), or gene amplification or translocation, but in many patients or cancer types, these single biomarkers are not sufficient to select patients for targeted therapies. One reason might be the fact that in many cases, multiple changes in tumor cells, rather than a single modification, lead to activation of selective and often interactive molecular pathways promoting tumor growth and survival. In addition, various targeted treatment regimens have been shown to result in the activation of alternative, compensatory molecular pathways that continue to promote cancer cell survival.

The development of new technologies such as protein and gene arrays has allowed researchers to screen the whole genome, proteome, transcriptome, and metabolome for new biomarkers in tumor tissue, serum, plasma, or other human body fluid and develop genetic, proteomic, or metabolic profiles, or "signatures," to better reflect the complex molecular aberrations within a single tumor [140–143]. Currently, most molecular discovery research in human tumors is performed retrospectively using residual tissue specimens obtained from surgical resection procedures for treatment or diagnostic intent. However, to succeed in developing more effective novel molecular targeted therapies and predictive molecular markers for personalized treatment of human cancer, our growing understanding of cancer biology and these powerful research tools must be directly applied to clinically relevant human tumor specimens. Therefore, for the most accurate molecular characterization of the disease at every stage of its evolution and discovery of new predictive biomarkers of sensitivity or resistance that can guide treatment selections for each patient, it is critical to sample and analyze tumors at each time point of clinical decision-making.

Given the paucity of effective predictive biomarkers in most cancers and the inherent harm in assigning patients to ineffective treatment regimens, biomarker discovery and validation should only be performed through rigorously controlled tissue/biomarker-based clinical trials; thus, new paradigms for clinical trial development must include mandated tissue and blood collection at the critical time points. However, much of this tissue is likely to be small specimens obtained from advanced metastatic lung tumors as core needle biopsies (CNB) and/or fine needle aspiration (FNA), which may limit molecular/genomic analysis with currently available methodologies and technologies. Therefore, there is a need to adapt the new emerging methodologies for molecular profiling to CNB and FNA specimens by improving the current technology or applying ancillary techniques such as the whole genome amplification for DNA sequencing analyses.

Most Relevant Molecular Pathology Methodologies

Immunohistochemistry (IHC)

Immunohistochemistry is a widely used technique to detect the presence and levels of expression of a specific protein. In lung cancer, the use of IHC is currently used for histopathology diagnosis and classification of tumors, particularly when small tissue specimens are examined. The most common IHC markers used to subtype NSCLC are cytokeratin 7 and TTF-1, which are positive in most adenocarcinomas, and p63, p40 and cytokeratins 5/6, which are positive in most SCCs [7]. In the research settings, the use of IHC markers has enabled the study of the correlation between the expression of biologically relevant proteins and clinicopathological features, including outcome and prediction of benefit to certain cytotoxic and molecularly targeted treatments. One example of these markers is the excision repair cross-complementation group 1 (ERCC1), a protein involved in repair of DNA platinum adducts and stalled DNA replication forks, which has been suggested as a potential marker to predict the response to platinum-based adjuvant therapy [144]; however, these findings have not validated in independent clinical datasets and not used in routine clinical practice in lung cancer.

The use of IHC to determine protein expression has several advantages. First, it is a technique widely used in pathology laboratories that can be used in formalin-fixed and paraffin-embedded (FFPE) tumor tissues. Second, it allows the identification of the protein expression in specific types of cells and distinct subcellular localization. Third, the levels of protein expression can be quantified. However, the utilization of IHC has some disadvantage, including the frequent presence of nonspecific staining due to antibodies cross-reactivity, the ample variety of methodologies and antibodies usually used and reported, and the diversity of scoring systems applied among laboratories. To overcome these problems, it is mandatory that proper relevant tissues or cells with known protein expression are used in the optimization of the IHC methodology, and it is highly recommended that trained pathologists interpret the IHC staining. The utilization of image analysis systems to assess IHC protein expression, although promising, has not shown to be useful in assessing protein expression in lung cancer tissue specimens for biomarker analysis.

Fluorescence In Situ Hybridization (FISH)

This is a cytogenetic technique that uses fluorescent-labeled probes to hybridize specific sequences of DNA on chromosomes [63]. It is applied to visualize chromosome deletions, amplification, and structural rearrangements. The main advantage of this technique is that it allows the in situ localization of the specific sequences and the simultaneous detection of multiple sites by using hybridization probes labeled with different fluorophores. The main disadvantage of FISH is the need for additional equipment for analysis such as dark-field microscopy and multiband fluorescent filters. Chromogenic in situ hybridization (CISH) is a variant of in situ hybridization technique that visualizes the specific DNA sequence by a peroxidase reaction and allows the visualization in a light microscope [145]. The main inconvenience of this method is that limits the use of different labeled probes to target multiple sites; however, recent advances in methodologies permit the use of dual colors to target two sequencing sites and enable the visualization of tissue architecture and cytomorphology [146].

Nucleic Acid Sequencing Techniques

Currently, the most used technique for DNA sequencing is direct sequencing previous PCR amplification of extracted DNA [147–150]. There are several sequencing methods available for mutation analysis applied to DNA extracted from tumor tissue specimens, including lung cancer.

Sanger Sequencing

Sanger sequencing is a chain terminator-based sequencing technique [148]. Currently, it is one of the preferred sequencing methods to detect mutations of clinically relevant genes, such as the *EGFR* hot-spot mutations for selection of EGFR TKI therapy [151]. It can detect essentially all base substitutions, small insertions, and deletions. However, the main disadvantage is the relatively low sensitivity of mutant alleles, estimated to be ~20 % of mutant versus wild-type alleles [151–153].

Pyrosequencing

The pyrosequencing methodology uses sequencing by synthesis method to sequence nucleic acids that relies on detection of pyrophosphate release on nucleotide incorporation [150]. Pyrosequencing is considered to be more sensitive than Sanger sequencing and detects ~5 % of mutant versus wild-type alleles [153–155]. Pyrosequencing detects short reads of DNA sequencing (300–500 base pairs), thus very suitable for DNA extracted from FFPE tissues, since this DNA is significantly fragmented. In lung cancer, this methodology is often applied to detect hot-spot mutations of known oncogenes such as *EGFR* and *KRAS* [153–155].

Allele-Specific Quantitative (q)PCR

This method combines allele-specific amplification with qPCR to detect hot-spot mutation of known mutant hot spot of genes [149, 156]. This method uses primers designated to anneal at sites of sequence variation, a primer whose sequence matches a specific variant selectively amplify only that variant [149, 156]. The main advantage of this method is that it is highly sensitive, with the potential to detect ≤1 % mutant alleles in DNA extracted from a tumor tissue, including DNA extracted from FFPE tissues [157]. Currently, it is widely used to detect hot-spot mutations of *EGFR* and *KRAS* hot-spot mutations [157, 158].

Quantitative PCR Melting Curve Analysis

This method detects differences among melting temperatures of a wild-type and a mutant DNA by using fluorescent probes [153]. This method is fast and has less risk of contamination; however, the main disadvantage is that it does not identify the specific mutation present or the percentage of mutated DNA [149, 153].

Matrix-Assisted Laser Desorption Ionization Time-of-Flight (MALDI-TOF) Mass Spectrometry (Sequenom™)

This is a high-throughput PCR-based sequencing assay to detect multiple hot-spot mutations simultaneously using small amounts of DNA obtained from small biopsy specimens [159]. It has been applied for mutation profiling of human cancer, detection of single nucleotide polymorphisms (SNPs) in germ-line DNA, and to find study disease susceptibility [149, 160]. It has a high level of sensitivity (~5 % of the mutant alleles) and allows quantification of the percentage of mutant DNA [159]. The Sequenom™ methodology is also useful to assess gene copy number variations such as CNG and amplification.

Primer Extension (SNaPshot) Assay (Applied Biosystems, Inc)

This is a primer extension-based method that allows simultaneous analysis of up to ten different mutations. It offers a specific sensitive, low-cost, and rapid method to screening for mutations and to analyze methylation. This assay utilizes an Applied Biosystems, Inc. SNaPshot Multiplex Kit that contains a reaction mix of four differentially fluorescently labeled ddNTPs, allowing the interrogation of each base at a mutation site [161, 162].

Quantitative Polymerase Chain Reaction (qPCR) and Reverse Transcriptase Polymerase Chain Reaction (RT-PCR)

Also called real-time PCR, qPCR is a method that combines the nucleic acid amplification with the detection step, so the amplicons are visualized during the amplification steps by using florescent reporter molecules in an instrument that monitors the amplification in real time and generates data for quantitative analysis using an appropriate software [62]. It is a specific and highly sensitive technique to detect and quantify nucleic acids (mainly used to quantify RNA: mRNA or microRNA), and it has been widely used to determine gene copy number gains and amplification and to detect gene hot-spot mutation (allele-specific qPCR) and translocations [46, 87, 88, 163]. Although this is a simple technique, the interpretation and reporting of the results may be subjective [164]. Additionally, the validation and reproducibility of the results require strict standardization protocols including, among others, adequate sample quality and quality controls, careful primer selection, adequate normalization, and regular calibration of the qPCR instrument [62, 164–166]. The main disadvantage of this technique is that contamination with stromal tumor cells limits the use of this technique to detect copy number gains and gene amplifications. RT-PCR is a variant of the PCR methodology in which small amounts of RNA strand are converted into its complementary DNA (cDNA) using the reverse transcriptase enzyme. The resulting cDNA is then amplified using specific primers by conventional PCR or quantitative PCR (qPCR) equipment [167].

Future Directions

The rapid development of technologies for large-scale sequencing (next-generation sequencing, NGS) has facilitated high-throughput molecular analysis holding various advantages over traditionally sequencing including the ability to fully sequence large numbers of genes in a single test and simultaneously detect deletions, insertions, copy number alterations, translocations, and exome-wide base substitutions (including known hot-spot mutations) in all known cancer-related genes [119, 168]. NGS involves successive methodological steps, including template preparation, sequencing per se and imaging, and data analysis [168]. One of the potential difficulties in this process is the large computing capacities needed to manage the billions of small sequence readouts generated and to assemble those with large databases to interpret the raw data. Another challenge for the NGS is the identification of meaningful driver mutations and the separation of "true" mutations among a background of intrinsic sequence variations [169, 170]. Verifying and validating the "driver" discovered mutations will require experimental and detailed classical molecular pathology studies to bring NGS into clinical context. Next-generation sequencing is greatly accelerating our understanding of the complexity of microRNAs and gene expression (mRNA). This technology has allowed the systematic detection of new microRNAs and experimental validation of novel or predicted miRNAs [171]. In addition, it provides great advantages over conventional methods for the whole RNA transcriptome analysis; it will potentially increase the sensitivity, reduce false positives, as well as increase the transcript coverage to detect novel transcripts, novel alternative splice isoforms, and direct measurement of transcript abundance [172, 173].

References

1. Jemal A, Siegel R, Ward E, Hao Y, Xu J, Murray T, et al. Cancer statistics, 2008. CA Cancer J Clin. 2008;58(2):71–96.
2. Bordoni R. Consensus conference: multimodality management of early- and intermediate-stage non-small cell lung cancer. Oncologist. 2008;13(9):945–53 [Consensus Development Conference Research Support, Non-U.S. Gov't].
3. Herbst RS, Heymach JV, Lippman SM. Lung cancer. N Engl J Med. 2008;359(13):1367–80.
4. Wistuba II, Gelovani JG, Jacoby JJ, Davis SE, Herbst RS. Methodological and practical challenges for personalized cancer therapies. Nat Rev Clin Oncol. 2011;8(3):135–41.
5. Hanahan D, Weinberg RA. Hallmarks of cancer: the next generation. Cell. 2011;144(5):646–74.
6. Weinstein IB, Joe A. Oncogene addiction. Cancer Res. 2008;68(9):3077–80; discussion 80.
7. Kerr KM. Personalized medicine for lung cancer: new challenges for pathology. Histopathology. 2012;60(4):531–46. Epub 2011 Sep 14.
8. Mok TS. Personalized medicine in lung cancer: what we need to know. Nat Rev Clin Oncol. 2011;8(11):661–8.
9. Travis WD, Brambilla E, Muller-Hemelink HK, Harris CC. World Health Organization Classification of tumours. In: Travis WD, editor. Pathology and genetics of tumours of the lung, pleura, thymus and heart. Lyon: IARC Press; 2004.
10. Arriagada R, Bergman B, Dunant A, Le Chevalier T, Pignon JP, Vansteenkiste J. Cisplatin-based adjuvant chemotherapy in patients with completely resected non-small-cell lung cancer. N Engl J Med. 2004;350(4):351–60. [Clinical Trial Multicenter Study Randomized Controlled Trial Research Support, Non-U.S. Gov't].
11. Minna JD, Roth JA, Gazdar AF. Focus on lung cancer. Cancer Cell. 2002;1(1):49–52.
12. Sun S, Schiller JH, Gazdar AF. Lung cancer in never smokers – a different disease. Nat Rev Cancer. 2007;7(10):778–90.
13. Subramanian J, Govindan R. Lung cancer in never smokers: a review. J Clin Oncol. 2007;25(5):561–70.
14. Dutt A, Ramos AH, Hammerman PS, Mermel C, Cho J, Sharifnia T, et al. Inhibitor-sensitive FGFR1 amplification in human non-small cell lung cancer. PLoS One. 2011;6(6):e20351.
15. Hammerman PS, Sos ML, Ramos AH, Xu C, Dutt A, Zhou W, et al. Mutations in the DDR2 kinase gene identify a novel therapeutic target in squamous cell lung cancer. Cancer Discov. 2011;1(1):78–89.
16. Hann CL, Rudin CM. Management of small-cell lung cancer: incremental changes but hope for the future. Oncology (Williston Park). 2008;22(13):1486–92 [Comment Research Support, Non-U.S. Gov't Review].
17. Dowell JE. Small cell lung cancer: are we making progress? Am J Med Sci. 2010;339(1):68–76.
18. D'Angelo SP, Pietanza MC. The molecular pathogenesis of small cell lung cancer. Cancer Biol Ther. 2010;10(1):1–10.
19. Wistuba II, Gazdar AF, Minna JD. Molecular genetics of small cell lung carcinoma. Semin Oncol. 2001;28(2 Suppl 4):3–13.
20. Motoi N, Szoke J, Riely GJ, Seshan VE, Kris MG, Rusch VW, et al. Lung adenocarcinoma: modification of the 2004 WHO mixed subtype to include the major histologic subtype suggests correlations between papillary and micropapillary adenocarcinoma subtypes, EGFR mutations and gene expression analysis. Am J Surg Pathol. 2008;32(6):810–27.
21. Travis WD, Brambilla E, Noguchi M, Nicholson AG, Geisinger KR, Yatabe Y, et al. International association for the study of lung cancer/american thoracic society/european respiratory society international multidisciplinary classification of lung adenocarcinoma. J Thorac Oncol. 2011;6(2):244–85.
22. Colby TV, Wistuba II, Gazdar A. Precursors to pulmonary neoplasia. Adv Anat Pathol. 1998;5(4):205–15 [Review].
23. Westra WH. Early glandular neoplasia of the lung. Respir Res. 2000;1(3):163–9 [Review].
24. Mascaux C, Iannino N, Martin B, Paesmans M, Berghmans T, Dusart M, et al. The role of RAS oncogene in survival of patients with lung cancer: a systematic review of the literature with meta-analysis. Br J Cancer. 2005;92(1):131–9 [Meta-Analysis Review].
25. Wistuba II. Genetics of preneoplasia: lessons from lung cancer. Curr Mol Med. 2007;7(1):3–14.
26. Chiosea SI, Sherer CK, Jelic T, Dacic S. KRAS mutant allele-specific imbalance in lung adenocarcinoma. Mod Pathol. 2011;24(12):1571–7. Epub 2011 Jul 8.
27. Ocque R, Tochigi N, Ohori NP, Dacic S. Usefulness of immunohistochemical and histochemical studies in the classification of lung adenocarcinoma and squamous cell carcinoma in cytologic specimens. Am J Clin Pathol. 2011;136(1):81–7.
28. Tang X, Kadara H, Behrens C, Liu DD, Xiao Y, Rice D, et al. Abnormalities of the TITF-1 lineage-specific oncogene in NSCLC: implications in lung cancer pathogenesis and prognosis. Clin Cancer Res. 2011;17(8):2434–43.
29. Hackett BP, Bingle CD, Gitlin JD. Mechanisms of gene expression and cell fate determination in the developing pulmonary epithelium.

Annu Rev Physiol. 1996;58:51–71 [Research Support, U.S. Gov't, P.H.S. Review].
30. Whitsett JA, Glasser SW. Regulation of surfactant protein gene transcription. Biochim Biophys Acta. 1998;1408(2–3):303–11 [Research Support, U.S. Gov't, P.H.S. Review].
31. Whitsett JA, Haitchi HM, Maeda Y. Intersections between pulmonary development and disease. Am J Respir Crit Care Med. 2011;184(4):401–6.
32. Perner S, Wagner PL, Soltermann A, LaFargue C, Tischler V, Weir BA, et al. TTF1 expression in non-small cell lung carcinoma: association with TTF1 gene amplification and improved survival. J Pathol. 2009;217(1):65–72.
33. Kwei KA, Kim YH, Girard L, Kao J, Pacyna-Gengelbach M, Salari K, et al. Genomic profiling identifies TITF1 as a lineage-specific oncogene amplified in lung cancer. Oncogene. 2008;27(25):3635–40.
34. Bustin SA. Developments in real-time PCR research and molecular diagnostics. Expert Rev Mol Diagn. 2010;10(6):713–5.
35. Shigematsu H, Gazdar AF. Somatic mutations of epidermal growth factor receptor signaling pathway in lung cancers. Int J Cancer. 2006;118(2):257–62.
36. Shigematsu H, Takahashi T, Nomura M, Majmudar K, Suzuki M, Lee H, et al. Somatic mutations of the HER2 kinase domain in lung adenocarcinomas. Cancer Res. 2005;65(5):1642–6.
37. Ahrendt SA, Decker PA, Alawi EA, Zhu Yr YR, Sanchez-Cespedes M, Yang SC, et al. Cigarette smoking is strongly associated with mutation of the K-ras gene in patients with primary adenocarcinoma of the lung. Cancer. 2001;92(6):1525–30 [Research Support, Non-U.S. Gov't Research Support, U.S. Gov't, P.H.S.].
38. Dacic S, Shuai Y, Yousem S, Ohori P, Nikiforova M. Clinicopathological predictors of EGFR/KRAS mutational status in primary lung adenocarcinomas. Mod Pathol. 2010;23(2): 159–68.
39. Koivunen JP, Kim J, Lee J, Rogers AM, Park JO, Zhao X, et al. Mutations in the LKB1 tumour suppressor are frequently detected in tumours from Caucasian but not Asian lung cancer patients. Br J Cancer. 2008;99(2):245–52.
40. Sanchez-Cespedes M, Parrella P, Esteller M, Nomoto S, Trink B, Engles JM, et al. Inactivation of LKB1/STK11 is a common event in adenocarcinomas of the lung. Cancer Res. 2002;62(13): 3659–62.
41. Kerr KM. Pulmonary preinvasive neoplasia. J Clin Pathol. 2001;54(4):257–71 [Review].
42. Wistuba II, Behrens C, Milchgrub S, Bryant D, Hung J, Minna JD, et al. Sequential molecular abnormalities are involved in the multistage development of squamous cell lung carcinoma. Oncogene. 1999;18(3):643–50 [Research Support, U.S. Gov't, P.H.S.].
43. Wistuba II, Behrens C, Virmani AK, Milchgrub S, Syed S, Lam S, et al. Allelic losses at chromosome 8p21-23 are early and frequent events in the pathogenesis of lung cancer. Cancer Res. 1999;59(8):1973–9 [Research Support, U.S. Gov't, P.H.S.].
44. Wistuba II, Lam S, Behrens C, Virmani AK, Fong KM, LeRiche J, et al. Molecular damage in the bronchial epithelium of current and former smokers. J Natl Cancer Inst. 1997;89(18):1366–73 [Research Support, U.S. Gov't, P.H.S.].
45. Bass AJ, Watanabe H, Mermel CH, Yu S, Perner S, Verhaak RG, et al. SOX2 is an amplified lineage-survival oncogene in lung and esophageal squamous cell carcinomas. Nat Genet. 2009;41(11): 1238–42.
46. Yuan P, Kadara H, Behrens C, Tang X, Woods D, Solis LM, et al. Sex determining region Y-Box 2 (SOX2) is a potential cell-lineage gene highly expressed in the pathogenesis of squamous cell carcinomas of the lung. PLoS One. 2010;5(2):e9112 [Research Support, N.I.H., Extramural Research Support, U.S. Gov't, Non-P.H.S.].
47. Sholl LM, Long KB, Hornick JL. Sox2 expression in pulmonary non-small cell and neuroendocrine carcinomas. Appl Immunohistochem Mol Morphol. 2010;18(1):55–61.
48. Wilbertz T, Wagner P, Petersen K, Stiedl AC, Scheble VJ, Maier S, et al. SOX2 gene amplification and protein overexpression are associated with better outcome in squamous cell lung cancer. Mod Pathol. 2011;24(7):944–53 [Research Support, Non-U.S. Gov't].
49. Khazaie K, Schirrmacher V, Lichtner RB. EGF receptor in neoplasia and metastasis. Cancer Metastasis Rev. 1993;12(3–4):255–74 [Review].
50. Normanno N, De Luca A, Bianco C, Strizzi L, Mancino M, Maiello MR, et al. Epidermal growth factor receptor (EGFR) signaling in cancer. Gene. 2006;366(1):2–16 [Research Support, Non-U.S. Gov't Review].
51. Janku F, Stewart DJ, Kurzrock R. Targeted therapy in non-small-cell lung cancer – is it becoming a reality? Nat Rev Clin Oncol. 2010;7(7):401–14.
52. Webb JD, Simon MC. Novel insights into the molecular origins and treatment of lung cancer. Cell Cycle. 2010;9(20):4098–105.
53. Lynch TJ, Bell DW, Sordella R, Gurubhagavatula S, Okimoto RA, Brannigan BW, et al. Activating mutations in the epidermal growth factor receptor underlying responsiveness of non-small-cell lung cancer to gefitinib. N Engl J Med. 2004;350(21):2129–39.
54. Ettinger DS, Akerley W, Bepler G, Blum MG, Chang A, Cheney RT, et al. Non-small cell lung cancer. J Natl Compr Canc Netw. 2010;8(7):740–801.
55. Hirsch FR, Scagliotti GV, Langer CJ, Varella-Garcia M, Franklin WA. Epidermal growth factor family of receptors in preneoplasia and lung cancer: perspectives for targeted therapies. Lung Cancer. 2003;41 Suppl 1:S29–42.
56. Cappuzzo F, Hirsch FR, Rossi E, Bartolini S, Ceresoli GL, Bemis L, et al. Epidermal growth factor receptor gene and protein and gefitinib sensitivity in non-small-cell lung cancer. J Natl Cancer Inst. 2005;97(9):643–55.
57. Hirsch FR, Varella-Garcia M, Cappuzzo F, McCoy J, Bemis L, Xavier AC, et al. Combination of EGFR gene copy number and protein expression predicts outcome for advanced non-small-cell lung cancer patients treated with gefitinib. Ann Oncol. 2007;18(4):752–60.
58. Tsao MS, Sakurada A, Cutz JC, Zhu CQ, Kamel-Reid S, Squire J, et al. Erlotinib in lung cancer – molecular and clinical predictors of outcome. N Engl J Med. 2005;353(2):133–44.
59. Sholl LM, Yeap BY, Iafrate AJ, Holmes-Tisch AJ, Chou YP, Wu MT, et al. Lung adenocarcinoma with EGFR amplification has distinct clinicopathologic and molecular features in never-smokers. Cancer Res. 2009;69(21):8341–8.
60. Hirsch FR, Varella-Garcia M, McCoy J, West H, Xavier AC, Gumerlock P, et al. Increased epidermal growth factor receptor gene copy number detected by fluorescence in situ hybridization associates with increased sensitivity to gefitinib in patients with bronchioloalveolar carcinoma subtypes: a Southwest Oncology Group Study. J Clin Oncol. 2005;23(28):6838–45.
61. Massarelli E, Varella-Garcia M, Tang X, Xavier AC, Ozburn NC, Liu DD, et al. KRAS mutation is an important predictor of resistance to therapy with epidermal growth factor receptor tyrosine kinase inhibitors in non-small-cell lung cancer. Clin Cancer Res. 2007;13(10):2890–6.
62. Dziadziuszko R, Hirsch FR, Varella-Garcia M, Bunn Jr PA. Selecting lung cancer patients for treatment with epidermal growth factor receptor tyrosine kinase inhibitors by immunohistochemistry and fluorescence in situ hybridization – why, when, and how? Clin Cancer Res. 2006;12(14 Pt 2):4409s–15.
63. Nakamura H, Kawasaki N, Taguchi M, Kabasawa K. Survival impact of epidermal growth factor receptor overexpression in patients with non-small cell lung cancer: a meta-analysis. Thorax. 2006;61(2):140–5.
64. Putnam EA, Yen N, Gallick GE, Steck PA, Fang K, Akpakip B, et al. Autocrine growth stimulation by transforming growth factor-alpha in human non-small cell lung cancer. Surg Oncol. 1992;1(1):49–60 [Research Support, Non-U.S. Gov't Research Support, U.S. Gov't, P.H.S.].

65. Rusch V, Baselga J, Cordon-Cardo C, Orazem J, Zaman M, Hoda S, et al. Differential expression of the epidermal growth factor receptor and its ligands in primary non-small cell lung cancers and adjacent benign lung. Cancer Res. 1993;53(10 Suppl):2379–85 [Comparative Study Research Support, Non-U.S. Gov't Research Support, U.S. Gov't, P.H.S.].
66. Menard S, Casalini P, Campiglio M, Pupa SM, Tagliabue E. Role of HER2/neu in tumor progression and therapy. Cell Mol Life Sci. 2004;61(23):2965–78 [Research Support, Non-U.S. Gov't Review].
67. Hirsch FR, Varella-Garcia M, Franklin WA, Veve R, Chen L, Helfrich B, et al. Evaluation of HER-2/neu gene amplification and protein expression in non-small cell lung carcinomas. Br J Cancer. 2002;86(9):1449–56.
68. Stephens P, Hunter C, Bignell G, Edkins S, Davies H, Teague J, et al. Lung cancer: intragenic ERBB2 kinase mutations in tumours. Nature. 2004;431(7008):525–6.
69. Tan D, Deeb G, Wang J, Slocum HK, Winston J, Wiseman S, et al. HER-2/neu protein expression and gene alteration in stage I-IIIA non-small-cell lung cancer: a study of 140 cases using a combination of high throughput tissue microarray, immunohistochemistry, and fluorescent in situ hybridization. Diagn Mol Pathol. 2003;12(4):201–11.
70. Jancik S, Drabek J, Radzioch D, Hajduch M. Clinical relevance of KRAS in human cancers. J Biomed Biotechnol. 2010;2010:150960 [Research Support, Non-U.S. Gov't Review].
71. Siegfried JM, Gillespie AT, Mera R, Casey TJ, Keohavong P, Testa JR, et al. Prognostic value of specific KRAS mutations in lung adenocarcinomas. Cancer Epidemiol Biomarkers Prev. 1997;6(10):841–7 [Research Support, Non-U.S. Gov't Research Support, U.S. Gov't, P.H.S.].
72. Capella G, Cronauer-Mitra S, Pienado MA, Perucho M. Frequency and spectrum of mutations at codons 12 and 13 of the c-K-ras gene in human tumors. Environ Health Perspect. 1991;93:125–31 [Research Support, Non-U.S. Gov't Research Support, U.S. Gov't, P.H.S.].
73. Riely GJ, Kris MG, Rosenbaum D, Marks J, Li A, Chitale DA, et al. Frequency and distinctive spectrum of KRAS mutations in never smokers with lung adenocarcinoma. Clin Cancer Res. 2008;14(18):5731–4 [Research Support, N.I.H., Extramural].
74. Eberhard DA, Johnson BE, Amler LC, Goddard AD, Heldens SL, Herbst RS, et al. Mutations in the epidermal growth factor receptor and in KRAS are predictive and prognostic indicators in patients with non-small-cell lung cancer treated with chemotherapy alone and in combination with erlotinib. J Clin Oncol. 2005;23(25):5900–9 [Clinical Trial Clinical Trial, Phase III Multicenter Study Randomized Controlled Trial Research Support, Non-U.S. Gov't].
75. Pao W, Wang TY, Riely GJ, Miller VA, Pan Q, Ladanyi M, et al. KRAS mutations and primary resistance of lung adenocarcinomas to gefitinib or erlotinib. PLoS Med. 2005;2(1):e17 [Research Support, N.I.H., Extramural Research Support, Non-U.S. Gov't Research Support, U.S. Gov't, P.H.S.].
76. Engelman JA, Chen L, Tan X, Crosby K, Guimaraes AR, Upadhyay R, et al. Effective use of PI3K and MEK inhibitors to treat mutant Kras G12D and PIK3CA H1047R murine lung cancers. Nat Med. 2008;14(12):1351–6 [Research Support, N.I.H., Extramural Research Support, Non-U.S. Gov't].
77. Kim ES, Herbst RS, Wistuba II, Lee JJ, Blumenschein GR, Tsao A, Stewart DJ, et al. The BATTLE trial: personalizing therapy for lung cancer. Cancer Discov. 2011;1(1):44–53.
78. Iwahara T, Fujimoto J, Wen D, Cupples R, Bucay N, Arakawa T, et al. Molecular characterization of ALK, a receptor tyrosine kinase expressed specifically in the nervous system. Oncogene. 1997;14(4):439–49 [Comparative Study].
79. Drexler HG, Gignac SM, von Wasielewski R, Werner M, Dirks WG. Pathobiology of NPM-ALK and variant fusion genes in anaplastic large cell lymphoma and other lymphomas. Leukemia. 2000;14(9):1533–59 [Research Support, Non-U.S. Gov't Review].
80. Lamant L, Pulford K, Bischof D, Morris SW, Mason DY, Delsol G, et al. Expression of the ALK tyrosine kinase gene in neuroblastoma. Am J Pathol. 2000;156(5):1711–21 [Research Support, Non-U.S. Gov't Research Support, U.S. Gov't, P.H.S.].
81. Griffin CA, Hawkins AL, Dvorak C, Henkle C, Ellingham T, Perlman EJ. Recurrent involvement of 2p23 in inflammatory myofibroblastic tumors. Cancer Res. 1999;59(12):2776–80 [Case Reports].
82. Soda M, Choi YL, Enomoto M, Takada S, Yamashita Y, Ishikawa S, et al. Identification of the transforming EML4-ALK fusion gene in non-small-cell lung cancer. Nature. 2007;448(7153):561–6.
83. Inamura K, Takeuchi K, Togashi Y, Hatano S, Ninomiya H, Motoi N, et al. EML4-ALK lung cancers are characterized by rare other mutations, a TTF-1 cell lineage, an acinar histology, and young onset. Mod Pathol. 2009;22(4):508–15.
84. Inamura K, Takeuchi K, Togashi Y, Nomura K, Ninomiya H, Okui M, et al. EML4-ALK fusion is linked to histological characteristics in a subset of lung cancers. J Thorac Oncol. 2008;3(1):13–7.
85. Rodig SJ, Mino-Kenudson M, Dacic S, Yeap BY, Shaw A, Barletta JA, et al. Unique clinicopathologic features characterize ALK-rearranged lung adenocarcinoma in the western population. Clin Cancer Res. 2009;15(16):5216–23.
86. Shaw AT, Yeap BY, Mino-Kenudson M, Digumarthy SR, Costa DB, Heist RS, et al. Clinical features and outcome of patients with non-small-cell lung cancer who harbor EML4-ALK. J Clin Oncol. 2009;27(26):4247–53.
87. Yoshida A, Tsuta K, Nakamura H, Kohno T, Takahashi F, Asamura H, et al. Comprehensive histologic analysis of ALK-rearranged lung carcinomas. Am J Surg Pathol. 2011;35(8):1226–34.
88. Choi YL, Takeuchi K, Soda M, Inamura K, Togashi Y, Hatano S, et al. Identification of novel isoforms of the EML4-ALK transforming gene in non-small cell lung cancer. Cancer Res. 2008;68(13):4971–6.
89. Takeuchi K, Choi YL, Soda M, Inamura K, Togashi Y, Hatano S, et al. Multiplex reverse transcription-PCR screening for EML4-ALK fusion transcripts. Clin Cancer Res. 2008;14(20):6618–24.
90. Koivunen JP, Mermel C, Zejnullahu K, Murphy C, Lifshits E, Holmes AJ, et al. EML4-ALK fusion gene and efficacy of an ALK kinase inhibitor in lung cancer. Clin Cancer Res. 2008;14(13):4275–83 [Research Support, N.I.H., Extramural Research Support, Non-U.S. Gov't].
91. Hemminki A, Markie D, Tomlinson I, Avizienyte E, Roth S, Loukola A, et al. A serine/threonine kinase gene defective in Peutz-Jeghers syndrome. Nature. 1998;391(6663):184–7 [Research Support, Non-U.S. Gov't].
92. Marignani PA. LKB1, the multitasking tumour suppressor kinase. J Clin Pathol. 2005;58(1):15–9 [Review].
93. Sanchez-Cespedes M. The role of LKB1 in lung cancer. Fam Cancer. 2011;10(3):447–53.
94. Sanchez-Cespedes M. A role for LKB1 gene in human cancer beyond the Peutz-Jeghers syndrome. Oncogene. 2007;26(57):7825–32.
95. Beenken A, Mohammadi M. The FGF family: biology, pathophysiology and therapy. Nat Rev Drug Discov. 2009;8(3):235–53 [Research Support, N.I.H., Extramural Review].
96. Turner N, Grose R. Fibroblast growth factor signalling: from development to cancer. Nat Rev Cancer. 2010;10(2):116–29 [Review].
97. Wesche J, Haglund K, Haugsten EM. Fibroblast growth factors and their receptors in cancer. Biochem J. 2011;437(2):199–213.
98. Weiss J, Sos ML, Seidel D, Peifer M, Zander T, Heuckmann JM, et al. Frequent and focal FGFR1 amplification associates with therapeutically tractable FGFR1 dependency in squamous cell lung cancer. Sci Transl Med. 2010;2(62):62ra93.
99. Turner NC, Seckl MJ. A therapeutic target for smoking-associated lung cancer. Sci Transl Med. 2010;2(62):62ps56.

100. Engelman JA, Luo J, Cantley LC. The evolution of phosphatidylinositol 3-kinases as regulators of growth and metabolism. Nat Rev Genet. 2006;7(8):606–19 [Research Support, N.I.H., Extramural Review].
101. Karakas B, Bachman KE, Park BH. Mutation of the PIK3CA oncogene in human cancers. Br J Cancer. 2006;94(4):455–9 [Research Support, N.I.H., Extramural Research Support, Non-U.S. Gov't Research Support, U.S. Gov't, Non-P.H.S. Review].
102. Samuels Y, Ericson K. Oncogenic PI3K and its role in cancer. Curr Opin Oncol. 2006;18(1):77–82 [Review].
103. Yamamoto H, Shigematsu H, Nomura M, Lockwood WW, Sato M, Okumura N, et al. PIK3CA mutations and copy number gains in human lung cancers. Cancer Res. 2008;68(17):6913–21 [Research Support, N.I.H., Extramural].
104. Kawano O, Sasaki H, Okuda K, Yukiue H, Yokoyama T, Yano M, et al. PIK3CA gene amplification in Japanese non-small cell lung cancer. Lung Cancer. 2007;58(1):159–60 [Letter].
105. Samuels Y, Waldman T. Oncogenic mutations of PIK3CA in human cancers. Curr Top Microbiol Immunol. 2010;347:21–41 [Review].
106. Samuels Y, Velculescu VE. Oncogenic mutations of PIK3CA in human cancers. Cell Cycle. 2004;3(10):1221–4.
107. Sequist LV, Waltman BA, Dias-Santagata D, Digumarthy S, Turke AB, Fidias P, et al. Genotypic and histological evolution of lung cancers acquiring resistance to EGFR inhibitors. Sci Transl Med. 2011;3(75):75ra26 [Research Support, N.I.H., Extramural Research Support, Non-U.S. Gov't].
108. Jiang BH, Liu LZ. PI3K/PTEN signaling in angiogenesis and tumorigenesis. Adv Cancer Res. 2009;102:19–65 [Research Support, N.I.H., Extramural Research Support, Non-U.S. Gov't Review].
109. Jia S, Roberts TM, Zhao JJ. Should individual PI3 kinase isoforms be targeted in cancer? Curr Opin Cell Biol. 2009;21(2):199–208 [Research Support, N.I.H., Extramural Research Support, Non-U.S. Gov't Research Support, U.S. Gov't, Non-P.H.S. Review].
110. Janku F, Tsimberidou AM, Garrido-Laguna I, Wang X, Luthra R, Hong DS, et al. PIK3CA mutations in patients with advanced cancers treated with PI3K/AKT/mTOR axis inhibitors. Mol Cancer Ther. 2011;10(3):558–65 [Research Support, N.I.H., Extramural].
111. Balsara BR, Testa JR. Chromosomal imbalances in human lung cancer. Oncogene. 2002;21(45):6877–83 [Research Support, Non-U.S. Gov't Research Support, U.S. Gov't, P.H.S. Review].
112. Burbee DG, Forgacs E, Zochbauer-Muller S, Shivakumar L, Fong K, Gao B, et al. Epigenetic inactivation of RASSF1A in lung and breast cancers and malignant phenotype suppression. J Natl Cancer Inst. 2001;93(9):691–9 [Research Support, Non-U.S. Gov't Research Support, U.S. Gov't, P.H.S.].
113. Gazdar AF, Zochbauer-Moller S, Virmani A, Kurie J, Minna JD, Lam S. RESPONSE: Re: promoter methylation and silencing of the retinoic acid receptor-beta gene in lung carcinomas. J Natl Cancer Inst. 2001;93(1):67–8.
114. Virmani AK, Rathi A, Zochbauer-Muller S, Sacchi N, Fukuyama Y, Bryant D, et al. Promoter methylation and silencing of the retinoic acid receptor-beta gene in lung carcinomas. J Natl Cancer Inst. 2000;92(16):1303–7 [Research Support, Non-U.S. Gov't Research Support, U.S. Gov't, P.H.S.].
115. Modi S, Kubo A, Oie H, Coxon AB, Rehmatulla A, Kaye FJ. Protein expression of the RB-related gene family and SV40 large T antigen in mesothelioma and lung cancer. Oncogene. 2000;19(40):4632–9 [Comparative Study].
116. Mogi A, Kuwano H. TP53 mutations in nonsmall cell lung cancer. J Biomed Biotechnol. 2011;2011:583929.
117. Kaiser U, Schilli M, Haag U, Neumann K, Kreipe H, Kogan E, et al. Expression of bcl-2 – protein in small cell lung cancer. Lung Cancer. 1996;15(1):31–40 [Comparative Study].
118. William Jr WN, Glisson BS. Novel strategies for the treatment of small-cell lung carcinoma. Nat Rev Clin Oncol. 2011;8(10):611–9.
119. Scagliotti G, Hanna N, Fossella F, Sugarman K, Blatter J, Peterson P, et al. The differential efficacy of pemetrexed according to NSCLC histology: a review of two phase III studies. Oncologist. 2009;14(3):253–63.
120. Scagliotti GV, Ceppi P, Capelletto E, Novello S. Updated clinical information on multitargeted antifolates in lung cancer. Clin Lung Cancer. 2009;10 Suppl 1:S35–40.
121. Rollins KD, Lindley C. Pemetrexed: a multitargeted antifolate. Clin Ther. 2005;27(9):1343–82 [Review].
122. Adjei AA. Pemetrexed (Alimta): a novel multitargeted antifolate agent. Expert Rev Anticancer Ther. 2003;3(2):145–56 [Review].
123. Lee SM. Is EGFR expression important in non-small cell lung cancer? Thorax. 2006;61(2):98–9.
124. Wu JY, Shih JY, Chen KY, Yang CH, Yu CJ, Yang PC. Gefitinib therapy in patients with advanced non-small cell lung cancer with or without testing for epidermal growth factor receptor (EGFR) mutations. Medicine (Baltimore). 2011;90(3):159–67.
125. Xu Y, Liu H, Chen J, Zhou Q. Acquired resistance of lung adenocarcinoma to EGFR-tyrosine kinase inhibitors gefitinib and erlotinib. Cancer Biol Ther. 2010;9(8):572–82 [Research Support, Non-U.S. Gov't Review].
126. Jackman D, Pao W, Riely GJ, Engelman JA, Kris MG, Janne PA, et al. Clinical definition of acquired resistance to epidermal growth factor receptor tyrosine kinase inhibitors in non-small-cell lung cancer. J Clin Oncol. 2010;28(2):357–60 [Research Support, Non-U.S. Gov't].
127. Takeda M, Okamoto I, Fujita Y, Arao T, Ito H, Fukuoka M, et al. De novo resistance to epidermal growth factor receptor-tyrosine kinase inhibitors in EGFR mutation-positive patients with non-small cell lung cancer. J Thorac Oncol. 2010;5(3):399–400 [Case Reports].
128. Balak MN, Gong Y, Riely GJ, Somwar R, Li AR, Zakowski MF, et al. Novel D761Y and common secondary T790M mutations in epidermal growth factor receptor-mutant lung adenocarcinomas with acquired resistance to kinase inhibitors. Clin Cancer Res. 2006;12(21):6494–501 [Research Support, N.I.H., Extramural Research Support, Non-U.S. Gov't].
129. Bean J, Brennan C, Shih JY, Riely G, Viale A, Wang L, et al. MET amplification occurs with or without T790M mutations in EGFR mutant lung tumors with acquired resistance to gefitinib or erlotinib. Proc Natl Acad Sci USA. 2007;104(52):20932–7 [Research Support, N.I.H., Extramural Research Support, Non-U.S. Gov't].
130. Engelman JA, Zejnullahu K, Mitsudomi T, Song Y, Hyland C, Park JO, et al. MET amplification leads to gefitinib resistance in lung cancer by activating ERBB3 signaling. Science. 2007;316(5827):1039–43 [Research Support, N.I.H., Extramural Research Support, Non-U.S. Gov't].
131. Morgillo F, Kim WY, Kim ES, Ciardiello F, Hong WK, Lee HY. Implication of the insulin-like growth factor-IR pathway in the resistance of non-small cell lung cancer cells to treatment with gefitinib. Clin Cancer Res. 2007;13(9):2795–803 [Research Support, N.I.H., Extramural Research Support, Non-U.S. Gov't Research Support, U.S. Gov't, Non-P.H.S.].
132. Yauch RL, Januario T, Eberhard DA, Cavet G, Zhu W, Fu L, et al. Epithelial versus mesenchymal phenotype determines in vitro sensitivity and predicts clinical activity of erlotinib in lung cancer patients. Clin Cancer Res. 2005;11(24 Pt 1):8686–98.
133. Zhan P, Wang J, Lv XJ, Wang Q, Qiu LX, Lin XQ, et al. Prognostic value of vascular endothelial growth factor expression in patients with lung cancer: a systematic review with meta-analysis. J Thorac Oncol. 2009;4(9):1094–103 [Meta-Analysis Research Support, Non-U.S. Gov't Review].

134. Meert AP, Paesmans M, Martin B, Delmotte P, Berghmans T, Verdebout JM, et al. The role of microvessel density on the survival of patients with lung cancer: a systematic review of the literature with meta-analysis. Br J Cancer. 2002;87(7):694–701 [Meta-Analysis Research Support, Non-U.S. Gov't].
135. Yang F, Tang X, Riquelme E, Behrens C, Nilsson MB, Giri U, et al. Increased VEGFR-2 gene copy is associated with chemoresistance and shorter survival in patients with non-small-cell lung carcinoma who receive adjuvant chemotherapy. Cancer Res. 2011;71(16):5512–21 [Research Support, N.I.H., Extramural Research Support, U.S. Gov't, Non-P.H.S.].
136. Kwak EL, Bang YJ, Camidge DR, Shaw AT, Solomon B, Maki RG, et al. Anaplastic lymphoma kinase inhibition in non-small-cell lung cancer. N Engl J Med. 2010;363(18):1693–703.
137. Choi YL, Soda M, Yamashita Y, Ueno T, Takashima J, Nakajima T, et al. EML4-ALK mutations in lung cancer that confer resistance to ALK inhibitors. N Engl J Med. 2010;363(18):1734–9 [Case Reports Research Support, Non-U.S. Gov't].
138. Katayama R, Khan TM, Benes C, Lifshits E, Ebi H, Rivera VM, et al. Therapeutic strategies to overcome crizotinib resistance in non-small cell lung cancers harboring the fusion oncogene EML4-ALK. Proc Natl Acad Sci USA. 2011;108(18):7535–40.
139. Zhang S, Wang F, Keats J, Zhu X, Ning Y, Wardwell SD, et al. Crizotinib-resistant mutants of EML4-ALK identified through an accelerated mutagenesis screen. Chem Biol Drug Des. 2011;78(6):999–1005 [Letter].
140. Chen G, Gharib TG, Wang H, Huang CC, Kuick R, Thomas DG, et al. Protein profiles associated with survival in lung adenocarcinoma. Proc Natl Acad Sci USA. 2003;100(23):13537–42 [Research Support, Non-U.S. Gov't Research Support, U.S. Gov't, P.H.S.].
141. Xie Y, Xiao G, Coombes KR, Behrens C, Solis LM, Raso G, et al. Robust gene expression signature from formalin-fixed paraffin-embedded samples predicts prognosis of non-small-cell lung cancer patients. Clin Cancer Res. 2011;17(17):5705–14 [Research Support, N.I.H., Extramural Research Support, U.S. Gov't, Non-P.H.S.].
142. Kadara H, Behrens C, Yuan P, Solis L, Liu D, Gu X, et al. A five-gene and corresponding protein signature for stage-I lung adenocarcinoma prognosis. Clin Cancer Res. 2011;17(6):1490–501 [Research Support, N.I.H., Extramural Research Support, Non-U.S. Gov't Research Support, U.S. Gov't, Non-P.H.S.].
143. Shedden K, Taylor JM, Enkemann SA, Tsao MS, Yeatman TJ, Gerald WL, et al. Gene expression-based survival prediction in lung adenocarcinoma: a multi-site, blinded validation study. Nat Med. 2008;14(8):822–7 [Multicenter Study Research Support, N.I.H., Extramural Research Support, Non-U.S. Gov't].
144. Olaussen KA, Dunant A, Fouret P, Brambilla E, Andre F, Haddad V, et al. DNA repair by ERCC1 in non-small-cell lung cancer and cisplatin-based adjuvant chemotherapy. N Engl J Med. 2006;355(10):983–91 [Multicenter Study Randomized Controlled Trial Research Support, Non-U.S. Gov't].
145. Tanner M, Gancberg D, Di Leo A, Larsimont D, Rouas G, Piccart MJ, et al. Chromogenic in situ hybridization: a practical alternative for fluorescence in situ hybridization to detect HER-2/neu oncogene amplification in archival breast cancer samples. Am J Pathol. 2000;157(5):1467–72 [Comparative Study Research Support, Non-U.S. Gov't].
146. Yoshida A, Tsuta K, Nitta H, Hatanaka Y, Asamura H, Sekine I, et al. Bright-field dual-color chromogenic in situ hybridization for diagnosing echinoderm microtubule-associated protein-like 4-anaplastic lymphoma kinase-positive lung adenocarcinomas. J Thorac Oncol. 2011;6(10):1677–86 [Research Support, Non-U.S. Gov't].
147. Lander ES, Linton LM, Birren B, Nusbaum C, Zody MC, Baldwin J, et al. Initial sequencing and analysis of the human genome. Nature. 2001;409(6822):860–921 [Research Support, Non-U.S. Gov't Research Support, U.S. Gov't, Non-P.H.S. Research Support, U.S. Gov't, P.H.S.].
148. Sanger F, Nicklen S, Coulson AR. DNA sequencing with chain-terminating inhibitors. Proc Natl Acad Sci USA. 1977;74(12):5463–7.
149. Ross JS, Cronin M. Whole cancer genome sequencing by next-generation methods. Am J Clin Pathol. 2011;136(4):527–39.
150. Ahmadian A, Ehn M, Hober S. Pyrosequencing: history, biochemistry and future. Clin Chim Acta. 2006;363(1–2):83–94 [Review].
151. Anderson SM. Laboratory methods for KRAS mutation analysis. Expert Rev Mol Diagn. 2011;11(6):635–42 [Review].
152. Pinto P, Rocha P, Veiga I, Guedes J, Pinheiro M, Peixoto A, et al. Comparison of methodologies for KRAS mutation detection in metastatic colorectal cancer. Cancer Genet. 2011;204(8):439–46.
153. Tsiatis AC, Norris-Kirby A, Rich RG, Hafez MJ, Gocke CD, Eshleman JR, et al. Comparison of Sanger sequencing, pyrosequencing, and melting curve analysis for the detection of KRAS mutations: diagnostic and clinical implications. J Mol Diagn. 2010;12(4):425–32 [Comparative Study].
154. Ogino S, Kawasaki T, Brahmandam M, Yan L, Cantor M, Namgyal C, et al. Sensitive sequencing method for KRAS mutation detection by pyrosequencing. J Mol Diagn. 2005;7(3):413–21 [Comparative Study Research Support, N.I.H., Extramural Research Support, Non-U.S. Gov't Research Support, U.S. Gov't, P.H.S.].
155. Dufort S, Richard MJ, de Fraipont F. Pyrosequencing method to detect KRAS mutation in formalin-fixed and paraffin-embedded tumor tissues. Anal Biochem. 2009;391(2):166–8 [Research Support, Non-U.S. Gov't].
156. Wu DY, Ugozzoli L, Pal BK, Wallace RB. Allele-specific enzymatic amplification of beta-globin genomic DNA for diagnosis of sickle cell anemia. Proc Natl Acad Sci USA. 1989;86(8):2757–60 [Research Support, Non-U.S. Gov't Research Support, U.S. Gov't, Non-P.H.S. Research Support, U.S. Gov't, P.H.S.].
157. Sundstrom M, Edlund K, Lindell M, Glimelius B, Birgisson H, Micke P, et al. KRAS analysis in colorectal carcinoma: analytical aspects of pyrosequencing and allele-specific PCR in clinical practice. BMC Cancer. 2010;10:660 [Comparative Study Evaluation Studies Research Support, Non-U.S. Gov't].
158. Kotoula V, Charalambous E, Biesmans B, Malousi A, Vrettou E, Fountzilas G, et al. Targeted KRAS mutation assessment on patient tumor histologic material in real time diagnostics. PLoS One. 2009;4(11):e7746 [Research Support, Non-U.S. Gov't].
159. Fumagalli D, Gavin PG, Taniyama Y, Kim SI, Choi HJ, Paik S, et al. A rapid, sensitive, reproducible and cost-effective method for mutation profiling of colon cancer and metastatic lymph nodes. BMC Cancer. 2010;10:101 [Research Support, N.I.H., Extramural Research Support, Non-U.S. Gov't].
160. Thomas RK, Baker AC, Debiasi RM, Winckler W, Laframboise T, Lin WM, et al. High-throughput oncogene mutation profiling in human cancer. Nat Genet. 2007;39(3):347–51 [Research Support, N.I.H., Extramural Research Support, Non-U.S. Gov't].
161. Pati N, Schowinsky V, Kokanovic O, Magnuson V, Ghosh S. A comparison between SNaPshot, pyrosequencing, and biplex invader SNP genotyping methods: accuracy, cost, and throughput. J Biochem Biophys Methods. 2004;60(1):1–12 [Comparative Study Research Support, Non-U.S. Gov't].
162. Hurst CD, Zuiverloon TC, Hafner C, Zwarthoff EC, Knowles MA. A SNaPshot assay for the rapid and simple detection of four common hotspot codon mutations in the PIK3CA gene. BMC Res Notes. 2009;2:66.
163. Nakagawa K, Yasumitu T, Fukuhara K, Shiono H, Kikui M. Poor prognosis after lung resection for patients with adenosquamous carcinoma of the lung. Ann Thorac Surg. 2003;75(6):1740–4.
164. Gustafson AM, Soldi R, Anderlind C, Scholand MB, Qian J, Zhang X, et al. Airway PI3K pathway activation is an early and reversible event in lung cancer development. Sci Transl Med. 2010;2(26):26ra5.

165. Miyamae Y, Shimizu K, Hirato J, Araki T, Tanaka K, Ogawa H, et al. Significance of epidermal growth factor receptor gene mutations in squamous cell lung carcinoma. Oncol Rep. 2011;25(4):921–8.
166. Cooke DT, Nguyen DV, Yang Y, Chen SL, Yu C, Calhoun RF. Survival comparison of adenosquamous, squamous cell, and adenocarcinoma of the lung after lobectomy. Ann Thorac Surg. 2010;90(3):943–8.
167. VanGuilder HD, Vrana KE, Freeman WM. Twenty-five years of quantitative PCR for gene expression analysis. Biotechniques. 2008;44(5):619–26 [Research Support, N.I.H., Extramural Research Support, U.S. Gov't, Non-P.H.S. Review].
168. Pfeifer GP, Hainaut P. Next-generation sequencing: emerging lessons on the origins of human cancer. Curr Opin Oncol. 2011;23(1):62–8 [Review].
169. Cronin M, Ross JS. Comprehensive next-generation cancer genome sequencing in the era of targeted therapy and personalized oncology. Biomark Med. 2011;5(3):293–305.
170. Bennett ST, Barnes C, Cox A, Davies L, Brown C. Toward the 1,000 dollars human genome. Pharmacogenomics. 2005;6(4):373–82 [Review].
171. Git A, Dvinge H, Salmon-Divon M, Osborne M, Kutter C, Hadfield J, et al. Systematic comparison of microarray profiling, real-time PCR, and next-generation sequencing technologies for measuring differential microRNA expression. RNA. 2010;16(5):991–1006 [Comparative Study Evaluation Studies Research Support, Non-U.S. Gov't Validation Studies].
172. Tariq MA, Kim HJ, Jejelowo O, Pourmand N. Whole-transcriptome RNAseq analysis from minute amount of total RNA. Nucleic Acids Res. 2011;39(18):e120 [Research Support, N.I.H., Extramural Research Support, U.S. Gov't, Non-P.H.S.].
173. Marioni JC, Mason CE, Mane SM, Stephens M, Gilad Y. RNA-seq: an assessment of technical reproducibility and comparison with gene expression arrays. Genome Res. 2008;18(9):1509–17 [Comparative Study Evaluation Studies Research Support, N.I.H., Extramural Research Support, Non-U.S. Gov't].

Index

A. Weissferdt, C.A. Moran, *Diagnostic Pathology of Pleuropulmonary Neoplasia*,
DOI 10.1007/978-1-4419-0787-5, © Springer Science+Business Media New York 2013

R

S

MIX
Papier aus verantwortungsvollen Quellen
Paper from responsible sources
FSC® C105338

If you have any concerns about our products,
you can contact us on
ProductSafety@springernature.com

In case Publisher is established outside the EU,
the EU authorized representative is:
Springer Nature Customer Service Center GmbH
Europaplatz 3, 69115 Heidelberg, Germany

Printed by Libri Plureos GmbH
in Hamburg, Germany